The GALE ENCYCLOPEDIA *of* CANCER

The GALE ENCYCLOPEDIA *of* CANCER

A GUIDE TO CANCER AND ITS TREATMENTS

VOLUME

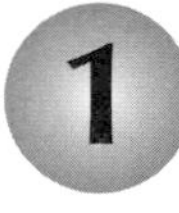

A-K

ELLEN THACKERY, EDITOR

GALE GROUP

THOMSON LEARNING

Detroit • New York • San Diego • San Francisco
Boston • New Haven, Conn. • Waterville, Maine
London • Munich

The GALE ENCYCLOPEDIA *of* CANCER

STAFF

Ellen Thackery, *Project Editor*

Christine B. Jeryan, *Managing Editor*
Donna Olendorf, *Senior Editor*
Stacey Blachford, *Associate Editor*
Kate Kretschmann, *Editorial Intern*

Mark Springer, *Technical Specialist*
Andrea Lopeman, *Programmer/Analyst*

Barbara Yarrow, *Manager, Imaging and Multimedia Content*
Robyn V. Young, *Project Manager, Imaging and Multimedia Content*
Randy Bassett, *Imaging Supervisor*
Dan Newell, *Imaging Specialist*
Pamela A. Reed, *Coordinator, Imaging and Multimedia Content*

Maria Franklin, *Permissions Manager*
Margaret A. Chamberlain, *Permissions Specialist*

Kenn Zorn, *Product Manager*
Michelle DiMercurio, *Senior Art Director, Page Design*
Pamela A. E. Galbreath, *Senior Art Director, Cover Design*

Mary Beth Trimper, *Manager, Composition and Electronic Prepress*
Evi Seoud, *Assistant Manager, Composition Purchasing and Electronic Prepress*
Dorothy Maki, *Manufacturing Manager*

Indexing provided by Synapse, the Knowledge Link Corporation.

This book is printed on recycled paper that meets Environmental Protection Agency standards.

The paper used in this publication meets the minimum requirements of American National Standard for Information Sciences-Permanence Paper for Printed Library Materials, ANSI Z39.48-1984.

ISBN 0-7876-5609-7 (set)
0-7876-5610-0 (Vol. 1)
0-7876-5611-9 (Vol. 2)

Printed in Canada
10 9 8 7 6 5 4 3 2 1

Library of Congress Cataloging-in-Publication Data
The Gale encyclopedia of cancer / Ellen Thackery.

p. cm.

Includes bibliographical references and index.

ISBN 0-7876-5610-0 (v. 1) — ISBN 0-7876-5611-9 (v.2) — ISBN 0-7876-5609-7 (set : hardcover)

1. Cancer—Encyclopedias. 2. Oncology—Encyclopedias. I. Thackery, Ellen, 1972-

RC254.5 .G353 2001
616.99'4'003—dc21
2001046015

CONTENTS

PLEASE READ—IMPORTANT INFORMATION

The *Gale Encyclopedia of Cancer* is a medical reference product designed to inform and educate readers about a wide variety of cancers, treatments, diagnostic procedures, side effects, and cancer drugs. The Gale Group believes the product to be comprehensive, but not necessarily definitive. It is intended to supplement, not replace, consultation with a physician or other health care practitioner. While the Gale Group has made substantial efforts to provide information that is accurate, comprehensive, and up-to-date, the Gale Group makes no representations or warranties of any kind, including without limitation, warranties of merchantability or fitness for a particular purpose, nor does it guarantee the accuracy, comprehensiveness, or timeliness of the information contained in this product. Readers should be aware that the universe of medical knowledge is constantly growing and changing, and that differences of medical opinion exist among authorities. Readers are also advised to seek professional diagnosis and treatment for any medical condition, and to discuss information obtained from this book with their health care provider.

INTRODUCTION

The *Gale Encyclopedia of Cancer: A Guide to Cancer and Its Treatments* is a unique and invaluable source of information for anyone touched by cancer. This collection of over 450 entries provides in-depth coverage of specific cancer types, diagnostic procedures, treatments, cancer side effects, and cancer drugs. In addition, entries have been included to facilitate understanding of common cancer-related concepts, such as cancer biology, carcinogenesis, and cancer genetics, as well as cancer issues such as clinical trials, home health care, fertility issues, and cancer prevention.

This encyclopedia minimizes medical jargon and uses language that laypersons can understand, while still providing thorough coverage that will benefit health science students as well.

Entries follow a standardized format that provides information at a glance. Rubrics include:

Cancer types	**Cancer drugs**
Definition	Definition
Description	Purpose
Demographics	Description
Causes and symptoms	Recommended dosage
Diagnosis	Precautions
Treatment team	Side effects
Clinical staging, treatments, and prognosis	Interactions
Coping with cancer treatment	
Clinical trials	
Prevention	
Special concerns	
Resources	

INCLUSION CRITERIA

A preliminary list of cancers and related topics was compiled from a wide variety of sources, including professional medical guides and textbooks, as well as consumer guides and encyclopedias. The advisory board, made up of medical doctors and oncology pharmacists, evaluated the topics and made suggestions for inclusion. Final selection of topics to include was made by the advisory board in conjunction with the Gale editor.

ABOUT THE CONTRIBUTORS

The essays were compiled by experienced medical writers, including physicians, pharmacists, nurses, and other health care professionals. The advisors reviewed the completed essays to ensure that they are appropriate, up-to-date, and medically accurate.

HOW TO USE THIS BOOK

The *Gale Encyclopedia of Cancer* has been designed with ready reference in mind.

- Straight **alphabetical arrangement** of topics allows users to locate information quickly.
- **Bold-faced terms** within entries direct the reader to related articles.
- **Cross-references** placed throughout the encyclopedia direct readers from alternate names and related topics to entries.
- A list of **key terms** is provided where appropriate to define unfamiliar terms or concepts.
- A list of **questions to ask the doctor** is provided whenever appropriate to help facilitate discussion with the patient's physician.
- The **Resources** section for non-drug entries directs readers to additional sources of medical information on a topic.
- Valuable **contact information** for organizations and support groups is included with each cancer type entry. Appendix II at the back of Volume II contains an extensive list of organizations arranged in alphabetical order.
- A comprehensive **general index** guides readers to all topics mentioned in the text.

- A note about **drug entries**: Drug entries are listed in alphabetical order by common **generic names**. However, because many oncology drugs have more than one common generic name, and because in many cases, the brand name is also often used interchangeably with a generic name, drugs can be located in one of three ways. The reader can: find the generic drug name in alphabetical order, be directed to the entry from an alternate name cross-reference, or use the **index** to look up a **brand name**, which will direct the reader to the equivalent generic name entry. If the reader would like more information about oncology drugs than these entries provide, the reader is encouraged to consult with a physician, pharmacist, or the reader may find helpful any one of a number of books about cancer drugs. Two that may be helpful are: D. Solimando's *Drug Information Handbook for Oncology*, or R. Ellerby's *Quick Reference Handbook of Oncology Drugs*.

GRAPHICS

The *Gale Encyclopedia of Cancer* contains over 200 full-color illustrations, photos and tables. Eleven illustrations of various body systems can be found in the front matter of the book, and these can help the reader to understand which cancers may affect which organs, and how the various systems interact.

ACKNOWLEDGMENTS

The editor would like to express appreciation to the following medical professionals who reviewed several entries within their areas of expertise for the *Gale Encyclopedia of Cancer*.

Linda Bressler, Pharm.D., B.C.O.P.
Clinical Associate Professor
College of Pharmacy
University of Illinois
Chicago, Illinois

Susan M. Mockus, Ph.D
Scientific Consultant
Seattle, Washington

James H. Morse, M.D.
Assistant Professor
Division of Gastroenterology
University of Virginia Health Sciences Center
Charlottesville, Virginia

PHOTO ACKNOWLEDGMENTS

On the cover, clockwise from upper left:

Colored computed tomography (CT) scan of a human brain. (Dept. of Clinical Radiology, Salisbury District Hospital, Science Source/Photo Researchers. Reproduced by permission.)

Color digitized image of the herpes simplex virus. (Custom Medical Stock Photo. Reproduced by permission.)

Colored CT scan revealing cancer of the liver. (Dept. of Clinical Radiology, Salisbury District Hospital, Science Source/Photo Reseachers. Reproduced by permission.)
False-color bone scan of the spine and ribs showing metastatic bone cancer of the spine. (CNRI, Science Source/Photo Researchers. Reproduced by permission.)

FOREWORD

Unfortunately, man must suffer disease. Some diseases are totally reversible and can be effectively treated. Moreover, some diseases with proper treatment have been virtually annihilated, such as polio, rheumatic fever, smallpox, and, to some extent, tuberculosis. Other diseases seem to target one organ, such as the heart, and there has been great progress in either fixing defects, adding blood flow, or giving medications to strengthen the diseased pump. Cancer, however, continues to frustrate even the cleverest of doctors or the most fastidious of health conscious individuals. Why?

By its very nature, cancer is a survivor. It has only one purpose: to proliferate. After all, that is the definition of cancer: unregulated growth of cells that fail to heed the message to stop growing. Normal cells go through a cycle of division, aging, and then selection for death. Cancer cells are able to circumvent this normal cycle, and escape recognition to be eliminated.

There are many mechanisms that can contribute to this unregulated cell growth. One of these mechanisms is inheritance. Unfortunately, some individuals can be programmed for cancer due to inherited disorders in their genetic makeup. In its simplest terms, one can inherit a faulty gene or a missing gene whose role is to eliminate damaged cells or to prevent imperfect cells from growing. Without this natural braking system, the damaged cells can divide and lead to more damaged cells with the same abnormal genetic makeup as the parent cells. Given enough time, and our inability to detect them, these groups of cells can grow to a size that will cause discomfort or other symptoms.

Inherited genetics are obviously not the only source of abnormalities in cells. Humans do not live in a sterile world devoid of environmental attacks or pathogens. Humans must work, and working environments can be dangerous. Danger can come in the form of radiation, chemicals, or fibers to which we may be chronically exposed with or without our knowledge. Moreover, man must eat, and if our food is contaminated with these environmental hazards, or if we prepare our food in a way that may change the chemical nature of the food to hazardous molecules, then chronic exposure to these toxins could damage cells. Finally, man is social. He has found certain habits that are pleasing to him because they either relax him or release his inhibitions. Such habits, including smoking and alcohol consumption, can have a myriad of influences on the genetic makeup of cells.

Why the emphasis on genes in the new century? Because they are potentially the reason as well as the answer for cancer. Genes regulate our micro- and macrosopic events by eventually coding for proteins that control our structure and function. If the above-mentioned environmental events cause errors in those genes that control growth, then imperfect cells can start to take root. For the majority of cases, a whole cascade of genetic events must occur before a cell is able to outlive its normal predecessors. This cascade of events could take years to occur, in a silent, undetected manner until the telltale signs and symptoms of advanced cancer are seen, including pain, lack of appetite, cough, loss of blood, or the detection of a lump. How did these cells get to this state where they are now dictating the everyday physical, psychological, and economic events for the person afflicted?

At this time, the sequence of genetic catastrophes is much too complex to comprehend or summarize because, it is only in the past year that we have even been able to map what genes we have and where they are located in our chromosomes. We have learned, however, that cancer cells are equipped with a series of self-protection mechanisms. Some of the altered genes are actually able to express themselves more than in the normal situation. These genes could then code for more growth factors for the transforming cell, or they could make proteins that could keep our own immune system from eliminating these interlopers. Finally, these cells are chameleons: if we treat them with drugs to try to kill them, they can "change their colors" by mutation, and then be resistant to the drugs that may have harmed them before.

Then what do we do for treatment? Man has always had a fascination with grooming, and grooming involves removal—dirt, hair, and waste. The ultimate removal involves cutting away the spoiled or imperfect portion. An abnormal growth? Remove it by surgery...make sure the edges are clean. Unfortunately, the painful reality of cancer surgery is that it is highly effective when performed in the early stages of the disease. "Early stages of the disease" implies that there is no spread, or, hopefully, before there are symptoms. In the majority of cases, however, surgery cannot eradicate all the disease because the cancer is not only at the primary site of the lump, but has spread to other organs. Cancer is not just a process of growth, but also a metastasizing process that allows for invasion and spread. The growing cells need nourishment so they secrete proteins that allow for the growth of blood vessels (angiogenesis); once the blood vessels are established from other blood vessels, the tumor cells can make proteins that will dissolve the imprisoning matrix surrounding them. Once this matrix is dissolved, it is only a matter of time before the cancer cells can migrate to other places making the use of surgery fruitless.

Since cancer cells have a propensity to leave home and pay a visit to other organs, therapies must be geared to treat the whole body and not just the site of origin. The problem with these chemotherapies is that they are not selective and wreak havoc on tissues that are not affected by the cancer. These therapies are not natural to the human host, and result in nausea, loss of appetite, fatigue, as well as a depletion in our cells that protect us from infection and those that carry oxygen. Doctors who prescribe such medications walk a fine line between helping the patient (causing a "response" in the cancer by making it smaller) or causing "toxicity" which, due to effects on normal organs, causes the patient problems. Although these drugs are far from perfect, we are fortunate to have them because when they work, their results can be remarkable.

But that's the problem—"when they work." We cannot predict who is going to benefit from our therapies, and doctors must inform the patient and his/her family about countless studies that have been done to validate the use of these potentially beneficial/potentially harmful agents. Patients must suffer the frustration that oncologists have because each individual afflicted with cancer is different, and indeed, each cancer is different. This makes it virtually impossible to personalize an individual's treatment expectations and life expectancy. Cancer, after all, is a very impersonal disease, and does not respect sex, race, wealth, age, or any other "human" characteristics.

Cancer treatment is in search of "smart" options. Like modern-day instruments of war, successful cancer treatment will necessitate the construction of therapies that can do three basic tasks: search out the enemy, recognize the enemy, and kill the enemy without causing "friendly fire." The successful therapies of the future will involve the use of "living components," "manufactured components," or a combination of both. Living components, white blood cells, will be educated to recognize where the cancer is, and help our own immune system fight the foreign cells. These lymphocytes can be educated to recognize signals on the cancer cell which make them unique. Therapies in the future will be able to manufacture molecules with these signature, unique signals which are linked to other molecules specifically for killing the cells. Only the cancer cells are eliminated in this way, hopefully sparing the individual from toxicity.

Why use these unique signals as delivery mechanisms? If they are unique and are important for growth of the cancer cell, it makes sense to target them directly. This describes the ambitious mission of gene therapy, whose goal is to supplement a deficient, necessary genetic pool or diminish the number of abnormally expressed genes fortifying the cancer cells. If a protein is not being made that slows the growth of cells, gene therapy would theoretically supply the gene for this protein to replenish it and cause the cells to slow down. If the cells can make their own growth factors that sustain them selectively over normal cells, then the goal is to block the production of this growth factor. There is no doubt that gene therapy is the wave of the future and is under intense investigation and scrutiny at present. The problem, however, is that there is no way to tell when this future promise will be fulfilled.

No book can describe the medical, psychological, social, and economic burden of cancer, and if this is your first confrontation with the enemy, you may find yourself overwhelmed with its magnitude. Books are only part of the solution. Newly enlisted recruits in this war must seek proper counsel from educated physicians who will inform the family and the patient of the risks and benefits of a treatment course in a way that can be understood. Advocacy groups of dedicated volunteers, many of whom are cancer survivors, can guide and advise. The most important component, however, is an intensely personal one. The afflicted individual must realize that he/she is responsible for charting the course of his/her disease, and this requires the above described knowledge as well as great personal intuition. Cancer comes as a series of shocks: the symptoms, the diagnosis, and the treatment. These shocks can be followed by cautious optimism or profound disappointment. Each one of these shocks either reinforces or chips away at one's resolve, and how an individual reacts to these issues is as unique as the cancer that is being dealt with.

While cancer is still life threatening, strides have been made in the fight against the disease. Thirty years ago, a young adult diagnosed with testicular cancer had few options for treatment that could result in cure. Now, chemotherapy for good risk Stage II and III testicular cancer can result in a complete response of the tumor in 98% of the cases and a durable response in 92%. Sixty years ago, there were no regimens that could cause a complete remission for a child diagnosed with leukemia; but now, using combination chemotherapy, complete remissions are possible in 96% of these cases. Progress has been made, but more progress is needed. The first real triumph in cancer care will be when cancer is no longer thought of as a life-ending disease, but as a chronic disease whose symptoms can be managed. Anyone who has been touched by cancer or who has been involved in the fight against it lives in hope that that day will arrive.

Helen A. Pass, M.D., F.A.C.S.
Dr. Pass is the Director of the Breast Care Center at William Beaumont Hospital in Royal Oak, Michigan.

ADVISORY BOARD

A number of experts in the medical community provided invaluable assistance in the formulation of this encyclopedia. The advisory board performed a myriad of duties, from defining the scope of coverage to reviewing individual entries for accuracy and accessibility. The editor would like to express appreciation to them for their time and for their contributions.

CONTRIBUTORS

Margaret Alic, Ph.D.
Science Writer
Eastsound, Washington

Lisa Andres, M.S., C.G.C.
Certified Genetic Counselor and Medical Writer
San Jose, California

Racquel Baert, M.Sc.
Medical Writer
Winnipeg, Canada

Julia R. Barrett
Science Writer
Madison, Wisconsin

Nancy J. Beaulieu, RPh., B.C.O.P.
Oncology Pharmacist
New Haven, Connecticut

Linda K. Bennington, C.N.S., M.S.N.
Clinical Nurse Specialist
Department of Nursing
Old Dominion University
Norfolk, Virginia

Kenneth J. Berniker, M.D.
Attending Physician
Emergency Department
Kaiser Permanente Medical Center
Vallejo, California

Olga Bessmertny, Pharm.D.
Clinical Pharmacy Manager
Pediatric Hematology/Oncology/Bone Marrow Transplant
Children's Hospital of New York
Columbia Presbyterian Medical Center
New York, New York

Patricia L. Bounds, Ph.D.
Science Writer
Zürich, Switzerland

Cheryl Branche, M.D.
Retired General Practitioner
Jackson, Mississippi

Tamara Brown, R.N.
Medical Writer
Boston, Massachusetts

Diane M. Calabrese
Medical Sciences and Technology Writer
Silver Spring, Maryland

Rosalyn Carson-DeWitt, M.D.
Durham, North Carolina

Lata Cherath, Ph.D.
Science Writer
Franklin Park, New York

Lisa Christenson, Ph.D.
Science Writer
Hamden, Connecticut

Rhonda Cloos, R.N.
Medical Writer
Austin, Texas

David Cramer, M.D.
Medical Writer
Chicago, Illinois

Tish Davidson, A.M.
Medical Writer
Fremont, California

Dominic De Bellis, Ph.D.
Medical Writer/Editor
Mahopac, New York

Tiffani A. DeMarco, M.S.
Genetic Counselor
Cancer Control
Georgetown University
Washington, DC

Lori De Milto
Medical Writer
Sicklerville, New York

Stefanie B. N. Dugan, M.S.
Genetic Counselor
Milwaukee, Wisconsin

Janis O. Flores
Medical Writer
Sebastopol, California

Paula Ford-Martin
Medical Writer
Chaplin, Minnesota

Rebecca J. Frey, Ph.D.
Research and Administrative Associate
East Rock Institute
New Haven, Connecticut

Jill Granger, M.S.
Senior Research Associate
University of Michigan
Ann Arbor, Michigan

David E. Greenberg, M.D.
Medicine Resident
Baylor College of Medicine
Houston, Texas

Maureen Haggerty
Medical Writer
Ambler, Pennsylvania

Kevin Hwang, M.D.
Medical Writer
Morristown, New Jersey

Michelle L. Johnson, M.S., J.D.
Patent Attorney and Medical Writer
Portland, Oregon

Paul A. Johnson, Ed.M.
Medical Writer
San Diego, California

Cindy L. A. Jones, Ph.D.
Biomedical Writer
Sagescript Communications
Lakewood, Colorado

Crystal H. Kaczkowski, M.Sc.
Medical Writer
Montreal, Canada

David S. Kaminstein, M.D.
Medical Writer
Westchester, Pennsylvania

Beth Kapes
Medical Writer
Bay Village, Ohio

Bob Kirsch
Medical Writer
Ossining, New York

Melissa Knopper
Medical Writer
Chicago, Illinois

Monique Laberge, Ph.D.
Research Associate
Department of Biochemistry and Biophysics
University of Pennsylvania
Philadelphia, Pennsylvania

Jill S. Lasker
Medical Writer
Midlothian, Virginia

G. Victor Leipzig, Ph.D.
Biological Consultant
Huntington Beach, California

Lorraine Lica, Ph.D.
Medical Writer
San Diego, California

John T. Lohr, Ph.D.
Utah State University
Logan, Utah

Warren Maltzman, Ph.D.
Consultant, Molecular Pathology
Demarest, New Jersey

Richard A. McCartney M.D.
Fellow, American College of Surgeons
Diplomat, American Board of Surgery
Richland, Washington

Sally C. McFarlane-Parrott
Medical Writer
Mason, Michigan

Monica McGee, M.S.
Science Writer
Wilmington, North Carolina

Alison McTavish, M.Sc.
Medical Writer and Editor
Montreal, Quebec

Molly Metzler, R.N., B.S.N.
Registered Nurse, Medical Writer
Seaford, Delaware

Beverly G. Miller
MT(ASCP), Technical Writer
Charlotte, North Carolina

Mark A. Mitchell, M.D.
Medical Writer
Seattle, Washington

Laura J. Ninger
Medical Writer
Weehawken, New Jersey

Nancy J. Nordenson
Medical Writer
Minneapolis, Minnesota

Teresa G. Norris, R.N.
Medical Writer
Ute Park, New Mexico

Melinda Granger Oberleitner, R.N., D.N.S.
Acting Department Head and Associate Professor
Department of Nursing
University of Louisiana at Lafayette
Lafayette, Louisiana

J. Ricker Polsdorfer, M.D.
Medical Writer
Phoenix, Arizona

Elizabeth J. Pulcini, M.S.
Medical Writer
Phoenix, Arizona

Kulbir Rangi, D.O.
Medical Doctor and Writer
New York, New York

Esther Csapo Rastegari, Ed.M., R.N., B.S.N.
Registered Nurse, Medical Writer
Holbrook, Masachusetts

Toni Rizzo
Medical Writer
Salt Lake City, Utah

Martha Floberg Robbins
Medical Writer
Evanston, Illinois

Richard Robinson
Medical Writer
Tucson, Arizona

Edward R. Rosick, D.O., M.P.H., M.S.
University Physician, Clinical Assistant Professor
Student Health Services
The Pennsylvania State University
University Park, Pennsylvania

Nancy Ross-Flanigan
Science Writer
Belleville, Michigan

Belinda Rowland, Ph.D.
Medical Writer
Voorheesville, New York

Andrea Ruskin, M.D.
Whittingham Cancer Center
Norwalk, Connecticut

Laura Ruth, Ph.D.
Medical, Science, & Technology Writer
Los Angeles, California

Kausalya Santhanam, Ph.D.
Technical Writer
Branford, Connecticut

Marc Scanio
Doctoral Candidate in Chemistry
Stanford University
Stanford, California

Joan Schonbeck, R.N.
Medical Writer
Nursing
Massachusetts Department of Mental Health
Marlborough, Massachusetts

Kristen Mahoney Shannon, M.S., C.G.C.
Genetic Counselor
Center for Cancer Risk Analysis
Massachusetts General Hospital
Boston, Massachusetts

Genevieve Slomski, Ph.D.
Medical Writer
New Britain, Connecticut

Anna Rovid Spickler, D.V.M., Ph.D.
Medical Writer
Salisbury, Maryland

Laura L. Stein, M.S.
Certified Genetic Counselor
Familial Cancer Program-Department of Hematology/Oncology
Dartmouth Hitchcock Medical Center
Lebanon, New Hampshire

Phyllis M. Stein, B.S., C.C.R.P.
Affiliate Coordinator
Grand Rapids Clinical Oncology Program
Grand Rapids, Michigan

Kurt Sternlof
Science Writer
New Rochelle, New York

Deanna M. Swartout-Corbeil
Registered Nurse, Freelance Writer
Thompsons Station, Tennessee

Jane M. Taylor-Jones, M.S.
Research Associate
Donald W. Reynolds Department of Geriatrics
University of Arkansas for Medical Sciences
Little Rock, Arkansas

Carol Turkington
Medical Writer
Lancaster, Pennsylvania

Marianne Vahey, M.D.
Clinical Instructor
Medicine
Yale University School of Medicine
New Haven, Connecticut

Malini Vashishtha, Ph.D.
Medical Writer
Irvine, California

Ellen S. Weber, M.S.N.
Medical Writer
Fort Wayne, Indiana

Barbara Wexler, M.P.H.
Medical Writer
Chatsworth, California

Wendy Wippel, M.Sc.
Medical Writer and Adjunct Professor of Biology
Northwest Community College
Hernando, Mississippi

Debra Wood, R.N.
Medical Writer
Orlando, Florida

Kathleen D. Wright, R.N.
Medical Writer
Delmar, Delaware

Jon Zonderman
Medical Writer
Orange, California

Michael V. Zuck, Ph.D.
Writer
Boulder, Colorado

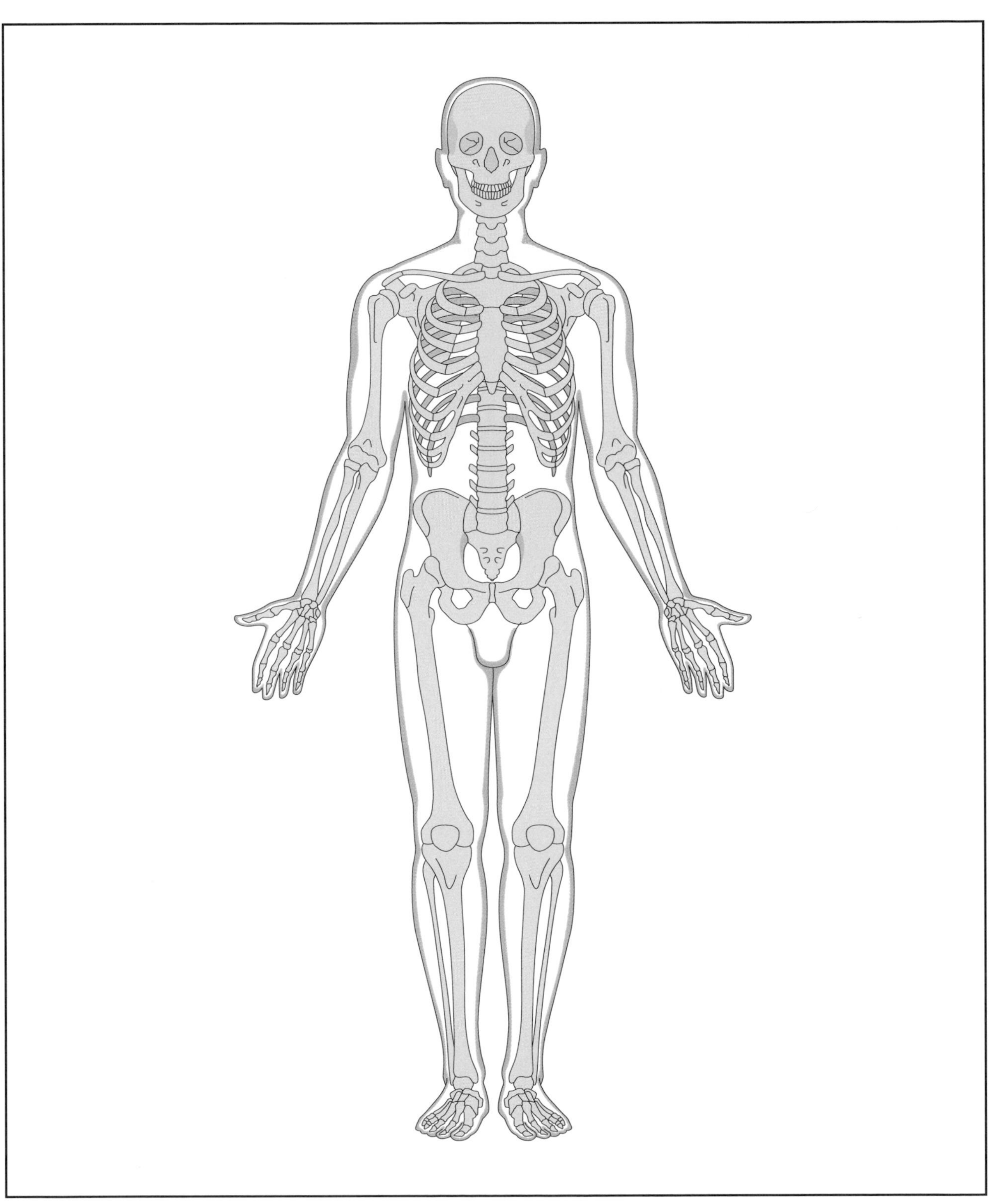

HUMAN SKELETON and SKIN. Some cancers that affect the SKELETON are: Osteosarcoma; Ewing's sarcoma; Fibrosarcoma (can also be found in soft tissues like muscle, fat, connective tissues, etc.). Some cancers that affect tissue near bones: Chondrosarcoma (affects joints near bones); Rhabdomyosarcoma (formed from cells of muscles attached to bones); Malignant fibrous histiocytoma (common in soft tissues, rare in bones). SKIN CANCERS: Basal cell carcinoma; Melanoma; Merkel cell carcinoma; Squamous cell carcinoma of the skin; and Trichilemmal carcinoma. Precancerous skin condition: Bowen's disease. Lymphomas that affect the skin: Mycosis fungoides; Sézary syndrome. *(Illustration provided by Argosy Publishing.)*

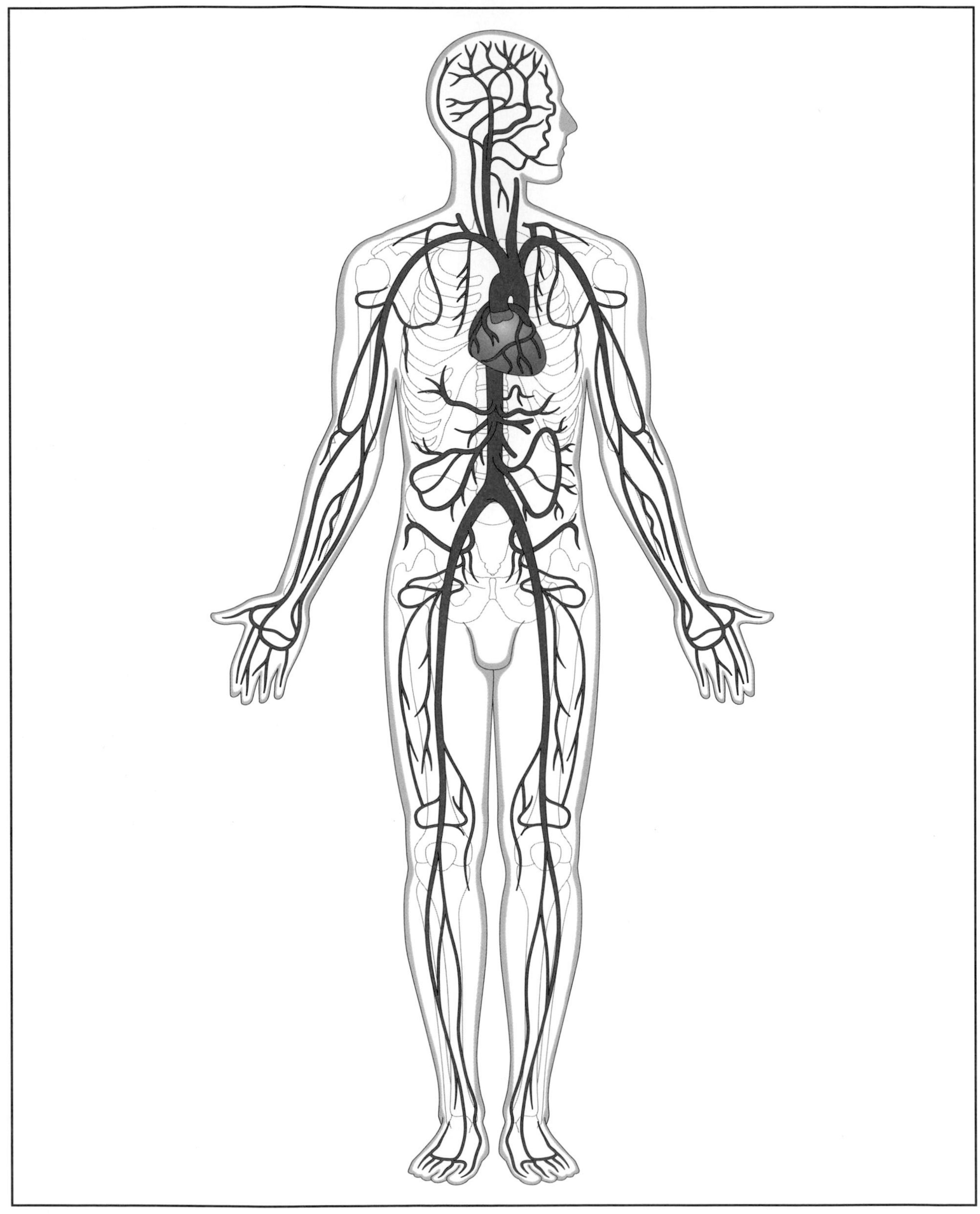

HUMAN CIRCULATORY SYSTEM. Some cancers of the blood cells are: Acute erythroblastic leukemia; Acute lymphocytic leukemia; Acute myelocytic leukemia; Chronic lymphocytic leukemia; Chronic myelocytic leukemia; Hairy cell leukemia; and Multiple myeloma. One condition associated with various cancers that affects blood is called Myelofibrosis. *(Illustration provided by Argosy Publishing.)*

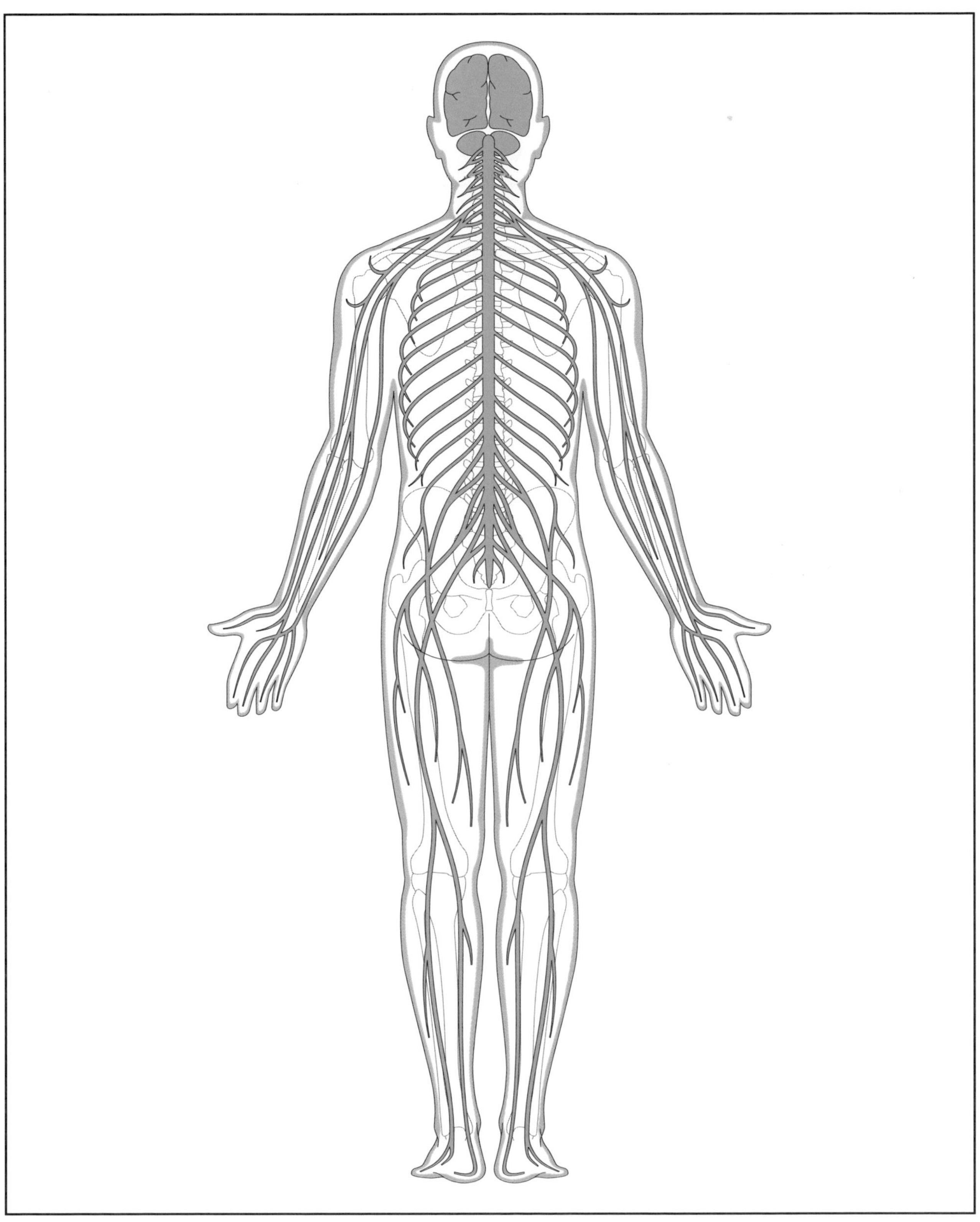

HUMAN NERVOUS SYSTEM. Some brain and central nervous system tumors are: Astrocytoma; Carcinomatous meningitis; Central nervous system carcinoma; Central nervous system lymphoma; Chordoma; Choroid plexus tumors; Craniopharyngioma; Ependymoma; Medulloblastoma; Meningioma; Oligodendroglioma; and Spinal axis tumors. One kind of noncancerous growth in the brain: Acoustic neuroma. *(Illustration provided by Argosy Publishing.)*

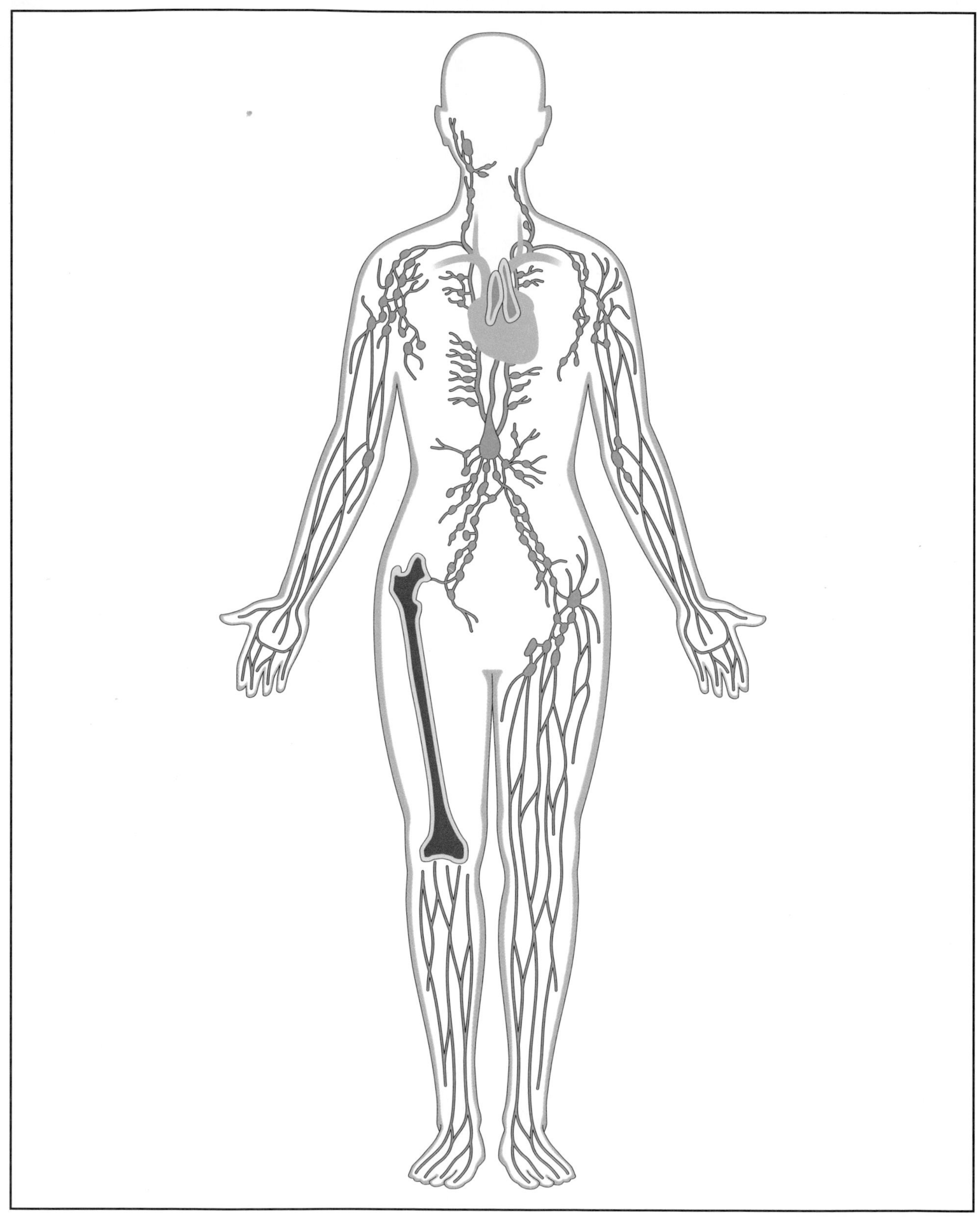

HUMAN LYMPHATIC SYSTEM. **The lymphatic system and lymph nodes are shown here in pale green, the thymus in deep blue, and one of the bones rich in bone marrow (the femur) is shown here in purple. Some cancers of the lymphatic system are: Burkitt's lymphoma; Cutaneous T-cell lymphoma; Hodgkin's disease; MALT lymphoma; Mantle cell lymphoma; Sézary syndrome; and Waldenström's macroglobulinemia.** *(Illustration provided by Argosy Publishing.)*

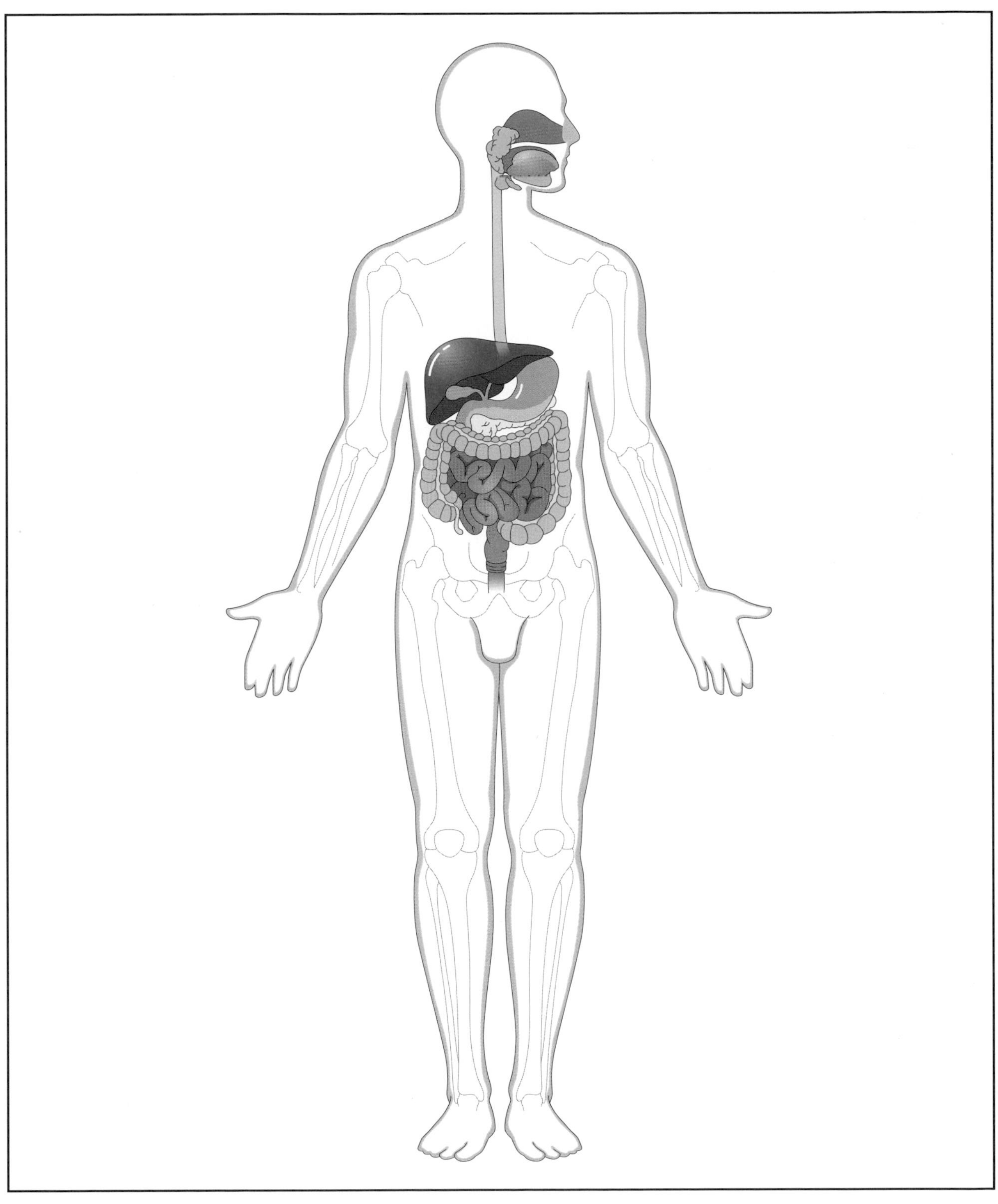

HUMAN DIGESTIVE SYSTEM. Organs and cancers of the digestive system include: Salivary glands (shown in turquoise): Salivary gland tumors. Esophagus (shown in bright yellow): Esophageal cancer. Liver (shown in bright red): Bile duct cancer; Liver cancer. Stomach (pale gray-blue): Stomach cancer. Gallbladder (bright orange against the red liver): Gallbladder cancer. Colon (green): Colon cancer. Small intestine (purple): Small intestinal cancer; can have malignant tumors associated with Zollinger-Ellison syndrome. Rectum (shown in pink, continuing the colon): Rectal cancer. Anus (dark blue): Anal cancer. *(Illustration provided by Argosy Publishing.)*

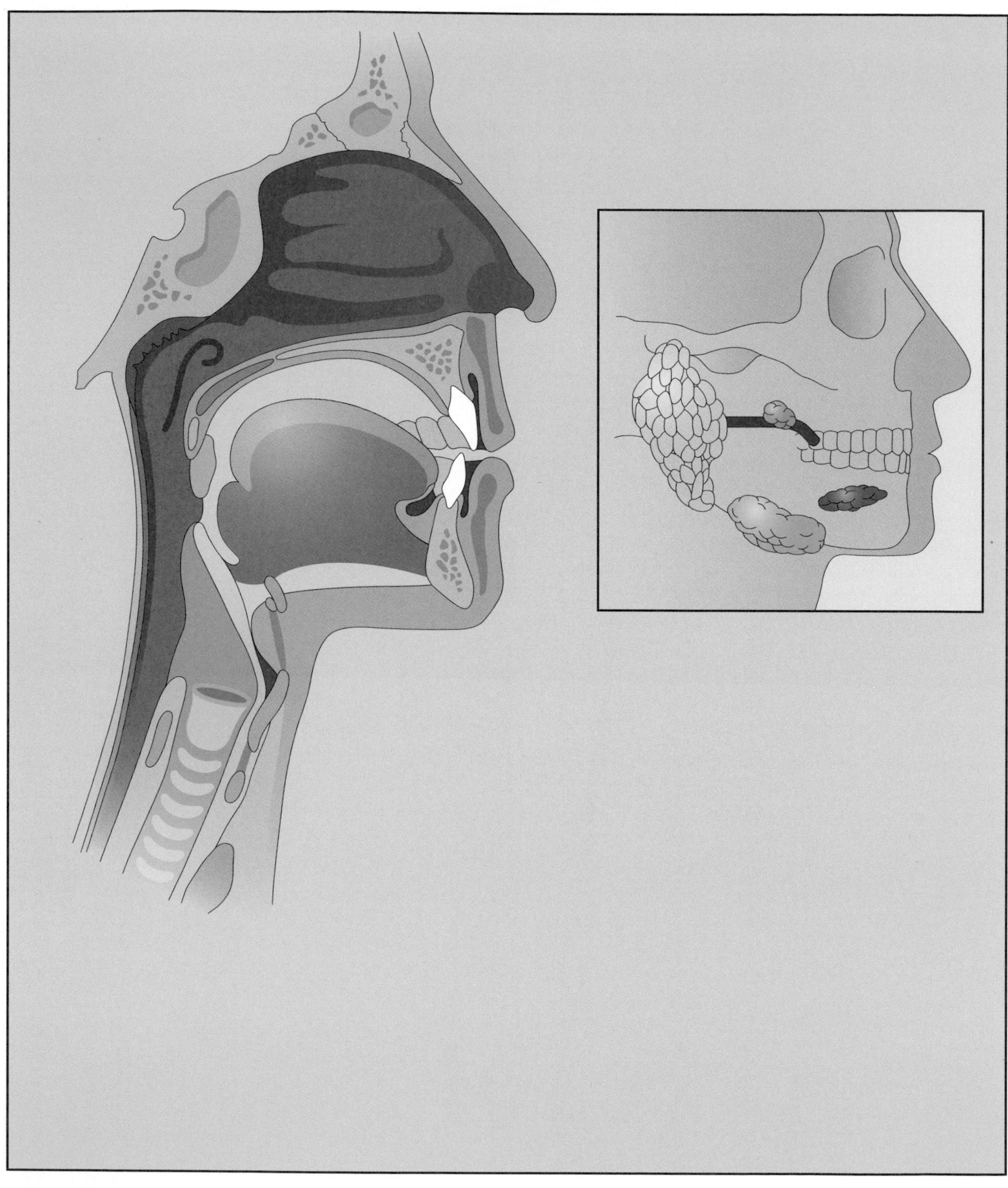

HEAD AND NECK. **The pharynx, the passage that leads from the nostrils down through the neck is shown in orange. This passage is broken into several divisions. The area posterior to (behind) the nose is the nasopharynx. The area posterior to the mouth is the oropharynx. The oropharynx leads into the laryngopharynx, which opens into the esophagus (still in orange) and the larynx (shown in the large image in medium blue). Each of these regions may be affected by cancer, and the cancers include: Nasopharyngeal cancer; Oropharyngeal cancer; Esophageal cancer; and Laryngeal cancer. Oral cancers can affect the lips, gums, and tongue (pink). Referring to the smaller, inset picture of the salivary glands, salivary gland tumors can affect the parotid glands (shown here in yellow), the submandibular glands (inset picture, turquoise), and the sublingual glands (purple).** *(Illustration provided by Argosy Publishing.)*

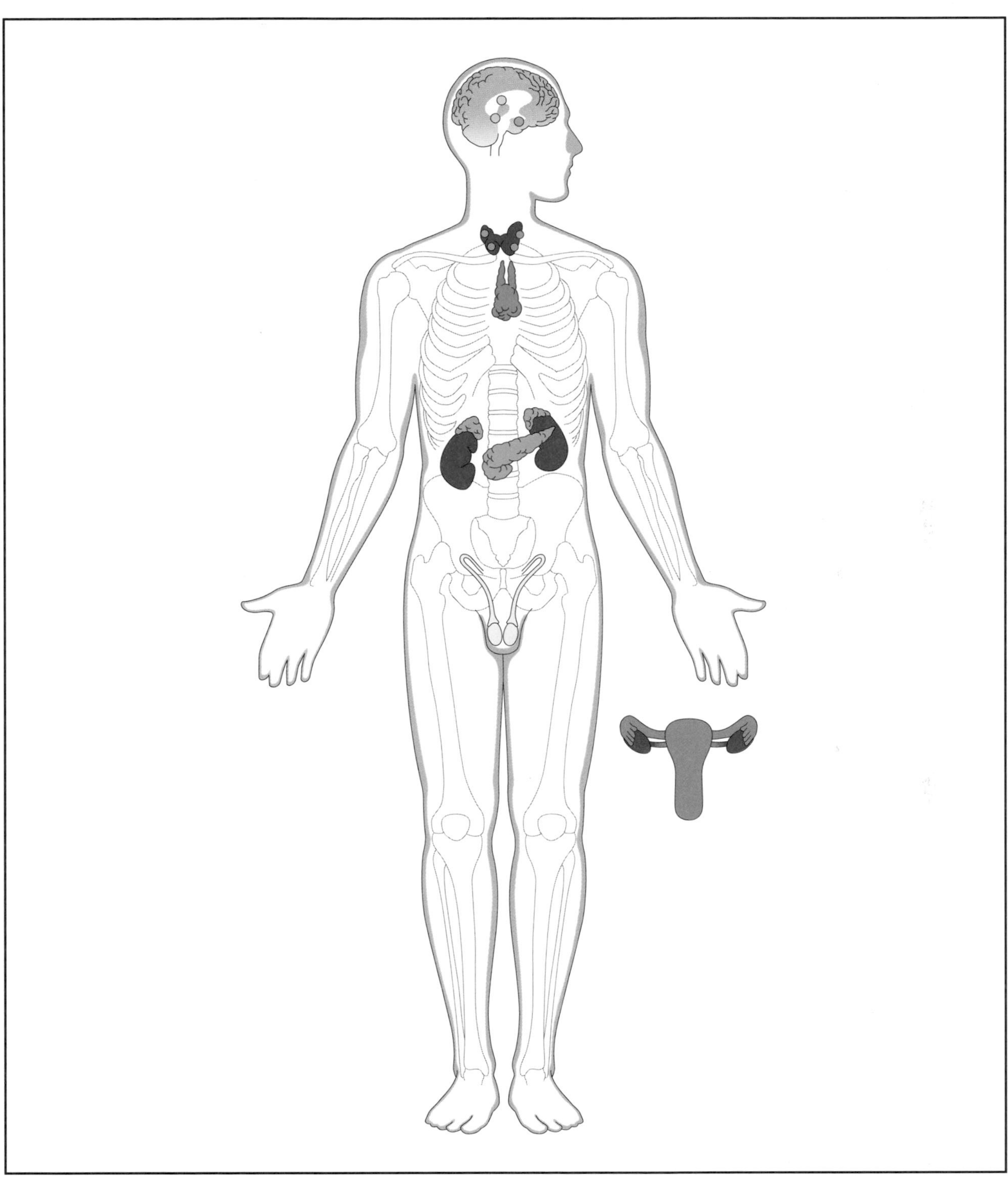

HUMAN ENDOCRINE SYSTEM. The glands and cancers of the endocrine system include: In the brain: the pituitary gland shown in blue (pituitary tumors), the hypothalamus in pale green, and the pineal gland in bright yellow. Throughout the rest of the body: Thyroid (shown in dark blue): Thyroid cancer. Parathyroid glands, four of them adjacent to the thyroid: Parathyroid cancer. Thymus (green): Thymic cancer; Thymoma. Pancreas (turquoise): Pancreatic cancer, endocrine; Pancreatic cancer, exocrine; Zollinger-Ellison syndrome tumors can be malignant and can be found in the pancreas. Adrenal glands (shown in apricot, above the kidneys): Neuroblastoma often originates in these glands; Pheochromocytoma tumors are often found in adrenal glands. Testes (in males, shown in yellow): Testicular cancer. Ovaries (in females, shown in dark blue in inset image): Ovarian cancer. *(Illustration provided by Argosy Publishing.)*

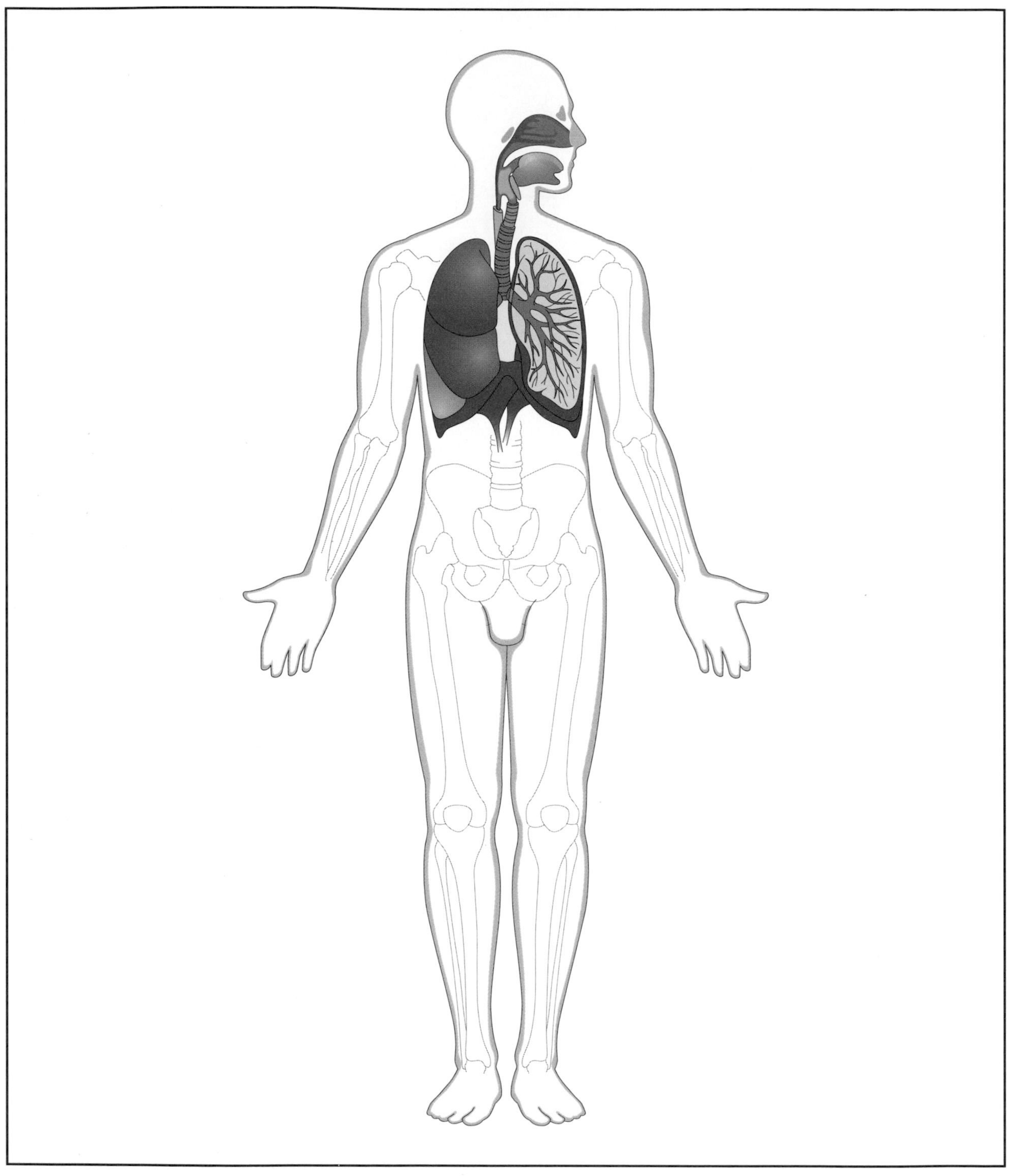

HUMAN RESPIRATORY SYSTEM. Air is breathed in through nose or mouth, enters the pharynx, shown here in orange, and passes through the larynx, shown here as a green tube with a ridged texture. (The smooth green tube shown is the esophagus, which is posterior to the larynx and which is involved in digestion instead of breathing.) The air then passes into the trachea (purple), a tube that divides into two tubes called bronchi. One bronchus passes into each lung, and continues to branch within the lung. These branches are called bronchioles and each bronchiole leads to a tiny cluster of air sacs called alveoli, where the exchange of gases occurs, so that the air and gases breathed in get diffused to the blood. The lungs (deep blue) are spongy and have lobes and can be affected by Lung cancer, both the non-small cell and small-cell types. *(Illustration provided by Argosy Publishing.)*

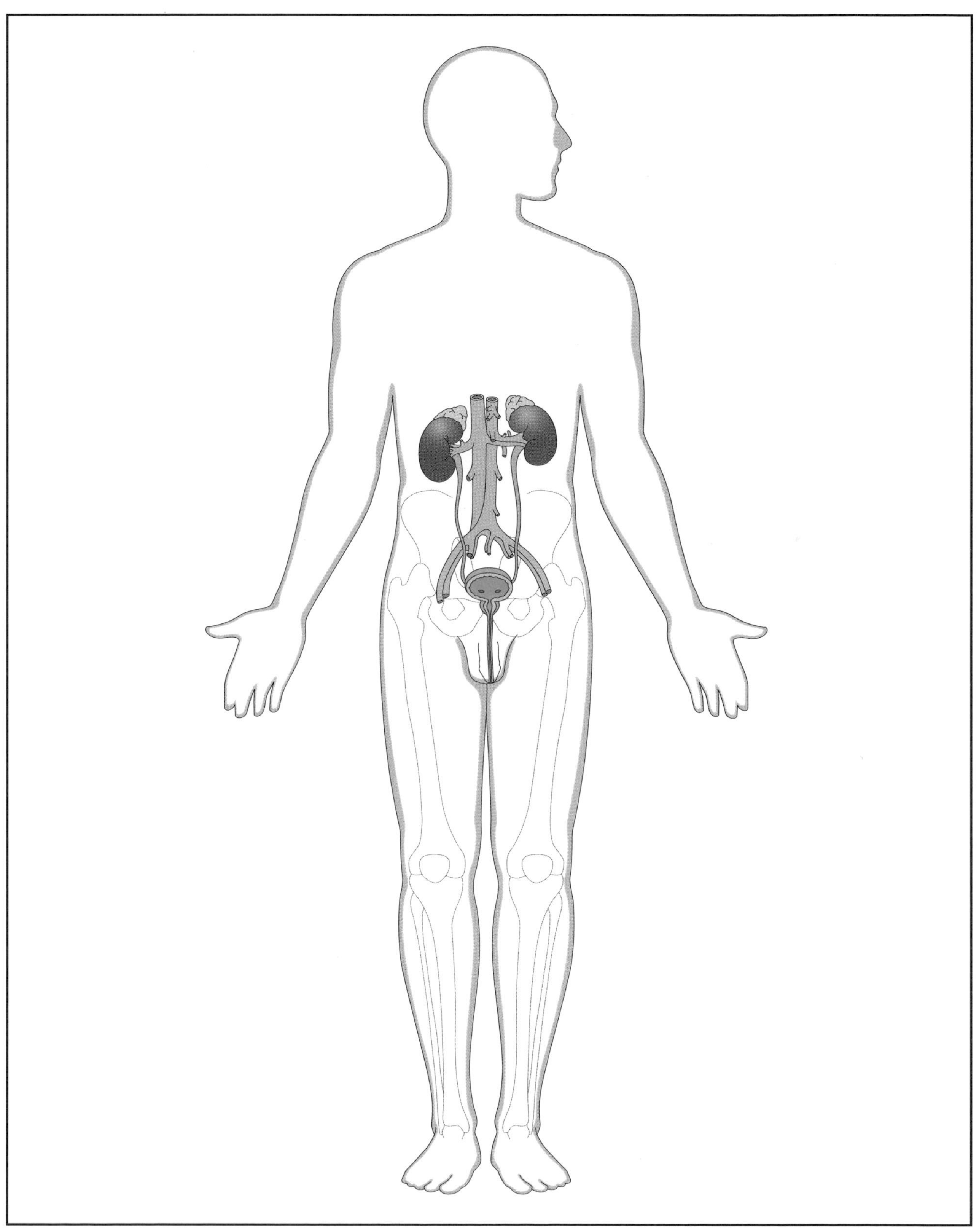

HUMAN URINARY SYSTEM. Organs and cancers of the urinary system include: Kidneys (shown in purple): Kidney cancer; Renal pelvis tumors; Wilms' tumor. Ureters are shown in green. Bladder (blue-green): Bladder cancer. The kidneys, bladder, or ureters can be affected by a cancer type called Transitional cell carcinoma. *(Illustration provided by Argosy Publishing.)*

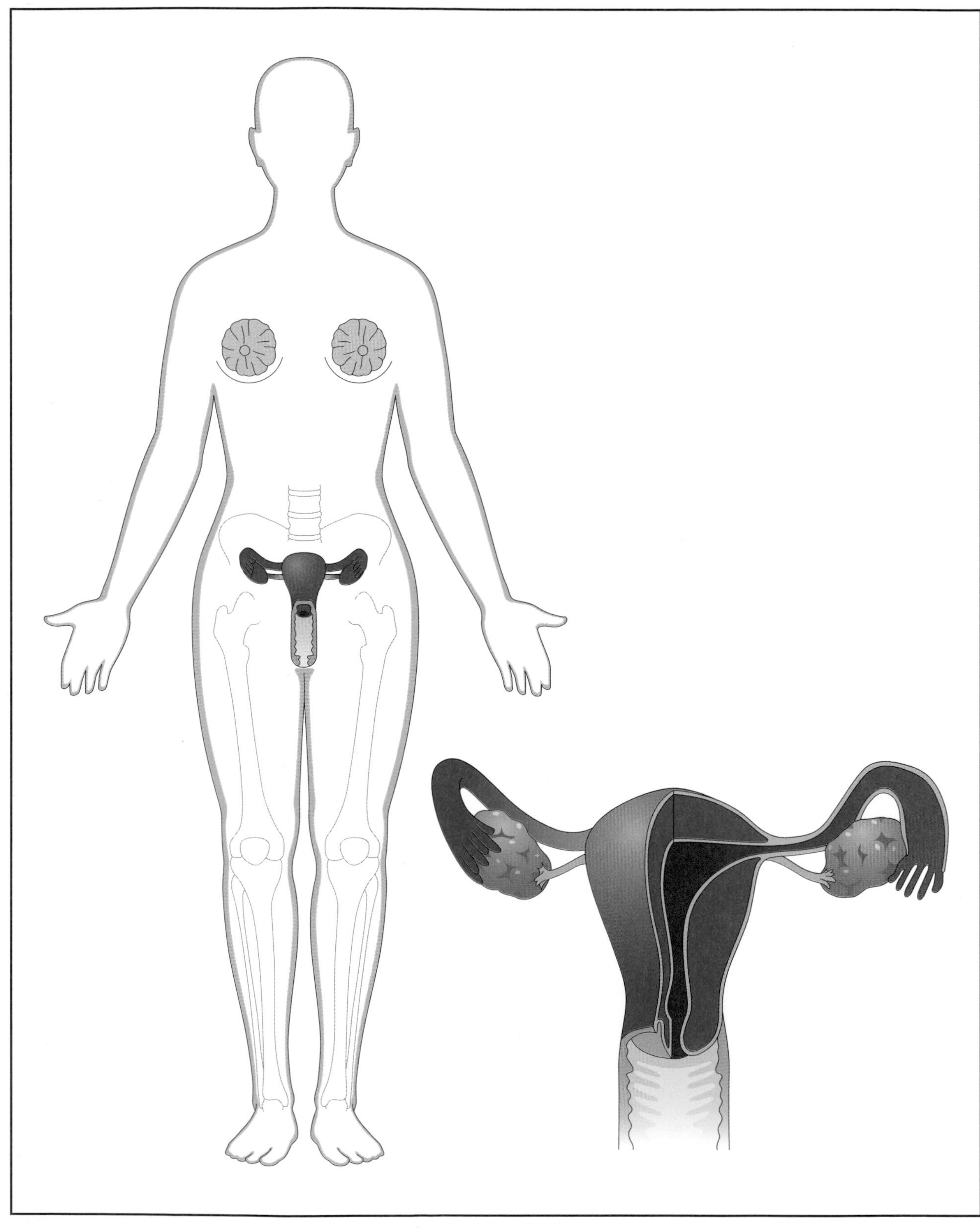

FEMALE REPRODUCTIVE SYSTEM. Organs and cancers of the female reproductive system include: Uterus, shown in red with the uterine or Fallopian tubes: Endometrial cancer. Ovaries (blue): Ovarian cancer. Vagina (shown in pink with a yellow interior or lining): Vaginal cancer. Breasts: Breast cancer; Paget's disease of the breast. Shown in detailed inset only in turquoise, Cervix: Cervical cancer. *(Illustration provided by Argosy Publishing.)*

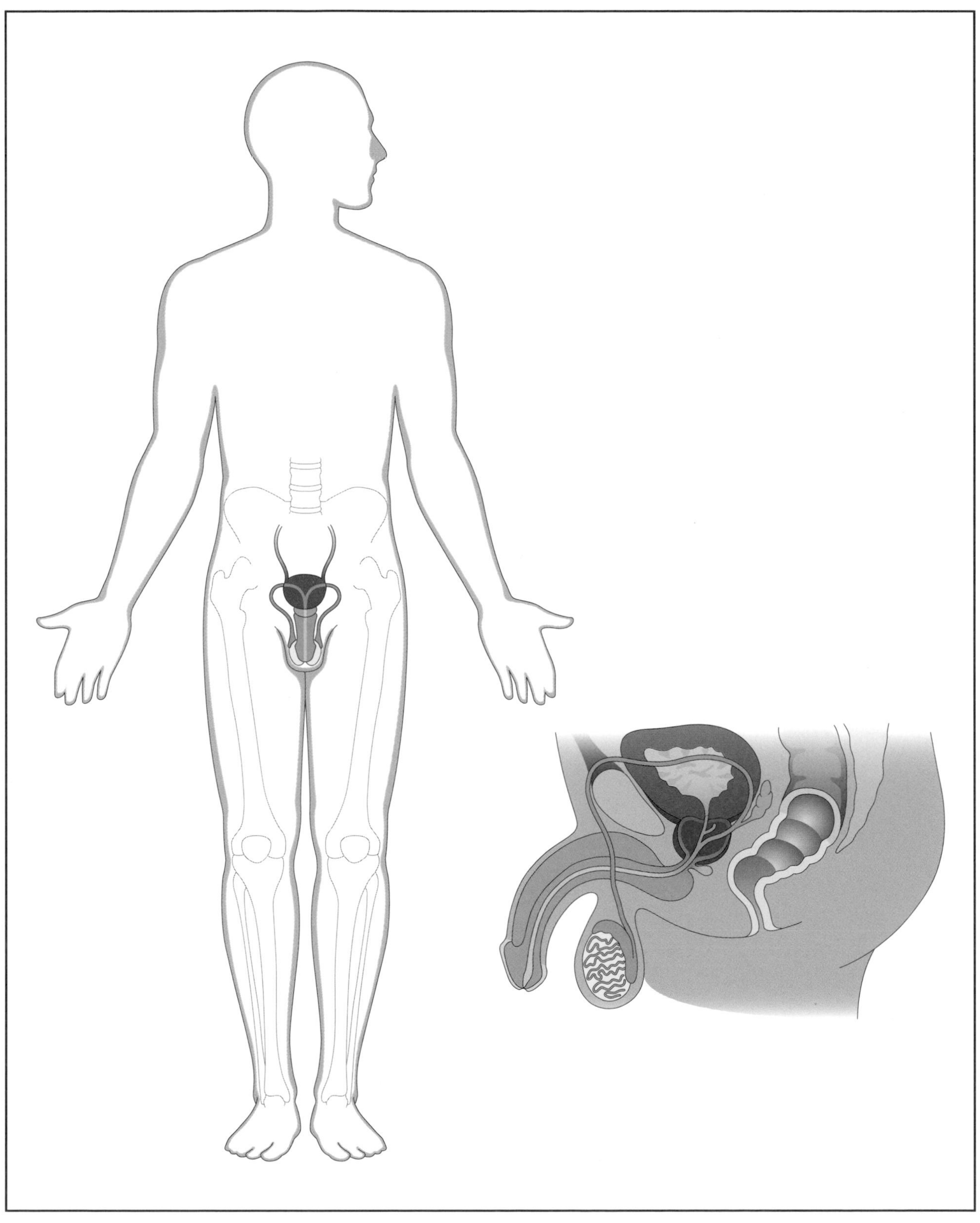

MALE REPRODCTIVE SYSTEM. Organs, glands, and cancers of the male reproductive system include: Penis (shown in pink): Penile cancer. Testes (shown in yellow): Testicular cancer. Prostate gland (shown in full-body illustration in a peach/ apricot color, and in the inset as the dark blue gland between the bladder and the penis): Prostate cancer. *(Illustration provided by Argosy Publishing.)*

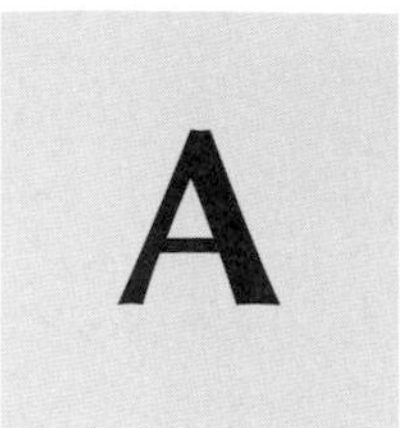

2-CdA *see* **Cladribine**
5-Azacitidine *see* **Azacitidine**
5-Fluorouracil *see* **Fluorouracil**
6-Mercaptopurine *see* **Mercaptopurine**
6-Thioguanine *see* **Thioguanine**

Acoustic neuroma

Definition

An acoustic neuroma is a benign tumor involving cells of the myelin sheath that surrounds the vestibulocochlear nerve (eighth cranial nerve).

Description

The vestibulocochlear nerve extends from the inner ear to the brain and is made up of a vestibular branch, often called the vestibular nerve, and a cochlear branch, called the cochlear nerve. The vestibular and cochlear nerves lie next to one another. They also run along side other cranial nerves. People possess two of each type of vestibulocochlear nerve, one that extends from the left ear and one that extends from the right ear.

The vestibular nerve transmits information concerning balance from the inner ear to the brain and the cochlear nerve transmits information about hearing. The vestibular nerve, like many nerves, is surrounded by a cover called a myelin sheath. A tumor, called a schwannoma, can sometimes develop from the cells of the myelin sheath. A tumor is an abnormal growth of tissue that results from the uncontrolled growth of cells. Acoustic neuromas are often called vestibular schwannomas because they are tumors that arise from the myelin sheath that surrounds the vestibular nerve. Acoustic neuromas are considered benign (non-cancerous) tumors since they do not spread to other parts of the body. They can occur anywhere along the vestibular nerve but are most likely to occur where the vestibulocochlear nerve passes through the tiny bony canal that connects the brain and the inner ear.

An acoustic neuroma can arise from the left vestibular nerve or the right vestibular nerve. A unilateral tumor is a tumor arising from one nerve and a bilateral tumor arises from both vestibular nerves. Unilateral acoustic neuromas usually occur spontaneously (by chance). Bilateral acoustic neuromas occur as part of a hereditary condition called Neurofibromatosis Type 2 (NF2). A person with NF2 has inherited a predisposition for developing acoustic neuromas and other tumors of the nerve cells.

Acoustic neuromas usually grow slowly and can take years to develop. Some acoustic neuromas remain so small that they do not cause any symptoms. As the acoustic neuroma grows it can interfere with the functioning of the vestibular nerve and can cause vertigo and balance difficulties. If the acoustic nerve grows large enough to press against the cochlear nerve, then hearing loss and a ringing (tinnitus) in the affected ear will usually occur. If untreated and the acoustic neuroma continues to grow, it can press against other nerves in the region and cause other symptoms. This tumor can be life threatening if it becomes large enough to press against and interfere with the functioning of the brain.

Causes and symptoms

Causes

An acoustic neuroma is caused by a change or absence of both of the NF2 tumor suppressor genes in a nerve cell. Every person possesses a pair of NF2 genes in every cell of their body including their nerve cells. One NF2 gene is inherited from the egg cell of the mother and one NF2 gene is inherited from the sperm cell of the father. The NF2 gene is responsible for helping to prevent the formation of tumors in the nerve cells. In particular the NF2 gene helps to prevent acoustic neuromas.

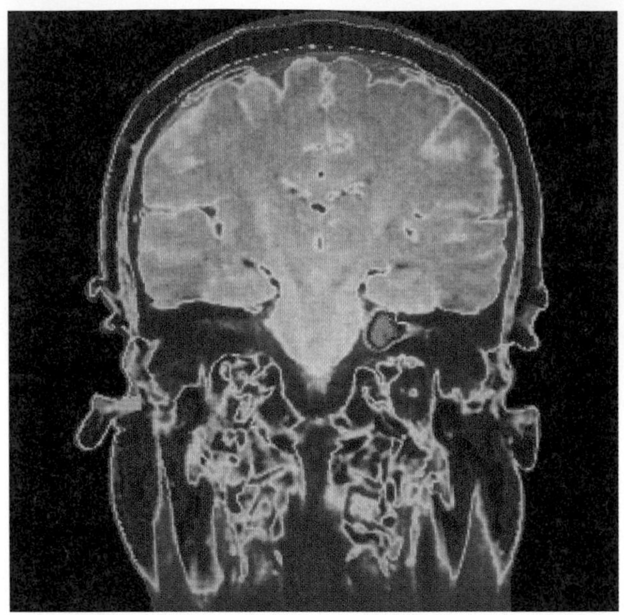

False-color magnetic resonance image (MRI) scan of a coronal section of the head & brain of someone suffering from an acoustic neuroma (green circular area). *(Photograph by Mehau Kulyk, Photo Researchers, Inc. Reproduced by permission.)*

Only one unchanged and functioning NF2 gene is necessary to prevent the formation of an acoustic neuroma. If both NF2 genes become changed or missing in one of the myelin sheath cells of the vestibular nerve, then an acoustic neuroma will usually develop. Most unilateral acoustic neuromas result when the NF2 genes become spontaneously changed or missing. Someone with a unilateral acoustic neuroma that has developed spontaneously is not at increased risk for having children with an acoustic neuroma. Some unilateral acoustic neuromas result from the hereditary condition NF2. It is also possible that some unilateral acoustic neuromas may be caused by changes in other genes responsible for preventing the formation of tumors.

Bilateral acoustic neuromas result when someone is affected with the hereditary condition NF2. A person with NF2 is typically born with one unchanged and one changed or missing NF2 gene in every cell of their body. Sometimes they inherit this change from their mother or father. Sometimes the change occurs spontaneously when the egg and sperm come together to form the first cell of the baby. The children of a person with NF2 have a 50% chance of inheriting the changed or missing NF2 gene.

A person with NF2 will develop an acoustic neuroma if the remaining unchanged NF2 gene becomes spontaneously changed or missing in one of the myelin sheath cells of their vestibular nerve. People with NF2 often develop acoustic neuromas at a younger age. The mean age of onset of acoustic neuroma in NF2 is 31 years of age versus 50 years of age for sporadic acoustic neuromas. Not all people with NF2, however, develop acoustic neuromas. People with NF2 are at increased risk for developing cataracts and tumors in other nerve cells.

Most people with a unilateral acoustic neuroma are not affected with NF2. Some people with NF2, however, only develop a tumor in one of the vestibulocochlear nerves. Others may initially be diagnosed with a unilateral tumor but may develop a tumor in the other nerve a number of years later. NF2 should be considered in someone under the age of 40 who has a unilateral acoustic neuroma. Someone with a unilateral acoustic neuroma and other family members diagnosed with NF2 probably is affected with NF2. Someone with a unilateral acoustic neuroma and other symptoms of NF2 such as cataracts and other tumors may also be affected with NF2. On the other hand, someone over the age of 50 with a unilateral acoustic neuroma, no other tumors and no family history of NF2 is very unlikely to be affected with NF2.

Symptoms

Small acoustic neuromas usually only interfere with the functioning of the vestibulocochlear nerve. The most common first symptom of an acoustic neuroma is hearing loss, which is often accompanied by a ringing sound (tinnitis). People with acoustic neuromas sometimes report difficulties in using the phone and difficulties in perceiving the tone of a musical instrument or sound even when their hearing appears to be otherwise normal. In most cases the hearing loss is initially subtle and worsens gradually over time until deafness occurs in the affected ear. In approximately 10% of cases the hearing loss is sudden and severe.

Acoustic neuromas can also affect the functioning of the vestibular branch of the vestibulocochlear nerve and van cause vertigo and dysequilibrium. Twenty percent of small tumors are associated with periodic vertigo, which is characterized by dizziness or a whirling sensation. Larger acoustic neuromas are less likely to cause vertigo but more likely to cause dysequilibrium. Dysequilibrium, which is characterized by minor clumsiness and a general feeling of instability, occurs in nearly 50% of people with an acoustic neuroma.

As the tumor grows larger it can press on the surrounding cranial nerves. Compression of the fifth cranial nerve can result in facial pain and or numbness. Compression of the seventh cranial nerve can cause spasms, weakness or paralysis of the facial muscles. Double vision is a rare symptom but can result when the sixth cranial nerve is affected. Swallowing and/or speaking difficulties can occur if the tumor presses against the ninth, tenth, or twelfth cranial nerves.

If left untreated, the tumor can become large enough to press against and affect the functioning of the brain stem. The brain stem is the stalk-like portion of the brain that joins the spinal cord to the cerebrum, the thinking and reasoning part of the brain. Different parts of the brainstem have different functions such as the control of breathing and muscle coordination. Large tumors that impact the brain stem can result in headaches, walking difficulties (gait ataxia) and involuntary shaking movements of the muscles (tremors). In rare cases when an acoustic neuroma remains undiagnosed and untreated it can cause nausea, vomiting, lethargy and eventually coma, respiratory difficulties and death. In the vast majority of cases, however, the tumor is discovered and treated long before it is large enough to cause such serious manifestations.

Diagnosis

Anyone with symptoms of hearing loss should undergo hearing evaluations. Pure tone and speech audiometry are two screening tests that are often used to evaluate hearing. Pure tone audiometry tests to see how well someone can hear tones of different volume and pitch and speech audiometry tests to see how well someone can hear and recognize speech. An acoustic neuroma is suspected in someone with unilateral hearing loss or hearing loss that is less severe in one ear than the other ear (asymmetrical).

Sometimes an auditory brainstem response (ABR, BAER) test is performed to help establish whether someone is likely to have an acoustic neuroma. During the ABR examination, a harmless electrical impulse is passed from the inner ear to the brainstem. An acoustic neuroma can interfere with the passage of this electrical impulse and this interference can, sometimes be identified through the ABR evaluation. A normal ABR examination does not rule out the possibility of an acoustic neuroma. An abnormal ABR examination increases the likelihood that an acoustic neuroma is present but other tests are necessary to confirm the presence of a tumor.

If an acoustic neuroma is strongly suspected then **magnetic resonance imaging** (MRI) is usually performed. The MRI is a very accurate evaluation that is able to detect nearly 100% of acoustic neuromas. **Computed tomography** (CT scan, CAT scan)is unable to identify smaller tumors; but it can be used when an acoustic neuroma is suspected and an MRI evaluation cannot be performed.

Once an acoustic neuroma is diagnosed, an evaluation by genetic specialists such as a geneticist and genetic

KEY TERMS

Benign tumor—A localized overgrowth of cells that does not spread to other parts of the body.

Chromosome—A microscopic structure, made of a complex of proteins and DNA, that is found within each cell of the body.

Cranial nerves—The set of twelve nerves found on each side of the head and neck that control the sensory and muscle functions of a number of organs such as the eyes, nose, tongue face and throat.

Computed tomography (CT)—An examination that uses a computer to compile and analyze the images produced by x rays projected at a particular part of the body.

DNA testing—Testing for a change or changes in a gene or genes.

Gene—A building block of inheritance, made up of a compound called DNA (deoxyribonucleic acid) and containing the instructions for the production of a particular protein. Each gene is found on a specific location on a chromosome.

Magnetic resonance imaging (MRI)—A test which uses an external magnetic field instead of x rays to visualize different tissues of the body.

Myelin sheath—The cover that surrounds many nerve cells and helps to increase the speed by which information travels along the nerve.

Neurofibromatosis type 2 (NF2)—A hereditary condition associated with an increased risk of bilateral acoustic neuromas, other nerve cell tumors and cataracts.

Protein—A substance produced by a gene that is involved in creating the traits of the human body such as hair and eye color or is involved in controlling the basic functions of the human body.

Schwannoma—A tumor derived from the cells of the myelin sheath that surrounds many nerve cells.

Tinnitus—A ringing sound or other noise in the ear.

Vertigo—A feeling of spinning or whirling.

Vestibulocochlear nerve (Eighth cranial nerve)—Nerve that transmits information, about hearing and balance from the ear to the brain.

counselor may be recommended. The purpose of this evaluation is to obtain a detailed family history and check for signs of NF2. If NF2 is strongly suspected then DNA testing may be recommended. DNA testing involves checking the blood cells obtained from a routine blood draw for the common gene changes associated with NF2.

Treatment

The three treatment options for acoustic neuroma are surgery, radiation, and observation. The physician and patient should discuss the pros and cons of the different options prior to making a decision about treatment. The patient's physical health, age, symptoms, tumor size, and tumor location should be considered.

Microsurgery

The surgical removal of the tumor or tumors is the most common treatment for acoustic neuroma. In most cases the entire tumor is removed during the surgery. If the tumor is large and causing significant symptoms, yet there is a need to preserve hearing in that ear, then only part of the tumor may be removed. During the procedure the tumor is removed under microscopic guidance and general anesthetic. Monitoring of the neighboring cranial nerves is done during the procedure so that damage to these nerves can be prevented. If preservation of hearing is a possibility, then monitoring of hearing will also take place during the surgery.

Most people stay in the hospital four to seven days following the surgery. Total recovery usually takes four to six weeks. Most people experience **fatigue** and head discomfort following the surgery. Problems with balance and head and neck stiffness are also common. The mortality rate of this type of surgery is less than 2% at most major centers. Approximately 20% of patients experience some degree of post-surgical complications. In most cases these complications can be managed successfully and do not result in long-term medical problems. Surgery brings with it a risk of stroke, damage to the brain stem, infection, leakage of spinal fluid and damage to the cranial nerves. Hearing loss and/or tinnitis often result from the surgery. A follow-up MRI is recommended one to five years following the surgery because of possible regrowth of the tumor.

Stereotactic radiation therapy

During stereotactic **radiation therapy**, also called radiosurgery or radiotherapy, many small beams of radiation are aimed directly at the acoustic neuroma. The radiation is administered in a single large dose, under local anesthetic and is performed on an outpatient basis. This results in a high dose of radiation to the tumor but little radiation exposure to the surrounding area. This treatment approach is limited to small or medium tumors. The goal of the therapy is to cause tumor shrinkage or at least limit the growth of the tumor. The long-term efficacy and risks of this treatment approach are not known. Periodic MRI monitoring throughout the life of the patient is therefore recommended.

Radiation therapy can cause hearing loss which can sometimes occurs even years later. Radiation therapy can also cause damage to neighboring cranial nerves, which can result in symptoms such as numbness, pain or paralysis of the facial muscles. In many cases these symptoms are temporary. Radiation treatment can also induce the formation of other benign or malignant schwannomas. This type of treatment may therefore be contraindicated in the treatment of acoustic neuromas in those with NF2 who are predisposed to developing schwannomas and other tumors.

Observation

Acoustic neuromas are usually slow growing and in some cases they will stop growing and even become smaller or disappear entirely. It may therefore be appropriate in some cases to hold off on treatment and to periodically monitor the tumor through MRI evaluations. Long-term observation may be appropriate for example in an elderly person with a small acoustic neuroma and few symptoms. Periodic observation may also be indicated for someone with a small and asymptomatic acoustic neuroma that was detected through an evaluation for another medical problem. Observation may also be suggested for someone with an acoustic neuroma in the only hearing ear or in the ear that has better hearing. The danger of an observational approach is that as the tumor grows larger it can become more difficult to treat.

Prognosis

The prognosis for someone with a unilateral acoustic neuroma is usually quite good provided the tumor is diagnosed early and appropriate treatment is instituted. Long-term hearing loss and tinnitis in the affected ear are common, even if appropriate treatment is provided. Regrowth of the tumor is also a possibility following surgery or radiation therapy and repeat treatment may be necessary. The prognosis can be poorer for those with NF2 who have an increased risk of bilateral acoustic neuromas and other tumors.

Resources

BOOKS

Filipo, R., and Barbara Maurizio *Acoustic neuroma: trends and controversies: proceedings of the Symposium Acoustic*

Neuroma: Trends and Controversies, Rome, Italy, November 13–15, 1997. The Hague, Netherlands: Kugler,1999.

Malis, Leonard *Acoustic Neuroma* New York: Elsevier, 1998.

Roland, Peter, and Bradley Marple.*Diagnosis and Management of Acoustic Neuroma (Sipac).* Alexandria, VA: American Academy of Otolaryngology—Head and Neck Survey Foundation, 1998.

PERIODICALS

Broad, R. W. "Management of Acoustic Neuroma." In *New England Journal of Medicine.* 340(14) (8 April 1999):1119.

Lederman G, E. Arbit, and J. Lowry. "Management of Acoustic Neuroma." *New England Journal of Medicine.* 340(14) (8 April 1999):1119–1120.

Levo H., I. Pyykko, and G. Blomstedt. "Non-surgical Treatment of Vestibular Schwannoma Patients." *Acta Oto-Laryngologica* 529 (1997): 56–8.

O'Donoghue G.M., T. Nikolopoulos and J. Thomsen. "Management of Acoustic Neuroma." In *New England Journal of Medicine* 340(14) (8 April 1999):1120–1121.

Rigby, P. L., et al. "Acoustic Neuroma Surgery: Outcome Analysis of Patient-Perceived Disability." In *American Journal of Otology* 18 (July 1997): 427–35.

van Roijen, L., et al. "Costs and Effects of Microsurgery versus Radiosurgery in Treating Acoustic Neuroma." In *Acta Neurochirurgica* 139 (1997): 942–48.

ORGANIZATIONS

Acoustic Neuroma Association. 600 Peachtree Pkwy, Suite 108, Cumming, GA 30041-6899. Phone:(770) 205-8211. Fax: (770) 205-0239. ANAusa@aol.com <http://anausa.org> 28 June 2001.

Acoustic Neuroma Association of Canada Box 369, Edmonton, AB T5J 2J6. 1-800-561-ANAC(2622). (780)428-3384. anac@compusmart.ab.ca. <http://www.anac.ca> 28 June 2001.

British Acoustic Neuroma Association. Oak House, Ransom Wood Business Park, Southwell Road West, Mansfield, Nottingham, NG21 0HJ. Tel: 01623 632143. Fax: 01623 635313. bana@btclick.com. <http://www.ukan.co.uk/bana> 28 June 2001.

Seattle Acoustic Neuroma Group. Emcityland@aol.com <http://acousticneuromaseattle.org/entryenglish.html> 28 June 2001.

OTHER

University of California at San Francisco (UCSF)*Information on Acoustic Neuromas* <http://itsa.ucsf.edu/~rkj/IndexAN.html> (18 March 1998). 28 June 2001.

National Institute of Health Consensus Statement Online*Acoustic Neuroma* 9(4)(11-13 December 1991). 28 June 2001. <http://text.nlm.nih.gov/nih/cdc/www/87txt.html>

Lisa Andres, M.S., CGC

Acquired Immune Deficiency syndrome *see* **AIDS-related cancers**

Actinomycin D *see* **Dactinomycin**

Acute erythroblastic leukemia

Definition

Acute erythroblastic leukemia, also called erythremic myelosis, DiGuglielmo syndrome, or erythroleukemia, results from uncontrolled proliferation of immature erythrocytes (red blood cells).

Description

Acute erythroblastic leukemia, a variant of **acute myelocytic leukemia**, originates in the blood and in the bone marrow. In this form of leukemia, a large number of abnormal, immature red blood cells are produced. The advanced phase is also called the blast crisis. At this stage, over 50% of the cells in the bone marrow are immature malignant cells (also called blast cells or promelocytes).

Demographics

There are no statistics available for this rare form of cancer.

Causes and symptoms

The causes of acute erythroblastic leukemia are largely unknown. However, acute erythroblastic leukemia constitutes 10–20% of leukemias secondary to radiation, alkylator therapy, or overexposure to benzene.

Patients with this type of leukemia have less than the normal amount of healthy red blood cells and platelets, which results in insufficient amounts of oxygen being carried through the body. This condition is called **anemia**, and causes patients to experience severe weakness and tiredness. Patients may have less than the normal number of white blood cells as well. Other symptoms include **fever**, chills, loss of appetite and weight, easy bleeding or bruising (due to lower than normal platelet levels), bone or joint pain, headaches, vomiting, and confusion. In addition, patients with leukemia may have hepatosplenomegaly, an enlargement of the liver and spleen. Enlargement of these organs is noticed as a fullness or swelling in the abdomen, and can be felt by a doctor during a physical examination. The occurrence of Sweet's syndrome, a rare skin disorder accompanied by fever, inflammation of the joints (arthritis), and the sudden onset of a rash, has also been associated with acute erythroblastic leukemia.

Diagnosis

Patients seeking treatment usually report a vague history of chronic general **fatigue**. Blood tests are used to establish the diagnosis. A sample of blood is examined

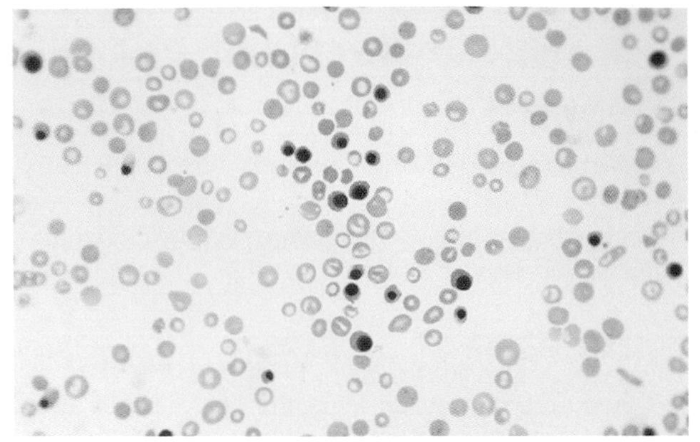

Erythroblastic leukemia cells. *(© Richard Green, Science Source/Photo Researchers, Inc. Reproduced by permission.)*

under a microscope to identify abnormal red cells—which are larger than healthy cells—and to count the number of mature cells and blasts present. Cancer red cell precursors predominate, myeloid blasts also are seen, and multinucleated red cell precursors are common. Bone marrow examinations are also performed, either by aspiration or **biopsy** to examine the cell types further.

Treatment

Treatment for acute erythroblastic leukemia depends on the features of the cancer cells present and on the extent of the disease, as well as on the age of the patient, his symptoms, and general health condition. This disease can have an indolent course and may only require observation in the early stages. The treatment strategy is based on **chemotherapy** and in some patients, bone marrow or cell transplantations are indicated as well. Chemotherapy is usually administered in combinations of two or more drugs. Post-remission therapy includes maintenance chemotherapy for most patients.

Clinical staging, treatments, and prognosis

Acute erythroblastic leukemia is a very aggressive form of leukemia and does not respond well to the types of therapy used for a related type of cancer known as acute myelocytic leukemia. However, recent advances in chemotherapy protocols and **bone marrow transplantation** techniques, either allogeneic or autologous, have been identified as a means to increase the cure rate. The patient's cancerous bone marrow is first purged using drugs and **radiation therapy** before being replaced by healthy bone marrow that is obtained from a suitable donor (allogeneic) or from the patient himself (autologous). In the case of an autologous transplant, the bone marrow is treated outside the patient's body to remove the cancer cells before transplantation.

KEY TERMS

Allogeneic bone marrow transplant—A bone marrow transplant using bone marrow obtained from a genetically matched healthy donor, such as a sister or a brother.

Autologous bone marrow transplant—A bone marrow transplant that uses the patient's own bone marrow.

Anemia—A condition in which the number of red blood cells is below normal

Blast cells—Immature cancer cells. Also called promelocytes.

Bone marrow aspiration—Common technique used to obtain a bone marrow sample from a patient. A needle is inserted into a marrow-containing bone, such as the hip (iliac crest) or sternum (breast bone) and a small amount of liquid bone marrow is removed for examination.

Bone marrow biopsy—Another common technique used to obtain a bone marrow sample from a patient. Like bone marrow aspiration, it is performed with a needle, but a larger one is used and a small piece of bone is removed as well as bone marrow.

Chemotherapy—The treatment of disease by means of chemicals. In cancer, the chemicals selectively destroy cancerous tissue. When cancer remission occurs, a course of maintenance chemotherapy is often prescribed so as to prevent recurrence.

Erythrocyte—Red blood cell.

Leukemia—Cancer of the blood-forming tissues.

Myeloid blast cell—Type of cancer cell originating in the bone marrow.

Platelet—A type of blood cell responsible for blood coagulation and for the repair of damaged blood vessels.

Proliferation—Rapid reproduction of tissue.

Remission—Complete or partial disappearance of the symptoms of cancer following treatment.

Coping with cancer treatment

Like all types of leukemias, patients with acute erythroblastic leukemia usually experience a number of specific complications and side effects resulting from treatment, as well as emotional concerns. They require supportive care to cope with these issues and to maintain their comfort and quality of life during treatment. As with every serious disease, psychological stress is increased and it is important for patients to be able to discuss their needs and concerns about tests, treatments, hospital stays, and financial consequences of the illness. Family, friends, doctors, nurses, and other members of the health care team are the best sources of support, as well as social workers, counselors, and members of the clergy.

Clinical trials

In 2001, no **clinical trials** for this leukemia were registered with the National Cancer Institute.

Prevention

Since this form of cancer is very rare and its causes are largely unknown, no specific preventive measures can be recommended.

Special concerns

Patients diagnosed with acute erythroblastic leukemia require special support in that they must deal with having a rare form of cancer about which there is very little specific information available. This creates additional anxiety and special care must be taken to explain to the patient that an uncommon cancer is not an untreatable one.

See Also Bone marrow aspiration and biopsy; Chronic myelocytic leukemia; Myeloproliferative diseases

Resources

BOOKS

Jandl, James H. *Blood. Textbook of Hematology.* Boston: Little, Brown, 1996.

PERIODICALS

Shichishima, T., "Minimally Differentiated Erythroleukemia: Recognition of Erythroid Precursors and Progenitors." *Internal Medicine* 39(October 2000): 843-46.

Mazzella, F.M., et al. "The Acute Erythroleukemias." *Clinical Laboratory Medicine* 20 (March 2000): 119-37.

Novik, Y., et al. "Familial Erythroleukemia: A Distinct Clinical and Genetic Type of Familial Leukemias." *Leuk. Lymphoma* 30 (July 1998): 395-401.

ORGANIZATIONS

National Cancer Institute, Public Inquiries Office, Building 31, Room 10A31, 31 Center Drive, MSC 2580, Bethesda, MD 20892-2580. (301)435-2848. <http://www.nci.nih.gov>.

National Cancer Information Center. 1-800-ACS-2345.

The Leukemia and Lymphoma Society of America. 1-800-955-4572. <http://www.leukemia-lymphoma.org/>.

OTHER

American Cancer Society's Consumer Guide to Cancer Drugs.Caregiving—A Step-by-Step Resource for Caring for the Person with Cancer at Home. Available from: American Cancer Society. (800) ACS-2345. <http://www.cancer.org.>.

Advanced Cancer: Living Day by Day.Chemotherapy and You: A Guide to Self-help During Treatment.Eating Hints for Cancer Patients.What You Need to Know About Leukemia. Available from: National Cancer Institute, National Institute of Health. (800) 4-CANCER. <http://www.nci.nih.gov>.

Monique Laberge, Ph.D.

QUESTIONS TO ASK THE DOCTOR

- How can I obtain information on a rare cancer such as acute erythroblastic leukemia?
- How are my chances of recovery affected by the fact that this cancer is so rare?

Acute leukemia

Definition

A rapidly progressing cancer that starts in the blood-forming cells of the bone marrow. Leukemia results from an abnormal development of leukocytes (white blood cells) and their precursors. Leukemia cells look different than normal cells and do not function properly.

Description

There are four main types of leukemia, which can be further divided into subtypes. When classifying the type of leukemia, the first steps are to determine whether the cancer is lymphocytic or myelogenous (cancer can occur in either the lymphoid or myeloid white blood cells) and whether it is acute or chronic (rapidly or slowly progressing).

In acute leukemia, the new or immature cells, called blasts, remain very immature and cannot perform their functions properly. The blasts rapidly increase in number and the disease progresses quickly. Major types of acute leukemia include **acute lymphocytic leukemia** (ALL) and **acute myelocytic leukemia** (AML; also known as acute myelogenous leukemia).

Kate Kretschmann

Acute lymphocytic leukemia

Definition

Acute lymphocytic leukemia is a cancer of the white blood cells known as lymphocytes.

Description

Leukemia is a cancer of white blood cells. In acute leukemia, the cancerous cells are immature forms called blasts that cannot properly fight infection; patients become ill in rapid fashion.

The cells that make up blood are produced in the bone marrow and the lymph system. The bone marrow is the spongy tissue found in the large bones of the body. The lymph system includes the spleen (an organ in the upper abdomen), the thymus (a small organ beneath the breastbone), and the tonsils (an organ in the throat). In addition, the lymph vessels (tiny tubes that branch like blood vessels into all parts of the body) and lymph nodes (pea-shaped organs that are found along the network of lymph vessels) are also part of the lymph system. The lymph is a milky fluid that contains cells. Clusters of lymph nodes are found in the neck, underarm, pelvis, abdomen, and chest.

The main types of cells found in the blood are the red blood cells (RBCs), which carry oxygen and other materials to all tissues of the body; white blood cells (WBCs), which fight infection; and the platelets, which play a part in the clotting of the blood. The white blood cells can be further subdivided into three main types: granulocytes, monocytes, and lymphocytes.

The granulocytes, as their name suggests, have particles (granules) inside them. These granules contain special proteins (enzymes) and several other substances that can break down chemicals and destroy microorganisms such as bacteria. Monocytes are the second type of white blood cell. They are also important in defending the body against pathogens. The lymphocytes form the third type of white blood cell. The two types of lymphocytes are B-cells, which make antibodies, and T-cells, which make other infection-fighting substances. Lymphocytic leukemia can arise in either B or T cells.

B-cell leukemia occurs more frequently than T-cell leukemia. It is the most common form of leukemia in children, but also occurs in adults. At diagnosis, leukemic cells can be found throughout the body, in the bloodstream, the lymph nodes, spleen, liver, occasionally in the central nervous system, and in T-cell ALL, the thymus gland.

Cancerous lymphoblasts take over the bone marrow, reducing both the number and the effectiveness of all types of blood cells. The cancerous cells reduce the ability of healthy white cells to fight infection. Fewer red cells are produced, causing **anemia**, and fewer platelets increases the risk of bleeding and bruising. The presence of the cancerous white cells in the central nervous system can produce headaches, confusion and seizures.

The type of treatment a person receives for ALL depends on the presence of risk factors for relapse. Children are at standard risk if they are between ages 1 and 9, have a total white cell count of less than 50,000 per microliter of blood, and have B-precursor cell leukemia. Children are at high risk if they are younger than 1 or older than 9, if their white blood cell count exceeds 50,000 per microliter, or if they have T-cell leukemia. Compared to children, adults are all at higher risk of relapse at the time of diagnosis, but younger adults (less than 25 years old) have a better prognosis.

B-cell ALL constitutes about 80% of all cases. The cancerous cells are either early pre-B cells, the most immature, pre-B cells, also somewhat immature, or B-cells. These B-lineage cells contain a variety of proteins called antigens. The presence of one of these antigens, called CALLA for common ALL antigen, carries a somewhat more favorable prognosis.

T-cell ALL has a less favorable prognosis than B-cell ALL. The presence of an antigen called CD2 indicates a more favorable prognosis.

ALL is also classified by karyotype, which is the number and composition of a cell's chromosomes. Normal human cells contain 46 chromosomes. One chromosomal abnormality often seen in ALL is a translocation, in which a piece of one chromosome becomes attached to a different chromosome. Different translocations carry different prognoses. One translocation, labeled t(9;22) is also called the Philadelphia chromosome and is found in 5% of childhood ALL and 20% of adult ALL cases. The Philadelphia chromosome carries a somewhat less favorable prognosis.

The number of chromosomes found in the leukemic cells, particularly in children, also impacts prognosis. The occurrence of more than 50 chromosomes in leukemic cells has a very favorable prognosis. Even the presence of one extra chromosome can be favorable.

Children whose leukemic cells have fewer than 45 chromosomes are at highest risk of treatment failure.

Demographics

ALL is less common than AML in adults; about 1500 adults are diagnosed with ALL each year, compared to 10,000 diagnosed with AML. About 1000 adults die of ALL each year and the overall five-year survival rate for adults with ALL is 58%.

About 1500 cases of ALL are diagnosed in children under 18 each year in the United States. ALL is by far the more common form of leukemia in children. The death rate for children with ALL has dropped nearly 60% in the last 30 years. The overall five-year survival rate for children with ALL is now 80%. Still, leukemia causes more deaths in children under 15, about 550 per year, than any other disease.

In the United States, ALL is highest among Caucasians and lowest among Asian-Americans. The incidence of ALL is about 50% higher for men than for women. Death rates in leukemia patients are highest in African-Americans and Caucasians and lowest in Asians.

In children, the highest leukemia rates in the US occur among those of Filipino descent; next highest are white Hispanics, then non-Hispanic whites, and the lowest incidence in children is in African-Americans. Survival is higher for Caucasians than African-Americans. The survival rate for girls is slightly higher, in part due to the risk of relapse occurring in the testicles and in part because boys appear to have a slightly higher risk of bone marrow relapse.

Causes and symptoms

Causes

While specific causes for ALL are not known, there are some known risk factors, including ionizing radiation. Exposure to certain chemicals, particularly benzene (used in the manufacture of plastics, rubber, and some medicines), has also been associated with an increased risk of developing ALL. ALL incidence in adults increases with age.

The causes of ALL in children are also unknown. Certain inherited genetic abnormalities, such as Down syndrome, increase the risk. Some studies have shown prenatal exposure to ionizing radiation increases a child's risk of ALL. Some contaminants of tap water, such as trihalomethanes, chloroform, zinc, cadmium, and arsenic are associated with an increased risk. A number of reports suggested an increased risk of ALL among children who lived in proximity to high voltage power lines, but several later analyses suggested that was not true. Studies continue in efforts to disprove or confirm this possible connection. ALL is more common in children who are not firstborn and among those whose mothers took **antibiotics** during their pregnancies. Breastfeeding has been found to be protective.

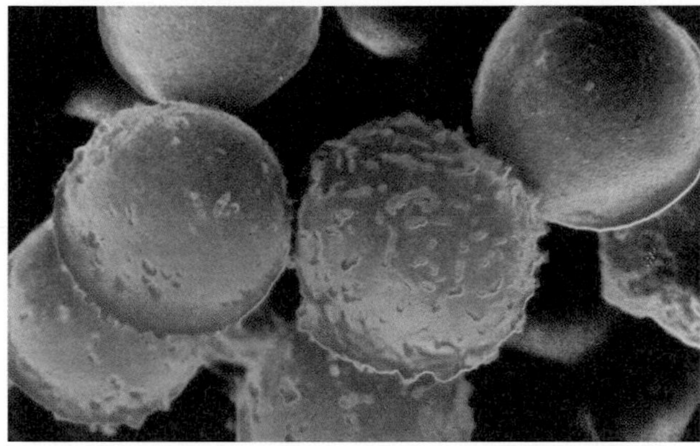

False-color scanning electron micrograph (SEM) of white blood cells from a patient with acute lymphocytic leukemia. In this disease, certain types of white blood cells are overproduced, and these abnormal cells suppress the normal function of white and red cells, increasing the susceptibility to infections. *(© Professor Aaron Polliack, Science Source/Photo Researchers, Inc. Reproduced by permission.)*

Symptoms

ADULTS. ALL in adults can cause any or all of the following symptoms:

- fevers, chills, sweats
- weakness, **fatigue**, shortness of breath
- frequent infections
- depressed appetite, weight loss
- enlarged lymph nodes
- easy bleeding or bruising
- rash of small, flat red spots (petechiae)
- bone and joint pain

Symptoms of central nervous system involvement include:

- headache
- **nausea and vomiting**
- confusion
- seizures

CHILDREN. Symptoms in children are similar, but young children may be unable to communicate them. They include:

- fevers

- frequent infections
- fatigue, irritability, decreased activity levels
- easy bruising or bleeding
- bone or joint pain
- a limp
- swollen belly
- enlarged lymph nodes

T-cell ALL can invade the thymus gland in the upper chest, which can cause compression of the windpipe, cough or shortness of breath, and **superior vena cava syndrome** (compression of a large vein that causes swelling of the head, neck, and arms).

Central nervous system involvement in children produces:

- headache
- nausea and vomiting
- blurred vision
- decline in school performance
- seizures

Spread to the testicles can cause painless swelling in them.

Diagnosis

There are no screening tests for leukemia. The patient's history and physical examination raise the physician's suspicions, triggering orders for appropriate tests. Pallor, swollen lymph nodes, bleeding, bruising, pinpoint red rashes, and in children, a swollen abdomen, will suggest the diagnosis. Testing is similar for adults and children.

The first test is a complete blood count (CBC), examining red cells, platelets and white cells. In early leukemia, the total white blood cell count might be normal, but there will usually be circulating lymphoblasts, which is always abnormal. The red cell and platelet counts may be low.

The abnormal CBC results trigger a referral to a hematologist/oncologist who will perform a **bone marrow aspiration and biopsy**, in which a small sample of marrow is removed with a hollow needle inserted in the hipbone. Although topical anesthetic will numb the skin and bone, most patients experience brief pain during this procedure. The sample will be examined microscopically for evidence of lymphoblasts. The marrow will be further studied to determine whether the lymphoblasts are of T-cell or B-cell origin and the cells tested for chromosomal abnormalities. A pathologist can examine the marrow and make the diagnosis immediately. The chromosome studies require several days to complete. The bone marrow aspirate will be repeated occasionally during treatment to confirm remission and to look for possible relapse.

A **lumbar puncture**, or spinal tap, will be performed to rule out spread of ALL to the central nervous system. A thin needle is inserted between two vertebrae in the lower back, and spinal fluid removed. This fluid is examined microscopically for the presence of lymphoblasts. Topical anesthetics eliminate most of the discomfort of a spinal tap, although many patients experience headaches afterwards. Remaining flat for 30 minutes after a spinal tap decreases the likelihood of headache.

A chest **x ray** will show enlargement of internal lymph nodes or the thymus gland.

No preparation is necessary for most of the testing done to diagnose ALL. Younger children will often receive mild sedatives before procedures like spinal taps and bone marrow studies. Topical anesthetic cream can be applied an hour in advance of either a bone marrow test or a spinal tap.

When treatment is complete, tests for minimal residual disease can be performed. These new tests detect the presence of lingering leukemic cells that would have been missed by standard testing. The presence of a certain amount of residual disease probably has an impact on prognosis and the likelihood of relapse.

Treatment team

The treatment team consists of a hematologist/oncologist who directs care, oncology nurses familiar with administering **chemotherapy**, and often social workers, who can address both insurance issues and psychological support. The patient's regular physician should be kept informed of all cancer-related care. Because treatment is so prolonged, most patients have long-term intravenous catheters placed by a surgeon.

In many hospitals, a Child Life specialist will participate in the care of children with ALL. They ensure that children with cancer are seen, first and foremost, as children, organizing play times, providing distraction during scary procedures and giving parents some much-needed respite.

Clinical staging, treatments, and prognosis

ALL does not have a formal staging system, but treatment is different in different phases of the disease. These phases are often divided into untreated ALL, ALL in remission, and recurrent ALL. Conventional treatment for ALL consists of chemotherapy for disease in the bone marrow and treatment aimed at preventing central nervous system disease.

ADULTS. The first phase of treatment is remission induction. The chemotherapeutic drugs typically include prednisone, **vincristine**, **cytarabine**, **cyclophosphamide** and **asparaginase**. Most are given intravenously and a few are given orally. Depending on the disease, these drugs can achieve a complete remission in 60% to 90% of adults. The relapse rate is higher in adults than in children. A 50% 3-year survival has been noted in some research series, and very aggressive treatment with multiple drugs has produced up to a 70% survival rate.

Adverse effects of these drugs include:

- bone marrow suppression
- anemia, pallor, fatigue, shortness of breath, and angina in older patients
- bleeding, bruising
- increased risk of infection
- hair loss **(alopecia)**
- mouth sores
- nausea and vomiting
- menopausal symptoms
- lower sperm counts
- **tumor lysis syndrome,** in which the dead cancer cells can harm healthy organs

Treatment that is directed at preventing central nervous system spread is called prophylactic. Because of the blood brain barrier, a physical and chemical barrier that prevents toxins from reaching the brain and spinal cord, chemotherapeutic drugs do not easily reach the central nervous system. Thus, chemotherapeutic drugs are administered directly into spinal fluid, which circulates around the brain and spinal cord. This is called intrathecal chemotherapy. The drugs are given by spinal tap or through an **Ommaya reservoir**, which is surgically inserted under the scalp. This reservoir empties into the spinal fluid around the brain.

Some patients receive prophylactic **radiation therapy** to the brain, in addition to or instead of intrathecal chemotherapy.

CHILDREN. The treatment of ALL in children represents one of the great success stories of modern oncology. In contrast to adults, most children with cancer enter into research protocols, strict treatment regimens with careful follow-up that are built on the most successful aspects of earlier treatments. Childhood ALL now has an 80% long-term survival rate, due in large part to the extensive and widely disseminated research on the disease. Within the United States, research on ALL was conducted for many years under the auspices of either the Children's Cancer Group or the Pediatric Oncology Group. In 1998, recognizing the benefits of cooperation and collaboration, these two groups joined forces with the National **Wilms' Tumor** Study Group and the Intergroup **Rhabdomyosarcoma** Study Group to form the Children's Oncology Group.

Remission induction chemotherapy for children includes **vincristine,** a steroid, and asparaginase. Children at higher risk of relapse are often given daunomycin as well. The adverse effects of these drugs include bone marrow suppression, risk of infection, nausea, vomiting, hair loss, and mouth sores. Although these drugs can reduce sperm counts, most survivors of childhood ALL grow up to have normal fertility. The drugs can be administered intravenously or as oral preparations. Oral prednisone has a particularly unpleasant taste that is hard to disguise and parents must be vigilant to ensure that their children are taking their proper doses.

Like adults, children also receive prophylaxis against central nervous system spread. They receive multiple doses of intrathecal chemotherapy, with the drugs delivered directly to the spinal fluid through a lumbar puncture or spinal tap. Cranial radiation as central nervous system prophylaxis for children is infrequently used. Though once standard, brain radiation produced a high incidence of cognitive and learning disabilities, especially among those younger than five years old. Cranial radiation is reserved for those children felt to be at high risk of central nervous system disease, including those older than ten at the time of diagnosis, those with initial white blood cell counts of more than 50,000 per microliter, and those with T-cell leukemia. Some high-risk children who enter remission rapidly with induction chemotherapy receive intrathecal chemotherapy alone, without radiation therapy.

Alternative and complementary therapies

ADULTS. Individuals with leukemia often employ alternative or complementary therapies. Some of these provide pain relief and improve psychological well being. No controlled studies have yet shown that alternative treatments offer cures for ALL, although some may hold promise of benefit.

Patients with ALL sometimes use acupuncture, which offers relief from generalized pain, nausea, and vomiting. Other methods that may help with the physical and often emotional side effects of treatment include hypnosis, guided imagery, and yoga.

Nutritional supplements and herbs are sometimes utilized by persons with leukemia. Coenzyme Q10 is an antioxidant, a substance that protects cells from toxic byproducts of metabolism. Early studies suggest, although it is not proven, that coenzyme Q10 can improve immune function and counteract some of the harmful effects of chemotherapy and radiation on healthy cells. Adverse effects of coenzyme Q10 include headache, rash, heartburn and **diarrhea**. Another supplement with potential benefit is polysaccharide K (PSK). A few studies have shown PSK to have some benefit in improving immunity.

Supplements that have not been proven to be of value or are potentially dangerous to those with leukemia include camphor, sometimes called 714-X. Green tea has received much press for its reported abilities to enhance the immune system and fight cancer, but studies have had conflicting results. Some show that green tea has preventive benefits and others show no effect. A few animal studies suggest that growth of tumors might be slowed by green tea, but this has not been shown in humans yet.

Hoxsey is another supplement touted as a cancer treatment, but no studies have confirmed any benefit. Some of its ingredients have serious adverse effects. Vitamin megadoses have long been advocated as beneficial in cancer, but no conclusive studies show benefit, and they have significant potential for adverse effects, such as diarrhea, kidney stones, iron overload, nerve damage and liver disease.

Laetrile, or amygdalin, was once touted as a cure for cancer and leukemia. No human or animal studies conducted in the decades since have shown any benefit other than relief of some pain. Laetrile can, however, cause cyanide poisoning.

CHILDREN. Complementary and alternative treatments are recommended less frequently for children. Real caution must be used in administering herbal remedies to children, whose metabolisms are very different from those of adults. For example, jin bu hua, a traditional Chinese medicine, can cause heart or breathing problems. Life root and comfrey can both cause fatal liver damage in children.

While many children are too young for formal guided imagery, they can be distracted from the fears and pain associated with some treatments by toys and videotapes. Reading favorite books during scary procedures can relieve some of their fears.

ALL in remission

ADULTS. Remission is achieved in many people within days of beginning treatment. Treatment does not end at that point, but rather enters into the next phases, called consolidation and maintenance. Several different approaches can be used in these. Some patients receive long-term chemotherapy with drugs that might include **cytarabine,** cyclophosphamide, **methotrexate**, 6-mercaptopurine, vincristine, prednisone, or **doxorubicin**. Other patients undergo high-dose chemotherapy or combination chemotherapy and radiation therapy to ablate or wipe out their own bone marrow, and then have bone marrow or stem cell transplants. Adverse effects of bone marrow transplant include significant risk of serious infection and graft versus host disease (GVHD), in which the transplanted cells fail to "recognize" the host's cells as self and attack the host cells. Medications to decrease this risk include those that suppress the immune system and steroids.

Central nervous system prophylaxis, as either intrathecal chemotherapy or radiation therapy or both, typically continues through at least a portion of the post-remission therapy.

Adults who receive intensive chemotherapy have a 40% likelihood of long-term survival.

CHILDREN. In children, remission induction therapy is followed by a phase termed consolidation or intensification, and then by a phase termed maintenance. During intensification, children receive intermediate or high-dose methotrexate, plus some of the same drugs that are used in induction, new drugs that do not cross-react with those used in induction, high-dose asparaginase, or some combination of these.

The maintenance phase of treatment for children with ALL continues for 18 to 30 months. Daily oral **mercaptopurine** and weekly oral or injected methotrexate are given on an outpatient basis, with frequent blood tests and examinations. Some protocols add pulses of vincristine and prednisone during the maintenance phase.

Recurrent ALL

ADULTS. Adults who relapse after initial remission and maintenance therapy often undergo reinduction chemotherapy and are then referred for bone marrow or stem cell transplant. Some receive transplants of umbilical cord blood. Such transplants carry the risk of graft versus host disease, but also carry the possibility of graft versus leukemia, in which the transplanted cells attack the residual leukemic cells. Unlike **graft-versus-host disease,** graft versus leukemia is useful.

New treatments for relapsed ALL include immunotherapies or biological response modifiers. Some reduce adverse effects of treatment and others are used to fight the leukemia. Some of these include cytokines, substances that stimulate the production of blood cells after treatment has suppressed the bone marrow, and colony-stimulating factors, which have the same effect. Other immunotherapies, such as **monoclonal antibodies** and interferon, have not yet been shown effective against ALL, but are still under study.

CHILDREN. The treatment and prognosis of children who relapse depends on the timing of that relapse. Relapse that occurs within six months is often treated with **bone marrow transplantation**. Early relapse carries the least favorable prognosis, with only 10% to 20% chance of long-term survival. Relapse that occurs more than a year after initial treatment is finished can be treated with another full round of chemotherapy, and bone marrow transplant reserved for those children who relapse a second time. Those with such late relapses have a 30% to 40% chance of long-term survival.

Recurrent disease may occur in a sanctuary site, or a part of the body difficult to penetrate with chemotherapeutic drugs. The central nervous system is the most common site of such recurrences. Children who have an isolated central nervous system relapse during the first 18 months of treatment have a 45% likelihood of long-term survival. Children with central nervous system relapse after the first 18 months of treatment have up to an 80% chance of long-term survival. Treatment for relapse in the central nervous system includes intrathecal chemotherapy, and for most children, the use of radiation therapy to the brain and spinal cord.

The testicles are the second most common site of relapse. Early testicular relapse (within the first 18 months of treatment) carries a 40% chance of long-term survival, and late testicular relapse carries an 85% chance of long-term survival. Another sanctuary site is the eye, but isolated relapse here is unusual.

Coping with cancer treatment

The treatment of ALL can be particularly draining, not only due to adverse effects but due to its prolonged time course. Although much of the treatment can be given on an outpatient basis, many protocols utilize lengthy intravenous infusions of chemotherapy and require hospitalization.

ADULTS. To prevent **nausea and vomiting**, adults can take oral anti-nausea medication an hour or so before scheduled treatments, including intrathecal treatments. To avoid headache, they should remain flat for at least 30 to 60 minutes after intrathecal chemotherapy. Nurses can give instructions in mouth care if mouth sores occur and skin care if rashes occur after radiation treatment. Books, music, and television can provide distraction and reduce anxiety during chemotherapy infusions.

KEY TERMS

Antiangiogenic drugs—Drugs that block the formation of new blood vessels.

Blasts—Immature blood cells.

CBC—Complete blood count, a blood test that measures red cells, white cells and platelets.

Graft versus host disease—After bone marrow transplant, the newly transplanted white blood cells can attack the patient's own tissues.

Intrathecal chemotherapy—Chemotherapeutic drugs instilled directly into the spinal fluid, either by spinal tap or through a special reservoir.

Karyotype—The number and type of chromosomes found within cells.

Lymphoblasts—The cancerous cells of ALL, immature forms of lymphocytes, white blood cells that fight infection.

Ommaya reservoir—A special device surgically placed under the scalp with a direct connection to spinal fluid. Medications to treat central nervous system disease are injected into the reservoir.

Petechiae—Pinpoint red spots seen on the skin with low platelet counts.

Philadelphia chromosome—An abnormal chromosome found in 20% of adults and 5% of children with ALL, the presence of which indicates a somewhat worse prognosis.

Sanctuary sites—Areas within the body which are relatively impermeable to medications such as chemotherapy but which can harbor cancerous cells. Some of these sites are the central nervous system, the testicles, and the eyes.

Thymus—A gland within the chest involved in the maturation of immune cells that can be invaded by T lymphocytes in T-cell ALL.

Patients scheduled for inpatient stays can bring their own pillows, pajamas and even food, with their doctor's approval. Temporary issuance of handicapped parking stickers are often helpful.

CHILDREN. The presence of parents during treatment is critical. While some hospitals exclude parents during treatments, others invite them to be present. Blood can be drawn and intravenous catheters placed while children sit in their parents' laps. If at all possible, a parent should spend the night during any hospitalizations.

QUESTIONS TO ASK THE DOCTOR

- What type of leukemia do I or does my child have?
- What characteristics of my or my child's illness are favorable? Which are unfavorable?
- What course of therapy do you recommend?
- What medications will you use and what side effects are anticipated?
- Will I or my child need to be hospitalized for those treatments?
- Should I or my child be enrolled in a clinical trial?
- Can I continue to work or can my child go to school?
- Can I stay with my child for procedures? For hospitalizations?
- How and what should we tell our child about this illness?
- What should we tell our other children?

Like adults, children can take anti-nausea drugs an hour or so before scheduled treatments. Children, and some adults, can apply topical anesthetic creams to sites of bone marrow aspirates or spinal taps. Favorite stuffed animals or blankets can be present for most procedures.

Play and fun are as important to children with cancer as to healthy children. Items such as board games, modeling clay, video games, dolls, and toy cars can be enjoyed even with intravenous lines in place. Play dates with friends should be encouraged, with proper screening to limit exposure to contagious illnesses.

School districts are required to accommodate the special needs of children. Children with ALL might require shorter school days or the provision of a tutor at home. Children who develop learning disabilities due to treatment might require the intervention of a special education team.

Clinical trials

There are numerous **clinical trials** looking at novel strategies for the treatment of ALL in adults and children. Most oncologists consider bone marrow transplants to be state-of-the-art in specific circumstances, and some insurance companies agree. Many still require extensive reviews before approving coverage for transplant.

A variety of biological agents are currently under study. These include antibodies that react specifically against leukemic cells, causing their death, and chemicals that interfere with the leukemic cells' normal DNA function or their ability to make proteins.

Researchers are developing second and third generation versions of established chemotherapeutic drugs, isolating the molecular components of those drugs that seem to be most useful in ALL and amplifying them. Some of these drugs include 9-aminocamptothecin, aminopterin, annamycin, Ara-G, codrycepin, decitabine, and **trimetrexate**. Quinine shows promise in reducing the incidence of **drug resistance** that is sometimes seen in leukemic cells.

Locating and enrolling in clinical trials has been made easier by listings on the Internet. A general search under "clinical trials and leukemia" will yield several listings. University-affiliated hospitals and oncologists participate in many trials and can refer patients to other sites if necessary.

Prevention

There are few preventive measures to take against ALL. Those who work with chemicals should be cautious, particularly around benzene. Pregnant women should avoid exposure to ionizing radiation to reduce the risk to their unborn children.

Special concerns

Parents of children with ALL have specific concerns regarding the long-term consequences of treatment for ALL, such as learning disabilities. Organizations devoted to childhood cancer, hospital social workers, pediatric oncologists and other parents can be important resources when advocating for the educational needs of the child with ALL.

When cranial radiation must be used, children have a risk of developing secondary cancers in the central nervous system years later. Some children are left infertile by the treatment. Chicken pox can be lethal in children with ALL. The introduction of the chicken pox vaccine has reduced this risk, but parents must still be vigilant.

Resources

BOOKS

Lackritz, Barb. *Adult Leukemia: A Comprehensive Guide for Patients and Families.* Sebastopol, CA: O'Reilly & Associates, 2001.

Keene, Nancy, and Linda Lamb.*Childhood Leukemia: A Guide for Families, Friends & Caregivers.* Sebastopol, CA: O'Reilly & Associates, 1999.

Laszlo, John, M.D.*The Cure of Childhood Leukemia: Into the Age of Miracles.* New Brunswick: Rutgers University Press, 1995.

McKay, Judith, and Nancee Hirano.*The Chemotherapy and Radiation Therapy Survival Guide.* Oakland: New Harbinger Publications, 1998.

Patenande, Robert.*Surviving Leukemia: A Practical Guide.* Quebec: Firefly Books, Ltd., 1999.

PERIODICALS

Gaynon, P.S., et al. "Children's Cancer Group Trials in Childhood Acute Lymphoblastic Leukemia: 1983–1995." *Leukemia* 14, no. 5 (December 2000): 2223–33.

Greaves, M.F. "Aetiology of Acute Leukaemia." *The Lancet* 349, no. 9048 (February 1997): 344–9.

Hasle, H., et al. "Risks of Leukaemia and Solid Tumours in Individuals with Down Syndrome." *The Lancet* 355, no. 9199 (January 2000): 165–9.

Pui, C.H. "Acute Lymphoblastic Leukemia in Children." *Current Opinions in Oncology* 12, no. 1 (January 2000): 3–12.

Weisdorf, D.J. "Bone Marrow Transplantation for Acute Lymphoblastic Leukemia (ALL)."*Leukemia* 11, Supp. 4 (May 1997): 420–2.

ORGANIZATIONS

The Leukemia and Lymphoma Society of America (formerly The Leukemia Society of America). 1311 Mamaroneck Ave., White Plains, NY 10605. (914) 949-5213. <http://www.leukemia-lymphoma.org>.

American Cancer Society. 1599 Clifton Rd., Atlanta, GA, 30329. (800) ACS-2345. <http://www.cancer.org>.

The National Cancer Institute. Cancer Information Service. Building 31, Room 10A31, 31 Center Dr., MSC 2580, Bethesda, MD 20892-2580. (301) 435-3848. <http://www.nci.nih.gov/>

Cancer Care, Inc. 1180 Avenue of the Americas, New York, NY 10036. (212) 302-2400 or (800) 813-4673. <http://www.cancercare.org>

National Marrow Donor Program. Suite 500, 3001 Broadway St. NE, Minneapolis, MN 55413-1753. (800) MARROW-2. <http://www.marrow.org/>

Candlelighters Childhood Cancer Foundation. 7910 Woodmont Ave., Suite 460, Bethesda, MD 20814. (800) 366-CCCF. <http://www.candlelighters.org>

National Childhood Cancer Foundation. 440 E. Huntington Dr., P.O. Box 60012, Arcadia, CA 91066-6012. (626) 447-1674. <http://www.nccf.org>

OTHER

PDQ (Physician Data Query). (800) 4-CANCER. 9 July 2001 <http://cancernet.nci.nih.gov>

GrannyBarb and Art's Leukemia Links. 9 July 2001 <http://www.acor.org/diseases/hematology/Leukemia/leukmain.html>

National Children's Cancer Society. 9 July 2001 <http://www.children-cancer.com>

Patient-centered Guides. <http://www.patientcenters.com/leukemia>

CancerNet Clinical Trials Listings. 9 July 2001 <http://www.cancernet.nci.nih.gov/index.html>

Veritas A service of Harvard Medical School, listing clinical trials throughout the US. 9 July 2001 <http://www.veritasmedicine.com/leukemia>

International clinical trials listings. 9 July 2001 <http://www.graylab.ac.uk/cancerweb/trials.html>

Why, Charlie Brown, Why? Videotape. Topper Books, 1990.

Marianne Vahey, M.D.

Acute myelocytic leukemia

Definition

Acute myelocytic leukemia (AML) is an acute cancer that affects white blood cells, primarily those of the granulocyte or monocyte types.

Description

Acute myelogenous leukemia and acute nonlymphocytic leukemia (ANLL)are other names for AML and refer to the identical disease.

The cells that make up blood are produced in the bone marrow and the lymph system. The bone marrow is the spongy tissue found in the large bones of the body. The lymph system includes the spleen (an organ in the upper abdomen), the thymus (a small organ beneath the breastbone), and the tonsils (an organ in the throat). In addition, the lymph vessels (tiny tubes that branch like blood vessels into all parts of the body) and lymph nodes (pea-shaped organs that are found along the network of lymph vessels) are also part of the lymph system. The lymph is a milky fluid that contains cells. Clusters of lymph nodes are found in the neck, underarm, pelvis, abdomen, and chest.

The main types of cells found in the blood are the red blood cells (RBCs), which carry oxygen and other materials to all tissues of the body; white blood cells (WBCs), which fight infection; and the platelets, which play a part in the clotting of the blood. The white blood cells can be further subdivided into three main types: granulocytes, monocytes, and lymphocytes.

The granulocytes, as their name suggests, have particles (granules) inside them. These granules contain special proteins (enzymes) and several other substances that can break down chemicals and destroy microorganisms such as bacteria. Monocytes are the second type of white blood cell. They are also important in defending the body against pathogens. The lymphocytes form the third type of white blood cell.

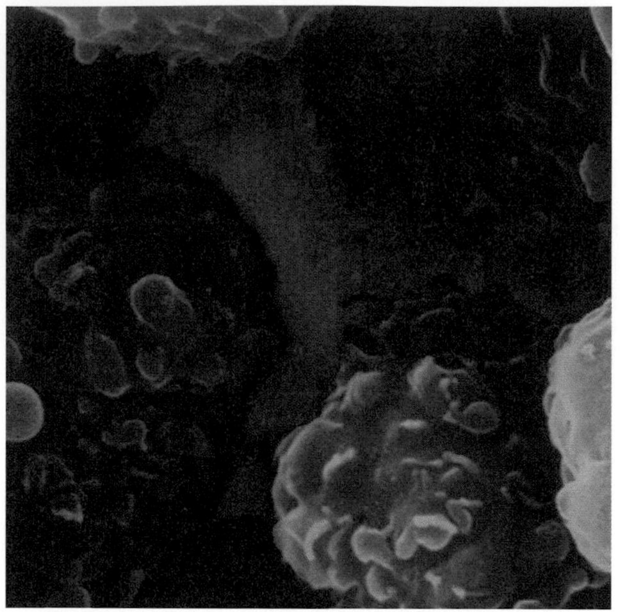

An enhanced scanning electron microscopy (SEM) image of acute myelocytic leukemia cells. *(Photograph by Robert Becker, Ph.D., Custom Medical Stock Photo. Reproduced by permission.*

The bone marrow makes stem cells, which are the precursors of the different blood cells. These stem cells mature through stages into either RBCs, WBCs, or platelets. In acute leukemias, the maturation process of the white blood cells is interrupted. The immature cells (or "blasts") proliferate rapidly and begin to accumulate in various organs and tissues, thereby affecting their normal function. This uncontrolled proliferation of the immature cells in the bone marrow affects the production of the normal red blood cells and platelets as well.

Acute leukemias are of two types: **acute lymphocytic leukemia** and acute myelogenous leukemia. Different types of white blood cells are involved in the two leukemias. In acute lymphocytic leukemia (ALL), it is the lymphocytes that become cancerous. AML is a cancer of the monocytes and/or granulocytes.

The reason certain leukemias are now called acute is because of names received decades ago. Before the discovery of modern methods of cancer treatment, these were illnesses that progressed rapidly. In contrast, chronic leukemias were, in this period before newer methods had been invented, illnesses that progressed more slowly.

Demographics

Approximately 23 new cases of AML appear per each million Americans each year. Men are somewhat more likely to develop AML than are women. Approximately 29 new cases appear per every million males while approximately 19 new cases appear per every million females per year.

Older persons are considerably more likely to develop AML. Approximately 13 people per million younger than 65 years of age will develop AML. In contrast, 122 people per million older than 65 years of age will develop the disease.

AML sometimes affects children. About 500 children develop AML in the United States every year. Approximately one in five of all children who develop leukemia develop AML. The disease affects boys and girls in roughly equal numbers. Children of all ethnic groups may develop the disease. If one of two identical twins develops AML, the chances are considerable that the other twin will develop it as well.

Causes and symptoms

AML is neither contagious nor inherited. However, people who suffer from certain genetic disorders, such as **Fanconi anemia**, Klinefelter syndrome, Patau syndrome, Bloom syndrome, and Down syndrome, are at greater risk of developing AML than the general population. A child with Down syndrome is roughly 14 times as likely as the average child to develop leukemia.

Any person who has been exposed to radiation at high doses is at heightened risk of developing AML, as are people exposed to benzene, a chemical used in the manufacture of plastics, rubber, medicines, and certain other chemicals. Another group of people at increased risk for developing AML are those who have been treated for cancer with certain medicines, for example, chloramphenicol, phenylbutazone, chloroquine, and methoxypsoralen.

The symptoms of AML are generally vague and non-specific. A patient may experience all or some of the following symptoms:

- weakness or chronic **fatigue**
- **fever** of unknown origin
- shortness of breath
- weight loss that is not due to dieting or exercise
- frequent bacterial or viral infections
- headaches
- skin rash
- non-specific **bone pain**
- easy bruising
- bleeding from gums or nose
- blood in urine or stools

- enlarged lymph nodes and/or spleen
- abdominal fullness

A small minority of patients with AML have a tumor of leukemic cells at diagnosis. Such a tumor may appear in the lung, breast, brain, uterus, ovary, stomach, prostate, or certain other places in the body.

Some children with AML present to their doctor with very few symptoms, while other children present with severe symptoms. **Anemia** is usually present. The symptoms of the anemia may include fatigue, dizziness, headache, paleness of the skin, or, infrequently, congestive heart failure. Easy bruising, bleeding gums, and nosebleeds may be present, as may fever. There may be swollen gums, bone pain or joint pain, or, rarely, an actual tumor. Some infants with AML have skin disorders.

Diagnosis

Like all cancers, acute leukemias are best treated when found early. There are no screening tests available.

A thorough diagnostic evaluation should be conducted. This is important because the doctor must determine more than whether or not AML is present. If it is suspected, has it affected the general health of the patient? Is the patient capable of undergoing rigorous treatment?

A doctor who suspects leukemia may start by obtaining a thorough medical history. The doctor may then conduct a very thorough physical examination to look for enlarged lymph nodes in the neck, underarm, and pelvic region. Swollen gums, enlarged liver or spleen, bruises, or pinpoint red rashes all over the body are among the signs of the disease. In addition, the physician may examine the teeth and look for dental abscesses, and may explore whether back pain is present.

Urine and blood tests may be ordered to check for microscopic amounts of blood in the urine and to obtain a complete differential blood count. This count will give the numbers and percentages of the different cells found in the blood. An abnormal blood test might suggest leukemia. Patients suffering from AML may have high leukocyte counts and typically have low counts of both red blood cells and platelets. Many patients with AML have low counts of all of the major components of the blood. A microscopic exploration of the blood will usually show that leukemic blast cells are present. However, the diagnosis has to be confirmed by more specific tests.

The doctor may perform a **bone marrow aspiration and biopsy** to confirm the diagnosis of leukemia. Aspiration involves the withdrawal of a liquid sample of marrow. During the **biopsy**, a cylindrical piece of bone and marrow is removed. The tissue is generally taken out of the hipbone. These samples are sent to the laboratory for examination. In addition to diagnosis, the aspiration and biopsy may be repeated during the treatment phase of the disease to see if the leukemia is responding to therapy.

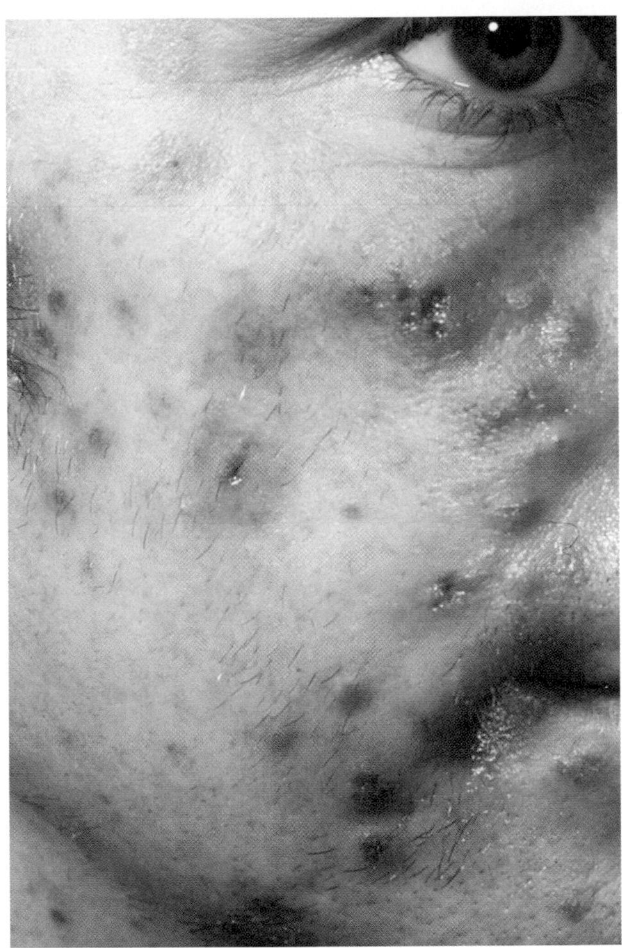

An acute myelocytic leukemia patient with a rash, one of the symptoms of the disease. *(Custom Medical Stock Photo. Reproduced by permission.)*

A chest **x ray** is taken. Cardiac tests, including an electrocardiogram, are conducted. The patient is examined for possible infection. These diagnostic procedures often disclose bleeding in the stomach or intestines, and there may be bleeding in the lungs, brain, or eyes. Anemia is often present and may be severe.

Cytogenetic studies, which examine the number and shape of the chromosomes in the DNA of individual blast cells, should be conducted in addition to the immunophenotyping of cells of the bone marrow. This procedure involves applying various stains to the marrow cells. These stains help doctors identify some of the proteins lying on the surface of the cells.

KEY TERMS

Blasts—An immature cell.

Bone marrow—Spongy tissue found in the large bones of the body.

Cytogenetic testing—Analysis of parts of the nucleus of blast cells.

Granulocytes—White blood cells containing particles or granules.

Immunophenotype—A test that involves placing various sorts of stains on bone marrow cells to help identify the chemicals located on the cell surfaces.

Monocytes—Another type of white blood cell, important in the defense against pathogens.

A spinal tap (**lumbar puncture**) is another procedure the doctor may order to diagnose leukemia. In this procedure, a small needle is inserted into the spinal cavity in the lower back to withdraw some cerebrospinal fluid and to look for leukemic cells.

Standard imaging tests such as x rays may be used to check whether the leukemic cells have invaded other areas of the body, such as the bones, chest, kidneys, abdomen, or brain. Other tests, such as **computed tomography** scans (CT scans), **magnetic resonance imaging** (MRI), or gallium scans, are not typical for AML but may also be performed.

Children with AML are given most of the same studies used for adults.

Clinical staging, treatments, and prognosis

Unlike several other cancers, AML is not staged. However, a classification system is used to separate different forms of AML. One of the most important classification systems, devised by a team of physicians, is known as the French-American-British (FAB) Classification System.

The goal of AML treatment is to achieve a complete remission (CR). What is a complete remission? It is a measure that indicates that the patient's disease has gotten markedly better in several ways. In general, it might be said that CR is achieved once the body has regained its ability to produce blood cells normally. At this point, the number of blood cells of various types should return to normal ranges, while none of the immature cells called leukemic blast cells should be present in the blood or the marrow.

Chemotherapy is the use of drugs to kill cancer cells. It is usually the treatment of choice and is used to relieve symptoms and achieve long-term remission of the disease. Generally, combination chemotherapy, in which multiple drugs are used, is more efficient than using a single drug for the treatment. Some drugs may be administered intravenously through a vein in the arm; others may be given by mouth in the form of pills. If the cancer cells have invaded the brain, then chemotherapeutic drugs may be put into the fluid that surrounds the brain and spinal cord. This is known as intrathecal chemotherapy. Chemotherapy should start soon after diagnosis.

Patients who are anemic or who have low platelet counts should receive transfusions. These transfusions should be sufficient to restore counts of various components of the blood to adequate levels.

There are two phases of treatment for leukemia. The first phase is called induction therapy. During this phase, the main aim of treatment is to reduce the number of leukemic cells as much as possible and induce a remission in the patient. A variety of chemotherapy agents may be used during the induction therapy portion of AML treatment. The chemotherapy agent Ara-C **(cytarabine)** is in 2001 often used in combination with either **daunorubicin** or **idarubicin** (Idamycin). Other doctors add **etoposide** to this combination of chemotherapy agents. For older patients, Ara-C and **mitoxantrone** may be used. Some patients benefit from receiving high doses of chemotherapy drugs. As of 2001,patients who do not achieve CR, as well as those who achieve CR but then relapse, may be given mitoxantrone plus etoposide.

The second phase of treatment is initiated once CR is achieved. This is called post-remission or consolidation therapy. The goal of therapy now becomes killing any remaining cells and maintaining the remission for as long as possible. There are various ways of attempting to reach this goal. One involves additional chemotherapy. Another involves **bone marrow transplantation** (BMT), also called stem cell transplant (SCT). Transplantation therapy has been studied very thoroughly. It involves taking blood-making cells, whether from the patient or from another person, and infusing them into the patient following removal of the diseased marrow, with either high doses of chemotherapy or total body irradiation. These procedures are potentially very effective because of the remarkable ability of these cells to create a sustained replacement of the patient's blood cells. Other strategies may also be applied. Approaches used for patients younger than 60 years of age may differ from those used for patients of older ages.

Because leukemia cells can spread to all the organs via the blood stream and the lymph vessels, surgery is not considered an option for treating leukemias.

Children with AML also receive induction therapy. Often two or three medicines are used in conjunction with one another. After remission is achieved in a young patient, postremission therapy is started. The type of postremission therapy depends largely on the type of AML the patient has. It may involve additional chemotherapy or, alternatively, bone marrow transplantation. Chemotherapy to the central nervous system (CNS) is given to most children, since without it, roughly one in five will develop CNS relapse. The CNS includes the brain and spinal cord.

The prognosis of patients with AML varies. A number of different matters should be examined before the prognosis of any individual patient is assessed. The most important of these is whether or not the patient attains a complete remission (CR). The most important consideration in terms of whether a patient is likely to achieve CR is the patient's age. However, it may be that chronological age is not what really matters. Rather, to a large extent, what is truly significant is the patient's ability to survive the difficulties associated with induction therapy. For example, the patient who has some other disease in addition to AML may have a more difficult time with the rigors of the therapy. Yet, it is also true that older patients are more likely to have AML that expresses certain characteristics associated with poorer outcomes.

Other factors also affect the patient's prognosis. For example, in the tests performed during diagnosis, the chromosomes of cells are examined. Some chromosomal findings are associated with a good prognosis. Others are only mildly good, while still others indicate the patient is less likely to achieve CR.

Other factors that may provide physicians with hints as to the patient's prognosis include: how long symptoms were present before the illness was diagnosed, and how quickly immature blast cells disappear after treatment is started.

Coping with cancer treatment

One of the most important aspects of treatment is guaranteeing that the patient will have the supportive care needed to come through the treatment period with physical and emotional strength intact. Part of what this means is that AML should be treated in major cancer centers, because only these centers have the expertise necessary to provide not only the right medicine but also the accompaniments of good treatment.

One way physicians help AML patients cope with treatment is to guarantee that adequate blood bank support is available. Many patients require platelet transfusions.

QUESTIONS TO ASK THE DOCTOR

- What type of AML do I have? What does it mean to have this variant of the disease?
- How can I obtain supportive care so I come through this not only alive but with my family and emotional life intact?
- Do I have any infections?
- What are the results of the cytogenetic testing?
- What are the results of the immunophenotyping?
- What is my prognosis?
- Are blasts present?
- Are blood counts returning to normal levels?
- Has complete remission been achieved?
- What can I do to lower my risk of infection during chemotherapy?

One of the great dangers to patients during induction treatment and other steps of treatment is the threat of serious infectious disease. These patients have weakened blood components and are therefore more susceptible to infectious illness than the average person is. The leading cause of death for patients receiving induction treatment and chemotherapy following remission is infectious illness.

To help build the patient's white cell count, doctors may prescribe growth factors. These encourage the body to produce certain types of blood cells. The types of growth factors prescribed most frequently are granulocyte-colony stimulating factor (G-CSF) and granulocyte-macrophage colony stimulating factor (GM-CSF).

The psychological aspects of cancer treatment are a major concern. Patients should ask their physician about local support groups and survivor networks that can help with the stresses associated with this disease.

Prevention

High doses of radiation and exposure to the chemical benzene (used in the manufacture of plastics, rubber, and medicines) are strong risk factors. With the exception of people with such rare genetic conditions as Fanconi anemia, Klinefelter syndrome, Patau syndrome, Bloom syndrome, and Down syndrome, there is no known genetic predisposition to AML.

Resources

BOOKS

Braunwald, Eugene, et al.*Harrison's Principles of Internal Medicine,*15th ed. New York: McGraw-Hill, 2001.

Pazdur, Richard, et al.*Cancer Management: A Multidisciplinary Approach: Medical, Surgical, & Radiation Oncology,* 4th ed. Melville, New York: PRR, 2000.

Steen, Grant, and Joseph Mirro.*Childhood Cancer: A Handbook from St. Jude Children's Research Hospital.* Cambridge, MA: Perseus Publishing, 2000.

PERIODICALS

Abramson, N., and B. Melton."Leukocytosis: Basics of Clinical Assessment."*American Family Physician* 63 (2000): 2053–60.

Hiddemann, W., et al. "Management of Acute Myeloid Leukemia in Elderly Patients." *Journal of Clinical Oncology* 17 (1999): 3569.

Lowenberg, B., et al. "Acute Myeloid Leukemia." *New England Journal of Medicine* 341 (1999): 1051.

Young, G., et al. "Recognition of Common Childhood Malignancies." *American Family Physician* 61 (2000): 2144–54

ORGANIZATIONS

Acute Myeloid Leukemia Treatment, Childhood.Acute Myeloid Leukemia Treatment, Adult. National Cancer Institute. (800) 4-CANCER. <http://www.nci.nih.gov>.

Acute Myelogenous Leukemia (AML).Emotional Aspects of Childhood Leukemia.Making Intelligent Choices About Therapy.Understanding Blood Counts.Patient Aid Program.Family Support Group.Information Resource Center. The Leukemia and Lymphoma Society. (800) 955-4572. <http://www.leukemia-lymphoma.org>.

Adult Acute Leukemia American Cancer Society. (800) ACS-2345. <http://www.cancer.org>.

Lata Cherath, Ph.D.
Bob Kirsch

Acute myelogenous leukemia *see* **Acute myelocytic leukemia**

Acyclovir *see* Antiviral therapy

Adenocarcinoma

Definition

Cancer that begins in the epithelial cells, which line certain internal organs and have glandular (secretory) properties. Some types of adenocarcinomas include cancers of the breast, thyroid, colon, stomach, pancreas, and prostate, as well as certain types of lung cancer.

Kate Kretschmann

Adenoma

Definition

A benign (noncancerous) tumor that forms from the cells lining the inside or the surface of an organ.

Description

Adenomas arise from cells that are specialized for secretion. These cells, called epithelial cells, are found throughout the body, but only a fraction is designed for secretion. This type of epithelial cell makes up specific organs and structures in the body known as glands. Glands produce sweat, saliva, mucus, milk, digestive juices, hormones, and an array of other substances. Hormone-secreting (endocrine) glands include the thyroid, pituitary, parathyroids, adrenals, and the ovaries and testes. Gland cells that secrete material outward through a duct, such as sweat glands and glands secreting digestive juices into the stomach and intestines, are called exocrine glands. Adenomas can arise from most of the gland cells in the body.

Adenomas result from excessive growth of normal epithelial cells. They arise in much the same way as malignant (cancerous) tumors but do not spread (metastasize) to nearby tissue or other parts of the body. New cells are normally created only when they are needed by the body. When the body does not need new cells and cell division continues, a mass or tumor is formed.

Tumors found on some glands are more likely to be adenomas than malignant tumors (carcinomas), including **adrenal tumors**, **pituitary tumors**, and **salivary gland tumors**. The adrenal tumor known as **pheochromocytoma** is benign in 90% of reported cases. The gastrinomas associated with **Zollinger-Ellison syndrome** are benign in 50% of patients with this condition. Adenomas are also associated with **Cushing's syndrome**, a disorder caused by excess levels of a hormone secreted by the adrenal glands. Although most cases are caused by a dysfunctional pituitary gland, 20–25% are due to adrenal adenomas.

The occurrence of an adenoma rarely indicates an increased chance for the later development of a **carcinoma**. However, **colon cancer** and **rectal cancer** are thought to arise from adenomas, and one type of lung adenoma—called a bronchial adenoma—can potentially develop into lung cancer.

Most adenomas affect the normal functioning of the organ or gland in which it arises, although some have no effect. Many secrete hormones, leading to elevated hormone levels in the blood and causing uncomfortable and sometimes life-threatening conditions.

Demographics

Certain types of adenomas are more common in women than in men (e.g., pituitary tumors and liver adenoma), and some are more common in older adults (e.g., adenomas of the colon). But specific demographics depend on the specific type of adenoma.

Causes and symptoms

The cause of adenomas is often unknown. Liver adenomas in women are linked to the use of oral contraceptives, and some conditions, such as pheochromocytomas and colon adenomas, can be inherited.

No single set of symptoms can be applied to all adenomas. Some disorders have similar or identical symptoms whether due to an adenoma or carcinoma. Ultimately, the signs and symptoms depend on the location of the adenoma:

- Adrenal glands: an adrenocortical adenoma often shows the same symptoms of an **adrenocortical carcinoma**, including abdominal pain and loss of weight. A benign and malignant pheochromocytoma also has the same symptoms, including headaches, sweating, and chest pains.
- Breast: a marble-like benign fibroadenoma causes no symptoms and is either too small to detect by touch or is several inches across and easily detected.
- Colon or rectum: persistent **diarrhea** can indicate villous adenomas of the rectum. Blood in stool samples can indicate adenomas in the colon or rectum.
- Liver: a hepatic adenoma causes pain and a mass that is detectable by touch.
- Lung: a chronic or bloody cough, **fever**, chills, and shortness of breath can indicate a bronchial adenoma.
- Pancreas: pain in the abdomen, diarrhea, stomach pain, persistent fatigue, fainting, and weight gain can indicate one of the various types of pancreatic adenomas or pancreatic cancer.
- Parathyroid: weakness, **fatigue**, constipation, kidney stones, loss of appetite, and **bone pain** are signs of a condition known as hyperparathyroidism, which occurs in patients with parathyroid adenomas or parathyroid cancer.

KEY TERMS

Adrenal glands—Two glands, one located above each kidney, that secrete hormones to prevent inflammation and to help regulate blood pressure, blood sugar levels, and metabolism.

Carcinoma—A malignant (cancerous) tumor that forms from the cells lining the inside or the surface of an organ. They tend to spread to other tissues and organs.

Colon—A section of the large intestine, occurring before the rectum, that functions to absorb water and minerals from material that passed undigested from the small intestines.

Epithelium—A type of tissue that is composed of epithelial cells. It covers the outer and internal surfaces of the body and forms glands and parts of the sense organs.

Parathyroid glands—Four glands found in the neck area, with a pair on either side of the thyroid. They produce parathyroid hormone, which controls the level of calcium in the blood.

Pituitary gland—A small gland found at the base of the brain. It is an important endocrine gland because it secretes many different hormones that control the activity of other endocrine glands.

Thyroid gland—A gland located at the base of the neck. It secretes hormones that are essential for the regulation of body temperature, heart rate, metabolism, the level of calcium in the blood, and the level of calcium absorption by the bones.

- Salivary gland: adenomas are small and usually painless but can cause swelling around the chin or jawbone, numbness of the face, and pain in the face, chin, or neck.
- Stomach and intestine: a gastrinoma causes a peptic ulcer in the intestines or stomach. The occurrence of many ulcers in the stomach, intestine, and pancreas that do not respond well to treatment can indicate Zollinger-Ellison syndrome.
- Sweat gland: adenomas may appear as many small, smooth, and firm bumps on the lower eyelids and upper parts of the cheek (syringomas), or as small bumps with bluish or dark-brown coloration on the head and neck area (hidrocystoma). Solitary adenomas (poromas) occur on the sole of the foot or palm of the hand.

QUESTIONS TO ASK THE DOCTOR

- Does the occurrence of this adenoma increase my chances of developing cancer?
- If I choose to have the adenoma surgically removed, what are the chances that I will develop another adenoma?
- Will all my symptoms disappear once the adenoma is removed?

- Thyroid: a lump in the neck region accompanied by a cough and difficulty swallowing or breathing often indicates a benign thyroid nodule; however, these are the same symptoms for thyroid cancer.

Diagnosis

A variety of techniques is used to diagnose adenomas. Blood and urine samples are taken to detect elevated levels of hormones or other substances associated with a specific adenoma. Tumors are located using a combination of **ultrasonography**, **computed tomography** scan (CT scan), **magnetic resonance imaging** (MRI), and possibly radionuclide imaging. A **biopsy** is performed to determine whether a tumor is benign or malignant.

Treatment team

A doctor who interprets tissue samples (a pathologist) and a doctor trained in examining x rays and computer images (a radiologist) will make an initial diagnosis. Adenomas are often surgically removed, so a surgical team consisting of an anesthesiologist, surgeon, and nurses is often associated with treatment.

Clinical staging, treatments, and prognosis

Surgical removal is the recommended treatment for most adenomas, although the symptoms of some adenomas, such as pituitary tumors, can be treated with medication. In most cases, treatment cures the condition.

Clinical trials

Two **clinical trials** completed in mid-2001 investigated treatments to prevent colon cancer in patients who have had surgery to remove adenomas of the rectum or colon. An 800 mg daily dose of **folic acid** may decrease the occurrence of colon cancer in patients who have had adenomas removed. The combined use of two drugs that are prescribed for other conditions, eflonithine and sulindac, may prevent the development of adenomas or the recurrence of colon cancer.

See Also Fibrocystic condition of the breast; Pancreatic cancer, endocrine; Pancreatic cancer, exocrine

Resources

BOOKS

DeVita, Vincent T. Jr., Samuel Hellman, and Steven A. Rosenberg, eds. *Cancer: Principles and Practice of Oncology.* Philadelphia: Lippincott-Raven Publishers, 1997.

Greenspan, Francis S., and Gordon J. Strewler.*Basic and Clinical Endocrinology.* Stamford, Connecticut: Appleton&Lange, 1997.

Monica McGee, M.S.

Adrenal tumors

Definition

Tumors that occur on one or both of the adrenal glands.

Description

The two small adrenal glands, one located just above each kidney, are among the many endocrine (hormone-secreting) glands in the body. All endocrine glands make and store hormones. Hormones are chemical messages that are sent from an endocrine gland and are received by an organ or a cell to trigger a specific reaction. When the body requires hormone levels to rise, endocrine glands secrete them into the bloodstream. Adrenal gland tumors often cause overproduction of one or a combination of the adrenal hormones.

An adrenal gland has two parts, each of which secretes different hormones. The inner part is called the adrenal medulla, and the outer part is the adrenal cortex.

The adrenal medulla secretes the hormones epinephrine and norepinephrine. These hormones help maintain normal blood pressure. In high-stress situations, they help prepare the body for quick action by increasing heartbeat and breathing rate, increasing the flow of blood to the heart and lungs, and increasing blood pressure.

The adrenal cortex secretes aldosterone and cortisol. They also make small amounts of androgens, which affect the expression of female and male sex characteristics.

Aldosterone helps maintain normal salt levels in the blood and the normal functioning of the kidneys. Cortisol (also called hydrocortisone) is the major adrenal hormone.

Cortisol is a steroid, an organic compound that affects metabolism. Many hormones and drugs used to relieve swelling and inflammation are steroids. Cortisol helps maintain blood pressure and is crucial in the breakdown of proteins, carbohydrates, and fats. It also raises blood sugar (glucose) when levels are too low, thus providing needed energy for the body's activities. Cortisol also prevents inflammation and is important for the normal response to stress.

The level of cortisol in the blood is carefully controlled. When the body needs cortisol, a small area of the brain called the hypothalamus releases coricotripoin-releasing hormone (CRH). The pituitary gland, located at the base of the brain, receives the message from the hypothalamus and begins secreting adrenocorticotropic hormone (ACTH). ACTH is received by the cortex of the adrenal glands, which responds by producing cortisol. When the level of cortisol meets the body's need, the pituitary stops producing ACTH, which then stops the adrenal cortex from secreting cortisol.

About 8% of people worldwide develop benign (noncancerous) adrenal tumors. Malignant (cancerous) tumors are very rare, occurring in two out of every one million people worldwide, and this cancer is more common in women than in men.

It is often difficult for a pathologist to distinguish between a benign and a malignant adrenal tumor. Several criteria are used to make a diagnosis, including the size and weight of the tumor, whether hormones are produced, and what hormones are produced. A benign tumor (**adenoma**) is usually less than 4–6 centimeters (1.57–2.3 inches) in diameter and likely causes changes in the blood level of only one hormone or may cause no changes at all. A malignant tumor is larger and may alter the level of several adrenal hormones. One reliable indicator for a malignant tumor is evidence that the cancer has spread (**metastasis**).

Types of cancers

Adrenal cortex

A disorder caused by an adrenal cortex tumor can occur alone, but often two or more conditions occur simultaneously. These disorders include

- **Cushing's syndrome**: a disorder resulting from prolonged exposure to high levels of cortisol. Most cases are the result of a pituitary gland dysfunction that causes excessive secretion of ACTH, but 20–25% are caused by a benign adrenal tumor, of which about 50% are malignant. Symptoms include obesity, moon-shaped face, increased fat in neck region, skin that bruises easily, severe **fatigue**, weak muscles, and high blood pressure. The common treatment is surgical removal of the affected gland. The outcome for a Cushing's syndrome patient with a benign adrenal adenoma is very good. Surgery usually results in a cure. The outcome is variable for malignant tumors.

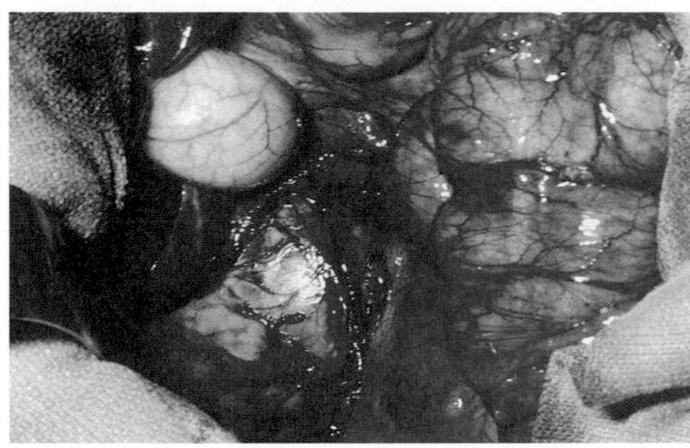

An adrenal tumor is shown at lower left. The gallbladder is white, and the nearby liver is deep red. *(Custom Medical Stock Photo. Reproduced by permission.)*

- Aldosteronism (also called Conn's disease or hypoaldosteronism): a condition resulting from an abnormally high level of the hormone aldosterone. It is usually caused by an adenoma and rarely is the result of a malignant adrenal tumor. Symptoms include headaches, weakness, fatigue, high blood salt levels, frequent urination, high blood pressure, and an irregular heartbeat. An adenoma is usually removed surgically, although medication that controls the secretion of aldosterone is an effective treatment in many cases.
- Virilization syndrome (also called adrenal virilism or adrenogenital syndrome): a disorder caused by an excessive secretion of androgen hormones, leading to high levels of the male hormone **testosterone**. Adenomas that cause virilization are rare. When the condition accompanies Cushing's syndrome it may indicate an **adrenocortical carcinoma**. In males, the symptom is early onset of puberty, whereas in females symptoms include deepening of voice, a masculine build, and abnormal hairiness. The recommended treatment depends on the cause. If the condition is caused by an adenoma, use of medications that surpress ACTH secretion by the pituitary is the preferred treatment.
- Adrenocortical carcinoma: a rare cancer that is often not detected until it has spread to the liver or lung. The symptoms can include that of Cushing's syndrome, aldosteronism, virilization, or a combination of each of these con-

KEY TERMS

Adenoma—A benign tumor.

Inherited disorder—A disease that has a tendency to occur within a family. A disorder may be acquired because of a gene or genes that are passed from parent to child.

Pathologist—A doctor specializing in the identification of diseases by studying cells and tissues under a microscope.

ditions. The preferred treatment depends on the stage of the cancer, but usually involves surgery to remove the tumor, **chemotherapy**, and **radiation therapy**. If the cancer is caught at an early stage, the long-term survival can be good. If found at a later stage, about 30% of patients will survive five years after the initial diagnosis.

Adrenal medulla

Only one type of tumor is associated with the adrenal medulla:

- Pheochromocytoma: a tumor that produces and secretes epinephrine and norepinephrine. Excessive secretion of these hormones can cause life-threatening hypertension and an irregular heartbeat. About 90% of these tumors are benign. Five percent of those diagnosed with this tumor have either **Von Hippel-Lindau syndrome**, type 2 of the **multiple endocrine neoplasia** (MEN) **syndromes, Von Recklinghausen's neurofibromatosis**, or another inherited disorder. Symptoms include headaches, sweating, and chest pains. Treatment involves medication to control hypertension and the surgical removal of the affected gland. Long-term survival depends on early detection of the tumor and whether the tumor is benign or malignant.

See Also Endocrine system tumors

Resources

BOOKS

DeVita, Vincent T. Jr., Samuel Hellman, and Steven A. Rosenberg, eds.*Cancer: Principles and Practice of Oncology* Philadelphia, Penn.: Lippincott-Raven Publishers, 1997.

Murphy, Gerald P., Lois B. Morris, and Dianne Lange.*Informed Decisions: The Complete Book of Cancer Diagnosis, Treatment, and Recovery.* New York: Viking, 1997.

PERIODICALS

Higgins, James C., and James M. Fitzgerald."Evaluation of Incidental Renal and Adrenal Masses."*American Family Physician* 63(2001): 288–294.

ORGANIZATIONS

American Association of Clinical Endocrinologists. 1000 Riverside Avenue Suite 205, Jacksonville, FL 32204. 904-353-7878. <http://www.aace.com>.

National Adrenal Diseases Foundation, 505 Northern Boulevard, Great Neck, NY 11021. 516-487-4992. <http://www.medhelp.org/nadf>.

Monica McGee, M.S.

Adrenocortical carcinoma

Definition

Adrenocortical carcinoma is a malignant growth that originates in the cortex, or the outer portion, of one of the two adrenal glands.

Description

There are two adrenal glands in the body. Each one is paired with a kidney. The adrenal gland rests atop the kidney, on the side of the kidney that is nearest to the head.

An adrenal gland has two parts. The inner part (medulla) produces hormones such as epinephrine (adrenaline) that increases the heart rate. The cortex, or outer part, is made up of layers of epithelial cells, the cells that form coverings for the surfaces of the body. The cortex produces cortical hormones that are essential to well-being, or homeostasis.

The hormones produced by the cortex include glucocorticoids, mineralocorticoids, and sex hormones. Among the many hormones the cortex makes, three—aldosterone, cortisol and adrenal sex hormones—are very important. Aldosterone helps regulate salt and water content in the body. Cortisol helps keep sugars, fats and proteins in balance. Adrenal sex hormones influence sex organ development and sex drive (libido).

Adrenocortical carcinoma is a cancer that originates in the cortex of the adrenal gland. When a tumor grows in the adrenal cortex, it interferes with the production of hormones. Consequently, the effects of adrenocortical carcinoma can be severe and are almost always a threat to life.

There are two types of adrenocortical carcinoma. In one type, a tumor functions—that is, it makes hormones. In the other type, the tumor does not function. If the tumor functions, it acts like the cells in the cortex from which it grew and thus, produces hormones. But since it grows large, it produces extra amounts of hormones and the body is thrown far out of balance in any one of a number of ways.

When a tumor functions

How excess hormones cause the symptoms they produce is complex because more than one hormone from the adrenal cortex can be involved in producing a single symptom. For example, both aldosterone and cortisol, when present in extra quantities, may contribute to the increase in blood pressure (hypertension) many patients experience. Extra amounts of adrenal sex hormones can cause children to begin to display the sexual characteristics (hair growth, genital maturation) of adults. And adults with extra amounts of sex hormones often begin to display the sexual characteristics of the opposite sex. A woman may grow excess facial hair. A man may begin to develop fatty tissue in his breasts. Large quantities of adrenal sex hormones coursing through the body disrupt what would be a normal loop of feedback from the pituitary area of the brain. The pituitary is geared to send information, via a stimulating hormone, to the adrenal cortex, to prompt the tissue to manufacture adrenal sex hormone. When there is an extra amount of adrenal sex hormone in the body, the pituitary stops sending instructions to the adrenal cortex, as well as to other organs that produce the hormones responsible for male features. Thus, a man can begin to look like a woman because he does not have enough male hormones. A woman can begin to look like a man because she has too much adrenal sex hormone.

When a tumor does not function

If the tumor does not function, it just grows large, and may go unnoticed for a long time. Sometimes a tumor that does not function is called dormant. Often, the tumor that does not function first gets attention when it grows large enough to push against the body wall or an organ and cause pain; or when it has spread (metastasized) to another organ.

The adrenocortical carcinoma that does not function has a high likelihood of metastasizing before it is discovered. The two most common sites for metastases are the lungs and liver. Thus, even a non-functioning tumor may cause serious complications.

Demographics

Adrenocortical carcinoma is rare. Fewer than two in one million people, and perhaps as few as one in four million people, are diagnosed in a year. Two age groups are most likely to be diagnosed: those between zero and ten years of age, and those between 40 and 50 years.

Causes and symptoms

Causes

The cause of adrenocortical carcinoma is not known. Infection with bacteria or parasites is linked to other conditions of the adrenal glands, and there could be a connection with adrenocortical carcinoma. There is also evidence that adrenocortical carcinoma in children is caused by some chemical to which they were exposed as fetuses—possibly a chemical that the women carrying the children were exposed to in food, drink, or in the air.

Many tumors of the adrenal cortex have cells with extra copies of chromosomes, the beads of genetic material or DNA. Chemicals in the environment that are known to affect cells and cause mutations are being investigated as possible causes for adrenocortical carcinoma.

Symptoms

Depending on whether or not the tumor interferes with the production of hormones, the tumor may or may not be linked to symptoms during its early growth. A

KEY TERMS

Biopsy—Tissue sample is taken from body for examination.

Carcinoma—A cancer that originates in cells that developed from epithelial tissue, a tissue found on skin and mucosal surfaces.

Computed tomography (CT)—X rays are aimed at slices of the body (by rotating equipment) and results are assembled with a computer to give a three-dimensional picture of a structure.

Homeostasis—Self-regulating mechanisms are working, body is in equilibrium, no uncontrolled cell growth.

Hormone—A chemical released by one organ of the body that affects the activity of another organ.

Inferior vena cava—The large vein that returns blood from the lower body to the heart.

Lymph nodes—Part of the lymphatic system, these clusters of tissue help to protect the body from foreign substances, organisms, and cancer cells.

Magnetic resonance imaging (MRI)—Magnetic fields used to provide images of the internal organs of the body.

Pituitary—A gland at the base of the brain that produces hormones.

Venography—Technique used for examining veins for blockage, using a dye to make the vein visible with scans similar to x ray.

QUESTIONS TO ASK THE DOCTOR

- In which stage is the carcinoma?
- With this type of carcinoma, what is the five-year survival rate for a person of my age and gender? What is the one-year survival rate?
- Is there a center that specializes in treating this type of cancer?
- Are there any clinical trials in which I might be eligible to participate?
- Does this health care institution have a support group for individuals with my type of carcinoma?
- What is your approach to relieving pain? (Do we agree?)

group of Japanese surgeons led by K. Kunieda reported the case of a 52-year-old man who had a tumor weighing more than two pounds at the time it was discovered. The tumor had not been producing extra hormones, and was not producing symptoms.

An adrenocortical tumor that functions produces many symptoms. Some of them are similar to those linked to other conditions, and many of these conditions have names that are based on a collection of symptoms and not on the cause. A combination of the following symptoms, known as **Cushing's syndrome**, could be caused by a tumor in the pituitary area of the brain, as well as by adrenocortical carcinoma:

- an abnormal accumulation of fatty pads in the face (creating the distinctive "moon face" of Cushing's syndrome); in the trunk (termed "truncal obesity"); and over the upper back and the back of the neck (giving the individual what has been called a "buffalo hump")
- purple and pink stretch marks across the abdomen and flanks
- high blood pressure
- weak, thinning bones (osteoporosis)
- muscle atrophy (due to protein loss)
- low energy
- thin, fragile skin, with a tendency toward both bruising and slow healing
- abnormalities in the processing of sugars (glucose), with occasional development of actual diabetes
- increased risk of infections
- irregular menstrual periods in women
- decreased sex drive in men and difficulty maintaining an erection
- abormal hair growth in women (in a male pattern, such as in the beard and mustache area), as well as loss of hair from the head (receding hair line)

Similarly, virilization syndrome, or the tendency of a child to exhibit adult sexual features, or a female adult to exhibit male features, can be caused by other conditions, such as tumors in the pituitary, or by adrenocortical carcinoma. So, too, with feminization, or the tendency of a male individual to exhibit female characteristics, such as enlarged breasts and fat deposits on the hips.

Diagnosis

Symptoms usually cause a patient to talk with a physician. Blood and urine samples are examined to learn whether hormones are out of balance. Venography, a way of getting a picture of the inside of veins, is a technique that is still used to examine the adrenal glands prior to any decision about surgery. But the **magnetic resonance imaging** (MRI) scan has replaced venography in many facilities. **Computed tomography** (CT) scan is also used to examine the adrenal cortex.

Treatment team

Depending on symptoms, the first specialized physician an individual consults may either be an endocrinologist (a physician who focuses on hormones) or a urologist (a physician who focuses on the study of the kidneys and nearby structures). Either one of them, or a medical oncologist (a physician who focuses on treating patients with cancer) will lead the treatment team. A surgeon will be on the team too because in almost all cases removal of the adrenocortical carcinoma to the fullest extent possible is standard procedure.

Nurses will be on the team to help with administering drugs and monitoring the status of the patient. And if the patient is given **chemotherapy**, technicians skilled in the treatment will be part of the team.

Clinical staging, treatments, and prognosis

Adrenocortical tumors are assigned to one of four stages.

- Stage I tumors have not spread beyond the cortex of the adrenal gland and are less than two in (5cm) in their greatest dimension.
- Stage II tumors have not spread beyond the cortex of the adrenal gland and are more than two inches.

- Stage III tumors have either spread into tissues around the adrenal cortex or they have spread into lymph nodes near the adrenal glands, or both.
- Stage IV tumors have spread to lymph nodes and other organs near the adrenal cortex or to other organs of the body.

A plan for treatment is based on the size and extent of the tumor. Surgical removal of the tumor, radiation and chemotherapy are all used. Method of treatment depends on how large the carcinoma is and whether it has spread to other organs. In some cases the treatment is strictly palliative (provides comfort) and is not expected to halt the course of the cancer. Palliative treatment can include surgery to reduce the size of tumor, as well the pain a large tumor causes by pushing against other organs.

Because adrenocortical carcinoma that metastasizes often moves into the renal (kidney) vein and then, the inferior vena cava, venography or MRI scan prior to surgical removal of all or part of the tumor is important. If the tumor has grown into a vein, a piece of it can be dislodged and become a dangerous object. The piece of tumor begins to move in the blood flow and it is capable of getting stuck in a small blood vessel in the heart or the brain, and causing a stroke.

The drug **mitotane** gives some good results is slowing tumor growth in certain patients. But the only therapy that provides relief in most patients is the removal of the tumor.

The outlook for individuals with adrenocortical carcinoma depends on the stage of the cancer. Because seven in ten individuals are diagnosed only after the cancer has reached stage III or stage IV the five-year survival rate for all stages is 40%. And for individuals with stage IV carcinoma it is much less, with most patients dying within nine months of diagnosis.

Alternative and complementary therapies

Yoga, biofeedback or other relaxation techniques may help manage pain.

Coping with cancer treatment

Being an active member of the treatment team is important. Premier cancer centers encourage patients to play such a role. A support group can also help.

Clinical trials

The Cancer Information Service at the National Institutes of Health, Bethesda, Md., offers information about **clinical trials** that are looking for volunteers. The Service offers a toll-free number at 1-800-422-6237.

Prevention

No prevention is known.

Special concerns

The excess production of hormones that indicate functioning tumors in adrenocortical carcinoma can also be symptoms of other conditions. A tumor in the pituitary gland can cause the pituitary to produce too much of the hormone that stimulates the adrenal cortex to make cortical hormones. The symptoms are identical to those for the adrenocortical tumor. A pituitary tumor must sometimes be ruled out when an adrenocortical carcinoma is suspected. Brain scans may be necessary.

Resources

PERIODICALS

Kunieda, K. et al. "Recurrence of giant adrenocortical carcinoma in the contralateral adrenal gland 6 years after surgery." *Surgery Today* 30(Mar. 2000):294-7.

Wajchenber, B. L. et al. "Adrenocortical carcinoma: clinical and laboratory observations." *Cancer* 88 (Feb. 15, 2000):711-36.

Diane M. Calabrese

Advance directives

Definition

An advance directive is a written document in which people clearly specify how medical decisions affecting them are to be made if they are unable to make them, or to authorize a specific person to make such decisions for them.

Description

Advance directives are recognized in most industrialized countries of the world. In the United States, by law, the creation of an advance directive is the right of all competent adults. The goal of this legislation is to empower all health care consumers to make their own judgments regarding medical decision-making, to approve of potential treatment they believe they would want, and to refuse care they do not perceive as being in their best interest. These directives are generally divided into living wills or durable powers of attorney.

Federal law requires that all health care providers (health maintenance organizations, or HMOs, skilled nursing care facilities, hospices, home health care providers, and hospitals) make information regarding

KEY TERMS

Competent—Duly qualified; having sufficient ability or authority; possessing all the requirements of law.

Dialysis—A technique used to remove waste products from the blood and excess fluid from the body as a treatment for kidney failure.

Hyperalimentation—The administration of a nutrient solution into a large, central vein near the heart. It is often used supplementary to eating, but can provide complete nourishment.

Tube feeding—Administration of nourishment, in nutritionally complete solutions, via tube into the stomach or intestines. Tubes can be either nasogastric, or inserted through the nose into the stomach via the esophagus, or surgically implanted directly into the stomach. These are usually used to sustain life when a person is unable to eat or take fluids by mouth.

advance directives available to all people in their care. Many states require that two people witness such advance directives.

Living wills

Living wills go into effect while the individual is still living, but is unable to communicate his/her wishes regarding care. Traditionally, a living will has specified the individual's wishes concerning procedures that would sustain life if he/she were terminally ill. Newer advance directives do not limit such preferences to terminal illness but instead go into effect whenever the individual is unable to speak for him/herself.

There are several ways of preparing a living will. Sometimes a preprinted form is provided, or people may create their own form, or may simply write down their wishes. Though all 50 states and the District of Columbia recognize the validity of advance directives, each state's laws have differences as to whether one or all of these types of preparation of the document are legal and binding in that state. It is recommended that people speak to their attorney or physician to ensure that their wishes are carried out.

Durable power of attorney for health care

A durable power of attorney for health care is the second type of advance directive. This is a signed, dated, and witnessed document that authorizes a designated person (usually a family member or close friend) to act as an agent, or proxy. This empowers the proxy to make medical decisions for a person when the person is deemed unable to make these decisions him/herself. Such a power of attorney frequently includes the person's stated preferences in regard to treatment. Several states do not allow any of the following people to act as a person's proxy:

- the person's physician, or other health care provider
- the staff of health care facilities that is providing the person's care
- guardians (often called conservators) of the person's financial affairs
- employees of federal agencies financially responsible for a person's care
- any person that serves as agent or proxy for 10 people or more

As in the case of living wills, regulations regarding such powers of attorney vary from state to state. Some states provide printed forms, and require witnesses, while other states do not.

Causes

As medical advances provide greater than ever means of extending life, it becomes increasingly important for people to evaluate which of the available means they would wish used. If this is not done, people run the risk of having health care providers make critical decisions regarding their care. The absence of advance directive information can also create dilemmas and increased stress for loved ones. Some of the terms describing now-routine medical interventions that can maintain life under dire circumstances include:

- cardiopulmonary resuscitation (CPR), the use of chest compressions and/or mouth-to-mouth resuscitation to restart heart beat and/or respirations
- ventilators or respirators that physically deliver oxygen via a tube into the windpipe when the lungs are unable to work on their own
- Life-sustaining care encompasses the use of machinery or equipment that prolongs life by keeping the body functioning. Examples of life-sustaining care include hyperalimentation, tube feedings, and kidney dialysis.

In contrast, life-enhancing care, sometimes referred to as Care and Comfort Only, involves the provision of high quality, but non-heroic medical care until death occurs naturally. Important examples of life-enhancing care include administration and monitoring of medications, carrying out other measures to control pain, comfort measures such as bathing and massage, and offering food and fluids.

Special concerns

Though specifics vary, all states have laws allowing people to spell out their health care wishes for a time when they might be unable to speak for themselves. But, as noted, there is a potential for disparity in how advance directives are interpreted. In most hospitals, an ethics committee is available to assist and support both patients and families faced with decisions regarding medical care. In 1995, the American Association of Retired Persons (AARP), with the help of the American Bar Association (ABA) and the American Medical Association (AMA), produced a combined living will and power of attorney for health care document that provides very specific and detailed statements of a person's wishes. Further information regarding the laws in individual states can be obtained from the AARP, ABA, or AMA.

The AARP recommends that those individuals considering making an advance directive address the following issues:

- What the person's goals for medical treatment are: Should treatment be used to sustain life, regardless of the quality of that life?
- Who should act as the person's proxy or agent? It is important for the person making an advance directive to actually speak with this designated person and make his/her wishes known.
- Though there is no formula for specificity, the AARP recommends that instructions be made as clear and specific as possible, but should not restrict the proxy from making informed decisions at the time that cannot be anticipated in advance.
- To ensure that an advance directive is carried out, copies of it should be given to a person's physician, proxy, family, or any other interested party.

Resources

BOOKS

Clayman, Charles A., M.D. *American Medical Association Home Medical Encyclopedia.* New York: Random House, 1989.

Doukas, David J., and William Reichel. *Planning for Uncertainty, A Guide to Living Wills and Other Advance Directives for Health Care.* Baltimore, MD: Johns Hopkins University Press, 1993.

ORGANIZATIONS

Choices In Dying, Inc., 200 Varick Street, New York, New York 10014-4810. (800) 989-WILL.

American Association of Retired Persons Legal Counsel for the Elderly., P.O. Box 96474, Washington, DC, 20090-6474.

American Medical Association. <http://www.ama-assn.org>.

American Bar Association. <http://www.abanet.org>.

Center for Healthy Aging. <http://www.careproject.net>.

Joan Schonbeck, R.N.

QUESTIONS TO ASK THE DOCTOR

- What is the prognosis for my type of cancer?
- What are the possible treatments?
- What are the side effects of these treatments?
- What are the laws in my state regarding living wills and durable powers of attorney for health care?
- How can I ensure that my wishes will be carried out regarding advance directives?

AIDS-related cancers

Definition

The AIDS-related cancers are a group of cancers that occur more frequently in persons with human immunodeficiency virus (HIV) infection than in the general population. The most common form of AIDS-related cancer, **Kaposi's sarcoma** (KS), was one of the first indications of the AIDS epidemic in the early 1980s. While the number of new cases of KS has been declining in recent years, the number of AIDS-related lymphomas has been increasing at a rate of 2% to 3% each year.

Description

In order to understand the causes and treatment of AIDS-related cancers, it is useful to begin with a basic description of HIV infection. AIDS, or acquired immunodeficiency syndrome, is a disease of the immune system that is caused by HIV. HIV is a retrovirus, a single-stranded virus containing ribonucleic acid (RNA) and an enzyme called reverse transcriptase. This enzyme enables the retrovirus to make its genetic material part of the DNA in the cells that it invades. HIV selectively infects and destroys certain subtypes of white blood cells called CD4 cells, which are an important part of the

KEY TERMS

Blood-brain barrier—A layer of tightly packed cells in the small blood vessels in the brain that prevent many medications and other substances from entering the brain.

Burkitt's lymphoma—A subtype of non-Hodgkin's lymphoma that is one thousand times more common in AIDS patients than in the general population.

Highly active antiretroviral therapy (HAART)—A combination drug therapy for AIDS, usually consisting of three or more medications.

Human herpesvirus (HHV)—A family of viruses that contain DNA and cause a number of diseases, including chickenpox, shingles, and genital herpes.

Human papilloma virus (HPV)—A type of tumor-causing virus that causes genital warts and is associated with AIDS-related cervical cancers in women.

Kaposi's sarcoma (KS)—The most common type of AIDS-related cancer. KS is characterized by purplish or brownish spots on the skin and may spread to the internal organs.

Lymphatic system—The system of glands, tissues, and vessels in the body that produces lymphocytes and circulates them through the body in a clear, yellowish fluid called lymph.

Lymphocyte—A type of white blood cell involved in the production of antibodies.

Non-Hodgkins lymphoma (NHL)—A type of cancer of the immune system that is the second most common form of AIDS-related cancer. It is sometimes called AIDS-related lymphoma.

Oncogenic—Producing or causing tumors. The most common types of AIDS-related cancers are associated with oncogenic viruses.

Monoclonal antibody—An antibody produced in the laboratory from a cloned cell rather than in the body.

Retrovirus—A virus that contains a single strand of RNA and a unique enzyme called reverse transcriptase.

Translocation—The movement of a gene or group of genes from one chromosome to another.

body's immune system. As an infected person's number of CD4 cells drops, he or she is at risk of developing opportunistic infections, disorders of the nervous system, or an AIDS-related cancer. HIV is transmitted through blood or blood products that enter the bloodstream—most commonly through sexual contact or contaminated hypodermic needles.

Kaposi's sarcoma

Kaposi's sarcoma is the most common type of cancer related to HIV infection. About 20% of patients diagnosed with AIDS will eventually develop KS. There are two other major subtypes of KS—so-called classic KS and African KS—with different causes that are not yet well understood. AIDS-related KS (also called epidemic KS) is characterized by purplish or brownish lesions (areas of diseased or injured tissue) on the skin, in the mouth, or in the internal organs. The lesions may take the form of small patches or lumps (nodular lesions), large patches that grow downward under the skin (infiltrating lesions), or lumpy swellings in the lymph nodes. Unlike other cancers that typically develop in one organ or area of the body, KS often appears simultaneously in many different parts of the body. It may be the first indication that the patient has AIDS.

Non-Hodgkin's lymphoma

Lymphomas are cancers of the immune system that develop when white blood cells called lymphocytes begin to grow and multiply abnormally. The increased numbers of lymphocytes cause the lymph nodes, the organs that produce these white blood cells, to swell and form large lumps that can be felt. Lymphomas are divided into two large categories: those that are related to **Hodgkin's disease** (HD), and non-Hodgkin's lymphoma (NHL). HD can be differentiated from NHL by the presence of Reed-Sternberg cells in the lymphatic tissue; these cells are not found in any other type of cancer.

Non-Hodgkin's lymphoma, or NHL, occurs more often than Hodgkin's disease; about 50,000 new cases are diagnosed annually in the United States. They may involve the spleen, liver, bone marrow, or digestive tract as well as the lymph nodes. Three important types of NHL are related to AIDS:

- Primary central nervous system lymphomas (PCNSL). This type accounts for about 20% of NHL cancers found in AIDS patients, but only 1% to 2% of NHL cancers in patients not infected by HIV. Lymphomas of this type start in the brain or the spinal cord. Their symptoms include headaches, paralysis, seizures, and changes in the patient's mental condition. Patients diagnosed with

PCNSL are more likely to suffer from advanced HIV infection than patients with other types of NHL.

- Systemic lymphomas. These are also called peripheral lymphomas. They begin in the lymph nodes or other parts of the lymphatic system and may spread throughout the body. **Burkitt's lymphoma** (BL) is a type of systemic lymphoma that is one thousand times more common in AIDS patients than in the general population.
- Primary effusion lymphomas, also called body cavity-based lymphomas (BCBL). This type of NHL is relatively rare, but seems to be related to infection by human herpesvirus 8 (HHV-8) in addition to HIV.

HIV-associated Hodgkin's disease

The symptoms of Hodgkin's disease include painless swelling of the lymph nodes of the neck, groin, and armpits; **itching**; **night sweats**; **weight loss**; and **fever**. While one study has indicated that HIV-positive gay men have a higher risk of developing Hodgkin's disease as well as non-Hodgkins lymphomas, the Centers for Disease Control and Prevention (CDC) has not defined Hodgkin's disease as an AIDS-related cancer as of early 2001. Hodgkin's disease appears to occur more frequently in HIV-positive intravenous drug users, however, than in other persons with HIV infection.

Cervical and anal cancers

In women, cancer of the cervix (the lower end of the uterus or womb) is more likely to occur in HIV-infected individuals than in the general female population. About 60% of women with HIV infection are found to have some kind of abnormal tissue growth or cell formation in the cervix when a **Pap test** is performed. The **human papilloma virus** (HPV) is thought to be a co-factor in the development of cervical cancers. Papilloma viruses are a group of tumor-causing viruses that also cause genital warts. Cervical cancers develop more rapidly in HIV-positive than in HIV-negative women, are harder to cure, and are more likely to recur.

Cancers of the anus represent less than 1% to 2% of cancers of the large bowel. There are about 10,000 cases of **anal cancer** annually in the United States. The high rates of occurrence of this type of cancer in gay men may be related more closely to the presence of HPV and to the practice of anal intercourse than to HIV infection by itself.

Other AIDS-associated cancers

Other cancers linked to HIV infection include **testicular cancer**, cancers of the mouth, and a type of cancer of the bone marrow called **multiple myeloma**. Some other cancers, including **breast cancer**, lung cancer, and **melanoma** (a type of skin cancer), are thought to occur more frequently among people with AIDS even though they are not identified as AIDS-associated cancers in the strict sense.

Demographics

The demographic distribution of AIDS-related cancers varies somewhat depending on the type of cancer. Epidemic KS is about 10 times more common among gay men than among members of other groups at risk for AIDS (hemophiliacs, intravenous drug users, etc.); it affects men eight times as frequently as women. AIDS-related Hodgkin's disease occurs more frequently among intravenous drug users. By contrast, AIDS-related lymphomas occur with equal frequency in members of all risk groups—including the children of persons with HIV infection.

Causes

The most common types of AIDS-related cancers have been linked to oncogenic (tumor-causing) viruses:

- Human herpesvirus 8 (HHV-8) is associated with KS and some of the less common types of AIDS-related lymphomas (ie. cancers of the lymphatic system).
- **Epstein-Barr virus** (EBV) is associated with the more common types of AIDS-related lymphomas, particularly PCNSL and Burkitt's lymphoma.
- Human papillomavirus (HPV) is associated with anal cancer and with **cervical cancer** in women.

Oncogenic viruses cause cancer by changing the genetic material inside tissue cells. When this genetic material is changed, the cells begin to grow and multiply uncontrollably. The abnormal tissue formed by this uncontrolled growth is called a tumor. A healthy human immune system has a greater ability to protect the body against oncogenic viruses and to stop or slow down tumor formation. Since the retrovirus that causes AIDS weakens the immune system, persons with AIDS are at greater risk of developing cancers caused by oncogenic viruses.

Some types of AIDS-related cancers, such as Burkitt's lymphoma, have been linked to changes in human chromosomes (translocations). In a translocation, a gene or group of genes moves from one chromosome to another. Burkitt's lymphoma is associated with exchanges of genetic material between chromosomes 8 and 14 or between chromosomes 2 and 22.

Special concerns

An important special concern for patients with AIDS-related cancers is the difficulty of combining cancer treatment—especially chemotherapy—with treatment for HIV infection. Since 1996, the standard treatment for AIDS is highly active antiretroviral therapy (HAART). HAART is a combination drug therapy involving three or four different medications. Because of the powerful side effects of these drugs, patients with AIDS-related cancers are usually put on low-dose **chemotherapy** for the cancer. The chemotherapy, however, increases the patient's risk of developing an AIDS-related infection, such as **thrush** or *Pneumocystis carinii* **pneumonia** (PCP).

Another special concern for patients with AIDS-related cancers is fear of rejection by friends and loved ones. Although the moral stigma attached to HIV infection is not as strong as it was at the beginning of the epidemic, some patients may still fear condemnation by others. Most hospitals have chaplains or spiritual counselors who can help patients with these concerns or put them in touch with someone from their own spiritual tradition.

Treatments

The different types of AIDS-related cancers have different treatment considerations.

Kaposi's sarcoma

KS differs from other solid tumors in that it lacks a stage or site of origin in which it can be cured. In addition, there is no relationship between the stage of KS and its response to treatment. Many doctors treat early KS with chemotherapy injections or treat localized lesions with **radiation therapy** rather than give the patient systemic chemotherapy. In 1999, the FDA approved alitretinoin (Panretin) gel as a topical treatment for KS. When systemic chemotherapy is used, the standard regimens are a combination of **vinblastine** (Velban) and **vincristine** (Oncovin) on a weekly schedule, or a combination of **doxorubicin**, **bleomycin**, and vincristine given every week. Surgery is not often used in the treatment of KS.

Non-Hodgkin's lymphoma

Patients with early, slow-growing forms of NHL are usually treated with radiation. The later stages of slow-growing **non-Hodgkin's lymphomas** may be treated with chemotherapy (single-agent or combination), or with a combination of radiation and chemotherapy. Common treatments for more aggressive AIDS-related lymphomas are the combination chemotherapy regimens known as CHOP (**cyclophosphamide**, doxorubicin, vincristine, and prednisone) or m-BACOD (intermediate-dose **methotrexate**, bleomycin, doxorubicin, cyclophosphamide, vincristine, and **dexamethasone**). In general, AIDS-related lymphomas are more aggressive than non-HIV-related lymphomas and do not respond as well to chemotherapy. PCNSL is usually treated with radiation therapy alone because most chemotherapy drugs cannot cross the blood-brain barrier and enter the central nervous system.

Newer forms of treatment for non-Hodgkin's lymphomas include bone marrow and stem cell transplants and immunotherapy with the use of **monoclonal antibodies** (MABs). MABs are antibodies produced by cloned mouse cells grown in a laboratory. They target cancer cells and bind to them, alerting cells of the immune system to destroy the abnormal cells. MABs are sometimes given together with chemotherapy.

HIV-associated Hodgkin's disease

HIV-associated Hodgkin's disease is usually treated with chemotherapy but does not respond as well to treatment as non-HIV-related Hodgkin's disease. Patients being treated with antiretroviral therapy may need to have it modified during a course of chemotherapy for Hodgkin's disease.

Cervical and anal cancers

Cervical and anal cancers are treated in the early stages with a combination of surgery and radiation. Larger or later-stage tumors are treated with chemotherapy (mitomycin or **cisplatin** and **fluorouracil**) in addition to surgery and radiation treatment.

Alternative and complementary therapies

In the early years of the AIDS epidemic, a variety of alternative approaches were used to treat the internal forms of KS as well as the external skin lesions: homeopathic preparations of periwinkle, poke root (phytolacca), and mistletoe; a mixture of selenium, aloe vera gel, and silica; Chinese patent medicines; periodic three- to seven-day grape fasts as part of an overall vegetarian diet; and castor oil packs.

The only alternative treatment for KS that has been evaluated by the National Institutes of Health (NIH) is shark cartilage. Shark cartilage products are widely available in the United States as over-the-counter (OTC) preparations. The use of shark cartilage to treat KS derives from a popular belief that sharks and other cartilaginous fish (skates and rays) do not get cancer. This therapy, however, has not been proven to be effective.

Other alternative treatments for AIDS-related KS include:

- Naturopathic remedies. High doses of vitamin C, zinc, echinacea, or goldenseal to improve immune function;

or preparations of astragalis, osha root, or licorice to suppress the HIV virus.

- Homeopathic remedies. These include a homeopathic preparation of **cyclosporine** and another made from a dilution of killed typhoid virus.
- Ozone therapy.

With regard to other categories of AIDS-related cancers, there have been reports of using hydrazine sulfate or laetrile to treat AIDS-related lymphomas. Some researchers in Germany are investigating mistletoe extracts as a treatment for AIDS-related cancers in women.

Complementary therapies are used in the treatment of AIDS-related cancers to help patients keep up their will to live; to cope with such side effects as **depression**, nausea caused by chemotherapy, concerns about disfigurement, and fear of rejection; and to gain comfort from supportive social groups. Specific complementary approaches that have been recommended for cancer patients include acupuncture, creative visualization, pet therapy, meditation, prayer, yoga, Reiki, aromatherapy, and some herbal remedies (St. John's wort for depression, peppermint or spearmint tea for nausea).

Clinical trials

As of early 2001, 39 **clinical trials** of treatments for AIDS-related lymphomas, 13 trials of treatment for KS, and 13 trials of treatments for PCNSL were being conducted in the United States. **Thalidomide**, a drug that made headlines in the 1960s for its role in causing birth defects, was shown to be effective in treating KS in July 2000. It is undergoing further study as of 2001.

See Also Immunologic therapies

Resources

BOOKS

Dollinger, Malin, Ernest H. Rosenbaum, and Greg Cable. *Cancer Therapy.* Kansas City, MO: Andrews and McMeel, 1994.

"Hematology and Oncology." Section 11 in *The Merck Manual of Diagnosis and Therapy*, edited by Mark H. Beers and Robert Berkow. Whitehouse Station, NJ: Merck Research Laboratories, 1999.

The Burton Goldberg Group. *Alternative Medicine: The Definitive Guide.* Fife, WA: Future Medicine Publishing, Inc., 1995.

PERIODICALS

San Francisco AIDS Foundation. *Bulletin of Experimental Treatments for AIDS.*

ORGANIZATIONS

AIDS Clinical Trials Group (ACTG). c/o William Duncan, Ph.D., National Institutes of Health. 6003 Executive Boulevard, Room 2A07, Bethesda, MD 20892.

American Cancer Society (ACS). 1599 Clifton Road, NE, Atlanta, GA 30329. (404) 320-3333 or (800) ACS-2345. Fax: (404) 329-7530. <http://www.cancer.org>.

National Cancer Institute, Office of Cancer Communications. 31 Center Drive, MSC 2580, Bethesda, MD 20892-2580. (800) 4-CANCER. TTY: (800) 332-8615. <http://www.nci.nih.gov>.

National Institutes of Health National Center for Complementary and Alternative Medicine (NCCAM) Clearinghouse. PO Box 8218, Silver Spring, MD 20907-8218. (888) 644-6226. TTY/TDY: (888) 644-6226. Fax: (301) 495-4957. <http://nccam.nih.gov>.

San Francisco AIDS Foundation (SFAF). 995 Market Street, #200, San Francisco, CA 94103. (415) 487-3000 or (800) 367-AIDS. Fax: (415) 487-3009. <http://www.sfaf.org>.

OTHER

<http://www.hivchannel.com>.

<http://www.oncologychannel.com>.

The Body: An AIDS and HIV Information Resource. <http://www.thebody.com>.

WEB SITES WITH INFORMATION IN SPANISH

Cancer Care. <http://www.cancercareinc.org>.

New York Online Access to Health (NOAH). <http://www.noah.cuny.edu>.

Rebecca J. Frey, Ph.D.

AJCC *see* **American Joint Commission on Cancer**

Alcohol consumption

Description

Alcohol (ethyl alcohol or ethanol) consumption has a social aspect to it, but it is often abused. The effect of alcohol consumption on the body depends on how often it is consumed, how much, and the alcohol content of the drinks. Frequent alcohol use may encourage alcohol dependence or alcoholism. Alcoholism is a chronic disease that progresses and is often fatal. It is a primary disorder and not only a symptom of other diseases or emotional disorders. Factors such as psychology, culture, genetics, and response to physical pain influence the severity of alcoholism.

KEY TERMS

Alcoholism—A primary disorder and chronic disease, progressive and often fatal where an individual is dependent on alcohol.

Anorexia—A condition frequently observed in cancer patients characterized by a loss of appetite or desire to eat.

Larynx—The enlarged upper end of the trachea below the root of the tongue and the primary organ that enables speech.

Pharynx—The passageway for air from the nasal cavity to the larynx and food from the mouth to the esophagus, also providing a place for resonance.

Satiation—A feeling of fullness or satisfaction during or after food intake.

Special concerns

Health concerns relating to alcohol consumption

Alcoholic liver disease may occur with chronic alcohol consumption. This disease is manifested in three forms: steatosis (fatty liver), alcoholic hepatitis, and cirrhosis. Alcohol abuse is responsible for 60% to 75% of cases of cirrhosis, which is a major risk factor for eventually developing primary liver cancer. Alcohol may further compromise the health of an individual through:

- Immune system suppression. People with alcoholism are prone to infections, in particular, pneumonia.
- Gastrointestinal problems; especially **diarrhea** and hemorrhoids.
- Mental and neurological disorders. Chronic use eventually leads to **depression** and confusion. In severe cases, gray matter in the brain is destroyed, possibly leading to psychosis and mental disturbances.
- Alcoholism increases levels of the female hormone estrogen and reduces levels of the male hormone **testosterone**, factors that contribute to impotence in men.
- Hypoglycemia (a drop in blood sugar) is particularly dangerous for diabetics taking insulin.
- Severe alcoholism is associated with osteoporosis.
- Drug interactions.

Alcohol's association with cancer

Alcohol consumption is an important risk factor for many types of cancer including: pharynx, larynx, mouth, breast, liver, lung, esophagus, gastric, pancreatic, urinary tract, prostrate, ovarian, colorectal, brain cancers, **lymphoma**, and leukemia.

The risk of **breast cancer** and other cancers rises as alcohol consumption increases. Risk increases with all types of alcoholic drinks: wine, beer and spirits; this suggests that cancer risk is related to alcohol consumption itself as opposed to the other compounds in the drinks. Approximately 75% of cancers of the esophagus and 50% of cancers of the mouth, throat, and larynx are due to alcoholism. Other research has demonstrated, however, that wine poses less danger for these cancers than beer or hard liquor. Alcohol, when combined with smoking, increases the chances of developing mouth, throat, pharynx, larynx and esophageal cancers significantly. For **esophageal cancer**, there is a 3 to 8 fold increase in risk in those who drink 40-100 grams of alcohol per day, and the risks are even greater with smoking.

Research has shown that women who consume only one alcoholic drink per day have a 30% higher risk of dying from breast cancer than nondrinkers. Even consuming small amounts of alcohol may increase breast cancer risk, particularly in postmenopausal women due to increased hormone levels circulating in the blood.

Cancer patients may find that alcohol consumption interferes with the effectiveness of anticancer therapy and may cause them to become even sicker.

Nutritional impact of alcohol consumption

Even moderate alcohol consumption can have detrimental effects on the health of cancer patients. If food intake is replaced by alcohol to a large extent, malnutrition is likely to occur. In fact, alcoholism is a major cause of malnutrition. The body requires protein, carbohydrate, fat, **vitamins**, and minerals, but these are often inadequate with heavy alcohol consumption. Nutritional status is thus further compromised in cancer patients who abuse alcohol.

Alcohol contains energy (or calories) just like food does, but it does not contain many of the nutrients required by the body. Furthermore, because few nutrients are provided in alcohol, the vitamin and mineral content of the diet may be poor, even if the total energy intake is adequate. Alcohol contains approximately 7 kilocalories (Kcal) per gram, while carbohydrate or protein contains about 4 Kcal per gram. Thus, the nutrients required by the body will not be obtained if alcohol replaces food intake to some extent. In fact, alcohol interferes with the body's mechanisms the regulate food intake, and therefore food intake decreases. When inadequate nutrients are consumed, the body may become weaker and less able to tolerate cancer therapies. As nutritional status declines, it becomes more difficult to fight off illness and infection.

In addition, the toxic effects of ethanol interfere with the absorption, metabolism, and storage of nutrients that are provided in foods. Several organs can be damaged in this process, primarily the liver and brain, but also the cardiovascular, endocrine, immune, and hematopoietic systems.

Alcohol may further compromise nutritional status of an individual through:

- malabsorption of vitamins and minerals and particularly folate, thiamine, Vitamins B6 and B12, calcium, magnesium, and fat-soluble vitamins (A, E, and K)
- inducing early satiation
- reduced absorption of amino acids (the building blocks of protein)
- immune suppression
- respiratory disorders
- liver, gastrointestinal tract, and pancreas damage

Dietary interactions relating to cancer

Alcohol has numerous influences on the nutritional status of the cancer patient which is often already compromised by the disease. Cancer often increases the body's energy (calorie) and protein requirements. These increased needs may be due to the effects of the tumor or the effects of treatment (surgery, radiation, or **chemotherapy**). At the same time, cancer patients tend to decrease their food intake, often due to **anorexia**, which can be characterized as a loss of interest in eating. Anorexia, cachexia, and **weight loss** are common side effects of cancer, so a cancer patient who consumes alcohol should be careful not to replace the needed energy and nutrients with too many calories from alcohol.

Recommendations regarding alcohol consumption

Although moderate alcohol consumption is recommended to reduce the risk of heart disease, other lifestyle factors such as a healthy diet and exercise reduce the risk of heart disease and cancer.

The American Cancer Society's (ACS) *Guidelines on Diet, Nutrition, and Cancer Prevention* recommend moderation in alcohol intake. Experts suggest that intake should be limited to no more than an average of two drinks daily for women and three drinks a day for men. One should consider, however, research reports that suggest that even one drink per day may be detrimental to breast cancer risk in women.

Treatments

Two of the most common forms of treatment for alcoholics are cognitive-behavioral and interactional group psychotherapy based on the Alcoholics Anonymous 12-step program. People with mild to moderate withdrawal symptoms are usually treated in outpatient programs and are treated through counseling, and/or support groups. Individuals may be treated in a general or psychiatric hospitals or substance abuse rehabilitation facilities if they: possess coexisting medical or psychiatric disorders; have a difficult home environment; are a danger to themselves or others; have not responded to other conservative treatments. Inpatient programs often include physical and psychiatric development, detoxification, psychotherapy or cognitive-behavioral therapy, and an introduction to Alcoholics Anonymous.

Crystal Heather Kaczkowski, M.S.

Aldesleukin

Definition

Aldesleukin is interleukin, or specific kind of biological response modifier, that is used to treat metastatic renal cell carcinoma (a form of kidney cancer) and metastatic **melanoma**. Aldesleukin is also known as interleukin-2, IL-2 and the trademarked name Proleukin.

Purpose

When renal cell carcinoma and metastatic melanoma (cancer of the skin that arises in the pigmented cells of the skin or eyes) do not respond to other therapies, they are candidates for treatment with aldesleukin.

Description

Aldesleukin is a biological response modifier (BMR). It promotes the development of T cells, or the cells in the lymphatic system that can fight cancer cells in cell-to-cell interaction. The human body produces aldesleukin naturally.

For use in therapy, aldesleukin is manufactured in a laboratory setting, using biotechnology methods, or methods that combine biological mechanisms and tools from technology. In the instance of aldesleukin, the compound is made in large quantities by using recombinant DNA technology. The DNA, or hereditary material, that provides instructions for making aldesleukin, is put in bacterial cells under laboratory confinement. The cells then produce large quantities of the human compound that are harvested, purified, and used for treatment.

KEY TERMS

Corticosteroids—Compounds that are made naturally by the body in the cortex of the adrenal glands and that are also made synthetically, or in the laboratory.

Intravenous line—A tube that is inserted directly into a vein to carry medicine directly to the blood stream, bypassing the stomach and other digestive organs that might alter the medicine.

Kilogram—Metric measure that equals 2.2 pounds.

Lymphatic system—The system that collects and returns fluid in tissues to the blood vessels and produces defensive agents for fighting infection and invasion by foreign bodies.

Metastatic—Spreading from one part of the body to another.

Milligram—One-thousandth of a gram, and there are one thousand grams in a kilogram. A gram is the metric measure that equals about 0.035 ounces.

Toxicity—The quality of acting as a poison.

T cell—A cell in the lymphatic system that contributes to immunity by attacking foreign bodies, such as bacteria and viruses, directly.

Treatment with aldesleukin is considered palliative, which means it provides comfort but does not produce a cure. In some cases, aldesleukin is used together with an anticancer drug.

Recommended dosage

Standard treatment with aldesleukin is via an intravenous line. The standard dose is 0.037 milligrams per kilogram of body weight every eight hours. For renal cancer, up to 15 doses can be repeated over 7-10 days every 5–6 weeks. But because the aldesleukin has such severe side effects, lower doses are being tried. And delivery of aldesleukin via an inhaler, or a mechanical device that puts the compound into the air passages when a person breathes, is being used in the case of metastatic melanoma that has invaded the lungs.

Precautions

Side effects from aldesleukin are generally very severe. No one who already has a metastatic growth in the central nervous system should take the treatment because aldesleukin will incite, or aggravate, symptoms from the tumor.

Side effects

Aldesleukin causes changes in the ways body fluids accumulate in the body that can lead to **ascites** and **pleural effusions.** Changes in personality are common due to the influence the drug has on the central nervous system. Among the most severe side effects is the possibility a patient will slip into a coma, or unconscious state. Other side effects may include alterations in liver function, skin reactions, such as rash, and infections may be severe and life threatening. Less serious, and almost always transient side effects, include flu-like symptoms, such as **nausea and vomiting**.

Interactions

Aldesleukin interacts with drugs that affect the central nervous system and it should not be taken with drugs that are used to modify moods or disposition (psychotropic agents). Many drugs, including those used to control blood pressure, heart beat and kidney function, increase the toxicity of aldesleukin and should not be taken in combination with it. **Corticosteroids** also interfere with the action of aldesleukin.

Physicians must be informed about every drug a patient is taking so interactions can be avoided.

Diane M. Calabrese

Alemtuzumab

Definition

Alemtuzumab is sold as Campath in the United States. Alemtuzumab is a humanized monoclonal antibody that selectively binds to CD52, a protein found on the surface of normal and malignant B and T cells, and that is used to reduce the numbers of circulating malignant cells of patients who have B-cell **chronic lymphocytic leukemia** (B-CLL).

Purpose

Alemtuzumab is a monoclonal antibody used to treat B-CLL, one of the most prevalent forms of adult **chronic leukemia**. It specifically binds CD52, a protein found on the surface of essentially all B and T cells of the immune system. By binding the CD52 protein on the malignant B cells, the antibody targets it for removal from the circulation. Scientists believe that alemtuzumab triggers antibody-mediated lysis of the B cells, a method that the immune system uses to eliminate foreign cells.

Alemtuzumab has been approved by the FDA for treatment of refractory B-CLL. For a patient's disease to be classified as refractory, both alkylating agents and **fludarabine** treatment must have been tried and failed. Thus, this drug gives patients who have tried all approved treatments for B-CLL another option. As most patients with B-CLL are in stage III or IV by the time both alkylating agents and fludarabine have been tried, the experience with alemtuzumab treatment are primarily with those stages of the disease. In **clinical trials**, about 30% of patients had a partial response to the drug, with 2% of these being complete responses.

This antibody has been tested with limited success in the treatment of non-Hodgkin's lymphoma (NHL) and for the preparation of patients with various immune cell malignancies for **bone marrow transplantation**. There is also a clinical trial ongoing to test the ability of this antibody to prevent rejection in kidney transplantation.

Description

Alemtuzumab is produced in the laboratory using genetically engineered single clones of B-cells. Like all antibodies, it is a Y-shaped molecule can bind one particular substance, the antigen for that monoclonal antibody. For alemtuzumab, the antigen is CD52, a protein found on the surface of normal and malignant B and T cells as well as other cells of the immune and male reproductive systems. Alemtuzumab is a humanized antibody, meaning that the regions that bind CD52, located on the tips of the Y branches, are derived from rat antibodies, but the rest of the antibody is human sequence. The presence of the human sequences helps to reduce the **immune response** by the patient against the antibody itself, a problem seen when complete mouse antibodies are used for cancer therapies. The human sequences also help to ensure that the various cell-destroying mechanisms of the human immune system are properly triggered with binding of the antibody.

Alemtuzumab was approved in May of 2001 for the treatment of refractory B-CLL. It is approved for use alone but clinical trials have tested the ability of the antibody to be used in combination with the purine analogs **pentostatin**, fludarabine, and **cladribine**, and **rituximab**, a monoclonal antibody specific for the CD20 antigen, another protein found on the surface of B cells.

Recommended dosage

This antibody should be administered in a gradually escalating pattern at the start of treatment and any time administration is interrupted for 7 or more days. The recommended beginning dosage for B-CLL patients is a daily dose of 3 mg of Campath administered as a 2-hour IV infusion. Once this amount is tolerated, the dose is increased to 10 mg per day. After tolerating this dose, it can be increased to 30 mg, administered three days a week. Acetominophen and **diphenhydramine** hydrochoride are given thirty to sixty minutes before the infusion to help reduce side effects.

Additionally, patients generally receive anti-infective medication before treatment to help minimize the serious opportunistic infections that can result from this treatment. Specifically, trimethoprim/sulfamethoxazole (to prevent bacterial infections) and famciclovir (to prevent viral infections) were used during the clinical trial to decrease infections, although they were not eliminated.

Precautions

Blood studies should be done on a weekly basis while patients are receiving the alemtuzumab treatment. Vaccination during the treatment session is not recommended, given the T cell depletion that occurs during treatment. Furthermore, given that antibodies like alumtuzumab can pass through the placenta to the developing fetus and in breast milk, use during pregnancy and breastfeeding is not recommended unless clearly needed.

Side effects

A severe side effect of alemtuzumab treatment is the possible depletion of one or more types of blood cells. Because CD52 is expressed on a patient's normal B and T cells, as well as on the surface of the abnormal B cells, the treatment eliminates both normal and cancerous cells. The treatment also seems to trigger autoimmune reactions against various other blood cells. This results in severe reduction of the many circulating blood cells including red blood cells (**anemia**), white blood cells (**neutropenia**), and clotting cells (**thrombocytopenia**). These conditions are treated with blood transfusions. The great majority of patients treated exhibit some type of blood cell depletion.

A second serious side effect of this drug is the prevalence of opportunistic infections that occurs during the treatment. Serious, and sometimes fatal bacterial, viral, fungal, and protozoan infections have been reported. Treatments to prevent **pneumonia** and herpes infections reduce, but do not eliminate these infections.

The majority of other side effects occur after or during the first infusion of the drug. Some common side effects of this drug include **fever** and chills, **nausea and vomiting**, **diarrhea**, shortness of breath, skin rash, and unusual **fatigue**. This drug can also cause low blood pressure (hypotension).

In patients with high tumor burden (a large number of circulating malignant B cells) this drug can cause a

KEY TERMS

Alkylating agent—A chemical that alters the composition of the genetic material of rapidly dividing cells, such as cancer cells, causing selective cell death; used as a chemotherapeutic agent to treat B-CLL.

Antibody—A protective protein made by the immune system in response to an antigen, also called an immunoglobulin.

Autoimmune—An immune reaction of a patient against their own cells.

Humanization—Fusing the constant and variable framework region of one or more human immunoglobulins with the binding region of an animal immunoglobulin, done to reduce human reaction against the fusion antibody.

Monoclonal—Genetically engineered antibodies specific for one antigen.

Tumor lysis syndrome—A side effect of some immunotherapies, like monoclonal antibodies, that lyse the tumor cells, due to the toxicity of flooding the bloodstream with such a quantity of cellular contents.

side effect called **tumor lysis syndrome**. Thought to be due to the release of the lysed cells' contents into the blood stream, it can cause a misbalance of urea, uric acid, phosphate, potassium, and calcium in the urine and blood. Patients at risk for this side effect must keep hydrated and can be given **allopurinol** before infusion.

Interactions

There have been no formal drug interaction studies done for alemtuzumab.

See Also Monoclonal antibodies; Rituximab

Michelle Johnson, M.S., J.D.

Allopurinol

Definition

This medication, also known as (Zyloprim), is used for the treatment and prevention of gout attacks and certain types of kidney stones. It is also used to treat elevated uric acid levels in the blood and urine, which can occur in patients receiving **chemotherapy** for the treatment of leukemia, **lymphoma** and other types of cancer. If left untreated, high uric acid levels in patients receiving cancer chemotherapy can cause kidney stones and kidney failure.

Description

Allopurinol decreases uric acid levels in the blood and urine by inhibiting a certain enzyme responsible for production of uric acid. It has been used for over three decades for prevention of gouty arthritis, kidney stones, and **tumor lysis syndrome** in cancer patients.

Recommended Dosage

Adults

GOUT. 200-300 mg per day for mild gout and 400-600 mg per day for severe gout. Patients greater than 65 years of age should be started at 100 mg per day. Their dose can be increased until desired uric acid levels in the blood are reached.

Children over 10 years of age and adults

PREVENTION OF URIC ACID KIDNEY STONES IN CANCER PATIENTS. 600-800 mg per day divided into several doses, usually starting 1-2 days before cancer chemotherapy and stopped two to three days after the chemotherapy is completed for that cycle.

Total daily dose greater than 300 mg should be given in divided doses.

Children less than 10 years of age

PREVENTION OF URIC ACID KIDNEY STONES IN CANCER PATIENTS. 10 mg per kg per day of allopurinol in two to three divided doses up to a maximum dose of 800 mg per day. Another alternative is to give 150 mg per day in three divided doses for children 6 years of age and 300 mg per day in two to three divided doses for children 6-10 years of age.

Administration

Allopurinol should be taken after meals to avoid stomach upset. Patients should drink plenty of fluids (at least eight glasses of water per day) while taking this medicine unless otherwise directed by a physician. Drinking a lot of water can prevent formation of kidney stones.

Precautions

The use of allopurinol in pregnant women should be avoided whenever possible because its effects on the human fetus are not known.

Allopurinol should be used with caution by the following populations:

- Patients who have had an allergic reaction to allopurinol in the past.
- Patients who are taking certain medicines for high blood pressure such as diuretics (water pills) or angiotensin converting enzyme (ACE) inhibitors (captopril, lisinopril, enalapril). These people may be at higher risk of hypersensitivity with allopurinol.
- Breast-feeding mothers.
- Children (except those who have high uric acid levels caused by cancer, chemotherapy, or genetic diseases).

Patients should call a doctor immediately if any of these symptoms develop:

- rash, **itching**, swelling of lips or mouth, trouble breathing (also known as hypersensitivity reaction)
- yellowing of the skin or eyes
- pain when urinating or blood in the urine
- unusual bleeding or bruising

Patients with kidney problems may need to use lower doses of allopurinol.

Patients taking allopurinol will need to see a physician before starting therapy and occasionally during therapy to do blood tests for monitoring of kidney and liver function and complete blood count.

Side effects

Allopurinol is usually well tolerated by most patients. The most common side effect is skin rash, hives and itching. Loss of hair, **fever**, and feelings of discomfort or uneasiness can happen alone or in combination with a rash. The risk of rash is higher in people with kidney disease or people taking amoxicillin or ampicillin. The use of allopurinol should be discontinued at first sign of a rash. Other side effects include nausea, vomiting, decreased kidney function and drowsiness (especially during the first few days of therapy). Because allopurinol can cause drowsiness, caution should be taken when performing tasks requiring alertness, such as cooking or driving.

Interactions

Patients should consult their doctor before drinking alcoholic beverages; alcohol can decrease the effectiveness of allopurinol. People consuming large amounts of vitamin C can be at an increased risk for kidney stones.

Allopurinol can prolong the effects of blood thinners such as **warfarin** (Coumadin) and put patients at risk for bleeding. It can also increase chances of low blood sugar with chlorpropamide (Diabinese) and nerve toxicity with vidarabine. Allopurinol can decrease breakdown of **azathioprine** (Imuran), **mercaptopurine** (6-MP), **cyclosporine** (Neoral, Sandimmune) and theophylline (Theo-Dur, Theolair, Theo-24) by the liver, increasing blood levels and side effects. Doses of azathioprine and mercaptopurine need to be reduced when they are used together with allopurinol. Mercaptopurine can be substituted for **thioguanine** (6-TG) to avoid this interaction altogether.

The use of amoxicillin and ampicillin should be avoided if possible in patients taking allopurinol because of increased risk of rash. Water pills such as hydrochlorthiazide (Diuril) can increase the risk of toxicity and allergic reaction when used with allopurinol.

Olga Bessmertny, Pharm.D.

KEY TERMS

ACE inhibitors—A group of drugs used to treat high blood pressure. These drugs work by decreasing production of a certain chemical in the kidneys that causes constriction of blood vessels.

Gout—A disease, especially common in men, in which patients may have high uric acid levels in the blood and sudden attacks of severe joint pain and swelling caused by the deposits of uric acid crystals in those joints. These gout attacks most commonly affect the big toe.

Kidney stone—A concretion in the kidney made of various materials, such as uric acid crystals, calcium, or lipids. These concretions, or stones, cause severe pain when they are transported from the kidney into the bladder and out of the body.

Tumor lysis syndrome—A potentially life-threatening condition caused by cancer chemotherapy associated with very high blood levels uric acid, phosphate, and potassium, low calcium, and acute kidney failure.

Uric acid—White, poorly soluble crystals found in the urine. Sometimes uric acid forms small solid stones or crystals that are deposited in different organs in the body, such as the kidney. High levels of uric acid can be seen in patients with gout or cancer.

Alopecia

Description

Alopecia, also called hair loss, baldness, and epilation, is a common side effect of **chemotherapy** and **radiation therapy**. Most patients undergoing chemotherapy, especially those who are being treated with more than one drug, will suffer from hair loss. Radiation therapy causes hair loss only in the area of skin being treated.

Although most often associated with head hair, alopecia can occur on any part of the body. Cancer treatments can also cause hair on the face (including the eyelashes and eyebrows), genitals, underarms, and body to fall out.

Alopecia usually occurs between two and three weeks after the first treatment. Most often, hair loss is gradual and occurs over a three-to-four week period. However, the chemotherapy drug **paclitaxel** can cause all the hair of the body to fall out within a 24-hour period. Loss of head hair usually begins on the top (crown) and sides of the head, presumably due to friction caused by pillows, bed linens, and hats.

Alopecia caused by chemotherapy is usually temporary. Hair loss caused by radiation therapy may be permanent. Hair regrows in about three to five months. Regrown hair may be a different color or type than before treatment.

Although alopecia is a harmless, painless condition, it can significantly affect **body image**, self esteem, and **sexuality**. As a result, alopecia may cause the patient to limit social activities. Hair loss can also cause **depression**.

Causes

To understand the cause of alopecia, it is helpful to understand how hair grows. Hair grows out of microscopic depressions in the skin called hair follicles. Normally, there are about 100,000 hairs on a person's head (scalp). Each hair is in one of three different growth stages. Eighty-eight percent of the hair on the head is in the growing (anagen) stage, which lasts for two to five years. Some of the hairs are no longer growing and are in a resting (telogen) stage. The telogen stage lasts for three to five months. The transitional (catagen) stage lies in between the growing and resting stages. At the end of the telogen stage, the hair falls out. Usually about 100 hairs fall out each day. Alopecia becomes noticeable only after about half of the hairs have fallen out.

Chemotherapy-induced alopecia

Chemotherapy drugs kill the rapidly growing cancer cells. However, certain normal cells of the body are rapidly growing and they, too, are affected by the chemotherapy drugs. Rapidly growing cells are found in the base of the hair (hair bulb), as well as other parts of the body. When the drug kills the cells of the hair bulb, the hair falls out. Alternatively, the drug affects the hair bulb, causing the hair to narrow. This weakened hair is prone to breakage during normal brushing or shampooing.

Although many chemotherapy drugs can cause alopecia, certain ones are highly prone to causing hair loss. In addition, the way in which the drug is administered, the dose, and the treatment schedule can all influence the ability of a drug to cause alopecia. For instance, the fast administration of large doses of drug (bolus-dosing) is more toxic to the hair bulb than administering lower doses more slowly. Chemotherapy drugs with a very high potential to cause alopecia include:

- **cyclophosphamide**
- **daunorubicin**
- **doxorubicin** (at doses higher than 50 mg)
- **etoposide**
- **ifosamide**
- **paclitaxel**
- **docetaxel**

Radiation-induced alopecia

Like chemotherapy, radiation kills rapidly dividing cells. Hair loss occurs only at the site where radiation is applied. High doses of radiation (greater than 6,000 cGy) usually causes permanent damage to hair follicles preventing hair from regrowing. If hair regrowth occurs, the hairs may be finer than before radiation therapy. However, hair usually regrows following low doses of radiation (less than 6,000 cGy).

Treatments

Methods to prevent chemotherapy-induced alopecia exist, although their safety and effectiveness remain questionable. One method puts pressure on the scalp (scalp tourniquet) to block blood flow, thereby preventing the drugs from damaging the hair follicles. Another method uses ice or cooling devices (scalp hypothermia) to decrease the amount of drug taken up by the hair cells. Lastly, certain medications have been used to prevent alopecia.

Alopecia resulting from cancer treatment is unavoidable and no treatments for it are available. Patients are encouraged to buy a wig before their hair falls out so that a good color and texture match can be made and the wig will be available when needed. Patients with long hair can have a wig made with their own hair. If a wig is covered by insurance, a doctor's prescription would be required to make an insurance claim. Some patients prefer to shave their head once hair loss begins.

Things that a cancer patient can do to treat an irritated and red scalp and minimize hair loss include:

- using a mild shampoo
- using hair brushes with soft bristles
- avoiding the use of hair dryers, hot curlers, and curling irons
- using the lowest setting on a hair dryer (if a dryer must be used)
- avoiding hair dyes
- avoiding permanent wave solutions
- wearing sunscreen or a hat when outdoors
- using a satin pillowcase

Alternative and complementary therapies

Patients suffering from alopecia may benefit from taking certain **vitamins** and minerals that promote healthy hair. These include zinc, selenium, magnesium, iron; and vitamins A, B-complex, C, and E. Vitamin E may be massaged into the scalp. Also, evening primrose oil and flaxseed oil are rich sources of omega-3 and omega-6 fatty acids, which are important for healthy hair.

Chinese medicinal herbs that promote hair growth include cornus, Chinese foxglove root, Chinese yam, lycium fruit, and polygonum. Herbalists recommend rinsing hair with sage tea or massaging the scalp with essential oil of rosemary to improve blood circulation and stimulate hair follicles.

It is important that patients check with their oncologist prior to taking any vitamin, mineral, or medicinal herb supplements as there is a possibility they may interfere with the effectiveness of the chemotherapy treatments.

KEY TERMS

Anagen stage—The growing stage in the growth cycle of hair.

Catagen stage—The intermediate stage in the hair-growth cycle during which proliferation ceases and regression of the hair follicle occurs.

Hair bulb—The base of a hair where living cells multiply causing the hair to grow.

Hair follicle—The depression in skin where a hair originates.

Scalp tourniquet—A process to prevent chemotherapy-induced alopecia in which a tight band is applied to the head.

Telogen stage—The resting stage in the growth cycle of hair.

Resources

BOOKS

De Vita, Vincent, Samuel Hellman, and Steven Rosenberg, eds. *Cancer, Principles & Practice of Oncology,* 6th ed. Philadelphia: Lippincott Williams & Wilkins, 2000. <http://www.LWWoncology.com>

Maleskey, Gale. *Nature's Medicines: from Asthma to Weight Gain, from Colds to High Cholesterol—The Most Powerful All-Natural Cures.* Emmaus, PA: Rodale Press, Inc., 1999.

Somerville, Robert, ed. *The Medical Advisor.* Alexandria, VA: Time-Life Books, 2000.

Yarbro, Connie Henke, Michelle Goodman, Margaret Hansen Frogge, and Susan L. Groenwald, eds. *Cancer Nursing, Principles and Practice,* 5th ed. Sudbury, MA: Jones and Bartlett Publishers, 2000.

Yarbro, Connie Henke, Margaret Hansen Frogge, and Michelle Goodman, eds. *Cancer Symptom Management,* 2nd ed. Sudbury, MA: Jones and Bartlett Publishers, 1999.

PERIODICALS

Dorr, Victoria J. "A Practitioner's Guide to Cancer-Related Alopecia." *Seminars in Oncology* 25, no. 5 (October 1998): 526-570.

OTHER

"How Do I Deal With Hair Loss?" *American Cancer Society, Inc.* 2000. 28 June 2001 <http://www3.cancer.org/cancerinfo>.

Belinda Rowland, Ph.D.

Alternative therapies *see* **Complementary cancer therapies**

Altretamine

Definition

Altretamine, also known by the brand name Hexalen, is an anticancer agent used to treat **ovarian cancer**.

Purpose

Altretamine is used to treat persistent or recurrent ovarian cancer, usually after treatment of the cancer with

KEY TERMS

Antiemetic—Agents used to alleviate nausea and vomiting, used during and sometimes following treatment with chemotherapy or radiotherapy.

Peripheral neuropathy—Symptoms resulting from damage to the peripheral nerves, that is, nerves not found in the spinal cord or brain.

cisplatin and/or an alkylating agent fails to effectively treat the tumor.

Description

The mechanism of action of altretamine is not known. However, it is thought that it may inhibit DNA and RNA synthesis.

Recommended dosage

Alretamine is administered orally. Doses for the drug may be different depending on the protocol that is used by the physician. Some example dosing regimens are: 4 to 12 mg per kg in three to four divided doses for 21 to 90 days; 240 to 320 mg per square meter of body surface area in three to four divided doses for 21 days, repeated every six weeks; 260 mg per square meter of body surface area per day for 14 to 21 days of a 28 days cycle in four divided doses; or 150 mg per square meter of body surface area in three to four divided doses for 14 days of a 28 day cycle. The dose of altretamine may be decreased if the patient has intolerable stomach side effects, low blood count of cells that fight infection (white blood cells) or cells that prevent bleeding (platelets), or if the patient has progressive toxicity affecting the nerves of the brain and body.

Precautions

Caution is usually taken in prescribing altretamine to patients with decreased kidney or liver function or damage to nerves due to previous **chemotherapy**. Careful monitoring of nerve, kidney, and liver function is required for these patients.

Pregnant women should be warned before taking this drug, as it may cause permanent harm to the fetus. Women who are of childbearing age should apply contraceptive methods to avoid pregnancy until they have discontinued drug use. Altretamine may also affect fertility. Additionally, although it is not known whether this drug is excreted in the breast milk, nursing mothers are cautioned not to breast feed while being treated with altretamine.

Side effects

Nausea and vomiting may gradually occur as patients receive continuous high dose of altretamine. In most instances, **antiemetics** can help control these side effects. However, some patients may experience severe nausea and vomiting that requires either reducing the dose or stopping treatment with altretamine. Other common side effects include loss of appetite (**anorexia**) and **diarrhea**. Patients may also experience nerve toxicity, which is described as numbness, tingling, and burning sensations in the fingers and toes. Patients can also have difficulty walking because of these sensation changes. Patients may also commonly experience: **thrombocytopenia**, a decrease of the platelet cells responsible for blood clotting; **anemia**, a decrease of the red blood cells responsible for oxygen transport to tissues and organs; and leukopenia, a decrease of the white blood cells responsible for fighting infections. Less common side effects include seizures, **depression**, dizziness, stomach cramps, liver toxicity, rash, and hair loss (**alopecia**).

Interactions

Persons taking altretamine and monoamine oxidase inhibitors (MAO inhibitors) may experience severe hypotension (low blood pressure) when standing up. Additionally, the drug cimetidine may increase the toxicity of altretamine. Prior to starting any over-the-counter medications, herbal medications, or new medications, patients should consult with their physician, nurse, or pharmacist to ensure that there are no potential drug interactions.

Michael Zuck, Ph.D.

Amenorrhea

Definition

Amenorrhea is the absence of menstruation and is a symptom, not a diagnosis.

Primary amenorrhea refers to the absence of the onset of menstruation by age 16 whether or not normal growth and secondary sexual characteristics are present, or the absence of menses after age 14 when normal growth and signs of secondary sexual characteristics are present. Secondary amenorrhea is the absence of menses for three cycles or six months in women who have previously menstruated.

In terms of the relationship of amenorrhea to cancer, amenorrhea may be a symptom of a gynecologic tumor, or the pause or cessation in menstruation may develop as a side effect of cancer treatment.

Demographics

The prevalence of primary amenorrhea is 0.3% and secondary amenorrhea occurs in approximately 1%–3% of women. However, among college students and athletes the incidence can range from 3%–5% and 5%–60%, respectively.

For cancer-related amenorrhea, one clinician noted that nine out of ten women under his care reported secondary amenorrhea following bone marrow transplants. **Chemotherapy** and abdominal-pelvic **radiation therapy** likewise produce similar outcomes.

Causes

Normal menstrual bleeding occurs between menarche and menopause and has an average length of 28 days but varies from woman to woman. The normal menstrual cycle depends on cyclic changes in estrogen and progesterone levels, as well as the integrity of the clotting system and the ability of the spiral arterioles in the uterus to constrict. Abnormalities in any of these components may cause bleeding to stop or increase.

Primary amenorrhea

There are multiple causes for primary amenorrhea once pregnancy, lactation and missed abortion are ruled out. These include:

- anorexia nervosa/bulimia/malnutrition
- extreme obesity
- hyperthyroidism/hypoglycemia
- congenital heart disease
- cystic fibrosis/Crohn's disease
- genetic abnormalities
- obstructions: imperforate hymen/vaginal or cervical absence
- ovarian, pituitary (**craniopharyngioma**) or adrenal tumors
- polycystic ovarian disease
- testicular feminization

It is rare for primary amenorrhea to be caused by tumors but it can be a cause and should always be a consideration if other factors are ruled out.

Gonadal failure (a nonfunctioning sex gland) is the most common cause of primary amenorrhea, accounting for almost half the patients with this syndrome. The second most common cause is uterovaginal agenesis (absence of a uterus and/or vagina) with an incidence of about 15% of individuals with this syndrome. One of the most important, and probably most common, causes of amenorrhea in adolescent girls is anorexia nervosa, which occurs in about 1 in 1,000 white women. It is uncommon in women older than 25 and rare in women of both African and Asian descent. When women lose weight 15% below ideal body weight, amenorrhea can occur due to central nervous system-hypothalamic dysfunction. When **weight loss** drops below 25% ideal body weight, pituitary gonadotrophin function (follicle stimulating hormone and luteinizing hormone) can also become abnormal.

Each year of athletic training before menarche (the beginning of menstrual function) delays menarche about four to five months. Amenorrhea associated with strenuous exercise is related to stress, not weight loss, and is most probably caused by an increase in central nervous system endorphins and other compounds which interfere with gonadotrophin-releasing hormone release.

Secondary amenorrhea

Once pregnancy, lactation and menopause are ruled out, the causes for secondary amenorrhea include:

- extreme obesity
- prolonged or extreme exercise
- anxiety or emotional distress
- non-oral contraceptives (Norplant/Depo-Provera)
- D & C (**dilatation and curettage**) (Asherman's syndrome)
- early menopause
- autoimmune dysfunction
- pituitary tumors and central nervous system lesions

Cancer and secondary amenorrhea

As mentioned, not only does amenorrhea occur as a symptom of a tumor and/or lesion, but it often develops in women undergoing treatment for cancer.

RADIATION. Radiation therapy is used in conjunction with chemotherapy in a number of clinical situations, including **Hodgkin's disease** and childhood leukemia and lymphomas. Ovarian damage occurs under these circumstances to varying degrees, depending upon the total dosage of radiation as well as the age of the patient at the time of exposure.

CHEMOTHERAPY. Premenopausal women receiving single or multi-agent chemotherapy are at risk for short-term amenorrhea, as well as ovarian damage. Even young women who resume menstruation following

KEY TERMS

Alkylating agents—A group of synthetic compounds that act on the deoxyribonucleic acid (DNA) in the nucleus of the cell and are used in cancer chemotherapy.

Aplastic anemia—Any form of anemia caused by defective development of bone marrow.

Asherman's syndrome—The presence of adhesions within the uterus following a D & C.

Autoimmune dysfunction—A disease associated with the production of antibodies directed against one's own tissues.

Craniopharyngioma—Tumor arising from the cells in the pituitary.

Crohn's disease—Inflammation of the gastrointestinal tract.

Imperforate hymen—The lack of an opening in the membranous fold partly or completely closing the opening to the vagina.

Intermenstrual—Time period between one menstrual cycle to another.

Luteinizing hormone—A hormone which acts with follicle-stimulating hormone to cause ovulation of mature follicles and secretion of estrogen from the ovary.

Menopause—The stage of life during which a woman passes from the reproductive to the nonreproductive stage and she experiences the cessation of menstruation.

Menses/Menstruation—The periodic discharge from the vagina of blood and tissues from a nonpregnant uterus.

Polycystic ovary disease—Also called Stein-Leventhal syndrome, it is the presence of many cysts in the ovaries.

Postcoital—Following intercourse.

Progestins—A steroid sex hormone that maintains the lining of the uterus.

Testicular feminization—An individual with female external development, including secondary sex characteristics, but with the presence of testes and absence of uterus and tubes.

chemotherapy are at risk for early menopause; therefore, those treated in childhood and adolescence should be counseled regarding the chance of early menopause in order to plan ahead for childbearing.

WEIGHT LOSS. Side effects of cancer as well as treatments can cause a decrease in appetite and **nausea and vomiting**, which, in turn, can cause severe weight loss as associated with malnutrition. Thus, menstruation may cease for the same reasons as it does in young adolescents with anorexia nervosa—hypothalamic dysfunction.

STRESS. Stress has always been noted to play a large role in the cause of amenorrhea, so the actual stress of having cancer and undergoing treatments may also cause amenorrhea to occur.

RETURN OF NORMAL OVARIAN FUNCTION FOLLOWING TREATMENT. Research on the recovery of normal ovarian function with young girls and/or young women has not revealed any reliable data. There are individual success stories especially with new advances in assisted reproductive technologies (ARTs), but overall, the return of normal ovarian function seems to be age-dependent. One researcher recently reported on ovarian function in 65 women who underwent high-dose chemotherapy and bone marrow transplants for aplastic anemia. All women younger than 26 years at the time of chemotherapy recovered ovarian function, while 7 of the 18 women aged 26 to 38 years did not recover ovarian function. Thus, the risk of ovarian dysfunction appears to increase with advancing age when ovarian reserve decreases. Additionally, the risk of dysfunction increases with the dose of alkylating agents, notably **cyclophosphamide**.

Treatments for amenorrhea

Even with the possibility of ovarian compromise, women previously treated for cancer have successfully achieved pregnancy via ART's. Advances in the area of ART's include the use of donor eggs, the possibility of freezing embryos, and eventual oocyte (immature ovum) pretreatment offer more options to young women facing cancer chemotherapy.

Special concerns

The need for effective contraception during and after cancer treatment is imperative. Normal menstrual cycles do not imply normal fertility and likewise, irregular menses or even amenorrhea does not imply a lack of fertility. Women with dysfunctional bleeding or amenorrhea are still capable of spontaneous ovulation and conception.

The most reliable form of birth control for any population of women is injectable progestins, which suppress luteinizing hormone secretion. Depo-Provera, 150 mg injected intramuscularly, will effectively block ovulation for four months. Norplant (six rubber capsules placed under anesthesia in the upper arm) will effectively block ovulation for five years. If the treatment or the specific cancer diagnosis contraindicates the use of either of these contraceptives, other options should be considered, i.e., sterilization for the woman or her partner, an intrauterine device (IUD), or barrier methods (condoms, diaphragm or spermicides).

See Also Fertility and cancer

Resources

BOOKS

Jarvis, Carolyn. *Physical Examination and Health Assessment.* Philadelphia: W. B. Saunders Company, 2000.

Trimble, E. *Cancer Obstetrics and Gynecology.* Philadelphia: Lippincott William & Wilkins, 1999.

Youngkin, Ellis Quinn and Marcia Davis Szmania. *Women's Health: A Primary Care Clinical Guide.* Stamford, CT: Appleton & Lange, 1998.

Linda K. Bennington, C.N.S., M.S.N.

American Joint Commission on Cancer

Definition

The American Joint Commission on Cancer (AJCC) is an organization dedicated to creating and promoting a universal system of classifying tumors according to their location in the body and involvement with surrounding tissues.

Description

Created in 1959, the AJCC works with the International Union Against Cancer (UICC), its European counterpart, and other organizations to standardize cancer-related information and data collection. The AJCC bases its classification on the TNM staging system, a universally accepted method of describing the extent of cancer, and other clinical information. The result is a standardized method of categorizing tumors that helps physicians to predict patient prognosis and develop treatment guidelines. The AJCC periodically publishes its *Cancer Staging Manual*, which is used widely by health care professionals in the diagnosis and treatment of cancer patients.

See Also Tumor staging

Tamara Brown, R.N.

Amifostine

Definition

Amifostine, also known as the brand name Ethyol and as ethiofos or WR2721, is a medicine that helps protect certain tissues of the body from damage caused by **chemotherapy** or **radiation therapy**.

Purpose

Amifostine is a protectant agent that is used in combination with the chemotherapy drug **cisplatin** or in combination with radiation therapy. Amifostine is approved by the Food and Drug Administration (FDA) to prevent kidney damage caused by repeat doses of the chemotherapy agent cisplatin in patients who have a diagnosis of **ovarian cancer** or non-small cell lung cancer. It is also FDA approved for patients with head and neck cancer who are receiving radiation therapy after surgery. In this group of patients, amifostine helps decrease radiation damage to the salivary glands, which can cause dry mouth.

Description

Amifostine has been on the market since the mid-1990s. A clear colorless solution, it is administered into a vein before chemotherapy and has been shown to decrease kidney damage by greater than 50% in advanced ovarian cancer patients who have received multiple cycles of cisplatin. It is also used before radiation therapy to prevent damage to the salivary gland known as the parotid gland.

When cisplatin is given to patients, it becomes broken down into toxic substances that destroy cancer cells and normal cells. When amifostine is administered into the body, it is broken down by an enzyme that occurs in large quantities in normal cells but not in cancerous cells. It then is converted into a substance called free thiol, which combines with the poisonous cisplatin by-products in the normal cells and makes them nontoxic.

KEY TERMS

Chemotherapy—Specific drugs used to treat cancer.

Enzyme—A protein in the body that breaks down substances, such as food or medicines, into simpler substances that the body can use.

Food and Drug Administration—A government agency that oversees public safety in relation to drugs and medical devices. The FDA gives approval to pharmaceutical companies for commercial marketing of their products.

Intravenous—To enter the body through a vein.

Radiation therapy—The use of high-energy beams focused to treat cancerous tumors.

In patients who receive radiation to the mouth area, including the salivary glands, the radiation causes the release of substances called free oxygen species, which damage cells of the mouth. An enzyme in cells of the mouth breaks down amifostine into a substance called free thiol. The free thiol blocks the free oxygen substances from damaging the salivary cells and decreases the amount of dry mouth patients suffer from when they receive radiation to the head and neck area.

Recommended dosage

Before dosing amifostine in chemotherapy or radiation therapy patients, intravenous fluids need to be given to keep the body well flushed with fluid and to maintain a normal blood pressure. All patients will receive amifostine lying down, sometimes with the head of the body lower than the feet. Patients should also receive medication to help prevent the **nausea and vomiting** that occurs due to amifostine.

Amifostine dosages can be determined using a mathematical calculation that measures a person's body surface area (BSA). This number is dependent upon a patient's height and weight. The larger the person, the greater the body surface area. Body surface area is measured in units known as square meter (m^2). To determine the actual dose a patient is to receive, the body surface area is calculated and then multiplied by the drug dosage in milligrams per squared meter (mg/m^2).

The recommended dosage of amifostine for protection of the kidney is 910mg/m^2 administered as a 15-minute infusion into a vein. This is to begin 30 minutes before chemotherapy administration. If a patient has difficulty with this dose, the dosage can be lowered to 740 mg/m^2.

The recommended dosage of amifostine for radiation therapy patients is 200 mg/m^2 administered once a day into a vein over a three-minute time period 15 to 30 minutes before the patient receives radiation treatment.

Precautions

Amifostine can cause a decrease in blood pressure when it is administered. During the 24 hours before receiving amifostine, patients need to drink a lot of liquids. When amifostine is being administered, medical personnel will be monitoring the patient's blood pressure. If the blood pressure drops significantly, the infusion of amifostine will be stopped until blood pressure returns to normal. The doctor will decide if the patient should receive any additional amifostine. Patients who have low blood pressure to begin with or patients who are not drinking a lot of fluids—referred to as being dehydrated—should not receive amifostine.

Patients with a known previous allergic reaction to aminothiol drugs should not receive amifostine.

Patients who may be pregnant, thinking of becoming pregnant, or who have a history of heart problems or strokes should tell their doctor before receiving amifostine.

Side effects

The most common side effect from receiving amifostine is a lowering of blood pressure, which occurs in approximately 62% of patients treated at a dose of 910mg/m^2. This lowering of blood pressure occurs within the first 15 minutes of administering the drug. Blood pressure is monitored throughout the infusion of amifostine. If the blood pressure drops to certain level then the drug is stopped and restarted only when blood pressure returns to normal.

Nausea and vomiting are common side effects. They occur rapidly and can be severe. Usually, patients are given medicines before receiving amifostine that can help prevent or decrease these side effects. Other side effects include sneezing, hiccups, a warm feeling and redness of the face, sleepiness and dizziness, metallic taste, **fever**, rash, and chills.

Rare side effects of amifostine are: a lowering of calcium levels in the blood, seizures, allergic reactions which include symptoms of fever, shaking chills, **itching**, low blood pressure, shortness of breath, and rashes. There have been rare reports of throat swelling, chest tightness, and heart stopping.

All side effects a patient experiences should be reported to their doctor.

Interactions

Amifostine causes a decrease in blood pressure and should be used with caution in patients who take blood pressure lowering medicines or other medications that may lower blood pressure. If patients are taking blood pressure medications, they may be asked to stop taking these medications for 24 hours before receiving amifostine.

Patients should tell their doctors if they have a known allergic reaction to amifostine or any other medications or substances, such as foods and preservatives. Before taking any new medications, including nonprescription medications, **vitamins**, and herbal medications, patients should notify their doctors.

Nancy J. Beaulieu, RPh., BCOP

Aminoglutethimide

Definition

Aminoglutethimide, also known by the brand name Cytadren, is a cancer drug which inhibits the formation of hormones like adrenal glucocorticoids, mineralocorticoids, estrogen, androgens, and aldosterone.

Purpose

Aminoglutethimide is used to treat Cushing's disease, **breast cancer**, or **prostate cancer**. It blocks the conversion of cholesterol to delta-5-pregnenolone, a precursor for the formation of the **corticosteroids**.

Description

Aminoglutethimide is used clinically to reduce the amount of the hormones that can sometimes cause tumors to grow more quickly or are necessary for the survival of the tumor. For example, estrogen is important for the growth of some breast tumors. Lowering estrogen production by the administration of aminoglutethimide might reduce tumor growth or contribute to the destruction of the tumor.

Recommended dosage

Aminoglutethimide is given orally and dosages vary from patient to patient based on a number of factors, including the underlying disease process.

Precautions

Because some corticosteroid is necessary for normal function, patients should receive steroid replacement in addition to aminoglutethimide. Patients may require more corticosteroid when undergoing surgery, illness, or other conditions that cause stress. Hormones that affect the balance of sodium in the body may also be affected by aminoglutethimide and might have to be replaced as a result. If they are not replaced, patients may experience constant low blood pressure or low blood pressure upon standing.

Pregnant women should be warned that aminoglutethimide administration could cause fetal abnormalities. Pregnant patients should consult their physician about the current state of knowledge regarding risks and alternatives before beginning administration of aminoglutethimide. Female patients of childbearing age should attempt to avoid pregnancy while taking this drug. Mothers who are nursing should discontinue nursing while taking this drug.

Side effects

Common side effects from the administration of aminoglutethimide is rash (possibly associated with **fever**) which usually occurs in the first two weeks of therapy. It is usually self-limiting and gets better in a about a week. If the rash continues after one week patient should contact his/her physician or nurse. **Fatigue** is another common side effect of the drug and usually occurs in the first week of therapy. It may take about a month before it gets better. It can be very severe in some patients and if this is the case the patient's physician or nurse should be notified. Female patients may experience masculinization: new and excessive hair growth, a deeper voice, and irregular, abnormal, or absent menstrual periods. Thyroid function may be decreased after several weeks of therapy and the patient's thyroid should be monitored by the physician. Mild **nausea and vomiting** may also occur, as well as dizziness, **depression**, shaking, difficulty speaking, and increased heart rate. Any of these effects, or other unusual symptoms, should be reported to the patient's physician.

Interactions

Dexamethasone, blood-thinning medications, theophylline, and digoxin doses for patients taking amino-

KEY TERMS

Hormone—A substance, such as cortisol or estrogen, that causes specific effects on target organs in the body. Hormones may be required for tumor growth or survival. Hormones usually travel in the bloodstream from the organ where they originate to a different organ where they have their effect.

glutethimide may need to be increased by the physician. Patients should tell their doctors if they have a known allergic reaction to aminoglutethimide medications or substances, such as foods and preservatives. Before taking any new medications, including nonprescription medications, **vitamins**, and herbal medications, patients should notify their doctors.

Michael Zuck, Ph.D.

Amitriptyline

Definition

Amitriptyline is a medication used to treat various forms of **depression**, pain associated with the nerves (neuropathic pain), and to prevent migraine headaches. It is sold in the United States under the brand name Elavil.

Purpose

Amitriptyline helps relieve depression and pain. It is often used to manage nerve pain resulting from cancer treatment. Such injury to nerves causes a burning, tingling sensation. This medication, usually given at bedtime, helps patients sleep better.

Description

This medication is one of several tricyclic antidepressants. Amitriptyline acts to block reabsorption of chemicals that transmit nerve messages in the brain.

Recommended dosage

Amitriptyline's usual adult dose for pain management is 10 mg to 150 mg at bedtime. Patients are generally started on a low dose. The amount of medication may be increased as needed. Side effects, such as a dry mouth and drowsiness, may make it difficult to increase the dose in older adults. Bedtime dosing helps the patient sleep. Doctors generally order 75 mg to 150 mg for depression. It is given at bedtime or in divided doses. It may take 30 days for the patient to feel less depressed. Pain relief is usually noticed sooner than the mood change. Teens and older adults usually receive a lower dose. If the nightly dose is missed, it should not be taken the next morning. Taking amitriptyline during waking hours could result in noticeable side effects. Patients should check with their doctor if the daily dose is missed. Those on more than one dose per day should take a missed dose as soon as it is noted. Patients should not take two doses at the same time. Injectable amitriptyline is available. It should not be used long-term. Patients should switch to tablets as soon as possible.

Precautions

Patients should not suddenly stop taking this medication. The dose should gradually be decreased, then discontinued. If the drug is abruptly stopped, the patient may experience headache, nausea, discomfort throughout the body, and a worsening of original symptoms. Amitriptyline's effects last for three to seven days after the medication has been stopped. Older adults usually are more prone to some side effects. These include drowsiness, dizziness, mental confusion, blurry vision, dry mouth, difficulty urinating, and constipation. Taking a lower dose may help resolve these problems. Patients may need to stop this medication before surgery.

Amitriptyline should not be given to anyone with allergies to the drug or to patients recovering from a heart attack. Patients taking MAO inhibitors, a different type of antidepressant, should not also use amitriptyline. It should be administered with caution to patients with glaucoma, seizures, urinary retention, an overactive thyroid, poor liver or kidney function, alcoholism, asthma, digestive disorders, an enlarged prostate, seizures, or heart disease. This medication should not be given to children under 12. Pregnant women should discuss the risks and benefits of this medication with their doctor. Fetal deformities have been associated with taking this drug during pregnancy. Women should not breastfeed while using amitriptyline.

Side effects

Common side effects associated with amitriptyline include dry mouth, drowsiness, constipation, and dizziness or lightheadedness when standing. Patients can suck on ice cubes or sugarless hard candy to combat the dry mouth. Increased fiber in the diet and additional fluids may help the constipation. The dizziness is usually caused by a drop in blood pressure when changing position. Patients should slowly rise from a sitting or lying position if dizziness is noticed. Amitriptyline may increase the risk of falls in older adults. Patients should not drive or operate machinery or appliances while under the influence of this drug. Alcohol and other central nervous system depressants can increase drowsiness. Amitriptyline may also produce blurry vision and an irregular or fast heartbeat. Amitriptyline also may raise or lower blood pressure, or cause palpitations. This medication may increase or decrease diabetic patients' blood sugar levels. Amitriptyline may make patients' skin more sensitive to the sun. Patients should avoid direct sunlight, wear protective clothing, and apply sunscreen with a protective factor of 15 or higher.

Amitriptyline may increase appetite, cause weight gain, or produce an unpleasant taste in the mouth. It may

KEY TERMS

MAO inhibitor—a type of antidepressant medication

also cause **diarrhea**, vomiting, or heartburn. Taking this medication with food may decrease digestive side effects. Other less likely side effects include muscle tremors, nervousness, impaired sexual function, sweating, rash, **itching**, hair loss, ringing in the ears, or changes in the make up of the patient's blood. Patients with schizophrenia may develop an increase in psychiatric symptoms.

Interactions

Patients should always tell all doctors and dentists that they are taking this medication. Amitriptyline may decrease the effectiveness of some drugs used to treat high blood pressure. Amitriptyline should not be taken with other antidepressants, epinephrine and other adrenaline-type drugs, or methylphenidate. Patients should not take over-the-counter medications without checking with their doctor. For instance, amitriptyline should not be taken with Tagamet (cimetidine) or Neo-Synephrine. Patients taking this drug should avoid the dietary supplements St. John's wort, belladonna, henbane and scopolia. Black tea may decrease the absorption of this drug. Patients should ingest the drug and tea at least two hours apart.

Debra Wood, R.N.

Amphotericin B *see* **Antifungal therapy**

Amputation

Definition

Amputation is the intentional surgical removal of a limb or body part. It is performed to remove diseased tissue or relieve pain.

Purpose

Arms, legs, hands, feet, fingers, and toes can all be amputated. Most amputations involve small body parts such as a finger, rather than an entire limb. More than 60,000 amputations are performed in the United States each year.

Amputation is performed for the following reasons:

- to remove tissue that no longer has an adequate blood supply
- to remove malignant cancers (almost exclusively in the case of osteogenic sarcoma or other sarcomas)
- as a result of severe trauma to the body part

The blood supply to an extremity can be cut off because of injury to the blood vessel, hardening of the arteries, arterial embolism, impaired circulation as a complication of diabetes mellitus, repeated severe infection that leads to gangrene, severe frostbite, Raynaud's disease, or Buerger's disease.

More than 90% of amputations performed in the United States are due to circulatory complications of diabetes, the most common cause of non-traumatic leg and foot amputations.

Precautions

Amputation cannot be performed on patients with uncontrolled diabetes mellitus, heart failure, or infection, and is also inadvisable for patients with blood clotting disorders.

Description

Amputations can be either planned or emergency procedures. Injury and arterial embolisms are the main reasons for emergency amputations. The operation is performed under regional or general anesthesia by a general or orthopedic surgeon in a hospital operating room.

Details of the operation vary slightly depending on what is to be removed. The goal of all amputations is twofold: to remove diseased tissue so that the wound will heal cleanly, and to construct a stump that will allow the attachment of a prosthesis or artificial replacement part.

The surgeon makes an incision around the part to be amputated. The part is removed, and the bone is smoothed. A flap is constructed of muscle, connective tissue, and skin to cover the raw end of the bone. The flap is then closed over the bone with sutures (surgical stitches) that remain in place for 3 to 4 weeks. Often, a rigid dressing or cast is applied that stays in place for about two weeks.

Preparation

Before an amputation is performed, extensive testing is done to determine the proper level of amputation. The goal of the surgeon is to find the place where healing is

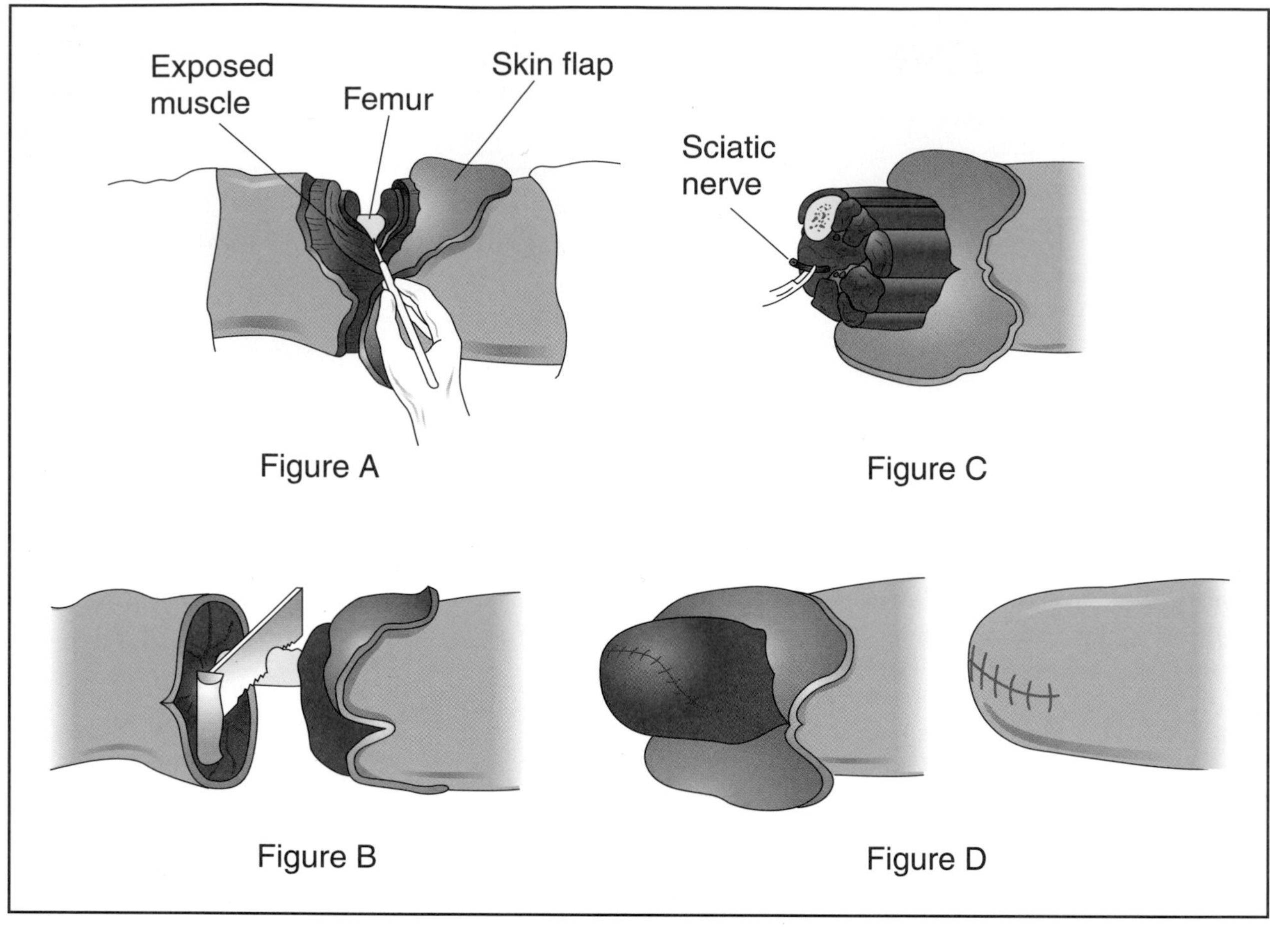

Amputation of leg. Figure A: After the surgeon creates two flaps of skin and tissue, the muscle is cut and the main artery and veins of the femur bone are exposed. Figure B: The surgeon severs the main artery and veins. New connections are formed beween them, restoring blood circulation. The sciatic nerve is then pulled down, clamped and tied, and severed. Figure C: The surgeon saws through the exposed femur bone. Figure D: The muscles are closed and sutured over the bone. The remaining skin flaps are then sutured together, creating a stump. *(Illustration by Electronic Illustrators Group.)*

most likely to be complete, while allowing the maximum amount of limb to remain for effective rehabilitation.

The greater the blood flow through an area, the more likely healing is to occur. These tests are designed to measure blood flow through the limb. Several or all of the following can be done to help choose the proper level of amputation:

- measurement of blood pressure in different parts of the limb
- Xenon 133 studies, which use a radiopharmaceutical to measure blood flow
- Oxygen tension measurements in which an oxygen electrode is used to measure oxygen pressure under the skin. If the pressure is 0, healing will not occur. If the pressure reads higher than 40ml Hg (40 milliliters of mercury), healing of the area is likely to be satisfactory.
- laser Doppler measurements of the microcirculation of the skin
- skin fluorescent studies that also measure skin microcirculation
- skin perfusion measurements using a blood pressure cuff and photoelectric detector
- infrared measurements of skin temperature

No one test is highly predictive of healing, but taken together, the results can give the surgeon a detailed idea of the best place to amputate.

Aftercare

After amputation, medication is prescribed for pain, and patients are treated with **antibiotics** to discourage infection. The stump is moved often to encourage good circulation. Physical therapy and rehabilitation are started as soon after surgery as possible. Studies have shown that there is a positive relationship between early rehabilitation and effective functioning of the stump and prosthesis. Length of stay in the hospital depends on the severity of the amputation and the general health of the amputee, but is usually less than one week.

Recovery from surgery takes about six weeks. Rehabilitation, however, is a long and arduous process, especially for above-the-knee amputees. The doctor and physical therapist decide how soon after surgery the patient can begin to exercise, and several sessions each day may be recommended. In addition, psychological counseling is an important part of rehabilitation. Many patients experience a sense of loss and grief when they lose a body part. Others are bothered by phantom limb syndrome, where they feel as if the amputated part is still in place. They may even feel pain in the limb that has been removed. Many amputees benefit from joining self-help groups and meeting others who are also living with amputation. Addressing the emotional aspects of amputation often speeds the physical rehabilitation process.

Risks

Amputation is a major surgery. All the risks associated with the administration of anesthesia exist, along with the possibility of heavy blood loss and the development of blood clots. Infection is of special concern to amputees. If the stump becomes infected, it is necessary to remove the prosthesis and sometimes to amputate a second time at a higher level.

Failure of the stump to heal is another major complication. Nonhealing is usually due to an inadequate blood supply. The rate of complications is generally lowest in centers that specialize in amputation.

As many as 80% of amputees experience some degree of sensation in the stump or phantom limb, and 5% to 10% seek medical attention for the pain. Although phantom pain is most common in the year following amputation, it can be a long-term problem that persists in spite of therapy. One final complication is that many amputees give up on the rehabilitation process and discard their prosthesis. Better-fitting prosthetics and earlier rehabilitation have decreased the incidence of this problem.

Normal results

Up to 50% of people who have one leg amputated because of diabetes will lose the other within five years. Amputees who walk using a prosthesis are likely to fall and break bones because of their unstable gait. Although the fractures can be treated, many of the amputees who suffer them remain wheelchair-bound.

KEY TERMS

Arterial embolism—A blood clot arising from another location that blocks an artery.

Buerger's disease—An episodic disease that causes inflammation and blockage of the veins and arteries of the limbs. It tends to be present almost exclusively on men under age of 40 who smoke, and may require amputation of the hand or foot.

Diabetes mellitus—A disease in which insufficient insulin is made by the body to metabolize sugars.

Raynaud's disease—A disease found mainly in young women that causes decreased circulation to the hands and feet. Its cause is unknown.

Abnormal results

The most common complications of amputation are:

- massive hemorrhage that occurs when a suture becomes loose
- infection
- rash, blisters, and skin breakdown caused by immobility, pressure, and other sources of irritation
- pneumonia, blood clots, and breathing problems associated with immobility
- formation of nerve cell tumors (neuromas) at severed nerve endings

Complications can develop immediately after surgery or after the patient has left the hospital. The doctor should be notified if a patient who has had an amputation experiences:

- increased pain, swelling, or drainage at the site of the surgery
- headache, muscle aches, dizziness, a general ill feeling, **fever**, or other signs of infection
- nausea
- vomiting
- chest pain
- constipation
- coughing
- shortness of breath
- changes in skin quality (certain areas become chalky or blackened)
- any new symptoms

Resources

BOOKS

Smertzer, Suzanne C., and Brenda G Bare. *Brunner & Budarth's Textbook of Medical-Surgical Nursing.* Philadelphia: Lippincott Williams & Wilkins, 2000.

Ignatavicius, Donna D., et al. *Medical-Surgical Nursing Across the Health Care Continuum,* 3rd ed. Philadelphia: W.B. Saunders Company, 1999.

Thompson, June M., et al. *Mosby's Clinical Nursing,* 4th ed. St. Louis: C.V. Mosby Company, 1997.

ORGANIZATIONS

American Diabetes Association. 1660 Duke St., Alexandria, VA 22314. <http://www.diabetes.org>

Amputation Information Resource Center. 6480 Wayzata Blvd., Minneapolis, MN 55426.

Amputation Prevention Global Resource Center. <http://www.diabetesresource.com>.

Cherub Association of Families and Friends of Limb Disordered Children, Inc. 8401 Powers Rd., Batavia, NY 14020.(716) 662-9997.

National Amputation Foundation. 73 Church St., Malverne, NY 11565. (516) 887-3600. <http://www.nationalamputation.org>

National Cancer Institute. (301) 435-3848. <http://www.nci.nih.gov>.

OTHER

Amputation. 14 May 2001. 6 July 2001 <http://community.healthgate.com>

Diabetes Facts and Figures. 11 May 2001. 6 July 2001 <http://www.diabetes.org>.

Tish Davidson, A.M.

Amsacrine

Definition

Amsacrine is an antitumor agent used to treat adult **acute leukemia**. It is no longer commercially available in the United States, although it is available in Canada.

Purpose

Amsacrine is an **investigational drug** used to treat refractory acute lymphocytic and nonlymphocytic leukemias, **Hodgkin's disease**, and **non-Hodgkin's lymphomas**. It may also have some activity against **head and neck cancers**.

Description

Amsacrine inhibits the synthesis of DNA. It also inhibits the enzyme responsible for cutting the strands of DNA, and untwists DNA so that replication of DNA can't occur.

Recommended dosage

The dose for amsacrine may be different depending on the protocol used by the physician. The drug is given through the vein as a 30- to 90- minute infusion or as a 24-hour continuous infusion. Example doses for adults are: 60 to 160 mg per square meter of body surface area every three to four weeks, or 40 to 120 mg per square meter of body surface area for five to seven days every three to four weeks. The dose for children is 120 to 150 mg per square meter of body surface area per day for five days. The dose of amsacrine is usually decreased in patients with decreased kidney or liver function.

Precautions

Amsacrine is usually given with caution to patients with underlying heart disease, severe kidney or liver disease, or to patients who have received high doses of anthracycline **chemotherapy** drugs, such as **doxorubicin**.

Although the effects of amsacrine treatment on children are currently unknown, caution is still indicated. Women of childbearing age should take precautions to prevent pregnancy while on this drug. Women should not breastfeed while taking this medication.

Side effects

Toxicity to the heart is a common side effect of amsacrine, and patients receiving this drug are usually very closely monitored by their physician. Other common side effects of amsacrine include **nausea and vomiting**, **diarrhea**, ulcerations of the mouth and the gastrointestinal tract, decreased white blood cells and platelets, and decreased liver function. Patients may notice orange-red discoloration of the urine, but should not be alarmed as this is normal. The urine will clear again once all the drugs have been eliminated from the body. Other common side effects include headache, dizziness, confusion, seizures, abnormal touch sensation such as burning and prickling, and blurred vision. As with any side effects that occur while taking any medications, patients should notify their doctor or nurse immediately.

Interactions

To prevent any drug interactions, patients should consult their physician, nurse, or pharmacist prior to taking any over-the-counter medications, herbal medications, or new medications. Many physicians recommend bringing the containers with the names of the drugs to an appointment.

Michael V. Zuck, Ph.D.

Anagrelide

Definition

Anagrelide, also known by the brand name Agrylin, is used to treat patients with thrombocytosis, a condition in which patients have too many platelet cells in their blood. Platelets are a cell type formed in the bone marrow that are involved in the blood clotting process.

Purpose and Description

Anagrelide reduces the platelet count in patients with blood disorders.

Recommended dosage

Adult patients taking anagrelide should receive 0.5 mg of the drug four times daily or one mg twice daily. Based on the response to therapy, the dose of anagrelide can be increased by 0.5 mg per day every seven to 14 days if necessary. The goal is to maintain platelets at a count of less than 600,000 at the lowest dose of the drug possible to keep side effects at a minimum.

Precautions

Patients with heart disease should be given anagrelide with caution. Anagrelide should be given with caution, if at all, in patients taking drugs that affect platelet aggregations such as aspirin, clopidrogel, ticlopodine, or non-steroidal agents.

Pregnant mothers should be warned that anagrelide administration may cause fetal abnormalities. Pregnant patients should consult their physician about the current state of knowledge regarding risks and alternatives before beginning administration of anagrelide. Female patients of childbearing age should attempt to avoid pregnancy while taking this drug. Mothers who are nursing should discontinue nursing while taking this drug.

Side effects

The most common side effects of anagrelide are palpitations, fluid gain resulting in swelling, headaches, dizziness, **diarrhea**, stomach discomfort, mild to moderate nausea, passing gas, weakness, shortness of breath, and decreased platelets. Less common side effects of anagrelide include increased heart rate and chest pain, malaise, rash, vomiting, and decreased appetite. As with all medications, patients should contact their physician or nurse if any of these side effects occur.

KEY TERMS

Platelets—A cell type found in the blood important for blood clotting.

Thrombocytosis—The condition of having too many platelet cells in the blood.

Interactions

There are no proven interactions between anagrelide and other drugs. The drug sucralfate may interfere with the absorption of anagrelide. Prior to starting any over-the-counter medications, herbal medications, or new medications, patients should consult their physician, nurse, or pharmacist to prevent drug interactions.

Michael Zuck, Ph.D.

Anal cancer

Definition

Anal cancer is an uncommon cancer occurring in the tissues that make up the opening through which stool passes out of the body.

Description

The anus is the opening at the end of the large intestine (rectum) through which solid waste passes out of the body. The anus is a junction between two types of tissues: mucosa, which lines the intestines, and skin. Cancer located at the junction between the rectum and anus is called "anal canal cancer" (also known as transitional-cell, squamous, epidermoid, or basal cell cancer). Cancer located near the external skin is called "anal margin cancer." Anal canal cancer is more common in women, and anal margin cancer is more common in men.

Approximately 3,400 cases of anal cancer were diagnosed in the United States in 2000. Anal cancer accounts for 1.5% of the cancers of the digestive system. The average age at diagnosis is 62 years. Most anal cancers are squamous cell carcinomas.

Demographics

Women are much more likely than men to develop anal cancer. Anal cancer is more prevalent in Caucasians than other races.

Causes and symptoms

The previously-held belief that anal cancer is caused by the chronic irritation associated with cracks (fissures), hemorrhoids, and abnormal passageways (fistulae), is falling out of favor. It is now believed that most cases of anal cancer are caused by **human papilloma virus** (HPV), a sexually-transmitted virus that can cause genital warts. Cancer is caused when the normal mechanisms that control cell growth become disturbed, causing the cells to grow continually without stopping. This may be the result of damage to the DNA in the cell or viral infection.

Symptoms of anal cancer may include:

- bleeding from the anus
- pain around the anus
- the sensation of anal pressure or a mass
- anal itching
- anal discharge
- straining to pass stool (rectal tenesmus)

Diagnosis

To diagnose anal cancer, the physician will first examine the skin of the anus and then will perform a **digital rectal examination** by inserting a greased, gloved finger into the rectum to feel for lumps. He or she will look for blood on the glove. If a lump is felt, a small sample of the lump will be removed (**biopsy**) through a small endoscope (flexible viewing instrument) to examine the tissue under a microscope. The biopsy may be performed using local anesthesia in the physician's office.

Although the diagnosis of anal cancer can be made by the examination alone, the cancer may be further evaluated by conducting other procedures. Endoscopic examinations of the anus (**anoscopy**) or rectum (proctoscopy) may be performed to see the tumor. **Endorectal ultrasound**, in which a wand-like ultrasound probe is inserted into the anus, enables the physician to determine how deep the tumor lies and whether or not nearby organs have been affected. Other possible diagnostic procedures include **x ray** and/or **computed tomography** (CT scan) to detect tumor spread (**metastasis**). It is common, however, for the cancer to be misdiagnosed at first as a benign lesion, such as a tissue lesion or hemorrhoid; due to this, treatment regimens may be delayed.

Treatment team

The treatment team for anal cancer may include a colorectal surgeon, gastroenterologist, oncologist, radiation oncologist, nurse oncologist, psychiatrist, psychological counselor, and social worker.

Clinical staging, treatments, and prognosis

Clinical staging

The American Joint Committee on Cancer and the Union Internationale Contra le Cancer developed a staging system for anal cancer. Anal cancer is categorized into five stages (0, I, II, III, and IV) which may be further subdivided (A and B) based on the depth or spread of cancerous tissue. This staging system does not apply to anal melanomas or **sarcomas**. Seventy-five percent of anal cancer patients have stage I or stage II disease. The stages of anal cancer are:

- Stage 0. Cancer has not spread below the limiting membrane of the first layer of anal tissue.
- Stage I. Cancer is 2 cm (approximately 0.75 in) or less in greatest dimension and has not spread anywhere else.
- Stage II. Cancer is between 2 and 5 cm in diameter and has spread beyond the topmost layer of tissue. There is no evidence of regional lymph node metastasis or distant metastasis.
- Stage IIIA. Cancer has spread to adjacent organs (e.g. vagina, bladder) or to the perirectal lymph nodes. Tumor may be of any size.
- Stage IIIB. Cancer has spread to nearby lymph nodes in the abdomen or groin or has spread to both adjacent organs and perirectal lymph nodes. Tumor may be of any size.
- Stage IV. Cancer has spread to distant abdominal lymph nodes or to distant organs in the body.

Treatments

The specific treatment depends on the stage of cancer, type of cancer, and the age and overall health of the patient. Anal cancer is most frequently treated with a combination of **radiation therapy** and **chemotherapy**.

Radiation therapy uses high-energy radiation from x rays and gamma rays to kill the cancer cells. Radiation given from a machine that is outside the body is called external radiation therapy. Radiation given internally is called internal radiation therapy or brachytherapy. Sometimes applicators containing radioactive compounds are placed directly into the cancerous lesion (interstitial radiation). The skin in the treated area may become red and dry and may take as long as a year to return to normal. **Fatigue**, upset stomach, **diarrhea**, and nausea are also common complaints of patients having radiation therapy. Women may develop vaginal narrowing (stenosis) caused by radiation therapy in the pelvic area, which makes intercourse painful. Radiation may injure the anal sphincter and may cause anal ulcers and anal stenosis.

Chemotherapy uses anticancer drugs to kill the cancer cells. The drugs are given by mouth (orally) or intravenously. They enter the bloodstream and can travel to all parts of the body to kill cancer cells. Generally, a combination of drugs is given because it is more effective than a single drug in treating cancer. The side effects of chemotherapy are significant and include stomach upset, vomiting, appetite loss (**anorexia**), hair loss (**alopecia**), mouth sores, and fatigue. Women may experience vaginal sores, menstrual cycle changes, and premature menopause. There is also an increased chance of infections.

Surgery may occasionally be employed in the treatment of advanced or recurrent anal cancer. Associated lymph nodes may be surgically removed (lymphadenectomy) if they contain metastatic disease. Most frequently, the cancerous tissue is removed by a procedure called a local resection. In this procedure, the muscle (sphincter muscle) that opens and closes the anus to allow the passage of stool is usually preserved. Alternatively, an abdominoperineal resection is rarely performed surgery in which the anus and lower portion of the rectum are removed. This procedure involves cutting into the abdomen and the perineum, which lies between the anus and vagina in women or between the anus and scrotum in men. An opening is created so that stool can pass out of the body (**colostomy**) and into a special bag (colostomy bag) affixed to the skin. Because of the success of radiation therapy and chemotherapy, abdominoperineal resection is infrequently performed. It is reserved for certain patients with recurrent cancer and cancer that is not responding to more conservative treatments.

Prognosis

Anal cancer is a curable disease. Tumors that are located in the anal canal, are less than 2 cm in diameter, and are well-differentiated have a favorable prognosis. Anal cancer patients treated with radiation therapy and chemotherapy (without surgery) have a five-year survival rate of approximately 80%. In the United States, approximately 500 people die from anal cancer each year.

Anal cancer can spread locally and invade other pelvic organs such as the vagina, prostate gland, and bladder. Anal cancer that spreads through the bloodstream (hematogenous spread) most often strikes the liver and lungs.

Alternative and complementary therapies

Although alternative and complementary therapies are used by many cancer patients, very few controlled studies on the effectiveness of such therapies exist. Mind-body techniques such as prayer, biofeedback, visualization, meditation, and yoga have not demonstrated any effect in reducing cancer but can reduce stress and have been shown to lessen some of the side effects of cancer treatments.

Clinical studies of hydrazine sulfate found that it had no effect on cancer and actually worsened the health and well-being of the study subjects. Laetrile, or amygdalin, is often suggested as a cure for cancer and leukemia. No human or animal studies conducted in the last few decades have shown any benefit other than relief of some pain. Laetrile can, however, cause cyanide poisoning.

Shark cartilage is another popular treatment, but has not shown anticancer activity in a clinical setting. Although the results are mixed, clinical studies suggest that the hormone melatonin may increase the survival time and quality of life for cancer patients.

Vitamin E, broccoli, and ellagic acid (found in raspberries, strawberries, cranberries, etc.) may help to prevent colorectal cancer. Selenium, in safe doses, may delay the progression of cancer. Laboratory and animal studies suggest that curcumin, the active ingredient of turmeric, has anticancer activity. According to laboratory and animal studies, maitake mushrooms may boost the immune system. Some laboratory studies suggest that mistletoe has anticancer properties; however, clinical studies have not been conducted.

Coping with cancer treatment

The patient should consult their treatment team regarding any side effects or complications of treatment. Many of the side effects of chemotherapy can be relieved by medications. Vaginal stenosis can be prevented and treated by vaginal dilators, gentle douching, and sexual

KEY TERMS

Anal sphincter—The muscle located between the rectum and anus that opens and closes to allow the passage of stool.

Colostomy—An opening created in the skin that allows stool to pass out of the body. A colostomy is necessary when the anus and rectum are removed.

Human papilloma virus (HPV)—A sexually-transmitted virus that causes genital and anal warts. It is associated with anal cancer and certain gynecologic cancers.

Stenosis—Narrowing of a passageway, such as radiation-induced narrowing of the vagina (vaginal stenosis) or anus (anal stenosis).

QUESTIONS TO ASK THE DOCTOR

- What type of cancer do I have?
- What stage of cancer do I have?
- What is the 5 year survival rate for persons with this type and stage of cancer?
- Has the cancer spread?
- What are my treatment options?
- What are the risks and side effects of these treatments?
- What medications can I take to relieve treatment side effects?
- Are there any clinical studies underway that would be appropriate for me?
- Is surgery necessary?
- Will my anal sphincter be affected by surgery?
- Are there any alternatives to abdominoperineal resection?
- What effective alternative or complementary treatments are available for this type of cancer?
- How debilitating is the treatment? Will I be able to continue working?
- Are there any local support groups for anal cancer patients?
- What is the chance that the cancer will recur?
- Is there anything I can do to prevent recurrence?
- How often will I have follow-up examinations?

intercourse. A water-soluble lubricant may be used to make sexual intercourse more comfortable. Patients should consult a psychotherapist and/or join a support group to deal with the emotional consequences of cancer and its treatment.

Clinical trials

As of 2001, there is one active clinical trial that is specifically studying anal cancer. The trial (protocol RTOG-9811) is sponsored by the National Cancer Institute and is open to patients with stage II or III anal cancer. This study aims to compare the effectiveness of radiation therapy with either of two different pairs of chemotherapeutic agents (**fluorouracil** and mitomycin versus fluorouracil and **cisplatin**). There are other trials underway that include all types of **gastrointestinal cancers**, which may include anal cancer. Patients should consult with their treatment team to determine if they are candidates for any ongoing studies. The National Cancer Institute also provides information on **clinical trials**, and can be reached at (800) 4-CANCER or at <http://www.nci.nih.gov>.

Prevention

There is moderately strong evidence linking anal cancer with human immunodeficiency virus (AIDS) infection, cigarette smoking, or long-term use of **corticosteroids**. Other factors that are strongly associated with the development of anal cancer include:

- Anogenital warts. Warts in and around the genitals and anus are found in 20% of women and heterosexual men and in 50% of homosexual men with anal cancer.
- Sexual activity. Having more than 10 sexual partners or being the recipient of anal intercourse increases the risk of developing anal cancer.
- Infections. Infection by sexually-transmitted microbes, such as human papilloma virus HPV, herpesvirus, *Neisseria gonorrhoeae*, or *Chlamydia trachomatis*, places one at a higher risk of developing anal cancer.
- Gynecologic cancer. Women with a history of vaginal, vulvar, or **cervical cancer** are at risk of developing anal cancer. This risk is not due to therapeutic radiation exposure for gynecologic cancer.
- Chronic immunosuppression. The long-term use of drugs by organ transplant recipients to suppress the immune system increases the chance of developing a squamous **carcinoma**, such as anal cancer.

Because anal cancer is believed to be caused by HPV, like cervical cancer, it may be a preventable disease. Practicing safe-sex methods should help to prevent anal cancer. Persons who are at a high risk of developing anal cancer may benefit from routine screening by a physician.

Special concerns

The effect of pelvic radiation therapy on fertility can be a concern for both men and women. The need for a colostomy raises many issues, including those related to **body image** and self esteem.

See Also Fertility issues

Resources

BOOKS

American Cancer Society's Guide to Complementary and Alternative Cancer Methods. Bruss, Katherine, Christina

Salter, and Esmeralda Galan, eds. Atlanta: American Cancer Society, 2000.

Minsky, Bruce, John Hoffman, and David Kelsen. "Cancer of the Anal Region." In *Cancer: Principles & Practice of Oncology.* DeVita, Vincent, Samuel Hellman, and Steven Rosenberg, eds. Philadelphia: Lippincott Williams & Wilkins, 2001.

PERIODICALS

Ryan, David, Carolyn Compton, and Robert Mayer. "Carcinoma of the Anal Canal." *New England Journal of Medicine* 342 (March 2000): 792–800.

ORGANIZATIONS

American Cancer Society. 1599 Clifton Rd. NE, Atlanta, GA 30329. (800) ACS-2345. <http://www.cancer.org>.

Cancer Research Institute, National Headquarters. 681 Fifth Ave., New York, NY 10022. (800) 992-2623. <http://www.cancerresearch.org>.

National Institutes of Health. National Cancer Institute. 9000 Rockville Pike, Bethesda, MD 20982. (800) 4-CANCER. <http://cancernet.nci.nih.gov>.

OTHER

"Anal Cancer."*Cancernet.* Dec. 2000. 13 Apr. 2001. 9 July 2001 <http://cancernet.nci.nih.gov>.

Belinda Rowland, Ph.D.

Anastrozole *see* **Aromatase inhibitors**

Anemia

Description

Anemia is characterized by an abnormally low number of red blood cells in the circulating blood. It frequently affects patients with cancer. In fact, in many cancer diagnoses such as **multiple myeloma** and **acute leukemia**, the presence of anemia may be what initially prompts a doctor to suspect an underlying tumor (neoplasm). Whether or not anemia develops depends on the type of cancer found, the treatment employed, as well as the presence or absence of other underlying medical disorders.

Symptoms of malignancy-associated anemia may range from weakness, pallor, and **fatigue** to shortness of breath and increased heart rate. Symptoms of anemia can compromise a patient's ability to tolerate treatment, and may severely interfere with activities of daily living. Anemia may be particularly problematic in older individuals with cancer. The incidence and severity of anemia tends to increase as the cancer progresses.

Blood is comprised of three major cell types: white blood cells, which help the body fight infection; platelets, which help the blood to clot when necessary; and red blood cells, which transport oxygen from the lungs to the tissues in the body, and then transport carbon dioxide from those tissues back to the lungs. This exchange is enabled by the most important component of red blood cells—the protein called hemoglobin that binds easily to oxygen and carbon dioxide.

Red blood cells are produced in the bone marrow through a process called erythropoiesis. When the bone marrow functions normally, it continuously replaces red blood cells to maintain a normal level that allows for adequate oxygenation of the tissues. The hormone erythropoietin stimulates red blood cell production and sends a message to the bone marrow to increase production when oxygen levels in the body are low. This mechanism is often impaired in patients with cancer.

Causes

The causes of anemia are multifactorial, and often those factors act in conjunction with one another. Generally, anemia may result from a direct effect of a cancerous tumor, or from an indirect effect of the tumor. The cancer process may directly cause anemia through two main mechanisms: blood loss or bone marrow replacement. However, most cases of anemia in cancer patients result from the indirect effects of the cancer.

Direct effects of the tumor

Anemia is a frequent complication of cancers due to bleeding. Cancers of the head and neck, the gastrointestinal and genitourinary system, and the cervix are frequently associated with endogenous bleeding, or bleeding that occurs outside the body. Bleeding occasionally develops within the tumor itself, particularly in **sarcomas**, melanomas, and ovarian and liver carcinomas.

A second direct cause of anemia in cancer is bone marrow replacement, which inhibits the body's ability to appropriately produce red blood cells. Certain cancers, such as acute leukemia, **lymphoma** and **myeloma**, directly suppress bone marrow function, thereby causing anemia. Other types of cancer, such as prostate or **breast cancer**, often spread to the bone marrow, inhibiting red blood cell production by actually replacing the bone marrow itself.

Indirect effects of the tumor

Anemia of chronic disease, also called anemia of malignancy, is the most common type of anemia seen in individuals with cancer. It is a diagnosis made only after other possible causes are ruled out and if very specific conditions are met. The presence of low levels of iron

KEY TERMS

Cytokines—Non-antibody proteins released by a group of cells that act as mediators in immune response.

Cytomegalovirus (CMV)—A virus sometimes present in blood products.

Erythropoiesis—The process in which red blood cells are produced in the bone marrow.

Erythropoietin—A hormone produced by the kidneys that stimulates the production of red blood cells in a process called erythropoiesis.

Hematocrit—The volume percentage of red blood cells in whole blood.

Hemoglobin—A protein in red blood cells that transports oxygen to tissues.

coupled with normal levels of storage iron helps distinguish anemia of chronic disease from iron deficiency anemia. Factors that cause anemia of chronic disease are not entirely clear. However, it is believed that cytokines (non-antibody proteins) produced by the tumor reduce production of and impair responsiveness to erythropoietin. Typically, this type of anemia develops slowly. Rapid development of anemia may indicate another cause.

Treatments used to manage cancer have been implicated in the development of anemia in cancer patients. **Radiation therapy** to large areas of bone marrow, as in the hip area, may suppress bone marrow function and lead to anemia. **Chemotherapy** can also cause bone marrow suppression, some drugs by specifically targeting red blood cell production. Studies have shown that 10 to 40% of patients taking **cisplatin** develop significant anemia. Cisplatin, a chemotherapy drug with potentially toxic effects to the kidneys, is believed to reduce the production of the hormone erythropoietin in the kidneys. Although most treatment-induced bone marrow suppression is short term, there is some evidence to support the possibility of long-term problems with blood cell production.

Treatment can increase the risk of anemia in other ways. Chemotherapy, for example, causes bone marrow suppression that may reduce the immune system's ability to fight off opportunistic infection. The resulting infections can impact the bone marrow's functioning, possibly leading to the development of anemia.

Hemolytic anemia is a type of anemia in which the red blood cell has a shortened life span (normal life span is 90-120 days). Because the bone marrow is not able to compensate by producing more red blood cells, anemia results. Abnormalities in the red blood cells may be intrinsic or may be caused by environmental factors such as auto-antibodies to red blood cells or damage from chemotherapy.

Although one factor may have a greater influence, it is important to realize that several factors may be causing anemia. For example, approximately 70% of patients with multiple myeloma are anemic at the time of diagnosis. Anemia in these cases is caused by a combination of mechanisms including bone marrow replacement with cancer cells, bone marrow suppression from chemotherapy, and impaired production of erythropoietin.

Treatments

Treatment of the anemia is directed at the underlying cause. In many cases, treating or removing the cancer corrects the red blood cell deficit. Management of autoimmune hemolytic anemia, which can be associated with **chronic lymphocytic leukemia**, may range from the administration of **corticosteroids** to the surgical removal of the spleen. More commonly, cancer-related anemias are treated with blood transfusions and/or a drug called epoetin alfa.

Blood transfusions

Blood transfusions have been the principle treatment for anemia for many years. Until the 1960s, only whole blood was given. Then, methods of separating whole blood were devised, allowing only particular components, such as platelets, red blood cells, or plasma, to be transfused.

Blood transfusions are not without risk, and must be used carefully. Many patients react to the white blood cell antigens by developing a **fever**. This is so common that patients are routinely premedicated to prevent fever from developing. Individuals with long-term transfusion needs, such as patients with leukemia, may be given blood products with a reduced number of white blood cells to reduce the risk of sensitization to transfused blood.

Cytomegalovirus (CMV) is a virus that may be present in blood products. Although it has no effect on individuals with normally functioning immune systems, cancer patients often have a diminished ability to fight infection. These patients may be at risk for CMV if they are CMV negative and receive CMV-positive blood.

Transfusion-associated **graft-versus-host disease** (TA-GvHD) is another risk factor associated with blood transfusions in cancer patients. Although it is very rare, it is often fatal. With TA-GvHD, the patient's immune system does not recognize the white blood cells in the donor blood as "nonself." The donor white blood cells, however, recognize the patient as "nonself," and an immune-mediated reaction ensues. To prevent this reaction in at-risk patients, blood may be irradiated prior to transfusion.

Epoetin alfa

As mentioned previously, erythropoietin is a protein produced in the kidneys that stimulates red blood cell production. Using DNA technology, this hormone has been replicated to create the drug epoetin alfa for the treatment of anemia in select cancer patients. (The drug is also called **erythropoietin.**) The use of this drug in the cancer setting has shown great promise, both in the treatment of cancer-related anemia, and in the reduction in the need for blood transfusion.

However, epoetin alfa therapy is not advisable for everyone. This drug is not recommended for use in cancer-related anemia caused by bleeding, hemolysis, or iron deficiencies. Nor is it recommended for patients with hypertension or albumin sensitivity. Because no human studies are available to determine its effect on a fetus, women taking epoetin alfa should take measures to prevent pregnancy.

Cancer patients with anemia who are undergoing chemotherapy may benefit from this drug. Studies have shown an increased hematocrit (the volume percentage of red blood cells in whole blood) level and a decreased need for blood transfusions after the first month of therapy in this population. Epoetin alfa is injected three times a week, and throughout therapy, blood cell counts are monitored closely.

Resources

BOOKS

Abeloff, M., et al. (Eds.) "Hematopoietic Dysfunction by Hematologic Lineage." In *Clinical Oncology, 2nd Ed.* New York: Churchill Livingstone Publishers, 2000.

Lee, G. and C. Bennett (Eds.) "Nonmetastatic Effects of Cancer: Other Systems." In *Cecil Textbook of Medicine, 21st Ed.* Philadelphia, PA: W. B. Saunders Co., 2000.

Lee, G., et al. (Eds.) *Wintrobe's Clinical Hematology.* Baltimore, MD: Williams & Wilkins Publishing, 1999.

Varricchio, C.,(Ed.) "Cytopenias." In *A Cancer Source Book for Nurses* Atlanta: Jones and Bartlett Publishers, 1997, pp.161-73.

PERIODICALS

Frenkel, E.P., et al. "Anemia of Malignancy."*Hematology Oncology Clinics of North America* (August 1996): 861-873.

Moniterno, A.R. "Anemia of Cancer."*Hematology Oncology Clinics of North America* (April 1996): 345-363.

Rytting, M., et al. "Hematologic Complications of Cancer."*Hematology Oncology Clinics of North America* (April 1996): 366-376.

Wuest, D. "Transfusion and Stem Cell Support in Cancer Treatment."*Hematology Oncology Clinics of North America* (April 1996): 397-429.

Tamara Brown, R.N.

Angiogenesis inhibitors

Definition

Angiogenesis inhibitors are medicines that stop the formation of new blood vessels in and around cancerous tumors.

Description

Angiogenesis inhibitors are a group of medicines that prevent the formation of tiny new blood vessels to the area of cancerous tumors. Angiogenesis refers to the ability of cancer cells to form new blood vessels that invade the tumor and other surrounding areas. Tumors need a blood supply to nourish the cancer cells; as tumors grow they must constantly form new blood vessels. These blood vessels are also used by the cancer cells to metastasize or spread the cancerous cells from one area to the next. Angiogenesis inhibitors are important because the scientific theory is that if one can remove and/or prevent the formation of new blood vessels in the tumors, the cancer cells will not be able to grow any further. This could cause the tumors to stay the same size or shrink. In addition, it may be possible to prevent the tumors from spreading by cutting off their ability to invade other surrounding areas through these newly formed blood vessels. There are a few drugs today thought to work as angiogenesis inhibitors, such as **thalidomide**. Additional agents being studied in ongoing oncology **clinical trials**.

Nancy J. Beaulieu, RPh.,BCOP

Angiography

Definition

Angiography is the x-ray study of the blood vessels. An angiogram uses a radiopaque substance, or dye, to make the blood vessels visible under **x ray**. Arteriography is a type of angiography that involves the study of the arteries.

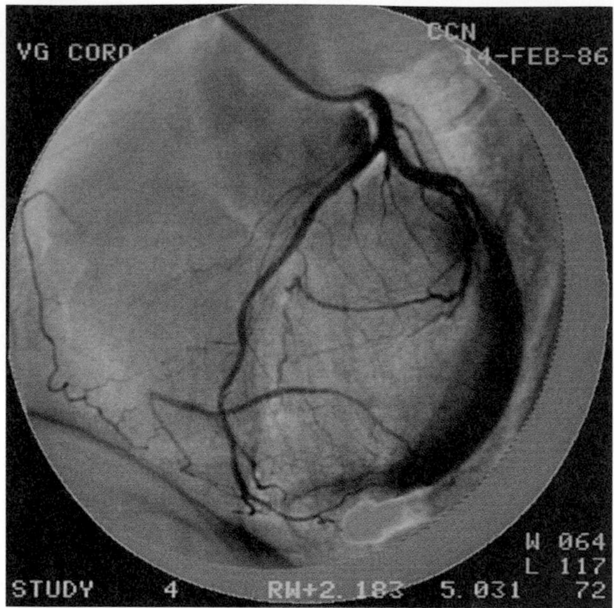

An angiogram of a coronary artery. *(© CNRI/Phototake NYC. Reproduced by permission.)*

Purpose

Angiography is used to detect abnormalities or blockages in the blood vessels (called occlusions) throughout the circulatory system and in some organs. The procedure is commonly used to: identify atherosclerosis; diagnose heart disease; evaluate kidney function and detect kidney cysts or tumors; detect an aneurysm (an abnormal bulge of an artery that can rupture and lead to hemorrhage), tumor, blood clot, or arteriovenous malformations (abnormal tangles of arteries and veins) in the brain; and to diagnose problems with the retina of the eye. It is also used to give surgeons an accurate "map" of the heart prior to open-heart surgery, or of the brain prior to neurosurgery.

Precautions

Patients with kidney disease or injury may suffer further kidney damage from the contrast mediums used for angiography. Patients who have blood clotting problems, have a known allergy to contrast mediums, or are allergic to iodine, a component of some contrast mediums, may also not be suitable candidates for an angiography procedure. Because x rays carry risks of ionizing radiation exposure to the fetus, pregnant women are also advised to avoid this procedure.

Description

Angiography is usually performed at a hospital by a trained radiologist and assisting technician or nurse. It takes place in an x-ray or fluoroscopy suite, and for most types of angiograms, the patient's vital signs will be monitored throughout the procedure.

Angiography requires the injection of a contrast dye that makes the blood vessels visible to x ray. Tissues such as bones and blood vessels absorb x rays as they pass through the body. They show up with a clear, white outline when captured on film. The dye is injected through a procedure known as arterial puncture. The puncture is usually made in the groin area, inside elbow, or neck. The site is cleaned with an antiseptic agent and injected with a local anesthetic. First, a small incision is made in the skin to help the needle pass. A needle containing an inner wire called a stylet is inserted through the skin into the artery. When the radiologist has punctured the artery with the needle, the stylet is removed and replaced with another long wire called a guide wire. It is normal for blood to spout out of the needle before the guide wire is inserted.

The guide wire is fed through the outer needle into the artery and to the area that requires angiographic study. A fluoroscopic screen that displays a view of the patient's vascular system is used to pilot the wire to the correct location. Once it is in position, the needle is removed and a catheter is slid over the length of the guide wire until it to reaches the area of study. The guide wire is removed and the catheter is left in place in preparation for the injection of the contrast medium, or dye.

Depending on the type of angiography procedure being performed, the contrast medium is either injected by hand with a syringe or is mechanically injected with an automatic injector connected to the catheter. An automatic injector is used frequently because it is able to propel a large volume of dye very quickly to the angiogram site. The patient is warned that the injection will start, and instructed to remain very still. The injection causes some mild to moderate discomfort. Possible side effects or reactions include headache, dizziness, irregular heartbeat, nausea, warmth, burning sensation, and chest pain, but they usually last only momentarily. To view the area of study from different angles or perspectives, the patient may be asked to change positions several times, and subsequent dye injections may be administered. During any injection, the patient or the camera may move.

Throughout the dye injection procedure, x-ray pictures and/or fluoroscopic pictures (moving x rays) will be taken. Because of the high pressure of arterial blood flow, the dye will dissipate through the patient's system quickly, so pictures must be taken in rapid succession. An automatic film changer is used because the manual changing of x-ray plates can eat up valuable time.

Once the x rays are complete, the catheter is slowly and carefully removed from the patient. Pressure is applied to the site with a sandbag or other weight for 10 to 20 minutes in order for clotting to take place and the arterial puncture to reseal itself. A pressure bandage is then applied.

Most angiograms follow the general procedures outlined above, but vary slightly depending on the area of the vascular system being studied. In addition to x rays, technological advances have allowed physicians to use other diagnostic tools for angiography, such as **computed tomography** (CT) scans and **magnetic resonance imaging** (MRI). A variety of common angiography procedures are outlined below:

Cerebral angiography

Cerebral angiography is used to detect aneurysms, blood clots, and other vascular irregularities in the brain. The catheter is inserted into the femoral artery (the main artery of the thigh) or the carotid artery in the neck, and the injected contrast medium travels through the blood vessels of the brain. Patients frequently experience headache, warmth, or a burning sensation in the head or neck during the injection portion of the procedure. A cerebral angiogram takes two to four hours to complete.

Coronary angiography

Coronary angiography is administered by a cardiologist with training in radiology or, occasionally, by a radiologist. The arterial puncture is typically given in the femoral artery, and the cardiologist uses a guide wire and catheter to perform a contrast injection and x-ray series on the coronary arteries (arteries that supply the heart with oxygenated blood). The catheter may also be placed in the left ventricle to examine the mitral and aortic valves of the heart. If the cardiologist requires a view of the right ventricle of the heart or of the tricuspid or pulmonic valves, the catheter will be inserted through a large vein and guided into the right ventricle. The catheter also serves the purpose of monitoring blood pressures in these different locations inside the heart. The angiogram procedure takes several hours, depending on the complexity of the procedure. Some cardiologists prefer to use a compbination of CT and x-ray angiography to study the heart.

Pulmonary angiography

Pulmonary, or lung, angiography is performed to evaluate blood circulation to the lungs. It is also considered the most accurate diagnostic test for detecting a pulmonary embolism, although some physicians prefer CT or MRI scans because they are less invasive. New technology has improved the accuracy of these alternative methods. The procedure differs from cerebral and coronary angiograms in that the guide wire and catheter are inserted into a vein instead of an artery, and are guided up through the chambers of the heart and into the pulmonary artery. Throughout the procedure, the patient's vital signs are monitored to ensure that the catheter does not cause arrhythmias, or irregular heartbeats. The contrast medium is then injected into the pulmonary artery where it circulates through the lung capillaries. The test typically takes up to 90 minutes.

Kidney angiography

Patients with chronic renal disease or injury can suffer further damage to their kidneys from the contrast medium used in a kidney angiogram, yet they often require the test to evaluate kidney function. These patients should be well-hydrated with a intravenous saline drip before the procedure, and may benefit from available medications (e.g., dopamine) that help to protect the kidney from further injury due to contrast agents. During a kidney angiogram, the guide wire and catheter are inserted into the femoral artery in the groin area and advanced through the abdominal aorta, the main artery in the abdomen, and into the renal arteries. The procedure will take approximately one hour.

Fluorescein angiography

Fluorescein angiography is used to diagnose retinal problems and circulatory disorders. It is typically conducted as an outpatient procedure. The patient's pupils are dilated with eye drops and he rests his chin and forehead against a bracing apparatus to keep it still. Sodium fluorescein dye is then injected with a syringe into a vein in the patient's arm. The dye will travel through the patient's body and into the blood vessels of the eye. The procedure does not require x rays. Instead, a rapid series of close-up photographs of the patient's eyes are taken, one set immediately after the dye is injected, and a second set approximately 20 minutes later once the dye has moved through the patient's vascular system. The entire procedure takes up to one hour.

Celiac and mesenteric angiography

Celiac and mesenteric angiography involves x-ray exploration of the celiac and mesenteric arteries, arterial branches of the abdominal aorta that supply blood to the abdomen and digestive system. The test is commonly used to detect aneurysm, thrombosis, and signs of ischemia in the celiac and mesenteric arteries, and to locate the source of gastrointestinal bleeding. It is also used in the diagnosis of a number of conditions, including portal hypertension and cirrhosis. The procedure can take up to three hours, depending on the number of blood vessels studied.

KEY TERMS

Arteriosclerosis—A chronic condition characterized by thickening and hardening of the arteries and the buildup of plaque on the arterial walls. Arteriosclerosis can slow or impair blood circulation.

Carotid artery—An artery located in the neck.

Catheter—A long, thin, flexible tube used in angiography to inject contrast material into the arteries.

Cirrhosis—A condition characterized by the destruction of healthy liver tissue. A cirrhotic liver is scarred and cannot break down the proteins in the bloodstream. Cirrhosis is associated with portal hypertension.

Computed tomography (CT)—A non-invasive diagnostic tool radiologists may use instead of x-ray angiography.

Embolism—A blood clot, air bubble, or clot of foreign material that travels and blocks the flow of blood in an artery. When blood supply to a tissue or organ is blocked by an embolism, infarction, or death of the tissue the artery feeds, occurs. Without immediate and appropriate treatment, an embolism can be fatal.

Femoral artery—An artery located in the groin area that is the most frequently accessed site for arterial puncture in angiography.

Fluorescein dye—An orange dye used to illuminate the blood vessels of the retina in fluorescein angiography.

Fluoroscopic screen—A fluorescent screen which displays moving x rays of the body. Fluoroscopy allows the radiologist to visualize the guide wire and catheter he is moving through the patient's artery.

Guide wire—A wire that is inserted into an artery to guide a catheter to a certain location in the body.

Ischemia—A lack of normal blood supply to a organ or body part because of blockages or constriction of the blood vessels.

Magnetic resonance imaging (MRI)—A non-invasive diagnostic tool radiologists may use instead of x-ray angiography. MRI scans use magnetic waves to create a picture of structures in the body.

Necrosis—Cellular or tissue death; skin necrosis may be caused by multiple, consecutive doses of radiation from fluoroscopic or x-ray procedures.

Plaque—Fatty material that is deposited on the inside of the arterial wall.

Portal hypertension—A condition caused by cirrhosis of the liver. It is characterized by impaired or reversed blood flow from the portal vein to the liver, an enlarged spleen, and dilated veins in the esophagus and stomach.

Portal vein thrombosis—The development of a blood clot in the vein that brings blood into the liver. Untreated portal vein thrombosis causes portal hypertension.

Splenoportography

A splenoportograph is a variation of an angiogram that involves the injection of contrast medium directly into the spleen to view the splenic and portal veins. It is used to diagnose blockages in the splenic vein and portal vein thrombosis and to assess the strength and location of the vascular system prior to liver transplantation.

Most angiography procedures are typically paid for by major medical insurance. Patients should check with their individual insurance plans to determine their coverage.

Preparation

Patients undergoing an angiogram are advised to stop eating and drinking eight hours prior to the procedure. They must remove all jewelry before the procedure and change into a hospital gown. If the arterial puncture is to be made in the armpit or groin area, shaving may be required. A sedative may be administered to relax the patient for the procedure. An IV line will also be inserted into a vein in the patient's arm before the procedure begins in case medication or blood products are required during the angiogram.

Prior to the angiography procedure, patients will be briefed on the details of the test, the benefits and risks, and the possible complications involved, and asked to sign an informed consent form.

Aftercare

Because life-threatening internal bleeding is a possible complication of an arterial puncture, an overnight stay in the hospital is sometimes recommended following an angiography procedure, particularly with cerebral and coronary angiograms. If the procedure is performed on an outpatient basis, the patient is typically kept under close observation for a period of six to twelve hours before being released. If the arterial puncture was performed in the femoral artery, the patient will be instructed to keep his leg straight and relatively immobile during the observation period. The patient's blood pressure and vital signs will be monitored and the puncture site observed closely. Pain medication may be prescribed if the patient is experiencing discomfort from the puncture, and a cold pack is applied to the site to reduce swelling. It is normal for the puncture site to be sore and bruised for several weeks. The patient may also develop a hematoma, a hard mass created by the blood vessels broken during the procedure. Hematomas should be watched carefully, as they may indicate continued bleeding of the arterial puncture site. Patients may be given intravenous fluids and may experience a frequent need to urinate due to the x-ray dye.

Angiography patients are also advised to enjoy a few days of rest and relaxation after the procedure in order to avoid placing any undue stress on the arterial puncture. Patients who experience continued bleeding or abnormal swelling of the puncture site, sudden dizziness, chest pains, chills, nausea, headaches, or numbness in the days following an angiography procedure should seek medical attention immediately.

Patients undergoing a fluorescein angiography should not drive or expose their eyes to direct sunlight for 12 hours following the procedure.

Risks

Because angiography involves puncturing an artery, internal bleeding or hemorrhage are possible complications of the test. As with any invasive procedure, infection of the puncture site or bloodstream is also a risk, but this is rare.

A stroke or heart attack may be triggered by an angiogram if blood clots or plaque on the inside of the arterial wall are dislodged by the catheter and form a blockage in the blood vessels or artery. The heart may also become irritated by the movement of the catheter through its chambers during pulmonary and coronary angiography procedures, and arrhythmias may develop.

Patients who develop an allergic reaction to the contrast medium used in angiography may experience a variety of symptoms, including swelling, difficulty breathing, heart failure, or a sudden drop in blood pressure. If the patient is aware of the allergy before the test is administered, certain medications can be administered at that time to counteract the reaction.

QUESTIONS TO ASK THE DOCTOR

- Did you see any abnormalities?
- How long will I need to stay in the hospital? How many days until I can resume normal activities?
- When can I resume any medications that were stopped?
- What future care will I need?

Angiography involves minor exposure to radiation through the x rays and fluoroscopic guidance used in the procedure. Unless the patient is pregnant, or multiple radiological or fluoroscopic studies are required, the small dose of radiation incurred during a single procedure poses little risk. However, multiple studies requiring fluoroscopic exposure that are conducted in a short time period have been known to cause skin necrosis (cell death) in some individuals. This risk can be minimized by careful monitoring and documentation of cumulative radiation doses administered to these patients.

Normal results

The results of an angiogram or arteriogram depend on the artery or organ system being examined. Generally, test results should display a normal and unimpeded flow of blood through the vascular system. Fluorescein angiography should result in no leakage of fluorescein dye through the retinal blood vessels.

Abnormal results

Abnormal results of an angiography may display a restricted blood vessel or arterial blood flow (ischemia) or an irregular placement or location of blood vessels. The results of an angiography vary widely by the type of procedure performed, and should be interpreted and explained to the patient by a trained radiologist.

Resources

BOOKS

Baim, Donald S., and William Grossman, eds. *Grossman's Cardiac Catheterization, Angiography and Intervention,* 6th ed. Philadelphia: Lippincott Williams & Wilkins, 2000.

OTHER

Angiography Fact Sheet. Beth Israel Hospital, 2001. 22 June 2001 <http://radiology.bidmc.harvard.edu/kinds_of_exams/angio/angio.html>.

Coronary Angiography Fact Sheet. American Heart Association, 2001. 22 June 2001 <http://www.americanheart.org/Heart_and_Stroke_A_Z_Guide/corang.html>.

Angiography Overview. Northwestern Memorial Hospital, 2001. 22 June 2001 <www.nmh.org/health_info/hlc.html>.

Coronary Angiography and angioplasty. Video. Timonium, MD: Milner-Fenwick, 1999.

Paula Anne Ford-Martin

Anorexia

Definition

Anorexia is characterized by a loss of appetite or lack of desire to eat.

Description

Anorexia is common in cancer patients with reported incidence between 15% and 40%. Primary anorexia is especially prevalent in patients with advanced malignancy, and is frequently a side effect of cancer treatments. Sometimes, early symptoms may remain undiagnosed, or will be masked by a more generalized wasting of the body from chronic disease, known as cachexia.

When patients experience appetite loss, decreased energy consumption will subsequently lead to **weight loss**. When inadequate calories are consumed, the body may become weaker and less able to tolerate cancer therapies. As body weight decreases, cachexia sets in, and a general failure to thrive may make it more difficult to fight off illness and infection. A poor response to cancer treatments, reduced quality of life, and death may result from substantial weight loss. The spiraling effect of a patient's reluctance to eat is a source of frequent anxiety for caregivers. Weight loss due to anorexia may be temporary or may continue at a life-threatening pace if the patient continues to consume inadequate energy to sustain bodyweight.

Causes

It is normal for a patient to consume less energy when not as active. It is also natural to lose interest in food when individuals are seriously ill. However, it is essential in anorexic patients to consider whether the loss of appetite is the result of a natural disinterest in eating (primary anorexia), or is due to some reversible cause (secondary anorexia).

Secondary anorexia may be a result of:

- nausea with or without fear of vomiting after food consumption
- fatigue
- constipation
- sores in the mouth or mouth pain
- candidiasis
- unappetizing food or change in food preference due to cancer-related treatments
- **depression**
- odors in the environment, or heightened sensitivity to odors as a result of cancer-related treatments
- early satiation
- metabolic causes such as **hypercalcemia** and uremia
- **radiation therapy** or **chemotherapy**
- drugs such as **antibiotics** or drugs that can cause nausea

Special concerns

In order to allow normal tissue repair following aggressive cancer therapies, patients require adequate energy and macronutrients in the form of protein, carbohydrates, and fat. Inadequate consumption of food and/or poor nutrition may impair the ability of a patient to tolerate a specific therapy. If a low tolerance to therapy necessitates a decrease in dose, the therapy's effectiveness could be compromised. Wound healing may also be impaired with poor nutrition and inadequate energy intake.

Individuals who experience pain, nausea, or **diarrhea** due to the side effects of radiation and chemotherapy may want to discuss treatments options with their doctor to ease these side effects.

Treatments

Dietary tips for managing anorexia

- Serve food when the patient is hungry. A microwave oven often helps.
- Have the patient eat small meals every one to two hours, or time meals corresponding to when the patient feels best (typically early in the day).
- If only a little food is consumed by the patient, it should ideally be high in protein and calories. Avoid empty calories (i.e. foods without protein and nutrients).

- Add extra calories and protein to foods with the use of butter, skim milk powder, commercially prepared protein powder, honey, or brown sugar.
- Try to tempt the patient with tiny portions on small plates.
- Serve food in an attractive manner.
- Food is more likely to be eaten if it is served at frequent intervals unrelated to standard meal times.
- Avoid strong aromas if the patient finds them bothersome.
- Avoid liquids with meals to decrease problems of early satiety
- A small alcoholic drink of the patient's choice may help unless contraindicated.
- Consider flavors, consistency and quantity of food when preparing meals.
- Encourage eating with friends or family members; a meal in a social setting may help the patient to eat.
- Stimulate appetite with light exercise.
- Treat any underlying cause and, if a particular drug appears to be the cause, modify drug regimen.
- Have the patient take medications with high-calories fluids, i.e. commercial liquid supplements unless medication necessitates an empty stomach.

Often, patients may experience difficulty with eating due to upper gastrointestinal blockage such as problems with swallowing, esophageal narrowing, tumor, stomach weakness, paralysis, or other conditions that preclude normal food intake. In those circumstances, enteral nutrition may be administered through a tube into the gastrointestinal tract via the nose, or through surgically placed tubes into the stomach or intestines. If the gastrointestinal tract is working and will not be affected by the cancer treatments, then enteral support by feeding directly into the gut is preferable. Parenteral nutrition (most often an infusion into a vein) can be used if the gut is not functioning properly or if there are other reasons that prevent enteral feeding.

An appetite stimulant may be given such as **megestrol acetate** or **dexamethasone**. In **clinical trials**, both these medications appear to have similar and effective appetite stimulating effects with megestrol acetate having a slightly better toxicity profile. **Fluoxymesterone** has shown inferior efficacy and an unfavorable toxicity profile.

Alternative and complementary therapies

Depression may affect approximately 15-25% of cancer patients, particularly if the prognosis for recovery is poor. If anorexia is due to depression, there are antidepressant choices available through a physician. Counseling may be also be sought through a psychologist or psychiatrist to deal with depression.

KEY TERMS

Anorexia—A condition frequently observed in cancer patients characterized by a loss of appetite or desire to eat.

Cancer—A term for diseases in which abnormal cells divide without control. Cancer cells can invade nearby tissues and can spread through the bloodstream and lymphatic system to other parts of the body.

Candidiasis—A yeast-like fungal infection occuring on the skin or mucous membranes, i.e. mouth.

Chemotherapy—Chemotherapy kills cancer cells using drugs taken orally or by needle in a vein or muscle. It is referred to as a systemic treatment due to fact that it travels through the bloodstream and kills cancer cells outside the small intestine.

Hypercalcemia—A high calcium blood concentration above 10.5 milligrams per deciliter of blood. Increased gastrointestinal tract absorption or increased intake of calcium may lead to hypercalcemia.

Malignant (also malignancy)—Meaning cancerous; a tumor or growth that often destroys surrounding tissue and spreads to other parts of the body.

Radiation therapy—Also called radiotherapy; uses high-energy x-rays to kill cancer cells.

Satiation—A feeling of fullness or satisfaction during or after food intake.

Uremia—An excess of nitrogenous substances in the blood that are toxic and usually excreted by the kidneys.

St. John's Wort has been used as a herbal remedy for treatment of depression, but it and prescription antidepressants is a dangerous combination that may cause symptoms such as nausea, weakness, and may cause one to become incoherent. It is important to check with a dietitian or doctor before taking nutritional supplements or alternative therapies because they may interfere with cancer medications or treatments.

Resources

BOOKS

Keane, Maureen et al. *What to Eat If You Have Cancer: A Guide to Adding Nutritional Therapy to Your Treatment*

Plan. Lincolnwood, IL: National Textbook Company/Contemporary Publishing Group, 1996.

Nixon, Daniel W., M.D., Jane A. Zanca, and Vincent T. DeVita, *The Cancer Recovery Eating Plan: The Right Foods to Help Fuel Your Recovery.* New York:Times Books, 1996.

Quillin, Patrick and Noreen Quillin. *Beating Cancer With Nutrition-Revised.* Sun Lakes, AZ: Bookworld Services, 2001.

PERIODICALS

Kant, Ashima et al. "A Prospective Study of Diet Quality and Mortality in Women." *JAMA* 283(16) (2000): 2109-2115.

Loprinzi, C.L. et al. "Randomized comparison of megestrol acetate versus dexamethasone versus fluoxymesterone for the treatment of cancer anorexia/cachexia." *Journal of Clinical Oncology* 17(10) (1999): 3299-306.

Singletary, Keith. "Diet, Natural Products and Cancer Chemoprevention." *Journal of Nutrition* 130 (2000): 465S-466S.

Willett, Walter C. "Diet and cancer." *The Oncologist* 5(5) (2000): 393-404.

ORGANIZATIONS

National Center for Complementary and Alternative Medicine (NCCAM), 31 Center Dr., Room #5B-58, Bethesda, MD 20892-2182. (800) NIH-NCAM, Fax (301) 495-4957. <http://nccam.nih.gov>.

The National Cancer Institute (NCI). For information contact the Public Inquiries Office: Building, 31, Room 10A31, 31 Center Drive, MSC 2580, Betheseda, MD 20892-2580 USA. (301) 435-3848, 1-800-4-CANCER. <http://cancer.gov/publications> , <http://cancernet.nci.nih.gov>.

American Institute for Cancer Research, 1759 R Street N.W., Washington, D.C. 20009. (800) 843-8114 or (202) 328-7744. <http://www.aicr.org, e-mail:support @aicr.org>.

Crystal Heather Kaczkowski, MSc.

Anoscopy

Definition

Anoscopy is a diagnostic procedure that allows a gastroenterologist or other physician to visually examine the rectum, anus, and anal canal.

Purpose

Doctors use anoscopy to diagnose **rectal cancer** and cancer of the anus. This procedure can also help the doctor:

- detect any lesions that could not be felt during a digital examination
- determine whether squamous cell carcinomas involving lymph nodes in or near the groin (inguinal lymph nodes) originated in the genital area or in or near the anus or rectum
- confirm the source of malignancies that have spread to the anorectal area from other parts of the body

Doctors also perform anoscopy to determine whether a patient has hemorrhoids or anal:

- growths or nodules (polyps)
- ulcer-like grooves (fissures)
- inflammation
- infection

Description

After removing underwear, the patient bends forward over the examining table or lies on one side with knees drawn up to the chest. The doctor performs a digital examination to make sure no tumor or other abnormality will obstruct the passage of a slender lubricated tube (anoscope). As the doctor gently guides the anoscope a few inches into the rectum, the patient is told to bear down as though having a bowel movement, then relax.

By tensing and relaxing, the patient makes it easier for the doctor to insert the anoscope, and discover growths in the lining of the rectum that could not be detected during the digital examination.

Directing a light into the anoscope gives the doctor a clear view of any tears or other irregularities in the lower anus or rectum. A doctor who suspects that a patient may have cancer will remove tissue for **biopsy** in the course of this procedure.

Slowly withdrawing the anoscope allows the doctor to thoroughly inspect the entire anal canal. As the procedure is being performed, the doctor explains what is happening, and why the patient feels pressure.

Removing tissue samples for biopsy can pinch, but anoscopy does not usually cause pain. Patients do experience the sensation of needing to have a bowel movement.

Preparation

The rectum should be emptied of fecal matter (stool) before the procedure is performed. The doctor may suggest using:

- a laxative,
- an enema,
- or some other preparation

to clear the rectum.

Aftercare

As soon as the procedure is completed, the doctor can tell the patient whether the results are normal or abnormal, and the patient can resume normal activities.

KEY TERMS

Anorectal—Pertaining to the anus and rectum

Anus—The opening of the rectum through which feces leave the body

Rectum—The portion of the large intestine where feces is stored before leaving the body

Risks

Removing tissue for biopsy may cause a little bleeding and some slight pain, but there are no significant risks associated with anoscopy.

Normal results

A normal anoscopy reveals no evidence of:

- tumor
- tissue irregularities
- polyps
- fissures
- hemorrhoids
- inflammation
- infection

or other abnormalities. The size, color, and shape of the anal canal look like they should.

Abnormal results

Abnormal results of anoscopy can indicate the presence of:

- cancer
- abscesses
- polyps
- inflammation
- infection
- fissures
- hemorrhoids

See Also Anal cancer; Digital rectal examination

Resources

BOOKS

Cahill, Matthew. *Everything You Need To Know About Medical Treatments.* Springhouse, PA: Springhouse Corporatioon, 1996.

QUESTIONS TO ASK THE DOCTOR

- Why do you want me to have an anoscopy?
- How long will this procedure take?
- What will the results of this test tell you?

OTHER

Anoscopy <http://www.thriveonline.oxygen.com/medical/library/article/003890.html>. 14 May 2001.

Maureen Haggerty

Antiandrogens

Definition

Antiandrogens, including flutamide (brand name Eulexin or Euflex), bicalutamide (brand name Casodex), and nilutamide (brand name Nilandron), are medicines used in the treatment of advanced **prostate cancer**.

Purpose

Antiandrogens are approved by the Food and Drug Administration (FDA) for the treatment of prostate gland cancer that has spread to other areas of the body.

Purpose

Antiandrogen therapy stops or blocks the effect androgen presence has on tumor cells of the prostate. Antiandrogens are combined with either surgery or drug therapy that shuts down male hormone production. The common drugs used with antiandrogens are known as leuteinizing hormone releasing hormone (LHRH) agonists, referred to by the brand names Lupron or Zoladex. The LHRH agonists produce side effects that the antiandrogens can keep under control and the combination of the two agents has improved survival in prostate cancer patients.

Description

Antiandrogens will not cure prostate cancer, but they will help improve some of the disease's symptoms. They may also increase survival time.

KEY TERMS

Adrenal gland—Small organ located above the kidneys that produce hormones.

Food and Drug Administration—A government agency that oversees public safety in relation to drugs and medical devices. The FDA gives approval to pharmaceutical companies for commercial marketing of their products

LHRH agonists—Luteinizing hormone-releasing hormone drugs that initially stimulate the testes to make and release testosterone. With time, as the amount of testosterone in the blood rises, it stops the production of luteinizing hormone, which results in stopping overall production of testosterone.

Androgens are made naturally in the body and include the hormone **testosterone** and its related compound, dihydrotestosterone. The testes produce the majority of testosterone. The adrenal glands also produce androgens in smaller amounts. Prostate cancer cells grow due to normal levels of androgens produced by the body. Some patients have prostate tumors that are extra-sensitive to androgens in the blood. The androgens attach to receptors on the tumor cells and send a signal to the tumor cells causing them to grow and multiply. Antiandrogen drugs block the receptors on the prostate cancer cell that are sensitive to the androgen hormones. By blocking these receptors, known as androgen-receptors, the cancer cells cannot be instructed to grow and multiply. Antiandrogens also cause the body to decrease production of androgens and, as a result, their effects.

Recommended dosage

Flutamide

Flutamide is an oral capsule dosed at 250 mg three times a day in combination with the LHRH agonist or surgical removal of the testis.

Bicalutamide

Bicalutamide is an oral tablet dosed at 50 mg once a day in combination with the LHRH agonist. The dose may need to be decreased in patients with decreased liver function.

Nilutamide

Nilutamide is an oral tablet dosed at 300 mg once a day for 30 days then 150 mg once a day in combination with surgical removal of the testis.

Precautions

Although antiandrogens are primarily given to men, women taking them should avoid pregnancy. Antiandrogens block the male hormone called testosterone and, as a result, can adversely affect the developing fetus. Blood counts will be monitored while on antiandrogen therapy.

Side effects

The most common side effects from all antiandrogens are due to the decreased levels of hormones. These commonly include hot flashes, loss of sex drive, and impotence (the inability of males to have sexual intercourse).

Antiandrogens can cause mild nausea, vomiting, **diarrhea**, loss of appetite, enlarged breasts or breast tenderness, skin reactions, muscle aches, liver problems, blood in the urine and generalized pain and decrease in blood counts. Nilutamide may cause visual disturbances, with patients having difficulty with the dark. Rarely, lung problems have occurred due to nilutamide or bicalutamide, including cough and shortness of breath.

Use with caution in patients who are receiving the blood-thinning drug **warfarin** or the drugs **phenytoin** and theophylline. Combining these drugs with antiandrogen therapy may increase the effects or side effects of these agents.

Interactions

Patients should tell their doctors if they have a known allergic reaction to antiandrogens or any other medications or substances, such as foods and preservatives. Before taking any new medications, including nonprescription medications, **vitamins**, and herbal medications, the patients should notify their doctors.

Nancy J. Beaulieu, RPh., BCOP

Antibiotics

Definition

Antibiotics are drugs that are used to treat infections caused by bacteria and other organisms, including protozoa, parasites, and fungi.

Purpose

Many treatments for cancer destroy disease-fighting white blood cells, thereby reducing the body's ability to fight infection. For example, bladder, pulmonary, and urinary tract infections may occur with **chemotherapy**. Single-celled organisms called protozoa are rarely a problem for healthy individuals. However, they can cause serious infections in individuals with low white blood cell counts. Because of the dangers that infections present for cancer patients, antibiotic treatment often is initiated before the exact nature of the infection has been determined; instead, the choice of antibiotic may depend on the site of the infection and the organism that is likely to be the cause. Often, an antibiotic that kills a broad spectrum of bacteria is chosen and several antibiotics may be used together.

Description

The common antibiotics that are used during cancer treatment include:

- Atovaquone (Mapren): antiprotozoal drug used to prevent and treat a very serious type of **pneumonia** called *Pneumocystis carinii* pneumonia (PCP), in individuals who experience serious side effects with SMZ-TMP (Sulfamethoxazole/Trimethoprim, brand name Bactrim).
- Aztreonam (Azactam): monobactam antibiotic used to treat gram-negative bacterial infections of the urinary and lower respiratory tracts and the female organs, and infections that are present throughout the body (systemic infections or septicemia).
- Cefepime (Maxipime), ceftazidime (Ceptaz, Fortaz, Tazicef, Tazidime), and ceftriaxone sodium (Rocephin): members of a group of antibiotics called cephalosporins used to treat bacterial infections of the urinary and lower respiratory tracts, and infections of the skin, bones, joints, pelvis, and abdomen.
- Ciprofloxacin (Cipro): fluoroquinolone antibiotic used to treat certain gram-negative and gram-positive bacteria and some mycobacteria.
- Clindamycin phosphate (Cleocin): used to treat gram-positive and gram-negative bacterial infections and, in individuals who are allergic to sulfadiazine, toxoplasmosis caused by a parasitic protozoa.
- Gentamicin (gentamycin) sulfate (generic name product, Garamycin, G-Mycin, Jenamicin): aminoglycoside antibiotic used to treat serious infections by many gram-negative bacteria that cannot be treated with other medicines.
- Metronidazole hydrochloride (Flagyl, Metric 21, Metro I.V., Protostat): used for anaerobic bacteria and protozoa.
- Pentamidine (generic name product, Pentam 300): used to treat PCP if serious side effects develop with SMZ-TMP.
- Pyrimethamine (Daraprim): antiprotozoal medicine used together with sulfadiazine to treat toxoplasmosis; or in combination with other medicines for treating mild to moderate PCP, in individuals who cannot tolerate the standard treatment.
- Sulfadiazine (generic name product): sulfonamide antibiotic used with pyrimethamine to treat toxoplasmosis.
- Sulfamethoxazole-Trimethoprim (SMZ-TMP) (generic name product, Bactrim, Cofatrim Forte, Cotrim, Septra, Sulfatrim): the sulfonamide antibiotic, sulfamethoxazole, used in combination with trimethoprim, to prevent and treat PCP and bacterial infections, such as bronchitis and middle ear and urinary tract infections.
- Trimethoprim (generic name product, Proloprim, Trimpex): primarily used to prevent or treat urinary tract infections.
- Vancomycin hydrochloride (generic name product, Vancocin): glycopeptide antibiotic used to treat a variety of serious gram-positive bacterial infections for which other medicines are ineffective, including strains of *Staphylococcus* that are resistant to most oral antibiotics.

Most of these antibiotics kill bacteria by preventing them from making protein for their cell walls. Ciprofloxacin and metronidazole prevent bacteria from reproducing by interfering with their ability to make new DNA. All of these drugs are approved for prescription by the U.S. Food and Drug Administration.

Recommended dosage

Dosages of antibiotics depend on the individual, the infection that is being treated, and the presence of other medical conditions. For children, the dosage usually is based on body weight and is lower than the adult dosage. To be effective, an entire treatment with antibiotics must be completed, even if the symptoms of infection have disappeared. Furthermore, it is important to keep the level of antibiotic in the body at a constant level during treatment. Therefore, the drug should be taken on a regular schedule. If a dose is missed, it should be taken as soon as possible. If it is almost time for the next dose, the missed dose should be skipped. Doubling up doses is generally not recommended.

Average adult dosages of common antibiotics for cancer patients are as follows:

- Atovaquone: for PCP treatment, 750 mg oral suspension twice a day, or tablets three times per day, for 21 days; for PCP prevention, 1,500 mg oral suspension, once a day; must be taken with balanced meals.

- Aztreonam: 1–2 gm every 6–12 hours, injected into a vein, over a 20–60 minute-period.
- Cefepime: 500 mg to 2 gm, injected into a vein or muscle, every 8–12 hours for 7–10 days.
- Ceftazidime: 250 mg to 2 gm, injected into a vein or muscle, every 8–12 hours.
- Ceftriaxone: 1–2 gm, injected into a vein or muscle, every 24 hours.
- Ciprofloxacin: 500–750 mg of the tablet or suspension, every 12 hours, for 3–28 days, taken two hours after meals with 8 oz of water; bone and joint infections usually are treated for at least 4–6 weeks; 200–400 mg injected every 8–12 hours.
- Clindamycin: 150–300 mg of capsule or solution, every six hours; 300–600 mg every six to eight hours or 900 mg every eight hours, injected into a vein or muscle.
- Gentamicin: dosage determined by body weight, every 8–24 hours for at least 7–10 days, injected into a vein or muscle.
- Metronidazole: for bacterial infections, 7.5 mg per kg (3.4 mg per lb) of body weight up to a maximum of 1 gm, every six hours for at least seven days (capsules or tablets); 15 mg per kg (6.8 mg per lb) for the first dose, followed by half that dosage every six hours for at least seven days (injected into a vein); for protozoal infections caused by amebas, 500–750 mg of oral medicine, three times per day for 5–10 days; for trichomoniasis, 2 gm for one day or 250 mg three times per day for seven days (oral medicine); extended-release tablets for vaginal bacterial infections, 750 mg once a day for seven days.
- Pentamidine: for treating PCP, 4 mg per kg (1.8 mg per lb) of body weight, once per day for 14–21 days, injected into a vein over one to two hours, while lying down.
- Pyrimethamine: for toxoplasmosis, 25–200 mg tablets, taken with other medicine, for several weeks.
- Sulfadiazine: for bacterial and protozoal infections, 2–4 gm for the first dose, followed by 1 gm every four to six hours (tablets).
- SMZ-TMP: 800 mg of sulfamethoxazole and 160 mg of trimethoprim, (tablet or oral suspension), every 12 hours for bacterial infections and every 24 hours for prevention of PCP; dosage based on body weight for PCP treatment; injections based on body weight, every six, eight or 12 hours for bacterial infections and every six hours for PCP treatment.
- Trimethoprim: 100 mg tablet every 12 hours for 10 days; for prevention of urinary tract infections, once a day for a long period.
- Vancomycin: 7.5 mg per kg (3.4 mg per lb) of body weight, or 500 mg–1 gram, injected or taken orally, every 6–12 hours.

Precautions

Stomach or intestinal problems or colitis (inflammation of the colon) may affect the use of:

- Atovaquone
- Cephalosporins
- Clindamycin

Kidney or liver disease may affect the use of:

- Aztreonam
- Cefepime
- Ceftazidime
- Ciprofloxacin
- Clindamycin
- Gentamicin
- Metronidazole
- Pentamidine
- Pyrimethamine
- Sulfadiazine
- SMZ-TMP
- Trimethoprim
- Vancomycin

Central nervous system or seizure disorders may affect the use of:

- Ciprofloxacin
- Metronidazole
- Pyrimethamine

Anemia (low red blood cell count) or other blood disorders may affect the use of:

- Metronidazole
- Pentamidine
- Pyrimethamine
- Sulfadiazine
- SMZ-TMP
- Trimethoprim

Ciprofloxacin may not be suitable for individuals with tendinitis or with skin sensitivities to sunlight. Gentamicin may not be suitable for people with hearing problems, **myasthenia gravis**, or Parkinson's disease. Metronidazole may not be suitable for individuals with heart disease, oral or vaginal yeast infections, or a history of alcoholism. Pentamidine may not be suitable for individuals with heart disease, bleeding disorders, or low blood pressure. Pentamidine may affect blood sugar levels, making control of diabetes mellitus or hypoglycemia (low blood sugar) difficult. Vancomycin may not be appropriate for individuals with hearing problems.

Many antibiotics should not be taken during pregnancy or while breast-feeding. Older individuals may be more susceptible to the side effects of sulfadiazine, SMZ-TMP, or trimethoprim.

Side effects

Some individuals may have allergic reactions to antibiotics. If symptoms of an allergic reaction (such as rash, shortness of breath, swelling of the face and neck), severe **diarrhea**, or abdominal cramping occur, the antibiotic should be stopped and the individual should seek medical advice.

Because antibiotics can affect bacteria that are beneficial, as well as those that are harmful, women may become susceptible to infections by fungi when taking antibiotics. Vaginal **itching** or discharge may be symptoms of such infections. All patients may develop oral fungal infections of the mouth, indicated by white plaques in the mouth.

Injected antibiotics may result in irritation, pain, tenderness, or swelling in the vein used for injection. Antibiotics used in cancer patients may have numerous side effects, both minor and severe; however, most side effects are uncommon or rare.

The more common side effects of atovaquone, aztreonam, cephalosporins, ciprofloxacin, clindamycin, gentamicin, metronidazole, and SMZ-TMP include:

- **nausea and vomiting**
- diarrhea
- loss of appetite

Eating active cultured yogurt may help counteract diarrhea, but if a patient has low white blood cells, this remedy is not recommended. For mild diarrhea with cephalosporins, only diarrhea medicines containing kaolin or attapulgite should be taken. With clindamycin, diarrhea medicines containing attapulgite should be taken several hours before or after the oral antibiotic. Diarrhea following antibiotics like clindamycin may indicate a bacterial infection that needs additional therapy, and a physician should be consulted.

Other side effects of atovaquone may include:

- **fever**
- skin rash

KEY TERMS

Gram-negative—Types of bacteria that do not retain Gram stain.

Gram-positive—Types of bacteria that retain Gram stain.

Mycobacteria—Rod-shaped bacteria, some of which cause human diseases such as tuberculosis.

***Pneumocystis carinii* pneumonia (PCP)**—Serious type of pneumonia caused by the protozoan *Pneumocystis carinii.*

Protozoa—Single-celled animals.

Toxoplasmosis—Infection caused by the protozoan parasite *Toxoplasma gondii,* affecting animals and humans with suppressed immune systems.

Trichomoniasis—Infection caused by a protozoan of the genus *Trichomonas;* especially vaginitis caused by *Trichomonas vaginalis*

- cough
- headache
- insomnia

Other side effects of ciprofloxacin may include:

- abdominal pain
- increase in blood tests for kidney function
- dizziness or light-headedness
- inflammation or tearing of a tendon
- drowsiness
- insomnia

Other common side effects of clindamycin include abdominal pain and fever. Side effects may occur up to several weeks after treatment with this medicine.

Gentamicin and vancomycin may cause serious side effects, particularly in elderly individuals and newborn infants. These include kidney damage and damage to the auditory nerve that controls hearing. Other, more common side effects of gentamicin may include:

- changes in urination
- increased thirst
- muscle twitching or seizures
- headache
- lethargy

When gentamicin is injected into a muscle, vein, or the spinal fluid, the following side effects may occur:

- leg cramps
- skin rash
- fever
- seizures

Side effects from gentamicin may develop up to several weeks after the medicine is stopped.

More common side effects of metronidazole include:

- mouth dryness
- unpleasant or metallic taste
- dizziness or light-headedness
- headache
- stomach pain

Sugarless candy or gum, bits of ice, or a saliva substitute may relieve symptoms of dry mouth.

Pentamidine, pyrimethamine, sulfonamides, SMZ-TMP, and trimethoprim can lower the number of white blood cells, resulting in an increased risk of infection. These drugs also can lower the number of blood platelets that are important for blood clotting. Thus, there is an increased risk of bleeding or bruising while taking these drugs.

Serious side effects of pentamidine may include:

- heart problems
- low blood pressure
- high or low blood sugar
- other blood problems
- decrease in urination
- sore throat and fever
- sharp pain in upper abdomen

Some of these symptoms may not occur until several months after treatment with pentamidine.

Pyrimethamine and trimethoprim may lower the red blood cell count, causing anemia. **Leucovorin** or the vitamin **folic acid** may be prescribed for anemia.

Some individuals become more sensitive to sunlight when taking sulfonamides, SMZ-TMP, or trimethoprim. Other common side effects of sulfonamides and SMZ-TMP include:

- dizziness
- itching
- skin rash
- headache
- mouth sores or swelling of the tongue
- fatigue

If vancomycin is injected into a vein too quickly, it can cause flushing and a rash over the neck, face, and chest, wheezing or difficulty breathing, and a dangerous decrease in blood pressure.

Interactions

Many prescription and non-prescription medicines can interact with these antibiotics. Therefore, it is important to consult a complete list of known drug interactions. Among the more common or dangerous interactions:

- Antibiotics that lower the number of blood platelets, with blood thinners (anticoagulants), such as warfarin
- Aztreonam and metronidazole with alcohol; it is important not to consume alcohol until at least three days after treatment with these antibiotics
- Ciprofloxacin with antacids, iron supplements, or caffeine
- Pentamidine or pyrimethamine with previous treatments with x rays or cancer medicines (increased risk of blood cell damage)
- Trimethoprim with diuretics to remove excess fluid in the elderly

Many medicines can increase the risk of hearing or kidney damage from gentamicin. These include:

- cisplatin
- combination pain medicine with acetaminophen and aspirin or other salicylates (taken regularly in large amounts)
- **cyclosporine**
- inflammation or pain medicine, except narcotics
- lithium
- methotrexate
- other medicines for infection

The following drugs may increase the risk of liver effects with sulfadiazine or SMZ-TMP:

- acetaminophen, long-term, high-dose (eg Tylenol)
- birth control pills containing estrogens
- disulfiram (Antabuse)
- other medicines for infection

Resources

BOOKS

American Cancer Society. *Consumers Guide to Cancer Drugs*. Atlanta: Jones and Bartlett, 2000.

Drum, David. *Making the Chemotherapy Decision*, 2nd ed. Los Angeles: Lowell House, 1998.

OTHER

American Cancer Society. *Cancer Drugs*. Cancer Resource Center. 2000. 27 May 2001. <http://www2.cancer.org/drug_reference/index.cfm?ct=1&language=english>.

American Cancer Society. *Infections in Individuals with Cancer*. Cancer Resource Center. 30 Sep. 1999. 27 May 2001. <http://www3.cancer.org/cancerinfo/load_cont.asp?ct=1&doc=12>.

MEDLINEplus Drug Information. U.S. National Library of Medicine. 24 Jan. 2001. 22 May 2001. <http://www.nlm.nih.gov/medlineplus/druginfo/>.

Margaret Alic, Ph.D.

Antidiarrheal agents

Definition

Antidiarrheal agents are prescription and non-prescription medicines that are used to treat **diarrhea**.

Purpose

Some types of cancer may cause diarrhea. In addition, diarrhea is a common side effect of **chemotherapy** treatments for cancer. This is because anticancer drugs can damage the cells of the intestines. Radiation treatment for cancer directed at the abdominal region also may cause diarrhea. Diarrhea can result in dehydration and the loss of minerals such as potassium. It may prevent the elimination of waste products in the urine, as the body attempts to conserve water.

Description

The common medicines for treating diarrhea that results from cancer and cancer treatments are:

- atropine and diphenoxylate
- loperamide
- octreotide
- opium tincture

Atropine and diphenoxylate are prescribed as a combination medicine with the brand names:

- Lofene
- Logen
- Lomocot
- Lomotil
- Lonox
- Vi-Atro

The generic name product also may be available. Atropine and diphenoxylate, antiperistaltic and anticholinergic agents, relax muscles and slow down the movements of the gastrointestinal tract. Diphenoxylate is similar to some narcotics and may be habit-forming if taken in dosages higher than prescribed. Since higher doses of atropine have unpleasant effects, it is unlikely that the combination medicine will be taken in high enough doses to cause diphenoxylate-dependence.

Loperamide slows down the movements of the intestines. The common brand names for this medicine are:

- Imodium
- Kaopectate II
- Maalox Anti-Diarrheal
- Pepto Diarrhea Control

Octreotide (brand name Sandostatin) is used to treat diarrhea and other symptoms of some types of intestinal cancers. It also is used to treat insulin-producing tumors of the pancreas and diarrhea caused by chemotherapy.

Opium tincture, also known as camphorated opium tincture or laudanum, is a narcotic that is used to treat severe diarrhea.

Except for loperamide liquid or tablets, all of these medicines require a prescription. Dosages vary with the individual.

Recommended dosage

The atropine-diphenoxylate combination is taken by mouth as a solution or a tablet. It may be taken with food to reduce stomach upset. The initial average dosage is 5 mg (2 tsp or two tablets) three to four times daily. Subsequent doses are once daily, as needed.

Loperamide is taken orally, as a liquid, tablet, or capsule. The usual dosage for adults and teenagers is 4 mg (2 capsules or tablets, 4 tsp of liquid) after the first loose bowel movement, followed by 2 mg after each successive loose bowel movement. The maximum dose is 16 mg of the capsules or 8 mg of the tablets or liquid in 24 hours. Loperamide should not be taken for more than two days unless ordered by a physician.

Following therapy with **irinotecan** (Camptosar), loperamide doses of 2 mg every two hours while awake and 4 mg every four hours at night are utilized at the onset of diarrhea to prevent severe dehydration and possible hospitalization.

Octreotide is packaged as a kit, for injection into a vein. For treating severe diarrhea from intestinal tumors, the average initial dosage of the long-acting form, for adults and teenagers, is 20 mg injected into the gluteal muscle of the buttocks, once every four weeks for two months. The dosage may then be adjusted by the physician. For the short-acting form, the average initial dose is 50 micrograms (mcg) injected under the skin, two to three times per day. The dosage may be gradually increased up to 600 mcg per day for the first two weeks. The average dosage after two weeks is 50–1500 mcg per day. For children, the usual dosage is 1–10 mcg per kg (0.45–4.5 mcg per lb) of body weight per day.

Opium tincture is taken orally, as a liquid. It may be taken with food to prevent stomach upset. The average adult dose is 5–16 drops, measured from the dropper in the bottle, four times per day, until diarrhea is controlled. It may be diluted with water. After several weeks of treatment, it may be necessary to lower the dosage gradually before stopping the medicine, to lessen the risk of side effects from opium withdrawal.

Precautions

Antidiarrheal agents may cause allergic reactions in some individuals. Atropine and diphenoxylate should not be given to children. Loperamide should not be given to children under six. Opium may cause breathing problems in children up to two years of age. Older adults are more sensitive to diphenoxylate and opium than younger individuals and these drugs may cause breathing problems. Diphenoxylate and loperamide may mask the symptoms of dehydration caused by diarrhea in older individuals, so it is very important to drink sufficient fluids.

Atropine and diphenoxylate

Other medical conditions may affect the use of atropine and diphenoxylate:

- alcohol or drug abuse may increase the risk of diphenoxylate addiction
- colitis (inflammation of the colon) may become more severe
- Down syndrome may cause more severe side effects
- dysentery may worsen
- emphysema, asthma, bronchitis, or other chronic lung diseases increase the risk of breathing problems
- enlarged prostate or urinary tract blockage may cause severe problems with urination
- gall bladder disease or gallstones may worsen
- glaucoma may result in severe eye pain (rare)
- heart disease may worsen
- hiatal hernia may worsen with atropine (rare)
- high blood pressure may increase (rare)
- intestinal blockage may worsen
- kidney disease may cause atropine to accumulate in the body, resulting in side effects
- liver disease may cause central nervous system side effects, including coma
- myasthenia gravis may become worse
- overactive or underactive thyroid may cause effects on breathing and heart rate
- incontinence may worsen

An overdose of atropine and diphenoxylate can lead to unconsciousness and death. Symptoms of overdose include:

- severe drowsiness
- breathing problems
- fast heartbeat
- warmth, dryness, and flushing of skin
- vision problems
- severe dryness of mouth, nose, and throat
- nervousness or irritability

Loperamide and octreotide

Other medical conditions may affect the use of loperamide:

- colitis (inflammation of the colon) may worsen
- dysentery may worsen
- liver disease may increase the risk of side effects

Loperamide should not be used in the presence of **fever** or blood or mucus in stools.

Medical conditions that may affect the use of octreotide include:

- diabetes mellitus, since octreotide may affect blood sugar levels
- gallbladder disease or gallstones, since octreotide may cause gallstones
- severe kidney disease that may cause octreotide to remain in the body longer

Opium tincture

Side effects of opium tincture may be increased or become dangerous when combined with the following medical conditions:

- alcohol or drug abuse
- colitis (inflammation of the colon)
- heart disease
- kidney disease
- liver disease
- underactive thyroid
- head injury or brain disease
- emphysema, asthma, bronchitis, or other chronic lung disease
- problems with urination or enlarged prostate
- gallbladder disease or gallstones
- seizures

Opium tincture may be habit-forming, causing mental or physical dependence that can lead to side effects of withdrawal when stopping the medicine. The use of opium tincture during pregnancy can cause dependency in the fetus and symptoms of drug withdrawal or breathing problems in the newborn infant.

Symptoms of opium overdose include:

- seizures
- confusion
- severe restlessness or nervousness
- severe dizziness
- severe drowsiness
- slow or irregular breathing
- severe weakness
- cold, clammy skin
- low blood pressure
- slow heartbeat
- contracted eye pupils

Side effects

Atropine and diphenoxylate

At low doses, taken for short periods of time, side effects of atropine and diphenoxylate are rare. However, serious side effects may include:

- bloating
- constipation
- loss of appetite
- stomach pain with nausea and vomiting

Other, less common or rare side effects of atropine and diphenoxylate include:

- dizziness
- drowsiness
- blurred vision
- confusion
- difficult urination
- dry skin or mouth
- fever
- headache
- depression
- numbness in hands or feet
- skin rash or itching
- swelling of gums

Rare side effects that may occur after stopping atropine and diphenoxylate include:

- sweating
- trembling or chills
- muscle cramps
- nausea or vomiting
- stomach cramps

Loperamide

Side effects are rare with low dosages of loperamide, taken for a short time. However, severe side effects may include:

- bloating
- constipation
- loss of appetite
- stomach pain with nausea and vomiting
- skin rash
- dry mouth
- dizziness or drowsiness

Octreotide

More common side effects of octreotide may include:

KEY TERMS

Anticholinergic agent—Drug that slows the action of the bowel by relaxing the muscles; reduces stomach acid.

Antiperistaltic agent—Drug that slows the contraction and relaxation (peristalsis) of the intestines.

- irregular or slow heartbeat
- constipation
- diarrhea
- flatulence
- discomfort at the site of injection

Less common or rare side effects of octreotide may include:

- dizziness or light-headedness
- fever
- flushing or redness of the face
- swelling of feet or lower legs
- inflammation of the pancreas with stomach pain, nausea, or vomiting
- hair loss
- seizures
- unconsciousness

Symptoms of high blood sugar (hyperglycemia) from octreotide include:

- blurred vision
- drowsiness and **fatigue**
- dry mouth
- flushed, dry skin
- fruity breath odor
- increased urination
- ketones in urine
- loss of appetite
- increased thirst
- nausea or vomiting
- stomach ache
- rapid, deep breathing

Symptoms of low blood sugar (hypoglycemia) from octreotide include:

- anxiety and nervousness
- confusion
- blurred vision
- cold sweats
- cool, pale skin
- drowsiness, fatigue, weakness
- hunger
- fast heartbeat
- headache
- nausea
- nightmares and restless sleep
- shakiness
- slurred speech

Opium tincture

Side effects of opium tincture that are more common with higher dosages may include:

- drowsiness
- dizziness, light-headedness, faintness
- nervousness
- weakness or fatigue
- painful or strained urination
- frequent urination
- decreased volume of urine

Lying down and rising slowly from a seated or lying position may help relieve dizziness.

Rare side effects of opium tincture include:

- bloating
- constipation
- loss of appetite
- nausea or vomiting
- stomach cramps
- fast or slow heartbeat
- sweating
- rash, hives, or itching
- redness or flushing of the face
- depression
- troubled breathing
- convulsions (seizures)

The following side effects may occur after stopping treatment with opium tincture:

- runny nose or sneezing
- body aches
- loss of appetite
- diarrhea
- stomach cramps
- nausea or vomiting
- fever
- sweating
- nervousness or irritability
- trembling
- insomnia

- dilated pupils
- severe weakness

Interactions

Atropine and diphenoxylate

Other drugs may interact with atropine and diphenoxylate:

- **Antibiotics** (cephalosporins, clindamycin, erythromycins, tetracyclines) can counteract the effects of atropine and diphenoxylate and make the diarrhea worse.
- Central nervous system depressants (alcohol, antihistamines, sedatives, pain medicines or narcotics, barbiturates, seizure medicine, muscle relaxants, anesthetics) may increase effects, such as drowsiness, from both the depressant and the antidiarrheal agent.
- Monoamine oxidase inhibitors may cause severe side effects if taken within two weeks of diphenoxylate and atropine.
- Opioid antagonists (naltrexone) may cause withdrawal from diphenoxylate addiction; naltrexone will counteract the antidiarrheal effects of the medicine.
- Other anticholinergics to reduce stomach acid or cramps may increase the effects of atropine.

Loperamide and octreotide

Antibiotics may interact with loperamide and make the diarrhea worse. Narcotic pain medicines in combination with loperamide may cause severe constipation.

Because octreotide may cause high or low blood sugar, it can interact with the following medicines:

- antidiabetic medicines, sulfonylurea
- diazoxide (Proglycem)
- glucagon
- insulin
- growth hormone

Opium tincture

The following medicines may increase side effects from opium tincture:

- anticholinergics for abdominal or stomach cramps
- other antidiarrheal medicines
- tricyclic antidepressants

Naltrexone (Trexan) makes opium less effective for treating diarrhea. Alcohol, narcotics, and other central nervous system depressants, including antihistamines, sedatives, prescription pain medicines, barbiturates, seizure medicines, muscle relaxants, or anesthetics, may lead to unconsciousness or death in combination with opium tincture.

Margaret Alic, Ph.D.

Antiemetics

Definition

Antiemetic drugs are drugs used to combat **nausea and vomiting**.

Purpose

Antiemetic drugs are used to prevent vomiting (emesis) in **chemotherapy** patients and postoperative patients. Aside from the difficulty of maintaining proper nutrition and a healthy weight, chronic vomiting can result in dehydration, which can be a medical emergency. Following are descriptions of antiemetic drugs in use as of 2001.

Description

Promethazine

Promethazine is also known as phenergan and mepergan. It is also used to treat motion sickness, reduce allergic symptoms, and for sedation. It is one of the drugs of the phenothiazine type. In addition to other qualities, it is an antihistamine.

Prochlorperazine

Prochlorperazine is also known as compazine. Like promethazine, it is a member of the class of phenothiazines. Unlike promethazine, however, prochlorperazine also belongs to the class of drugs known as antipsychotics, or neuroleptics. Antipsychotic drugs are used to treat psychoses and other psychiatric disorders. In addition to its use as an antiemetic and anti-psychotic drug, prochlorperazine is also used to treat non-psychotic anxiety.

Serotonin receptor antagonists

The serotonin receptor antagonists include granisetron (kytril), dolasetron (anzemet), and ondansetron (zofran). These drugs are used for postoperative nausea and emesis as well as nausea and vomiting associated with chemotherapy, and are often used in combination with a corticosteroid. Ondansetron is approved for nausea and vomiting associated with **radiation therapy**.

Dronabinol

Dronabinol (marinol) is used to combat **anorexia** in AIDS patients, and emesis in cancer patients who haven't responded to other antiemetics. Marinol is the synthetic or extracted form of the active ingredient found in **marijuana**.

Other antipsychotic (neuroleptic) drugs

The other neuroleptic (antipsychotic) drugs used to treat nausea and emesis are droperidol (inapsine), haloperidol (haldol), chlorpromazine (thorazine), and perphenazine (trilafon). One other antipsychotic, triethylperazine (torecan or norzine), was used as an antiemetic, but is no longer widely available. Some of the antipsychotics are also used to treat aggressive or violent behavior or intractable hiccups (chlorpromazine). These drugs are similar to prochlorperazine in terms of their actions and potentially severe side effects.

There are some additional precautions and side effects associated with each of these drugs. Patients should be sure to notify their physician of any health concerns (including pregnancy) or medications they are taking. Patients should also ask about potential side effects for each individual medication before receiving any of these drugs.

Dosage

Promethazine

Promethazine is given in doses of 12.5 to 25 mg every 4 hours if injected into the muscle or as a suppository. As a syrup, 25 mg should be given every 4 to 6 hours. Doses for children vary by age, weight, and severity of condition.

Prochlorperazine

Generally, the dose is 5 to 10 mg, 3 to 4 times per day. However, the effect of medication varies widely from patient to patient, so the dose should be tailored to each individual. Prochlorperazine is available as a syrup, tablet, 25 mg slow-release capsule, and in injectable form.

Dronabinol

The effective dose of dronabinol varies widely from patient to patient and should be monitored and tested by the physician. The basic dose is $5mg/m^2$ given 4 to 6 times per day.

Precautions

Promethazine

Patients with cardiovascular disease or impaired liver function should either use this drug with caution or not at all. Children should also use this drug cautiously for two reasons. First, some side effects may suggest, or mask, underlying disease, such as Reye's syndrome. Second, large doses of this drug, or any antihistamine, may cause convulsions, hallucinations, or death in children. Patients taking this medication should not drive, operate heavy machinery, or engage in any hazardous activity while under the influence of this drug. This drug has not been established as safe for use during pregnancy, or in nursing mothers.

Prochlorperazine

Persons allergic to any other phenothiazine (such as promethazine) should not take prochlorperazine. Patients who have heart problems, glaucoma or bone marrow depression should take this drug with caution, or not at all, and inform their physician of their condition. Persons who will be around high temperatures should also avoid this drug. In addition, persons who experience seizures should be aware that administration of this drug makes seizures more likely.

Breast cancer patients may wish to avoid this drug because it increases levels of prolactin in the blood. Increased prolactin may help some types of breast cancer to thrive.

Prochloroperazine, like promethazine, may mask symptoms of Reye's disease in children. It may also mask symptoms of intestinal obstructions or brain disease. In addition, children who are acutely ill, under two years of age, or under 20 pounds should not be given this drug.

This drug has not been established as safe for use during pregnancy and is found in the breast milk of lactating mothers. Therefore, caution should be used when administering this drug to pregnant women and extreme caution should be used when administering to nursing women.

Serotonin receptor antagonists

Patients with allergies to any drug in this category should not take any other drug in this category. Also, patients with hypokalemia, hypomagnesia, or certain heart problems should avoid taking these drugs. The effect of these drugs on the children or fetuses of nursing or pregnant mothers is not known, so they should be used with caution.

Dronabinol

Dronabinol is inadvisable for patients with a known allergy to either sesame oil or any part of the cannabis plant. Patients taking this drug should not drive, operate heavy machinery, or engage in hazardous tasks until used to this medication.

This medication also should be used cautiously, if at all, for persons with depression, mania, or schizophrenia, elderly patients, patients with cardiac disorders, and for pregnant and nursing women. It is especially inadvisable for nursing women, since marinol is concentrated in the breast milk.

Side effects

Promethazine

Patients taking promethazine may experience a large number of side effects, including drowsiness, ringing in the ears, a lack of coordination, problems with vision, **fatigue**, euphoria, nervousness, tremors, seizures, a catatonic-like state, and hysteria. These effects are usually reversible. At high doses, patients may also exhibit extrapyramidal reactions. Extrapyramidal reactions can briefly be described as agitation (jitteriness, sometimes insomnia), muscle spasms, and/or pseudo-Parkinson's (a group of symptoms including, but not limited to, drooling, tremors, and a shuffling gait).

Patients may also experience rashes, asthma, jaundice, abnormally low production of white blood cells, and abnormalities in how fast or slow their heart beats. Patients may sometimes experience unusual side effects not known as typical for the medication they are taking. These should be reported to the physician.

Prochlorperazine

Prochlorperazine has many side effects, including low blood pressure, dizziness, blurred vision, skin reactions, jaundice, lack of production of white cells, damage to the DNA in sperm, problems in the regulation of body temperature, impotence, **amenorrhea** (a lack of menstruation), and gynecomastia (the growth of female-like breasts in males). However, the most severe side effects stem from damage to the brain. Patients may suffer from extrapyramidal reactions. These symptoms may be reversed by treating the patient with drugs effective in treatment of Parkinson's patients (except levodopa). A reduction or elimination in the amount of the antipsychotic medication may also be necessary to eliminate these symptoms.

Two other (rare) disorders, tardive dyskinesia and neuroleptic malignant syndrome (NMS), are also associated with antipsychotic drug use. Patients with NMS have high temperatures, rigid muscles, an altered mental state, and symptoms such as excessive sweating and irregular blood pressure or heart rhythm. Patients with NMS usually respond to treatment. Patients with tardive dyskinesia have involuntary movement of muscles in the chest, arms, and legs, or in the muscles in and around the face (including the tongue). Tardive dyskinesia may be irreversible.

KEY TERMS

Depersonalization—An alteration in the perception of self.

Tardive dyskinesia—A disorder brought on by antipsychotic medication use, and is characterized by uncontrollable muscle spasms.

Serotonin receptor antagonists

Side effects include rashes, increased sweating, problems with taste or vision, flushing, agitation, sleep disorder, depersonalization, headache, fatigue, nausea, weakness, abdominal pain, constipation, **diarrhea**, hypertension, dizziness, chills and shivering, and dry mouth. Patients may also have abnormal liver function tests.

Dronabinol

Possible side effects are fatigue, weakness, abdominal pain, nausea, vomiting, heart palpitations, fast heart rate, facial flushing, amnesia, anxiety, an abnormal mental state, depersonalization, confusion, dizziness, and euphoria.

Interactions

Promethazine

Promethazine interacts with central nervous system depressants, like alcohol and barbiturates. Therefore, the physician should alerted to any medications the patient is taking, and doses of the drugs should be adjusted accordingly. Alcohol should be avoided. It has not been proven, but promethazine may interfere with the action of epinephrine.

Prochlorperazine

Like promethazine, prochlorperazine should be used cautiously, or not at all, with central nervous system depressants like alcohol and barbiturates. Prochlorperazine has also been shown to interact with anticonvulsant medication, guanethidene, propanolol, thiazide diuretics, and oral anticoagulants (like **warfarin** and coumadin).

Serotonin receptor antagonists

These drugs may have very negative effects on the patient when combined with diuretics, anti-arrhythmia drugs, or high doses of anthracycline.

Dronabinol

Dronabinol interacts with the antiemetic prochlorperazine synergistically. Therefore, the use of these two drugs in combination results in a greater antiemetic effect. Patients taking central nervous system depressants, such as barbiturates or alcohol should notify their physician before taking marinol, since marinol may increase their effect. Although no drugs have been shown to interact with marinol, many drugs similar to marinol do interact with a number of other drugs, including central nervous system depressants such as alcohol or barbiturates, or drugs like flouxetine or disulfiram. Again, the physician should alerted to any medications the patient is taking before beginning a course of dronabinol.

See Also Corticosteroids; Lorazepam; Metoclopramide; Scopolamine

Michael Zuck, Ph.D.

Antiestrogens

Definition

Antiestrogens are a group of medications that block the effect that estrogen has on the growth of a tumor.

Description

Antiestrogens refer to a group of drugs that are used to treat advanced hormone-sensitive breast cancers. Many **breast cancer** tumors grow due to normal levels of estrogen, a hormone found in the bloodstream. Some patients have tumors that are extra-sensitive to this normal estrogen level. The estrogen attaches to the area on the outside of the tumor cells and sends a signal to the cell that causes it to grow and multiply. Antiestrogens block the protein on the outside wall of the estrogen-sensitive breast cancer cell. By blocking this protein, known as the estrogen receptor, the free-floating estrogen cannot stimulate the cancer cells to grow and multiply any further.

The drug **tamoxifen** is a common antiestrogen that has proven to have a positive effect in breast cancer patients for both treatment and prevention.

Nancy J. Beaulieu, RPh.,BCOP

Antifungal therapy

Definition

Antifungal drugs are used to treat infections caused by fungus and to prevent the development of fungal infections in patients with weakened immune systems.

Purpose

Fungal infections

A fungus is a living organism that can cause infection when it grows in the human body. In healthy people, fungal infections tend to be mild and treatable. For cancer patients, however, fungal infections can become severe and must be treated quickly. Cancer patients, particularly those with leukemia or **lymphoma**, tend to have weakened immune systems as a result of **chemotherapy** or the disease. Once they are infected, their weak immune system allows the fungus to grow quickly. Because of this risk, some cancer patients with no obvious fungal infection are given antifungal therapy to help prevent infection from developing.

Fungal infection can occur in two ways. Some fungi, such as candida, are usually found in the bodies of healthy people and cause little or no harm. When the immune system is weak, however, these fungi begin to grow and cause infection. Other fungi, such as aspergillus and cryptococcus, are found in the air. Infection occurs when the fungus is either inhaled into the lungs or comes into contact with an operative wound. The most common fungal infections found in patients with weakened immune systems are candidiasis, aspergillosis and cryptococcosis.

Treatment

The treatment of a fungal infection depends on the type and location of infection. Superficial infections that affect the skin, hair, and nails can be treated with topical (cream or ointment) or oral antifungal drugs. Systemic infections that affect the internal organs require aggressive treatment with either oral or intravenous drugs.

Description

There are three classes of drugs typically used to treat fungal infections: polyenes, azoles, and echinocandins.

Polyenes

Polyenes are drugs that work by attaching to the sterol component found in the fungal membrane, causing the cells to become porous and die. The two polyenes most commonly used are nystatin (Mycostatin) and amphotericin B (Fungizone). Nystatin is often used as a topical agent to treat superficial infections, or is taken orally to treat candidal infections such as oral or esophageal candidiasis.

Amphotericin B was the first antifungal drug to be approved for use, and it is still the standard therapy for the most severe systemic fungal infections. Recently, several new types of amphotericin B (Abelcet, Amphotec and AmBisome) have been introduced. These drugs, called lipid formulations, cause fewer side effects than traditional amphotericin B but are more expensive.

Azoles

Azoles stop fungal growth by preventing fungi from making an essential part of their cell wall. Three typical azoles are ketoconazole (Nizoral), fluconazole (Diflucan), and itraconazole (Sporanox). Ketoconazole is the oldest of these three drugs, and has been used since the 1970s. It is slightly more toxic than the other azoles and does not work for aspergillosis and many candidiasis infections.

Although fluconazole is effective against both superficial and systemic candidiasis, some strains of this fungus have now become resistant to the drug. Itraconazole, the newest of the azoles, is effective against a range of different fungal infections. Unlike ketoconazole or fluconazole, it can be used to treat aspergillosis.

Echinocandins

Echinocandins are a new class of antifungal drugs that work by disrupting the wall that surrounds fungal cells. Caspofungin (Cancidas) is the first of this new class of drugs to be approved. It is an effective treatment for severe, systemic fungal infections, and is given to patients who do not respond to other therapies.

Recommended dosage

Although dosages differ for the various antifungal treatments, most therapies continue even after there is no sign of infection.

Polyenes

Topical nystatin should be liberally applied two to three times daily. Liquid formulations of the drug are usually taken in doses of 400,000 to 600,000 units four times a day for adults and children. The dose for the oral tablets is 500,000 to 1 million units every 8 hours. Both traditional amphotericin B and the new lipid formulations of the drug are given intravenously. Dosages are adjusted according to each patient's tolerance and the severity and location of the infection. Patients receiving amphotericin B treatment are usually hospitalized.

Azoles

Ketoconazole is available as a tablet and as a topical treatment. Both treatments are usually given once daily. Treatment can last for several weeks for superficial infections, or up to a year for more serious infections. Fluconazole and itraconazole are both administered either orally or intravenously. The dose depends on the type of fungal infection, the patient's condition and the response to treatment.

Echinocandins

Caspofungin is given intravenously once daily, and most patients receive the same dose.

Precautions

Patients who are given topical or oral antifungal therapy should make sure they use their medication regularly, and for as long as their doctor thinks is necessary. Infections that are not completely eradicated frequently recur.

Side effects

Antifungal drugs that are applied topically rarely cause side effects unless the patient is allergic to the drug. Side effects are more common when drugs are taken orally or intravenously. The most common reactions from azole drugs are nausea, **diarrhea** and other gastrointestinal symptoms. These symptoms usually affect less than 10% of patients. Caspofungin also produces few side effects. The most common side effect is a rash.

Amphotericin B can be quite toxic and most patients experience side effects. These include **fever**, rigors, and chills. Premedication with acetaminophen, **diphenhydramine**, hydrocortisone, and sometimes meperidine can be given to prevent these side effects. Amphotericin B can also seriously damage the kidneys. However, patients are carefully monitored while taking this drug. If symptoms develop, the liposomal alternative is usually given. Lipid formulations of amphotericin B are far less damaging to the kidneys.

KEY TERMS

Aspergillosis—A fungal infection that can be life-threatening to patients with a weakened immune system.

Candidiasis—A fungal infection that can be mild or very serious depending on what part of the body it infects.

Cryptococcosis—A fungal infection that can cause meningitis.

Intravenous—A treatment that is given directly into the bloodstream.

Topical—A treatment that is applied on the skin.

Interactions

Drug interactions are significant with antifungal treatment. Patients taking amphotericin B should not take any other drug that can cause kidney damage. Potentially serious reactions can occur when patients taking azole antifungal therapies also take certain antihistamines such as astemizole (Hismanal) or the statin drug lovastatin (Mevacor). Patients on antifungal therapy who plan to take other prescribed, over the counter, or alternative medicines should always check with their doctor first.

Alison McTavish, M.Sc.

Antimicrobials

Definition

Antimicrobial drugs are used to fight infections caused by bacteria, fungi, and viruses.

Description

Antimicrobial drugs are drugs designed to kill, or prevent the growth of microorganisms (bacteria, fungi, and viruses). Bacteria, fungi, and viruses are responsible for almost all of the common infectious diseases found in North America from athlete's foot, to AIDS, to ulcers (as of 2001). Interestingly enough, many disorders formerly thought to be caused by other factors, like stress, are now known to be caused by bacteria. For example, it has been shown that many ulcers are caused by the bacteria *Helicobacter pylori*, and not by stress, as many originally thought. Thus, antimicrobials represent an important part of medicine today.

The history of antimicrobials begins with the observations of Pasteur and Joubert, who discovered that one type of bacteria could prevent the growth of another. They did not know at that time that the reason one bacteria failed to grow was that the other bacteria was producing an antibiotic. Technically, **antibiotics** are only those substances that are produced by one microorganism that kill, or prevent the growth, of another microorganism. Of course, in today's common usage, the term antibiotic is used to refer to almost any drug that cures a bacterial infection. Antimicrobials include not just antibiotics, but synthetically formed compounds as well.

The discovery of antimicrobials like penicillin and tetracycline paved the way for better health for millions around the world. Before 1941, the year penicillin was discovered, no true cure for gonorrhea, strep throat, or **pneumonia** existed. Patients with infected wounds often had to have a wounded limb removed, or face death from infection. Now, most of these infections can be easily cured with a short course of antimicrobials.

However, the future effectiveness of antimicrobial therapy is somewhat in doubt. Microorganisms, especially bacteria, are becoming resistant to more and more antimicrobial agents. Bacteria found in hospitals appear to be especially resilient, and are causing increasing difficulty for the sickest patients–those in the hospital. Currently, bacterial resistance is combated by the discovery of new drugs. However, microorganisms are becoming resistant more quickly than new drugs are being found, Thus, future research in antimicrobial therapy may focus on finding how to overcome resistance to antimicrobials, or how to treat infections with alternative means.

Michael Zuck, Ph.D.

Antineoplastic agents

Definition

Antineoplastic agents are a group of specialized drugs used primarily to treat cancer (the term "neoplastic" refers to cancer cells).

Description

The first antineoplastic agents, used in the 1940s, were made from either synthetic chemicals or natural plants. Antineoplastic agents are classified by origin and by how they work to destroy cancer cells. There are over fifty of these agents approved by the Food and Drug Administration (FDA) to be used in the United States. These include: **methotrexate**, **fluorouracil, doxorubicin**, **paclitaxel**, and **cyclophosphamide**.

Antineoplastic agents can be administered to patients alone or in combination with other antineoplastic drugs. They can also be given before, during or after a patient receives surgery or **radiation therapy**. The treatment plan is disease-specific. It is important that patients receive treatment on schedule.

Antineoplastic agents travel the body and destroy cancer cells. Side effects are expected to occur when treated with these agents, and can include nausea, mouth sores, hair loss, and lowering of the blood counts. Many of the side effects associated with antineoplastic agents occur because **chemotherapy** treatment destroys the body's normal cells in addition to cancerous cells.

Healthcare providers should be able to assist patients in managing these side effects so that antineoplastic therapy is a tolerable treatment.

Nancy J. Beaulieu, RPh., BCOP

Antioxidants

Definition

Antioxidants are chemical compounds that can bind to free oxygen radicals preventing these radicals from damaging healthy cells.

Purpose

Preliminary studies have suggested that antioxidants are useful in a number of ways in regards to cancer. For instance, they may improve the effectiveness of **chemotherapy**, decrease side effects of chemotherapy and radiotherapy, and prevent some types of cancer. Sufficient epidemiological studies have shown that ingesting foods high in antioxidants, such as fruits and vegetables, can decrease the risk of many types of cancer. Studies have also found that cancer patients have lower levels of antioxidants in their blood. The American Cancer Society suggests eating five servings of fruits a day to decrease the risk of cancer.

Precautions

Studies of antioxidant supplements to decrease the risk of cancer have not been conclusive. Most antioxidant research has centered around **vitamins** A (and its provitamin, beta-carotene), C, E (alpha-tocopherol), and the trace element selenium. While some studies have shown positive effects for antioxidants in preventing cancer, they have been conducted mostly in underfed populations or persons otherwise deficient in these antioxidants. The CARET studies in the early 1990s found that if smokers take beta-carotene and vitamin A supplements they actually increase their risk of developing lung cancer. Rather than isolated antioxidants found in supplements, it may be the combination of antioxidants found in foods that are responsible for decreasing the risk of cancer. The American Institute of Cancer Research warns that antioxidant supplements cannot substitute for whole foods. Individuals who may want to consider supplements include those who are underfed, have certain medical conditions, chronic dieters, some vegetarians, some seniors, and newborns.

Concern has developed about potential negative interactions between high doses of antioxidants and chemotherapy. Anthracycline antitumor **antibiotics** used as chemotherapy act by creating free oxygen radicals to kill tumor cells through a process known as apoptosis. Although patients taking antioxidants may improve their tolerance to chemotherapy drugs, they may be decreasing the effectiveness of treatment and risking a recurrence of the tumor in the long run. This viewpoint is theoretical, however, and no clinical studies have as yet addressed it. Patients interested in using antioxidants during chemotherapy or radiotherapy should discuss this option with their physicians.

High doses of vitamins and minerals can be toxic. The National Academy of Sciences has suggested safe upper intake levels for adults for some antioxidants. These limits are 2,000 milligrams of vitamin C per day from both foods and supplements combined, 1,000 milligrams of vitamin E per day, and 400 micrograms per day of selenium from both supplements and foods. It is not known how higher levels than these will affect healthy persons.

Side effects of vitamin E overdose may include **fatigue**, intestinal cramping, breast soreness, thrombophlebitis, acne, and **diarrhea**, and increase in blood pressure in certain people. Blood clotting time has been shown to increase. Also, with 1,800 IU per day, and vitamin E is antagonistic to iron and patients with **anemia** who are taking iron supplements should not take the two supplements at the same time. Vitamin E may also interfere with vitamin K. Selenium toxicity is characterized by dermatologic lesions; brittle hair, fragile or black fingernails, metallic taste, dizziness, and nausea.

Description

Free radicals are naturally produced in the body through the normal metabolism of amino acids and fats. These free radicals are unstable molecules that can freely react with and destroy healthy cells. They can bind to and alter the structure of DNA thus leading to mutations and eventually to cancer. Besides cancer, this oxidative stress on the cells can lead to heart, eye, and neurological diseases.

Glutathione, lipoic acid, and CoQ10 are antioxidants formed naturally by the body but their levels decline with age. Vitamins C and E are necessary antioxidants but not produced by the body and must be obtained from the diet. The most common antioxidants are the vitamins A, C, and E. Additional antioxidants are natrol, found in grapes and wine; selenium; and melatonin. Flavonoids consist of a large family of antioxidant compounds found in fruits and vegetables. Among the well-studied flavonoids in terms of **cancer prevention** are catechins from green tea, genistein from soy, curcumin from turmeric, anthocyanosides from blueberries, and quercetin from yellow vegetables.

KEY TERMS

Apoptosis—A type of cell death. A mechanism by which one cell dies if it becomes severely mutated as a means of protecting the entire organism.

Cisplatin—An anticancer drug.

Doxorubicin—An anticancer antibiotic therapy. Its trade name is Adriamycin

Fluorouracil—An anticancer drug. Its trade names include Adrucil, 5-FU, Efudex, and Fluoroplex.

Mutation—A change in the genetic structure of the cell.

Oxidative stress—A condition where the body is producing an excess of oxygen-free radicals.

Although controversy will surround the topic of supplemental antioxidants for some time, there is little if any controversy that dietary levels of antioxidants are useful in preventing cancer. Because of this evidence, the American Cancer Society suggests five servings of fruits and vegetables each day.

Resources

BOOKS

Moss, Ralph W. *Antioxidants Against Cancer.* Brooklyn, NY: Equinox Press, Inc., 2000.

PERIODICALS

Kelly, Kara M. "The Labriola/Livingston Article Reviewed." *Oncology* 13,no. 7 (1999):1008-1011.

Labriola, Dan, and Robert Livingston. "Possible Interactions Between Dietary Antioxidants and Chemotherapy."*Oncology* 13, no. 7 (1999): 1003-1008.

Lamson, Davis W, and Matthew S. Brignall. "Antioxidants in Cancer Therapy: Their Actions and Interactions with Oncologic Therapies."*Alternative Medicine Review* 4, no. 5 (1999): 304-329.

ORGANIZATIONS

American Cancer Society. <http://www.cancer.org>

American Institute for Cancer Research. 1759 R Street, NW, PO Box 97167, Washington, DC 20090-7167. (800)843-8114. <http://www.aicr.org>

National Academy of Science. <http://www.nas.edu>

OTHER

<http://clinical.caregroup.org/altmed/interactions/Nutrients/Vitamin_E.htm>

<http://www.medical.com.hk/english_site/pharmacy_site/vitamins_s/selenium/selenium_m.htm>

Cindy Jones, Ph.D.

Antiviral therapy

Definition

Antiviral therapy is often used by cancer patients to treat viral infections. Commonly used antiviral medications include acyclovir, famciclovir, ganciclovir, valacyclovir, and foscarnet.

Description

Viral infections occur in almost all people at some time in their lives. The common cold is the most easily recognizable example of a virus that can be unpleasant but generally does not cause serious problems. For people with cancer, however, viruses can often cause life-threatening illnesses.

Viral infections in cancer patients can be much more serious and debilitating than in patients without cancer. Cancer patients will often have weakened immune systems from **chemotherapy** or from the cancer itself. Cancer patients who have bone marrow transplants are at especially high risk for life-threatening viral infections. Immediately after the transplant, the patient will have very few, if any, white blood cells, which are the body's main infection fighters. Viral infections such as **herpes simplex** virus (HSV), **herpes zoster** virus (HZV), and cytomegalovirus are often seen in cancer patients, and all can cause serious, life-threatening infections.

Until the development of the antiviral drug acyclovir 1974, no relatively safe and effective anti-viral medications for cancer patients were available. By the mid-1980s, acyclovir was being routinely used for cancer patients with herpes infections. Besides treating the infection itself, acyclovir can be taken on a daily basis to prevent infection from occurring. This can be especially important in people with very depressed immune systems, such as cancer patients who have undergone a bone marrow transplant.

Since the introduction of acyclovir, other anti-viral medications have been developed that have been very useful in the treatment of viral illnesses. For reasons that are still unknown, certain herpes infections in certain cancer patients do not respond to acyclovir. Fortunately, two other newer medications similar to acyclovir, called famciclovir and valaciclovir, are helpful in treating herpes infections, especially ones that are resistant to acyclovir.

While antiviral drugs such as acyclovir have made a large difference in treating herpes infections in cancer patients, there are other viral infections that do not respond to acyclovir. Cytomegalovirus is a common viral infection among cancer patients, and especially common among cancer patients who have had bone marrow transplants. Some antiviral medications like acyclovir are not effective against cytomegalovirus. Fortunately, two other antiviral medications known as ganciclovir and foscarnet are both effective against cytomegalovirus.

Recommended dosage

The recommended dosage for the various antiviral medications can vary considerably, depending on the health of the patient and how the medication is administered. For the treatment of herpes simplex and herpes zoster, the drugs acyclovir, famciclovir, and valacyclovir can be used. The recommended oral dosage ranges from 500 mg twice a day for valacyclovir, 500 mg three times a day for famciclovir, to 800 mg every four hours for acyclovir. There is also a formulation for the drug to be given administered though the vein. The dose for injection is different than the dose for oral therapy.

For the treatment of cytomegalovirus, ganciclovir or foscarnet can be used. Both medications are generally given intravenously, although there is an oral formulation available for ganciclovir. The dosage is 5 mg per kg of body weight every 12 hours for 14 to 21 days, followed by maintenance therapy at a dose of 5 mg per kg per day as a single daily dose. The dosage for foscarnet ranges from 40 mg per kg to 90 mg per kg, depending on the diagnosis.

Precautions

The drugs acyclovir, famciclovir, valcyclovir, ganciclovir and foscarnet should all be used with caution by patients with kidney problems. With higher doses of these drugs, patients who do have kidney problems should have their kidney functioning monitored closely on a daily basis. The dosage is usually decreased depending on the degree of decreased kidney function. Kidney failure has been reported in patients taking high doses of foscarnet.

Ganciclovir should be used with extreme caution in women who may be pregnant, since it is teratogenic (causes abnormalities), as well as toxic, to developing embryos. There are no well-controlled studies of the other antiviral agents in pregnant women and it is not known whether these agents are excreted in breast milk. Therefore, it is not recommended that these antiviral agents be given to pregnant or nursing mothers unless the benefit outweighs the risk.

Side effects

Side effects common to all the antiviral medications include nausea, vomiting, **diarrhea**, headaches, and dizziness, rash, and decreased kidney function. Of the drugs used to treat herpes simplex, acyclovir seems to have more reported side effects than the other medications.

The two drugs that are used to treat cytomegalovirus, ganciclovir and foscarnet, have very different side effect profiles. Ganciclovir's major side effect is the lowering of white blood cells, a condition known as **neutropenia**. Because of this, a patient on ganciclovir should have their white blood cell count monitored closely. Foscarnet, while generally not causing a marked decrease in white blood cells, can cause sudden kidney failure. Patients who are taking foscarnet should make sure they maintain their fluid intake and have their kidney functions monitored closely.

Interactions

The antiviral drugs used to treat herpes simplex and zoster should be used with caution with other drugs that cause kidney problems. Also, they all interact with probenecid, a medication commonly used to treat gout.

Drug interactions with foscarnet and ganciclovir are more numerous and potentially dangerous. Both, especially foscarnet, must be used with caution with other drugs that cause kidney problems. Both must also be used with caution with other medications that lower seizure thresholds. Patients should notify their physician or consult with their pharmacist prior to starting any over the counter or herbal medications due to the numerous drug interactions that can occur with these agents.

Edward R. Rosick, DO, MPH, MS

KEY TERMS

Herpes simplex virus—An infectious, contagious viral disease, caused by herpes simplex virus type one or two. It is characterized by fluid-filled lesions that can recur.

Herpes zoster virus—An acute, infectious viral disease, characterized by painful, fluid-filled lesions.

Cytomegalovirus—A viral disease caused by a herpes virus, generally rare but often seen in cancer patients. It can cause life-threatening pneumonia as well as blindness.

Teratogenic—Causes abnormalities to occur in developing embryos.

Gout—A condition, most often occurring in men, caused by a buildup of uric acid crystals deposited in joints, commonly the big toe.

Aromatase inhibitors

Definition

Aromatase inhibitors are a class of hormone drugs. They inhibit aromatase, an enzyme that regulates the production of estrogen.

Purpose

The aromatase inhibitors decrease blood and tumor levels of estrogen in postmenopausal women. They are used to treat advanced forms of **breast cancer** in postmenopausal women whose disease has progressed following therapy with other antiestrogen therapy.

Description

Aromatase inhibitors lower a postmenopausal woman's estrogen levels, thereby preventing the cancer cells that are dependent on estrogen from growing.

Anastrazole (trade name Arimidex)

Anastrazole is a non-steroidal aromatase inhibitor that lowers blood levels of estradiol to prevent the rapidly growing cancerous cells. It is usually used in postmenopausal women as a treatment for advanced breast cancer that has not responded to other therapies, or it can be used as first-line therapy in these patients.

Exemestane (trade name Aromasin)

Exemestane is an aromatase inhibitor that reduces the concentration of estradiol in the bloodstream. It is also called an aromatase inactivator because it inactivates aromatase irreversibly, potentially providing continued benefits after treatment is stopped. It is used to treat advanced breast cancers in postmenopausal women whose cancers have not responded to other antiestrogen therapies.

Letrozole (trade name Femara)

Letrozole is a non-steroidal aromatase inhibitor that lowers blood estrogen levels by hindering the conversion of androgens to estrogens. It is used in postmenopausal women with advanced breast cancer that has progressed while on other antiestrogen therapy.

Recommended dosage

- Anastrazole: The adult dose is 1 mg a day by mouth
- Exemestane: The adult dose is 25 mg a day by mouth, after a meal
- Letrozole: The adult dose is 2.5 mg a day by mouth

Precautions

Aromatase inhibitors are not used in pregnant women because of the risk to the fetus. Since these drugs are generally prescribed for postmenopausal women, pregnancy is not usually an issue.

Except in life-threatening conditions, anastrazole, exemestane, and letrozole are not used in pregnancy because of risks to the fetus. These drugs should be avoided by those allergic to it and by nursing mothers.

Side effects

The aromatase inhibitors are generally tolerated quite well. Side effects are similar to the effects of decreased estrogen, such as hot flashes. The specific side effects are discussed in this section. People should report any side effects to the doctor.

Anastrazole

Rash is the most common side effect of anastrazole. Less common side effects include:

- hot flashes
- headache, light-headedness, dizziness, confusion
- depression, insomnia, anxiety
- chest pain, high blood pressure, obstruction of blood vessels
- **nausea and vomiting**, **diarrhea**, constipation, abdominal pain
- dry mouth, altered taste, appetite loss
- vaginal bleeding, vulvar itching
- hair thinning
- bone pain, tumor pain, weakness, muscle aches
- cough, sinusitis
- abnormally low red blood cell levels (**anemia**)
- abnormally low white blood counts (leukopenia)

Exemestane

Side effects include:

- hot flashes
- headache, **fatigue**, insomnia
- depression, anxiety
- high blood pressure
- nausea, vomiting
- increase in appetite
- diarrhea, constipation, abdominal pain
- cough, difficulty breathing

KEY TERMS

Estradiol—A steroid that has some of the properties of estrogen.

Letrozole

Common side effects include:

- headache
- nausea, vomiting
- lethargy
- appetite loss (**anorexia**)
- rash, itching

Less common side effects include:

- drowsiness, dizziness
- depression, anxiety
- high blood pressure
- constipation, diarrhea, heartburn
- hair loss
- hot flashes, sweating
- cough, difficulty breathing

Interactions

Patients who are taking any kind of prescription drug, over-the-counter drug, or herbal remedy should notify their physician before beginning any treatment with aromatase inhibitors.

See Also Megestrol acetate; Tamoxifen

Rhonda Cloos, R.N.

Arsenic trioxide

Definition

Arsenic trioxide, also known by the trade name Trisenox, is an antitumor agent used for a specific type of leukemia known as acute promyelocytic leukemia.

Purpose

Arsenic trioxide is used to treat acute promyelocytic leukemia in patients who have not responded to standard treatment.

Description

Arsenic trioxide, like many other antineoplastic (antitumor) agents, acts by interfering with the growth of cells. Unfortunately, these drugs affect the growth of normal cells and tumor cells. In some patients the drug may have to be discontinued because normal cell growth is too severely affected. For example, a patient taking a large dose of arsenic trioxide might see tumor growth stop. However, the dosage might be high enough to also stop the body's normal growth of platelet cells. The loss of platelets might cause severe internal bleeding–a consequence more immediately toxic than the tumor.

Recommended dosage

Doses vary from individual to individual and depend on body weight as well as other medications the patient is taking. For acute promyelocytic leukemia dosages for adults and children five years of age and older are up to 60 injections of 0.15 mg/kg of body weight until bone marrow remission occurs.

Precautions

Arsenic trioxide has been shown to cause fetal abnormalities and miscarriage in animals. Women who might become pregnant should take precautions to ensure they do not become pregnant while taking this drug. Women who are nursing their infants should discontinue nursing while this medication is in their system.

Patients with bone marrow problems, heart problems, kidney problems, or low levels of magnesium or potassium in the blood should notify their physician before taking any of this medicine. Patients should notify their physician of any illnesses they may have before taking arsenic trioxide.

Because persons taking arsenic trioxide may have decreased immunity, it is important for them to avoid infection. Caution should be taken to avoid unnecessary exposure to crowds and people with infections.

Patients may experience unusual or excessive bruising and/or bleeding and should avoid situations in which it is likely they could cut or bruise themselves. Patients should consult their physician immediately if they have any indication of excessive bleeding or bruising, including black and tarry stools, blood in the urine or stools, unusual bleeding or bruising, pinpoint red marks on their skin, vomit containing blood or what appears to be coffee grounds (dried blood). Severe symptoms may indicate a medical emergency.

KEY TERMS

Antineoplastic—A substance used to help prevent tumor growth.

Side effects

Symptoms include unusual heartbeat (fast, slow, irregular, or pounding), chest pain, high blood pressure, trouble breathing, bluish lips, skin, palms, or skin underneath the fingernails, muscle cramps, numbness or tingling, headache, acting or feeling drunk, confusion, fainting, dizziness, eye pain, blurred vision, excessive weakness, excessive **fatigue**, or excessive drowsiness.

Patients should also contact their physician immediately if they experience a fruity odor in their mouth, a dry mouth, excessive sweating, flushing, urine retention, excessive urination, increased appetite or thirst, abdominal pain, loss of appetite, unexplained weight gain or loss, or severe nausea.

Patients may have vomiting, nausea, **diarrhea**, insomnia, sour stomach, heartburn, constipation, gas, neck pain, back pain, **bone pain**, bloating, swelling, pain or swelling at the injection site, joint, muscle, or limb pain, **depression**, or nosebleeds.

Patients should always notify their physician about any unusual symptoms they experience while on medication.

Interactions

Patients should tell their doctors if they have a known allergic reaction to arsenic trioxide or any other medications or substances, such as foods and preservatives. Before taking any new medications, including nonprescription medications, **vitamins**, and herbal medications, the patients should notify their doctors.

Michael Zuck, Ph.D.

Arteriography, *see* **Angiography**

Ascites

Description

Ascites is defined as an excessive amount of fluid built up within the peritoneal cavity. Both the abdominal organs and the abdomen itself are lined with membranes called the peritoneum. Between these two linings is a space referred to as the peritoneal cavity. In pathological conditions that result in edema, or excessive fluid accumulation in bodily tissues, fluid can build up in the peritoneal cavity.

Smaller abdominal fluid amounts usually do not produce symptoms. However, larger accumulations can cause:

- rapid weight gain
- abdominal discomfort and distention
- shortness of breath and actual dyspnea, or difficulty breathing
- swollen ankles

Severe cases of ascites can result in the retention of literally gallons (each gallon equals nearly four liters) of liquid in the peritoneal cavity. If fluid retention is sufficiently severe, the abdomen becomes swollen and even painful. Breathing can be affected as the fluid-filled peritoneal cavity presses upon the diaphragm, a very necessary component of respiration. The diaphragm is made up of a dome-shaped sheet of muscles that separates the thoracic, or chest, cavity from the abdomen. When the muscle fibers of the diaphragm contract, the space in the chest cavity is enlarged, and air enters the lungs to fill the enlarged space. When pressure on the diaphragm from fluid build-up occurs, it lessens the ability of these diaphragm muscular fibers to expand and contract, and results in impaired breathing.

Ascites, in itself, is not a disease, but rather a symptom of several other pathological conditions. These include:

- Cirrhosis of the liver, which is responsible for 80% of all instances of ascites in the United States.
- Pancreatic ascites develops when a cyst that has thick, fibrous walls (pseudocyst) bursts and permits pancreatic juices to enter the abdominal cavity.
- Chylous ascites, which has a milky appearance caused by lymph that has leaked into the abdominal cavity. Although chylous ascites is sometimes caused by trauma, abdominal surgery, tuberculosis, or another peritoneal infection, it is usually a symptom of **lymphoma** or some other cancer.
- Cancer causes 10% of all occurrences of ascites in the United States. It is most commonly a consequence of disease that originates in the peritoneum (peritoneal carcinomatosis) or of cancer that spreads (metastasizes) from another part of the body. Tumors especially prone to malignant ascites formation include **ovarian cancer** and metastatic gastrointestinal tumors.

- Endocrine and renal ascites are rare disorders. Endocrine ascites, sometimes a symptom of an endocrine system disorder, also affects women who are taking fertility drugs. Renal ascites develops when blood levels of albumin dip below normal. Albumin is the major protein in blood plasma. It functions to keep fluid inside the blood vessels.

Causes

The two most important factors in the production of ascites due to chronic liver disease are low levels of albumin in the blood and an increase in the pressure within the branches of the portal vein that run through liver (portal hypertension). Low levels of albumin in the blood cause a change in the pressure necessary to prevent fluid exchange (osmotic pressure). This change in pressure allows fluid to seep out of the blood vessels. The scarring that occurs in cirrhosis causes portal hypertension. Blood that cannot flow through the liver because of the increased pressure leaks into the abdomen and causes ascites.

Other conditions that contribute to ascites development include:

- hepatitis
- heart or kidney failure
- inflammation and fibrous hardening of the sac that contains the heart (constrictive pericarditis)

Persons who have systemic lupus erythematosus but do not have liver disease or portal hypertension occasionally develop ascites. Depressed thyroid activity sometimes causes pronounced ascites, but inflammation of the pancreas (pancreatitis) rarely causes significant accumulations of fluid.

Treatments

Reclining minimizes the amount of salt the kidneys absorb, so treatment generally starts with bed rest and a low-salt diet. Urine-producing drugs (diuretics) may be prescribed if initial treatment is ineffective. The weight and urinary output of patients using diuretics is normally carefully monitored, often on a daily basis. This scrutiny involves watching for signs of:

- Hypovolemia (massive loss of blood or fluid) that can often result in drastic drops in blood pressure.
- Azotemia (abnormally high blood levels of nitrogen-bearing materials).
- Potassium imbalance that can result in cardiac arrhythmia.
- High sodium concentration. Sodium should be restricted from the diet as much as possible.

Because of the discomfort and respiratory difficulty moderate-to-severe accumulations of fluid can produce, fluid removal, or **paracentesis**, is often the treatment of choice. Paracentesis involves the extraction of fluid from the abdominal cavity via a needle that is usually inserted into the peritoneum under local anesthesia. This is a relatively safe and painless method of relieving fluid build-up. It is considered safer than diuretic therapy, resulting in fewer complications and requiring shorter hospital stays.

Large-volume paracentesis is also the preferred treatment for massive ascites. Diuretics are sometimes used to prevent new fluid accumulations, and the procedure may need to be repeated periodically.

In cases of ascites that do not respond appropriately to the treatments described above, a **peritoneovenous shunt** may be inserted. This device is equipped with a one-way valve that allows fluid from the peritoneal cavity to pass into the venous blood circulatory system. From there the fluid is eliminated by the kidneys. In cases of malignant ascites, there is a concern that the use of such a shunt could enhance the spread of the cancer. This relatively small risk must be balanced against the positive effect the shunt can have on the individual's quality of life as well as against his or her expected survival period.

Alternative and complementary therapies

Dietary alterations, focused on reducing salt intake, are an important facet of treatment. Potassium-rich foods like low-fat yogurt, mackerel, cantaloupe, and baked potatoes help balance excess sodium intake and help ensure proper heart function. Such complementary therapies should always be considered an adjunct to, not a substitute for, the conventional treatments described above.

Resources

BOOKS

Berkow, Robert, ed. *The Merck Manual of Medical Information.* Whitehouse Station, NJ: Merck Research Laboratories, 1997.

PERIODICALS

Bieligk, S.C., B.F. Calvo, and D.G. Coit. "Peritoneovenous Shunting for Nongynecologic Malignant Ascites." *Cancer* 91, no. 7 (April 2001): 1247–9.

ORGANIZATIONS

National Cancer Institute, National Institute of Health. 31 Center Drive, MSC 2580, Bethesda, MD 20892-2580. (800) 4-CANCER. <http://www.nci.nih.gov>.

Joan Schonbeck

Asparaginase

Definition

Asparaginase (also known as L-asparaginase, and sold under the brand name Elspar) is a medicine used to stop growth of cancer and formation of new cancer cells.

Purpose

Asparaginase is used as part of an induction regimen for the treatment of **acute lymphocytic leukemia** (ALL) in children.

Description

Asparaginase is an enzyme made from the bacteria *escherichia coli* (E. coli). In this country, two forms of asparaginase are available: one made from E. coli, and a slightly changed version of the E.Coli form linked to polyethylene glycol (PEG) molecule. This PEG-linked asparaginase is called **pegaspargase**. This version was made available in 1994, is more expensive than the other form, and is mainly used in patients who have developed an allergy to E. Coli. Another natural form of asparaginase made from the plant bacteria *erwinia carotovora* is known by the brand name Erwinar and can be specially obtained for patients who develop a severe allergy to E. coli asparaginase. Asparaginase kills cancer cells by depleting a certain protein in the blood (L-asparagine) that is necessary for survival and growth of tumor cells in patients with ALL. Fortunately, normal cells are not dependent on L-asparagine for survival.

Asparaginase is mainly given in combination with **vincristine** and steroids (either prednisone or **dexamethasone**) for the first three weeks of therapy.

Recommended Dosage

Adults and children

INDUCTION CHEMOTHERAPY FOR ALL. Doses vary between different **chemotherapy** protocols. The usual dose is 6,000-10,000 units per square meter of body surface area given for 10 days. Patients should refer to individual protocol for recommended dose.

Administration

This medicine can be given directly into the muscle (intramuscular) or into the vein (intravenous). Intramuscular injection of asparaginase lowers the risk of severe allergic reactions (also known as hypersensitivity or anaphylaxis). The risk of hypersensitivity reaction is higher with the second and third dose of the drug.

KEY TERMS

Acute lymphocytic leukemia (ALL)—This is the most common cancer in children. Patients with ALL can present with fever, weakness, fatigue, pallor, unusual bleeding and easy bruising, pinpoint dots on the skin, large lymph nodes, large liver and spleen. ALL in children has a much better prognosis than in adults, with over 90% of children going into remission and an 80% cure rate with chemotherapy.

Anaphylaxis—An immediate kind of an allergic reaction that usually happens after a second exposure of a body to a drug, toxin, or some types of foods. A person may experience a dangerous drop in blood pressure, skin rash, itching, puffiness of the face, and difficulty breathing. Anaphylaxis is a medical emergency and can result in death.

Induction therapy—The first stage in treatment of ALL. The purpose of this stage is to quickly cause remission of the disease. The combination of vincristine, asparaginase, and steroids make up the foundation of induction regimen.

Precautions

The use of this medication should be avoided in patients with active pancreatitis (inflammation of the pancreas) or history of pancreatitis, and in patients with serious allergic reaction to asparaginase in the past.

Asparaginase should only be given in a hospital. A patient's blood pressure will need to be monitored every 15 minutes for the first hour. A small test dose may be given to check if patient is allergic to this medicine.

This medication can lower the body's ability to fight infections. Patients should avoid contact with crowds or any individual that may have an infection.

Breast-feeding mothers should use asparaginase with caution. It is not yet known whether this drug crosses into breast milk. Women who are pregnant or may become pregnant should avoid this drug unless the benefits to the mother outweigh the risks to the child.

Contact a doctor immediately if any of these symptoms develop:

- **fever**, chills, sore throat
- yellowing of the skin or eyes
- puffy face, skin rash, trouble breathing, joint pain
- drowsiness, confusion, hallucinations, convulsions
- unusual bleeding or bruising

- stomach pain with nausea, vomiting and loss of appetite

A physician will perform blood tests before starting therapy and during therapy to monitor complete blood count, blood sugar, and pancreas, kidney, and liver functions.

Side effects

Asparaginase is a very potent medicine that can cause serious side effects. An allergic reaction with skin rash, **itching**, joint pain, puffy face, and difficulty breathing can occur very quickly after injection with his drug. This side effect is managed by having the drugs epinephrine, **diphenhydramine**, and steroids available near the bedside to counter the allergic reaction if it occurs. Other common side effects include nausea, vomiting, **diarrhea**, loss of appetite, stomach cramps, and yellowing of the eyes or skin. Less frequent side effects include high blood sugar, drowsiness, confusion, hallucinations, convulsions, decreased kidney function, increased blood clotting, mouth sores, and decreased ability to fight infections. Usually the side effects of asparaginase are more severe in adults than in children.

Interactions

Asparaginase can decrease effectiveness of **methotrexate** in killing cancer cells when given right before and together with methotrexate. The use of these two medicines together should be avoided.

Asparaginase can decrease breakdown and increase toxicity of **cyclophosphamide**.

Risk of liver disease may be increased in patients receiving both asparaginase and **mercaptopurine**.

This medicine can increase blood sugar especially when given in together with steroids.

Asparaginase should be given after vincristine instead of before or with vincristine because it can increase the risk of numbing, tingling and pain in hands and feet.

Olga Bessmertny, Pharm.D.

Astrocytoma

Definition

Astrocytoma is a tumor that arises from astrocytes, star-shaped cells that play a supportive role in the brain.

Description

The brain acts as a computer that controls all of the functions of the body. It stores information, memories, and with the use of hormones and electrical impulses, regulates and sends instructions to the rest of the body. Because of the brain's importance, cancers in the brain can affect many of the body's functions. The location of a tumor within the brain determines which effects it will have. Astrocytomas may occur in the cerebrum, the site of thought and language, the cerebellum, the area responsible for movement and muscle co-ordination, or the brainstem, the location that regulates critical activities like breathing and heartbeat. Childhood astrocytomas are most commonly located in the cerebellum, while adults usually develop astrocytoma in the cerebrum.

Astrocytomas rarely metastasize (spread) outside the brain to other parts of the body; however, they may grow and spread within the brain. As there is no extra room in the skull, the presence of a brain tumor causes an increase in intracranial (within the skull) pressure, resulting in headaches and possibly affecting normal brain function by compressing delicate brain tissue.

Astrocytomas are a type of glioma, a tumor of glial cells (specialized cells that give physical support and electrical insulation between neurons). They are sometimes called gliomas, anaplastic astrocytomas, or glioblastoma multiforme. Oligoastrocytomas are a type of mixed glioma similar to astrocytomas. They usually contain cells that originate from oligodendrocytes as well as astrocytes, and are usually low grade (grading is an estimate of the tumor's malignancy and aggressiveness; lower-grade tumors require less drastic therapy than high-grade tumors).

Demographics

Astrocytoma occurs slightly more often in males than in females. It is also slightly more common in Caucasians than in those of African or Asian descent. Although it affects both adults and children, children usually develop a less serious form with a better prognosis. The total incidence of all types of brain cancer, including astrocytomas, is approximately 13 people out of every 100,000.

Causes and symptoms

The cause of astrocytoma is not known. Brain cancer may occasionally be caused by previous radiation treatments; however, x rays are not believed to play a role. As of 2001, studies have indicated that the moderate use of handheld cellular phones does not cause brain cancer; ongoing research will determine if long-term cellular phone use causes an increase in cancer incidence.

Some studies suggest that brain tumors may occur more frequently in people who have occupational expo-

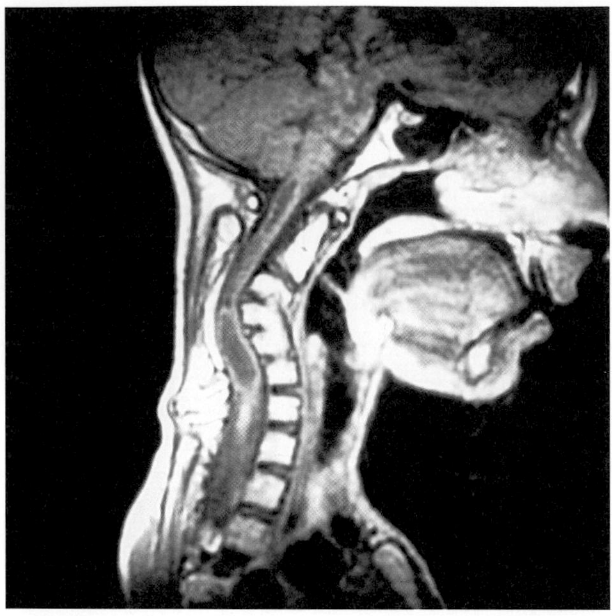

Magnetic resonance image (MRI) of the head and neck of a 15-year-old boy showing the recurrence of an astrocytoma of the spinal cord. The tumor appears about halfway down the neck. *(© Simon Fraser, Neuroradiology Dept., Newcastle General Hospital, Science Source/Photo Researchers, Inc. Reproduced by permission.)*

sure to certain chemicals, including some pesticides, formaldehyde, vinyl chloride, phenols, acrylonitrile, N-nitroso compounds, polycyclic aromatic hydrocarbons, lubricating oils, and organic solvents. The greatest risk is associated with exposure before birth or during infancy.

There is a slightly higher incidence of astrocytoma in the siblings and parents of people with this tumor; however, only one type of astrocytoma is known to have a genetic cause. The rare subependymal giant cell astrocytoma occurs in conjunction with tuberous sclerosis, a hereditary disorder.

A wide variety of symptoms develop as a result of astrocytoma, including the following:

- headache
- **nausea and vomiting**
- neck stiffness or pain
- dizziness
- seizures
- unsteadiness in walking or unusual gait
- lack of coordination, decreased muscle control
- visual problems such as blurring, double vision, or loss of peripheral vision
- weakness in arms or legs
- speech impairment
- altered behavior
- loss of appetite

Because there are several different types of astrocytoma, not all patients will show the same symptoms. The location of the tumor within the brain will determine which symptoms a patient will experience. Because the tumor causes an increase in intracranial pressure, most people with astrocytoma will develop headaches and nausea and vomiting.

Diagnosis

In the first stage of diagnosis the doctor will take a history of symptoms and perform a basic neurological exam, including an eye exam and tests of vision, balance, coordination and mental status. The doctor will then require a computerized tomography (CT) scan and **magnetic resonance imaging** (MRI) of the patient's brain. During a CT scan, x rays of the patient's brain are taken from many different directions; these are combined by a computer, producing a cross-sectional image of the brain. For an MRI, the patient relaxes in a tunnel-like instrument while the brain is subjected to changes of magnetic field. An image is produced based on the behavior of the brain's water molecules in response to the magnetic fields. A special dye may be injected into a vein before these scans to provide contrast and make tumors easier to identify.

If a tumor is found it will be necessary for a neurosurgeon to perform a **biopsy** on it. This simply involves the removal of a small amount of tumor tissue, which is then sent to a neuropathologist for examination and staging. The biopsy may take place before surgical removal of the tumor or the sample may be taken during surgery. Staging of the tumor sample is a method of classification that helps the doctor to determine the severity of the astrocytoma and to decide on the best treatment options. The neuropathologist stages the tumor by looking for atypical cells, the growth of new blood vessels, and for indicators of cell division called mitotic figures.

Treatment team

Treatment of astrocytoma will involve a neurosurgeon to remove the tumor, a neuropathologist to examine the tumor sample, and an oncologist to monitor the patient's health and coordinate **radiation therapy** and **chemotherapy** if necessary. Nurses and radiation therapists will also play a role. After treatment, the patient may be followed up by a neurologist to ensure that the tumor does not grow or recur.

Clinical staging, treatments, and prognosis

There are several different systems for staging astrocytomas. The World Health Organization (WHO) system is the most common; it has four grades of increasing severity based on the appearance of the astrocytoma cells. Other methods of staging correspond fairly closely to the WHO system. Grades I and II are sometimes grouped together and referred to as low-grade astrocytomas. Over time, tumors may progress from a low-grade form with a relatively good prognosis to a higher grade form and poorer prognosis. Additionally, tumors may recur at a higher grade.

KEY TERMS

Anaplastic—Undifferentiated, appearing to have an immature cell type.

Biopsy—A sample of tissue taken from the tumor.

Glioma—A tumor of the brain's glial cells.

Primary tumor—An original tumor, not a metastatic tumor resulting from cancer's spread.

Grade I Pilocytic Astrocytoma

This is also sometimes referred to as juvenile astrocytoma because it occurs more frequently in children than adults. Under a microscope, the astrocytes are thin and elongated, and known as pilocytes. They are accompanied by Rosenthal fibers. The tumor mass does not invade surrounding tissues and is sometimes enclosed in a cyst. In children, pilocytic astrocytoma often occurs in the cerebellum, but may also occur in the cerebrum.

Treatment of this grade depends on the patient's age and the location of the tumor. Surgery is the preferred treatment for this type of astrocytoma; it is performed by a procedure known as a **craniotomy**. An incision is made in the skin and an opening is made in the skull. After the tumor is removed, the bone is normally replaced and the incision closed. The neurosurgeon may also insert a shunt (drainage system) to relieve intracranial pressure; this involves inserting a catheter into a cavity inside the brain called a ventricle, then threading the other end under the skin to a drainage area where the fluid is absorbed.

If the tumor can be completely surgically removed, the patient may not need further therapy and may be monitored only for recurrence. If the tumor cannot be completely removed, patients may be given chemotherapy as well. If the tumor is not completely resected or if it continues to grow after chemotherapy, radiation therapy may be necessary. Radiation therapy is not normally given to children under the age of three in order to prevent permanent damage to the child's healthy brain tissue. Radiation treatment may cause swelling in the brain; steroids may be prescribed to reduce the swelling.

The best indicator for prognosis is complete removal of the tumor. With complete tumor removal, 80% of patients are alive ten years later. Location of the tumor in the cerebellum also suggests a better prognosis than other locations.

Grade II Low-Grade Diffuse Astrocytoma

These astrocytomas spread out and invade surrounding brain tissues but grow very slowly. Under the microscope, fibrous structures are present. Grade II astrocytomas may occur anywhere in the brain, in the cerebellum and brain stem, or in the cerebrum, including the optic pathways. Genetic studies indicate that mutations of the tumor suppressor gene p53 occur frequently in these tumors.

Surgical removal of the tumor is the first choice for treatment, but it may not be possible due the tumor's location. Surgery is usually followed by radiation. Patients under 35 years of age have a better prognosis than older patients; in older patients, low-grade tumors progress to higher grades more rapidly. Overall median survival is four to five years.

Pleimorphic xanthoastrocytoma, a tumor originating in cells of a mixture of glial and neuronal origin, is often considered a grade II astrocytoma. It is relatively benign and treated only with surgery.

Grade III Anaplastic Astrocytoma

Anaplastic astrocytoma occurs most frequently in people aged 50 to 60. The term anaplastic means that the cells are not differentiated; they have the appearance of immature cells and cannot perform their proper functions. Researchers believe this is due to a gradual accumulation of genetic alterations in these cells. These tumor cells invade surrounding healthy brain tissue.

Anaplastic astrocytomas may be inoperable because of their location and their infiltration into normal tissue; in this case radiation therapy is recommended. Chemotherapy may include various combinations of alkylating agents and other drugs, including **carmustine**, **cisplatin**, **lomustine**, **procarbazine** and **vincristine**. These tumors tend to recur more frequently than grade I and II tumors. Following treatment, median survival is 12 to 18 months. The five-year survival rate for these patients is approximately 10% to 35%.

Grade IV Glioblastoma Multiforme

Glioblastoma Multiforme (GBM) is the most common primary brain tumor in adults. These tumors

QUESTIONS TO ASK THE DOCTOR

- Where inside my brain is the cancer located and where will it spread?
- What types of treatment are recommended?
- What are the possible side effects of this treatment?
- How can the side effects be minimized?
- Am I eligible for any clinical trials?
- Are there any alternatives to this treatment?
- What are the chances that the cancer will return?
- Will this cause any disabilities?
- How will this affect my daily life?

aggressively invade adjacent tissue and may even spread throughout the central nervous system. They frequently occur in the frontal lobes of the cerebrum. Tumor biopsies may show large areas of necrosis, or dead cells, surrounded by areas of rampant growth. There may also be a mixture of cell types within the biopsy. Genetic studies show that a number of different types of mutations can take place in genes for tumor suppressor p53 and other proteins that play a role in controlling the normal growth of cells.

Often GBM cannot be entirely surgically removed because it affects large areas of the brain. Radiation therapy will be given regardless of whether surgery is possible, except to very young children. Conventional radiation may be performed, but more specialized types, such as stereotactic radiosurgery, which uses imaging and a computer to treat the tumor very precisely, or interstitial radiation, which delivers radiation by placing radioactive material directly on the tumor, may also be used. Chemotherapy will follow radiation; it may include carmustine, lomustine, procarbazine, and vincristine.

GBM is most common in patients over 50 years of age and rarely occurs in patients under 30. Increasing age is associated with a poorer prognosis. Median survival is 9 to 11 months following treatment. Fewer than 5% of patients are alive five years later. Because of the poor prognosis of GBM, it is treated more aggressively than low-grade astrocytomas; many **clinical trials** take place to test new treatments.

Alternative and complementary therapies

While no specific alternative therapies have become popular for this particular type of brain cancer, patients interested in pursuing complementary therapies should discuss the idea with their doctor. A doctor may be able to provide information about the efficacy of certain techniques and whether they may interfere with conventional treatment.

Coping with cancer treatment

Patients may experience unpleasant side effects due to their treatment. Patients should discuss any side effects they experience with their doctors; occasionally an effect may be unexpected or dangerous and dosages may need to be adjusted. Doctors can help alleviate nausea with antinausea medications and may prescribe antidepressants to help the patient deal with the cancer on a psychological level. Joining support groups will also help patients deal with the psychological effects of treatment. Cancer survivors can help provide encouragement and offer advice for coping with cancer on a day-to-day basis.

Clinical trials

Clinical trials are an important treatment possibility, especially for patients with tumors that are inoperable or do not respond well to treatment. Participation in clinical trials also gives patients an opportunity to make contributions to the search to find a cure for their cancer. A wide variety of clinical trials are available, particularly for the higher-grade astrocytomas. Trials for higher-grade astrocytomas may test new drugs, new combinations of drugs, drug implants, and higher doses of drugs, possibly in combination with different methods of radiation therapy. Some studies may examine the use of gene therapy or immune therapy, including **vaccines**.

Trials for lower-grade astrocytomas focus on finding chemotherapy that causes fewer side effects. Some studies may also feature new combinations of drugs while others may attempt to treat the tumor by using lower dosages of drugs spread out over a longer period of time.

Prevention

Currently, scientists do not know what causes the majority of brain cancers. There may be a slight genetic predisposition, as family members of astrocytoma patients have a slightly increased incidence of the disease. Clinical studies show that a large number of genetic alterations take place in the higher grade astrocytomas; although this helps to explain what is going wrong in the cells, it does not explain what is causing these genetic mutations to take place.

While it is known that ionizing radiation can cause brain tumors, most people are not exposed to this type of radiation unless they are being treated for cancer. Ongoing studies are examining the long-term risks of other types of radiation, but as of 2001, neither x rays, electromagnetic fields, or cellular phones appear to increase the likelihood of brain cancers.

Although evidence is not yet conclusive, some studies suggest that some brain tumors may be caused by environmental exposure to certain organic chemicals. Exposure is most harmful to the developing fetus and infants, so pregnant women may wish to consider whether they have any occupational exposure to organic chemicals. Parents of infants should be aware of pesticides and any other potentially harmful chemical their child could come into contact with.

Additionally there is some evidence that supplements containing **vitamins** A, C, E, and folate may have a protective effect when taken during pregnancy. The children of women who take these supplements during pregnancy are half as likely to develop brain tumors before age five.

Special concerns

Children who develop astrocytoma should be monitored regularly by their physicians to ensure that the tumor does not recur. A follow-up schedule should be discussed with the doctor; the child may be examined twice a year initially, then tested annually afterwards. In addition to the possibility of recurrence, other health problems due to treatment may arise in the child. The child may have lower levels of growth hormone or thyroid hormone or delayed growth as a result of radiation. There may also be decreased intellectual capacity or learning or physical disabilities that can be detected during follow-up. Parents can then arrange for rehabilitation or special education for their child.

Adults may also experience permanent negative effects as a result of their treatment. Radiation damage to healthy tissue may occasionally cause delayed effects such as decreased intellect, impaired memory, changes in personality, and confusion. These types of side effects should be reported to a health professional; the patient can be referred to rehabilitation specialists who can help with regaining abilities.

See Also Brain and central nervous system tumors; Childhood cancers; Tumor grading

Resources

PERIODICALS

Inskip, Peter D., et al. "Cellular Telephone Use and Brain Tumors." *New England Journal of Medicine* 344 (2001): 79–86.

Pencalet, Phillipe, et al. "Benign Cerebellar Astrocytomas in Children." *Journal of Neurosurgery* 90 (1999): 265–73.

Yu, John S., et al. "Vaccination of Malignant Glioma Patients with Peptide-pulsed Dendritic Cells Elicits Systemic Cytotoxicity and Intracranial T-cell Infiltration." *Cancer Research* 61 (2001): 842–7.

ORGANIZATIONS

American Brain Tumor Association. 2720 River Rd., Des Plaines, IL 60018. (800) 886-2282. <http://www.abta.org>.

National Brain Tumor Foundation. 414 13th St., Suite 700, Oakland, CA 94612-2603. (800) 934-2873. <http://www.braintumor.org>.

The Brain Tumor Society. 124 Watertown St., Suite 3-H, Watertown, MA 02472. (800) 770-8287. <http://www.tbts.org>.

OTHER

BRAINTMR T.H.E. Brain Trust. Electronic mailing list. (June 22, 2001) <http://www.braintrust.org>.

Racquel Baert, M.S.

ATG *see* **Lymphocyte immune globulin**

Atropine *see* **Antidiarrheal agents**

Azacitidine

Definition

Azacitidine, is an antineoplastic (antitumor) agent that acts by interfering with the growth of cells.

Purpose

Azacitidine is a **chemotherapy** drug used primarily to treat adults and children with **acute myelocytic leukemia** that have not responded to traditional therapy. It is also used to treat myelodysplastic syndrome. There is limited data that azacitidine may be useful for chronic myelogenous leukemia, sickle cell anemia, and cancers that have spread to other organs in the body. It should also be noted that azacitidine does not appear on the FDA's approved drug list. Currently, azacitidine is prescribed only as an experimental drug.

Description

DNA can be thought of as the blueprint for the cell, and RNA as the messenger to carry out the instructions of the DNA. RNA, or ribonucleic acid, is a close relative of DNA, deoxyribonucleic acid. Both are made up of four different bases, adenine, guanine, cytosine, and thymine.

KEY TERMS

Gene—A functional unit of DNA.

Azacitidine pretends to be cytosine, and is incorporated into the RNA and DNA of cells, inhibiting them from carrying out their normal functions and causing cell death.

Recommended dosage

The dose of azacitidine depends on the reason it is being administered and whether any other drugs are involved in treatment. The usual dose for azacitidine is 50 to 200 mg per square meter of body surface area per day for five to 10 days. This is repeated at two to three week intervals. Azacitidine is administered either through the vein or injected under the skin. It may be injected under the skin at a dose of 75 mg per square meter of body surface area per day for seven days, to be repeated every 4 weeks.

Precautions

Pregnant women should not take this drug, and should be aware that this drug has been shown to cause death or abnormality in the fetuses of laboratory animals. Women who might become pregnant while taking this medication should take steps to ensure that they do not. Nursing mothers should discontinue nursing while taking this medication. All patients should have this drug administered by a health care professional and their progress regularly monitored.

Side effects

The most common side effect of azacitidine is the decreased production of white blood cells, which are important in fighting infections, and platelets, which are important in preventing bleeding. Nausea, vomiting, and **diarrhea** are also very common with this drug.

Other side effects include **fever**, general muscle pain, weakness, and lethargy. Decreased liver function, low blood pressure, and changes in kidney function have also been reported with azacitidine. Also, injections of the drug under the skin can cause redness, swelling, or mild pain.

Interactions

Azacitidine has no known interactions with other drugs. However, prior to initiating any over-the-counter, herbal, or new medications, patients should consult their physician, nurse, or pharmacist to prevent possible drug interactions.

Michael Zuck, Ph.D.

Azathioprine

Definition

Azathioprine is a non-specific immunosuppressant antimetabolite that can be used as a chemotherapeutic agent to inhibit lymphocyte purine metabolism. In the United States, azathioprine is also known by the brand name Imuran.

Purpose

In 1968 the Food and Drug Administration approved azathioprine for use after an organ transplant to decrease the chance of the body rejecting the transplanted organ. However, azathioprine is an experimental drug that can be used during treatment of cancers such as leukemia and lymphomas. In the body, azathioprine is converted to **mercaptopurine** (6-MP) and thus has the same effects as that **chemotherapy** drug. They both are purine analogs that interfere with the metabolism of purine-based nucleotides found in DNA.

The use of azathioprine results in killing cells such as T-lymphocytes. This is important in cancers such as lymphocytic leukemia. The idea is that if T-lymphocyte reproduction is inhibited by interfering with DNA synthesis, then the cancer cell reproduction will also be inhibited. Certain types of leukemia and lymphomas are treated with radiation and chemotherapy, which destroy dividing cells such as those in the bone marrow. As a result, the patient is no longer able to produce blood cells. To combat the loss of blood cells, a bone marrow transplant may be performed to provide the patient with healthy marrow. The body may react against the foreign bone marrow. Therefore, an additional benefit of azathioprine use as an immunosuppressant could be to produce fewer white blood cells, thus interfering with the body's natural **immune response** to foreign proteins, such as those found on the cell surfaces of bone marrow coming from a bone marrow donor.

Description

Azathioprine is a derivative of mercaptopurine, a purine analog antimetabolite, which interferes with the enzymatic pathways for biosynthesis of nucleic acids by substituting for normal metabolites. In this way, it can act as an immunosuppressant by interfering with the production of white blood cells such as lymphocytes.

Recommended dosage

Azathioprine can be taken either orally (50 milligram scored tablets) or through an injection (100 milligram vials for intravenous use). Dosing is based on body weight and size of the patient. Initially, the oral dosage is approximately 3 to 5 milligrams per kilogram of body weight, while the injection dosage is approximately 1 milligram per kilogram of body weight. At time goes on, the physician may decrease the dosage. Patients can take this medicine in a single dose per day. The duration of treatment will continue until the fear of transplant rejection has passed.

Precautions

Since this medication is an immunosuppressant and results in a lower white blood cell count, there is a higher risk of developing infection. Therefore, patients using azathioprine should limit their contact with people that have existing infections, they should not have dental work done while on this medication, and they should not touch their eyes or inside of their nose unless they have just washed their hands. Patients should also take care not to cut themselves and should be careful when using a regular toothbrush and dental floss.

Pregnant women should not take this drug since it can cross the placenta and can have serious side effects. Women who are breastfeeding should not take this drug. Azathioprine can pass through the breast milk to the baby and can result in serious problems.

Side effects

The most common and less serious side effects include **fatigue**, weakness, loss of appetite (**anorexia**), **nausea and vomiting**, and upset stomach. Upset stomach can be alleviated if azathioprine is taken with food or milk.

Other side effects may occur that require the attention of a medical professional. These include:

- cough or hoarseness
- **fever** or chills
- lower back or side pain
- extreme fatigue
- black tarry stools
- blood in the urine
- red spots on the skin
- fast heartbeat
- shortness of breath
- liver problems

Since the immune system is depressed when azathioprine is used, the result can be pancytopenia, including leukopenia and **thrombocytopenia** as well as macrocytic **anemia**. The severity of these is dependent on the dose, and the dose may be lowered by the physician as needed.

Azathioprine has been used in children and has not been shown to induce side effects different than those found in adults. However, as with many medications there have not been any specific tests done with the elderly. It is not expected to cause any different side effects than those encountered in younger adults.

Interactions

There are medications and other medical conditions that can interact with azathioprine. A medication called **allopurinol** is used to treat gout and can increase the

KEY TERMS

Analog—A chemical compound with a structure similar to another chemical, but differing in a certain way.

Antimetabolite—A drug that resembles a substance that occurs naturally in a metabolic pathway, interfering with metabolism.

Bone marrow—The soft tissue inside of bones that produces blood cells.

Gout—A form of arthritis that involves ureic acid.

Leukopenia—Decrease in the amount of white blood cells.

Lymphocytes—A type of white blood cell and part of the immune system.

Macrocytic anemia—Anemia where blood cells are much larger than normal.

Myelosuppression—Decrease in the proliferation of bone marrow cells.

Pancytopenia—Decrease in all the cellular components of the blood.

Purine—A base found in nucleotides and nucleic acids that are used to make DNA.

effects and toxicity of azathioprine because it interferes with the removal of azathioprine from the body.

Both kidney disease and liver disease can increase the effects and toxicity of azathioprine. Both diseases interfere with the removal of azathioprine from the body. If the patient has either of these diseases, the physician may make adjustments in the dosage given.

Sally C. McFarlane-Parrott

Aztreonam *see* **Antibiotics**

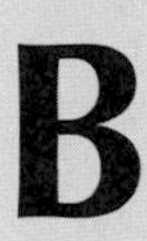

Bacillus Calmette Guérin

Definition

BCG, or bacillus Calmette Guérin, is a genetically engineered bacterium that is used to treat **bladder cancer**. BCG is also known by the brand names ImmuCys, TheraCys and TICE BCG.

Purpose

Excision (cutting out) of bladder tumors can lead to extreme discomfort in patients because of the damage done to the bladder, the organ that collects and holds urine until it can be released from the body. In certain kinds of bladder cancers, treatment with BCG seems to cause cancers to shrink or disappear. Thus, when BCG treatment is effective, it is possible to preserve the bladder.

Description

BCG is made by altering the DNA, or hereditary material, of a bacterium. The bacterium that is altered is one that has been used for decades to vaccinate against tuberculosis. There are several different ways in which BCG has been modified by genetic engineering. In each case, however, the DNA added to the BCG from human cells gives instructions for the production of compounds that stimulate the immune system. The compounds are all proteins and are known by the scientific category name of cytokines.

Even BCG that has not been modified by genetic engineering seems to reduce the growth of superficial tumors in the bladder. But when the BCG introduced to the bladder contains DNA that gives instructions for cytokines, the tumor-fighting ability it confers on the organ is greater.

The live BCG is put inside the bladder where it causes an inflammatory response. This means that the bladder responds as though an infection were present and mounts an attack from the body's immune system. Somehow the response inhibits, or stops, tumor growth, but the way it does so is not understood.

Recommended dosage

BCG is delivered directly to the bladder via a catheter, or a tube that is inserted in the urethra. The method of delivery is called intravesical, which means it is sent directly into the cavity, or holding space, of the bladder.

The patient takes treatment once a week for six weeks and then once a month for six to twelve months. Large quantities of BCG are used. One standard dose of TheraCys calls for 81 milligrams in the first series of treatments.

Precautions

Care providers who have an immune system that is not functioning optimally should not handle BCG. Patients with HIV are at high risk for infection from BCG. All materials from BCG administration are considered biohazards.

Side effects

Most side effects fall into the category of flu-like symptoms and include chills, **fever**, and **nausea and vomiting**. There is also discomfort related to the inflammation of the bladder, particularly the feeling of an urgent need to urinate.

In a very few individuals BCG has spread throughout the body and caused infection and death.

Interactions

Antibiotics, or drugs given to fight infection, can stop the activity of the BCG and should not be given at the same time. Chemicals that suppress the immune sys-

KEY TERMS

Catheter—An artificial tube that is inserted in the urethra to introduce substances to the bladder, or under some circumstances, to drain the bladder.

Genetically engineered—An organism that has been modified by the intervention of humans, usually by the addition of DNA, or hereditary material, from one species to the DNA of another species.

Kilogram—Metric measure that equals 2.2 pounds.

Milligram—One-thousandth of a gram. There are one thousand grams in a kilogram. A gram is the metric measure that equals about 0.035 ounces.

Urethra—Tube that connects the bladder to the outside of the body.

tem can also interfere with the action of BCG, as can **radiation therapy**.

Diane M. Calabrese

Barium enema

Definition

A barium enema, also known as a lower GI (gastrointestinal) exam, is a diagnostic test using x-ray examination to view the large intestine (colon and rectum). There are two types of this test: the single-contrast technique, in which barium sulfate solution is injected into the rectum to gain a profile view of the large intestine; and the double-contrast (or air contrast) technique, in which air and barium sulfate are injected into the rectum.

Purpose

A barium enema may be performed to assist in diagnosing or detecting:

- colon or **rectal cancer** (colorectal cancer)
- inflammatory diseases such as ulcerative colitis
- polyps (small benign growths in the tissue lining of the colon and rectum)
- diverticula (pouches pushing out from the colon)
- structural changes in the large intestine

The double-contrast barium enema is more accurate than the single-contrast technique for detecting small polyps or tumors, early inflammatory disease, and bleeding caused by ulcers because it gives a better view of the intestinal walls.

The decision to perform a barium enema is based on the patient's history of altered bowel habits. These alterations may include **diarrhea**, constipation, lower abdominal pain, blood, mucus or pus in the stool. It is also recommended that this exam be used every five to 10 years beginning at age 50 to screen healthy people for **colon cancer**, the second most deadly type of cancer in the United States. Those who have a close relative with colon cancer or who have had a precancerous polyp are considered to be at an increased risk for the disease and should be screened more frequently to detect abnormalities.

Precautions

Although the barium enema is an effective screening method and may lead to a timely diagnosis of a variety gastrointestinal diseases, the test may not detect all abnormalities present in the colon and rectum. In addition, the barium enema visualizes only the large intestine; the small intestine may also require examination with an **upper GI series** to rule out abnormalities in that area of the digestive tract. Another drawback is that intestinal gas may hinder the accuracy of test results.

As of 2001, numerous studies have shown that a **colonoscopy** performed by an experienced gastroenterologist is a more accurate initial diagnostic tool for detecting early signs of colorectal cancer than a barium enema. Colonoscopy allows a physician to examine the entire colon and rectum for polyps. In addition, if abnormalities such as polyps are observed during the procedure, these often-precancerous growths may be removed during the procedure and later examined (**biopsy**). One additional difference between a barium enema and a colonoscopy is that a colonoscopy almost always involves conscious sedation, while the barium enema is an unsedated procedure. Some physicians use flexible **sigmoidoscopy** (proctosigmoidoscopy) plus a barium enema instead of colonoscopy. However, sigmoidoscopy only visualizes the rectum and the portion of the colon immediately above it (sigmoid colon) and does not allow the physician to remove polyps but only to obtain tissue or stool samples.

Description

To begin a barium enema, the patient lies flat on his or her back on a tilting radiographic table in order to have x rays of the abdomen taken. After being assisted to a different position, a well-lubricated rectal tube is inserted through the anus. This tube allows the physician or assistant to slowly administer the barium sulfate into the intestine. While this filling process is closely monitored, it is important for the patient to keep the anus tightly contracted against the rectal tube to help maintain its position and prevent the barium from leaking. This step is important because the test may be inaccurate if the barium leaks. A rectal balloon may also be inflated to help retain the barium. The table may be tilted or the patient moved to different positions to aid in the filling process.

As the barium fills the intestine, x rays of the abdomen are taken to distinguish significant findings. There are many ways to perform a barium enema. One way is that shortly after filling, the rectal tube is removed and the patient expels as much of the barium as possible. Upon completing this expulsion, an additional **x ray** is taken, and a double-contrast enema exam may follow. If this procedure is done immediately, a thin film of barium will remain in the intestine, and air is then slowly injected to expand the bowel lumen (space in the intestine). Sometimes no x rays will be taken until after the air is injected. The entire test takes about 20-30 minutes.

Preparation

In order to conduct the most accurate barium enema test, the large intestine must be empty. Thus, patients must follow a prescribed diet and bowel preparation instructions prior to the test. This preparation commonly includes restricted intake of dairy products and a liquid diet for 24 hours prior to the test, in addition to drinking large amounts of water or clear liquids 12–24 hours before the test. Patients may also be given **laxatives** and asked to give themselves a cleansing enema.

In addition to the prescribed diet and bowel preparation prior to the test, the patient can expect the following during a barium enema:

- The patient will be well draped with a gown and secured to a tilting x-ray table.
- As the barium or air is injected into the intestine, the patient may experience cramping pains or the urge to defecate.
- The patient will be instructed to take slow, deep breaths through the mouth to ease any discomfort.

Aftercare

Patients should follow several steps immediately after undergoing a barium enema, including:

- Drinking plenty of fluids to help counteract the dehydrating effects of bowel preparation and the test.

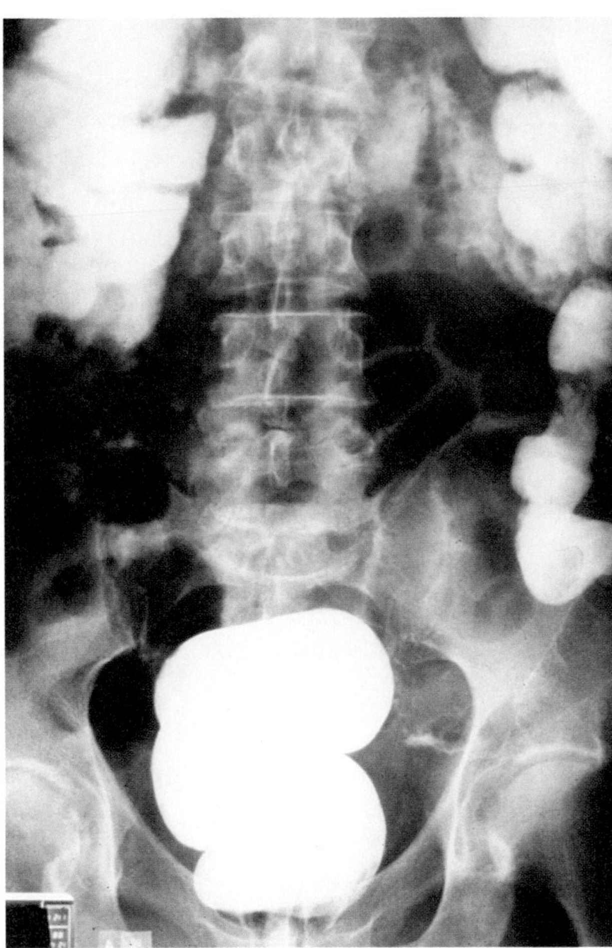

X ray of sigmoid colon after implementation of a barium enema. *(Custom Medical Stock Photo. Reproduced by permission.)*

- Taking time to rest because a barium enema and the bowel preparation taken before it can be exhausting.
- Administering a cleansing enema may help to eliminate any remaining barium. Light-colored stools will be prevalent for the next 24-72 hours following the test.

Risks

Although a barium enema is generally considered a safe **screening test**, it can cause complications in certain people. For example, patients with a rapid heart rate, severe ulcerative colitis, toxic megacolon (acute dilation of the colon that may progress to rupture), or a presumed perforation in the intestine should not undergo a barium enema. Patients with a known blocked intestine, diverticulitis, or severe bloody diarrhea may be tested with caution on the advice of a physician. Also, administering a barium enema to a pregnant woman is not advisable because of radiation exposure to the fetus.

KEY TERMS

Barium sulfate—A barium compound used during a barium enema to block the passage of x rays during the exam.

Colonoscopy—An examination of the upper portion of the rectum performed with a colonoscope or elongated speculum.

Diverticula—A diverticulum of the colon is a sac or pouch in the colon walls which is usually asymptomatic (without symptoms) but may cause difficulty if it becomes inflamed.

Diverticulitis—A condition of the diverticulum of the intestinal tract, especially in the colon, in which inflammation may cause pain and distended sacs extending from the colon.

Sigmoidoscopy—A visual examination of the rectum and sigmoid colon using an instrument called a sigmoidoscope.

Ulcerative colitis—An ulceration or erosion of the mucosa (lining) of the colon.

Although the barium enema may cause minor stomach or abdominal discomfort in some people, more serious complications include:

- severe cramping
- nausea and vomiting
- perforation of the colon
- water intoxication
- barium granulomas (inflamed nodules)
- allergic reactions

These complications, however, are all very rare.

Normal results

When the patient undergoes a single-contrast enema, the intestine is steadily filled with barium to differentiate the colon's markings. A normal result displays uniform filling of the colon. As the barium is expelled, the intestinal walls collapse. A normal result on the x ray after the barium is expelled shows an intestinal lining with a standard, feathery appearance and no abnormalities.

The double-contrast enema expands the intestine, which is already lined with a thin layer of barium; however, the addition of air displays a detailed image of the mucosal pattern. Varying positions taken by the patient allow the barium to collect on the dependent walls of the intestine by way of gravity.

QUESTIONS TO ASK THE DOCTOR

- How long will the test take?
- Will the test be painful?
- Is barium safe?
- Can I take my usual medications the day before the test?
- How many days will the barium be in my system?
- When will I get the test results?

Abnormal results

A barium enema visualizes abnormalities appearing on a series of x rays, thus aiding in the diagnosis of a variety of gastrointestinal disorders and the early signs of cancer. However, most colon cancers occur in the rectosigmoid region, or upper part of the rectum and adjoining portion of the sigmoid colon, and are better detected with flexible sigmoidoscopy or colonoscopy.

Abnormal findings on a barium enema examination may include polyps, lesions or tumors, diverticulae, inflammatory disease, such as ulcerative colitis, obstructions, or hernias. Structural changes in the intestine, gastroenteritis, and the size, position, and motility of the appendix may also be apparent.

Resources

BOOKS

Fischbach, Frances Talaska. *A Manual of Laboratory and Diagnostic Tests, 6th ed.* Philadelphia: Lippincott Williams and Wilkins, 2000.

Pagana, Kathleen Deska, and Timothy James Pagana. *Mosby's Manual of Diagnostic and Laboratory Tests.* St. Louis, Mo: Mosby,1998.

Schull, Patricia, ed. *Illustrated Guide to Diagnostic Tests, 2nd ed.* Springhouse, PA: Springhouse Corporation, 1998.

Segen, Joseph C., and Joseph Stauffer. "Barium Enema (lower GI series)." In *The Patient's Guide To Medical Tests: Everything You Need To Know About The Tests Your Doctor Prescribes.* New York, NY: Facts On File, Inc., 1998: 44-45.

PERIODICALS

Fletcher, Robert H. "The End of Barium Enemas?" *The New England Journal of Medicine* 342 (June 15, 2000): 1823–1824.

Winawer, Sidney J., R. H. Fletcher, L. Miller, et al. "Colorectal Cancer Screening Clinical Guidelines and Rationale." *Gastroenterology* 112 (1997):594-642.

Winawer, Sidney J., Edward T. Stewart, Ann Zauber et al. "A Comparison of Colonoscopy and Double-Contrast Barium Enema for Surveillance After Polypectomy." *The New England Journal of Medicine* 342 (June 15, 2000): 1766–1772.

Zoorob, Roger, Russell Anderson, Charles Cefalu, and Modamed Sidari. "Cancer Screening Guidelines." *American Family Physician* 63 (March 15, 2001): 1101–1112.

ORGANIZATIONS

American Cancer Society. 1599 Clifton Road, NE, Atlanta, GA 30329-4251. Phone: 1-800-ACS-2345. <http://www.cancer.org>.

American College of Gastroenterology. 4900 B South 31st Street, Arlington, VA 22206. Phone: 703-820-7400. Health Hotline: 1-800-978-7666. <http://www.acg.gi.org>.

American College of Radiology, <http://www.acr.org>.

Beth Kapes

Barrett's esophagus

Definition

Barrett's esophagus is pre-cancerous condition in which normal cells lining the esophagus are replaced with abnormal cells that, in some people, develop into a type of cancer of the esophagus called **adenocarcinoma**.

Description

The esophagus is a tube 10–13 inches (25–33 cm) long and about 1 inch (2.5 cm) wide that carries food from the mouth to the stomach. Normally, the esophagus is lined with squamous epithelial cells. These cells are similar to skin cells, and look smooth and pinkish-white.

The stomach makes acid to help digest food. A different type of cell that is resistant to acid lines the stomach. These cells look red and velvety. At the place where the esophagus meets the stomach, there is a ring of muscle called the lower esophageal sphincter (LES) muscle that normally keeps acid stomach juices from backflowing into the esophagus. When this sphincter is not working correctly, due to a hiatal hernia or medications or loss of muscle tone, acid material enters the bottom portion of the esophagus. This backflow is called reflux. When reflux occurs frequently over an extended period of time, it is called gastroesophageal reflux disease (GERD).

Acid and digestive enzymes from the stomach irritate the cells lining the esophagus. The result is inflammation of the esophagus called esophagitis, or heartburn.

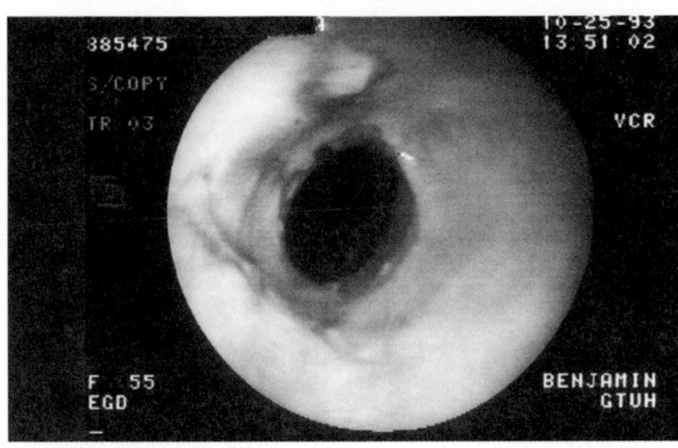

Endoscopic view of a mid-esophageal stricture in a patient with Barrett's esophagus. *(Custom Medical Stock Photo. Reproduced by permission.)*

When the cells lining the lower esophagus are frequently exposed to stomach juices, they erode and are replaced with abnormal cells. These new cells are more resistant to stomach acids and, while they look similar to the cells lining the stomach, they are different. Under the microscope, they appear as a pre-cancerous type of cell not normally found in the body.

These new, pre-malignant cells are called specialized columnar cells. Once specialized columnar cells appear, even if the GERD is controlled and the esophagus heals, the abnormal cells remain and are not replaced with normal cells. The presence of patches of these abnormal red cells in the esophagus is known as Barrett's esophagus. The condition is named after British surgeon Norman Barrett (1903–1979).

Cancer that develops from Barrett's esophagus is called adenocarcinoma. It is one of two types of cancer of the esophagus. This type of cancer cannot occur unless the normal cells lining the esophagus have been damaged and replaced with abnormal cells.

Heartburn is an extremely common complaint. About 10% of people in the United States, or more than 20 million Americans, experience severe or frequent symptoms. Of those people who have frequent heartburn for five years or more, 10–20% develop Barrett's esophagus. From this group, approximately 5–10% go on to develop cancer. Overall, people with Barrett's esophagus have a 30- to 125-fold higher risk of developing adenocarcinoma than the general population.

Demographics

White men over age 45 who experience frequent heartburn for more than 10 years are at highest risk of developing adenocarcinoma arising from Barrett's esophagus. Adenocarcinoma is one of the most rapidly increasing types of cancer in the United States and Western Europe. Often, when the esophagus is damaged by stomach acid, the lining at the entrance to the stomach becomes thick and hard and the opening of the esophagus into the stomach narrows (stricture). People with strictures appear to be at higher risk of developing Barrett's esophagus than other people with GERD. Barrett's esophagus is rare in children.

Causes and symptoms

Barrett's esophagus is caused by gastroesophageal reflux disease that allows the stomach's contents to damage the cells lining the lower esophagus. However, every person who has GERD does not develop Barrett's esophagus. Researchers have thus far been unable to predict which people who have heartburn will develop Barrett's esophagus. While there is no relationship between the severity of heartburn and the development of Barrett's esophagus, there is a relationship between chronic heartburn and the development of Barrett's esophagus. Sometimes people with Barrett's esophagus will have no heartburn symptoms at all. In rare cases, damage to the esophagus may be caused by swallowing a corrosive substance such as lye.

The change from normal to pre-malignant cells that indicates Barrett's esophagus does not cause any particular symptoms. However, warning signs that should not be ignored include:

- frequent and long-standing heartburn
- trouble swallowing (dysphagia)
- vomiting blood
- pain under the breast bone where the esophagus meets the stomach
- unintentional **weight loss** because eating is painful

Diagnosis

Tissue biopsies and an endoscopy are used to diagnose Barrett's esophagus. An endoscopy is normally done in a clinic under sedation or light anesthesia. A flexible fiber-optic tube is inserted through the mouth and down into the esophagus, which allows a doctor to observe the lining of the esophagus.

Sometimes the line dividing the esophagus from the stomach is not clear. Many people who have trouble with heartburn have a condition called hiatal hernia. A hiatal hernia is a stretching, or dilation, of the hole of the diaphragm that allows a bit of the stomach to bulge up into the esophagus. Because the abnormal cells that develop with Barrett's esophagus look like the cells that normally line the stomach, simply looking at the esophagus during an endoscopy is often not enough to diagnose Barrett's esophagus.

Depending on what is observed, the doctor will use tiny clips at the end of the endoscope to collect samples of tissue. This is a painless procedure. The samples are sent to the laboratory where they are examined under the microscope. Microscopic findings that abnormal cells have replaced normal cells are the only definitive diagnosis of Barrett's esophagus.

Currently, trials are underway on alternate ways to recognize abnormal esophageal cells. One trial involves the use of laser-induced spectroscopy to visually pinpoint abnormal cells during endoscopy. This has the advantage of requiring no tissue biopsies, and allows the doctor to make an immediate diagnosis rather than wait several days for laboratory results. The technique, however, is still in the experimental stage and is not part of normal clinical practice.

Treatment team

A gastroenterologist (a specialist in diseases of the digestive system) will diagnose and monitor Barrett's esophagus. Should the pre-malignant cells of Barrett's esophagus develop into adenocarcinoma, an oncologist (cancer specialist) or a cancer surgeon will take over treatment of the cancer.

Clinical staging, treatments, and prognosis

The American College of Gastroenterologists (ACG) recognizes five stages of cellular changes in **biopsy** samples obtained from the esophagus. These are (in increasing severity):

- Negative: No abnormal changes in the cells.
- Indefinite: A few cellular changes; often difficult to distinguish from low-grade dysplasia.
- Low-grade dysplasia: Some signs of cellular abnormality are present.
- High-grade dysplasia: Many signs of cellular abnormality are present.
- Carcinoma: Malignant cells are present.

Treatment and monitoring of Barrett's depends on the results of the biopsies. First-line treatment is aimed at stopping stomach acid from entering the esophagus and giving the lining of the esophagus a chance to heal. Two categories of drugs are used to prevent the stomach from producing acid. Histamine $_2$ blockers include cimetidine (Tagamet), ranitidine (Zantac), and nizatidine (Axid). Proton pump inhibitors include omeprazole (Prilosec) and lansoprazole (Prevacid). Lifetime therapy is usually necessary to control GERD, and higher than normal doses of these drugs may be necessary for people with Barrett's esophagus. Surgery to control GERD is recommended only when these drugs are ineffective or if the patient is unwilling or unable to continue taking them.

Monitoring by endoscopy with biopsies has been the standard approach to Barrett's esophagus. However, there is some debate about the effectiveness of the monitoring in detecting adenocarcinomas and about how cost-effective the monitoring is. Research in this area continues, but ACG guidelines (1999) suggest the following monitoring program:

- Negative or indefinite biopsies: At least two follow-up endoscopies and biopsies at two- to three-year intervals.
- Low-grade dysplasia: Endoscopies and biopsies every six months for a year, then every year if low-grade dysplasia continues.

Treatment of high-grade dysplasia is controversial. Diagnosis of high-grade dysplasia requires confirmation by at least one expert pathologist, with two experts' opinions recommended. One treatment choice is surgery to remove the esophagus (esophagectomy). About 40–45% of people who have high-grade dysplasia also have previously-undetected adenocarcinoma. The advantage of surgically removing the esophagus is that the cancerous cells are also removed.

The alternative to surgery is to continue to monitor cellular changes with endoscopies and biopsies every three months. The choice of treatment depends both on the health of the patient and on the patient's preference.

Surgical removal of the esophagus is the only effective way known to treat adenocarcinoma. The survival rate for people who progress from Barrett's esophagus to adenocarcinoma is poor, with fewer than 10% surviving five years. However, the earlier the cancer is detected and the esophagus removed, the greater the chances of survival.

Alternative and complementary therapies

Several non-medical ways to prevent GERD can be used effectively along with drug treatments that block the production of stomach acid. These include:

- raising the head of the bed a few inches on bricks to encourage gravity to keep the stomach contents from rising into the esophagus
- eliminating caffeine, acidic foods such as orange juice, and spicy foods from the diet
- eating smaller, more frequent meals, rather than large meals
- not eating within three hours of going to bed

None of these methods have any reported adverse side effects.

KEY TERMS

Diaphragm—The muscle that separates the abdominal cavity (stomach and intestines) from the thoracic cavity (heart and lungs).

Dysplasia—The abnormal change in size, shape, or organization of adult cells.

Clinical trials

Since adenocarcinoma arising from Barrett's esophagus is one of the fastest-growing cancers in the United States and Europe, it has sparked new research activity concerning the more sensitive ways to identify high-grade dysplasia, the best methods of monitoring Barrett's esophagus, and the techniques to remove adenocarcinoma without removing the entire esophagus. One of these **clinical trials** involves using drugs to make cancer cells more sensitive to light, and then using a laser to kill these cells in the esophagus. Another clinical trial involves determining if genetic markers can be used to predict which people with Barrett's esophagus are at risk for developing cancer.

The selection of clinical trials underway changes frequently. Current information on what clinical trials in process and where they are being held is available by entering the search term "Barrett's esophagus" at the following Web sites:

- National Cancer Institute <http://cancertrials.nci.nih.gov> or 1-800-4-CANCER.
- National Institutes of Health Clinical Trials <http://clinicaltrials.gov>.
- Center Watch: A Clinical Trials Listing <http://www.centerwatch.com>.

Prevention

People cannot get esophageal adenocarcinoma unless the cells lining the esophagus are damaged. Prevention, therefore, involves prompt treatment of GERD. Some studies have found that factors that increase the risk of a person with the Barrett's esophagus condition developing into adenocarcinoma include heavy smoking, being overweight, and a family history of gastric cancer.

Special concerns

People who are diagnosed with Barrett's esophagus should expect to eliminate caffeine from their diet as caffeine stimulates the production of stomach acid. Other

QUESTIONS TO ASK THE DOCTOR

- How would you characterize the changes in the cells in my esophagus?
- What kind of drugs will you prescribe to control my reflux?
- What frequency of endoscopic monitoring do you propose?
- What are the chances of my Barrett's esophagus progressing to adenocarcinoma?
- If high-grade dysplasia is present, where can I get a second opinion?
- If high-grade dysplasia is present, what is involved in a esophagectomy?
- What is daily life like after an esophagectomy?
- Where can I find out more about clinical trials using drugs and light from a laser (called endoscopic laser photablation) to treat adenocarcinoma?
- What changes in my lifestyle can I make to help control my reflux?
- If my GERD cannot be controlled with medication, what is involved in surgery to control reflux?
- Are there any particular signs or symptoms that suggest that I should see a doctor immediately rather than waiting until my next scheduled endoscopy?

foods that may need to be eliminated include citrus fruits and juices, tomatoes, and spicy foods.

People with high-grade dysplasia are faced with the stressful decision of whether to undergo surgical removal of the esophagus and endure the lifestyle changes that loss of the esophagus involves, or whether to proceed with intensive monitoring, realizing that monitoring is not totally effective and that cancer may not always be detected early. People faced with this decision should discuss the matter with their doctors, their loved ones, and support group members to get a balanced picture of how their lives may be changed by their choices.

Resources

BOOKS

Sharma, Prateek, Richard E. Sampliner, and Bradley Marino.*Barrett's Esophagus and Esophageal Adenocarcinoma, 2nd ed.* Boston: Blackwell Science, 2001.

PERIODICALS

D'Eprio, Nancy. "Barrett's Esophagus: Put Guidelines Into Practice."*Patient Care* 33 (September 1999): 73.

Jankowski, Janusz, et. al. "Barrett's Metaplasia."*The Lancet* 356 (December 2000): 2079.

McGarrity, Thomas. "Barrett's Oesophagus: The Continuing Conundrum."*British Medical Journal* 321 (November 2000): 1238.

Morales, Thomas G. and Richard E. Sampliner. "Barrett's Esophagus."*Archives of Internal Medicine.* 159 (July 1999): 1411.

ORGANIZATIONS

American Cancer Society. (800) ACS-2345. <http://www.cancer.org>.

OTHER

Cancerlinksusa. <http:cancerlinksusa.com>.

OncoLink University of Pennsylvania Cancer Center. <http://cancer.med.upenn.edu/disease/esophageal>.

Tish Davidson, A.M.

Basal cell carcinoma

Definition

A basal cell carcinoma is a skin cancer that originates from basal keratinocytes in the top layer of the skin, the epidermis. Sometimes these tumors are called "rodent ulcers."

Description

Basal keratinocytes are unpigmented skin cells found deep in the epidermis, hair follicles, and sweat glands. When they become cancerous, these cells invade the dermis (the layer of skin just below the epidermis) and spread out into the normal skin. They become visible as a small growth or area of change in the skin's appearance. These tumors can appear anywhere on the body, but most become evident on the face and neck.

Most basal cell carcinomas are small tumors that can be cured with simple surgeries. They usually grow quite slowly. However, neglected or aggressive tumors can invade vast amounts of skin. These cancers can also spread along bones, cartilage, muscles, and, more rarely, nerves. Some tumors may eventually reach the eye or brain or become large enough to significantly disfigure the face. These serious consequences are more likely if the tumor lies close to bone and cartilage—for instance, at the corner of the eye. Very few basal cell carcinomas spread to more distant organs; no more than five out of every 10,000 of these tumors metastasize.

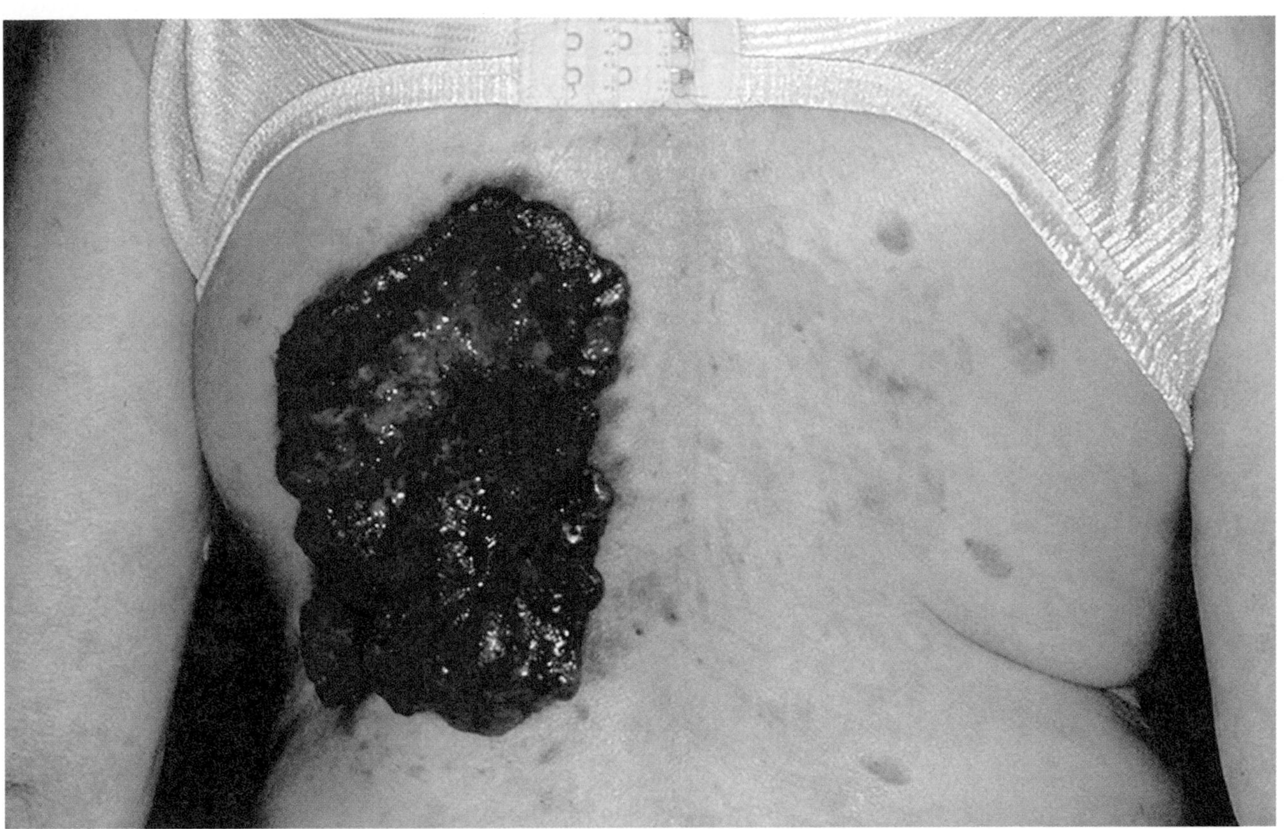

A basal cell carcinoma tumor. *(Custom Medical Stock Photo. Reproduced by permission.)*

Most that do are very large, deep cancers that have been visible for years.

Demographics

Basal cell carcinomas are most common from middle age until old age. They are more frequent in men than women. These cancers seem to be associated with exposure to ultraviolet light; they tend to develop on sun-exposed areas and are more common in people living near the equator. Those who have lighter skin are more susceptible; fair-haired blonds are more likely to develop tumors than people with darker complexions. In the United States, Caucasians have a 28% to 33% chance of developing a basal cell carcinoma over a lifetime.

Weakened immunity may also play a role. Those who have had an organ transplanted or who have contracted acquired immune deficiency syndrome (AIDS) are more likely to develop one of these cancers.

Basal cell carcinomas are particularly common among individuals with a rare genetic disease called nevoid basal cell carcinoma syndrome (Gorlin's syndrome). Individuals with this disease can be born with basal cell carcinomas or begin to develop them in childhood. Some have few or no cancers; others have more than 250. These tumors seldom grow much before puberty, but during and after adolescence they can spread rapidly. Other symptoms include small pits in the palms and soles, cysts in the jaw, and other abnormalities in the bones.

Causes and symptoms

Basal cell carcinomas are caused by genetic damage to a skin cell. Exposure to ultraviolet light and x rays, suppression of the immune system, and genetic factors seem to increase the risk that this will happen. The exact cause, however, is rarely known.

Several types of basal cell carcinomas exist. Nodular basal cell carcinomas are the most common form. These tumors begin as a tiny red or clear bump on the skin. Over time, they develop into a growth with clear or white "pearly" raised edges and, often, a depressed area in the middle. A network of tiny blood vessels usually crisscrosses the surface, and the tumor may bleed repeatedly or crust over. Morpheaform (sclerosing, morpheic) basal cell carcinomas are more difficult to detect. These tumors are usually pale, firm, flat growths that can blend into the normal skin around them. Many look just like a scar. Superficial basal cell carcinomas are flat, red, scaly plaques that can look like psoriasis or eczema. Unlike other basal cell carcinomas, they are usually found on the arms, legs, and torso. Pigmented basal cell carcinomas are brown, black, or blue; they are usually of the nodular type and can look like a **melanoma**.

Some general characteristics of skin cancers include:

- irregular or ragged borders
- non-symmetrical shape
- a change in color
- a size greater than 0.2 inches (6 mm)

Diagnosis

Basal cell carcinomas are usually diagnosed with a skin **biopsy** taken in the doctor's office. This is generally a brief and simple procedure. After numbing the skin with an injection of local anesthetic, the doctor snips out a tiny piece of the tumor. The skin sample must be sent to a trained pathologist to be analyzed. It may take up to a week for the biopsy results to come back. Sometimes the tumor is removed immediately after the biopsy, before the results are known.

Treatment team

Primary care physicians remove some basal cell carcinomas; other cancers, including larger or more complicated tumors, may be referred to a dermatologist. The services of a plastic surgeon are occasionally necessary. In the rare event that a tumor metastasizes, an oncologist and full cancer treatment team become involved.

Clinical staging, treatments, and prognosis

Basal cell carcinomas very rarely spread into the lymph nodes and internal organs. For this reason, doctors tend not to stage them. If staging is needed, the TNM (tumor, lymph node, and metastases) system is usually used. For basal cell carcinomas, this can be simplified into the following five categories:

- Stage 0: The cancer is very small and has not yet spread from the epidermis to the dermis.
- Stage 1: The cancer is less than 2 cm (0.8 inches) in diameter. No cancer cells can be found in lymph nodes or other internal organs.
- Stage 2: The cancer is more than 2 cm (0.8 inches) in diameter. No cancer cells can be found in lymph nodes or other internal organs.
- Stage 3: Cancer cells have been found either in nearby lymph nodes or in the bone, muscle, or cartilage beneath the skin (or in both locations).
- Stage 4: Cancer cells have been discovered in internal organs, most often the lungs or lymph nodes, that are distant from the skin. A stage four cancer can be any size.

Treatment options for non-metastatic, non-staged tumors

For most tumors—non-metastatic, non-staged cancers—there may be several treatment options. Which treatment is recommended depends on the size and type of tumor, its location, and cosmetic considerations. The cure rates for most of the following techniques are approximately 85% to 95%, but vary with tumor size and other factors. Mohs' micrographic surgery has a five-year cure rate of 96%. Success rates for recurrent tumors are approximately 50% with most techniques and 90% with **Moh's surgery**.

In conventional surgery, the doctor numbs the area with an injection of local anesthetic, then cuts out the tumor and a small margin of normal skin around it. The wound is closed with a few stitches. One advantage to conventional surgery is that the wound usually heals quickly. Another benefit is that the complete cancer can be sent to a pathologist for evaluation. If the skin around the tumor is not completely free of cancer cells, the tumor can be treated again immediately.

Mohs' micrographic surgery is a variation of conventional surgery. In this procedure, the surgeon examines each piece of skin under the microscope as it is removed. If any cancer cells remain, another slice is taken from that area and checked. These steps are repeated until the edges of the wound are clear of tumor cells, then the wound is closed. The advantage to this technique is that all of the visible cancer cells are removed but as much normal skin as possible is spared. Mohs' surgery is often used for larger or higher risk tumors and when cosmetic considerations are important. The main disadvantage is that it takes much longer than conventional surgery and requires a specially trained surgeon.

A laser is sometimes used as a cutting instrument instead of a scalpel. Laser light can also destroy some cancer cells directly. A disadvantage to laser surgery is that the wounds from some lasers heal more slowly than cuts from a scalpel. The advantage is that bleeding is minimal.

In electrodessication and curettage, the physician scoops out the cancer cells with a spoon-shaped instrument called a curette. After most of the tumor is gone, the remaining cancerous tissue is destroyed with heat from an electrical current. The wound is left open to heal like an abrasion. It leaks fluid, crusts over, and heals during the next two to six weeks. This is a safe and easy method for removing many basal cell carcinomas. One disadvan-

KEY TERMS

Albinism—A genetic disease characterized by the absence of the normal skin pigment, melanin.

Biopsy—A sample of an organ taken to look for abnormalities. Also, the technique used to take such samples.

Dermis—A layer of skin sandwiched between the epidermis and the fat under the skin. It contains the blood vessels, nerves, sweat glands, and hair follicles.

Epidermis—The thin layer of skin cells at the surface of the skin.

Fluorouracil—A cancer drug.

Hair follicles—The structures in the skin that make each hair.

Imiquimod—A drug, approved by the FDA to treat warts, that may destroy basal cell carcinomas by stimulating the immune system. Also known by its trade name Aldara.

Interferon alpha—A chemical made naturally by the immune system and also manufactured as a drug.

Local anesthetic—A liquid used to numb a small area of the skin.

Lymph node—A small organ full of immune cells, found in clusters throughout the body. Lymph nodes are where reactions to infections usually begin.

Nonsteroidal anti-inflammatory drugs (NSAIDS)—A class of drugs that suppresses inflammation. Includes a wide variety of drugs, including aspirin.

Oncologist—A doctor who specializes in the treatment of cancer.

Pathologist—A doctor who specializes in examining cells and other parts of the body for abnormalities.

Premalignant skin lesion—An abnormal change in the skin that has a good chance of turning into skin cancer but is not yet cancerous.

Selenium—A mineral needed in extremely small quantities by the body. Large amounts can be very toxic.

Squamous cell carcinoma—A type of skin cancer.

Sweat glands—Tiny glands scattered throughout the skin that produce sweat.

TNM system—A commonly used staging system that examines the main tumor (T), the lymph nodes (N), and metastases (M).

Xeroderma pigmentosum—A genetic disease characterized by the inability to repair damaged DNA. Individuals with this disease develop an excessive number of skin cancers.

tage is that there is no skin sample to confirm that the tumor is completely gone. The electrical current used during this surgery can interfere with some pacemakers and larger tumors may heal with a noticeable scar.

In cryosurgery, liquid nitrogen is used to freeze the tumor and destroy it. This treatment is another type of blind destruction; there is no skin sample to make sure the cancer cells have all been killed. Patients report swelling and pain after cryosurgery, and a wound appears a few days later where the cells were destroyed. When the site heals, it has usually lost its normal pigment. There is a risk of nerve damage with this technique.

Radiation therapy is an uncommon treatment for basal cell carcinoma. One disadvantage is the inconvenience: multiple treatments, over a period of weeks, are necessary. Tumors that return after radiation also tend to grow more quickly than the original cancer. In addition, x rays may promote new skin cancers. Radiation therapy may be an option for patients who cannot undergo even minor surgery. It is also used occasionally as an adjunct to surgery. One advantage is that the cosmetic results can be very good.

Occasionally a lotion containing **fluorouracil** is applied to the tumor. This drug cannot penetrate very far and cancer cells in the deeper parts of the tumor may not be destroyed. The main advantage to this treatment is its simplicity.

Treatment options for metastatic cancers

Cancers that have spread to internal organs are treated with a combination of surgery, radiation, and **chemotherapy**.

Prognosis

The prognosis for small, uncomplicated basal cell carcinomas is very good. The vast majority of these tumors can be successfully removed. However, cancers that were not completely destroyed may regrow. If the

QUESTIONS TO ASK THE DOCTOR

- What treatment(s) would you recommend for my tumor?
- How effective would you expect each of them to be, for a tumor of this size and in this location?
- How much cosmetic damage am I likely to see with each treatment?
- Are there any alternatives?
- How should I prepare for the procedure?
- What is the risk that my tumor in particular will regrow?

edges of the removed skin contain cancer cells, the chance that the tumor will return within the next five years is about 40%. Regrowth is more likely with cancers larger than 0.8 inches (2 cm), those on the face (particularly around the nose, eye, and ear), and higher risk types such as morpheaform tumors. Tumors can redevelop in the scar from the surgery, on the edges of the surgery site, or deep in the skin. These cancers may not look like the original tumor. Patients should be particularly watchful for minor changes in the appearance of the scar or sores that appear nearby.

Cancers that metastasize spread most often to the lymph nodes and lungs. The prognosis for metastatic cancers is poor, even with treatment. Survival after spread of the cancer to internal organs is eight months on the average and seldom more than a year and a half.

Coping with cancer treatment

Most basal cell carcinomas are removed with techniques that cause few, if any, lasting side effects. Patients who have cosmetic concerns may wish to discuss them with their doctor.

Clinical trials

In photodynamic laser therapy, a dye activated by laser light destroys the cancer. This dye is spread onto the skin, injected, or drunk. During a waiting period, normal cells clear the dye, then a laser activates the remainder. As of 2001, this technique was only useful for cancers very near the surface of the skin. One side effect after treatment is a period of excessive sun-sensitivity. Several **clinical trials** are in progress.

In 1999, researchers first reported that imiquimod 5% cream, spread onto the skin several times a week, could destroy small nodular or superficial basal cell carcinomas. The side effects from this treatment were mainly local skin reactions such as **itching**, rashes, and redness. Ongoing studies are promising.

Interferon alpha injected into the tumor is sometimes effective for basal cell carcinomas. This experimental treatment is mainly used for less dangerous forms such as the nodular type.

Retinoids, drugs related to vitamin A, may have some effect on basal cell carcinomas. These drugs are taken internally and can have significant serious side effects.

Prevention

The risk factors for basal cell carcinoma include:

- ethnic background
- complexion
- geographic location
- increasing age
- exposure to x rays and ultraviolet light (both UVA and UVB)
- a history of premalignant skin lesions or skin cancer
- genetic disorders such as nevoid basal cell carcinoma syndrome, xeroderma pigmentosum, and albinism
- suppression of the immune system by AIDS or an organ transplant

Some important preventative steps are to wear protective clothing and hats in the sun, use a sunscreen, avoid the sun between 10 A.M. and 4 P.M., and stay away from suntanning booths. Checking the skin for early signs of cancer is also critical.

Drugs related to vitamin A (including beta-carotene, retinol, and isotretinoin), vitamin E, nonsteroidal anti-inflammatory drugs (NSAIDS), and selenium might be able to prevent basal cell carcinoma. As of 2001, their effectiveness was still in question.

Special concerns

Because many basal cell carcinomas are found on the face and neck, cosmetic concerns are a priority for many patients. If there is a risk of noticeable scarring or damage, a patient may wish to ask about alternative types of removal or inquire about the services of a plastic surgeon.

After treatment, it is important to return to the doctor periodically to check for regrowth or new skin cancers. Approximately 36% of all patients find a new basal cell or squamous cell carcinoma within the next five years. Having a basal cell carcinoma before the age of 60 may also increase the chance of developing other cancers in internal organs.

See Also chemoprevention; familial cancer syndromes; reconstructive surgery

Resources

BOOKS

Keefe, Kristin A., and Frank L. Meyskens, Jr. "Cancer Prevention." In *Clinical Oncology.* 2nd ed. Abeloff, M., J. Armitage, A. Lichter, and J. Niederhuber, eds. Philadelphia: Churchhill Livingstone, 2000.

Rohrer, Thomas E. "Cancer of the Skin." In *Conn's Current Therapy; Latest Approved Methods of Treatment for the Practicing Physician.* 52nd ed. Rakel, R., et al, eds. Philadelphia: W. B. Saunders, 2000.

Wolfe, Jonathan. "Nonmelanoma Skin Cancers: Basal Cell and Squamous Cell Carcinoma." In *Clinical Oncology*, 2nd ed. Abeloff, M. J. Armitage, A. Lichter, and J. Niederhuber. Philadelphia: Churchhill Livingstone, 2000.

PERIODICALS

Beutner, Karl R., John K. Geisse, Donita Helman, Terry L. Fox, Angela Ginkel, and Mary L. Owens. "Therapeutic Response of Basal Cell Carcinoma to the Immune Response Modifier Imiquimod 5% Cream." *Journal of the American Academy of Dermatology* 41, no. 6 (December 1999): 1002-7.

Garner, Kyle L., and Wm. Macmillian Rodney. "Basal and Squamous Cell Carcinoma." *Primary Care; Clinics in Office Practice* 27, no. 2 (June 2000): 477-58.

"Is Sunscreen an Enabler?" *Harvard Health Letter* 25, no. 9 (July 2000): 1-3.

Jerant, Anthony F., Jennifer T. Johnson, Catherine Demastes Sheridan, and Timothy J. Caffrey. "Early Detection and Treatment of Skin Cancer." *American Family Physician* 62 (15 July 2000): 357-68, 375-6, 381-2.

Keller, Karen Laszlo, and Neil A. Fenske. "Use of Vitamins A, C, and E and Related Compounds in Dermatology: A Review." *Journal of the American Academy of Dermatology* 38, no. 4 (October 1998): 611-25.

ORGANIZATIONS

Nevoid Basal Cell Carcinoma Syndrome Support Network. 162 Clover Hill Street, Marlboro, MA 01752. (800) 815-4447. souldansur@aol.com.

Skin Cancer Foundation. 245 Fifth Ave., Suite 2402, New York, NY 10016. (212) 725-5176. <http://www.skincancer.org>.

OTHER

"Nonmelanoma Skin Cancer Treatment—Health Professionals." *CancerNet, National Cancer Institute.* Aug. 2000. 25 June 2001 <http://cancernet.nci.nih.gov/pdq.html>.

"Non-Melanoma Staging." *Oncology Channel.* Mar. 2001. 29 June 2001 <http://oncologychannel.com/nonmelanoma/staging.shtml>.

"Skin Cancer." *CancerLinksUSA.* 1999. 29 June 2001 <http://www.cancerlinksusa.com/skin/index.htm>.

Anna Rovid Spickler, D.V.M.,Ph.D.

BCG *see* **Bacillus Calmette Guérin**

Bexarotene

Definition

Bexarotene, also known by the brand name Targretin, is an antitumor agent of the class known as retinoids.

Purpose

Bexarotene is used to treat cutaneous T-cell lymphomas that have not responded to therapy with other drugs commonly used to treat this disease. A **cutaneous T-cell lymphoma** is a tumor found on the skin and originates from cells of the immune system.

Description

Bexarotene is one of a group of drugs called retinoids, a derivative of vitamin A. Retinoids are involved with the process of stimulating some cells to mature to normal cells, and with inhibiting some cells from growing. It is thought that bexarotene binds to the retinoic acid receptors on cells. This binding ultimately results in the regulation of the growth and maturation of the cells.

Recommended dosage

Doses vary from individual to individual and depend on body weight and other factors. Bexarotene is taken by mouth in capsule form. The initial dose is usually 300 mg per square meter of body surface area per day. The maintenance dose is 300 to 400 mg per square meter of body surface area per day.

Precautions

Pregnant women should not take bexarotene. The risks of fetal abnormality are high, and women should take precautions to ensure they do not become pregnant.

Patients should limit their intake of vitamin A supplements to avoid additive toxic effects with bexarotene, which is a vitamin A derivative. Patients with diabetes and who are receiving insulin or oral medications for their diabetes are usually prescribed bexarotene with caution, and their blood sugar should be frequently monitored. Bexarotene may enhance the effects of the medications for diabetes, and patients may have low blood sugar levels.

KEY TERMS

Anorexia—Loss of appetite.

Lipids—Fatlike substances stored in the body that serve as a source of fuel and are important constituents of cell structure.

Photosensitivity—An abnormal cutaneous response to sunlight or filtered or artificial light.

Patients taking bexarotene may experience photosensitivity, or increased sensitivity to sunlight. In order to prevent rash, **itching**, or severe sunburn, patients should avoid direct sunlight exposure, avoid sunlamps or tanning beds, use sunblock lotion that is SPF 15 or greater, and wear a lip balm that is SPF 15 or greater. Patients should also wear sunglasses, a hat, and garments covering as much skin as possible when outside.

Side effects

The most common side effects of bexarotene increased levels of triglycerides, cholesterol, and high-density lipoprotein cholesterol. Some patients may require medications to control this rise in lipids. Decreased thyroid function also occurs frequently, and thyroid hormone replacement therapy may be necessary in some patients. Other common side effects include headaches, rash, red and scaly inflammation of the skin, hair loss (**alopecia**), decreased red and white blood cells, and cataracts of the eyes. Patients should have eye examinations if they have any visual difficulties. Patients may be at increased risk of infections due to decreased white blood cells and experience **fatigue** due to decreased red blood cells. Other less common side effects include fluid gain causing swelling of extremities, insomnia, chills, **fever**, **anorexia**, **nausea and vomiting**, abdominal pain, back pain, flu-like symptoms, and dry skin. As with all medications, patients experiencing any of these (or other) side effects should notify their physician.

Interactions

There are an extremely large number of drugs that interact with bexarotene. Patients should consult their physician, nurse, or pharmacist about any medications they are taking before beginning a course of Bexarotene. Many physicians recommend bringing the containers with the names of all the drugs the patient is taking to their appointment with the physician.

Michael Zuck, Ph.D.

Bicalutamide *see* **Antiandrogens**

Bile duct cancer

Definition

Bile duct cancer, or cholangiocarcinoma, is a malignant tumor of the bile ducts within the liver (intrahepatic), or leading from the liver to the small intestine (extrahepatic). It is a rare tumor with poor outcome for most patients.

Description

Bile is a substance manufactured by the liver that aids in the digestion of food. Bile ducts are channels that carry the bile from the liver to the small intestine. Like the tributaries of a river, the small bile ducts in the liver converge into two large bile ducts called the left and right hepatic ducts. These exit the liver and join to form the common hepatic duct. The gallbladder, which concentrates and stores the bile, empties into the common hepatic duct to form the common bile duct. Finally, this large duct connects to the small intestine where the bile can help digest food. Collectively, this network of bile ducts is called the biliary tract.

Bile duct cancer originates from the cells that line the inner surface of the bile ducts. A tumor may arise anywhere along the biliary tract, either within or outside of the liver. Bile duct tumors are typically slow-growing tumors that spread by local invasion of neighboring structures and by way of lymphatic channels.

Demographics

Bile duct cancer is an uncommon malignancy. In the United States, approximately one case arises per 100,000 people per year, but it is more common in Southeast Asia. It occurs in men only slightly more often than in women. The most common time of diagnosis is during the fifth and sixth decades of life.

Causes and symptoms

A number of risk factors are associated with the development of bile duct cancer:

- Primary sclerosing cholangitis. This disease is characterized by extensive scarring of the biliary tract, sometimes associated with inflammatory bowel disease.

- Choledochal cysts. These are abnormal dilatations of the biliary tract that usually form during fetal development. There is evidence that these cysts may rarely arise during adulthood.
- Hepatolithiasis. This is the condition of stone formation within the liver (not including gallbladder stones).
- Liver flukes. Parasitic infection with certain worms is thought to be at least partially responsible for the higher prevalence of bile duct cancer in Southeast Asia.
- Thorotrast. This is a chemical that was previously injected intravenously during certain types of x rays. It is not in use anymore. Exposure to Thorotrast has been implicated in the development of cancer of the liver as well as the bile ducts.

Symptoms

Jaundice is the first symptom in 90% of patients. This occurs when the bile duct tumor causes an obstruction in the normal flow of bile from the liver to the small intestine. Bilirubin, a component of bile, builds up within the liver and is absorbed into the bloodstream in excess amounts. This can be detected in a blood test, but it can also manifest as yellowish discoloring of the skin and eyes. The bilirubin in the bloodstream also makes the urine appear dark. Additionally, the patient may experience generalized **itching** due to the deposition of bile components in the skin. Normally, a portion of the bile is excreted in stool; bile actually gives stool its brown color. But when the biliary tract is obstructed by tumor, the stools may appear pale.

Abdominal pain, **fatigue**, **weight loss**, and poor appetite are less common symptoms. Occasionally, if obstruction of the biliary tract causes the gallbladder to swell enormously yet without causing pain, the physician may be able to feel the gallbladder during a physical examination. Sometimes the biliary tract can become infected, but this is normally a rare consequence of invasive tests. Infection causes **fever**, chills, and pain in the right upper portion of the abdomen.

Diagnosis

Certain laboratory tests of the blood may aid in the diagnosis. The most important one is the test for elevated bilirubin levels in the bloodstream. Levels of alkaline phosphatase and CA 19-9 may also be elevated.

When symptoms, physical signs, and blood tests point toward an abnormality of the biliary tract, then the next step involves radiographic tests. Ultrasound and **computed tomography** (CT scan) are noninvasive and rapid. These tests can often detect the actual tumor as well as dilatation of the obstructed biliary tract. If these tests indicate the presence of a tumor, then cholangiography is required. This procedure involves injecting dye into the biliary tract to obtain anatomic images of the bile ducts and the tumor. The specialist that performs this test can also insert small tubes, or stents, into a partially obstructed portion of the bile duct to prevent further obstruction by growth of the tumor. This is vitally important since it may be the only intervention that is possible in certain patients. Cholangiography is an invasive test that carries a small risk of infection of the biliary tract. The objective of these radiological tests is to determine the size and location of the tumor, as well as the extent of spread to nearby structures.

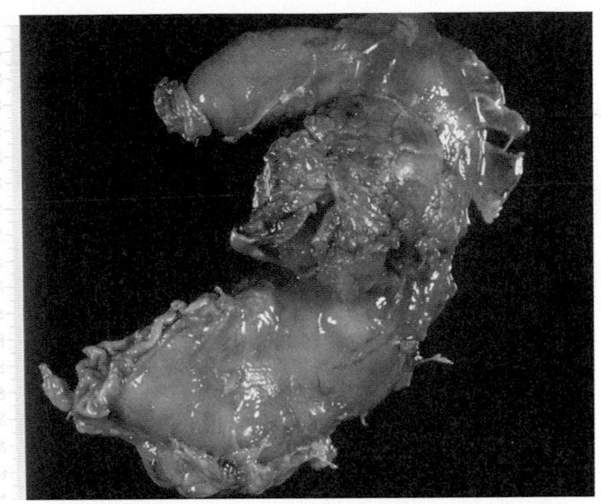

Cancer of the bile duct. *(© Biophoto Associates, Science Source/Photo Researchers, Inc. Reproduced by permission.)*

The treatment of bile duct tumors is usually not affected by the specific type of cancer cells that comprise the tumor. For this reason, some physicians forego **biopsy** of the tumor.

Treatment team

The treatment team may include the patient's primary physician, a surgeon, and a gastroenterologist who specializes in the **stenting** technique described above for palliation of bile duct strictures.

Clinical staging, treatments, and prognosis

Staging

Bile duct tumors are staged according to the tumor-node-metastasis (TNM) system of the **American Joint Commission on Cancer**. This staging scheme assesses the invasiveness of the tumor, the involvement of nearby lymph nodes, and the extent of distant **metastasis**.

KEY TERMS

Angiography—Radiographic examination of blood vessels after injection with a special dye

Cholangiography—Radiographic examination of the bile ducts after injection with a special dye

Computed tomography—Radiographic examination by which images of cross-sectional planes of the body are obtained

Jaundice—Yellowish staining of the skin and eyes due to excess bilirubin in the bloodstream

Lymphatic—Pertaining to lymph, the clear fluid that is collected from tissues, flows through special vessels, and joins the venous circulation

Metastasis—The spread of tumor cells from one part of the body to another

Resection—To surgically remove a part of the body

Stent—Slender hollow catheter or rod placed within a vessels for duct to provide support or maintain patency

Ultrasound—Radiographic imaging technique utilizing high frequency sound waves

- Stage I tumors are confined to the bile duct itself.
- Stage II tumors extend to the immediately adjacent tissues.
- Stage III tumors have spread to associated lymph nodes.
- Stage IV tumors have invaded local structures or have metastasized to distant structures.

A higher stage signifies worse prognosis.

Treatment

The only hope for cure lies with surgical resection (removal) of the tumor and all involved structures. Unfortunately, sometimes the cancer has already spread too far when the diagnosis is made. Thus, in the treatment of bile duct cancer, the first question to answer is if the tumor may be safely resected by surgery with reasonable benefit to the patient. If the cancer involves certain blood vessels or has spread widely throughout the liver, then resection may not be possible. Sometimes further invasive testing is required.

Angiography can determine if the blood vessels are involved. **Laparoscopy** is a surgical procedure that allows the surgeon to directly assess the tumor and nearby lymph nodes without making a large incision in the abdomen. Only about 45% of bile duct cancers are ultimately resectable.

QUESTIONS TO ASK THE DOCTOR

- Has my cancer spread?
- What is the stage of my cancer and what does that mean for my prognosis?
- What treatment choices do I have?
- What are the risks or side effects of the treatment you recommend?
- What are the chances my cancer will come back after treatment?

If the tumor is resectable, and the patient is healthy enough to tolerate the operation, then the specific type of surgery performed depends on the location of the tumor. For tumors within the liver or high up in the biliary tract, resection of part of the liver may be required. Tumors in the middle portion of the biliary tract can be removed alone. Tumors of the lower end of the biliary tract may require extensive resection of part of the pancreas, small intestine, and stomach to ensure complete resection.

Unfortunately, sometimes the cancer appears resectable by all the radiological and invasive tests, but is found to be unresectable during surgery. In this scenario, a bypass operation can relieve the biliary tract obstruction, but does not remove the tumor itself. This does not produce a cure but it can offer a better quality of life for the patient.

Chemotherapy and **radiation therapy** have not been proven effective in the treatment of bile duct cancer.

Prognosis

Prognosis depends on the stage and resectability of the tumor. If the patient cannot undergo surgical resection, then survival is expected to be less than one year. If the tumor is resected, survival improves but is still dismal. Only 20% of these patients survive past five years.

Clinical trials

Studies of new treatments in patients are known as **clinical trials**. These trials seek to compare the standard method of care with a new method, or the trials may be trying to establish whether one treatment is more beneficial for certain patients than others. Sometimes, a new treatment that is not being offered on a wide scale may be available to patients participating in clinical trials, but participating in the trials may involve some risk. To learn more about clinical trials, patients can call the National Cancer Institute (NCI) at 1-800-4-CANCER or visit the NCI web site for patients at <http://www.cancertrials.nci.nih.gov>.

Prevention

Other than the avoidance of infections caused by liver flukes, there are no known preventions for this cancer.

Resources

BOOKS

Ahrendt, Steven A. and Henry A. Pitt. "Biliary Tract." In *Sabiston Textbook of Surgery*, edited by Courtney Townsend Jr., 16th ed. Philadelphia: W.B. Saunders Company, 2001, pp. 1076-1111.

Callery, Mark P. and William C. Meyers. "Bile Duct Cancer." In *Current Surgical Therapy*, edited by John L. Cameron, sixth ed. St Louis: Mosby, 1998, pp.455-161.

"Cholangiocarcinoma." In *Clinical Oncology*, edited by Abeloff, Martin D., second ed. New York: Churchill Livingstone, 2000, pp.1722-1723.

ORGANIZATIONS

The American Cancer Society. Phone: 1-800-ACS 2345. Web site: <http://www.cancer.org>.

National Cancer Institute Cancer Information Service. Phone: 1-800-4-CANCER. Web site: <http://www.nci.nih.gov>.

American Liver Foundation. Phone: 1-800-GO-LIVER (1-800-465-4837). Web site: <http://www.liverfoundation.org>.

Kevin O.Hwang, M.D.

Biliary tract cancers *see* **Bile duct cancer; Gallbladder cancer**

Biology of cancer *see* **Cancer biology**

Biopsy

Definition

Biopsy is a diagnostic procedure in which a piece of tissue and/or cells are removed to be examined under a microscope by a pathologist.

Purpose

Biopsies are performed to determine the presence of cancer cells, establish **tumor grading**, and provide more information for treatment.

Precautions

Most biopsies should not be done on patients with blood clotting problems. If the patient has a low blood platelet count, a platelet transfusion can be given as a temporary relief measure, and a biopsy can then be performed. The physician should be notified of any bleeding problems—as well as any allergies, current medications, or pregnancy—well in advance.

Patients receiving IV sedation for a biopsy procedure will continue to feel drowsy for several hours, and should refrain from cooking, driving, or operating any equipment that requires careful attention. A ride home from the clinic should be arranged in advance.

Description

There are several different types of biopsies, and the decision on which one is most effective depends on where the tumor is located and the general health of the patient. Four common categories of biopsy are fine needle aspiration, core needle biopsy, excisional biopsy, and incisional biopsy.

Fine needle aspiration biopsy

Fine needle aspiration biopsy, also known as suction biopsy or needle aspiration biopsy, involves applying negative pressure through the use of a syringe and hollow, hypodermic needle. This type of biopsy is often used as a diagnostic procedure on neck and thyroid masses. It results in the removal of tissue that is fragmented into cells, as opposed to one sample of undamaged tissue. Fine needle aspiration biopsy is a frequently performed procedure that results in minimum discomfort and is less costly than many other types of biopsy.

Core needle biopsy

Core needle biopsy, also know as wide-core needle biopsy or cutting core biopsy, involves the use of a large-bore needle and is the simplest method of pathologic diagnosis of cancer. It results in minimal disturbance of surrounding tissues and a solid, intact sample. Tumors located in the liver and breast are commonly biopsied with this technique.

Incisional biopsy

This refers to the removal of part of the tumor from the larger tumor mass. An incisional biopsy is employed for tumors located deep within the body and after an initial needle biopsy has failed to supply enough tissue for diagnosis. Biopsies of this type are the preferred technique for diagnosing soft tissue cancers and osteosarcomas.

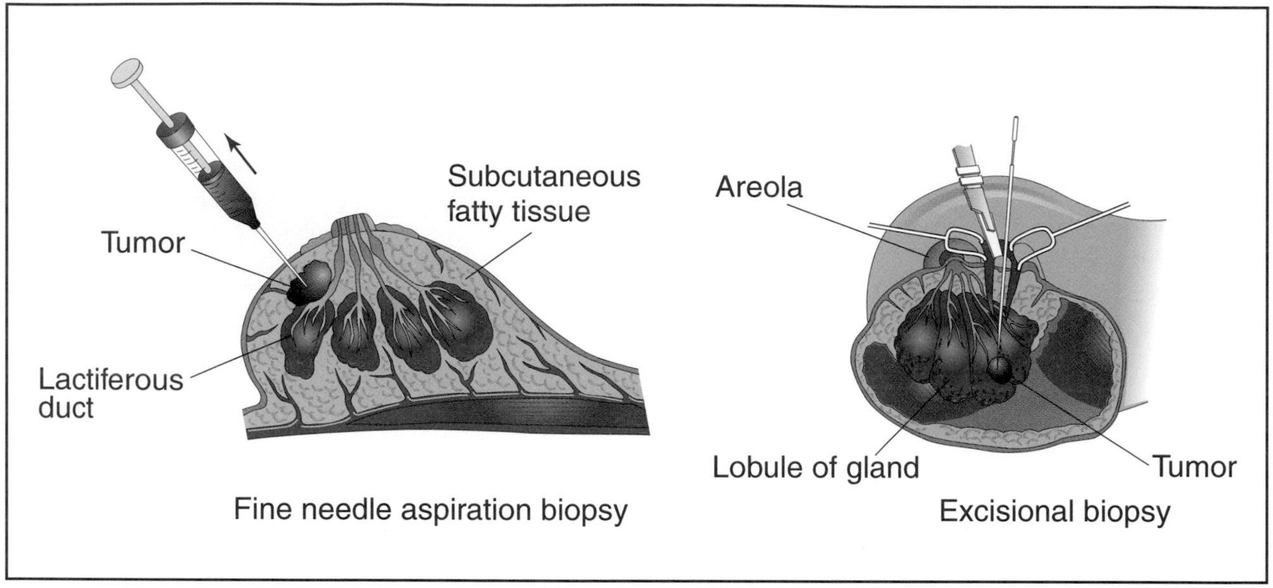

Of the four different types of biopsy discussed, two are shown here: Fine needle aspiration biopsy and Excisional biopsy. A fine needle aspiration biopsy uses a very thin needle to withdraw fluid and cells from the growth to be examined. An excisional biopsy is a surgical procedure in which the entire area of concern and some surrounding tissue is removed for analysis. *(Illustration by Electronic Illustrators Group.)*

Excisional biopsy

Also known as surgical biopsy, the excisional biopsy entails the surgical removal of the entire tumor mass and is a diagnostic technique that simultaneously serves as a treatment. For example, a **lumpectomy** removes the entire primary tumor mass associated with **breast cancer**. Excisional biopsy is also useful for diagnosing and removing surface tumors of the skin, such as those associated with squamous cell **carcinoma**, **basal cell carcinoma**, and malignant **melanoma**.

Preparation

Many biopsies can be performed in the doctor's office or in the hospital on an outpatient basis. Most do not require much special preparation on the part the patient, but patients should ask their physician for special instructions. Prior to the procedure, most require the use of anesthesia. Prior to and during a biopsy, special imaging techniques may be employed to assist in locating the tumor and guidance of biopsy procedures using a needle. Such imaging techniques include **computed tomography** scan (CT guided biopsy), fluoroscopy, **magnetic resonance imaging** (MRI), nuclear medicine scan, and ultrasound (ultrasound guided biopsy). Patients who undergo imaging scans may be injected with or asked to drink a contrast agent (dye) prior to biopsy.

Fine needle aspiration biopsy

Some routine blood work (blood counts, clotting profile) should be completed two weeks prior to biopsy. Patients may be asked not to eat for a specified time before the procedure. Those taking blood thinners (anticoagulants) or aspirin should talk to their physicians about whether they should discontinue using them prior to biopsy.

Core needle biopsy

Women undergoing breast biopsy should not wear talcum powder, deodorant, lotion, or perfume under their arms or on their breasts on the day of the procedure (since these may cause image artifacts or other problems). A comfortable two-piece garment should be worn. Patients may be asked not to eat for a specified time before the procedure. Those taking blood thinners or aspirin should talk to their physicians about whether they should discontinue using them prior to core needle biopsy.

Incisional biopsy

Patients should follow instructions provided by their doctor and give notification of any allergies. Those expecting general anesthesia should not eat or drink for at least 8 hours before an incisional biopsy. Patients should also bathe thoroughly before the procedure and allow time to rest afterward.

Excisional biopsy

Patients may be asked to: sign a consent form allowing the physician to perform this test; refrain from eating or drinking for at least 8 hours prior to surgery; and arrange for a ride home from the hospital (most patients can go home on the same day as the surgery). Those taking insulin, aspirin, non-steroidal anti-inflammatory drugs, or any medicines that affect blood clotting should notify their doctor well before the procedure.

Aftercare

Fine needle aspiration biopsy

After the biopsy, patients should be able to drive home, return to work, or perform any other routine activity. This biopsy does not affect medication schedules.

Core needle biopsy

Most patients can resume normal activities right after the biopsy. If there is excessive redness, pain, or drainage from the puncture site, patients should call their doctor immediately.

Incisional biopsy

After recovering from anesthesia, the patient will be observed for a few hours before returning home. During this time, an analysis may come back from the lab and the doctor may explain the nature of the abnormality. This analysis is the result of only one test and will not be 100% accurate. In about two days, lab testing should be complete. Patients should call their doctor immediately if there is drainage from the wound or a **fever** develops.

Excisional biopsy

Depending on the invasiveness of the procedure, the patient may receive varied instructions for aftercare. The incision site should be kept clean, dry, and free of lotion, medication, or ointments. The patient may be required to remain in a certain position until sufficient time has passed to warrant the release of the patient from medical care. For example, patients are required to remain on their right side for approximately four hours to allow for healing to occur after a liver punch biopsy. Some patients, however, may be able to return to normal activities on the same day. Those who develop a fever, or notice bleeding, drainage, strong pain, or redness and warmth at the biopsy site should contact their doctor immediately.

Risks

Although most biopsies end with success, there are a certain number of risks to keep in mind. For example, complications can arise if other organs are nicked during a biopsy using a long needle. As with any procedure, there is a slight risk of allergic reaction to anesthesia. To be well informed, patients should consult with their physician about the risks prior to undergoing the procedure.

Fine needle aspiration biopsy

This biopsy poses no significant risks. Some minor bleeding may occur and some patients report a mild, dull, and throbbing sensation in the area of the biopsy, which usually subsides within 30 to 60 minutes. The risk of infection exists any time the skin is penetrated, but is extremely rare with this procedure. The error rate of diagnosis, however, is substantially higher than that of other biopsy procedures; major surgical resections should not be undertaken solely on the basis of the evidence of aspiration biopsy.

Core needle biopsy

A lumpy scar called a keloid may form in the area of puncture. Infection and bleeding may also occur at or under the biopsy site; however, this risk is uncommon. Core needle biopsy, like fine needle aspiration, only removes samples of a mass and not the entire area of concern. Therefore, it is possible that a more serious diagnosis may be missed by limiting the sampling of an abnormality.

Incisional biopsy

A keloid may form in the incision area. In rare cases, infection and bleeding may occur.

Excisional biopsy

Some patients may experience infection, bleeding, or bruising around the biopsy site. The physician should

KEY TERMS

Contrast agent—A substance introduced into the body that allows radiographic visualization of certain tissues. Often used in MRI and CT imaging scans to emphasize the contrast between healthy and cancerous cells.

Excision—Surgical removal.

Incision—A surgical cut or gash.

Platelets—Small blood cells that play a role in the blood clotting process.

Tumor grading—Tumor grade refers to the degree of abnormality of cancer cells compared with normal cells. Establishing a grade allows the physician to determine further courses of treatment.

be consulted about any risks that may be related to a patient's medical history.

Normal results

The tissue sample obtained from the biopsy needs to be prepared for examination by a pathologist, and results usually are reported to the patient within a few days of the procedure. Normal (negative) results indicate that no malignancy is present.

Abnormal results

Abnormal results indicate that a malignancy or other abnormality is present. In some cases, results are indeterminate and patients are subject to further diagnostic procedures.

See Also Bone marrow aspiration and biopsy; CT-guided biopsy; Liver biopsy; Pleural biopsy; Stereotactic needle biopsy

Resources

BOOKS

Bast, Robert C., et al. *Cancer Medicine,* 5th ed. Hamilton, ON: B.C. Decker Inc., 2000.

DeVita, Vincent T., Jr. *Cancer: Principles and Practice of Oncology.* Philadelphia, PA: Lippincott-Raven Publishers, 1997.

OTHER

"An Alternative to Excisional Breast Biopsy: Core Needle Breast Biopsy." *Washington Radiology Associates* 25 June 2001 <http://www.wrapc.com/corenedl.htm>.

Harvard Health Online 25 June 2001 <http://www.health.harvard.edu>.

National Cancer Institute. 25 June 2001 <http://www.nci.nih.gov>.

Sally C. McFarlane-Parrott

Bisacodyl *see* **Laxatives**

Bisphosphonates

Definition

Bisphosphonates are a class of drugs that lower calcium levels in the blood and can slow down bone loss that results from cancer or other causes.

Purpose

Bisphosphonates are used to slow down the loss of bone that results from **multiple myeloma** or from **breast cancer** that has spread, or metastasized, to the bones. These cancers cause bone to dissolve, in a process called resorption. This results in bone weakness and fractures. Bisphosphonates can prevent the holes that form in the bones from multiple myeloma. They can ease **bone pain** caused by cancer. They also help to prevent bone fractures and compression of the spinal cord, as well as the high calcium levels in the blood (**hypercalcemia**) caused by bone loss. Hypercalcemia can cause kidney failure and death. Bisphosphonates may help prevent breast cancer from spreading to the bones and other organs. **Clinical trials** are evaluating bisphosphonates for the treatment of bone metastases from other types of cancers.

Description

The most commonly used bisphosphonates are pamidronate disodium (APD; brand name Aredia) and etidronate disodium (EHDP; brand name Didronel). Both drugs are approved by the U.S. Food and Drug Administration. These drugs are classified as antihypercalcemics, meaning that they can lower blood calcium levels. They also are classified as bone resorption inhibitors, meaning that they can prevent bone from dissolving.

Other bisphosphonates include cladronate and alendronate. Cladronate is used less frequently because it is not completely absorbed by the digestive system and can cause stomach upset. Zoledronate and ibandronate are new, much more powerful bisphosphonates that are being evaluated, but are not yet available for routine use.

For cancer treatment, bisphosphonates may be used in conjunction with **chemotherapy**. Treatment with bisphosphonates may be accompanied by the injection of fluids into a vein (intravenous) so that large amounts of urine are excreted.

Recommended dosage

Pamidronate and etidronate are solutions that are injected into a vein. For the treatment of hypercalcemia, 30–90 mg of pamidronate are injected over a period of 2–24 hours. For the treatment of bone metastases from breast cancer, 90 mg are injected over a two-hour period every 3–4 weeks. For multiple myeloma, the 90-mg injection is over a four-hour period once a month. The usual dosage of etidronate is 7.5 mg per kg (3.4 mg per pound) of body weight, injected over two hours, for two or more days. The treatment may be repeated after at least one week off.

Etidronate also may be taken as a tablet, with water, on an empty stomach. The usual dosage for the treatment of hypercalcemia is 20 mg per kg (9.1 mg per pound) of body weight per day for 30 days. The maximum length of treatment usually is 90 days, but the treatment may be repeated after at least 90 days off of the drug. Cladronate is also taken as a pill.

Precautions

The amount of calcium in the diet may be important when taking bisphosphonates. Too much calcium in the diet may prevent absorption of oral etidronate. However, it is important to consume adequate amounts of calcium and vitamin D.

Other medical problems that may affect the use of bisphosphonates include:

- heart problems that may be aggravated by fluid retention
- kidney disease that could result in high levels of bisphosphonate in the blood
- intestinal problems or bowel disease, because etidronate can cause diarrhea
- bone fractures, particularly of the arm or leg, since etidronate can increase the risk of fractures

Bisphosphonates may cause allergic reactions in some individuals. Children may experience temporary changes in bone growth while being treated with etidronate and they should not take pamidronate. Older individuals may suffer from fluid retention if bisphosphonates are given with large amounts of fluid. Bisphosphonates should not be taken during pregnancy. It is not known whether these drugs pass into breast milk.

Side effects

Although bisphosphonates usually are well tolerated, some patients may experience side effects. The most common side effects include:

- **fatigue**
- **fever**
- nausea
- vomiting
- abdominal cramps
- low red blood cell levels (anemia)
- bone or joint pain
- muscle stiffness or pain
- pain or swelling at the site of injection or in the vein

However, some of these symptoms may result from the cancer or from other treatments for the cancer. A mild pain reliever can reduce or prevent the muscle and joint pain. Bisphosphonates that are taken by mouth can cause irritation and ulcers in the esophagus (the tube between the mouth and the stomach).

Additional side effects that may occur with pamidronate, particularly at dosages above 60 mg, include:

- chills
- confusion
- muscle spasms
- sore throat
- constipation
- decreased appetite

Additional side effects that may occur with etidronate include:

- decreased levels of magnesium and phosphorus in the blood
- **diarrhea**
- bone fracture, particularly of the thigh
- increases in test results for kidney function
- hives, skin rash, or **itching** (rare)
- swelling of the arms, legs, face, lips, tongue, or throat (rare)
- loss or altered sense of taste (with drug injection)

Interactions

Substances that may interact or interfere with bisphosphonates include:

- mineral supplements, antacids, or other substances containing calcium, iron, magnesium, or aluminum, particularly if taken within two hours of taking etidronate
- substances containing vitamin D

Margaret Alic, Ph.D.

KEY TERMS

Antihypercalcemic—Drug that lowers the levels of calcium in the blood.

Hypercalcemia—High levels of calcium in the blood.

Metastasis—Spread of cancer from its point of origin to other parts of the body.

Resorption—Dissolving of bone, as with multiple myeloma or bone metastases from other cancers.

Bladder cancer

Definition

Bladder cancer is a disease in which the cells lining the urinary bladder lose the ability to regulate their growth and start dividing uncontrollably. This abnormal growth results in a mass of cells that form a tumor.

Description

The urinary bladder is a hollow muscular organ that stores urine from the kidneys until it is excreted out of the body. Two tubes called the ureters bring the urine from the kidneys to the bladder. The urethra carries the urine from the bladder to the outside of the body.

Bladder cancer has a very high rate of recurrence following treatment. Even after superficial tumors are completely removed, there is a 75% chance that new tumors will develop in other areas of the bladder. Hence, patients need very frequent and thorough follow-up care. When detected at the early stages, the prognosis for bladder cancer is excellent. At least 94% of patients survive five years or more after initial diagnosis. If the disease has spread to the nearby tissues, however, the survival rates drop to 49%. If it has metastasized to distant organs such as the lung or liver, only 6% of patients will survive five years or more.

Demographics

Bladder cancer is the sixth most common cancer in the United States. The American Cancer Society (ACS) estimated that in 2001, approximately 54,300 new cases of bladder cancer would be diagnosed (about 39,200 men and 15,100 women), causing approximately 12,400 deaths.

The highest occurrences of bladder cancer are found in industrialized countries such as the United States, Canada, France, Denmark, Italy, and Spain. In all countries, the incidence of bladder cancer is higher for men than women. Among men, the highest rates occur in white non-Hispanic males (33.1 per 100,000). The rates for men of African descent and Hispanic men are similar and are approximately one-half of the rate among white non-Hispanic men. The lowest rate of bladder cancer occurs in the Asian population. Among women, the highest rates also occur in white non-Hispanic females and are approximately twice the rate for Hispanics. Women of African descent have higher rates of bladder cancer than Hispanic women.

Age is also an important factor: bladder cancer is significantly more common in older men and women in all populations. Bladder cancer rates for people aged 70 years and older are two to three times higher than for people in the 55 to 69 age group, and approximately 15 to 20 times higher than for people between the ages of 30 and 54.

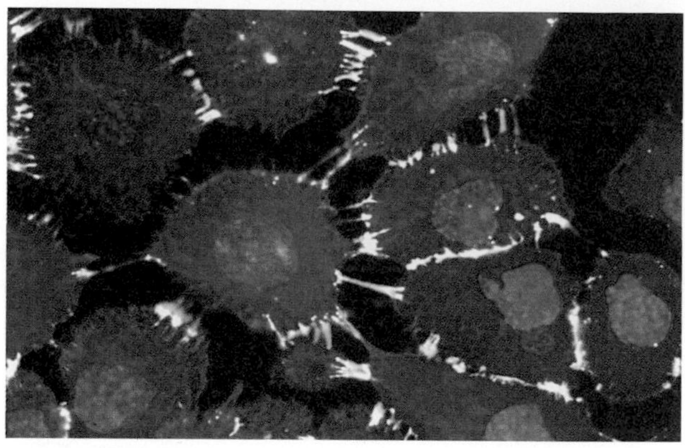

An immunofluorescent light micrograph of cells cultured from squamous carcinoma of the bladder. *(Photograph by Nancy Kedersha, Photo Researchers, Inc. Reproduced by permission.)*

Causes and symptoms

Although the exact cause of bladder cancer is not known, smokers are twice as likely to get the disease as are nonsmokers. Smoking is subsequently considered to be the greatest risk factor for bladder cancer. Workers who are exposed to certain chemicals that are used in the dye, rubber, leather, textile, and paint industries are also believed to be at a higher risk for bladder cancer.

Frequent urinary infections, kidney and bladder stones, and other conditions that cause long-term irritation to the bladder may increase the risk of getting bladder cancer. A past history of tumors in the bladder also increases one's risk of developing new tumors.

One of the first warning signals of bladder cancer is blood in the urine. There may be enough blood in the urine to change its color to a yellow-red or dark red. At other times, the color of the urine appears normal but chemical testing of the urine reveals the presence of blood cells. Painful urination, increased frequency, and increased urgency (the sensation of having to urinate immediately but being unable to do so) are other possible signs of bladder cancer. All of these symptoms may also be caused by conditions other than cancer, so it is important to see a doctor to have the symptoms evaluated.

Diagnosis

If a doctor has any reason to suspect bladder cancer, several tests may be used to find out if the disease is present. A complete medical history will be taken to check for any risk factors. A thorough physical examination will be conducted to assess all the signs and symptoms. Laboratory testing of a urine sample will help to rule out the presence of a bacterial infection. In a urine **cytology** test, the urine is examined under a microscope to look for any abnormal or cancerous cells. A catheter (tube) can be advanced into the bladder through the urethra and a salt solution passed through it to wash the bladder. The solution can then be collected and examined under a microscope to check for the presence of any cancerous cells.

A test known as the intravenous pyelogram (IVP) is an x-ray examination performed after a dye is injected into a vein in the arm. The dye travels through the blood stream and reaches the kidneys to be excreted, clearly outlining the kidneys, ureters, bladder, and urethra. Multiple x rays are taken to detect any abnormalities in the lining of these organs.

The physician may use a procedure known as a **cystoscopy** to view the inside of the bladder. A thin hollow lighted tube is introduced into the bladder through the urethra. If any suspicious-looking masses are seen, a small piece of the tissue can be painlessly removed using a pair of **biopsy** forceps. The tissue is then examined microscopically to verify if cancer is present, and if so, the type of cancer will be identified.

If cancer is detected and there is evidence showing that it has metastasized to distant sites in the body, imaging tests such as chest x rays, **computed tomography** scans (CT scans), and **magnetic resonance imaging** (MRI) may be done to determine which organs are affected. Bladder cancer tends to spread to the lungs, liver, and bone.

Treatment team

Treatment for bladder cancer depends on the stage of the disease and how deeply the cancer has penetrated the bladder wall. It also depends on the grade of the cancer and on the patient's general health status and personal preferences. Most likely, a team of specialists including a urologist, an oncologist, a surgeon, and a radiation oncologist will be responsible for treatment. The treatment team will develop a plan tailored to the individual patient and may recommend one treatment method or a combination of methods.

Clinical staging, treatments, and prognosis

Staging

The following stages are used by health care providers to classify the location, size, and spread of the cancer, according to the TNM (tumor, lymph node, and metastases) staging system:

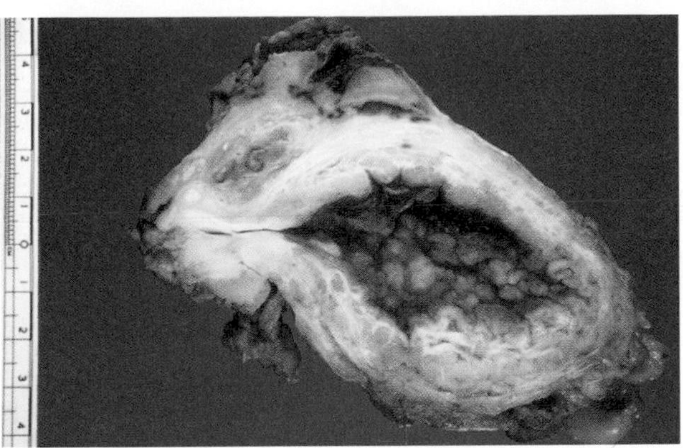

Excised specimen of a cancerous human bladder, showing a large tumor mass. *(© Science Photo Library, Science Source/Photo Researchers, Inc. Reproduced by permission.)*

- Stage 0: Cancer is found only on the inner lining of the bladder (a noninvasive **carcinoma**).
- Stage I: Cancer has spread to the layer of tissue beyond the inner lining of the bladder but not to the bladder muscles.
- Stage II: Cancer has spread to the muscles in the bladder wall but not to the fatty tissue surrounding the bladder.
- Stage III: Cancer has spread to the fatty tissue surrounding the bladder and potentially to the prostate, vagina, or uterus, but not to the lymph nodes or other organs.
- Stage IV: Cancer has spread to the lymph nodes, pelvic or abdominal wall, and/or other organs.
- Recurrent: Cancer has recurred in the bladder or at another site after having been treated.

Standard treatments

The three standard modes of treatment that are available for bladder cancer are surgery, **radiation therapy**, and **chemotherapy**.

Surgery is considered to be an option only when the disease is in its early stages. If the tumor is localized to a small area and has not spread to the outer layers of the bladder, then the surgery is done without entering the abdomen. A cystoscope is introduced into the bladder through the urethra, and the tumor is removed. This procedure is called a transurethral resection (TUR). Passing a high-energy laser beam through the cystoscope to burn cancer cells, a procedure known as electrofulguration, may treat any remaining cancer.

If the cancer has invaded the wall of the bladder, surgery will be done through an incision in the abdomen.

KEY TERMS

Biopsy—The surgical removal and microscopic examination of living tissue for diagnostic purposes.

Chemotherapy—Treatment with drugs that selectively destroy cancer cells.

Computed tomography (CT) scan—A medical procedure in which a series of x rays are taken and analyzed by a computer in order to form detailed pictures of areas inside the body.

Cystoscopy—A diagnostic procedure in which a hollow lighted tube, (cystoscope) is used to look inside the bladder and the urethra.

Electrofulguration—A procedure in which a high-energy laser beam is used to burn the cancerous tissue.

Immunotoxins—Antibodies produced in the laboratory that recognize specific substances which are more abundant in cancer cells than in normal cells; immunotoxins identify cancer cells and deliver a powerful toxin that kills the cells.

Intravenous pyelogram (IVP)—A procedure where an injected dye outlines the urinary system on an x ray to help reveal potential abnormalities.

Magnetic resonance imaging (MRI)—A medical procedure used for diagnostic purposes where pictures of areas inside the body can be created using a magnet linked to a computer.

Partial cystectomy—A surgical procedure where the cancerous tissue is removed by cutting out a small piece of the bladder.

Photodynamic therapy—A combination of special light rays and drugs that are used to destroy the cancerous cells.

Radiation therapy—Treatment using high-energy radiation from x-ray machines, cobalt, radium, or other sources.

Radical cystectomy—A surgical procedure that removes the entire bladder and occasionally other adjoining organs.

Stoma—An artificial opening between two cavities or between a cavity and the surface of the body.

Transurethral resection—A surgical procedure to remove abnormal tissue from the bladder using an instrument called a cystoscope.

Urostomy—A surgical procedure in which the ureters are disconnected from the bladder and connected to an opening (see stoma) on the abdomen, allowing urine to flow into a collection bag.

Cancer that is not very large can be removed by partial cystectomy, a procedure where a part of the bladder is removed. If the cancer is large or is present in more than one area of the bladder, a radical cystectomy is done. The entire bladder is removed in this procedure; adjoining organs may also be removed. In men, the prostate is removed, while in women, the uterus, ovaries, and fallopian tubes are removed.

If the entire urinary bladder is removed, then an alternate storage place must be created for urine before it is excreted out of the body. To do this, a piece of intestine is converted into a small bag and attached to the ureters. This is connected to an opening (stoma) that is made in the abdominal wall. The procedure is called a **urostomy**. In some urostomy procedures, the urine from the intestinal sac is routed into a bag that is placed over the stoma in the abdominal wall. The bag is hidden by clothing and has to be emptied occasionally by the patient. In a different procedure, the urine is collected in the intestinal sac, but there is no bag on the outside of the abdomen. The intestinal sac has to be emptied by the patient by placing a drainage tube through the stoma.

Radiation therapy that uses high-energy rays to kill cancer cells is generally used after surgery to destroy any remaining cancer cells. If the tumor is in a location that makes surgery difficult or if it is large, radiation may be used before surgery to shrink the tumor. In cases of advanced bladder cancer, radiation therapy is used to ease the symptoms such as pain, bleeding, or blockage. External beam radiation focuses a beam of radiation on the area of the tumor. Alternatively, a small pellet of radioactive material may be placed directly into the cancer. This is known as interstitial radiation therapy.

Chemotherapy uses anticancer drugs to destroy the cancer cells that may have migrated to distant sites. The drugs are injected into the intravenously or taken orally in pill form. Generally a combination of drugs is more effective than any single drug in treating bladder cancer. Chemotherapy may be given following surgery to kill any remaining cancer cells. It may also be given even when no remaining cancer cells can be seen (adjuvant chemotherapy). Anticancer drugs, including **thiotepa**, **doxorubicin**, and mitomycin, may also be instilled directly into the bladder (intravesicular chemotherapy) to treat superficial tumors.

Immunotherapy or biological therapy uses the body's own immune cells to fight the disease. To treat superficial bladder cancer, **bacillus Calmette-Guérin** (BCG) may be instilled directly into the bladder. BCG is a weakened (attenuated) strain of the tuberculosis bacillus that stimulates the body's immune system to fight the cancer. This therapy has been shown to be effective in controlling superficial bladder cancer.

Photodynamic treatment is a novel mode of treatment that uses special chemicals and light to kill the cancerous cells when the bladder cancer is in its early stages. First, a drug is introduced into the bladder that makes the cancer cells more susceptible to light. A special light is then shone on the bladder in an attempt to destroy the cancerous cells.

Alternative and complementary therapies

Gene therapy is a new method being tested as a complementary therapy for bladder cancer. Research has shown that mutations in tumor suppressor genes can cause abnormal growth of bladder cells. Gene therapy involves infecting bladder cancer cells with specially designed viruses that contain a normal gene in order to restore a normal cell growth process.

Immunotherapy is another area that is expected to contribute new complementary treatment methods. Immunotoxins are antibodies produced in the laboratory that recognize specific substances that are more abundant in cancer cells than in normal cells. Once the immunotoxins identify a cancer cell, they deliver a powerful toxin attached to the antibody which enters and kills the cell.

Coping with cancer treatment

As with any cancer, shock and stress are natural reactions to a confirmed bladder cancer diagnosis. Coping is often made easier with access to helpful information and support services. Many patients want to learn all they can about the disease and their treatment choices so as to be fully involved in the decisions that are being made concerning their medical care. The national cancer organizations are an important source of medical information. Many associations have also been organized to allow patients the opportunity to meet others undergoing similar experiences in support groups.

Patients are often uncomfortable during the first few days after bladder surgery. They may also experience **fatigue** and weakness. Those undergoing radiation therapy or chemotherapy may experience side effects such as pain, fatigue, rashes, or bleeding. Pain can be controlled with medication and patients should feel free to discuss aspects of pain relief with their physician or nurse.

QUESTIONS TO ASK THE DOCTOR

- Why do I need to have a biopsy?
- How long will it take? Will I be awake? Will it hurt?
- How soon will I know the results?
- If I do have bladder cancer, who will talk with me about treatment? When?

Clinical trials

In 2001 the National Cancer Institute (NCI) supported over 50 bladder cancer **clinical trials** to evaluate a variety of anticancer drugs. Some trials study new treatments involving radiation therapy, chemotherapy, biological therapies, and new combinations of various therapies. Other trials study ways to lower the side effects of treatment. Patients who take part in these studies often have the chance to benefit from promising new drugs and developments. Those interested in taking part in a trial should discuss the possibility with their physician and consult an NCI booklet entitled, "Taking Part in Clinical Trials: What Cancer Patients Need To Know" (NIH Publication #97-4250).

Prevention

Since it is not known what exactly causes bladder cancer, there is no certain way to prevent its occurrence. Avoiding risk factors whenever possible is the best alternative. Since smoking doubles one's risk of getting bladder cancer, avoiding tobacco may prevent at least half the deaths that result from bladder cancer. Taking appropriate safety precautions when working with organic cancer-causing chemicals is another way of reducing one's risk.

Those with a history of bladder cancer, kidney stones, urinary tract infections, and other conditions that cause long-term irritation to the bladder are advised to undergo regular screening tests such as urine cytology, cystoscopy, and x rays of the urinary tract, so that cancer may be detected at an early stage and treated appropriately.

Special concerns

Special concerns may arise for those who have undergone partial or radical cystectomy. For example, if the bladder has to be removed, the patient will need to learn a new way to store and pass urine. Women who have had a radical cystectomy are not able to have children because their uterus has also been removed. Men who have had a radical cystectomy will become impotent (unable to sustain an erection) if their prostrate and seminal vesicles have also been removed.

See Also Intravenous urography; Metastasis; Tumor staging

Resources

BOOKS

Berkow, Robert, ed. *Merck Manual of Diagnosis and Therapy.* 16th ed. Rahway, NJ: Merck Research Laboratories, 1992.

Dollinger, Malin, Ernest H. Rosenbaum, and Greg Cable. *Everyone's Guide to Cancer Therapy.* Kansas City: Andrews and McMeel, 1994.

Murphy, Gerald P., Lois B. Morris, and Dianne Lange. *Informed Decisions: The Complete Book of Cancer Diagnosis, Treatment and Recovery.* New York: Viking, 1997.

PERIODICALS

Lamm, D. L., and M. Allaway. "Current trends in bladder cancer treatment." *Annales Chirurgiae et Gynaecologiae* 89 (2000): 234-241.

Lockyer, C. R., and D. A. Gillatt. "BCG immunotherapy for superficial bladder cancer." *Journal of the Royal Society of Medicine* 94 (March 2001): 119-23.

Oosterlinck, W. "The management of superficial bladder cancer." *BJU International* 87 (January 2001): 135-40.

Petrovich, Z., G. Jozsef, and L. W. Brady. "Radiotherapy for carcinoma of the bladder: a review." *American Journal of Clinical Oncology* 24 (February 2001): 1-9.

Ryan, C. W., and N. J. Vogelzang. "Gemcitabine in the treatment of bladder cancer." *Expert Opinions in Pharmacotherapy* 1 (March 2000): 547-53.

ORGANIZATION

American Cancer Society. 1599 Clifton Rd. NE, Atlanta, GA 30329. (800) 227-2345. <http://www.cancer.org.>.

American Foundation for Urologic Disease. 300 W. Pratt St., Suite 401, Baltimore, MD 21201. (800) 828-7866. <http://www.afud.org>.

Cancer Research Institute. 681 Fifth Ave., New York, NY 10022. (800) 992-2623. <http:://www.cancerresearch.org>.

National Cancer Institute. 9000 Rockville Pike, Building 31, Room 10A16, Bethesda, MD 20892. (800) 422-6237. <http://www.nci.nih.gov>.

National Kidney and Urologic Diseases Information Clearinghouse. 3 Information Way, Bethesda, MD 20892. (301) 651-4415. <http://www.niddk.nih.gov/health/kidney/nkudic.htm>.

Oncolink, University of Pennsylvania Cancer Center. <http://cancer.med.upenn.edu>.

OTHER

"Bladder Cancer." *American Cancer Society's Urinary Bladder Cancer Resource Center.* 2000. 26 June 2001 <http://www3.cancer.org/cancerinfo/res_home.asp?ct=44>.

"Bladder Cancer: FAQ." *American Cancer Society.* 11 July 2000. 26 June 2001 <http://www3.cancer.org/cancerinfo>.

"Staging: Stages of cancer of the bladder." *University of Pittsburgh Cancer Institute.* June 2001. 28 June 2001 <http://www.upci.upmc.edu/internet/prostate/cancer/bladder/stage.cfm>.

"Taking Part in Clinical Trials: What Cancer Patients Need To Know (NIH Publication #97 4250)." *National Institutes of Health & National Cancer Institute.* May 1998. 26 June 2001 <http://www.cancernet.nci.nih.gov/peb/taking_part_treatment/index.html>.

Lata Cherath, Ph.D.
Monique Laberge, Ph.D.

Bleomycin

Definition

Bleomycin (Blenoxane) kills cancer cells by damaging the genetic material known as DNA, thus preventing cells from repairing themselves.

Purpose

Bleomycin is used in the treatment of a number of different cancers, including cancer of the head and neck, skin, esophagus, lung, testis, penis, vulva, cervix, and genitourinary tract. In addition, it is used in the treatment of **Hodgkin's disease** and **non-Hodgkin's lymphomas**. It may also be used to treat **Kaposi's sarcoma**.

Because bleomycin is used in the treatment of so many different cancers, only a sampling of its uses can be provided here. In the treatment of Hodgkin's disease, one **chemotherapy** regimen used is the so-called ABVD, which consists of **doxorubicin**, bleomycin, **vinblastine**, and **dacarbazine**. Another regimen is called MOPP/ABV, which consists of **mechlorethamine**, **vincristine**, prednisone, **procarbazine**, doxorubicin, bleomycin, and vinblastine.

A treatment used for stage III and IV non-Hodgkin's **lymphoma** is the CHOP-bleomycin regimen, which consists of **cyclophosphamide**, hydroxydaunomycin, vincristine, prednisone, and bleomycin. Another approach to the same illness involves the m-BACOD chemotherapy regimen, which consists of **methotrexate**, bleomycin, doxorubicin, cyclophosphamide, vincristine, and **dexamethasone**. Yet another approach to treating this disease is called ProMACE-CytaBOM, and consists of cyclophosphamide, doxorubicin, **etoposide**, prednisone, **cytarabine**, bleomycin, vincristine, methotrexate, and **leucovorin**.

Description

Bleomycin is an antitumor antibiotic that fights cancer by attacking the DNA in cancerous cells, thus interfering with cell growth.

Recommended dosage

A dose of 0.25-0.50 units/kg (10-20 units per square meter) is given once or twice a week either intravenously, intramuscularly, or subcutaneously. A small test dose should be given first to test for a possible severe allergic reaction.

Precautions

Patients who receive certain forms of oxygen therapy while taking bleomycin or who receive anesthesia while taking bleomycin are at increased risk for developing serious lung problems.

Patients given bleomycin may develop an acute allergic reaction that may be fatal in rare cases. Therefore, a patient should only receive a small test dose of bleomycin the first time the drug is administered. After this initial dose the patient is observed carefully for one hour. Assuming no further problems appear, the patient may then receive a standard dose.

The likelihood that lung damage will occur increases if a patient receives more than 450–500 units of the drug during an entire lifetime. So, it is prudent to limit the amount of this medication given. Furthermore, it may be unwise to give bleomycin in regimens containing cyclophosphamide, as this combination also increases the likelihood that lung damage will occur.

Side effects

Lung problems are a serious side effect affecting some patients who receive bleomycin. While lung problems can appear regardless of how much of the medicine is given, they are more likely to appear if a patient receives more than a certain amount of the medicine—250 units according to some authorities and 450–500 units according to others. The appearance of a dry cough may indicate the development of lung problems. Lung damage can be assessed by measuring the rate at which the patient is able to transfer gas across the lung membranes (DLCO or diffusion lung capacity).

KEY TERMS

DNA—DNA is a nucleic acid found inside of cells that carries genetic information.

Raynaud's phenomenon—Raynaud's phenomenon, which affects the fingers and toes, may involve pain, pale color, and abnormal sensation (e.g., burning or prickling).

Other side effects of bleomycin may include skin problems and alteration of skin color, allergic reactions, Raynaud's phenomenon, and hair loss. In addition, headache, and **nausea and vomiting** may occur. Rheumatoid arthritis may worsen during bleomycin therapy. Patients with testicular tumors who receive multiple chemotherapy agents including bleomycin may develop Raynaud's phenomenon and cardiovascular disease. Raynaud's phenomenon, which affects the fingers and toes, may involve pain, pale color, and abnormal sensation (for instance, burning or prickling).

Approximately 1 out of every 100 patients who takes bleomycin experiences a reaction that involves chills, **fever**, wheezing, low blood pressure, and mental confusion. Unlike many other cancer drugs, bleomycin is not likely to cause any damage to the bone marrow.

Patients may be given steroids before bleomycin therapy is started in an effort to reduce the side effects of the drug.

Interactions

Bleomycin is often given in combination with with other anticancer drugs, for example **cisplatin**, vinblastine, and etoposide. Such combinations have been found to be more effective than single drug therapy.

Bob Kirsch

Blood dyscrasias *see* **Multiple myeloma; Waldenström's macroglobulinemia**

Blood transfusion *see* **Transfusion therapy**

Body image/self image

Description

Body image refers to a person's internal picture of his or her external physical appearance. Self image is a broader category that refers to one's inner perception of his or her physical, mental, interpersonal, and spiritual characteristics and abilities. The distinction is important because cultures vary significantly regarding the amount of emphasis given to body image as one aspect of self image. In Japan, for example, body image is a much smaller part of most people's self-image than it is in the United States. Both forms of self-perception, however, may be affected by cancer treatment.

Specific body image or self image concerns vary according to age and gender. Children being treated for cancer have different issues from adults because their self and body images are still being formed. Children and adolescents with cancer sometimes internalize a picture-of themselves as disfigured or unattractive, or as physically weak and incompetent. Even when the cancer has been successfully treated, the child's self image may still reflect feelings of being "sick" or "damaged." A distorted self image in turn can cause difficulties in social relationships as the child grows older. The Candlelighters programs offer practical advice and social support for children with cancer and their families.

Self image problems in adults tend to reflect (and reinforce) American society's patterns of gender socialization. Studies indicate that many women tend to be openly concerned about damage to their external appearance caused by cancer treatments. For many women, anxiety about losing their looks is directly related to fear of losing their husband or partner. Men's concern about outward appearance is less obvious but may be expressed as a need to look "healthy" in order to keep their job. Although there are not as many studies of men's reactions to cancer treatment as there are of women's, recent research indicates that men are still more concerned about losing physical strength or specific physical abilities required by their work than about their looks as such.

Causes

Cultural context

It is important to situate body image/self image issues related to cancer treatment within the larger context of contemporary emphasis on physical perfection. Advertising in the mass media encourages people to feel dissatisfied with their bodies. One study of the effects of television advertising on college youth found that as little as half an hour of ideal-body commercials has a negative impact on a person's body image. Another study found that a majority of American adults, men as well as women, believe that people are judged on the basis of appearance first and talent or personality second. In a cultural setting in which healthy people often feel they cannot measure up to media standards of attractiveness, it is not surprising that cancer patients are concerned about the effects of therapy on their appearance.

Surgery

Surgery on the face or the parts of the body associated with sexual performance or attractiveness has a more severe impact on self image than surgery on the hands, feet, or back. Breast surgery in women and surgical treatment of **prostate cancer** in men are often accompanied by changes in the patient's self image, particularly with respect to sexual relations. Sexual responsiveness can also be affected if the surgeon has had to remove tissue containing nerve endings that are sensitive to touch.

Radiation and chemotherapy

Radiation and **chemotherapy** can affect a cancer patient's body image because they often cause hair loss, radiation burns, and unattractive changes in the patient's complexion. While hair loss caused by chemotherapy is usually a temporary condition, hair loss caused by radiation treatment may be permanent. In addition, both radiation and chemotherapy can cause nausea, vomiting, fatigue, **depression**, and other reactions that affect the patient's sense of competence as well as their relationships with others. Self image often suffers when a person feels that job performance and valued relationships are being strained by these side effects of cancer treatment.

Treatments

Cosmetic

Since 1989, the American Cancer Society, the Cosmetic, Toiletry, and Fragrance Association Foundation, and the National Cosmetology Association have sponsored the "Look Good... Feel Better" (LGFB) program, which offers classes in a number of medical centers. These classes help female cancer patients with self image issues as well as teaching them special grooming techniques to manage the side effects of cancer therapy. LGFB has been available in Canada since 1992.

Hair loss can be covered by a variety of wigs, partial hairpieces, and scarves or turbans. The American Hair Loss Council offers more detailed information about these and other ways to cope with hair loss caused by cancer treatment. Doctors who specialize in plastic surgery can suggest ways to treat facial scars or other types of surgical disfigurement, including the loss of body parts. A prosthesis, which is an artificial replacement for a missing or damaged body part, can be made to order for the patient.

Counseling and support

Cancer patients who are experiencing serious emotional problems related to changes in appearance may benefit from counseling or support groups. Individual psychotherapy guides people to look at the reasons for focusing on their looks as well as ways to cope with the changes. Pastoral or spiritual counseling can help remind patients that they are more than just their bodies. Support groups for cancer patients are good places to share feelings and useful tips about dress and grooming with others who are in the same situation.

Alternative and complementary therapies

Alternative and complementary therapies may help patients to deal with changes in self and body image through developing a fuller self image, finding new interests, or learning new skills. Meditation and prayer can help patients put physical appearance inside a larger framework of values. Some cancer patients find yoga, t'ai chi, and dance or movement therapy are interesting to learn as well as good forms of exercise. Lastly, massage, calming or uplifting music, and aromatherapy allow patients to balance the side effects of cancer treatment with relaxing and pleasant experiences.

See Also Sexuality; Alopecia

Resources

BOOKS

Chapkis, Wendy. *Beauty Secrets: Women and the Politics of Appearance.* Boston: South End Press, 1986.

Dollinger, Malin, M.D., Ernest H. Rosenbaum, M.D., and Greg Cable. *Cancer Therapy.* Kansas City, MO: Somerville House, 1994.

Johnston, Joni E., Psy. D. *Appearance Obsession:Learning to Love the Way You Look.* Deerfield Beach, FL: Health Communications, Inc. 1994.

Peiss, Kathy. *Hope in a Jar: The Making of America's Beauty Culture.* New York: Metropolitan Books, Henry Holt and Company, 1998.

PERIODICALS

Clark, Jack A., Nelda Wray, Baruch Brody, Carol Ashton,Brian Giesler, and Herbert Watkins. "Dimensions of Quality of Life Expressed by Men Treated for Metastatic Prostate Cancer." *Soc. Sci. Med,* 45, no. 8 (1999): pp 1299–1309.

PROGRAMS AND ASSOCIATIONS

American Hair Loss Council. (888) 873-9719. <http://www.ahlc.org>.

Candlelighters Childhood Cancer Foundation. 7910 Woodmont Avenue, Suite 460, Bethesda, MD 20814. (301) 657-8401 or (800) 366-CCCF.

Look Good... Feel Better (LGFB). 1100 Connecticut Avenue N. W., Washington, DC 20036. (800) 395-5665. In Canada: Look Good... Feel Better, 420 Britannia Road East, Suite 102, Mississaugua, Ontario L4Z 3L5 (905) 890-5161. Fax: (905) 890-2607. Web site: <http://www.lgfb.ca>.

National Cancer Institute of the National Institutes of Health. *Chemotherapy and You: A Guide to Self-Help During Cancer Treatment.* NIH Publication #99-1136. Can be downloaded from <http://cancernet.nci.nih.gov>.

OTHER

"For Women:Body Image Issues." *Gillette Women's Cancer Connection.* 1999. 16 March 2001. <http://www.gillettecancerconnect.org>.

Rebecca J. Frey, Ph.D.

KEY TERMS

Body image—A term that refers to a person's inner picture of his or her outward appearance.

Prosthesis (plural, prostheses)—An artificial substitute for a missing or defective body part. Prostheses are usually designed to look and feel as natural as possible.

Self image—A wider term that includes a person's perception of his or her talents, character traits, interests, spirituality, and other aspects of their being as well as outward physical appearance.

Bone marrow aspiration and biopsy

Definition

Bone marrow aspiration, also called bone marrow sampling, is the removal by suction of fluid from the soft, spongy material that lines the inside of most bones. Bone marrow **biopsy**, or needle biopsy, is the removal of a small piece of bone marrow.

Purpose

Bone marrow aspiration is used to:

- pinpoint the cause of abnormal blood test results
- confirm a diagnosis or check the status of severe **anemia** (abnormally low numbers of red blood cells in the bloodstream) of unknown cause, or other irregularities in the way blood cells are produced or become mature
- evaluate abnormalities in the blood's ability to store iron

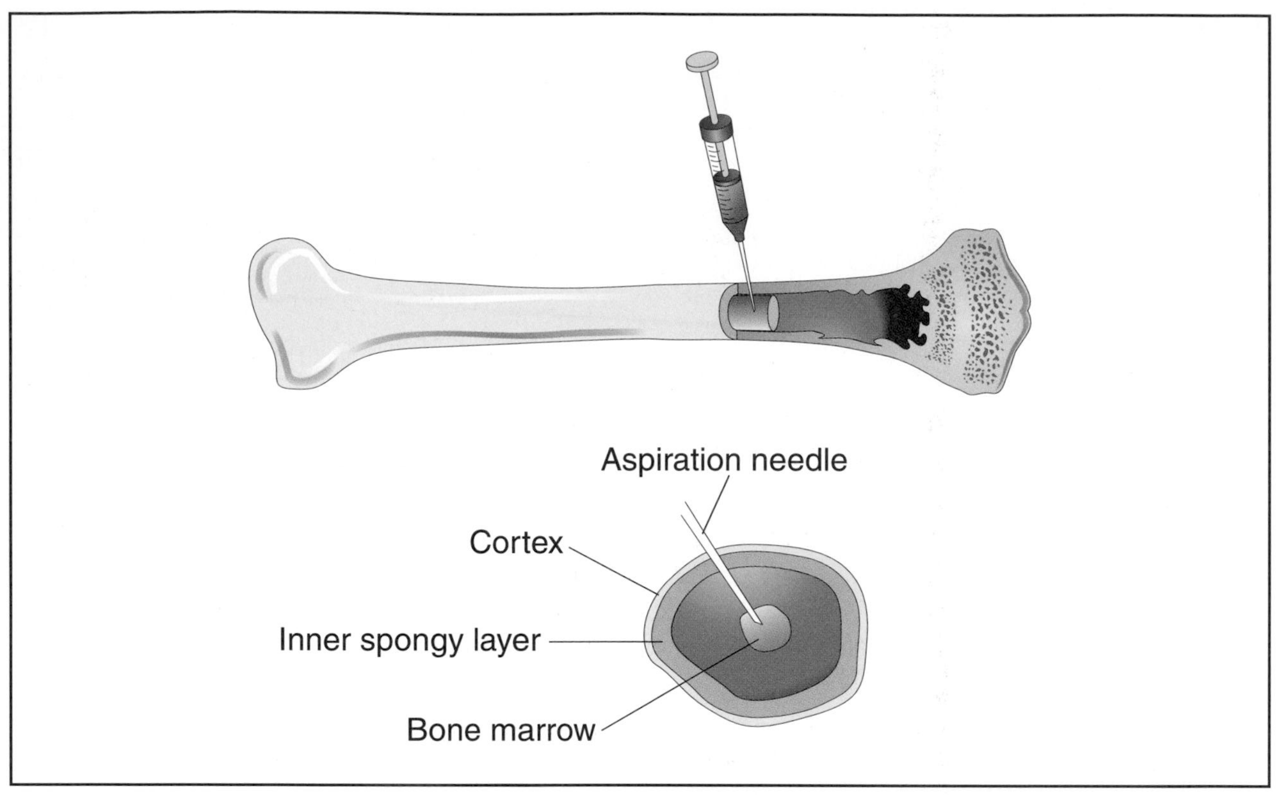

In a bone marrow aspiration, a needle is inserted beneath the skin and rotated until it penetrates the cortex, or outer covering, of the bone. A small amount of marrow is suctioned out of the bone by a syringe attached to the needle. *(Illustration by Electronic Illustrators Group.)*

- diagnose infection

Bone marrow biopsy is used to:

- obtain intact bone marrow for laboratory analysis
- diagnose and stage some types of cancer or anemia and other blood disorders
- identify the source of an unexplained fever
- diagnose fibrosis of bone marrow or **myeloma** (a tumor composed of cells normally found in the bone marrow) when bone marrow aspiration has failed to provide an appropriate specimen

Bone marrow aspiration and bone marrow biopsy are also used to gauge the effectiveness of **chemotherapy** and other medical treatments. These procedures are often used together to ensure the availability of the best possible bone marrow specimen.

Precautions

Allergies or previous adverse reactions to medications should be discussed with the doctor. Any current medications, including herbal or nutritional supplements, should be evaluated for the potential to interfere with proper coagulation (clot formation). These would include coumadin, aspirin, and other agents used as blood thinners. Caution should be used when the herbs gingko, ginger, garlic, or ginseng have been utilized as supplements, due to a risk of bleeding.

Pregnancy, lactation (production and secretion of milk), and preexisting platelet or bleeding disorders should be evaluated before either procedure is undertaken.

Description

Bone marrow aspiration and biopsy should be performed by a physician or nurse clinician. Each procedure takes about 20 to 30 minutes and is usually performed on an outpatient basis, but can be done in a hospital if necessary.

The skin covering the biopsy site is cleansed with an antiseptic, and the patient may be given a mild sedative. A local anesthetic is administered. The hematologist or nurse clinician performing the procedure will not begin until the anesthetic has numbed the area from which the specimen is to be extracted. In both adults and children, aspiration and biopsy are most commonly performed on the rear bone of the hip (posterior iliac crest). In adults, sampling from the sternum (breastbone) is sometimes done. The latter location is technically easier, but is somewhat more painful for the patient and presents the risk of heart injury. On rare occasions, a long bone of the leg (tibia) may be used as a sample site for an infant.

In a bone marrow aspiration, a special needle is inserted beneath the skin and rotated until it penetrates the cortex, or outer covering of the bone. At least half a teaspoon of marrow is withdrawn from the bone by a syringe attached to the needle. The patient may experience discomfort when the needle is inserted or when the marrow is aspirated. If more marrow is needed, the needle is repositioned slightly, a new syringe is attached, and a second sample is taken. The samples are transferred from the syringes to slides and vials, then sent to a laboratory for analysis.

Bone marrow biopsy may be performed immediately before or after bone marrow aspiration. The procedure utilizes a special large-bore needle that is used to drill out a core of marrow. In bone marrow biopsy, the needle is inserted, rotated from side to side, withdrawn, and reinserted at a different angle. This procedure is repeated if needed until a small core, about 0.4 inches (1 cm) long, is separated from the bone marrow. The needle is again removed, and a piece of fine wire threaded through its tip transfers the specimen onto sterile gauze. The patient may feel discomfort or pressure when the needle is inserted and experience a brief, pulling sensation when the marrow is withdrawn. Unlike aspiration specimens, which are smeared, these samples contain structurally intact bone marrow. Microscopic examination can show what material its cells contain and how they are alike or different from one another. The bone may either be embedded intact in paraffin (a type of wax), or be decalcified (a process which takes place overnight) for a different type of staining and examination. Each type of preparation has certain advantages.

Preparation

A current history and physical are obtained from the patient, along with proper consent. The patient is generally placed in a prone position (lying face down) for preparation, and local anesthetic, with or without sedation, is administered.

Aftercare

After the needle is removed, the biopsy site will be covered with a clean, dry bandage. Pressure is applied to control bleeding. The patient's pulse, breathing, blood pressure, and temperature are monitored until they return to normal, and the patient may be instructed to remain in a supine position (lying face up) for half an hour before getting dressed.

The patient should be able to leave the clinic and resume normal activities immediately. Patients who have received a sedative often feel sleepy for the rest of the day; driving, cooking, and other activities that require clear thinking and quick reactions should therefore be avoided.

The biopsy site should be kept covered and dry for several hours. Walking or taking prescribed pain medications usually ease any discomfort felt at the biopsy site, and ice can be used to reduce swelling.

A doctor should be notified if the patient:

- Feels severe pain more than 24 hours after the procedure.
- Experiences persistent bleeding or notices more than a few drops of blood on the wound dressing.
- Has a temperature above 101°F (38.3°C). Inflammation and pus at the biopsy site and other signs of infection should also be reported to a doctor without delay.

KEY TERMS

Aspiration—A procedure to withdraw fluid from the body.

Connective tissue—Material that links one part of the body with another.

Fibrosis—A condition characterized by the presence of scar tissue or fiber-containing tissues that replace normal tissues.

Hematologist—A medical specialist who treats diseases and disorders of the blood and blood-forming organs.

Hematoma—Blood that collects under the skin and causes swelling.

Hemorrhage—Heavy bleeding.

Myeloma—A tumor that originates in bone marrow and usually spreads to more than one bone.

Nurse practitioner—A registered nurse who is qualified to perform some specialized duties.

QUESTIONS TO ASK THE DOCTOR

- What will this tell me about my condition?
- What should I do to prepare for this procedure?
- What are my chances of infection or other complications?
- What future care will I need?

Risks

Bleeding and discomfort often occur at the biopsy site. Infection and hematoma may also develop. In rare instances, the heart or a major blood vessel is pierced when marrow is extracted from the sternum during bone marrow biopsy. This can lead to severe hemorrhage.

Normal results

Healthy adult bone marrow contains yellow fat cells, connective tissue, and red marrow that produces blood. The bone marrow of a healthy infant is primarily red due to active production of red cells necessary for growth.

Abnormal results

Culture of bone marrow aspirate may yield information about an infectious agent. Microscopic examination of bone marrow can reveal granulomas, **myelofibrosis**, lymphomas, leukemias, or other cancers. Analyzing specimens can help doctors diagnose iron deficiency, vitamin B_{12}deficiency, and folate deficiency, as well as anemia.

Obesity can affect the ease with which a bone marrow biopsy can be done, and the results of either procedure can be affected if the patient has had **radiation therapy** at the biopsy site.

Resources

BOOKS

Bain, Barbara, et al. *Bone Marrow Pathology.* Oxford, UK: Blackwell Science, Ltd., 1996.

Gatter, Kevin, and David Brown. *An Illustrated Guide to Bone Marrow Diagnosis.* Oxford, UK: Blackwell Science, Ltd., 1997.

Zaret, Barry L., et al. *The Yale University Patient's Guide to Medical Tests.* Boston: Houghton Mifflin Company, 1997.

ORGANIZATION

Leukemia Society of America. 600 Third Ave., New York, NY 10016. (800) 955-4572. <http://www.leukemia.org>.

National Cancer Institute Cancer Information Service. 9000 Rockville Pike, Bethesda, MD 20892. (800) 422-6237. <http://cis.nci.nih.gov>.

National Marrow Donor Program. 3433 Broadway St. NE, #400, Minneapolis, MN 55413. (800) 627-7692. <http://www.marrow.org>.

The Wellness Community. 35 E. Seventh St., Suite 412, Cincinnati, OH 45202. (888) 793-WELL. <http://www.wellness-community.org>.

Maureen Haggerty

Bone marrow transplantation

Definition

The bone marrow—the sponge-like tissue found in the center of certain bones—contains stem cells that are the precursors of white blood cells, red blood cells, and platelets. These blood cells are vital for normal body functions, such as oxygen transport, defense against infection and disease, and clotting. Blood cells have a limited lifespan and are constantly being replaced; therefore, healthy stem cells are vital.

In association with certain diseases, stem cells may produce too many, too few, or otherwise abnormal blood cells. Also, medical treatments may destroy stem cells or alter blood cell production. The resultant blood cell abnormalities can be life threatening.

Bone marrow transplantation involves extracting bone marrow containing normal stem cells from a healthy donor, and transferring it to a recipient whose body cannot manufacture proper quantities of normal blood cells. The goal of the transplant is to rebuild the recipient's blood cells and immune system and hopefully cure the underlying ailment.

Purpose

A person's red blood cells, white blood cells, and platelets may be destroyed or may be abnormal due to disease. Also, certain medical therapies, particularly **chemotherapy** or **radiation therapy**, may destroy a person's stem cells. The consequence to a person's health is severe. Under normal circumstances, red blood cells carry oxygen throughout the body and remove carbon dioxide from the body's tissues. White blood cells form the cornerstone of the body's immune system and defend it against infection. Platelets limit bleeding by enabling the blood to clot if a blood vessel is damaged.

A bone marrow transplant is used to rebuild the body's capacity to produce these blood cells and bring their numbers to normal levels. Illnesses that may be treated with a bone marrow transplant include both cancerous and noncancerous diseases.

Cancerous diseases may or may not specifically involve blood cells; but, cancer treatment can destroy the body's ability to manufacture new blood cells. Bone marrow transplantation may be used in conjunction with additional treatments, such as chemotherapy, for various types of leukemia, **Hodgkin's disease**, **lymphoma**, breast and **ovarian cancer**, and other cancers. Noncancerous diseases for which bone marrow transplantation can be a treatment option include aplastic anemia, sickle cell disease, thalassemia, and severe immunodeficiency.

Precautions

Bone marrow transplants are not for everyone. Transplants are accompanied by a risk of infection, transplant rejection by the recipient's immune system, and other complications. The procedure has a lower success rate the greater the recipient's age. Complications are exacerbated for people whose health is already seriously impaired as in late-stage cancers. Therefore, a person's age or state of health may prohibit use of a bone marrow transplant. The typical cut-off age for a transplant ranges from 40 to 55 years; however, a person's general health is usually the more important factor.

Even in the absence of complications, the transplant and associated treatments are hard on the recipient. Bone marrow transplants are debilitating. A person's ability to withstand the rigors of the transplant is a key consideration in deciding to use this treatment.

Description

Autologous and allogeneic transplants

Two important requirements for a bone marrow transplant are the donor and the recipient. Sometimes, the donor and the recipient may be the same person. This type of transplant is called an autologous transplant. It is typically used in cases in which a person's bone marrow is generally healthy but will be destroyed due to medical treatment for diseases such as **breast cancer** and Hodgkin's disease. Most bone marrow transplants are autologous. If a person's bone marrow is unsuitable for an autologous transplant, the bone marrow must be derived from another person in an allogeneic transplant.

Allogeneic transplants are more complicated because of proteins called human lymphocyte antigens (HLA) that are on the surface of bone marrow cells. If the donor and the recipient have very dissimilar antigens, the recipient's immune system regards the donor's bone marrow cells as invaders and launches a destructive attack against them. Such an attack negates any benefits offered by the transplant.

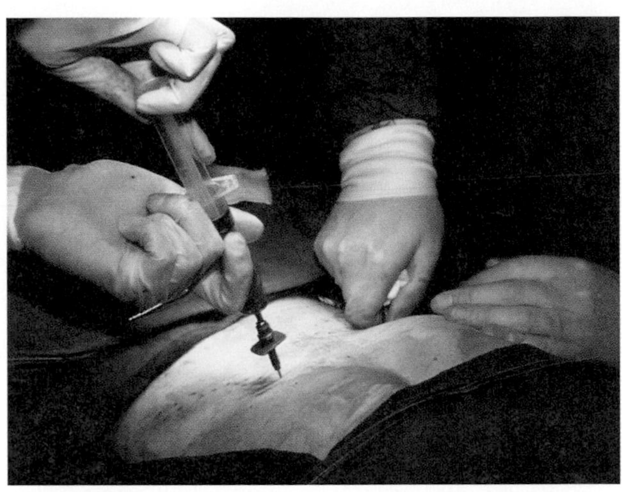

Treatment of acute leukemia by bone marrow transplant. *(© Dr. Rob Stepney, Science Source/Photo Researchers, Inc. Reproduced by permission.)*

HLA matching

There are only five major HLA classes or types—designated HLA–A,–B, –C,–D, and class III—but much variation within the groupings. For example, HLA–A from one individual may be similar to, but not the same as, HLA–A in another individual; such a situation can render a transplant from one to the other impossible.

HLA matching is more likely if the donor and recipient are related, particularly if they are siblings; however, an unrelated donor may be a potential match. Only in rare cases is matching HLA types between two people not an issue: if the recipient has an identical twin. Identical twins carry the same genes; therefore, the same antigens. A bone marrow transplant between identical twins is called a syngeneic transplant.

Peripheral blood stem cell transplants

A relatively recent development in stem cell transplantation is the use of peripheral blood stem cells instead of cells from the bone marrow. Peripheral blood stem cells (PBSCs) are obtained from circulating blood rather than from bone marrow, but the amount of stem cells found in the peripheral blood is much smaller than the amount of stem cells found in the bone marrow. Peripheral blood stem cells can be used in either autologous or allogeneic transplants. The majority of PBSC transplants are autologous. However, recent clinical

KEY TERMS

ABO antigen—Protein molecules located on the surfaces of red blood cells that determine a person's blood type: A, B, or O.

AML—Acute myelogenous leukemia, also called acute myelocytic leukemia. Malignant disorder where myeloid blast cells accumulate in the marrow and bloodstream.

Allogeneic—Referring to bone marrow transplants between two different, genetically dissimilar people.

Anemia—Decreased red cell production which results in deficiency in oxygen-carrying capacity of the blood.

Antigen—A molecule that is capable of provoking an immune response.

Aplastic anemia—A disorder in which the body produces inadequate amounts of red blood cells and hemoglobin due to underdeveloped or missing bone marrow.

Autologous—Referring to bone marrow transplants in which recipients serve as their own donors.

Blank—If an individual has inherited same HLA antigen from both parents, the HLA typing is designated by the shared HLA antigen followed by a "blank"(–).

Blast cells—Blood cells in early stage of cellular development.

Blast crisis—Stage of chronic myelogenous leukemia where large quantities of immature cells are produced by the marrow and is not responsive to treatment.

Bone marrow—A spongy tissue located within flat bones, including the hip and breast bones and the skull. This tissue contains stem cells, the precursors of platelets, red blood cells, and white blood cells.

Bone marrow transplant—Healthy marrow is infused into people who have had high-dose chemotherapy for one of the many forms of leukemias, immunodeficiencies, lymphomas, anemias, metabolic disorders, and sometimes solid tumors.

Chemotherapy—Medical treatment of a disease, particularly cancer, with drugs or other chemicals.

Chronic myelogenous leukemia (CML)—Also called chronic myelocytic leukemia, malignant disorder that involves abnormal accumulation of white cells in the marrow and bloodstream.

Cytomegalovirus (CMV)—Virus that can cause pneumonia in post bone marrow transplant patients

Conditioning—Process of preparing patient to receive marrow donation, often through the use of chemotherapy and radiation therapy

Confirmatory typing—Repeat tissue typing to confirm the compatibility of the donor and patient before transplant

Donor—A healthy person who contributes bone marrow for transplantation.

Graft versus host disease—A life-threatening complication of bone marrow transplants in which the donated marrow causes an immune reaction against the recipient's body.

Histocompatibility—The major histocompatibility determinants are the human leukocyte antigens

studies indicate that PBSCs are being used more frequently than bone marrow for allogeneic bone marrow transplantation.

The advantages of PBSC transplants when compared to bone marrow transplants are: in allogeneic transplantation, haematopoietic and immune recovery are faster with PBSCs. In autologous transplantation, the use of PBSCs can result in faster blood count recovery. Also, some medical conditions exist in which the recipient cannot accept bone marrow transplants, but can accept PBSC transplants. Some possible disadvantages to PBSC transplant versus bone marrow transplantation are: so much more fluid volume is necessary to collect enough PBSCs that, at the time that the new stem cells are infused into the recipient, the fluid can collect in the lungs. Also, the time commitment for the donor for a PBSC transplant is considerable. When the PBSCs are being collected, several outpatient sessions are needed and each session lasts approximately two–four hours.

The transplant procedure

BONE MARROW TRANSPLANTATION. The bone marrow extraction, or harvest, is the same whether for an autologous or allogeneic transplant. Harvesting is done under general anesthesia (i.e., the donor sleeps through the procedure), and discomfort is usually minimal after-

KEY TERMS (CONTINUED)

(HLA) and characterize how well the patient and donor are matched.

HLA (human leuckocyte antigen)—A group of protein molecules located on bone marrow cells that can provoke an immune response. A donor's and a recipient's HLA types should match as closely as possible to prevent the recipient's immune system from attacking the donor's marrow as a foreign material that does not belong in the body.

Hodgkin's disease—A type of cancer involving the lymph nodes and potentially affecting nonlymphatic organs in the later stage.

Immunodeficiency—A disorder in which the immune system is ineffective or disabled either due to acquired or inherited disease.

Leukemia—A type of cancer that affects leukocytes, a particular type of white blood cell. A characteristic symptom is excessive production of immature or otherwise abnormal leukocytes.

Lymphoma—A type of cancer that affects lymph cells and tissues, including certain white blood cells (T cells and B cells), lymph nodes, bone marrow, and the spleen. Abnormal cells (lymphocyte/leukocyte) multiply uncontrollably.

Match—How similar the HLA typing, out of a possible six antigens, is between the donor and the recipient.

Mixed lymphocyte culture (MLC)—Test that measures level of reactivity between donor and recipient lymphocytes.

Neuroblastoma—Solid tumor in children, may be treated by BMT.

Platelets—Fragments of a large precursor cell, a megakaryocyte found in the bone marrow. These fragments adhere to areas of blood vessel damage and release chemical signals that direct the formation of a blood clot.

Recipient—The person who receives the donated blood marrow.

Red blood cells—Cells that carry hemoglobin (the molecule that transports oxygen) and help remove wastes from tissues throughout the body.

Sickle cell disease—An inherited disorder characterized by a genetic flaw in hemoglobin production. (Hemoglobin is the substance within red blood cells that enables them to transport oxygen.) The hemoglobin that is produced has a kink in its structure that forces the red blood cells to take on a sickle shape, inhibiting their circulation and causing pain. This disorder primarily affects people of African descent

Syngeneic—Referring to a bone marrow transplant from one identical twin to the other.

Thalassemia—A group of inherited disorders that affects hemoglobin production. (Hemoglobin is the substance within red blood cells that enables them to transport oxygen.) Because hemoglobin production is impaired, a person with this disorder may suffer mild to severe anemia. Certain types of thalassemia can be fatal.

White blood cells—A group of several cell types that occur in the bloodstream and are essential for a properly functioning immune system.

wards. Bone marrow is drawn from the iliac crest (the part of the hip bone to either side of the lower back) with a special needle and a syringe. Several punctures are usually necessary to collect the needed amount of bone marrow, approximately 1–2 quarts. (This amount is only a small percentage of the total bone marrow and is typically replaced within four weeks.) The donor remains at the hospital for 24–48 hours and can resume normal activities within a few days.

If the bone marrow is meant for an autologous transplant, it is stored at –112 to –320°F (–80 to –196°C) until it is needed. Bone marrow for an allogeneic transplant is sometimes treated to remove the donor's T cells (a type of white blood cell) or to remove ABO (blood type) antigens; otherwise, it is transplanted without modification.

The bone marrow is administered to the recipient via a catheter (a narrow, flexible tube) inserted into a large vein in the chest. From the bloodstream, it migrates to the cavities within the bones where bone marrow is normally stored. If the transplant is successful, the bone marrow begins to produce normal blood cells once it is in place, or engrafted.

PERIPHERAL BLOOD STEM CELL TRANSPLANTATION. Before collection for a PBSC transplant, donors receive daily four injections of the drug G-CSF, or **filgrastim**. (Patients can give it to themselves at home if need be.) These pretreatments stimulate the body to release stem cells into the blood. After these pretreatments, the donors' experience is similar to that of a whole blood donor's experience—PBSC donors' blood is collected at a clinic or hospital as an outpatient procedure. The differences are that several sessions will be needed over days or weeks and the blood is collected in a process called apheresis. The blood travels from one arm into a blood cell separator that removes only the stem cells, and the rest of the blood is returned back to the donor, in the other arm. The cells are then frozen for later use.

The PBSCs are administered to the recipient using the same methods as those used in bone marrow transplantation. As stated, the amount of fluid with PBSCs infused into the recipient's body can be an issue.

Costs

Bone marrow transplantation is an expensive procedure. (Bone marrow donors are volunteers and do not pay for any part of the procedure.) Insurance companies and health maintenance organizations (HMOs) may not cover the costs.

Preparation

A bone marrow transplant recipient can expect to spend 4–8 weeks in the hospital. In preparation for receiving the transplant, the recipient undergoes "conditioning"—a preparative regimen in which the bone marrow and abnormal cells are destroyed. Conditioning rids the body of diseased cells and makes room for the marrow to be transplanted. It typically involves chemotherapy and/or radiation treatment, depending on the disease being treated. Unfortunately, this treatment also destroys healthy cells and has many side effects such as extreme weakness, nausea, vomiting, and **diarrhea**. These side effects may continue for several weeks.

Aftercare

A two– to four–week waiting period follows the marrow transplant before its success can begin to be judged. The marrow recipient is kept in isolation during this time to minimize potential infections. The recipient also receives antibiotic medications and blood and platelet transfusions to help fight off infection and prevent excessive bleeding. Further side effects, such as **nausea and vomiting**, can be treated with other medications. Once blood counts are normal and the side effects of the transplant abate, the recipient is taken off **antibiotics** and usually no longer needs blood and platelet transfusions.

Following discharge from the hospital, the recipient is monitored through home visits by nurses or out-patient visits for up to a year. For the first several months out of the hospital, the recipient needs to be careful in avoiding potential infections. For example, contact with other people who may be ill should be avoided or kept to a minimum. Further blood transfusions and medications may be necessary, but barring complications, the recipient can return to normal activities about six to eight months after the transplant.

Risks

Bone marrow transplants are accompanied by serious and life-threatening risks. Furthermore, they are not always an absolute assurance of a cure for the underlying ailment; a disease may recur in the future. Approximately 30% of people receiving allogeneic transplants do not survive. Autologous transplants have a much better survival rate—nearly 90%—but are not appropriate for all types of ailments requiring a bone marrow transplant. Furthermore, they have a higher failure rate with certain diseases, specifically leukemia.

In the short term, there is the danger of **pneumonia** or other infectious disease, excessive bleeding, or liver disorder caused by blocked blood vessels. The transplant may be rejected by the recipient's immune system, or the donor bone marrow may launch an immune-mediated attack against the recipient's tissues. This complication is called acute **graft-vs.-host disease**, and it can be a life-threatening condition. Characteristic signs of the disease include **fever**, rash, diarrhea, liver problems, and a compromised immune system.

Approximately 25–50% of bone marrow transplant recipients develop long-term complications. Chronic graft-versus-host disease symptoms include skin changes such as dryness, altered pigmentation, and thickening; abnormal liver function tests; dry mouth and eyes; infections; and **weight loss**. Other long-term complications include cataracts (due to radiation treatment), abnormal lung function, hormonal abnormalities resulting in reduced growth or hypothyroidism, secondary cancers, and infertility.

Normal results

In a successful bone marrow transplant, the donor's marrow migrates to the cavities in the recipient's bones and produces normal numbers of healthy blood cells. Bone marrow transplants can extend a person's life, improve quality of life, and may aid in curing the underlying ailment.

Resources

BOOKS

Armitage, J. O. "Bone Marrow Transplantation." *Harrison's Principles of Internal Medicine* 14th Ed. New York, NY: McGraw Hill, Inc., 1998: 724-730.

Lonergan, Jean Nelson, et al. *Homecare Management of the Bone Marrow Transplant Patient.* 2nd ed. Boston: Jones and Bartlett Publishers, 1996.

Treleaven, Jennifer, and Peter Wiernik, editors. *Color Atlas and Text of Bone Marrow Transplantation.* St. Louis: Mosby-Wolfe, 1995.

PERIODICALS

Dreger, P. and N. Schmitz. "Allogeneic transplantation of blood stem cells: coming of age?" *Annals of Hematology* (March, 2001) 80(3):127-36.

Nuzhat, Iqbal, Donna Salzman, Audrey J. Lazenby, et al. "Diagnosis of Gastrointestinal Graft-Versus-Host Disease." *The American Journal of Gastroenterology* (November, 2000) 95:3034- 3038.

ORGANIZATIONS

American Society for Blood and Marrow Transplantation (ASBMT) 85 W. Algonquin Road, Suite 550 Arlington Heights, IL 60005. (847) 427-0224. mail@asbmt.org. Founded in 1990, a national professional association that promotes advancement of the field of blood and bone marrow transplantation in clinical practice and research.

Blood & Marrow Transplant Newsletter (Formerly BMT Newsletter). 2900 Skokie Valley Road, Suite B, Highland Park, IL 60035 (847) 433-3313. 1-888-597-7674. help@bmtinfonet.org. <http://www2.bmtnews.org>. Blood & Marrow Transplant Newsletter is a not-for-profit organization that provides publications and support services to bone marrow, peripheral blood stem cell, and cord blood transplant patients and survivors.

International Bone Marrow Transplant Registry/Autologous Blood and Marrow Transplant Registry N. America, Health Policy Institute, Medical College of Wisconsin, 8701 Watertown Plank Road, P.O. Box 26509, Milwaukee, WI 53226 USA, 414-456-8325, ibmtr@mcw.edu. Voluntary organizations of more than 400 institutions in 47 countries that submit data on their allogeneic and autologous blood and marrow transplant recipients to the IBMTR/ABMTR Statistical Center at the Medical College of Wisconsin in Milwaukee.

Health Resources and Services Administration. 5600 Fishers Lane, Rm. 14-45, Rockville, MD 20857, 301-443-3376, comments@hrsa.gov. <http://www.hrsa.gov>. HRSA manages contracts for the Organ Procurement and Transplantation Network, Scientific Registry of Transplant Recipients and National Marrow Donor Program and provides public education and technical assistance to increase donation. HRSA also monitors the performance of the nation's transplant centers and provides potential transplant recipients with survival rates and other vital information.

Leukemia & Lymphoma Society, Inc. 1311 Mamaroneck Avenue White Plains, NY 10605, 914-949-5213 <http://www.leukemia-lymphoma.org/>. National voluntary health agency dedicated to curing leukemia, lymphoma, Hodgkin's disease and myeloma, and to improving the quality of life of patients and their families.

National Marrow Donor Program. Suite 500, 3001 Broadway Street Northeast, Minneapolis, MN 55413-1753. (800) MARROW-2. <http://www.marrow.org>. Founded in 1986, The National Marrow Donor Program (NMDP) is a non-profit international leader in the facilitation of unrelated marrow and blood stem cell transplantation.

BMT Information <http://www.bmtinfo.org/>. Web site, sponsored by a variety of other bone marrow transplant organizations, lists basic information and resources about bone marrow transplants.

National Organ and Tissue Donation Initiative <http://www.organdonor.gov/> Created by Health Resources and Services Administration (HRSA) Department of Health and Human Services (DHHS) <http://www.os.dhhs.gov/>. Provides information and resources on organ donation and transplantation issues.

Julia Barrett
Laura Ruth, Ph.D.

QUESTIONS TO ASK THE DOCTOR

- What is allogenic bone marrow transplantation (BMT)?
- What is syngenic bone marrow transplantation?
- What is autologous bone marrow transplantation?
- What is Graft-versus-Host disease (GVHD) and can it be prevented?
- What diseases are treated by BMT?
- What is HLA/histocompatibility matching?

Bone metastasis *see* **Metastasis**

Bone pain

Description

Bone pain represents one of the most debilitating side effects of the metastases of high-incidence cancers such as breast, prostate, lung, and **multiple myeloma** (myelomatosis). Severe bone pain is frequent, reported by greater than 65% of patients suffering with bone metastases. The most common sites affected include the pelvis, femur,

KEY TERMS

Calcitonin—A hormone produced by the thyroid that causes a reduction of calcium ions in the blood.

Cognitive distraction and reframing—Techniques to teach the patient to focus on things not associated with pain.

Hypercalcemia—The presence of abnormally high concentrations of calcium compounds in the bloodstream.

Magnetic resonance imaging (MRI)—A diagnostic technique that makes images of internal structures of the body, often superior to a normal x ray.

Metastases—Cancer that starts from cancer cells that originate in a different location in the body.

Multiple myeloma—Multiplying plasma cells that often replace all other cell types found in the bone marrow and frequently cause the loss of the bone cortex.

Nociceptors—Peripheral pain receptors that are sensitive to movement, extreme heat and cold, and chemical stimuli.

Opioid—Any morphine-like compound producing bodily effects that may include relief from severe pain, respiratory depression, or sedation.

Osteoclast—Cells responsible for the breakdown of bone tissue.

Radionuclide scintography—The process of injecting a radionuclide to capture an image of a particular area of the body for diagnostic purposes.

Radiopharmaceuticals—Compounds used as radiation sources for radiotherapy and for diagnostic procedures.

skull, and vertebra. The patient often describes the pain as dull and aching, localized at the site affected; however, some patients experience short, shooting pain that radiates out from the torso to the extremities. Movement typically aggravates the pain. Bone pain can signal disease progression, a new infection, or a complication from treatment. Pain is a reliable early indicator of complications from metastases-osteoporosis, **hypercalcemia**, fractures, and **spinal cord compression**. These conditions not only adversely affect the patient's quality of life, but in some cases may create such a decline that death results not from the metastases, but solely from bone- and skeletal-related complications. Patient complaints of bone pain require diagnostic confirmation, usually by radiographic techniques. Plain-film radiography may adequately detect typical lesions from metastatic causes, but may not be sensitive enough to detect certain complications. In these cases, radionuclide scintigraphy and **magnetic resonance imaging** (MRI) are the preferred diagnostic tools.

Causes

Bone pain may be the result of direct tumor involvement. Pain is produced when the tumor infiltrates the skeletal structures. The tumor may compress surrounding blood vessels, nerves, and soft tissue, or may be activating nociceptors (pain receptors) located at the site. Pain may also be a result of tissue compression caused by fibrosis (a condition caused by an increase in tissue) after the patient has undergone **radiation therapy**; this type of bone pain tends to be tolerable. A predominant source of bone pain in the cancer patient is due to pathologic fracture and to osteoclast-induced bone resorption by the tumor. This condition promotes bone loss and, at the same time, provides growth factors for the tumor to increase in size.

Treatments

Pain management for bone metastases has multiple options for the health care team to draw upon. The primary treatment for the majority of patients is external beam radiotherapy, either localized or wide field. These treatments provide excellent relief of the bone pain. Localized radiation treatments target specific sites for pain relief and the promotion of healing and prevention of fractures. Spinal cord compression from vertebral collapse requires immediate and localized radiation therapy, possibly in conjunction with surgical intervention to prevent paralysis or loss of life. Wide-field radiation therapy treats multiple disease sites and is appropriate for more diffuse bone pain. One half of the body receives radiation in a single treatment. Studies report relief of the bone pain in 55-100% of patients. Analgesics (pain relievers) are typically given in conjunction with radiotherapy. Severity of the bone pain and general health of the patient will determine the prescribed medication. The spectrum of medications prescribed range from over-the-counter pain medication to **opioids** for extreme bone pain management.

Radiopharmaceuticals may be an effective choice for bone pain management. Iodine-131 is used in the treatment of multiple bone metastases from **thyroid cancer**. Phosphorus-32 orthophosphate has a success rate of about 80% in bone pain management in patients suffering with breast and **prostate cancer**. Strontium-89 provides partial or complete pain relief in approximately 65% of patients. Other radiopharmaceuticals are being tested internationally but have not yet received FDA approval for use in the United States. In treatments for bone resorption-induced pain, a group of chemical agents, known as **bisphosphonates** and **calcitonin**, acts to strongly block the bone resorption process. These agents are used in the management of hypercalcemia and have the added effect of reducing the prescribed amount of analgesics and shortening the duration of bone pain.

Alternative and complementary therapies

Comprehensive management of bone pain includes non-clinical choices. Patients should be encouraged to participate in complementary therapies, and some patients may choose to investigate more alternative therapies. More conventional complementary therapies may include relaxation and imagery therapy, cognitive distraction and reframing, support group and pastoral counseling, skin stimulation, biofeedback, nerve blocks, immobilization and stabilization techniques, and surgical intervention. Less well-defined alternative therapies may include acupuncture, body massage with pressure and vibration techniques, hypnosis, menthol preparations, and holistic or herbal medical practices. No conclusive data exist of the effectiveness of these therapies used alone; however, in conjunction with conventional methods of bone pain management, they do not appear to hinder therapy and may provide the patient with increased goodwill and a positive outlook.

Resources

PERIODICALS

Coleman, Robert E. "Management of Bone Metastases."*The Oncologist* 5 (September 2000): 463-470.

Jane Taylor-Jones, M.S., Research Associate

Bone scan *see* **Nuclear medicine scans**

Bone survey

Definition

A bone survey is an **x ray** to check the health and status of a person's bones. It is an important tool for diagnosing the presence of **multiple myeloma** lesions in bone.

Purpose

The bone survey is the standard method for determining if there is bone involvement in multiple myeloma. Multiple myeloma lesions may not show up in other bone studies. However, if the lesions are present, they are likely to appear on a bone survey, making this an important diagnostic tool.

In patients who have been treated for multiple myeloma, bone surveys should be repeated to see if the disease has responded to treatment, or if it has progressed further. While the repeated bone survey may show that bone healing has occurred, this is not usually the case. Only 30% of patients whose multiple myeloma is responding to treatment show an improvement on their bone surveys. Multiple myeloma patients whose disease is progressing, or who have new areas of **bone pain**, can benefit from repeat bone surveys because this procedure can locate sites of potential fractures that may then be prevented by radiation or surgery.

KEY TERMS

Radiologic procedure—A medical procedure, such as an x ray, that uses radiation or other sources to create images useful in diagnosis.

Radiologist—A medical doctor who specializes in interpreting radiologic (imaging) studies. Imaging studies include x ray, computed tomography (CT), and magnetic resonance imaging (MRI).

Precautions

The dose of radiation in diagnostic x rays is very small, and this procedure is considered relatively safe. However, x rays are generally not advised for pregnant women. These women should inform their physician or the x-ray technician of their pregnancy (or suspected pregnancy) prior to the procedure.

Description

A bone survey in people with multiple myeloma includes x rays of the skull, spine, pelvis, and long bones of the legs and arms because the disease may spread to these particular areas. The procedure may be done in the radiology department of a hospital (for inpatients or outpatients) or in an imaging facility.

Patients may be given a hospital gown and asked to remove clothing that could interfere with the image, such as buttons or snaps. A lead shield for protection from radiation may be placed over the parts of the body that are not undergoing an x ray.

QUESTIONS TO ASK THE DOCTOR

- How long will the bone survey take?
- Where will the procedure be done?
- What is the risk from radiation?
- Who will examine the x rays?
- When will I get the results?
- If the results are abnormal, what treatment will be given?

An x ray creates a two dimensional (flat) image shown on film. Since the human body is three-dimensional, at least two different angles of the same area will be x-rayed. The radiology technician helps the patient achieve the proper position. Most imaging centers have special tables that help position the patient.

When the patient is properly positioned, the technician will leave the room to activate the x-ray machine. It is important that the patient remain completely still while the x ray is being taken. The x ray does not cause any pain or other sensation, and gives off no smell, sound, or taste, although it is penetrating the body. The patient may hear a sound, but this is the equipment and not the x ray itself.

The x ray creates shadows on film, and the film is viewed by a physician (radiologist) who specializes in **imaging studies**. The film will have contrasts that appear as varying shades of gray.

Preparation

Because the procedure in non-invasive, no specific preparation is necessary.

Aftercare

Bone surveys do not require any aftercare.

Risks

While radiation in high doses may present a cancer risk, the dosage for diagnostic purposes is very low. New technology has increased the safety of radiologic procedures. As in any procedure, the risk must be weighed against the benefit. In patients with multiple myeloma, the bone survey is needed to determine bone involvement, which could then dictate treatment. Pregnant women generally do not receive x rays, and should discuss this with their physician.

Normal results

Bone structure that is free of disease, fracture, or other problem areas is a normal result.

Abnormal results

Areas where multiple myeloma is present show up as destructive bone lesions. Parts of the bone may appear moth-eaten, and fractures may be present.

Resources

BOOKS

Bos, Gary D., and H. Robert Brashear. "Tumors." In *General Orthopaedics*. Wilson, F., amd Lin, P., eds. New York: McGraw-Hill, 1997, pp. 316-18.

Helms, Clyde A. "Malignant Bone and Soft-Tissue Tumors" In *Fundamentals of Diagnostic Radiology,* 2nd ed. Brant, W., and Helms, C., eds. Philadelphia: Williams & Wilkins, 1999, pp. 991–3.

Hosley, Julie B., et al. *Lippincott's Textbook for Medical Assistants.* Philadelphia, PA: Lippincott-Raven Publishers, 1997.

Kyle, Robert A., and Joan Blade. "Multiple Myeloma and Related Disorders." In *Clinical Oncology.* Abeloff, M., et al, eds. Philadelphia: Churchill Livingstone, 2000, pp. 2601–3.

Vescio, Robert A., and James R. Berenson. "Myeloma, Macroglobulinemia, and Amyloidosis." In *Cancer Treatment*, 5th ed. Haskell, C., ed. Philadelphia: W. B. Saunders, 2001, pp. 1503-4.

Wolbarst, Anthony Brinton. *Looking Within: How X-Ray, CT, MRI, Ultrasound, and Other Medical Images Are Created and How They Help Physicians Save Lives.* Berkeley, CA: University of California Press, 1999.

Rhonda Cloos, R.N.

Bowen's disease

Definition

A superficial precancerous squamous cell cancer, slow growing (i.e. has not started spreading) skin malignancy.

Description

Red-brown, scaly or crusty patch on the skin that resembles psoriasis, dermatitis or eczema that can occur on any part of the body.

Demographics

Bowen's disease affects both males and females. Women are affected in the genital area three times as

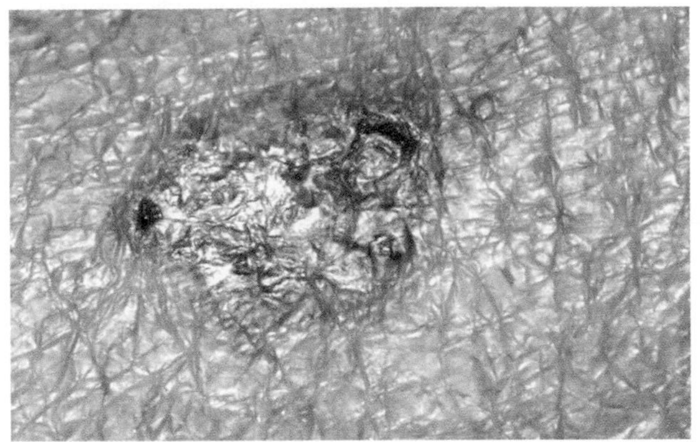

Close-up of a dark, bruise-like lesion on the leg of an elderly woman, caused by Bowen's disease. *(© Dr. P. Marazzi, Science Source/Photo Researchers, Inc. Reproduced by permission.)*

often as men. The disease can occur at any age, but is rare in children.

Causes and symptoms

The exact cause of Bowen's disease is unknown. Like many forms of cancer, long-term sun exposure may be a cause. The skin usually indicates sun damage, such as wrinkling, changes in pigmentation, and loss of elasticity. Ingestion of arsenic has been associated with cases of Bowen's disease found in skin areas unexposed to light or mucous membranes. Human papillomavirus 16 DNA is found repeatedly in Bowen's disease lesions, which suggests that this virus might be a cause. The role of heredity is not well understood. There are cases of Bowen's disease for which a cause cannot be determined.

Symptoms

The symptoms of Bowen's disease include:

- plaque located on or within the skin (intraepidermal)
- open sore that bleeds and crusts and persists for weeks
- wart-like growth that crusts and occasionally bleeds
- persistent, scaly red patch with irregular borders that sometimes crusts or bleeds
- pinkish or brownish raised areas of skin

Diagnosis

Bowen's disease can be confused with the other common skin disorders, such as psoriasis or types of dermatitis. **Paget's disease of the breast** and malignant **melanoma** are other types of cancer which may be confused for Bowen's disease. A medical history, physical examination, and **biopsy** establish the diagnosis.

KEY TERMS

Cancer—General term for abnormally growing (malignant) cells.

Dermatitis—Inflammation of the skin that may be due to an allergic reaction.

Melanoma—Abnormal growth in melanin cells which are most commonly found in the skin or in the eye.

Paget's disease of the breast—Cancer of breast nipples which occurs in both men and women. Paget's is characterized by oozy and crusty skin inflammation (dermatitis).

Psoriasis—Common inherited condition that is characterized by reddish, slivery-scaled maculopapules, predominantly on the elbows, knees, scalp, and trunk.

Squamous cell carcinoma—Type of skin cancer

Clinical staging, treatments, and prognosis

Treatment usually involves surgical removal of the lesion. Curettage and cautery methods,which include carbon dioxide lasers, liquid nitrogen, and topical **fluorouracil** (5-FU) compose the most efficient treatment for management of small solitary lesions.

There can be difficulties with the liquid nitrogen, 5-FU (Efudex, fluoroplex), scraping and burning because Bowen's lesions can hide deep in pores, and cells may extend into the surrounding area where lesion is visible.

Clinical trials

Dr. Colin Morton and colleagues at the Western Infirmary in the UK have been developing a photodynamic therapy using topical 5-aminolaevulinic acid(5-ALA).

Dr. Lee and colleagues at the University College of Medicine in Korea have been developing a specially designed radioactive skin patch.

Prevention

As with most skin cancers, prolonged exposure to the sun can increase the risk of developing the disease.

Special concerns

All treatment options have a recurrence rate of 5 to 10%, and no treatment modality seems superior for all clinical situations.

QUESTIONS TO ASK THE DOCTOR

- How do I know I have Bowen's disease rather than psoriasis, Paget's disease, dermatitis or another skin cancer?
- Is surgical removal of the affected skin area the best treatment?
- What other treatments for Bowen's disease are available other than surgical removal?

Resources

BOOKS

Fauci, Anthony, S. *Harrison's Principles of Internal Medicine,* 14th Ed. New York, NY: McGraw Hill, Inc., 1998: 303, 548, 1099T.

PERIODICALS

Ahmed, I., J., S. Berth-Jones, Charles Holmes, C. J. O. Callaghan, and A. Ilcyhyshyn. "Comparison of cryotherapy with curettage in the treatment of Bowen's disease: a prospective study." *British Journal of Dermatology* (2000)143:759–766.

Bell, H. K. and L. E. Rhodes. "Bowen's disease—a retrospective review of clinical management." *Clinical and Experimental Dermatology* 24(1999):336–339.

Chung, Y. L., J. D. Lee, D. Bang, J. B. Lee, K. B. Park, and M. G. Lee. "Treatment of Bowen's disease with a specially designed radioactive skin patch." *European Journal Nuclear Medicine* (July 2000)27(7):842–6.

Clavel, C. E., Valerie Pham Huu, Anne P. Durlach, Philippe L. Birembaut, Philippe M., Bernard, and Christian G. Derancourt. "Mucosal Oncogenic Human Papillomaviruses and Extragenital Bowen Disease." *Cancer* (July 1999)86: 282–287.

Cox, N. H."Bowen's disease: where now with therapeutic trials?" *British Journal of Dermatology* (2000)143:699–700.

Cox N. H., D. J. Eedy, C. A. Morton. "Guidelines for management of Bowen's disease. British Association of Dermatologists." *British Journal of Dermatologists* (October, 1999):633–4.

Morton, Colin, A., Colin Whitehurst, John H. McColl, James V. Moore, and Rona M. MacKie."Photodynamic Therapy for Large or Multiple Patches of Bowen Disease and Basal Cell Carcinoma." *Archives Dermatology* (March 2001)137:319–324.

ORGANIZATIONS

American Cancer Society, Inc. 1599 Clifton Road NE, Atlanta, GA 30329, (404)320-3333, <http://www.cancer.org>. The American Cancer Society (ACS) is a nationwide community-based voluntary health organization dedicated to eliminating cancer as a major health problem and the largest source of private, nonprofit cancer funds. The ACS hopes to prevent cancer, save lives, and diminish suffering from cancer, through research, education, advocacy, and service. 2 July 2001.

NIH/National Arthritis and Musculoskeletal and Skin Diseases Information Clearinghouse One AMS Circle, Bethesda, MD, 20892-3675.(301)495-4484. <http://www.nih.gov/niams>. The NIAMS conducts and supports basic, clinical, and epidemiologic research and research training and disseminates information on diseases that include many forms of arthritis and diseases of the musculoskeletal system and the skin. 2 July 2001.

NIH/National Cancer Institute (NCI) Office of Communications-Public Inquiries Office, Building 31, Rm 10A03, 9000 Rockville Pike, Bethesda, MD 20892.(800)422-6237. <http://www.cancer.gov.>. Specializes in different aspects of cancer which includes cancer biology, cancer control and population sciences, cancer epidemiology and genetics, cancer prevention, and cancer treatment and diagnosis. 2 July 2001.

National Organizations of Rare Disorders (NORD) PO Box 8923, Fairfield, CT, 06812-8923, (800)999-6673; <http://www.rarediseases.org.>. NORD is a voluntary health organization dedicated to helping people with rare diseases and assisting the organizations that serve them. 2 July 2001.

Skin Cancer Foundation 245 Fifth Avenue, Suite 1403, New York, NY 10016.(212)725-5176; <http://www.skincancer.org.> National and international organization that is concerned exclusively with skin cancer. 2 July 2001.

OTHER

Skincancerinfor.com Detailed summary of information about Bowen's disease. <http://www.skincancerinfo.com/sectionc/bowen.html>. 2 July 2001.

Laura Ruth, Ph.D.

Brain and central nervous system tumors

Definition

Like all other parts of the body, the brain and central nervous system are made up of cells that ordinarily grow and divide to create new cells as needed. This is usually an orderly process; but when cells lose their ability to grow normally or to die off naturally, they divide too often and produce tumors that are made up of these extra cells.

Description

The brain and spinal cord together comprise what is known as the central nervous system (CNS). Like all tumors in the body, CNS tumors are either benign or malignant. Benign tumors are called non-cancerous because they have precise borders, are not invasive, and the cells that make up the growth are similar to other normal cells and grow relatively slowly. However, benign CNS tumors can press on a specific region of the spinal cord or brain and, thereby, cause symptoms. However, when such a benign tumor develops in an area that interferes with essential nervous system functioning, it is treated as malignant.

Malignant, or cancerous, tumors of the central nervous system are likely to be fast-growing, are invasive into surrounding healthy tissue, and the cells are very different from normal cells. These tumors can create a life-threatening situation by stopping vital functions of the brain. Some cancerous CNS tumors do not put out roots nor do they grow rapidly. These tumors are described as being encapsulated.

Another way that brain and central nervous system tumors are classified is by site of origin. Those that actually develop in the brain or spinal cord are called primary CNS tumors. **Metastasis** to the brain or spinal cord is, for the most part, a one-way street, meaning these tumors almost never metastasize to other areas in the body. The tumors that develop elsewhere in the body and metastasize, or spread, to the central nervous system are considered to be secondary CNS tumors. Such metastatic cells do not resemble other CNS cells. Instead, they have the same appearance as the cancer cells at the original cancer site elsewhere in the body.

Frequently observed signs of a brain tumor are the following:

- severe headaches
- an ataxic, or stumbling, gait
- **nausea and vomiting**
- lack of coordination
- unusual drowsiness
- weakness or loss of feelings in the arms and legs
- changes in personality or memory
- changes in speech
- changes in vision or abnormal eye movements
- seizures

Approximately 1 1/2% of all diagnosed cancers are CNS cancers, and they account for about 2 1/2% of all cancer deaths. The American Cancer Society (ACS) estimates that in 2001 17,200 malignant tumors of the brain or spinal cord will be diagnosed in adults and children in the United States. Of those people diagnosed, ACS projects that 13,100 will die from malignant CNS tumors.

Brain and Central nervous system tumors

Gliomas	Non-glial tumors
Astrocytomas	Medulloblastomas
Brain stem gliomas	Meningiomas
Ependymomas	Schwannomas
Oligodendrogliomas	Craniopharyngiomas
	Germinomas
	Pineal region tumors

Typically, diagnosis of CNS tumor is made by a physician who does a complete physical examination, including a family history and neurological examination. Computerized tomography (CT) scans, **magnetic resonance imaging** (MRI) scans, skull x rays, brain scans, angiograms, or myelograms are among the means of visualizing the brain or spinal cord to search for tumors.

General categories of treatment methods for CNS tumors include surgery, **radiation therapy**, and **chemotherapy**, with surgery being the single most commonly used therapy. Steroids are usually given prior to treatment to decrease swelling, and anti-convulsant drugs may be given to prevent seizures.

Types of cancers

Primary brain tumors are also classified by their site of origin. Gliomas, occurring in the glial, or supportive tissues around the brain, are the most common. Gliomas are further broken down into the following variations:

- **Astrocytomas** are named for the star-shaped, small cells that they are comprised of. Children may develop these in their brain stem, cerebrum, or cerebellum, while adults commonly develop them in the cerebrum.
- Brain-stem gliomas are usually astrocytomas that originate in the bottom, stem-like portion of the brain. Because this area controls many essential bodily functions, such tumors often cannot be removed.
- **Ependymomas** occur in the linings of the four brain ventricles, or chambers, or along the spinal cord. These are more common in children.
- **Oligodendrogliomas** are very rare and, when seen, are usually found in middle-aged adults. They grow slowly and ordinarily do not invade surrounding brain or spinal cord tissue. They originate in the cells responsible for the manufacture of myelin, a fatty covering for nerve tissue.

Other CNS tumors do not originate in glial tissue. Among these are:

- **Medulloblastomas**, tumors of the cerebellum, are most common in male children. Studies have shown these to

KEY TERMS

Angiogram—A diagnostic test that makes it possible for blood vessels to be seen on film by filling them with a contrast substance or dye that appears on x rays.

Anti-convulsant drugs—A group of medications used in the treatment of seizures.

Brain scan—A general term that can include CT scans, MRIs, seldom-used radionuclide scanning (use of radioactive isotopes), or ultrasounds.

Computerized tomography (CT) scan—The combined use of a computer and x rays that are passed through the body to produce clear, cross-sectional images.

Magnetic resonance imaging (MRI)—An imaging technique that produces good cross-sectional images without x rays or other radiation sources.

Myelogram—X-ray examination of the spinal cord after injection of a contrast substance or dye that shows up on x rays.

Neurological exam—A physical examination that focuses on the patient's nerves, reflexes, motor and sensory functions, and muscle strength and tone.

Seizures—Sudden, uncontrolled electrical activity in the brain resulting in characteristic twitching, or spastic, movements that may be accompanied by loss of consciousness.

Steroids—A group of drugs that are similar to the hormones produced by the cortex of the adrenal gland.

Ventricles of the brain—The four fluid-filled chambers, or cavities, found in the two cerebral hemispheres of the brain, at the center of the brain, and between the brain stem and cerebellum, and linked by channels, or ducts, allowing cerebral fluid to circulate through them.

originate in primitive nerve cells that normally would have disappeared soon after birth.

- **Meningiomas** are usually benign. They develop in the meninges, or brain linings, and grow very slowly. Because of this slow growth, they may go undetected for years. Meningiomas are more common in women between the ages of 30 and 50.
- Schwannomas are also benign tumors, specific to the myelin-producing cells (Schwann cells) for the acoustic, or hearing, nerve. These, too, are more common in women than men.
- **Craniopharyngiomas** are usually benign, but because of their location near the pituitary gland and hypothalmus, they can easily affect vital functions and are therefore treated as if malignant. They occur more frequently in children and teenagers.
- Germinomas, or **germ cell tumors**, develop from primitive sex cells called germ cells.
- Pineal-region tumors originate in the area near the pineal gland, a small central brain gland that secretes melatonin, a brain chemical. These can be either fast-growing pineoblastoma, or slow-growing pineocytoma.

Resources

BOOKS

Clayman, Charles, M.D. *The American Medical Association Home Medical Encyclopedia.* New York: Random House, 1989.

Diamond, John W., MD, Cowden, W. Lee, M.D., and Burton Goldberg. *An Alternative Medicine Definitive Guide to Cancer.* Tiburon, CA: Future Medicine Publishing, Inc., 1997.

ORGANIZATIONS

National Cancer Institute. <http://cancernet.nci.nih.gov>.

The American Cancer Society's Resource Center for Brain/Central Nervous System Tumors in Children. (800) ACS-2345.

Cancer Care, Inc. (800) 813-4673. <http://www.cancercare.org>.

Joan Schonbeck, R.N.

Brain metastasis *see* **Metastasis**

Breast cancer

Definition

Breast cancer is caused by the development of malignant cells in the breast. The malignant cells originate in the lining of the milk glands or ducts of the breast (ductal epithelium), defining this malignancy as a cancer. Cancer cells are characterized by uncontrolled division leading to abnormal growth and the ability of these cells to invade normal tissue locally or to spread throughout the body, in a process called **metastasis**.

Description

Breast cancer arises in the milk-producing glands of the breast tissue. Groups of glands in normal breast tissue are called lobules. The products of these glands are secreted into a ductal system that leads to the nipple. Depending on where in the glandular or ductal unit of the breast the cancer arises, it will develop certain characteristics that are used to sub-classify breast cancer into types. The pathologist will denote the subtype at the time of evaluation with the microscope. Ductal carcinoma begins in the ducts, and lobular carcinoma has a pattern involving the lobules or glands. The more important classification is related to the evaluated tumor's capability to invade, as this characteristic defines the disease as a true cancer. The stage before invasive cancer is called *in situ*, meaning that the early malignancy has not yet become capable of invasion. Thus, ductal carcinoma in situ is considered a minimal breast cancer.

How breast cancer spreads

The primary tumor begins in the breast itself but once it becomes invasive, it may progress beyond the breast to the regional lymph nodes or travel (metastasize) to other organ systems in the body and become systemic in nature. Lymph is the clear, protein-rich fluid that bathes the cells throughout the body. Lymph will work its way back to the bloodstream via small channels known as lymphatics. Along the way, the lymph is filtered through cellular stations known as nodes, thus they are called lymph nodes. Nearly all organs in the body have a primary lymph node group filtering the tissue fluid, or lymph, that comes from that organ. In the breast, the primary lymph nodes are under the armpit, or axilla. Classically, the primary tumor begins in the breast and the first place to which it is likely to spread is the regional lymph nodes. Cancer, as it invades in its place of origin, may also work its way into blood vessels. If cancer gets into the blood vessels, the blood vessels provide yet another route for the cancer to spread to other organs of the body.

Breast cancer follows this classic progression though it often becomes systemic or widespread early in the course of the disease. By the time one can feel a lump in the breast it is often 0.4 inches, or one centimeter, in size and contains roughly a million cells. It is estimated that a tumor of this size may take one to five years to develop. During that time, the cancer may metastasize, or spread by lymphatics or blood to areas elsewhere in the body.

When primary breast cancer spreads, it may first go to the regional lymph nodes under the armpit, the axillary nodes. If this occurs, regional metastasis exists. If it proceeds elsewhere either by lymphatic or blood-borne spread, the patient develops systemic metastasis that may involve a number of other organs in the body. Common sites of systemic involvement for breast cancer are the lung, bones, liver, and the skin and soft tissue. As it turns

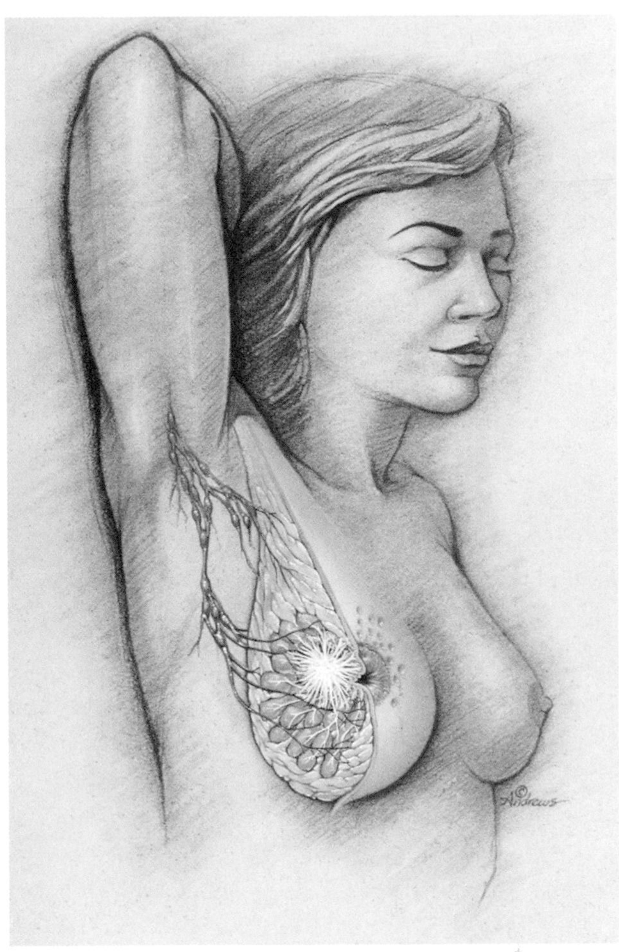

The woman in this illustration has breast cancer. The tumor is visible in the breast, and the axillary lymph nodes reveal cancer as well. *(Custom Medical Stock Photo. Reproduced by permission.)*

out, the presence of, and the actual number of, regional lymph nodes containing cancer remains the single best indicator of whether or not the cancer has become widely metastatic. Because tests to discover metastasis in other organs may not be sensitive enough to reveal minute deposits, the evaluation of the axilla for regional metastasis becomes very important in making treatment decisions for this disease.

If breast cancer spreads to other major organs of the body, its presence will compromise the function of those organs. Death is the result of extreme compromise of vital organ function.

Demographics

Every woman is at risk for breast cancer. If she lives to be 85, there is a one out of nine chance that she will develop the condition sometime during her life. As a woman ages, her risk of developing breast cancer rises dramatically regardless of her family history. The breast cancer risk of a 25-year-old woman is only one out of 19,608; by age 45, it is one in 93. In fact, less than 5% of cases are discovered before age 35 and the majority of all breast cancers are found in women over age 50.

In 1999, there were 180,000 new cases of breast cancer diagnosed. About 45,000 women die of breast cancer each year, accounting for 16% of deaths caused by cancer in women. For the first time ever, mortality rates decreased an average of 1.7% per year from 1995 through 1999, a reflection of earlier diagnosis and improving therapies.

Causes and symptoms

There are a number of risk factors for the development of breast cancer, including:

- family history of breast cancer in mother or sister
- early onset of menstruation and late menopause
- reproductive history: women who had no children or have children after age 30 and women who have never breastfed have increased risk
- history of abnormal breast biopsies

Though these are recognized risk factors, it is important to note that more than 70% of women who get breast cancer have no known risk factors. Having several risk factors may boost a woman's chances of developing breast cancer, but the interplay of predisposing factors is complex. In addition to those accepted factors listed above, some studies suggest that high-fat diets, obesity, or the use of alcohol may contribute to the risk profile. Another factor that may contribute to a woman's risk profile is hormone replacement therapy (HRT).

HRT provides significant relief of menopausal symptoms, prevention of osteoporosis, and possibly protection from cardiovascular disease and stroke. However, studies show that there is a small increased risk of developing breast cancer with HRT use. Thus, the use of hormone replacement therapy should be based on personal risk factors.

Of all the risk factors listed above, family history is the most important. In *The Biological Basis of Cancer*, the authors estimate that probably about half of all familial breast cancer cases (families in which there is a high breast cancer frequency) have mutations affecting the tumor suppressor gene BRCA-1. Another gene (BRCA-2) also appears to confer inherited vulnerability to early-onset breast cancers. However, breast cancer due to heredity is only a small proportion of breast cancer cases; only 5%–10% of all breast cancer cases will be women who inherited a susceptibility through their genes. Nevertheless, when the family history is strong for development of breast cancer, a woman's risk is increased.

Not all lumps detected in the breast are cancerous. Fibrocystic changes in the breast are extremely common. Also known as **fibrocystic condition of the breast**, fibrocystic changes are a leading cause of non-cancerous lumps in the breast. Fibrocystic changes also cause symptoms of pain, swelling, or discharge and may become evident to the patient or physician as a lump that is either solid or filled with fluid. Complete diagnostic evaluation of any significant breast abnormality is mandatory because though women commonly develop fibrocystic changes, breast cancer is common also, and the signs and symptoms of fibrocystic changes overlap with those of breast cancer.

Diagnosis

The diagnosis of breast cancer is accomplished by the **biopsy** of any suspicious lump or mammographic abnormality that has been identified. (A biopsy is the removal of tissue for examination by a pathologist. A mammogram is a low-dose, 2-view, x-ray examination of the breast.) The patient may be prompted to visit her doctor upon finding a lump in a breast, or she may have noticed skin dimpling, nipple retraction, or discharge from the nipple. Or, the patient may not have noticed anything abnormal, and a lump is detected by the mammogram.

When a patient has no signs or symptoms

Screening involves the evaluation of women who have no symptoms or signs of a breast problem, so when the screening mammogram leads to the evaluation, the patient has no symptoms and may not have any abnormality on examination of the breast. **Mammography** has been very helpful in detecting breast cancer that one cannot identify on physical examination. However, 10%–13% of breast cancer does not show up on mammography, and a similar number of patients with breast cancer have an abnormal mammogram and a normal physical examination. These figures emphasize the need for examination as part of the screening process.

Screening

It is recommended that women get into the habit of doing monthly breast self examinations to detect any lump at an early stage. If an uncertainty or a lump is found, evaluation by an experienced physician and mammography is recommended. The American Cancer Society (ACS) has made recommendations for the use of mammography on a screening basis. There has been controversy about the tim-

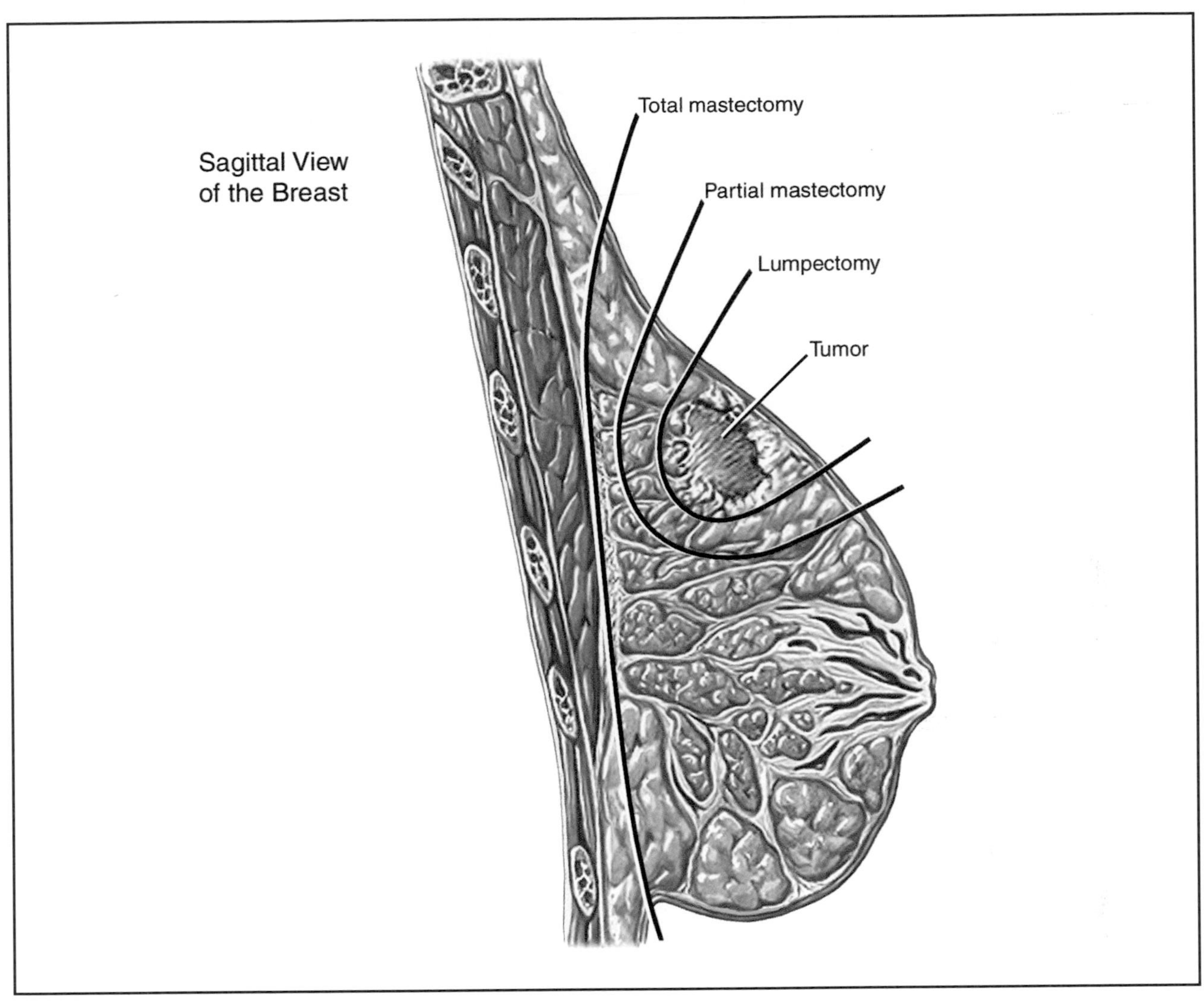

The varying degrees of breast cancer surgery. *(Copyright 2001 adam.com, Inc. Reproduced by permission.)*

ing and appropriate frequency of mammography when used as a screening tool, but the ACS recommendations are as follows: Women should get annual mammograms after age 40. Those with a significant family history (one or more first-degree relatives who have been treated for breast cancer), should start annual mammograms 10 years younger than the youngest relative was when she was diagnosed, but not earlier than 35.

Because of the greater awareness of breast cancer in recent years, screening evaluations by examinations and mammography are performed much more frequently than in the past. The result is that the number of breast cancers diagnosed increased, but the disease is being diagnosed at an earlier stage than previously. The earlier the stage of disease at the time of presentation, the better the long-term outcome after treatment, or prognosis, becomes.

When a patient has physical signs or symptoms

A very common finding that leads to diagnosis is the presence of a lump within the breast. Skin dimpling, nipple retraction, or discharge from the nipple are less frequent initial findings prompting biopsy. Though bloody nipple discharge is distressing, it is most often caused by benign disease. Skin dimpling or nipple retraction in the presence of an underlying breast mass on examination is a more advanced finding. Actual skin involvement, with edema or ulceration of the skin, are late findings.

A very common presenting sign is the presence of a breast lump. If the lump is suspicious and the patient has not had a mammogram by this point, a study should be done on both breasts prior to anything else so that the original characteristics of the lesion can be studied. The opposite breast should also be evaluated mammographically to determine if other problems exist that were undetected by physical examination.

Whether an abnormal screening mammogram or one of the signs mentioned above followed by a mammogram prompted suspicion, the diagnosis is established by obtaining tissue by biopsy of the area. There are different types of biopsy, each utilized with its own indication depending on the presentation of the patient. If signs of widespread metastasis are already present, biopsy of the metastasis itself may establish diagnosis.

Biopsy

Depending on the situation, different types of biopsy may be performed. The types include incisional and excisional biopsies. In an incisional biopsy, the physician takes a sample of tissue, and in excisional biopsy, the mass is removed. Fine needle aspiration biopsy and core needle biopsy are kinds of incisional biopsies.

FINE NEEDLE ASPIRATION BIOPSY. In a fine needle aspiration biopsy, a fine-gauge needle may be passed into the lesion and cells from the area suctioned into the needle can be quickly prepared for microscopic evaluation (**cytology**). (The patient experiencing nipple discharge can have a sample taken of the discharge for cytological evaluation, also.) Fine needle aspiration is a simple procedure that can be done under local anesthesia, and will tell if the lesion is a fluid-filled cyst or whether it is solid. The sample obtained will yield much diagnostic information. Fine needle aspiration biopsy is an excellent technique when the lump is palpable and the physician can easily hit the target with the needle. If the lesion is a simple cyst, the fluid will be evacuated and the mass will disappear. If it is solid, the diagnosis may be obtained. Care must be taken, however, because if the mass is solid and the specimen is non-malignant, a complete removal of the lesion may be appropriate to be sure.

CORE NEEDLE BIOPSY. Core needle biopsies are also obtained simply under local anesthesia. The larger piece of tissue obtained with its preserved architecture may be helpful in confirming the diagnosis short of open surgical removal. An open surgical incisional biopsy is rarely needed for diagnosis because of the needle techniques. If there remains question as to diagnosis, a complete open surgical biopsy may be required.

EXCISIONAL BIOPSY. When performed, the excisional, (complete removal) biopsy is a minimal outpatient procedure often done under local anesthesia.

NON-PALPABLE LESIONS. As screening increases, non-palpable lesions demonstrated only by mammography are becoming more common. The use of x rays and computers to guide the needle for biopsy or to place markers for the surgeon performing the excisional biopsy are commonly employed. Some benign lesions can be fully removed by multiple directed core biopsies. These techniques are very appealing because they are minimally invasive; however, the physician needs to be careful to obtain a good sample.

Other tests

If a lesion is not palpable and has simple cystic characteristics on mammography, ultrasound may be utilized both to determine that it is a cyst and to guide its evacuation. Ultrasound may also be used in some cases to guide fine needle or core biopsies of the breast.

Computed tomography (CT scan, CAT scans), and **magnetic resonance imaging** (MRI) have only a very occasional use in the evaluation of breast lesions.

Clinical staging, treatments, and prognosis

Staging

Once diagnosis is established, before treatment is rendered, more tests are done to determine if the cancer has spread beyond the breast. These tests include a chest **x ray** and blood count with liver function tests. Along with the liver function measured by the blood sample, the level of alkaline phosphatase, an enzyme from bone, is also determined. A radionuclear bone scan may be ordered. This test looks at the places in the body to which breast cancer usually metastasizes. A CT scan may also be ordered. The physician will do a careful examination of the axilla to assess likelihood of regional metastasis but unfortunately this exam is not very accurate. Since the axillary node status is the best reflection of possible widespread disease, these nodes in part or all will be removed at the time of surgical treatment.

Using the results of these studies, clinical stage is defined for the patient. This helps define treatment protocol and prognosis. After surgical treatment, the final, or pathologic, stage is defined as the true axillary lymph node status is known. Detailed staging criteria are available from the American Joint Commission on Cancer Manual and are generalized here:

- Stage 1—The cancer is no larger than 2 cm (0.8 in) and no cancer cells are found in the lymph nodes.
- Stage 2—The cancer is between 2 cm and 5 cm, and the cancer has spread to the lymph nodes.
- Stage 3A—Tumor is larger than 5 cm (2 in) or is smaller than 5 cm, but has spread to the lymph nodes, which have grown into each other.
- Stage 3B—Cancer has spread to tissues near the breast, (local invasion), or to lymph nodes inside the chest wall, along the breastbone.

KEY TERMS

Adjuvant therapy—Treatment involving radiation, chemotherapy (drug treatment), or hormone therapy, or a combination of all three given after the primary treatment for the possibility of residual microscopic disease.

Aneuploid—An abnormal number of chromosomes in a cell.

Aspiration biopsy—The removal of cells in fluid or tissue from a mass or cyst using a needle for microscopic examination and diagnosis.

Benign—Not malignant, noncancerous.

Biopsy—A procedure in which suspicious tissue is removed and examined by a pathologist for cancer or other disease. For breast biopsies, the tissue may be obtained by open surgery, or through a needle.

Estrogen-receptor assay—A test to see if a breast cancer needs estrogen to grow.

Hormones—Chemicals produced by glands in the body which circulate in the blood and control the actions of cells and organs. Estrogens are hormones which affect breast cancer growth.

Hormone therapy—Treating cancers by changing the hormone balance of the body, instead of by using cell-killing drugs.

Lumpectomy—A surgical procedure in which only the cancerous tumor in the breast is removed, together with a rim of normal tissue.

Lymph nodes—Small, bean-shaped masses of tissue scattered along the lymphatic system that act as filters and immune monitors, removing fluids, bacteria, or cancer cells that travel through the lymph system. Breast cancer cells in the lymph nodes under the arm or in the chest are a sign that the cancer has spread, and that it might recur.

Malignant—Cancerous.

Mammography—X-ray imaging of the breast that can often detect lesions in the tissue too small or too deep to be felt.

Oncogene—A gene that has to do with regulation of cell growth. An abnormality can produce cancer.

- Stage 4—Cancer has spread to skin and lymph nodes beyond the axilla or to other organs of the body.

Treatment

Surgery, radiation, and **chemotherapy** are all utilized in the treatment of breast cancer. Depending on the stage, they will be used in different combinations or sequences to effect an appropriate strategy for the type and stage of the disease being treated.

SURGERY. Historically, surgical removal of the entire breast and axillary contents along with the muscles down to the chest wall was performed as the lone therapy, (radical **mastectomy**). In the last twenty-five years, as it has been appreciated that breast cancer is often systemic early in its course, the role of surgery is still primary but of less and less magnitude.

Today, surgical treatment is best thought of as a combination of removal of the primary tumor and staging of the axillary lymph nodes. If the whole breast is removed along with the entire axillary contents, but the muscles of the chest wall are not, the modified radical mastectomy has been performed.

If the tumor is less than 4 cm (1.5 in) in size and located so that it can be removed without destroying a reasonable cosmetic appearance of the residual breast, just the primary tumor and a rim of normal tissue will be removed. The axillary nodes will still be removed for staging purposes, usually through a separate incision. Because of the risk of recurrence in the remaining breast tissue, radiation is used to lessen the chance of local recurrence. This type of primary therapy is known as **lumpectomy**, (or segmental mastectomy), and axillary dissection.

Currently the necessary extent of the axillary dissection is being questioned. Sentinel lymph node biopsy, a technique for identifying which nodes in the axilla drain the tumor, has been developed to provide selective sampling and further lessen the degree of surgical trauma the patient experiences.

When patients are selected appropriately based on the preoperative clinical stage, all of these surgical approaches have been shown to produce similar results. In planning primary surgical therapy, it is imperative that the operation is tailored to fit the clinical circumstance of the patient.

The pathologic stage is determined after surgical treatment absolutely defines the local parameters. In addition to stage, there are other tests that are very necessary to aid in decisions regarding treatment. Handling of the surgical specimen is thus very important. The tissue needs to be analyzed for the presence or absence of hormone receptors and a receptor called HER-2. The presence of these receptors will influence additional therapies. Microscopic evaluation may also include the assessment of lymphatic or blood vessel invasion as these predict a worse outcome. The DNA of the tumor cells is quantitatively analyzed to help decide the biologic aggressiveness of the tumor. These parameters will be utilized collectively along with the axillary lymph node status to define the anticipated aggressiveness of the cancer. This assessment, along with the age and general condition of the patient, will be considered when planning the adjuvant therapies. Adjuvant therapies are treatments utilized after the primary treatment to help ensure that no microscopic disease exists and to help prolong patients' survival time.

RADIATION. Like surgical therapy, **radiation therapy** is a local modality—it treats the tissue exposed to it and not the rest of the body. Radiation is usually given post-operatively after surgical wounds have healed. The pathologic stage of the primary tumor is now known and this aids in treatment planning. The extent of the local surgery also influences the planning. Radiation may not be needed at all after modified radical mastectomy for stage I disease, but is almost always utilized when breast-preserving surgery is performed. If the tumor was extensive or if multiple nodes were involved, the field of tissue exposed will vary accordingly. Radiation is utilized as an adjunct to surgical therapy and is considered an important modality in gaining local control of the tumor. The use of radiation therapy does not affect decisions for adjuvant treatment. In the past, radiation was used as an alternative to surgery on occasion. However, now that breast-preserving surgical protocols have been developed, primary radiation treatment of the tumor is no longer performed. Radiation also has an important role in the treatment of the patient with disseminated disease, particularly if it involves the skeleton. Radiation therapy can effect pain control and prevention of fracture in this circumstance.

DRUG THERAPY. Many breast cancers, particularly those originating in post-menopausal women, are responsive to hormones. These cancers have receptors on their cells for estrogen and progesterone. Part of primary tumor assessment after removal of the tumor is the evaluation for the presence of these estrogen and progesterone receptors. If they are present on the cancer cells, altering the hormone status of the patient will inhibit tumor growth and have a positive impact on survival. The drug **tamoxifen** binds up these receptors on the cancer cells so that the hormones can't have an effect and, in so doing, inhibits tumor growth. If the patient has these receptors present, tamoxifen is commonly prescribed for five years as an adjunct to primary treatment. Adjuvant hormonal therapy with tamoxifen has few side effects but they have to be kept in mind, particularly the need for yearly evaluation of the uterus. Other agents directed at altering hormone environment are under study. Because of these agents, there is rarely any need for surgical removal of hormone-producing glands, such as the ovary or adrenal gland, that was sometimes necessary in the past.

Shortly after the modified radical mastectomy replaced the radical mastectomy as primary surgical treatment, it was appreciated that survival after local treatment in stage II breast cancer was improved by the addition of chemotherapy. Adjuvant chemotherapy for an interval of four to six months is now standard treatment for patients with stage II disease. The addition of systemic therapy to local treatment in patients who have no evidence of disease is performed on the basis that some patients have metastasis that are not currently demonstrable because they are microscopic. By treating the whole patient early, before widespread disease is diagnosed, the adjuvant treatment improves survival rates from roughly 60% for stage II to about 75% at five years after treatment. The standard regimen of cytoxan, **methotrexate**, and **fluorouracil** (CMF), is given for six months and is well tolerated. The regimen of cytoxan, adriamycin (**doxorubicin**), and floururacil, (CAF), is a bit more toxic but only requires four months. (Adriamycin and cytoxin may also be used alone, without the fluorouracil.) The two methods are about equivalent in results. Adjuvant hormonal therapy may be added to the adjuvant chemotherapy as they work through different routes.

As one would expect, the encouraging results from adjuvant therapy in stage II disease have led to the study of similar therapy in stage I disease. The results are not as dramatic, but they are real. Currently, stage I disease is divided into categories a, b, and c on the basis of tumor size. Stage Ia is less than a centimeter in diameter. Adjuvant hormonal or chemotherapy is now commonly recommended for stage Ib and Ic patients. The toxicity of the treatment must be weighed individually for the patient as patients with stage I disease have a survivorship of over 80% without adjuvant chemotherapy.

If patients are diagnosed with stage IV disease or, in spite of treatment, progress to a state of widespread disease, systemic chemotherapy is utilized in a more aggressive fashion. In addition to the adriamycin-containing regimens, **docetaxel** and **paclitaxel** have been found to be effective in inducing remission.

On the basis of prognostic factors such as total number of involved nodes over 10, aneuploid DNA with a high synthesis value, or aggressive findings on microscopic evaluation, some patients with stage II or III disease can be predicted to do poorly. If their performance status allows, they can be considered for treatment with highly aggressive chemotherapy. The toxicity is such that bone marrow failure will result. To get around this anticipated side effect of the aggressive therapy, either the patients will be transplanted with their own stem cells, (the cells that will give rise to new marrow), or an allogeneic **bone marrow transplantation** will be required. This therapy can be a high-risk procedure for patients. It is given with known risk to patients predicted to do poorly and then only if it is felt they can tolerate it. Most patients who receive this therapy receive it as part of a clinical trial. At present, it is unclear that such aggressive therapy can be justified and it is under study.

For patients who are diagnosed with advanced local disease, surgery may be preceded with chemotherapy and radiation therapy. The disease locally regresses allowing traditional surgical treatment to those who could not receive it otherwise. Chemotherapy and sometimes radiation therapy will continue after the surgery. The regimens of this type are referred to as neo-adjuvant therapy. This has been proven to be effective in stage III disease. Neo-adjuvant therapy is now being studied in patients with large tumors that are stage II in an effort to be able to offer breast preservation to these patients.

A drug known as Herceptin (**trastuzumab**), a monoclonal antibody, is now being used in the treatment of those with systemic disease. The product of the Human Epidermal Growth Factor 2 gene, (HER-2) is overexpressed in 25%–30% of breast cancers. Herceptin binds to the HER-2 receptors on the cancer, resulting in the arrest of growth of these cells.

Prognosis

The prognosis for breast cancer depends on the type and stage of cancer. Over 80% of stage I patients are cured by current therapies. Stage II patients survive overall about 70% of the time, those with more extensive lymph nodal involvement doing worse than those with disease confined to the breast. About 40% of stage III patients survive five years, and about 20% of stage IV patients do so.

Coping with cancer treatment

Surgery for breast cancer is physically well-tolerated by the patient, especially those undergoing minimal surgery in the axilla. Most patients can return to a normal lifestyle within a month or so after surgery. Exercises can help the patient regain strength and flexibility. Arm, shoulder, and chest exercises help, and complete recovery of activity is to be expected.

About 5-7% of patients undergoing complete axillary lymph node resection as part of their therapy may develop clinically significant lymphedema, or swelling in the arm on the side of involvement. If present, elevation and massage may be needed intermittently. Though usually not serious, on occasion this complication may interfere with complete physical recovery. The incidence of lymphedema is less with less axillary surgery. This is the reason for the enthusiasm for sentinel node biopsy as the surgical staging procedure in the axilla.

It is common after breast cancer treatment to be depressed or moody, to cry, lose appetite, or feel unworthy or less interested in sex. The breast is involved with a woman's identity and loss of it may be disturbing. For some, counseling or a support group can help. Many women have found a support group of breast cancer survivors to be an invaluable help during this stage. Involvement with volunteers from the local chapter of the Reach to Recovery program may be very helpful.

Nearly all patients undergo some form of adjuvant therapy for breast cancer. The magnitude of the toxicity of these adjuvant therapies is usually small and many patients receiving chemotherapy on this basis are capable of normal activity during this time. Certainly, those who progress to advanced disease are treated with more toxic chemotherapeutic regimens in an attempt to induce remission.

Clinical trials

The use of tamoxifen and other agents which alter the hormone status of the patient are under study. The National Surgical Adjuvant Breast and Bowel Project (NSABP) with support from the National Cancer Institute began a study in 1992 (called the Breast Cancer Prevention Trial, or BCPT) studying the use of tamoxifen as a breast cancer preventative for high-risk women. The results yielded from the study showed that tamoxifen significantly reduced breast cancer risk, and the U.S. Food and Drug Administration approved the use of tamoxifen to reduce breast cancer risk for high-risk patients in 1998. Another NSABP study, known as STAR, is seeking to understand if another drug, **raloxifene**, is as effective as tamoxifen in reducing breast cancer risk in high-risk patients. That study was begun in 1999, and participants are to be monitored for five years.

Neo-adjuvant therapies to allow the use of breast preservation in those with more advanced local disease are under investigation.

Immune therapies have not been helpful to date though there are **vaccines** being developed against proteins such as that produced by HER-2 that may be beneficial in the future.

QUESTIONS TO ASK THE DOCTOR

- Has my cancer spread?
- What is the stage of my cancer? What does that mean?
- What treatment choices do I have?
- What treatment do you recommend? Why?
- What are the advantages and disadvantages of this treatment?
- Will I lose my hair? If so, what can be done about it?
- What are the chances my cancer will come back after this treatment?
- What should I do to be ready for treatment?

High-dose chemotherapy with bone marrow rescue remains controversial. Factors can be identified that predict certain patients will develop metastatic disease. This treatment has been offered to this select group of patients but the toxicity is such that defining a clear indication for this treatment remains under study.

Prevention

As mentioned above, because of the results yielded from the BCPT clinical trial, tamoxifen can now be prescribed to high-risk women to help prevent breast cancer.

And, while most breast cancer can't be prevented, it can be diagnosed from a mammogram at an early stage when it is most treatable. The results of awareness and routine screening have allowed earlier diagnosis, which results in a better prognosis for those discovered.

Special Concerns

Though breast-preserving therapy is being done more frequently than in years past, modified radical mastectomy remains an option when selecting therapy for the primary tumor. This option may allow treatment without radiation in earlier stage patients, or may be necessary if the presentation of the tumor does not allow breast preservation. Loss of the breast is disfiguring and many patients so treated desire reconstruction of the breast. Breast reconstruction is performed either at the time of initial surgery (immediate) or it may be delayed. Alternatives include placement of implants or the rotation of muscle flaps from the abdomen or back. Most agree that breast preservation gives superior results to any form of reconstruction. When the breast is removed as part of primary therapy, these reconstructions are available and do produce very reasonable results.

See Also Breast ultrasound; Sentinel lymph node mapping; Tumor staging

Resources

BOOKS

Abelhoff, Armitage, Lichter, Niederhuber. *Clinical Oncology Library.* Philadelphia: Churchill Livingstone 1999.

American Joint Committee on Cancer. *AJCC Clinical Staging Manual.* Philadelphia: Lippincott-Raven, 1997.

Love, Susan and Karen Lindsey. *Dr. Susan Love's Breast Book.* Reading, MA: Addison-Wesley, 1995.

Mayers, Musa. *Holding Tight, Letting Go: Living with Metastatic Breast Cancer.* Sebastopol, CA: O'Reilly & Associates, 1997.

McKinnell, Robert G., Ralph E. Parchment, Alan O. Perantoni, and G. Barry Pierce. *The Biological Basis of Cancer.* New York: Cambridge University Press, 1998.

Schwartz, Spencer, Galloway, Shires, Daly, Fischer. *Principles of Surgery.* New York: McGraw Hill, 1999.

PERIODICALS

Esteva and Hortobagyi. "Adjuvant Systemic Therapy for Primary Breast Cancer." *Surgical Clinics of North America* Volume 79 No. 5 (October 1999) p 1075-1090.

Krag, et al, "The Sentinel Node in Breast Cancer." *New England Journal of Medicine* Volume 339 No. 14 (October 1, 1998), p 941-946.

Margolese, R. G., M.D. "Surgical Considerations For Invasive Breast Cancer." *Surgical Clinics of North America* Volume 79 No. 5 (October 1999), p 1031-1046.

Munster and Hudis. "Adjuvant Therapy for Resectable Breast Cancer." *Hematology Oncology Clinics of North America* Volume 13 No. 2 (April 1999) p 391-413.

Shuster, et al. "Multidisciplinary Care For Patients With Breast Cancer." *Surgical Clinics of North America* Volume 80 No. 2 (April, 2000) p 505-533.

ORGANIZATIONS

American Cancer Society. (800) ACS-2345. <http://www.cancer.org>.American Cancer Society's Reach to Recovery Program: <http://www2.cancer.org/bcn/reach.html>.

Cancer Care, Inc. (800) 813-HOPE. <http://www.cancercareinc.org>.

Cancer Information Service of the NCI. (1-800-4-CANCER). <http://wwwicic.nci.nih.gov>.

National Alliance of Breast Cancer Organizations. 9 East 37th St., 10th floor, New York, NY 10016. (888) 80-NABCO.

National Coalition for Cancer Survivorship. 1010 Wayne Ave., 5th Floor, Silver Spring, MD 20910. (301) 650-8868.

National Women's Health Resource Center. 2425 L St. NW, 3rd floor, Washington, DC 20037. (202) 293-6045.

OTHER

Breast Cancer Online <http://www.bco.org/>

National Alliance of Breast Cancer Organizations <http:// www.nabco.org/>

National Cancer Institute <http://rex.nci.nih.gov/PATIENTS/ INFO_PEOPL_DOC.html>

Richard A. McCartney, M.D.
Carol A. Turkington

Breast self-exam

Definition

Breast self-examination (BSE) is a diagnostic technique regularly performed by a woman, independent from a physician, both by feeling for anything suspicious in her breasts and by observing any changes through the use of a mirror.

Purpose

BSE should be performed monthly in order to discover changes in breast tissue, discharge from the nipple, or the onset of pain in the breast area. While 80% of lumps are not cancerous, such discoveries can ultimately lead to the detection of **breast cancer**.

Precautions

BSE is an effective self-diagnostic procedure, but it must not take the place of having a mammogram and having a health care provider check the breasts for abnormal changes. Make sure to schedule an annual clinical breast examination with a licensed medical care provider to supplement the BSE.

Description

It is important that BSEs are performed routinely so that a woman knows what her breasts normally feel and look like, resulting in quicker identification of anything abnormal. Self-exams take less than five minutes to perform and should be done a few days after the end of menstruation. Women that menstruate irregularly should choose a day of the month that is easy to remember, such as the date of their birth, and perform the exams on the same day each month.

The first phase of the BSE is to disrobe and stand in front of a mirror, observing the breast area in four different positions. First, with the arms down to the sides, look at the color, shape, outline, and direction of the breasts and nipples, taking note of anything atypical. Then, press the hands on the hips in order to flex the chest muscles, making the same observations. Next, observe the breasts while leaning forward. Finally, raise the arms overhead and notice anything abnormal such as color changes, dimpling of the skin, or nipple discharge.

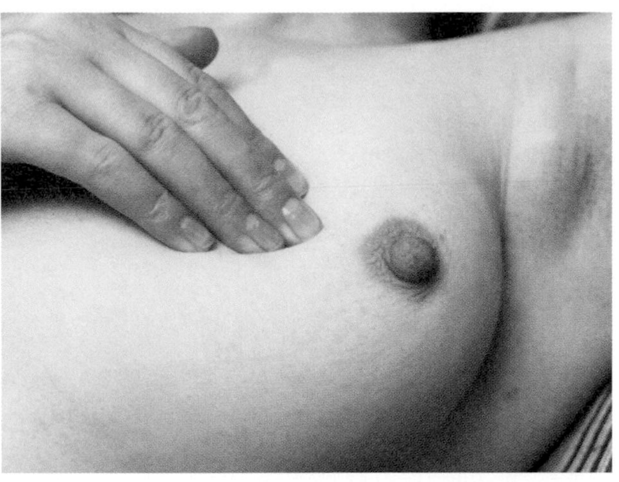

Woman examining her breast for abnormalities. *(© Francoise Sauze, Science Source/Photo Researchers, Inc. Reproduced by permission.)*

The second phase of the BSE is performed lying down. First, put a pillow under the right shoulder and place the right hand under the head so that the elbow is positioned at a 90-degree angle. This is done in order to flatten the breast as much as possible, making the examination easier and more effective.

Then, using the pads of the fingers of the left hand, press firmly around the breast using a small circular motion about the size of a penny. A small amount of lotion or petroleum jelly can make it easier to feel for lumps. Three types of pressure should be used. The first pressure should be enough to examine the surface, typically just to move the skin and feel for changes in the top layer of tissue. The second level of pressure is a deeper pressure, probing into the tissue. The final pressure level is applied deep into the breast tissue so that the rib cage can be felt and a minor amount of discomfort is experienced. Choose a comfortable pattern such as circles, lines, or wedges to make sure that the entire breast and armpit area are thoroughly examined with each level of pressure.

Finally, tenderly squeeze the area around the nipple and check for fluid discharge. After the right breast has been thoroughly examined, repeat the above steps on the left breast.

Although it is uncommon, forms of breast cancer can also occur in men. The breast self-exam can be modified to be effective for men. Men can utilize the visual exam and can also feel for any changes in the tissue.

QUESTIONS TO ASK THE DOCTOR

- When should a mammogram be performed to complement the BSE?
- Do breast implants interfere with BSE?
- Do hormone supplements interfere with BSE?

Preparation

Since the patient performs BSE in the comfort of her own home, there are not many preparations that need to be made. The patient should remove any distractions that could interfere with the performance of a thorough exam. It is also advisable to disrobe and to use lotion or lubricant when palpating the breast area.

Aftercare

BSE is not an invasive procedure. Therefore there is not any significant aftercare that needs to take place. Individuals should simply remember to perform the exam monthly and inform their doctor of any changes.

Risks

There are no known risks associated with the breast self-exam as long as the individual schedules regular exams with a physician and immediately reports anything unusual.

Normal results

Patients who perform BSE regularly know what their breast tissue normally feels like. Typically, there will not be any detectable anomalies in their breast tissue, unless they carry out the exam just prior to menstruation or during pregnancy when breasts may seem more lumpy and tender. In these cases, it is likely that abnormal lumps and tenderness are not associated with cancerous tumors. However, if a woman finds anything that makes her uneasy, she should consult with her physician.

Abnormal results

Women should consult with their physician if they notice dimpling of the skin, any change in outline or shape of their breasts, unusual lumps, areas of thickening, or pain during the palpation of the breasts. If milky white or bloody discharge from the nipple is observed, then the patient should call the doctor. Generally, if there are any observations that make a person uneasy, it is advisable to contact a doctor.

KEY TERMS

Palpate—Examination by feeling and touching with the hands.

Resources

OTHER

"An Ounce of Prevention...How to Do Self-Exams." *Sister: Columbia University's Feminist Magazine* April 2001. 27 June 2001 <http://www.columbia.edu/cu/sister/Self Exams.html>.

"Breast Self-Exam (BSE) Why, When and How." *Breast Cancer Information Service* April 2001. 29 June 2001 <http://trfn.clpgh.org/bcis/GeneralInfo/bse.html>

"Breast Self Examination: Your Key to Better Breast Health." *Y-ME National Breast Cancer Organization* April 2001. 27 June 2001 <http://www.y-me.org/images/breast_self_exam.pdf>.

"BSE Breast Self Examination." *Info Breast Cancer* April 2001. 27 June 2001 <http://www.infobreastcancer.cyberus.ca/bse2.htm>.

Sally C. McFarlane-Parrott

Breast ultrasound

Definition

Breast ultrasound (or sonography) is an imaging technique for diagnosing breast disease, such as cancer. It uses harmless, high-frequency sound waves to form an image (sonogram). The sound waves pass through the breast and bounce back or echo from various tissues to form a picture of the internal structures. It is not invasive and involves no radiation.

Purpose

Breast ultrasound may be used in several ways. The most common application is to investigate a specific area of the breast where a problem is suspected. A palpable lump and/or a lump or density discovered by **x ray** (mammogram) can be further evaluated by ultrasound. It is especially helpful in distinguishing between a fluid-filled cyst and a solid mass. It can also identify small lesions that are too tiny to be felt.

Breast ultrasound is often the first study performed to evaluate masses in women under 35 whose mammograms can be difficult to interpret due to the density of their breast tissue. The lack of radiation used with ultrasound makes it ideal for studying breast abnormalities in women who are pregnant. Assessing breast implants for leakage or rupture is another way ultrasound is used. Breast inflammation, where pockets of infection or abscesses may form, can be diagnosed and monitored by ultrasound.

Thickened and swollen breast skin may be a sign of inflammatory **breast cancer**. Ultrasound can sometimes identify a cancerous growth within the breast causing the thickened skin. These cases are usually followed by a core **biopsy** guided by ultrasound (described below).

Breast ultrasound is employed to observe and guide a needle for several interventional procedures. These include cyst aspiration, fine needle aspiration, large core needle biopsy (as a first step in determining treatment for a lesion that is likely to be cancerous), and needle localization in surgical breast biopsy. Biopsies guided by ultrasound have distinct advantages. The ultrasound guides the needle so that a lesion can be removed for the biopsy. Patients usually find that the procedure is less traumatic and more comfortable than surgical biopsies. Ultrasound is known for its accuracy in determining how far a cancerous growth extends into the surrounding tissue in lesions that cannot be felt. Biopsies guided by ultrasound are generally less costly than surgical biopsies. Additionally, if the abnormality that requires biopsy can be seen on both a mammogram and ultrasound, an ultrasound-guided biopsy is often more comfortable for the patient as no compression is necessary.

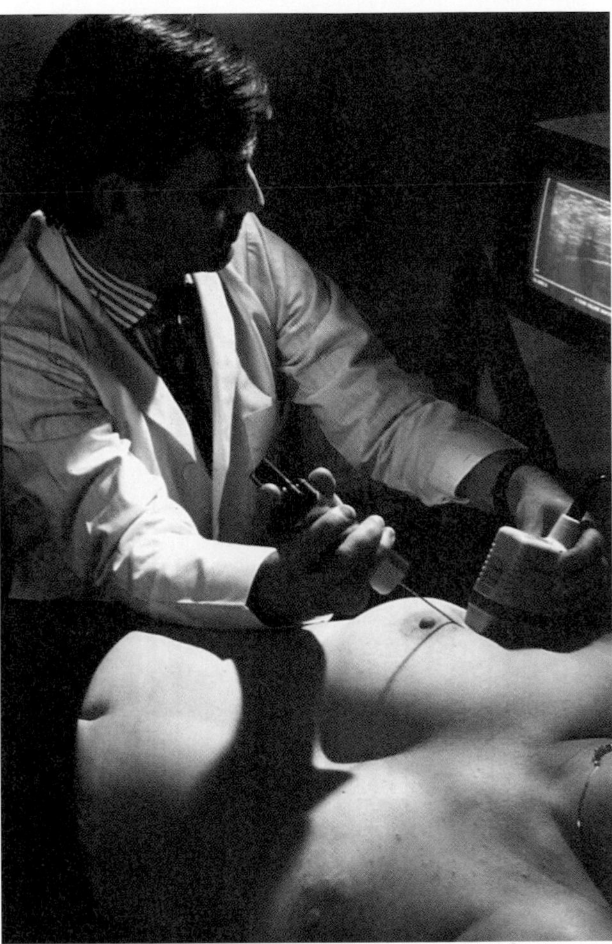

This woman is having her breast scanned by ultrasound while a tissue biopsy is being taken. In breast scanning, ultrasound is used to distinguish between solid lumps and fluid-filled cysts. *(Photo by Geoff Tompkinson. Photo Researchers, Inc. Reproduced by permission.)*

Description

Ultrasound can be done in a doctor's office or another outpatient setting, such as a hospital or imaging center.

The patient removes her clothing from the waist up and puts on a hospital gown, open in the front. She lies on her back or side on an examining table. A gel that enhances sound transmission is spread over the area to be examined. The technologist then places a transducer, an instrument about the size of an electric shaver, against the skin. The images from reflected sound waves appear on a monitor screen.

A good ultrasound study is difficult to obtain if the patient is unable to remain quietly in one position. Obesity may hinder clear viewing of internal structures, and the accuracy of an ultrasound study is highly dependent on the skill of the person performing the examination. The images recorded vary with the angle and pressure of the transducer and the equipment settings. The examination may take from 30 to 45 minutes. Most insurance plans cover the cost of an ultrasound examination.

Normal results

An ultrasound examination may reveal either normal tissue or a benign condition such as a cyst. Ultrasound can confidently diagnose a benign structure that has certain characteristics of a simple cyst. In the case of a simple cyst with no symptoms, additional treatment beyond continued observation is usually not needed.

Abnormal results

A potentially malignant mass can be identified by breast ultrasound. Abnormal results fall into the following categories: benign fibrous nodule, complex cyst, suspicious lesion, and lesion highly suggestive of cancer. In cases where ultrasound shows the presence of a complex cyst or fibrous nodule, a biopsy is justified because 10% to 15% of these growths are malignant. Lesions falling into

KEY TERMS

Cyst—A thin-walled, fluid-filled benign structure in the breast.

Ductal carcinoma—A type of cancer that accounts for as much as 80% of breast cancers. These tumors feel bigger than they look on ultrasound or mammogram.

Fibroadenoma—A benign breast growth made up of fibrous tissue. It is the most common mass in women under 35 years of age, and is found in both breasts in 3% of cases.

Infiltrating lobular carcinoma—A type of cancer that accounts for 8% to 10% of breast cancers. In breasts that are especially dense, ultrasound can be useful in identifying these masses.

Microcalcifications—Tiny flecks that are too small to be felt. They are important markers of cancer that show up on ultrasound and mammogram.

Mucinous (colloid) carcinoma—A type of cancer that accounts for 1% to 2% of breast cancers. Resembles medullary carcinoma in ultrasound and mammogram, but usually affects older women.

Nonpalpable—Cannot be felt by hand. In cancer, growths that are nonpalpable are too small to be felt, but may be seen on ultrasound or mammogram.

Papillary carcinoma—A type of breast cancer that primarily occurs in older women. On ultrasound, this type of tumor may look like a solid or complex mass, or it may show up as solid tissue protruding into a cyst.

Tubular carcinoma—A type of cancer that accounts for approximately 1% to 2% of breast cancers. Can appear small on ultrasound or mammogram.

the last two categories (suspicious or highly suggestive of cancer) have a higher chance of being cancerous, and should be investigated further, either by biopsy or surgery.

Breast cancers such as the following may be identified on ultrasound: ductal **carcinoma**, infiltrating lobular carcinoma, medullary carcinoma, mucinous (colloid) carcinoma, tubular carcinoma, and papillary carcinoma. On ultrasound, the shape of a lesion and the type of edges it has can sometimes indicate if it is benign or cancerous, but there are exceptions. For example, benign fibroadenomas are usually oval, and some cancers can be similarly shaped. Cancerous tumors usually have jagged edges, but some benign growths can have these edges as well. Ultrasound is not a definitive test. Tissue diagnosis is often required.

QUESTIONS TO ASK THE DOCTOR

- Why is/was this procedure necessary?
- How long will the ultrasound take?
- What are the chances of finding an abnormal growth?
- Will the results be given during the procedure?
- If an abnormal growth is found, what is the next step?

See Also Biopsy; Breast cancer; Breast self–exam

Resources

BOOKS

Love, Susan M., with Karen Lindsey. *Dr. Susan Love's Breast Book.* 2nd ed. Reading, MA: Addison-Wesley, 1995.

Rumack, Carol M. et al., ed. *Diagnostic Ultrasound* St. Louis: Mosby–Year–Book, Inc., 1998.

PERIODICALS

Jackson, Valerie. "The Current Role of Ultrasonography in Breast Imaging." *Radiologic Clinics of North America* 33 (November 1995): 1161-70.

Rubin, Eva, et al. "Reducing the Cost of Diagnosis of Breast Carcinoma: Impact of Ultrasound and Imaging–Guided Biopsies on a Clinical Breast Practice." *Cancer* 91 (January 2001) 324-31.

Smith, LaNette F. et al. "Intraoperative Ultrasound–guided Breast Biopsy." *The American Journal of Surgery* 180 (December 2000): 419-23.

Velez, Nitzet et al. "Diagnostic and Interventional Ultrasound for Breast Disease." *The American Journal of Surgery* 180 (October 2000): 284-7.

Ellen S. Weber

Bronchoscopy

Definition

Bronchoscopy is a procedure in which a cylindrical fiberoptic scope is inserted into the airways. This scope contains a viewing device that allows the visual examination of the lower airways.

Purpose

During a bronchoscopy, a physician can visually examine the lower airways, including the larynx, trachea, bronchi, and bronchioles. The procedure is used to examine the mucosal surface of the airways for abnormalities that might be associated with a variety of lung diseases. Its use includes the visualization of airway obstructions such as a tumor, or the collection of specimens for the diagnosis of cancer originating in the bronchi of the lungs (bronchogenic cancer). It can also be used to collect specimens for culture to diagnose infectious diseases such as tuberculosis. The type of specimens collected can include sputum (composed of saliva and discharges from the respiratory passages), tissue samples from the bronchi or bronchioles, or cells collected from washing the lining of the bronchi or bronchioles. The instrument used in bronchoscopy, a bronchoscope, is a slender cylindrical instrument containing a light and an eyepiece. There are two types of bronchoscopes, a rigid tube that is sometimes referred to as an open-tube or ventilating bronchoscope, and a more flexible fiberoptic tube. This tube contains four smaller passages—two for light to pass through, one for seeing through and one that can accommodate medical instruments that may be used for **biopsy** or suctioning, or that medication can be passed through.

Bronchoscopy may be used for the following purposes:

- to diagnose cancer, tuberculosis, lung infection, or other lung disease
- to examine an inherited deformity of the lungs
- to remove a foreign body in the lungs, such as a mucus plug, tumor, or excessive secretions
- to remove tissue samples, also known as biopsy, to test for cancer cells, help with staging the advancement of the lung cancer, or to treat a tumor with laser therapy
- to allow examination of a suspected tumor, obstruction, secretion, bleeding, or foreign body in the airways
- to determine the cause of a persistent cough, wheezing, or a cough that includes blood in the sputum
- to evaluate the effectiveness of lung cancer treatments

Precautions

Patients not breathing adequately on their own due to severe respiratory failure may require mechanical ventilation prior to bronchoscopy. It may not be appropriate to perform bronchoscopy on patients with an unstable heart condition. All patients must be constantly monitored while undergoing a bronchoscopy so that any abnormal reactions can be dealt with immediately.

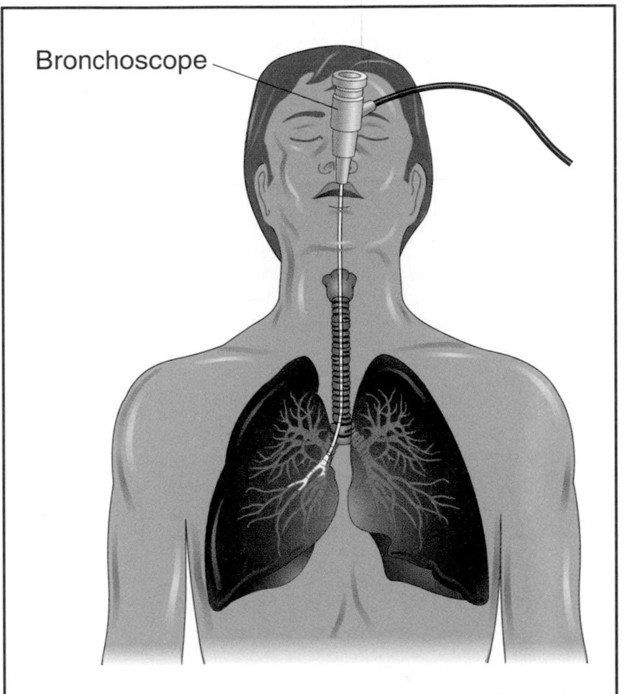

Bronchoscopy is a procedure in which a hollow, flexible tube is inserted into the airways, allowing the physician to visually examine the lower airways, including the larynx, trachea, bronchi, and bronchioles. It can also be used to collect specimens for bacteriological culture to diagnose infectious diseases such as tuberculosis. *(Illustration by Electronic Illustrators Group.)*

Description

There are two types of bronchoscopes, a rigid tube and a fiberoptic tube. Because of its flexibility, the fiberoptic tube is usually preferred. However, if the purpose of the procedure is to remove a foreign body caught in the windpipe or lungs of a child, the more rigid tube must be used because of its larger size. The patient will either lie face-up on his/her back or sit upright in a chair. Medication to decrease secretions, lessen anxiety, and relax the patient are often given prior to the procedure. While breathing through the nose, anesthesia is sprayed into the mouth or nose to numb it. It will take 1-2 minutes for the anesthesia to take effect. Once this happens, the bronchoscope will be put into the patient's mouth or nose and moved down into the throat. While the bronchoscope is moving down the throat, additional anesthesia is put into the bronchoscope to numb the lower parts of the airways. Using the eyepiece, the physician then observes the trachea and bronchi, and the mucosal lining of these passageways, looking for any abnormalities that may be present.

If the purpose of the bronchoscopy is to take tissue samples or biopsy, forceps or a bronchial brush are used

KEY TERMS

Anesthesia—A drug used to induce loss of sensation. It is used to lessen the pain of surgery and medical procedures.

Bronchi—The network of tubular passages that carry air to the lungs and allow air to be expelled from the lungs.

Bronchioles—Small airways extending from the bronchi into the lobes of the lungs.

Bronchoalveolar lavage—Washing cells from the air sacs at the end of the bronchioles.

Trachea—The windpipe.

to obtain cells. If the purpose is to identify an infectious agent, a bronchoalveolar lavage (BAL) can be used to gather fluid for culture purposes. Also, if any foreign matter is found in the airways, it can be removed.

Another procedure using bronchoscopy is called fluorescence bronchoscopy. This can be used to detect precancerous cells present in the airways. By using a fluorescent light in the bronchoscope, precancerous tissue will appear dark red, while healthy tissue will appear green. This technique can help detect lung cancer at an early stage, so that treatment can be started early.

Alternative procedures

Depending upon the purpose of the bronchoscopy, alternatives might include a **computed tomography** scan (CT) or no procedure at all. Bronchoscopy is often performed to investigate an abnormality that shows up on a chest **x ray** or CT scan. If the purpose is to obtain biopsy specimens, one option is to perform surgery, which carries greater risks. Another option is percutaneous (through the skin) biopsy guided by computed tomography.

Preparation

The doctor should be informed of any allergies and all the medications that the patient is currently taking. The doctor may instruct the patient not to take medications like aspirin or anti-inflammatory drugs, which interfere with clotting, for a period of time prior to the procedure. The patient needs to fast for 6 to 12 hours prior to the procedure and refrain from drinking any liquids the day of the procedure. The bronchoscopy takes about 45 to 60 minutes, with results usually available in one day. Prior to the bronchoscopy, several tests may be done, including a chest x ray and blood work. Sometimes a bronchoscopy is done under general anesthesia. Patients usually have an intravenous (IV) line in the arm. Most likely, the procedure will be done under local anesthesia, which is sprayed into the nose or mouth. This is necessary to decrease the gag reflex. A sedative may also be used to help the patient relax. It is important that the patient understands that at no time will the airway be blocked and that oxygen can be supplied through the bronchoscope. A signed consent form is necessary for this procedure.

Aftercare

After the bronchoscopy, the patient will be monitored for vital signs such as heart rate, blood pressure, and breathing, while resting in bed. Sometimes patients have an abnormal reaction to anesthesia. All saliva should be spit into a basin so that it can be examined for the presence of blood. If a biopsy was taken, the patient should not cough or clear the throat as this might dislodge any blood clot that has formed and cause bleeding. No food or drink should be consumed for about two hours after the procedure or until the anesthesia wears off. Diet is gradually progressed from ice chips and clear liquids to the patient's regular diet. There will also be a temporary sore throat and hoarseness that may last for a few days.

Risks

Minor side effects arise from the bronchoscope causing abrasion of the lining of the airways. This results in some swelling and inflammation, as well as hoarseness caused from abrading the vocal cords. If this abrasion is more serious, it can lead to respiratory difficulty or bleeding of the airway lining. A more serious risk involved in having a bronchoscopy performed is the occurrence of a pneumothorax, due to puncturing of the lungs, which allows air to escape into the space between the lung and the chest wall. These risks are greater with the use of a rigid bronchoscope than with a fiberoptic bronchoscope. If a rigid tube is used, there is also a risk of chipped teeth.

Normal results

Normal tracheal appearance consists of smooth muscle with C-shaped rings of cartilage at regular intervals. The trachea and the bronchi are lined with a mucous membrane.

Abnormal results

Abnormal bronchoscopy findings may involve abnormalities of the bronchial wall such as inflamma-

QUESTIONS TO ASK THE DOCTOR

- Did you see any abnormalities?
- How soon will you know the results of the biopsy (if one was done)?
- When can I resume any medications that were stopped?
- What future care will I need?
- For what type of problems should I call you?

tion, swelling, ulceration, or anatomical abnormalities. The bronchoscopy may also reveal the presence of abnormal substances in the trachea and bronchi. If samples are taken, the results could indicate cancer, disease-causing agents or other lung disease. Other abnormalities include constriction or narrowing (stenosis), compression, dilation of vessels, or abnormal branching of the bronchi. Abnormal substances that might be found in the airways include blood, secretions, or mucus plugs. Any abnormalities are discussed with the patient.

Resources

BOOKS

Bone, Roger C., ed. *Pulmonary & Critical Care Medicine, 1998 ed.* St. Louis, MO: Mosby-Year Book, Inc., 1998.

Fauci, Anthony S. *Harrison's Principles of Internal Medicine,* 14th Edition. New York: McGraw-Hill, 2000.

PERIODICALS

"Fluorescence Bronchoscopy Technology Used in Early Detection." *Cancer Weekly Plus* (Feb 3, 1997): 17.

ORGANIZATION

American College of Chest Physicians. 3300 Dundee Rd., Northbrook, IL 60062. (800) 343-2227. <www.chestnet.org>.

Cindy L. Jones, Ph.D.

Burkitt's lymphoma

Definition

Burkitt's lymphoma (BL) is a type of non-Hodgkin's lymphoma (NHL) that is sometimes called a B-cell lymphoma or small noncleaved cell lymphoma. It is an endemic (characteristic of a specific place) disease in central Africa but sporadic (occurring in scattered instances) in other countries. Burkitt's lymphoma is one of the most rapidly growing forms of human cancer. In addition, the number of new cases of this tumor is rising in most countries.

Description

Burkitt's lymphoma was first described in 1957 by Denis Parsons Burkitt, an Irish surgeon. While this type of lymphoma is still relatively rare in the United States, it is responsible for 50% of cancer deaths in children in Uganda and central Africa. The endemic form of Burkitt's lymphoma is characterized by rapid enlargement of the patient's jaw, loosening of the teeth, protruding eyeballs, or an abdominal tumor in the region of the kidneys or ovaries.

In the sporadic form of Burkitt's, the patient may have a facial tumor but is much more likely to have an abdominal swelling, often in the area of the ileocecal valve (the valve between the lower portion of the small intestine and the beginning of the large intestine). About 90% of American children with Burkitt's have abdominal tumors. Others may develop tumors in the testes, ovaries, skin, nasal sinuses, or lymph nodes. In adults, Burkitt's lymphoma frequently produces a bulky abdomen and may involve the liver, spleen, and bone marrow.

Demographics

In Western countries, Burkitt's lymphoma is more common in male than in female children. While the average age of patients with endemic Burkitt's is seven years, outside Africa the average age is closer to 11 years. In the United States, the **non-Hodgkin's lymphomas** as a group account for about 7% of cancers in persons under 20 years of age. Between 40% and 50% of these cases are Burkitt's lymphoma.

In adults, Burkitt's lymphoma is again more common in males than in females. It is 1,000 times more common in persons with AIDS than in the general population. Currently, about 2% of AIDS patients develop Burkitt's lymphoma. The majority of these patients have stage IV disease by the time the tumor is diagnosed.

Causes and symptoms

Causes

ONCOGENES. Burkitt's lymphoma affects a part of the immune system known as the lymphatic or lymphoid system. The lymphatic system is a network of tissues, glands, and channels that produces lymphocytes, a type of white blood cell. Some lymphocytes remain in clusters

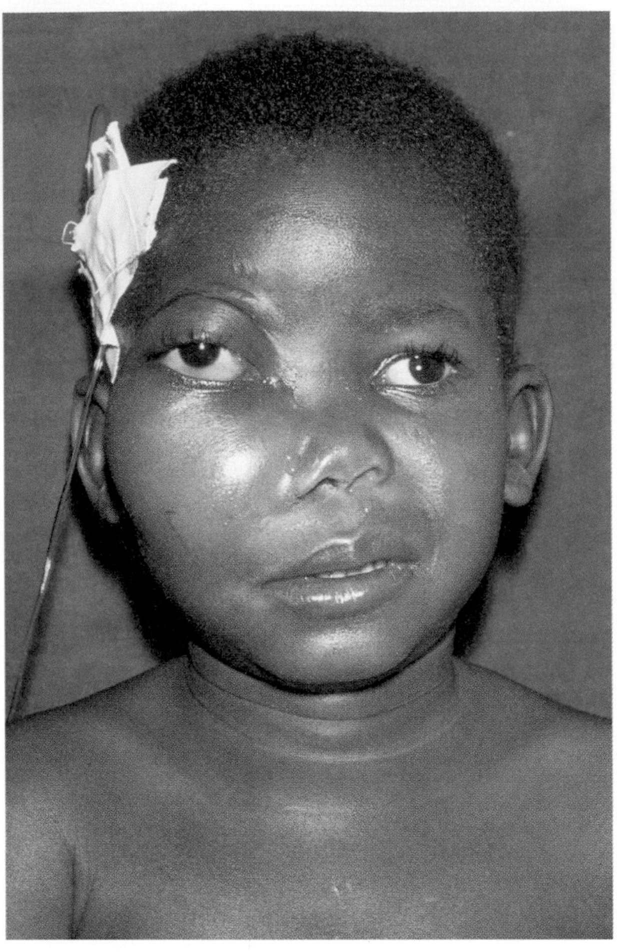

African child with facial disfigurement caused by Burkitt's lymphoma. *(Custom Medical Stock Photo. Reproduced by permission.)*

within the lymph nodes, while others circulate throughout the body in the bloodstream or in the lymph, which is a clear yellowish fluid carried by the lymphatic channels. Lymphocytes fall into two groups: T-cells, which regulate the immune system; and B-cells, which produce antibodies. Burkitt's lymphoma involves the B-cell lymphocytes. In 1982, researchers discovered an oncogene (a gene that can release cells from growth constraints, possibly converting them into tumors) in 90% of patients with Burkitt's lymphoma. Called the C-*myc* oncogene, it is responsible for the uncontrolled production of B-lymphocytes. It results from a translocation, or exchange, of genetic material between the long arm of human chromosome 8 and the long arm of human chromosome 14. In a smaller number of patients with Burkitt's, the translocation involves chromosomes 2 and 22 or chromosomes 2 and 8.

In the summer of 2000, researchers reported that a gene called the HMG-I/Y gene is also involved in the development of Burkitt's lymphoma. The C-*myc* oncogene appears to stimulate the HMG-I/Y gene, which then triggers the changes in normal B-cells that cause them to multiply rapidly and form tumors.

VIRUSES. In addition to translocations of genetic material, Burkitt's lymphoma is also associated with oncogenic viruses—the **Epstein-Barr virus** (EBV) in endemic Burkitt's and human immunodeficiency virus (HIV) in the sporadic form. EBV, or human herpesvirus 4, is the virus that causes infectious mononucleosis. The presence of EBV in patients with endemic Burkitt's has been interpreted as a side effect of the high rates of malaria in central Africa. African children may have immune systems that cannot fight off infection with EBV because they have been weakened by malaria. The children's B-lymphocytes then reproduce at an unusually high rate. Currently, however, the precise role of EBV in Burkitt's lymphoma is still being investigated, because the virus is less common in patients outside Africa. In the United States, about 25% of children and 40% of adult AIDS patients with Burkitt's have the Epstein-Barr virus.

Symptoms

In children, symptoms may appear as soon as four to six weeks after the lymphoma begins to grow. The more common symptom pattern is a large tumor in the child's abdomen accompanied by fluid buildup, pain, and vomiting. If the lymphoma begins in the blood marrow, the child may bleed easily and become anemic.

In adults, the first symptoms of Burkitt's lymphoma may include swelling in a lymph node in the upper body or a swollen and painful abdomen. If the tumor is located in the chest, it may put pressure on the airway and cause difficulty in breathing. There may be unexplained **itching** or **weight loss**. Other patients may have more general symptoms, such as **fever** or a loss of energy. Adults with AIDS often have tumors developing in several different locations in the body by the time they are diagnosed.

Diagnosis

Burkitt's lymphoma is usually diagnosed by examining a piece of tissue from a surgical **biopsy** of a swollen area in the patient's body—often the jaw area in endemic Burkitt's or the abdomen in the sporadic form. The tissue is examined under a microscope by a pathologist, who is a physician with special training in the study of tissue or body fluid samples. In Burkitt's lymphoma, the tumor cells will show a very high rate of cell division and a characteristic "starry sky" pattern. The pathologist may also test the tissue sample for the presence of EBV, which is found in about 30% of patients diagnosed with Burkitt's lymphoma in the United States.

KEY TERMS

Ann Arbor system—A system of tumor staging used to classify non-Hodgkin's lymphomas in adults. It specifies four stages, which can be further defined by the use of letters to identify general physical symptoms and the parts of the body affected by the lymphoma. The corresponding staging system in children is the St. Jude Children's Research Hospital system.

B-cell—A type of lymphocyte that produces antibodies. Burkitt's lymphoma is a cancer of the immune system in which the B-cells multiply at an extremely fast rate.

Endemic—Natural to or characteristic of a specific place. In central Africa, Burkitt's lymphoma is an endemic disease.

Epstein-Barr virus (EBV)—A type of herpesvirus (human herpesvirus 4), first identified in 1964, that causes infectious mononucleosis. It is found in most patients with the endemic form of Burkitt's lymphoma, though its role in the disease is still unclear.

International Prognostic Index (IPI)—A system for predicting the prognosis of lymphoma patients on the basis of five factors.

Intrathecal chemotherapy—A form of treatment in which the drug is injected directly into the patient's spinal fluid. It is given to prevent a lymphoma from spreading to the brain and spinal cord, or to treat one that has already spread.

Lymphatic system—The system of glands, tissues, and vessels in the body that produces lymphocytes and circulates them through the body in a clear, yellowish fluid called lymph.

Lymphocyte—A type of white blood cell involved in the production of antibodies.

Monoclonal antibody—An antibody produced in the laboratory from a cloned cell rather than in the body.

Non-Hodgkin's lymphoma (NHL)—One of two major subdivisions of lymphomas. Burkitt's lymphoma is a subcategory of NHL.

Oncogene—A gene that causes the uncontrolled cell growth characteristic of cancer.

Sporadic—Occurring in isolated or scattered instances. Burkitt's lymphoma is a sporadic disease in most countries.

Translocation—The movement of a gene or group of genes from one chromosome to another. Burkitt's lymphoma is associated with a genetic translocation.

In addition to a tissue biopsy, the patient is also given a complete blood count (CBC) test, a platelet count, and a **lumbar puncture** (spinal tap). A small sample of bone marrow is usually taken as well. Most cases of Burkitt's lymphoma do not require extensive x rays, although CT (**computed tomography**) scans of the chest and abdomen are usually taken, as well as a **gallium scan**. This scan involves being injected with the radioactive isotope gallium, which is attracted to cancerous cells. Thus, when technicians scan images the body, they are able to pinpoint those cells.

Treatment team

Because cancer in children and adolescents is rare, young people with cancer should be referred to pediatric cancer centers with multidisciplinary teams that specialize in treating cancers in this age group. The specialty teams usually include primary care doctors, pediatric oncologists (pediatricians who specialize in the treatment of **childhood cancers**), radiation oncologists, social workers, pediatric nurses, and rehabilitation specialists.

Adult AIDS patients who develop Burkitt's lymphoma require specialists in treating HIV infection on their treatment team as well as oncologists, radiologists, and nursing specialists.

Clinical staging, treatments, and prognosis

Staging

The most common system of staging for non-Hodgkin's lymphomas in adults, including Burkitt's lymphoma, is the Ann Arbor system. It specifies four stages as follows:

- Stage I: The lymphoma is either limited to one group of lymph nodes either above or below the diaphragm, or is in an organ or part of the body other than the lymph nodes, but has not spread to other organs or lymph nodes.
- Stage II: The lymphoma is either in two or more lymph node groups on the same side of the diaphragm, or is in only one organ or site other than the lymph nodes but has spread to the lymph nodes near that organ or site.

- Stage III: The lymphoma is present in groups of lymph nodes on both sides of the diaphragm. It may involve an organ or site outside the lymph nodes, the spleen, or both.
- Stage IV: The lymphoma is disseminated (spread) throughout one or more organs outside the lymph nodes. There may or may not be involvement of lymph nodes that are remote from the affected organs.

At each stage, the patient's condition may be described in more detail by using letters to denote the presence of specific general symptoms and/or the body organs that have been affected by the disease. A is used to designate patients who do not have general symptoms; B is used for patients with any of the following:

- unexplained loss of more than 10% of body weight in the last six months
- unexplained fever higher than 38 degrees C (101 degrees F)
- drenching night sweats

The letter E is added if the patient has developed malignancies outside the lymph nodes in areas of the body other than the lymphatic system. Other sites in the body are identified with additional letters, such as D for the skin or H for the liver.

The most commonly used staging system for NHL in children is that of the St. Jude's Children's Research Hospital. It separates patients with a single tumor or diseased lymph node (Stage I) or two or more tumors or diseased lymph nodes on the same side of the diaphragm (Stage II) from those with a large chest or abdominal tumor (Stage III) or involvement of the bone marrow and central nervous system (Stage IV).

Treatment

Because of the rapid rate of tumor growth in this lymphoma, it is important to begin treatment as soon as possible after diagnosis. Bulky abdominal tumors or chest tumors are sometimes removed surgically before the patient begins **chemotherapy**.

Children with Burkitt's lymphoma are treated with chemotherapy and **radiation therapy**. The drug used most often to treat endemic Burkitt's is **cyclophosphamide** (Cytoxan), a drug that suppresses the immune system but has severe side effects. It may be given orally or intravenously. Radiation therapy is used to treat lymphomas that affect the jaw and the area around the eyes. Children with sporadic Burkitt's are treated with a short course of high-dose chemotherapy, usually cyclophosphamide in combination with **methotrexate** (MTX), **vincristine** (Oncovin), prednisone (Meticorten), and **doxorubicin** (Adriamycin). To prevent the spread of the lymphoma to the central nervous system, the patient's head and spine may be treated with radiation therapy and intrathecal methotrexate. In intrathecal chemotherapy, the drug is injected directly into the patient's spinal fluid.

Adults with sporadic Burkitt's lymphoma are treated with a combination of radiation therapy and chemotherapy. A newer high-dose chemotherapy regimen called CODOX-M/IVAC, which is a combination of cyclophosphamide, vincristine, doxorubicin, methotrexate, **ifosfamide** (Ifex), **etoposide** (VePesid), and **cytarabine** (ARA-C), appears to produce good results. Adults with AIDS are usually given low-dose chemotherapy because their immune systems are already damaged. They do not respond as well to treatment as patients without HIV infection.

Newer methods of treatment include bone marrow or stem cell transplantation and **monoclonal antibodies** (antibodies produced by cloned mouse cells grown in a laboratory). One monoclonal antibody, **rituximab** (Rituxan), has been approved by the FDA for treatment of non-Hodgkin's lymphomas, including Burkitt's lymphoma. **Clinical trials** in France indicate that rituximab combined with standard chemotherapy improves the rates of remission and survival in high-risk patients.

Prognosis

The prognosis for children with Burkitt's lymphoma is generally good, as this type of lymphoma responds well to chemotherapy. Children with African Burkitt's often show a significant improvement after only one dose of cyclophosphamide. In the United States, 80% of children treated for early-stage Burkitt's lymphoma remain free from relapse three years after treatment. The newer CODOX-M/IVAC combination chemotherapy has been credited with a cure rate above 90% in both children and adults.

The prognosis for adults depends on a number of factors. In recent years, the International Prognostic Index, or IPI, has been used to predict a specific patient's chance of recurrence and length of survival on the basis of five factors. Each of the following factors is given one point:

- age over 60 years
- the lymphoma is classified as Stage III or Stage IV
- the lymphoma has spread to more than one site outside the lymph nodes
- high levels of lactate dehydrogenase (an enzyme used to measure tumor burden)
- poor general health

An IPI score of 0 or 1 is associated with a 70% rate of disease-free survival at the end of five years and an overall survival rate of 73% at the end of five years. An IPI score of 5, on the other hand, is associated with five-year rates of 40% disease-free survival and 26% overall survival respectively.

In patients with AIDS, the factors that affect the prognosis include: the CD4 lymphocyte count; the presence of opportunistic infections (AIDS-defining illnesses); involvement of the bone marrow; spread of the lymphoma beyond the lymph nodes; age; and the patient's overall strength. A history of opportunistic infections, a CD4 count below 200, age above 35, and being too weak to walk indicate a poor prognosis. The average length of survival of HIV-positive patients with Burkitt's lymphoma is six months.

Alternative and complementary therapies

Alternative and complementary treatments that have been reported as helpful to lymphoma patients include yoga, therapeutic massage, meditation, creative visualization, acupuncture, Reiki, journaling, and art therapy.

Coping with cancer treatment

Adults being treated for Burkitt's lymphoma are most likely to be affected by the side effects of chemotherapy (nausea, hair loss, etc.). Patients with AIDS have the additional concern of increased vulnerability to other AIDS-related infections (**thrush**, **pneumonia**, etc.).

Children

Children being treated for Burkitt's lymphoma share many of the concerns of children with other types of cancer, such as changes in appearance (hair loss caused by chemotherapy), continuing a normal schedule (school, sports participation), and coping with such other side effects of treatment as nausea or **fatigue**. One useful resource is the Candlelighters programs, which offer support and practical information to the parents of children with cancer.

Clinical trials

As of 2001, 39 clinical trials of treatments for AIDS-related lymphomas in adults were being conducted at research centers in the United States. Because Burkitt's lymphoma is relatively rare in children, the National Cancer Institute (NCI) requests that all children with Burkitt's (or other non-Hodgkin's lymphomas) be considered as possible subjects for clinical trials. Information about current clinical trials is available at (800) 4-CANCER or <http://www.cancernet.nci.nih.gov/trialsrch>.

Prevention

Prevention of the endemic form of Burkitt's lymphoma is complicated by the high incidence of malaria in central Africa combined with inadequate medical care. In other countries, some risk factors associated with the sporadic form can be lowered, most particularly lifestyle behaviors that increase the risk of HIV infection. In addition, patients with Burkitt's lymphoma may want to consider genetic counseling because of the role of the C-*myc* oncogene in their disorder.

QUESTIONS TO ASK THE DOCTOR

- Should I consider bone marrow transplant or monoclonal antibodies as treatment options?
- What are the best treatment options in case of a relapse?
- (for AIDS patients) How can I best protect myself against AIDS-related infections during chemotherapy for Burkitt's lymphoma?

Special concerns

Patients diagnosed with Burkitt's lymphoma should be followed up at regular intervals after chemotherapy because of the possibility of long-term relapse. Follow-up examinations should include a general physical examination, a complete blood count, and radiologic examinations.

See also AIDS-related cancers; Alopecia; Chromosome rearrangements; nausea and vomiting.

Resources

BOOKS

Dollinger, Malin, MD, Ernest H. Rosenbaum, MD, and Greg Cable. *Cancer Therapy.* Kansas City, MO: Andrews and McMeel, 1994.

"Hematology and Oncology." In *The Merck Manual of Diagnosis and Therapy*, edited by Mark H. Beers, MD, and Robert Berkow, MD. Whitehouse Station, NJ: Merck Research Laboratories, 1999.

Kabat-Zinn, Jon. *Full Catastrophe Living: Using the Wisdom of Your Body and Mind to Face Stress, Pain, and Illness.* New York: Dell Publishing, 1990. A useful resource on mindfulness meditation in pain control and living with cancer.

Lyon, Jeff, and Peter Gorner. *Altered Fates: Gene Therapy and the Retooling of Human Life.* New York and London: W. W. Norton & Co., Inc., 1996.

PERIODICALS

Burkitt, Denis P. "The Discovery of Burkitt's lymphoma." *Cancer* (May 15, 1983): 1777-86.

ORGANIZATIONS

American Cancer Society (ACS). 1599 Clifton Road, NE, Atlanta, GA 30329. (404) 320-3333 or (800) ACS-2345. Fax: (404) 329-7530. <http://www.cancer.org>.

Candlelighters Childhood Cancer Foundation. 7910 Woodmont Avenue, Suite 460, Bethesda, MD 20814. (301) 657-8401 or (800) 366-CCCF.

National Cancer Institute, Office of Cancer Communications. 31 Center Drive, MSC 2580, Bethesda, MD 20892-2580. (800) 4-CANCER. TTY: (800) 332-8615. <http://www.nci.nih.gov>.

NIH National Center for Complementary and Alternative Medicine (NCCAM) Clearinghouse. P.O. Box 8218, Silver Spring, MD 20907-8218. TTY/TDY: (888) 644-6226. Fax: (301) 495-4957.

OTHER

Lymphoma Information Network 21 June 2001 <http://www.lymphomainfo.net>.

Oncology Channel 21 June 2001 <http://www.oncology channel.com>.

Rebecca J. Frey, Ph.D.

Buserelin

Definition

Buserelin is a synthetic analog of natural gonadotropin-releasing hormone and is used to treat **prostate cancer**. Buserelin, also called buserelin acetate, is sold under the brand name Suprefact in Canada. It is not commercially available in the U.S. for human use.

Purpose

Androgens, particularly **testosterone**, appear to play a major role in prostate cancer. Buserelin inhibits production of luteinizing hormone from the pituitary gland which decreases the levels of testosterone. Prostate cancer is often sensitive to testosterone levels, thus, a reduction in testosterone may influence the rate of cancer growth progression and affect the size of the tumor. Hormone therapy with buserelin cannot cure prostate cancer but may decrease symptoms and improve the quality of life for most patients.

Breast cancer may also treated with buserelin. A research study examined combined treatment with buserelin and **tamoxifen** in women with premenopausal metastatic breast cancer. Together, these drugs were more effective and resulted in longer overall survival than treatment with either drug alone.

Description

Buserelin indirectly decreases the testosterone levels in the body. Testosterone is produced in the testes and the adrenal glands, but the testes will only produce testosterone if adequate levels of luteinizing hormone are present. Buserelin reduces the production of luteinizing hormone, thus causing a drop in testosterone levels. When buserelin administration is started, a brief increase in the hormone levels in the first few days or weeks may occur.

Recommended dosage

Two dosage forms of buserelin are available. Either as an injection (1 mg/mL multidose vial) or as an intranasal spray (100 mcg/spray).

A dose of 500 mcg (0.5 milligrams [mg]) is injected under the skin three times per day for seven days every eight hours. The doctor may lower the dose to 200 micrograms (mcg) or 0.2 mg once a day with time if required. Treatment with the nasal spray form of the drug is administered at 200 mcg, (2 sprays) into each nostril every eight hours. The doctor determines the duration of treatment.

Precautions

Buserelin induces a temporary rise in sex hormones at the start of treatment, but they usually remain within the normal range. This rise may be associated with an increase in disease symptoms in some patients. Symptoms such as **bone pain**, impaired urination, and muscular weakness in the legs may occur with the temporary increase in tumor activity. These symptoms usually ease gradually, although they can be avoided altogether by prescribing an antiandrogen such as cyproterone acetate or flutamide at the same time.

Due to these effects, it is advisable for patients to also take an antiandrogen with buserelin if a temporary increase in the size of the tumor may lead to: urinal tract obstruction, increased intracranial pressure (in rare cases with brain metastases), or paresis (slight or incomplete paralysis) due to increased pressure on the spinal cord. Antiandrogen treatment should be started about five days before buserelin and for three to four weeks along with buserelin therapy until the sex hormones have returned to an acceptable level.

Buserelin causes sterility in men and menopause in women which may be permanent. It is not known if buserelin is safe to use during pregnancy. Due to the secretion into breast milk, breast-feeding is not recommended. In addition, it is not known if buserelin is mutagenic or carcinogenic.

Alert doctors or dentists about buserelin therapy before receiving any treatment.

Side effects

Many people have very few side effects with buserelin, while others may experience more.

KEY TERMS

Androgens—A male hormone necessary for the normal sexual development of males. Some androgens are produced naturally in the body.

Antiandrogens—A drug that decreases the level of male hormones in the body. Nonsteroidal antiandrogens (eg, flutamide, bicalutamide, nilutamide) counteract the effect of testosterone within prostate cancer cells.

Luteinizing hormone—A hormone that comes from part of the brain known as the pituitary gland. The testes will only produce testosterone if adequate levels of luteinizing hormone are present.

Testosterone—A male hormone, an androgen, produced in the testes and the adrenal glands. Testosterone is responsible for many male sex characteristics such as facial hair.

Tumor—An abnormal mass of tissue that serves no purpose. Tumors may be either benign (non-cancerous) or malignant (cancerous).

The most common side effects are:

- Nasal irritation.
- Skin reaction at the injection site. The injection may be slightly uncomfortable, and redness might occur at the injection site following administration.
- Hot flushes.
- Headache (when administered through the nasal passage).
- Burning, swelling, and/or **itching** at place of injection.
- Loss of libido and impotence during treatment.
- Breast tenderness or fullness. Slight breast swelling and tenderness may occur. This side effect can be reduced with medication.
- Weight gain.
- Fatigue.
- Depressive moods.
- Feelings of sickness and **diarrhea**. They are usually mild and controlled easily.
- Dry nose (when administered through the nasal passage).
- Tumor flare. Because buserelin may temporarily increase testosterone levels for the first few days or weeks of treatment, an increase in symptoms may be experienced. Serious disease flare reactions may occur such as an increase in bone pain, **spinal cord compression**, or urinary tract obstruction.
- Thrombosis with pulmonary embolism.
- Calcium loss in the skeleton (women).

Interactions

There are no known interactions between buserelin and any other medication reported to date.

Crystal Heather Kaczkowski, M.S.

Busulfan

Definition

Busulfan (also known by the brand name Myleran) is a **chemotherapy** medicine used to treat cancer by destroying cancerous cells.

Purpose

Busulfan is approved by the Food and Drug Administration (FDA) to treat chronic myelogenous leukemia (also called **chronic myelocytic leukemia**). It has also been less commonly used for other acute leukemias and a blood disease known as polycythemia vera, in which there are too many red blood cells. Busulfan is also used in combination with other chemotherapy drugs for a procedure known as **bone marrow transplantation**.

Description

Busulfan a member of the group of chemotherapy drugs known as alkylating agents. Alkylating agents interfere with the genetic material (DNA) inside the cancer cells and prevent them from further dividing and producing more cancer cells. Busulfan is taken orally and comes in tablet form.

Recommended dosage

Busulfan can be taken following several different dosing schedules, depending on the disease. Busulfan is a 2mg oral tablet, and patients may need to take more than one tablet at a time depending on the dose. The induction or starting dose is 4mg up to 12mg per day. This may then be decreased to 1mg to 3mg per day as a maintenance dose. The dose of busulfan for use in combination with other chemotherapy drugs before a bone

KEY TERMS

Anemia—A red blood cell count that is lower than normal

Bone marrow transplant—A procedure that destroys all of a patients' diseased bone marrow and replaces it with healthy bone marrow

Cataract—Formation on the lens of the eye that causes cloudy vision

Chemotherapy—Specific drugs used to treat cancer

Food and Drug Administration—A government agency that oversees public safety in relation to drugs and medical devices

Gout—A disease caused by a buildup of uric acid in the joints causing pain

Hemoglobin—A respiratory pigment in the red blood cells that combines with and transports oxygen around the body

Intravenous—To enter the body through a vein

Metastatic—Cancer that has spread to one or more parts of the body

Neutropenia—A white blood cell count that is lower than normal

Polycythemia vera—A blood disease in which too many red blood cells exist in the body

Thalassemia—A genetic form of anemia that prevents affected individuals from synthesizing hemoglobin properly

marrow transplant is much larger than leukemia dosing. Busulfan, when used for bone marrow transplants, is dosed by patient body weight. Busulfan is usually given at a dose of 4mg per kilogram of body weight each day for 4 days before **bone marrow transplantation**.

Precautions

Blood counts are monitored regularly while on busulfan therapy. During a certain period of time after receiving busulfan, there is an increased risk of contracting infections. Caution should be taken to avoid unnecessary exposure to bacteria and viruses. All patients should increase their daily fluid intake while receiving this drug.

Patients who are pregnant or are trying to become pregnant should notify their physician before taking busulfan (or any chemotherapy medication). Busulfan causes a high incidence of sterility in males, and has been known to cause sterility in females as well.

Patients with a known previous allergic reaction to chemotherapy drugs, or who suffer from gout, thalassemia, or seizure problems, should notify their physician before beginning treatment. The physician should also be consulted before receiving live virus **vaccines** while on chemotherapy.

Side effects

The most common side effect expected from taking busulfan is low blood counts, referred to as **myelosuppression**. Lowering of the white count, or **neutropenia**, is common and lasts for some time before the white count returns to normal levels. When the white blood cell count is low, patients are at an increased risk of developing a **fever** and infections. The platelet blood count can also be decreased due to busulfan administration. Platelets are blood cells in the body that cause clots to form; the purpose of these clots is to control bleeding. When the platelet count is low, patients are at an increased risk for both bruising and bleeding. If the platelet count remains too low, a platelet blood transfusion may be an option for treatment. Busulfan also causes low red blood cell counts, or **anemia**. Low red counts make patients feel tired, dizzy, and fatigued. **Erythropoietin** is a drug that can be used to increase red blood cell count.

In bone marrow transplant patients, the dose of busulfan that is given in combination with other chemotherapy drugs is intended to cause complete bone marrow destruction prior to bone marrow transplant.

Nausea, vomiting, loss of appetite, mouth sores, and **diarrhea** are rare side effects from busulfan at normal doses, but are common at the higher doses used for bone marrow transplant. If **nausea and vomiting** are a problem, patients can be given medications known as **antiemetics** before receiving busulfan to help prevent or decrease these side effects. Taking busulfan on an empty stomach may also decrease nausea and vomiting.

Damage to nerves and nervous system tissues is uncommon with standard busulfan therapy. However, at high doses, some reports do exist of seizures, dizziness, confusion, and visual disturbances.

Busulfan can also cause severe lung problems known as "busulfan lung". Symptoms include a nonstop cough, shortness of breath, fever, and difficulty breathing.

Less common side effects caused by busulfan include skin rashes or reactions (including darkening of the skin), dryness of the skin, **itching**, and hair loss (**alopecia**).

Although it is uncommon, severe liver problems may occur due to busulfan administration at higher doses. Rare reactions to busulfan include: lung problems, cataracts, fatigue, heart problems, low blood pressure, development of another type of cancer or leukemia, enlarged breast tissue (referred to as gynecomastia), and increased uric acid levels (which can lead to kidney problems and gout).

Any side effects experienced by a patient should be reported to the physician.

Interactions

Busulfan used for transplant purposes, when given in high doses with the chemotherapy drug **cyclophosphamide**, caused an increase in serious heart problems.

Patients who have taken busulfan with the drug **thioguanine** over long periods of time have shown an increase in enlarged veins in the esophagus and liver problems.

Nancy J. Beaulieu, RPh.,BCOP

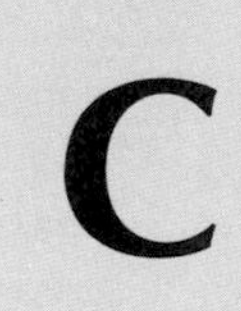

Calcitonin

Definition

Calcitonin is a hormone involved in regulating calcium metabolism. The hormone calcitonin is produced by the thyroid gland. A synthetic human product is available.

Purpose

Calcitonin is often ordered for cancer patients experiencing **bone pain** due to **metastasis**. Calcitonin is also used to treat Paget's disease, post-menopausal osteoporosis and increased levels of calcium in the blood.

Description

Calcitonin reduces breakdown of bone. It causes less bone tissue to be reabsorbed. It slows the rate of bone destruction and decreases the amount of calcium released into the blood. Most calcitonin ordered for patients is derived from salmon. Calcitonin is not effective when given orally, and is available for injection or in a nasal spray. It is sold under the brand name Calcimar in the United States.

Recommended dosage

The usual dose for patients receiving Calcitonin-salmon for bone metastases is 200 IU given through the vein twice daily. It is important to take this drug exactly as ordered. If a dose is missed and is noticed within two hours, the drug should be taken. If it is not noted until later, the patient should skip the dose and return to the regular schedule. Patients should not take additional or double doses. When using calcitonin to lower calcium levels, therapy is limited to approximately 5 days. Extended use of calcitonin results in a loss of effect at lowering the calcium.

Precautions

Calcitonin-salmon solution should be stored in the refrigerator, not frozen. Patients should allow a new bottle of nasal spray to warm to room temperature. It may be kept at room temperature for two to four weeks. The nasal spray pump should be primed before using. Patients should push the plunger until a mist is observed. This usually occurs within several pushes. Before using, the patient should blow his or her nose. The patient should alternate nostrils with each dose. The head should be kept upright. The pump should be pressed toward the bottle one time. The patient should not inhale when spraying. The patient should then inhale through the nose and exhale through the mouth. The nosepiece should be wiped clean after each use. Patients giving themselves an injection should check that the contents are clear. Patients should not inject medication that is colored or grainy.

Calcitonin should be used cautiously when breast feeding, as it may decrease the amount of available milk. Its use during pregnancy has not been adequately studied. However, animal studies indicated a risk for low birth weight offspring.

Side effects

Calcitonin is a protein. It may cause a severe allergic reaction. The doctor should be notified if a rash or hives develop. Patients should have supplies on hand to manage an allergic reaction. Skin testing may be done prior to treatment. Allergic reactions are rarer in the human product than in the salmon product.

Diarrhea, red skin, poor appetite, nausea, vomiting, stomach pain, and back and joint pain are common side effects. Other side effects include increased or decreased appetite, gas, constipation, or an unusual taste in the mouth. Nausea is usually mild and temporary. Giving calcitonin at bedtime may decrease **nausea and vomiting**. Patients may experience dizziness, difficulty sleeping, anxiety, headache, agitation, palpitations, or other

KEY TERMS

Osteoporosis—Disease causing bone tissue to become brittle.

Paget's disease—Chronic inflammation of the bone, with the bones becoming thinner and softer. Long bones bow.

heart problems. Redness, swelling and soreness may occur at the injection site. Patients using the nasal spray may develop crusting or patches in the nose, as well as nasal dryness, redness, swelling or irritation. Less often, those using the nasal spray may experience difficulty with urination, breathing problems, loss of smell, or cold symptoms. Some patients injecting the drug may develop frequent urination, chills, dizziness, headache, chest pressure, a congested nose, tingling or discomfort in the hands and feet, difficulty breathing or weakness. Patients should notify the doctor if side effects occur. Side effects may subside as the patient's body becomes accustomed to the drug. Patients should receive regular medical checks and lab work to assess for adverse reactions and changes in urine content.

Interactions

At present, there are no known interactions with other drugs.

Debra Wood, RN

Cancer biology

Definition

Cancer is the second leading cause of death in the United States, with one out of every three Americans falling victim to it at some point in their lives. It is a disease of unregulated cell growth. The knowledge gained in cancer biology over the past 20 years has allowed for the discovery of new, highly targeted drugs to treat cancer.

Causes of cancer

The molecular cause of cancer involves mutations in the nuclear DNA (the genetic material in cells) that can be caused by chemicals, viruses, radiation or spontaneous mutations. Although much importance has been put on chemicals and environmental pollutants as carcinogens (agents that cause cancer), it actually turns out that the predominant factors in determining cancer are associated with lifestyle. For instance, cigarette smoking accounts for 30% of cancers in males. Dietary factors are associated with another 35% of all human cancers. It is estimated that with dietary improvements there could be a 50% reduction in colon and rectal cancers, a 25% reduction in **breast cancer** and 15% reductions each in prostate, endometrial and gallbladder cancers. Other cancers that might be decreased by dietary improvements include cancer of the stomach, esophagus, pancreas, ovaries, liver, lung and urinary bladder. This adds up to 9% reduction in overall deaths. It is estimated that if Americans doubled their intake of fruits and vegetables and fiber and decreased their fat intake by 25%, significant advances could be made. Obesity also puts an individual at an increased risk of death for uterus, gallbladder, kidney, stomach, colon, and breast cancers. Obese women have a 55% greater risk of mortality from cancer than women of normal weight, while men are at a 33% greater risk of mortality. Alcohol and lack of exercise are also associated with increased risk for cancer.

Cell growth

Normal growth of cells is a highly regulated cellular function. The stimulus to begin cell division comes from growth factors that react with growth factor receptors on the surface of the cell. After the binding of growth factor to a growth factor receptor, the growth message is carried from the surface of the cell to the nucleus through a cascade of biochemical reactions referred to as signal transduction. Once the signal reaches the nucleus, transcription factors bind to the DNA, which turns on the production of proteins involved in growth and division of the cells.

DNA contains genetic information that encodes proteins involved in all aspects of cell metabolism. If a gene is damaged or mutated, the protein it encodes will be affected. DNA mutations can result in an altered expression of protein; either too much or too little, or in altered forms of a protein that either do not perform their function or perform it differently. Damage to genes that encode for proteins regulating cell growth such as oncogenes, tumor suppressor genes and DNA repair genes can result in alterations in cell growth and thus cancer.

Oncogenes

Oncogenes are altered forms of normal genes called proto-oncogenes. There have been over 100 oncogenes identified so far. Their primary role in the cell is in regulation of growth. They encode growth factors, growth factor receptors, transcription factors that regulate the manufacturing of new proteins and signal transduction proteins. Signal transduction refers to the process of transmitting a signal from the outside layer of the cell, through the cytoplasm into the nucleus of the cell and begins with a growth factor and receptor interaction. Cancer cells sometimes have altered levels of growth factors or their receptors or factors involved in signal transduction. For example, the K-*ras* oncogene is an example of a mutated signal transduction protein involved in cancers such as colon and lung cancer, and the HER2/neu oncogene is a mutated receptor associated with breast cancer. Finally, this series of biochemical reactions reaches the nucleus to affect gene transcription, or the reading of genes into RNA and protein. This occurs via transcription factors. Mutations in transcription factors result in abnormal levels of certain proteins that can result in cancer. *Myc* is an example of a transcription factor mutated in lung cancer.

Tumor suppressor genes

Also called anti-oncogenes, tumor suppressor genes code for proteins that halt cell growth. In the normal cell, when DNA has become damaged, the cell stops growing to devote time to repairing DNA. Factors responsible for allowing this repair to take place are tumor suppressor genes. If tumor suppressor genes malfunction, the cells do not stop dividing when DNA is damaged and the mutation is then carried over to the daughter cells after cell division. This increases the risk of developing cancer. In hereditary cancers it is often a malfunctioning tumor suppressor gene that is inherited. Although there are two copies of each tumor suppressor gene, the second gene can take over the role if it is not mutated. A mutation in the second copy of the gene is required for total loss of tumor suppressor function. There are dozens of tumor suppressor genes identified that are involved in cancer including p53 (identified with many cancers) and APC in **colon cancer**, and BRCA-1 in breast cancer.

Characteristics of cancer cells

Cancer cells appear differently than normal cells do under the microscope. Their nucleus is much larger than in normal cells, their chromosomes are irregular in distribution and the nucleoli in the nucleus are very prominent. When cancer cells are grown in culture in the lab they also appear different than normal cells. Rather than growing in neat single-layer sheets with one next to the other they grow more haphazardly. They have long processes that extend from the cells, they overlap one another and their shape is more rounded. Normal cells will continue to divide and grow in a culture plate until they touch a neighboring cell where they receive a signal to stop growing. Cancer cells, on the other hand, do not receive this signal and grow on top of each other forming piles of growing cells that resemble a tumor.

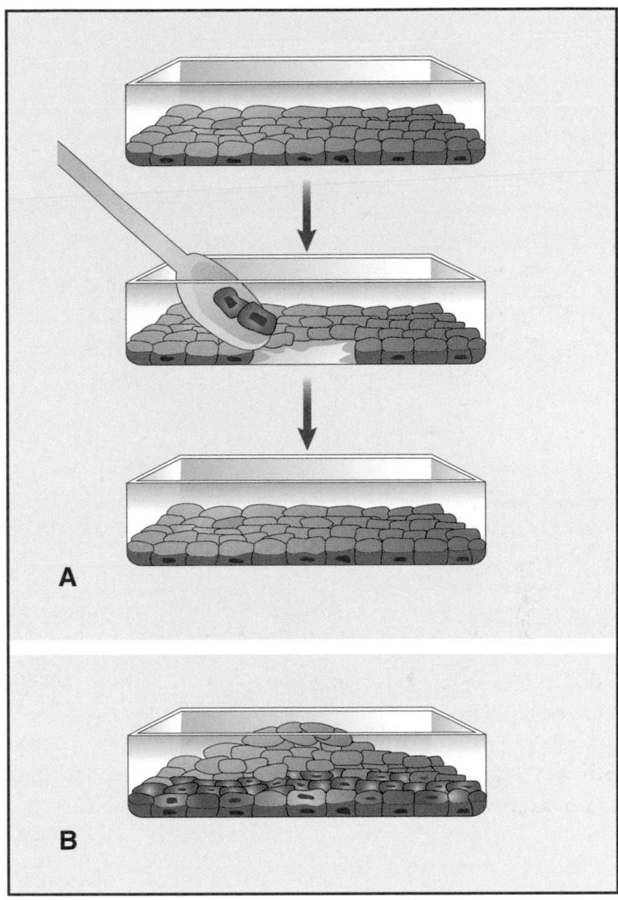

A. When normal cells in a culture plate are scraped away, the cells on the plate divide to replace them. The cells on the plate grow until they touch a neighboring cell and receive a signal to stop growing. B. Cancer cells do not receive this signal and grow on top of each other, forming piles of cells, or tumors. *(Illustration by Argosy Publishing.)*

Normal cells require growth factors added to their growth medium to enable them to grow in culture. Cancer cells do not require the same amount of growth factors, possibly because they are able make their own growth factors. Normal human cells will grow for a short amount of time in culture and then die, while cancer cells tend to keep on growing. The term given for this ability is immortalization. Cancer cells in culture are immortalized or have unlimited growth potential.

Cancer cells also have a more immature appearance compared to normal cells. This is referred to as dedifferentiation, or they lack differentiation. As an embryo matures and develops, its cells differentiate. This means they take on more specific roles that are reflected in their appearance—kidney cells begin to look different than

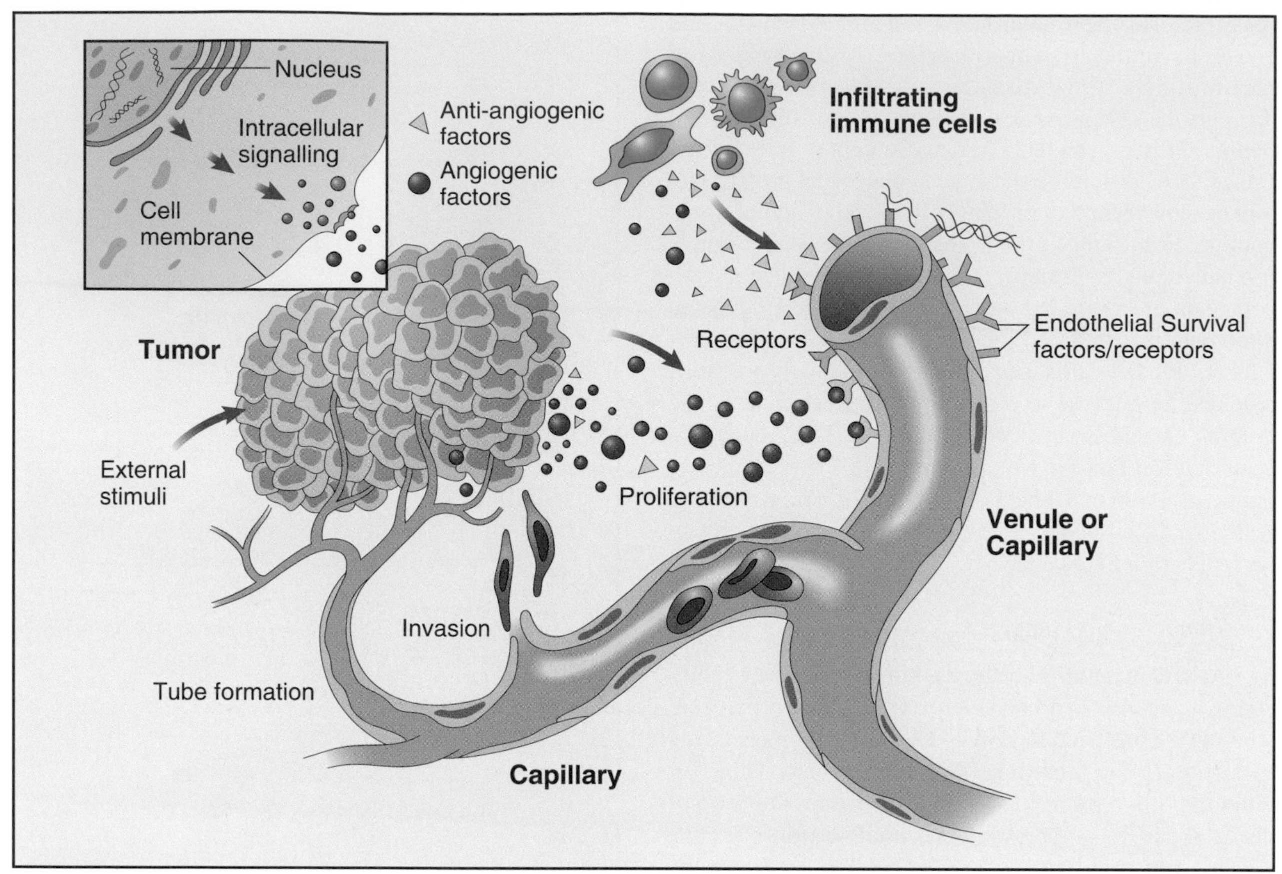

Angiogenesis. To keep up with the demand for blood vessels, the tumor releases factors called angiogenic factors. (An individual tumor cell is shown in the inset.) These factors initiate the growth of more blood vessels into the tumor. The rich supply of blood vessels also gives the tumor more opportunity to metastasize (spread) to distant sites by traveling through the blood. *(Illustration by Argosy Publishing.)*

skin cells or breast cells. Cancer cells look less and less like the tissue they are part of and more like embryonic cells. They also produce embryonic proteins that are used as **tumor markers** such as carcinoembryonic antigen (CEA) and alpha fetoprotein (AFP).

Pathology

Tumors are either malignant or benign depending upon their invasiveness. Benign tumors are less aggressive, less likely to invade the surrounding tissue, less likely to metastasize (spread) and are slower growing. Although it sounds as if they pose no threat to the individual, this is not always the case. A tumor in the brain especially can be life threatening and put pressure on the brain as it grows. A benign tumor may also secrete hormones that in high levels can be toxic to the individual.

A malignant tumor is more aggressive, more invasive into the surrounding tissue, faster growing and more likely to metastasize. Malignant tumors usually kill the individual if they are not removed. The diagnosis as to whether a tumor is benign or malignant is done on a small sample of the tumor, called a **biopsy**. A pathologist will microscopically examine a thin, stained slice of the tissue. The tumor is graded, or given a number from 1 - 4 that corresponds to its degree of malignancy, with 4 being the most malignant and 1 being benign. The more malignant the tumor, the less organized the cells of the tissue are and the more anaplastic or dedifferentiated they appear.

The tumor is also staged which refers to the amount it has spread. This is done both by gross examination of the patient and by microscopic examination of the tissue. The staging relates to the patient's prognosis. The best prognosis is if the tumor is confined to the epithelial layer of an organ and not spread into the basement membrane. The prognosis is worse if the tumor cells have spread to adjacent lymph nodes. As a tumor grows, it becomes capable of both invasion and **metastasis**.

An organ of the body consists of epithelial cells that are supported by a basement membrane. (Epithelial cells are cells that form the tissue that covers internal and external surfaces of the body and is found on skin and mucosal surfaces.) The basement membranes separate the epithelial cells from connective tissues that are rich in blood vessels. As the tumor enlarges, it can grow into the surrounding tissue, through the basement membrane and into blood or lymph vessels. This is a critical point in the growth of a tumor. Now, a small piece of tumor can break off and travel through the circulation until it receives a signal to attach to the vessel wall. It can then move through the vessel, into the tissue bed, where it grows to become a secondary tumor. This is termed metastasis. Two common locations for metastasizing tumors are the lungs and the liver.

Cancer can also involve the immune system and individuals with weakened immune systems are often at increased risk for developing cancer. AIDS patients, for example, are at increased risk for developing some cancers, such as **Kaposi's sarcoma**. As a cell becomes cancerous, it develops different antigens on its cell surface that should be recognized by the immune system and removed. For some reason, the immune system does not remove tumors. Probably, many cancer cells do develop in the body that are identified and removed by the immune system. It is not understood why this happens occasionally but not consistently. There have been documented cases of spontaneous tumor regression which may be due to activation of the immune system.

These unique antigens expressed on the surface of cancer cells can be used to the patient's advantage in treating cancer. **Monoclonal antibodies** are proteins produced in the laboratory from a single clone of a B cell, the type of cells of the immune system that make antibodies. Antibodies, also known as immunoglobulins, are proteins that help identify foreign substances to the immune system, such as bacteria or a virus. Antibodies work by binding to the foreign substance to mark it as foreign. The substance that the antibody binds to is called an antigen. Monoclonal antibodies that can recognize and attach to the specific antigens found on cancer cells are now being used to target cancer cells directly.

Unfortunately, cancer may go undiagnosed until it is quite advanced. This is because the body has many ways to adapt itself to damage and so symptoms are reduced for some time. Metastasis may be present by the time cancer is diagnosed. Symptoms of cancer include pain emanating from the organ being stretched, as well as **fever** and weakness. As the disease progresses, cachexia (the wasting that occurs due to starvation and debilitation caused by the cancer) may occur. The patient becomes unable to mount an anti-inflammatory response and infections occur. These infections become the cause of death in most cancer patients.

Factors that favor the progression of cancer

Genetic susceptibility
Age
Mutations
Abnormal cell growth
Aneuploidy (abnormal numbers of chromosomes)
Growth and survival factors
Angiogenesis
Loss of heterozygosity (Having only one version of a gene instead of the usual two different versions)
Gene amplification

Carcinogenesis

How does a cancer cell become a cancer cell? Most scientists agree that cancer is a "multi-hit" process—a process that requires a series of genetic mutations that occur either spontaneously, are inherited or are caused by specific carcinogens. There are several stages in the development of cancer: initiation, promotion and progression.

- Initiation. During initiation, a carcinogen interacts with and damages the DNA. Repair can occur after this point and the process can be reversed.
- Promotion. Promotion causes reproduction or proliferation of these damaged cells, forming a mass of cells or a benign **adenoma**. This stage is still reversible and removal of the promoting agent can stop the expansion of the tumor mass.
- Progression. Progression, however, is irreversible and involves a number of sequential mutations in genes including oncogenes and tumor suppressor genes. The end result of progression is a late adenoma that eventually converts to a malignant carcinoma.

This entire process can take 20 years or more.

A specific multistep **carcinogenesis** scheme has been outlined for colon cancer that involves the following sequence of events:

- mutation of the APC tumor suppressor gene causing loss of its function
- activation of the K-*ras* oncogene
- loss of function of the DCC ("Deleted for Colon Cancer") tumor suppressor gene followed by loss of function of the p53 tumor suppressor gene

Such defining of the process of carcinogenesis can identify tumor markers used for diagnosis and monitoring of cancers. Also, an understanding of pathways involved in carcinogenesis can provide information to better design and target drugs, making them more specific to decrease their effects on normal cells. Information

Factors that help to protect the body from cancer

Genetic resistance
Nutrition
Metabolism
DNA repair
Tumor suppressor genes
Cell differentiation
Death of damaged tissue
Programmed cell death
Immune system

gained on carcinogenesis pathways can also be used to research targets for gene replacement therapy.

Angiogenesis

As the tumor grows, its need for a blood supply increases. A tumor larger than 1 mm diameter (0.03 in) cannot continue to grow without access to circulation. Blood supplies the nutrients the tumor requires and can remove the toxic metabolites that are built up in the tumor tissue. To keep up with the demand for blood vessels, the tumor releases factors called angiogenic factors. One such factor is termed vascular endothelial growth factor (VEGF). These factors initiate the growth of more blood vessels into the tumor. This process of increased blood vessel growth is termed angiogenesis. The rich supply of blood vessels also gives the tumor more opportunity to metastasize to distant sites by traveling through the blood. Using drugs that can block angiogenesis is a newly developing field of cancer treatment.

Apoptosis

Apoptosis is a way the organism has of removing genetically damaged cells from itself to prevent cancer. It is different from another process of death called necrosis where damaged tissue dies for various reasons. When DNA damage occurs to the cell, the body has many opportunities to repair this damage and thus to prevent cancer. If the DNA repair does not occur, however, the last chance the organism has to protect itself from cancer is to eradicate the entire cell. This programmed cell death, or selective destruction of a cell, is called apoptosis. Precancerous cells receive signals that activate this self-destruct program. Genes that are involved in apoptosis include bcl-2 (breast cancer tumor suppressor genes 1 and 2) and p53. When these genes are mutated, apoptosis is limited and the risk of a cell becoming cancerous is increased. Some anti-cancer drugs act by stimulating the apoptotic pathway.

Tumor markers

Tumor markers may be soluble factors secreted by cancer cells, altered proteins retained by cancer cells, or mutated genes in the cancer cells. They are typically identified in the blood of patients but sometimes tissue from a biopsy is necessary. Tumor markers can be used as an aid in diagnosing cancer but, more importantly, they can give information on the prognosis of the cancer and aid the clinician in determining appropriate treatment. For instance, if the tumor marker HER-2/neu associated with breast cancer is identified in a patient, specific **chemotherapy** that is directly targeted to the HER-2/neu protein can be used giving the patient a better prognosis. Some tumors secrete high levels of hormones that are used as tumor markers to help identify the cancer. For instance, choriocarcinoma (a malignancy that originates inside the uterus) produces large amounts of human chorionic gonadotropin (hCG). The presence of hCG in the blood helps identify the tumor. Other common tumor markers include prostate-specific antigen associated with **prostate cancer** and CA 125 associated with **ovarian cancer**.

Genetics

Cancer is basically thought of as a genetic disease. (That is not to say, however, that all cancers are inherited.) Genes are sequences of DNA located on chromosomes within the nucleus. The genes contain information that encodes proteins involved in all aspects of cell metabolism. Genes involved in cell growth and division are the most important in regards to cancer. These genes are oncogenes, tumor suppressor genes and DNA repair genes. Before science had the ability to identify specific genes it was noted that some cancers were associated with chromosomal abnormalities. For instance, chronic myeloid leukemia (CML) is associated with a fragmented chromosome termed the Philadelphia chromosome. The Philadelphia chromosome results from a translocation of part of chromosome 22 to chromosome 9. Using newer molecular techniques, we now know that this translocation results in a fusion between two oncogenes: *bcr* and *abl.*

We now know of many hereditary conditions that result in an increased risk of cancer. Although hereditary cancers are actually quite rare, they are notable because individuals who inherit a predisposition for cancer become afflicted with cancer at a much earlier age than those without an inherited susceptibility. Cancer results from a series of genetic mutations that may take 20 years or more to accumulate. If one of these mutations is inherited, it shortens the time for cancer to develop. Individuals with hereditary predispositions tend to get cancer at a much earlier age than those who get non-hereditary cancer.

Familial colon cancer and breast cancer are two widely known examples of inherited cancers. One percent of individuals with colon cancer has an inherited condition called familial adenomatous polyposis (FAP).

Individuals with FAP inherit a mutation of the adenomatous polyposis coli (APC) gene, a tumor suppressor gene that is involved in apoptosis. Patients with FAP tend to have many benign polyps of the colon and are likely to develop colon cancer by the age of 40. Mutation of the APC gene is an early event in non-hereditary colon cancer as well. The difference is that in non-hereditary colon cancer, this mutation is a spontaneous event, and the accumulation of mutations that result in cancer occur later in life than with hereditary colon cancer.

There are two genes associated with hereditary breast cancer, the BRCA1 gene and the BRCA2 gene. About 80% of families with cases of early onset breast cancer have mutations in the BRCA1 gene. This gene is also associated with increased risk of ovarian cancer. The BRCA2 gene, associated with hereditary breast cancer is related to ovarian cancer to a lesser extent than BRCAI. Both genes act as tumor suppressor genes.

The **Li-Fraumeni syndrome** is a hereditary syndrome that puts individuals at an increased risk for a number of cancers including breast cancer, soft tissue **sarcomas**, osteosarcomas, brain tumors, leukemias and adrenocortical carcinomas. Individuals with this syndrome have mutations in the tumor suppressor gene, p53. Mutations in this gene are associated with 50% of all cancers. The protein associated with p53 is found in the nucleus of the cell and regulates cell functions such as cell cycle, DNA repair, and apoptosis. Mutations in p53 are also noted in colon cancer.

Other hereditary cancer syndromes include **retinoblastoma** in which a mutated Rb gene is inherited and neurofibromatosis in which a mutated NF1 gene is inherited. The K-*ras* gene is an oncogene that is commonly mutated in many types of cancer including colon and lung cancer. Individuals who are part of families with high rates of these types of cancers can choose to be genetically tested to determine if they are at an elevated risk for developing cancer.

Treatment

Most cancer treatments center around three modalities, surgical removal of the tumor, radiotherapy, and chemotherapy to kill the cancer cells. If the cancer has not spread and is isolated, surgery is the best option as it can physically remove the entire tumor. The location of all tumor tissue must be able to be identified for this procedure, however. There are risks of surgery that include those associated with anesthesia and infection.

Radiation therapy uses x rays directed at the tumor to cause damage that kills the cells. Radiation therapy will also affect normal tissue that lies in the radiation field. These side effects will vary depending upon the part of the body undergoing treatment.

Chemotherapy involves using drugs that circulate through the body to affect the tumor. The first drugs that were used to treat cancer are the antimetabolite drugs such as **methotrexate** and **mercaptopurine**. These drugs were designed to interfere in cell division and kill rapidly dividing cells. Unfortunately, they cannot differentiate between rapidly dividing tumor cells and rapidly dividing normal cells. The toxic effects on non-tumor cells account for many of the side effects of chemotherapy, including loss of hair and gastrointestinal problems. Calculating the correct dosage of these drugs is very important to minimize side effects. Although these drugs cause more side effects because they are delivered to the entire body, this is the only way to treat tumors that have metastasized from the main tumor.

Knowledge gained about cancer over the past 20 years or so have brought about cancer therapies more directly targeted at proteins known to be involved in carcinogenesis. For instance, small molecules that can specifically inhibit signal transduction proteins can slow cancer growth. A new drug known as **imatinib mesylate** (formerly known as STI-571) deactivates the enzyme called tyrosine kinase, which allows the growth of **chronic myelocytic leukemia** cells.

Monoclonal antibodies can be made in the lab that are able to recognize specific antigens on cancer cells.

KEY TERMS

Anaplastic—The undifferentiated appearance common to a cancer cell.

Antisense—An RNA sequence that can prevent the synthesis of a specific protein.

Chromosomes—Structures within the nucleus of the cell that contain DNA.

Genome—All the genetic information of an organism.

Immortal—To grow and divide indefinitely.

Metastasis—Cancer growth at a secondary site.

Nucleus—The cellular compartment containing the chromosomes.

Nucleoli—Structures within the nucleus of the cell that are associated with chromosomes.

Phenotype—The physical expression of the DNA, or the appearance of an organism.

These antibodies can in turn be joined to cancer drugs and be used to deliver the drug directly to the cancer cell. Being able to deliver the cytotoxic drug to the cancer cell decreases the side effects on normal tissue.

New categories of cancer treatment have also evolved including hormone therapy and immunotherapy, also called biological therapy or biological response modifiers. Biological therapy takes advantage of the body's own immune system to recognize the cancer and remove it. Cytokines are immunoregulatory substances secreted by the cells of the immune system. Immunotherapy can use cytokines that are naturally produced by the body and affect immune cells and blood cells. These cytokines include **interferons**, interleukins and colony stimulating factors, such as **filgrastim** and **sargramostim**. For instance, interferon-alpha and interleukin-2 are now used to treat metastatic **melanoma**.

Hormonal treatment of cancer aims to interfere with some hormonal action on cancer cells. This therapy is mostly used on breast cancer and prostate cancer. Some breast cancers grow in response to estrogen. The anti-estrogen **tamoxifen** can reduce the amount of growth in breast cancer. Prostate cancer grows in response to **testosterone**. Drugs can be used to decrease the amount of testosterone produced by the testes.

Finally, gene therapy has potential to directly target genetic abnormalities found in cancer cells. The tumor suppressor protein p53 is found mutated in a large number of cancers. By introducing the appropriate DNA sequence into a cell, this protein can be replaced bringing back the ability of the cancer cell to undergo apoptosis.

Tumor growth

A tumor that can be clinically identified is typically at least one gram in size and has undergone 30 population doublings. It is before this point that tumor growth has been its fastest and now growth has slowed down significantly. This growth curve of cancer is expressed mathematically by the Gompertzian equation. According to this growth curve, most tumors originate two years before detection. Why does tumor cell growth slow down after it reaches the one-gram size? Factors that contribute to this decline in growth include lack of oxygen, decreased availability of nutrients, accumulation of toxic metabolites and lack of communication between cells.

Understanding the Gompertzian growth curve mathematics can help with decisions about cancer treatment. Most chemotherapy drugs target fast-growing cells and so they work best when a tumor is growing quickly. If at the time a tumor is detected, its cells are growing slower, then chemotherapy is less effective. If initial treatment involves surgery or radiation therapy, then the number of tumor cells will be decreased enough that cells will begin to reproduce again at a faster rate of growth. This makes chemotherapy more effective following surgery or radiation therapy to reduce the tumor load. This might also explain why some patients seem to go into remission only to have their cancer recur later. During remission, the cell number was too low to be detected, but cell growth was rapid during that period.

Many times a patient's response to chemotherapy is very good only to be followed by a relapse with a drug-resistant tumor. Combination chemotherapy, or the use of more than one drug at a time, is often more effective that single drug therapy. This is because cancer cells can spontaneously mutate and become resistant to drugs. This ability to mutate was mathematically explained by Goldie and Coldman and named the Goldie-Coldman model. This model predicts that spontaneous mutations in cancer cells that are capable of leading to **drug resistance** occur every 10,000 to 1,000,000 cell divisions. Basically this model implies that smaller tumors are less likely to be drug-resistant and are easier to cure. By treating tumors early and aggressively, the chance of recurrence with a drug-resistant cancer decreases. The combination of active drugs is also more effective in reducing the initial cancer.

This model of combination chemotherapy has proven useful in treating childhood **acute lymphocytic leukemia**, **Hodgkin's disease**, and **testicular cancer**. However, it has not proven useful in treating some solid tumors. These tumors seem to have a much higher capacity to develop drug resistance. The drugs used to treat these cancers are actually capable themselves of promoting resistance in the tumors. Resistance to one of these drugs often results in resistance to another drug and is referred to as multi-drug resistance. Multi-drug resistance is due to a decreased uptake and increased elimination of the drugs from the tumor cells. A specific pump has been identified in cancer cells that is responsible for multi-drug resistance.

Resources

BOOKS

American Cancer Society, ed: Osteen, Robert T. *Cancer Manual.* Framingham, MA: The American Cancer Society, 1996.

McKinnell, Robert G, Ralph E. Parchment, Alan O. Perantoni, and G. Barry Pierce. *The Biological Basis of Cancer.* New York: Cambridge University Press, 1998.

Templeton, Dennis J., and Robert A. Weinberg. "Principles of Cancer Biology." In *Clinical Oncology,* edited by Gerald P. Murphy, Walter Lawrence, and Raymond E. Lenhard. Atlanta, GA: The American Cancer Society, 1995.

Weinberg Robert A.*One Renegade Cell: How Cancer Begins.* New York: Basic Books, 1998.

PERIODICALS

Lowe Scott W. and Athena W. Lin. "Apoptosis in Cancer." *Carcinogenesis* 2000; 21:485-495.

Gibbs, Jackson B. "Mechanism-Based Target Identification and Drug Discovery in Cancer Research." *Science* 2000; 287:1969-1973.

Caldas, Carlos. "Science, Medicine, and the Future: Molecular Assessment of Cancer." *British Medical Journal* 1998; 316:1360-1363.

ORGANIZATIONS

American Cancer Society. 1599 Clifton Road NE, Atlanta, GA, 30329. (800) 227-2345. <http://www.cancer.org>.

American Society of Clinical Oncology. 225 Reinekers Lane, Suite 650, Alexandria, VA 22314. (703) 299-0150. <http://www.asco.org>.

National Cancer Institute. 9000 Rockville Pike, Building 31, Bethesda, MD 20892.(800) 4-CANCER. <http://www.nci.nih.gov>.

OTHER

DeNittis, Albert, Thomas J. Dilling, Joel W. Goldwein. "The Biology of Cancer." *OncoLink, University of Pennsylvania* December 21, 2000, <http://www.oncolink.upenn.edu/specialty/med_onc/nature_cancer1.htm>

Mellors, Robert C. "Etiology of Cancer: Carcinogenesis." *Neoplasia.* Weill Medical College of Cornell University, July 1999. <http://edcenter.med.cornell.edu/CUMC_PathNotes/Neoplasia/Neoplasia_04.html>

"Oncogenes and Tumor Suppressor Genes." *Cancer Resource Center, American Cancer Society* January 19, 2001, <http://www3.cancer.org>

Cindy L. A. Jones, Ph.D.

Cancer genetics

Definition

A continuous process in which multiple alterations occur in genes that control cell division and differentiation that leads to cancer—the uncontrolled division and proliferation of cells. These genetic alterations are referred to as mutations, which are changes in the normal DNA sequence of a particular gene. Mutations may include deletions, chromosomal translocations, inversions, amplifications, or point mutations.

Cancer genetics is the understanding of the genetic processes underlying the actual disease occurrence. This understanding plays a significant role in early detection, therapy, prevention, and prognosis.

Description

Nearly all cancers originate from a single cell and are the result of genetic alterations, although most of them are not inherited. Individuals who are genetically predisposed to a particular cancer will not necessarily develop the disease in the absence of somatic mutations. Somatic mutations occur in non–sex determining cells, meaning they will not be passed on to offspring. These mutations can be influenced by environment and other causes, such as an individual's habits (i.e. smoking). A single genetic error or mutation in a cell does not typically induce malignancy; instead it develops after a series of mutations over a period of time.

Regulation of cell death and survival

A balance between cell division and death of the old, degenerated cells is essential for proper cellular functioning of any organism. Cells that can no longer replicate or that have sustained injuries (like hypoxia, heat, extreme cold, or ultraviolet radiation) are candidates for cell death. Alternatively, cells can be killed if infected by intracellular organisms (pathogens), or damaged cells may be engulfed by a host's lymphocytes (white blood cells involved in cellular defense mechanisms). Another form of cell death in the disease process is a suicide mechanism initiated by cells known as apoptosis. In this process, extracellular or intracellular signals may trigger the degradation of nuclear material resulting in cell death. Some of the apoptotic genes like bcl2 family members (bcl-X, A1, bax, bad) are shown to be involved in various cancers. Studies to alter the activity of bcl2 family members and related genes will be of potential use in designing cancer therapies.

Oncogenes and tumor suppressor genes

The incessant cell proliferation in cancer may either be due to over-activation of a specific gene that promotes cell division or due to the improper functioning of a gene that will otherwise restrain growth. Genes that promote cell division are proto-oncogenes—positive regulators of cell division. Overexpression of proto-oncogenes results in uncontrolled cell growth. Genes that suppress or restrain growth are tumor suppressor genes and loss of their function results in unregulated cell division. An alteration in the function of genes in each of these classes is due to a change, or mutation, in the DNA within the cell. The different types of mutations include point mutations, amplifications, and chromosomal alterations.

Point mutations

DNA is composed of a string of nucleotides, each containing a phosphate group, deoxyribose, and one of four bases; adenine (A), guanine (G), cytosine (C), and thymine (T). These bases are paired as either A-T or C-G and these pairs compose the "rungs" in the double helix

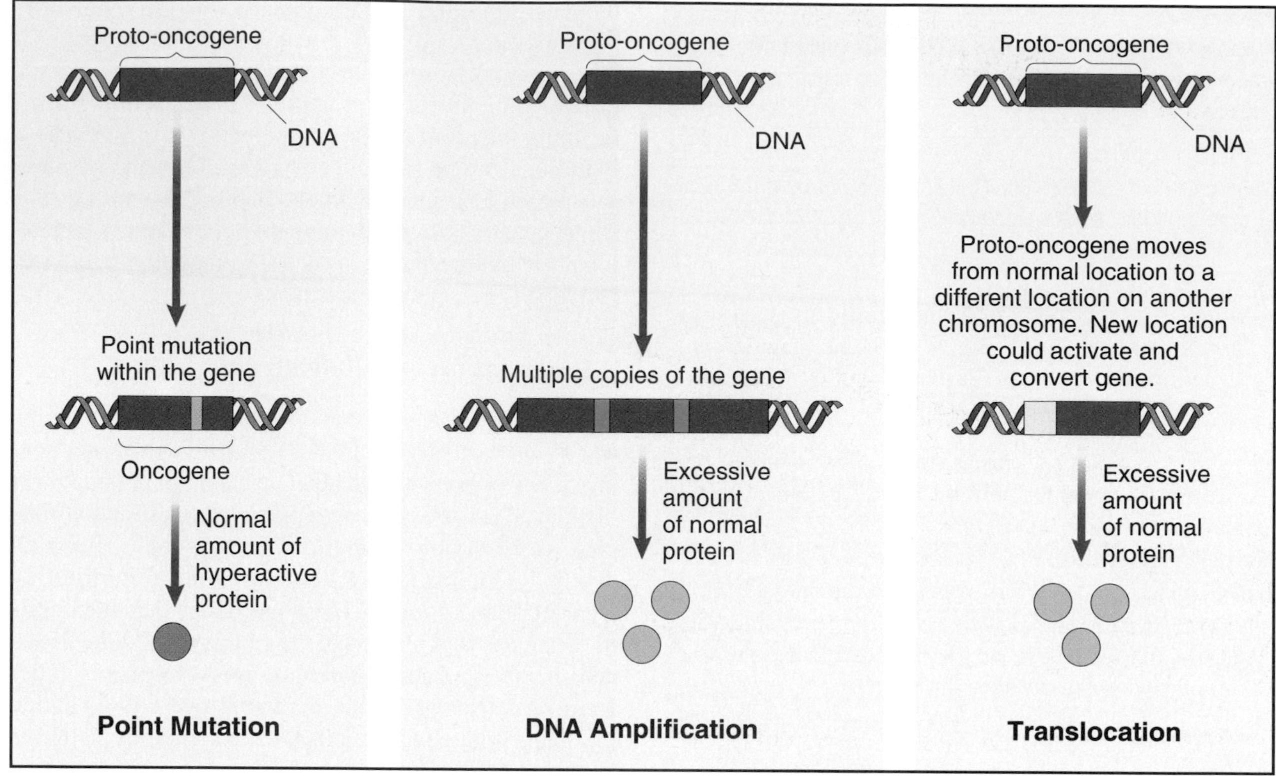

Point mutation, DNA amplification, and chromosomal alterations (like translocations) are three examples of mutations that can turn proto-oncogenes into oncogenes. *(Illustration by Argosy Publishing.)*

structure of DNA. The order of the bases creates the genetic code for development. A sample genetic code is CAG-TAA-CCA-GCG, etc. These triplets code for synthesis of specific proteins.

A point mutation is a single nucleotide change in a DNA strand. This may alter the genetic code, thus altering the function of the protein. In the above example, a point mutation in the thymine base of the second triplet would look like: CAG-AAA-CCA-GCG. Changing the code from TAA to AAA could alter the function of a protein and thus could cause a predisposition to disease such as cancer. One example of a point mutation that has been identified is the *ras* family of oncogenes (such as H*ras*, K-*ras*, N-*ras*), present in 15% of all human cancers.

DNA amplification

Another mechanism of oncogene activation—DNA amplification—results in an increase in the amount of DNA in the cell. A large number of genes are amplified in human cancers.

DNA amplification can be detected by cytological staining (a method in which the amplified DNA is stained), or by another fluorescent technique called comparative genomic hybridization (CGH). CGH allows the specific recognition of regions of gene amplifications in tumor DNA and is a more sensitive diagnostic tool.

Chromosomal alteration

Chromosomal alteration may involve translocations and is often seen in lymphoid tumors. Translocation is the transfer of one part of a chromosome to another chromosome during cell division and may involve transcription factors (i.e., nuclear factors), signal transduction proteins, and cellular regulatory molecules.

DNA repair genes

In addition to oncogenes and tumor suppressor genes, DNA repair genes may lead to cancer. DNA repair genes are capable of correcting the errors that occur during cell division. Malfunction of these repair genes, either through inherited mutation or acquired mutation, may affect cell division resulting in malignancies.

RNA and DNA viruses

Malignancies are known to be associated with RNA or DNA viruses. A retrovirus is an RNA virus that possesses a single-stranded RNA as its genetic material, in contrast to the double-stranded DNA. Retroviruses are known to induce malignancies in animals, and one known human

Childhood cancers associated with congenital syndromes or malformations

Syndrome or Anomaly	Tumor
Aniridia	Wilms' tumor
Hemihypertrophy	Wilms' tumor Hepatoblastoma Adrenocortical carcinoma
Genito-urinary abnormalities (including undescended testicles)	Wilms' tumor Ewing's sarcoma Nephroblastoma Testicular cancer
Beckwith–Wiedmann syndrome	Wilms' tumor Neuroblastoma Adrenocortical carcinoma
Dysplastic nevus syndrome	Melanoma
Nevoid basal cell carcinoma syndrome	Basal cell carcinoma Medulloblastoma Rhabdomyosarcoma
Poland syndrome	Leukemia
Trisomy-21 (Down syndrome)	Leukemia Retinoblastoma
Bloom syndrome	Leukemia, gastrointestinal carcinoma
Severe combined immune deficiency disease	EBV-associated B-lymphocyte lymphoma/leukemia
Wiscott-Aldridge syndrome	EBV-associated B-lymphocyte lymphoma
Ataxia telangiectasia	EBV-associated B-lymphocyte lymphoma Gastric carcinoma (stomach cancer)
Retinoblastoma	Wilms' tumor Osteosarcoma Ewing's sarcoma
Fanconi anemia	Leukemia Squamous cell carcinoma
Multiple endocrine neoplasia syndromes (MEN I, II, III)	Adenomas of islet cells, pituitary, parathyroids, and adrenal glands Submucosal neuromas of the tongue, lips, eyelids Pheochromocytomas Medullary carcinoma of the thyroid (thyroid cancer, a specific type) Malignant schwannoma Non-appendiceal carcinoid
Neurofibromatosis (von Recklinghausen syndrome)	Rhabdomyosarcoma Fibrosarcoma Pheochromocytomas Optic glioma Meningioma

malignancy is T-cell **lymphoma** or leukemia caused by human T-cell lymphotropic virus (HTLV) type I.

DNA viruses are implicated in human malignancies more often than RNA viruses. **Human papilloma virus** is related to human **cervical cancer**, and hepatitis B and C are related to hepatocellular carcinoma (liver cancer). In addition, the **Epstein-Barr virus** that causes the commonly known infectious mononucleosis also causes **Burkitt's lymphoma** in Africa and nasopharyngeal carcinoma in parts of Asia.

Mendelian cancer syndromes

Some forms of cancer are classified as hereditary cancers, or familial cancers, because they follow the Mendelian pattern of inheritance, the more familiar form of inheritance in which genetic material is passed from the mother or father to the offspring during reproduction. Cancer-related genes may be inherited as autosomal dominant, autosomal recessive, or x-linked traits.

About 100 syndromes have been identified as hereditary cancers although not all of them are common. Some of the known tumor suppressor genes responsible for **familial cancer syndromes** are *BRCA1*, which is associated with breast, ovarian, colon, or prostate cancers; *BRCA2* involved in **breast cancer**, male breast cancer, and **ovarian cancer**; *TSC2* associated with angiofibroma; and *RB* associated with **retinoblastoma** and **osteosarcoma**. The discovery of these genes that are associated with hereditary cancer syndromes is also beneficial in understanding the normal control of cell growth.

KEY TERMS

KEY TERMS

Autosomal recessive—A pattern of genetic inheritance where two copies of an abnormal gene must be present to display the trait or disease.

Autosomal dominant—A pattern of genetic inheritance where only one abnormal gene is needed to display the trait or disease.

Gene—A building block of inheritance, which contains the instructions for the production of a particular protein, and is made up of a molecular sequence found on a section of DNA. Each gene is found on a precise location on a chromosome.

Hypoxia—Lack of oxygen to the cells that may lead to cell injury and ultimately cell death.

Infectious mononucleosis—A common viral infection caused by Epstein-Barr virus with symptoms of sore throat, fever, and fatigue. This infection is not in any way related to cancer.

Malignant—A tumor growth that spreads to another part of the body, usually cancerous.

Nucleotides—Building blocks of genes, which are arranged in specific order and quantity.

Oncogene—Genes that allow the uncontrolled division and proliferation of cells that lead to tumor formation and usually cancer.

Translocation—The transfer of one part of a chromosome to another chromosome during cell division. A balanced translocation occurs when pieces from two different chromosomes exchange places without loss or gain of any chromosome material. An unbalanced translocation involves the unequal loss or gain of genetic information between two chromosomes.

X-linked traits—Genetic conditions associated with mutations in genes on the X chromosome. A male carrying such a mutation will contract the disorder associated with it because he carries only one X chromosome. A female carrying a mutation on just one X chromosome, with a normal gene on the other chromosome, will not be affected by the disease.

Complex inherited cancer syndromes

Several types of cancer do not follow a simple Mendelian pattern of inheritance. In many instances, environmental factors can affect the outcome of disease expression in conjunction with genetic alterations. One such example is lung cancer. Cigarette smoke is an environmental factor that may result in lung cancer for individuals frequently exposed to the toxins in the smoke. However, individuals who possess a gene that predisposed them to lung cancer are genetically more susceptible than the rest of the population to these toxins, and may develop cancer with less exposure or none at all. Individuals without a predisposing gene may not develop the cancer as readily.

It is estimated that less than 10% of the breast and ovarian cancers are the result of mutations in the *BRCA1* or *BRCA2* genes. The remaining 90% of breast cancer incidences are not usually dependent on inherited factors, although family history should be investigated.

Genetic counseling

Genetic counselors comprehend the medical aspects of hereditary cancer syndromes and can educate the affected family regarding available management options. The counselors communicate the risk for disease development to individuals and their families and actively participate in guiding the course of action from an unbiased perspective. Genetic counselors also aid in providing updated information regarding **genetic testing** for cancer risk, especially with the discovery of hereditary cancer–associated genes. Genetic counseling efforts may involve a team of health professionals anchored by the genetic counselor which includes a medical geneticist with appropriate background, mental health professional, a physician specializing in cancer (oncologist), and a surgeon (if the type of cancer requires surgery).

Genetic testing

Genetic testing examines the genetic information contained inside an individual's DNA, to determine if that person has a certain disease, is at risk to develop a certain disease, or could pass a genetic alteration to his or her offspring. Individuals who seek genetic testing are usually family members believed to have a predisposition or susceptibility to cancer as known from the personal family medical history. The identification of genes associated with certain types of cancers such as *BRCA1*, *BRCA2*, *HNPCC* (**colon cancer**), and *RB* improves the accuracy of DNA testing to predict cancer risk.

Often a positive test result indicates that the individual does carry the abnormal gene and is more likely to get the disease for which the test was performed than the rest of the population. A negative test result can signify the absence of the abnormal gene and a lesser chance of developing the disease. However, a negative test result cannot guarantee that the person will never develop cancer at any point in his or her lifetime. This is because

Chromosomes and cancer

Cancer type	Associated gene mutation
Chronic myelocytic leukemia	translocation resulting in the Philadelphia chromosome (Ph)
Burkitt's lymphoma	translocation involving the c-*myc* proto-oncogene
Retinoblastoma	mutation in chromosome 13; mutation can be inherited
Wilms' tumor	mutation in chromosome 11; mutation can be inherited
Colon cancer (occurs sporadically, but also occurs as a familial cancer syndrome)	mutation in adenomatous polyposis coli (APC) gene followed by further mutations
Breast cancer (occurs sporadically and also as a familial cancer syndrome)	mutation affecting the gene *BRCA1*, or mutation in *BRCA2*

many mutations are induced by environmental factors and accumulate over a period of time.

It is necessary for the individual undergoing genetic testing to know that assessing the mutations is challenging and false-positive results are possible. False-positive results are those that indicate the presence of an abnormal gene that may not really exist, or the abnormal gene may result in a disorder other than the one for which the testing was performed. If the tests administered are not sensitive and specific, they may detect sequence variations that could be benign variants rather than the disease-causing mutations.

Genetic testing is recommended for individuals of higher risk of cancer based on the family medical history.

Genetic testing is also performed for individuals who have survived cancer at an earlier time in their lives. It may be performed to determine one or more of the following:

- risk to offspring
- necessity of prophylactic surgery in appropriate cases
- surveillance purposes
- personal cancer etiology (cause of disease)

Genetic counseling professionals can assist in the decision to perform genetic testing and in understanding the associated risks. Some individuals find it difficult to cope with the knowledge of their own genetic predisposition. These patients should consider addressing these issues with appropriate health care professionals.

Future potential of genetics in cancer

In 2000, researchers finished successfully sequencing the draft of the entire human genome, in which 30,000 to 40,000 genes have been identified. Each gene codes for a specific protein with a unique function in cellular metabolism. Genomic scientists are examining the draft sequence to identify novel genes in an attempt to decipher their functionality. This research to understand the role of a particular gene in cancer development may lead to improved early diagnostic tools and advancements in therapeutic intervention.

See Also Cancer biology; Carcinogenesis; Chromosome rearrangements

Resources

BOOKS

Harrison's Principles of Internal Medicine, Volume 1, 14th edition. New York: McGraw-Hill, 1998.

DeVita Jr., Vincent T., et al. (Eds). *Cancer: Principles and Practice of Oncology*. J.B. Lippincott Company, 1997.

PERIODICALS

"Hereditary common cancers: molecular and clinical genetics." *Anticancer Research* 20 (November-December 2000): 4841-4851.

Venter, J. Craig, et al. "The sequence of the Human Genome." *Science* 291 (February 16, 2001): 1304-1351.

OTHER

American Academy of Family Physicians. *Genetic Testing: What you should know*. <http://family doctor.org/handouts/462.htm>. (Rev. June 2001).

National Cancer Institute. "Cancer genetics." *CancerNet.* <http://cancernet.nci.nih.gov/prevention/genetics.shtml>. (December 1999).

Kausalya Santhanam, Ph.D.

Cancer prevention

Definition

Preventing the incidence of cancer is complex and involves many factors which ultimately work by avoiding or limiting exposure to carcinogens. Known carcinogens in humans include physical, chemical, viral, and bacterial carcinogens. Physical carcinogens include the hydrocarbon byproducts of cigarette smoke, radiation, and asbestos. Benzene and vinyl chloride are examples of chemical carcinogens. The human papillomaviruses, which play a role in the development of **cervical cancer**, are viral carcinogens. A bacterial carcinogen is the bacteria, *Helicobacter pylori*, which has been linked to the cancer B-cell **lymphoma**, unique to the gastric mucosa. Familial (hereditary) **carcinogenesis** plays a role in as many as 15% of all human cancers and has been implicated as the cause of some cases of **melanoma**, breast, colon, and other cancers.

Some factors that place individuals at high risk for the development of cancer can be modified to decrease risk for development. For example, lifestyle and environmental changes can be made to decrease risk. Behavior modification such as dietary changes, exercise, and avoiding exposure to known carcinogens are primary prevention measures that everyone should adopt.

An evolving field, **chemoprevention**, is the use of **vitamins** or medicines to prevent cancer development. Chemopreventive agents have the ability to potentially delay and even reverse the sequence of events at the cellular level that change a normal cell to a cancer cell. An example of a chemopreventive agent is **tamoxifen**, a drug that is effective in preventing **breast cancer** in women who are at high risk for the development of breast cancer. **Vaccines** for Hepatitis B virus will not only prevent primary Hepatitis B and liver failure, but also liver cancer.

Preventive surgery may be an option for those individuals who are considered to be at very high risk of developing cancer because of a genetic or inherited predisposition. Examples of preventive surgery are prophylactic **mastectomy** to reduce risk for breast cancer, and colon polyp removal in individuals at high risk for the development of **colon cancer**.

In 1999 the American Cancer Society (ACS) estimated that 173,000 cancer deaths were caused by cigarette smoking, and an additional 20,000 cancer deaths were due to excessive **alcohol consumption**. All cancers caused by smoking **cigarettes** and by excessive use of alcohol can be completely prevented. According to the ACS, up to one-third of the more than 550,000 cancer deaths expected to occur in the United States in 2001 are related to poor nutrition or insufficient physical exercise. Many of the more than one million skin cancers which develop annually could be prevented by adopting protective measures from ultraviolet radiation caused by the sun.

Different cancers are associated with different risk factors. While modification of risk factors plays an important role in the prevention of cancer, it is known that some individuals who have one or more risk factors never develop cancer. Others, however, who have no known risk factors, are eventually diagnosed with cancer. Research aimed at identifying additional risk factors for specific cancers continues.

Lifestyle and cancer

Nutrition

The relationship between food intake and cancer is complex and not well understood. Research does seem to indicate that certain foods may have either protective or promoting effects on the development of cancer. Foods that have a protective effect seem to play a role in the prevention of certain types of cancers. Foods that have promoting effects are associated with an increased risk of developing certain types of cancers. According to the American Cancer Society, the single most important dietary intervention to lower risk for cancer is eating five or more servings of fruits and vegetables daily. Adopting a diet rich in plant sources provides phytochemicals that are nonnutritive substances in plants that possess health protective benefits. Dietary recommendations related to reducing risk of cancer include the recommendation to choose most of the foods eaten from plant sources such as fruits and vegetables. Five or more servings of fruits and vegetables should be consumed every day. Fruits and vegetables should be eaten at every meal and as snacks. Other foods from plant sources that should be included in the diet several times a day include breads, cereals, grain products (preferably whole grain), rice, and pasta. Beans should be eaten as an alternative to meat. The foods and herbs with the highest anticancer activity include garlic, soybeans, cabbage, ginger, licorice root, and the umbelliferous vegetables such as carrots. Citrus foods also contain a host of active phytochemicals.

A diet rich in foods from plant sources reduces the risk for development of cancers of the gastrointestinal tract, respiratory tract, and colon. Vegetables that seem to play a strong role in protecting against colon cancer include green and dark yellow vegetables, vegetables in the cabbage family, soy products, and legumes. Increased consumption of fruits and vegetables reduce risk for lung cancer, even for those individuals who smoke. Forms of fruits and vegetables that appear to provide the greatest protection include foods in fresh, frozen, canned, dried, or juice forms. Extractions from fruits and vegetable do not provide protective effects.

Diets high in fat have been associated with increased risk for colon, rectal, prostate, and endometrial (uterine) cancers. The association between high-fat diets and the development of breast cancer is much weaker. Specific dietary recommendations are to replace high-fat foods with fruits and vegetables, eat smaller portions of high fat foods, and limit consumption of meats, especially those that are considered high-fat.

Foods from animal sources remain a staple in American diets. Consumption of meat, especially red meats such as beef, pork, and lamb, have been associated with increased risk of colon and **prostate cancer**. Cooking methods have also been linked to the development of cancer. Mutagenic compounds are produced when proteins such as meat protein are cooked at high temperatures. These compounds may be responsible for the association between meat consumption and increased risk for colon cancer.

Obesity is often the result of meat-based, high-fat diets. Obesity has been linked to cancers at several sites including colon and rectum, prostate, kidney, and endometrium and breast cancer in postmenopausal women.

Physical activity

Recommendations related to physical exercise include engaging in moderate levels of activity for at least 30 minutes on most days of the week. Studies have revealed an association between physical activity and a reduced risk of the development of certain types of cancers, including colon, breast, and prostate cancer. For example, physical activity is thought to stimulate the movement of stool through the bowel, resulting in less exposure of the bowel lining to mutagens in the stool.

Consumption of alcohol

Drinking alcohol increases the risk of developing cancers of the mouth, esophagus, pharynx, larynx, and liver in both men and women, and increases the risk of breast cancer in women. Cancer risk increases as the amount of alcohol consumed increases. An individual who both smokes and drinks alcohol greatly increases the risk of developing cancer when compared to either smoking or drinking alone. Risk increases significantly for cancers of the mouth, esophagus, and larynx when more than two drinks per day are consumed. A drink is defined as 5 ounces (141.75 grams) of wine, 12 ounces (340.20 grams) of regular beer, or 1.5 ounces (42.52 grams) of 80-proof distilled spirits. Women who drink are at increased risk for the development of breast cancer. Studies have shown that the risk of breast cancer increases with just a few drinks per week.

Consumption of tobacco

Smoking-related illnesses account for more than 400,000 deaths each year in the United States. These deaths occur 12 years earlier than would be expected on average. Tobacco is known as one of the most potent human carcinogens. Tobacco causes more than 148,000 deaths each year in the form of various cancers. Most of the cancers of the lung, trachea, bronchus, larynx, pharynx, oral cavity, and esophagus diagnosed each year are caused by tobacco. Smoking is also associated with cancers of the pancreas, kidney, bladder, and cervix. Smoking is known to affect the health of nonsmokers through environmental or secondhand smoke, which is implicated in causing lung cancer. Cigarette smoking is more common among men; however, because of the increase in the number of women who smoke, more women die from lung cancer each year than from breast cancer. Mortality from lung cancer for men appears to have peaked and has been declining since the 1980s. This decline in mortality is attributed to a decrease in tobacco product use among men.

Substantial health benefits occur once an individual stops smoking. If a smoker stops smoking before the age of 50 years, that individual's risk of dying in the next 15 years is half of what a continuing smoker's risk of dying is. Even if the smoker stops smoking after the age of 70 years, the risk of dying is still reduced substantially. After 10 years of not smoking, an ex-smoker's risk of lung cancer is reduced by 30-50%. After five years of not smoking, an ex-smoker's risk of oral and **esophageal cancer** is reduced by 50%. Risk for cervical and **bladder cancer** is also reduced once smoking is stopped.

The three treatment elements identified as particularly effective in **smoking cessation** treatment include pharmacotherapy, such as nicotine replacement patches and gums, social support from physicians and other clinicians, and skills training and problem solving, particularly in the areas of smoking cessation and abstinence techniques.

Radiation exposure

Only high-frequency radiation such as ionizing radiation (IR) and ultraviolet (UV) radiation has been proven to cause cancer in humans. A source of ultraviolet radia-

KEY TERMS

Carcinogens—Cancer-causing agents.

Gastric mucosa—Lining of the stomach.

Legumes—Foods such as peas and beans.

Mutagens/mutagenic—Capable of causing changes or mutations at the chromosome or gene level.

Umbelliferous vegetables—Vegetables from the carrot family.

tion is sunlight. Prolonged, unprotected exposure to UV radiation is the major cause of basal and squamous cell skin cancers. UV radiation is also a major cause of melanoma. Disruption of Earth's ozone layer by pollution is thought to result in increasing levels of UV radiation reaching the earth's surface which has been linked to the rise in the incidence of skin cancers and melanomas.

IR has cancer-causing capability as proven by studies on atomic bomb survivors and other groups. Virtually any part of the body can be affected by IR, but the areas most affected are the bone marrow and the thyroid gland. IR is released in very low levels from diagnostic equipment such as medical and dental X-ray equipment. Much higher levels of IR are released from machines delivering **radiation therapy**. Great precautions are taken during treatment not to expose patients or staff unnecessarily to the effects of IR. Another occupational group affected by IR includes uranium miners. Exposure to radon, a naturally occurring gas which is a form of IR, can increase risk for lung cancer, especially among smokers.

See Also Antioxidants; Familial cancer syndromes; Occupational exposures and cancer

Resources

BOOKS

National Research Council *Carcinogens and Anticarcinogens in the Human Diet* Washington, D.C.: National Academy Press, 1996.

U.S. Department of Health and Human Services *Physical Activity and Health: A Report of the Surgeon General* Atlanta, GA: Centers for Disease Control and Prevention, National Center for Chronic Disease Prevention and Health Promotion, President's Council on Physical Fitness and Sports, 1996.

Yarbro, J.W. "Carcinogenesis" *Cancer Nursing Principles and Practice*, edited by C.H. Yarbro, M.H. Frogge, M. Goodman, and S.L. Groenwald. Boston: Jones and Bartlett, 2000, pp.48-59.

PERIODICALS

Craig, W., and L. Beck. "Phytochemicals: Health Protective Effects." *Canadian Journal of Dietetic Practice and Research* 60(1999): 78-84.

Glade, M.J. "Dietary fat and cancer: Genetic and molecular interactions annual research conference, American Institute for Cancer Research." *Nutrition* 13(1997): 75-77.

OTHER

"Prevention and Early Detection." *American Cancer Society, Inc.* 2000 29 June 2001 <http://www2.cancer.org/prevention/Prevention.cfm.>

"Prevention of Cancer PDQ." *CancerNet*2000 National Cancer Institute. 29 June 2001 <http://cancernet.nci.nih.gov.>

Melinda Granger Oberleitner, RN, DNS

Capecitabine

Definition

Capecitabine (brand name Xeloda) is a drug that interferes with the growth of cancer cells.

Purpose

Capecitabine is used to treat **breast cancer** and cancer of the colon and rectum (colorectal cancer) that have spread to other parts of the body (metastasized).

Description

Capecitabine is a recently developed drug. It is a type of medicine called an antimetabolite because it interferes with the metabolism and growth of cells. Capecitabine is an unusual anti-cancer drug in that it is most active in cancer cells; normal cells are exposed to far lower concentrations of the drug. Cancer cells convert capecitabine into another anti-cancer drug called 5-fluorouracil (**fluorouracil**). This substance prevents cells from growing and reproducing by interfering with the production of DNA and RNA. Eventually the cells die.

Capecitabine has been approved by the U.S. Food and Drug Administration for the treatment of metastasized breast cancer that is resistant to standard **chemotherapy**. Capecitabine may be used in combination with the drug **docetaxel** (Taxotere). A study completed in 2000 found that 56% of women receiving this combination therapy survived at least one year, with an average survival time of 14 months.

A study completed in 2001 found that capecitabine is as effective as 5-fluorouracil for treating metastasized colorectal cancer, and has fewer and less severe side effects. However, it does not increase the average survival time of approximately 13 months.

Recommended dosage

The dosage of capecitabine depends on a number of factors including body size. The average dosage is 2500 mg per square meter of body surface area per day. Capecitabine is a pill that is taken with water within 30 minutes after a meal. It may be taken every 12 or 24 hours. For colorectal cancer, capecitabine may be administered for two weeks, followed by one week off, for a total of 30 weeks.

Precautions

Capecitabine can temporarily reduce the number of white blood cells, thus reducing the body's ability to fight infection. Thus, it is very important to avoid exposure to infections and to receive prompt medical treatment. Immunizations (vaccinations) should be avoided during or after treatment with capecitabine. It also is important to avoid contact with individuals who have recently taken an oral polio vaccine.

Capecitabine may temporarily reduce the number of blood platelets that are necessary for blood clotting. The risk of bleeding may be reduced by:

- using caution when cleaning teeth
- avoiding dental work
- avoiding cuts, bruises, or other injuries

Capecitabine can cause birth defects and fetal death in animals. Therefore this drug should not be taken by pregnant women or by either the man or the woman at the time of conception. Because capecitabine may cause serious side effects, women usually are advised against breast-feeding while taking this drug.

Some individuals may have an allergic reaction to capecitabine. Allergies to foods, preservatives, or dyes, or to the drug 5-fluorouracil must be considered before this drug is prescribed.

Side effects

Common side effects of capecitabine may include:

- loss of appetite (**anorexia**)
- **diarrhea**
- **nausea and vomiting**
- stomach or abdominal pain
- swelling, peeling, redness, or blistering of hands and feet
- numbness, pain, **itching**, or tingling in hands and feet
- pain, swelling, or sores in the mouth or on the lips
- rashes or dry skin
- fatigue or weakness due to reduced red blood cell count

The treatment is stopped if side effects are severe enough to interfere with eating or other normal activities.

Less common or rare side effects of capecitabine may include:

- constipation
- cough or hoarseness
- difficulty swallowing
- shortness of breath
- chest pain
- blood pressure changes

KEY TERMS

Colorectal cancer—Cancer of the colon and rectum.

Metastasis—Spread of cancer from its point of origin to other parts of the body.

Platelet—Blood component that aids in clotting.

- fast or irregular heartbeat
- pain or swelling of the ankles, legs, or stomach
- poor coordination, dizziness
- changes in fingernails or toenails
- headache
- heartburn
- sensitivity to sunlight
- muscle pain
- eye irritation
- insomnia
- lower back or side pain
- painful or difficult urination

Side effects of capecitabine may include symptoms of infection, such as **fever**, chills, sore throat, or swollen glands, or symptoms of liver malfunction. Side effects also may include unusual bleeding or bruising due to the reduction in blood platelets.

Other diseases or medical conditions may increase the side effects associated with capecitabine. Chicken pox or shingles (**Herpes zoster**) may become very severe and spread to other parts of the body. If heart, kidney, or liver disease is present, the side effects related to these organs may be more severe. In addition, in the presence of liver disease, the amount of capecitabine in the body may be higher. Individuals over the age of 80 often experience more severe side effects with capecitabine.

Interactions

Other drugs that may interact with capecitabine include:

- Amphotericin B (Fungizone)
- Antithyroid drugs that are used to treat an overactive thyroid
- Azathioprine (Imuran)
- Chloramphenicol (Chloromycetin)

- Colchicine
- Flucytosine (Ancobon)
- Ganciclovir (Cytovene)
- Interferon (Intron A, Roferon-A)
- Plicamycin (Mithracin)
- Zidovudine (AZT, Retrovir)

Coumarin-type anticoagulants that are used to thin the blood and medicines containing aspirin can increase the chances of bleeding. **Folic acid**, alone or in a multivitamin, may increase the side effects of capecitabine. Finally, capecitabine can increase the effects on the blood of other cancer medicines or **radiation therapy**.

Margaret Alic, Ph.D.

Capsaicin

Definition

Capsaicin is the active ingredient in chili peppers, the substance that gives chili and cayenne its heat.

Purpose

Research on the use of capsaicin for cancer patients has focused on several areas:

- its ability to decrease pain
- its potential to be carcinogenic
- any chemoprotective capacity
- any antimicrobial and detoxification properties

Description

Folk accounts of capsaicin's medicinal properties in the form of cayenne have included aiding digestion, promoting the sweating process to create cooling (for reducing a **fever**), fighting infections, and stimulating the function of the kidneys, lungs, stomach, and heart. Research on capsaicin's ability to decrease pain has been in the areas of chronic pain, arthritic pain, migraine pain, and neuropathic cancer pain. It appears to interfere with chemicals that facilitate pain messages to the brain. Capsaicin has a hyperemic effect, which means that it increases blood flow similar to when an area is inflamed. When applied to the skin in cream form, the area becomes red, warm, and may become slightly swollen. Many individuals experience a localized burning sensation when a cream containing capsaicin is applied to the skin. However, with repeated use, the burning sensation usually disappears, and pain relief is noted. The burning or stinging sensation may last a few weeks for some. Capsaicin appears to work through a mechanism that initially causes a hypersensitivity to pain, and then ends in pain relief.

Several clinical studies performed on the effectiveness of various formulations of capsaicin have demonstrated that a majority of patients experience a reduction in pain and few or minor side effects. Capsaicin has been reported to have an effect against *H. pylori*, and also some antimicrobial properties. It appears to protect the lining of the digestive tract from harm due to aspirin use. Capsaicin has also showed an inhibitory effect on skin **carcinogenesis** in mice and a suppression of proliferation of human cancer cells.

Early studies on capsaicin raised the concern that capsaicin could be carcinogenic. However, further studies reported that capsaicin was not carcinogenic, and in fact might have chemoprotective properties. Studies investigating its potential to promote tumor development indicate it does not have this ability.

Recommended dosage

The Physician's Desk Reference (PDR) for Herbal Medicines indicates the availability of the following dosages of cayenne:

- Capsules: 400, 445, 450, 455, and 500 mg strengths
- Cream containing 0.25% and 0.75% capsaicin
- Liquid alcohol-based extract

The average daily dose in capsule form for cayenne (capsicum annum) is 30 to 120 mg. Individuals wishing to use capsaicin should do so under the guidance of a practitioner knowledgeable about its properties, to ensure proper monitoring for any adverse reactions.

Precautions

Capsaicin's fiery nature requires some precautions to be used when handling it in its natural form or when applying it topically as a cream. Thorough hand washing after contact with it is necessary, as it can cause an intense burning or stinging sensations. Avoid any contact with mucous membranes, such as eyes or mouth, or any open wounds, until hands have been washed. Bottles storing capsaicin or cayenne should be well sealed and kept out of the light. It should not be refrigerated.

The National Cancer Institute (NCI) cautions that it is not known whether capsaicin used by a breast feeding mother will pass into the breast milk. Individuals who have had an allergic reaction to hot peppers should speak

KEY TERMS

Bioavailability.—A term used in describing the amount of a medication taken that is actively available to the targeted body area. Bioavailability can be affected by factors such as the rate at which a tablet or capsule dissolves, binding products using in formulating the medication, and the person's ability to break down and use the medication.

Carcinogenic—A substance that can cause cancer to develop.

Mucositis.—An inflammation of the lining of the digestive tract, often accompanied by mouth and throat lesions.

Neuropathic pain.—Pain that is felt near the surface of the skin, along nerve pathways.

Neurotoxic.—A substance that is harmful to the nervous system.

to their health care provider before using capsaicin. Some individuals may experience a prolonged burning sensation with topical capsaicin. However, the NCI states that reducing the number of doses per day will not result in decreasing the sensation, and may prolong the time period over which the sensation is experienced. In addition, a reduction in the number of doses may also reduce the degree of pain relief. Patients taking capsaicin should not double-up on a dose if a dose is missed.

Side effects

Research on capsaicin is still in the early stages, but the following has been reported:

- hypersensitivity reaction such as anaphylaxis and rhinoconjunctivitis
- abnormal blood clotting ability
- an increase in bowel function, leading to diarrhea
- blister formation on the skin
- contact dermatitis
- increase in cough with extended exposure to chili peppers
- long-term use of high dosages can lead to kidney and liver damage, chronic gastritis, and neurotoxic effects

Interactions

If aspirin and capsicum annum extract (in the form of 100 mg of capsaicin) are taken at the same time, decreased bioavailability of aspirin may occur. This treatment may interfere with MAO inhibitors and antihypertensive therapy. As with any medication, patients should notify their physician of any prescription, over-the-counter, or herbal remedies they are taking prior to receiving treatment.

Resources

INFORMATION ON CLINICAL STUDIES

Anesthesia and Analgesia 86, no. 3 (March 1998): 579–83.
Annals of the New York Academy of Sciences 889 (1999): 157–92.
Cancer Letters 120, no. 2 (9 December 1997): 235–41.
Cancer Letters 164, no. 2 (26 March 2001): 119–26
Mutation Research 428, no. 1–2 (16 July 1999): 305–27.

Esther Csapo Rastegari, R.N., B.S.N., Ed.M.

Carbamazepine

Definition

Carbamazepine (Tegretol, Carbatrol) may be administered to cancer patients as a pain medicine.

Purpose

Carbamazepine is given to cancer patients primarily as a pain medication. The drug may, for example, be prescribed for stabbing pain that moves along a nerve. For noncancer patients, it is often used to treat epilepsy or bioplar disorder (manic-depressive illness).

Description

Carbamazepine suppresses some of the activities of the nerves. It does this by delaying the amount of time it takes for certain passageways in the nerves to recover after they have sent out a message.

Recommended dosage

Carbamazepine comes in several forms. There are 200 mg tablets, 100 mg chewable tablets, and a liquid containing 20 mg per milliliter that may be swallowed. There are extended-release tablets of carbamazepine containing 100, 200, or 400 mg and extended release capsules of the medication containing 200 and 300 mg.

Some authorities recommend starting with 100 to 200 mg twice a day. This strategy helps to minimize side effects. Then, the dose may be gradually increased every week. Adults may eventually receive 600 to 1200 mg a

KEY TERMS

Bone marrow—The spongy tissue found in the large bones of the body.

Trigeminal neuralgia—A nerve problem associated with pain.

day, while 20 to 30 mg per kg of body weight per day is appropriate for children.

Side effects

Carbamazepine may exhibit side effects to the nervous system, for example, drowsiness, dizziness, blurred vision, unsteadiness, **depression**, impaired concentration, and headache. Patients should be cautious about operating machinery or performing tasks requiring alertness until tolerant of the side effects. After several weeks of treatment, these side effects may disappear. To minimize these side effects, doctors may start carbamazepine at a low dose and may recommend that it be taken before bedtime. As carbamazepine may cause stomach upset and nausea, the medicine should be taken with meals.

Effects of carbamazepine may include bone marrow suppression, which involves a low white blood cell and platelet count, but this is usually not severe. Very rarely, a dangerous **anemia** may occur during carbamazepine therapy. Blood counts should be monitored for patients using this drug. Some patients with previously diagnosed depression of the bone marrow should not be given carbamazepine.

Carbamazepine may cause birth defects and should be avoided in women who are pregnant. An appropriate contraceptive method should be used while on carbamazepine. Carbamazepine can cross into breast milk and should be avoided in women who are breastfeeding. Carbamazepine may also cause rash or sensitivity to the sun.

Interactions

Carbamazepine may affect the activity of other medicines, for example, oral contraceptives, **warfarin**, theophylline, doxycycline, haloperidol, **corticosteroids**, valproate, clonazepam, ethosuximide, lamotrigine, felbamate, and thyroid hormones. Oral contraceptives may become less effective if a patient is taking carbamazepine. Some doctors recommend that the form of birth control pill be altered or that a different method of contraception be used. If **phenytoin** and phenobarbital are taken at the same time as carbamazepine, the capacity of carbamazepine to interact with additional medications may increase. Side effects may occur if a patient is taking carbamazepine and one of the following medications simultaneously: **danazol**, dextropropoxyphene, erythromycin, clarithromycin, isoniazid, verapamil, or diltiazem. Due to the numerous potential of interactions with other drugs, patients should consult with their physician or pharmacist prior to starting any new medications either bought over the counter or initiated by another physician. Patients taking carbamazepine should not drink grapefruit juice.

Bob Kirsch

Carboplatin

Definition

Carboplatin is a chemotherapeutic agent used to treat cancer by interfering with the growth of cancer cells. Carboplatin is marketed under the brand name Paraplatin; it may also be referred to as CBDCA, JM-8, or carboplatinum.

Purpose

Carboplatin is approved by the Food and Drug Administration (FDA) to treat **ovarian cancer**. It has also been useful for other types of cancer including head and neck cancer, **cervical cancer**, lung cancer, **endometrial cancer**, **testicular cancer**, and brain tumors.

Description

Carboplatin is a member of the group of **chemotherapy** drugs known as heavy metal-like alkylating agents. Alkylating agents interfere with the genetic material (deoxyribonucleic acid, or DNA) inside the cancer cells and prevent them from further dividing and growing more cancer cells.

Recommended dosage

The dose of carboplatin can be calculated using several methods. A carboplatin dose can be determined using a mathematical calculation that measures a person's body surface area (BSA). This number is dependent upon a patient's height and weight: the larger the person, the greater the body surface area. BSA is measured by the square meter (m^2). The body surface area is calculated and then multiplied by the drug dosage in milligrams per square meter (mg/m^2). This calculates the actual dose a patient is to receive.

A common dosage of carboplatin alone for the treatment of patients with recurrent ovarian cancer is 360 mg/m^2 given on day one into a vein every four weeks. When given in combination with the chemotherapeutic agent **cyclophosphamide** for the treatment of recurrent ovarian cancer, a dose of 300 mg/m^2 administered intravenously is typical. This combination is repeated every four weeks for six cycles.

The second way to determine the dose of carboplatin is for the physician to measure or estimate how well the patient's kidneys work. The patient may be asked to collect all of their urine in a bottle for a 24-hour period. The sample will then be sent to a laboratory and analyzed. A mathematical calculation is performed to determine how well the patient's kidneys are working and subsequently to determine the carboplatin dose.

Precautions

Blood counts will be monitored regularly while on carboplatin therapy. During a certain time period after receiving carboplatin there is an increased risk of getting infections. Caution should be taken to avoid unnecessary exposure to infectious agents. Patients should also check with their doctors before receiving live virus **vaccines** while on chemotherapy.

Patients who may be pregnant or trying to become pregnant should talk to their doctor before receiving carboplatin. Men and women undergoing chemotherapy are at risk of becoming sterile.

Patients with known previous allergic reactions to chemotherapy drugs should notify their doctors.

Side effects

Nausea and vomiting are among the most common side effects from receiving carboplatin. Nausea and vomiting can begin up to six hours after treatment and can last as long as 24 hours. Patients are given medicines known as **antiemetics** before receiving carboplatin to help prevent or decrease this side effect. **Diarrhea**, loss of appetite, constipation, pain, and weakness have also been reported to occur.

Myelosuppression, or a suppression of bone marrow activity resulting in a low blood cell count, is expected to occur following carboplatin administration. When a patient's white blood cell count drops below normal (leukopenia), there is an increased risk of developing a **fever** and infections. Neupogen, a drug used to increase the white blood cell count, may be administered.

KEY TERMS

Anemia—An abnormally low red blood cell count.

Chemotherapy—Specific drugs used to treat cancer.

DNA—Deoxyribonucleic acid; the genetic material inside of cells.

Electrolytes—Natural salt substances in the body that move in and out of cells to maintain cell function.

Food and Drug Administration—A government agency that oversees public safety in relation to drugs and medical devices. The FDA gives the approval to pharmaceutical companies for commercial marketing of their products.

Intravenous—Entering the body through a vein.

Leukopenia—An abnormally low white blood cell count.

Metastatic—Cancer that has spread to one or more parts of the body.

A decrease in platelet count is most notable following carboplatin administration. Platelets are blood cells that aid for the formation of clots. When the platelet count becomes abnormally low, patients are at an increased risk for bruising and bleeding. If the platelet count remains too low a platelet blood transfusion is an option. Low red blood cell counts (**anemia**) may also occur following many cycles of carboplatin administration; during the first cycles this is usually not a common problem. Low red blood cell counts may result in dizziness and **fatigue** and can be treated with the drug **erythropoietin**.

A less common side effect of carboplatin is damage to nerves and nervous system tissues. Patients may feel tingling and numbness of the fingers and toes. This side effect is more common in patients over 65 years of age or those who have previously received the chemotherapy drug **cisplatin**. Other less common side effects include rash, **itching**, hair loss (**alopecia**), mouth sores, hearing problems, kidney problems, liver problems, vision problems, swelling, redness and pain at the site of injection, allergic reactions, heart problems, and breathing problems.

Carboplatin has caused allergic reactions. The symptoms of an allergic reaction include difficulty breathing, drop in blood pressure, rash, itching, sweating, redness of the face, dizziness, and increased heart rate. These symptoms occur within minutes of administering the drug and appear to be more common in patients previously treated with platinum medicines.

Carboplatin may cause the body to waste certain normal electrolytes that circulate in the body. Low levels of magnesium, calcium, phosphate, or sodium can be found in patients who have received carboplatin. These rarely cause difficulties and are monitored by the doctor.

Interactions

Patients should avoid other drugs that may cause damage to the kidneys or hearing.

Nancy J. Beaulieu, RPh.,BCOP

Carcinogenesis

Definition

Also called tumorigenesis, carcinogenesis is the molecular process by which cancer develops.

Description

The development of cancer is a complicated process in which a large number of factors interact to disrupt normal cell growth and division. Cancer can be caused by a number of internal factors such as heredity, immunology, and hormones as well as external factors such as chemicals, viruses, diet, and radiation. Although attention is often focused on environmental chemicals (such as asbestos and coal tar) as a cause of cancer, only 5% of cancers can be linked to chemical exposure. We now know that the chief causes of cancer are lifestyle factors such as diet, cigarette smoke, alcohol, and sun exposure. In fact, dietary factors are associated with 35% of all human cancers and cigarette smoke for another 30%.

Whatever the cause of cancer, its development is a multi-stage process involving damage to the genetic material of cells (deoxyribonucleic acid, or DNA). This damage occurs in genes regulating normal cell growth and division. Because several stages or several mutations are required for cancer to develop, there is usually a long latent period before cancer appears.

Carcinogens

Agents that cause cancer (carcinogens) can be classified as genotoxic or nongenotoxic (also referred to as epigenetic). Genotoxins cause irreversible genetic damage or mutations by binding to DNA. Genotoxins include chemical agents like N-methyl-N-nitrosourea (MNU) or non-chemical agents such as ultraviolet light and ionizing radiation. After the carcinogen enters the body, the body makes an attempt to eliminate it through a process called biotransformation (a series of reactions in which the chemical structure of a compound is altered). The purpose of these reactions is to make the carcinogen more water-soluble so that it can be removed from the body. But these reactions can also convert a less toxic carcinogen into a more toxic one. Certain viruses can also act as carcinogens by interacting with DNA.

Nongenotoxins do not directly affect DNA but act in other ways to promote growth. These include hormones and some organic (carbon-based) compounds.

Stages of carcinogenesis

Cancer develops through four definable stages: initiation, promotion, progression and malignant conversion. These stages may progress over many years. The first stage, initiation, involves a change in the genetic makeup of a cell. This may occur randomly or when a carcinogen interacts with DNA causing damage. This initial damage rarely results in cancer because the cell has in place many mechanisms to repair damaged DNA. However, if repair does not occur and the damage to DNA is in the location of a gene that regulates cell growth and proliferation, DNA repair, or a function of the immune system, then the cell is more prone to becoming cancerous.

During promotion, the mutated cell is stimulated to grow and divide faster and becomes a population of cells. Eventually a benign tumor becomes evident. In human cancers, hormones, cigarette smoke, or bile acids are substances that are involved in promotion. This stage is usually reversible as evidenced by the fact that lung damage can often be reversed after smoking stops.

The progression phase is less well understood. During progression, there is further growth and expansion of the tumor cells over normal cells. The genetic material of the tumor is more fragile and prone to additional mutations. These mutations occur in genes that regulate growth and cell function such as oncogenes, tumor suppressor genes, and DNA mismatch-repair genes. These changes contribute to tumor growth until conversion occurs, when the growing tumor becomes malignant and possibly metastatic. Many of these genetic changes have been identified in the development of **colon cancer** and thus it has become a model for studying multi-stage carcinogenesis.

Cancer genes

Oncogenes

Normal cell proliferation is controlled by growth factors and cytokines (mediating proteins) that act on the cell

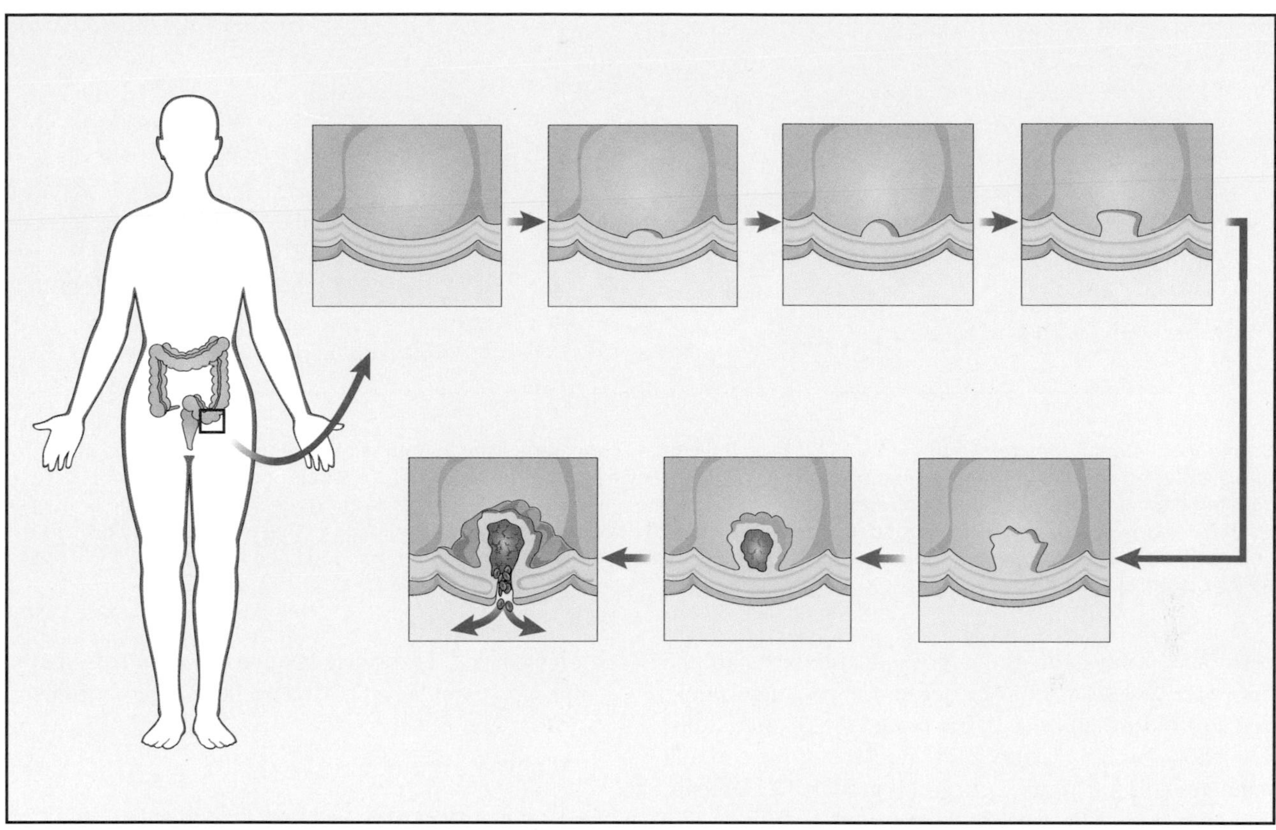

Colon cancer has become a model for studying multi-stage carcinogenesis. Four distinct sequential mutations have been described in the development of colon cancer: mutations of the APC (adenomatous polyposis coli), K-ras, DCC (deleted in colon cancer), and p53 genes. With each mutation, progressive changes are seen in the colonic epithelium (the cells on the internal surface of the colon). Normal epithelium is shown in first panel. Mutation of APC typically occurs early and is sometimes inherited. Mutations in APC lead to dysplasia or formation of a polyp (panel 2). When one cell in this polyp develops a second mutation, in the K-ras gene, it grows at a faster rate resulting in a benign Class I adenoma (panel 3). Subsequent mutations in DCC and p53 genes lead to late adenoma (panels 4 and 5) and finally carcinoma (panel 6). Once cancer forms, it can eventually break through the colon's cellular surface (panel 7) and spread through blood to other sites in the body. *(Illustration by Argosy Publishing.)*

membrane, triggering a cascade of biochemical signals (a process called signal transduction). These signals control, among others, the genes that regulate cell growth and division. Oncogenes are altered forms of normal cellular genes called proto-oncogenes that are involved in this cascade of events. They may mutate spontaneously, through interaction with viruses, or by chemical or physical means.

When a proto-oncogene is altered to become an oncogene, the pathway of cell growth and proliferation become altered. This may lead to the abnormal growth of cells (neoplastic transformation). More than 100 oncogenes have been identified. An example of an oncogene is the K-ras gene that is mutated in colon cancer cells.

Genes are the means by which a cell produces proteins, each of which have a very specific role. A mutated gene can cause overproduction of a protein, underproduction of a protein, or alteration of a protein that may be unable to carry out its purpose. Oncogenes typically produce more of their protein product when mutated, while tumor suppressor genes typically produce less of their protein product when mutated.

Tumor suppressor genes

Both the activation of oncogenes and the inactivation of tumor suppressor genes appear to be necessary for cancer to occur. Tumor suppressor genes are typically associated with cell growth and differentiation and cell suicide (apoptosis). More than a dozen tumor suppressor genes have been identified. Proteins produced by tumor suppressor genes typically inhibit a cell from reproducing during times when growth is inappropriate such as during DNA repair; they are considered the "brakes" of the cell.

Mutations that inactivate the tumor suppressor gene p53 are the most common mutations seen in human can-

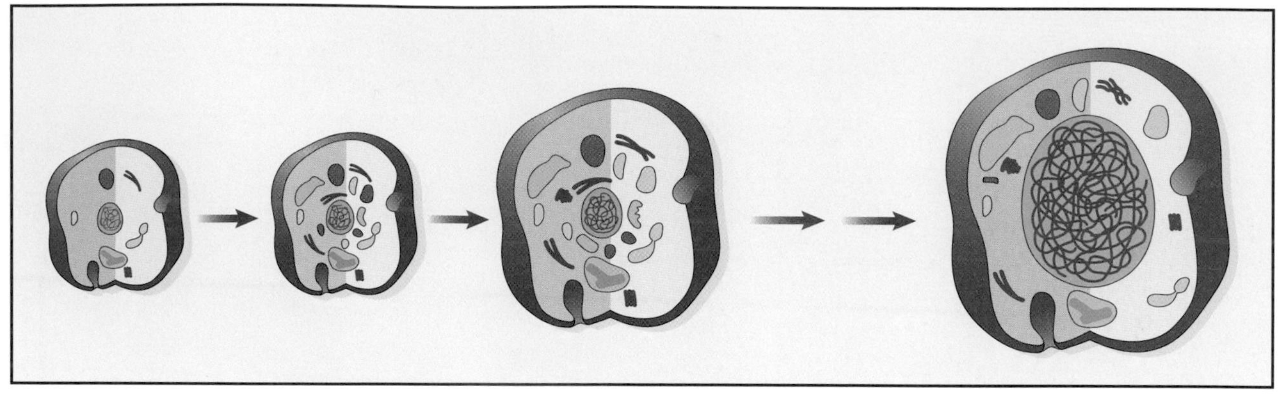

Carcinogenesis. After several mutations, a normal cell becomes cancerous. The first stage of carcinogenesis, called initiation, involves a change in the genetic makeup of a cell. This may occur randomly or when a carcinogen interacts with DNA causing damage. This initial damage rarely results in cancer because the cell has in place many mechanisms to repair damaged DNA. However, if repair does not occur and the damage to DNA is in the location of a gene that regulates cell growth and proliferation, DNA repair, or a function of the immune system, then the cell is more prone to becoming cancerous. *(Illustration by Argosy Publishing.)*

cers, accounting for about 50%. Carcinomas of the breast, colon, stomach, bladder and testis; **melanoma**; and soft tissue sarcoma all are linked to p53 mutations. The p53 protein is found in the nucleus of the cell and regulates cell functions such as cell growth, DNA repair, and apoptosis. The most notable role for p53 is to halt cell growth to allow the cell time to repair damaged DNA. If p53 is mutated, it loses this function, apoptosis does not occur, and unregulated cell growth results. In **Li-Fraumeni syndrome** a mutation of the p53 gene is inherited. This puts the individual at a high risk for a number of cancers such as early onset breast carcinoma, childhood **sarcomas**, and other tumors. Other tumor suppressor genes include the **retinoblastoma** gene and the DCC gene that is mutated in colon cancer.

DNA mismatch-repair genes

This more recently discovered class of cancer susceptibility genes is associated with the genetic instability of cancer cells that allows for multiple mutations to occur. This instability hastens the course of cancer. The normal function of these genes is to repair damage to the DNA. Mutations in DNA mismatch-repair genes are most notable in hereditary non-polyposis colorectal cancer (HNPCC).

Apoptosis

Apoptosis, also called cell suicide, refers to the death of a damaged cell. It is not random but occurs in cells with damaged DNA. When a cell becomes mutated and does not repair itself, it can be sacrificed to prevent that mutation from being passed on to the next generation of cells. Inhibition of apoptosis can be an essential step in carcinogenesis. Two genes involved in apoptosis are the tumor suppressor gene p53 and the bcl-2 proto-oncogene.

Colon carcinogenesis

Colon cancer has become a model for studying multi-stage carcinogenesis. Four distinct sequential mutations have been described in the development of colon cancer. These are mutations of the APC (adenomatous polyposis coli), K-ras, DCC (deleted in colon cancer), and p53 genes. With each mutation, progressive changes are seen in the colonic epithelium (the cells on the internal surface of the colon).

Mutation of APC typically occurs early and is sometimes inherited. Mutations in APC lead to dysplasia (abnormalities in adult cells) or polyp formation (usually benign growths on the surface of mucous membranes). These polyps can remain dormant for many decades. When one cell in this polyp develops a second mutation, in the K-ras gene, it grows at a faster rate resulting in a larger tumor or intermediate **adenoma**. Subsequent mutations in DCC and p53 lead to late adenoma and finally carcinoma.

These mutations result in both the overexpression of oncogenes and the deletion of anti-oncogenes, the combination of which results in cancer. This is, however, just a model and not all genes are altered in all cases of colon cancer; additional mutations are likely. Individuals with the hereditary predisposition to colon cancer known as familial adenomatous polyposis (FAP) typically have inherited mutations of the APC gene, the first step of colon cancer. Only 15% of colon cancer cases are due to hereditary factors, however, with 85% due to sporadic mutations.

KEY TERMS

Apoptosis—A process of cell death performed by a damaged cell.

Differentiation—A change to a more mature phenotype or appearance.

Dysplasia—A abnormal appearance of cells caused by cancer.

Malignant—A cancerous or invasive tumor.

Metastatic—A tumor with the ability to break off and grow in a distant location.

Mutation—A change in the genetic code that can be inherited or acquired.

Oncogene—A gene involved in normal cell growth that when mutated can lead to unregulated cell growth or cancer.

Proliferation—Reproduction of a cell. It differs from growth in that it is a change in number rather than size.

Tumor suppressor gene—A gene involved in slowing down cell growth so that if inactivated allows growth to progress without control.

Resources

BOOKS

Kinzler, Kenneth W., and Bert Vogelstein. "Colorectal Tumors." In*The Genetic Basis of Human Cancer.* Volgelstein, B., and K. Kinzler, eds. New York: McGraw-Hill, 1998.

McKinnell, Robert G., Ralph E. Parchment, Alan O. Perantoni, and G. Barry Pierce. *The Biological Basis of Cancer.* New York: Cambridge University Press, 1998.

Templeton, Dennis J., and Robert A. Weinberg. "Principles of Cancer Biology" In *Clinical Oncology.* Murphy, G., W. Lawrence, and R. Lenhard, eds. Atlanta: The American Cancer Society, 1995.

Weinberg, Robert A.*One Renegade Cell: How Cancer Begins.* New York: Basic Books, 1998.

PERIODICALS

Weinstein, I. Bernard. "Disorders in Cell Circuitry During Multistage Carcinogenesis: The Role of Homeostasis." *Carcinogenesis* 21 (2000): 857-64.

OTHER

Mellors, Robert C. "Etiology of Cancer: Carcinogenesis." *Neoplasia* Weill Medical College of Cornell University. July 1999. 27 June 2001 <http://edcenter.med.cornell.edu/CUMC_PathNotes/Neoplasia/Neoplasia_04.html>.

Cindy L. A. Jones, Ph.D.

Carcinoid tumors, gastrointestinal

Definition

Gastrointestinal carcinoid tumors are rare malignancies in which cancer develops in hormone-producing cells that line the appendix, bronchus, esophagus, intestines, liver, ovary, pancreas, rectum, stomach, testes, and thymus.

Description

Gastrointestinal carcinoid tumors are also called:

- carcinoids
- endocrine tumors, carcinoid type
- metastatic carcinoid tumors
- neuroendocrine tumors
- neuroendocrine cancers

Types of gastrointestinal carcinoids

Doctors describe gastrointestinal carcinoids according to the part of the gastrointestinal tract in which they originate. Foregut tumors start in the cells of the esophagus, bronchus, thymus, and stomach.

Midgut tumors originate in the: appendix, liver, ovary, small intestine, and parts of the large intestine.

Hindgut tumors originate in the rest of the colon or in the rectum.

About 75% of all carcinoid tumors originate in the digestive system. Most of them develop in the:

- small intestine (ileum)
- appendix
- rectum

Atypical tumor behavior

Most cancers cause symptoms in the organs in which they start or to which they spread (metastasize), but carcinoids can release chemicals (hormones) that travel through the bloodstream and cause symptoms in many parts of the body. These substances can damage heart valves, causing weakness, heart murmur, and shortness of breath.

Some gastrointestinal carcinoids stimulate the adrenal glands to produce abnormally high levels of the hormones that regulate the balance of water and salt in the body. Overproduction of these hormones causes weakness, weight gain, secondary diabetes, and excessive facial and body hair.

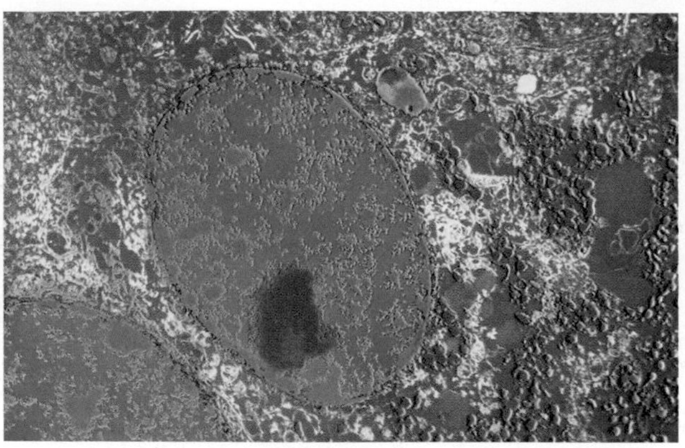

Colored transmission electron micrograph of a cancer cell from a carcinoid tumor of the human gut. The large oval is the cell nucleus. The red patch inside it is the nucleolus, often prominent in cancer cells. The small red granules in the cytoplasm are packed with the hormone serontonin. High levels of this hormone can cause symptoms like wheezing and diarrhea. *(© Science Photo Library/Photo Researchers, Inc. Photo reproduced by permission.)*

Carcinoid syndrome

Although gastrointestinal carcinoids behave differently in different people, tumors that originate in the appendix don't usually spread to other organs. Tumors that develop in the colon or rectum hardly ever produce hormones. Tumors that originate in the small intestine or other parts of the gastrointestinal tract and spread to the liver generally cause carcinoid syndrome. Flushing of the face and neck is the most common symptom of this rare malignant disease that affects the small intestine, stomach, and pancreas, and fewer than 10% of patients with gastrointestinal carcinoids.

Carcinoid syndrome is also characterized by:

- abdominal cramps
- breathlessness
- cyanosis
- **diarrhea**
- rapid heart beat (tachycardia)
- swelling around the eyes
- tearing
- wheezing

Stress, strenuous exercise, eating spicy foods, or drinking alcohol can intensify these symptoms.

Disease progression

Gastrointestinal carcinoids originate as small growths called tumorlets. These miniature tumors grow very slowly and few of them develop into carcinoid tumors.

The hormones that gastrointestinal carcinoids release generally cause more problems than the tumors themselves. Death usually results from heart or liver failure or from complications associated with tumor growth.

Demographics

About 2,500 carcinoids are diagnosed in the United States every year. African Americans develop carcinoids more often than Caucasians, and African-American women develop them more often than African-American men. Caucasian men and women are equally likely to develop these tumors.

The average age of patients diagnosed with carcinoid tumor of the appendix is 40. The average age of patients diagosed with carcinoid tumor of the stomach, small intestine, colon, and rectum is 55–65.

Causes and symptoms

The cause of gastrointestinal carcinoids is unknown, some risk factors have been identified. The risk factors that increase a person's risk of developing gastrointestinal carcinoids include:

- Having certain diseases that damage the stomach and decrease production of stomach acid. (Some of these diseases include chronic atrophic gastritis associated with pernicious anemia, chronic gastric infection with the *H. pylori* bacteria, auto-immune gastritis, or AIDS.)
- Having a family history of multiple endocrine neoplasia, type 1. (The multiple endocrine neoplasia (MEN) syndromes are three related disorders in which two or more of the hormone-secreting (endocrine) glands of the body develop tumors. Commonly affected glands are the thyroid, parathyroids, pituitary, adrenals, and pancreas. Patients diagnosed with this syndrome are at a higher risk for developing a variety of cancers, and require more frequent monitoring than the average patient might.)

Symptoms

Early-stage gastrointestinal carcinoids rarely cause symptoms. About half of these tumors are discovered during tests or surgical procedures performed to diagnose or treat other diseases of the digestive system.

The most common early symptom of gastrointestinal carcinoids is uncomfortable flushing of the face and neck. Most people who have gastrointestinal carcinoids eventually experience:

- abdominal cramps
- changes in bowel habits

- other symptoms similar to those of other intestinal cancers

Some gastrointestinal carcinoids cause:

- intestinal bleeding
- asthmatic wheezing
- impotence
- loss of interest in sex (libido)

Most patients develop abnormal connective tissue on the right side of the heart (endocardial fibrosis).

Diagnosis

If a patient has any abnormality that could be a symptom of a gastrointestinal carcinoid, the doctor asks about other symptoms that could be associated with carcinoid syndrome or caused by a tumor in the stomach, intestines, or rectum.

Diagnostic techniques

Doctors use a variety of diagnostic techniques to locate gastrointestinal carcinoids and determine how far the disease has spread:

- barium enemas and x rays highlight abnormalities in the lining of the esophagus, stomach, and intestines
- blood and urine tests measure amounts of substances that carcinoids secrete
- **colonoscopy** provides a view of the entire length of the colon
- endoscopic ultrasound shows how deeply tumors have penetrated the wall of the esophagus, stomach, intestines, or rectum and whether they have spread to nearby tissues
- octreoscan detects the spread of gastrointestinal carcinoids by using a special camera to track the path of injected radioactive hormone-like substances that are attracted to these tumors

Provocative testing designed to cause the patient to flush can help doctors diagnose some gastrointestinal carcinoids, can provoke potentially serious reactions, and must be performed in a hospital, under close medical supervision.

Biopsy

Diagnostic tests can indicate that a patient has a gastrointestinal carcinoid, but only **biopsy** can confirm the diagnosis. Endoscopic biopsy is the most common way to remove a sample of a suspected gastrointestinal carcinoid.

A doctor performs this procedure by passing a flexible lighted tube topped with a tiny video camera (endoscope) down the patient's throat or up through the anus to examine the lining of the organs of the digestive tract. After locating a tumor, the doctor manipulates pincers or tongs (biopsy forceps) through the endoscope to remove a tissue sample.

Clinical staging, treatments, and prognosis

Staging

Doctors divide gastrointestinal carcinoids into three categories.

- Localized cancer is found in the appendix, colon, rectum, small intestine, and stomach, but has not spread beyond the wall of the organ in which it originated.
- Regional spread describes tumors that have penetrated the wall of the organ in which they originated and have involved nearby fat cells, ligaments, muscles, and lymph nodes.
- Distant spread, or metastatic disease, refers to gastrointestinal carcinoids that have spread to the liver, bones, lungs, or other tissues or organs far from the original tumor.

Recurrent gastrointestinal carcinoid is disease that has returned after having been treated. Recurrent disease can develop at the site of the original tumor or in another part of the body.

Treatment

Treatment of gastrointestinal carcinoids is based on:

- where the tumor originated

KEY TERMS

Adrenal gland—Either of two glands that secrete hormones that maintain the balance of water and salt in the body and regulate the functions of other organs. Also called suprarenal glands.

Cyanosis—Bluish discoloration of the skin.

Heart murmur—Abnormal heart sound heard through a stethoscope.

Hormone—Chemical that is produced in certain cells of the body and that controls the activity of other cells.

Secondary diabetes—Form of diabetes resulting from damage to the pancreas.

- whether the cancer has spread beyond the gastrointestinal system
- the patient's general health

Surgery

Surgery cures most gastrointestinal carcinoids. What type of operation a patient undergoes depends on the size and location of the tumor, whether the patient has serious disease of any other organ, and whether the tumor is causing carcinoid syndrome.

TREATING LOCALIZED GASTROINTESTINAL CARCINOIDS. A surgeon can usually remove all of a tumor that has not spread (is localized). This procedure, called local excision, consists of removing the tumor and nearby normal tissue, and sewing together the affected ends of the remaining tissue.

If a carcinoid originates in the appendix, doctors usually remove the appendix (appendectomy). If the tumor is larger than 3/4" (cm) and the patient is under the age of 60 and otherwise in good health, the doctor may also remove the third of the colon closest to the appendix, and nearby blood vessels and lymph nodes.

When a carcinoid tumor originates in the small intestine, doctors usually remove part of the bowel, and may remove nearby lymph nodes to see if they contain cancer cells. Local excision is used to remove carcinoids that are not much larger than 3/8" (cm). Surgery for larger tumors removes a greater amount of normal surrounding tissue and some nearby blood vessels and lymph nodes.

Doctors usually treat localized carcinoids that originate in the stomach, pancreas, and colon by removing the affected organ.

Local excision is used to treat carcinoids that are limited to areas of the large intestine other than the appendix or to the rectum. Doctors use a flexible lighted instrument (colonoscope) to remove small tumors from these sites and remove larger tumors through an incision in the patient's abdomen.

Electrofulguration, a surgical procedure sometimes used to cure rectal carcinoids, destroys the tumor by heating it with electrical current. Doctors use electrofulguration to burn away rectal carcinoids no larger than 3/8" (cm). Tumors measuring 3/4" (cm) or more are apt to grow and metastasize and must be surgically removed.

Segmental colon resection (also called hemicolectomy) removes between one-third and one-half of the large intestine, and blood vessels and lymph nodes near the affected tissue.

Abdominoperineal resection is used for very large or very invasive carcinoids of the lower rectum. A patient who has this operation also has a **colostomy**. Deeply invasive rectal carcinoids that measure less than 3/4" are treated like larger tumors. Mildly invasive tumors of comparable size are treated with local excision and careful monitoring to check for recurrence.

Lower anterior resection is used for some carcinoids in the upper part of the rectum. This procedure removes some of the rectum before the remaining ends are sewn together, and has little lasting effect on the digestive system.

TREATING REGIONAL SPREAD. When a gastrointestinal carcinoid has spread to organs or tissues close to the original tumor (regional spread), doctors usually remove the affected organ. Some nearby organs and tissues may also be removed.

If it is not possible to completely remove a gastrointestinal carcinoid that has spread to another part of the body, surgeons remove as much of the cancer as they can without damaging vital organs or causing severe side effects. Surgery cannot cure gastrointestinal carcinoids that have spread to parts of the body far from the original tumor, but it can relieve symptoms and slow the progression of the disease.

Liver resection removes one or more metastases (secondary tumors) from the liver. This procedure does not cure cancer but can relieve symptoms of carcinoid syndrome. Doctors destroy gastrointestinal carcinoids that have spread to the liver by:

- using images generated by a CT scan (**computed tomography** scan) to guide a long thin needle into tumors and injecting them with concentrated alcohol
- cooling the needle with liquid nitrogen to freeze carcinoid tumor cells (cryosurgery)

TREATING METASTATIC DISEASE. Doctors treat gastrointestinal carcinoids that have spread to distant parts of the body by:

- freezing and killing cancer cells
- performing surgery or administering radiation or **chemotherapy** to relieve symptoms
- using biological therapy to stimulate the patient's immune system to attack tumor cells

Neither radiation nor chemotherapy can cure gastrointestinal carcinoids. Doctors sometimes use external beam radiation to treat patients who are too ill or frail to withstand surgery, and to relieve pain caused by tumors that have spread to the bones.

Doctors may use several different chemotherapy drugs or combine a chemotherapy drug with other medication to slow tumor growth and relieve symptoms. Chemotherapy is generally used only for gastrointestinal carcinoids that have spread to other organs, cause severe symptoms, and have not responded to other treatments.

Doctors sometimes treat gastrointestinal carcinoids that have spread to the liver by injecting chemotherapy drugs directly into the artery that supplies blood to the liver (hepatic artery). This technique (intra-arterial chemotherapy):

- exposes liver tumors to high doses of cancer-killing drugs
- prevents side effects by shielding healthy tissues from these powerful medications

When doctors also inject material that blocks the hepatic artery, this treatment is called **chemoembolization**.

Octreotide is a hormone-like drug that can prevent or relieve flushing, wheezing, diarrhea, and other symptoms that sometimes occur during surgery or when gastrointestinal carcinoids release high levels of hormones. Octreotide can temporarily shrink these tumors but does not cure the cancer. Some patients experience pain at the site where the medication is injected, cramps, **nausea and vomiting**, dizziness, and **fatigue**.

Doctors also prescribe other medications to relieve specific symptoms.

Biological therapy, or Interferon-alpha therapy may stimulate the patient's immune system to attack the tumor, shrink metastatic gastrointestinal carcinoids, and may relieve symptoms of carcinoid syndrome. This technique, which is also called immunotherapy, is sometimes used to treat tumors that have not responded to chemotherapy or octreotide, but can cause severe flu-like side effects.

TREATING RECURRENT DISEASE. Treatment of recurrent disease depends on where the new tumor is located and what treatment the patient has already received.

TREATING CARCINOID SYNDROME. Treatments for carcinoid syndrome include surgically removing the cancer, blocking the hepatic artery or injecting chemotherapy drugs into it, medication to relieve symptoms, and stimulating the patient's immune system to attack the tumor.

LONG-TERM SURVEILLANCE. After completing treatment, patients with certain types of gastrointestinal carcinoids must continue to have regular physical examinations, x rays, and blood and urine tests to help doctors detect recurrence during the earliest stages of disease.

Because some gastrointestinal carcinoids recur many years after initial treatment, high-risk patients should continue to see their doctor regularly. Any patient who has had a gastrointestinal carcinoid should immediately notify the doctor of any new symptoms. These symptoms could be side effects of treatment or a sign that the cancer has returned.

Prognosis

The only way to cure gastrointestinal carcinoids is to remove the tumors surgically. But because these cancers grow so slowly, it is not unusual for a patient to survive 10–15 years after being diagnosed with metastatic disease.

5-YEAR SURVIVAL RATES. For patients whose carcinoid tumor originates in the stomach, the 5-year survival rate is:

- 64% for localized disease
- 40% for regional spread
- 10% for mestatatic disease

When tumors originate in the small intestine, the 5-year survival rate is:

- 65% for localized disease
- 66% for regional spread
- 36% for metastatic disease

For carcinoids that originate in parts of the colon other than the appendix, the 5-year survival rate is:

- 71% for localized disease
- 44% for regional spread
- 21% for metastatic disease

For carcinoids that originate in the appendix, the 5-year survival rate is:

- 94% for localized disease
- 85% for regional spread
- 34% for metastatic disease

For carcinoids that originate in the rectum, the 5-year survival rate is:

- 81% for localized disease
- 47% for regional spread
- 18% for metastatic disease

Having a gastrointestinal carcinoid increases a patient's risk of developing other cancers in the digestive system.

Clinical trials

Researchers are investigating:

- how changes in cells transform normal tissues into gastrointestinal carcinoid tumors
- how effectively specific chemotherapy drugs and surgical procedures treat gastrointestinal carcinoids

QUESTIONS TO ASK THE DOCTOR

- What kind of gastrointestinal carcinoid do I have?
- What kind of treatment should I have?
- Will this treatment cure my disease?
- What are the side effects of this treatment?

- new ways of slowing or preventing growth of gastrointestinal carcinoids by blocking or shrinking the blood vessels that nourish them
- how nuclear medicine can contribute to early detection of gastrointestinal carcinoids

Prevention

There is no known way to prevent gastrointestinal carcinoids or to reduce the risk of developing them, but avoiding the following can prevent symptoms of carcinoid syndrome from becoming more intense:

- alcoholic drinks
- hot, spicy foods
- strenuous exercise
- stress

See Also Cryotherapy; Gastrointestinal cancers; Hepatic arterial infusion; Neuroendocrine tumors

Resources

BOOKS

Goldman, Lee and J. Claude Bennett. *Cecil Textbook of Medicine,* 21st ed., vol, 2. Philadelphia, PA: W.B.Saunders Company, 2000.

ORGANIZATIONS

National Carcinoid Support Group, Inc. 6666 Odana Rd., #146, Madison, WI 53719-1012. <http://members.aol.com/thencsg/info.html>

OTHER

"Gastrointestinal Carcinoid Tumor." *CancerNet.* November 2000. 31 March 2001 <http://cancernet.nci.nih.gov>.

"Gastrointestinal Carcinoid Tumors." *Gastrointestinal Carcinoid Tumors Resource Center.* 12 February 1999. April 2001 <http://www3.cancer.org>

"Carcinoid May Be Rare—But If You have It, You Are Not Alone." *National Carcinoid Suport Group.* 15 May 1999. 31 March 2001 <http://members.aol.com/thencsg>

"Carcinoid Research:There Is Hope." *National Carcinoid Support Group* 31 March 2001 <http://members.aol.com/thencsg>.

"Carcinoid Treatment:More Than One Option to Consider." *National Carcinoid Support Group.* 31 March 2001 <http://members.aol.com/thencsg/treatment.html>.

National Carcinoid Support Group *Questions & Answers About Carcinoid* 31 March 2001<http://members.aol.com/thencsg/info.html>.

Maureen Haggerty

Carcinoid tumors, lung

Definition

Lung carcinoid tumors are rare malignant growths that develop from cells that help regulate the flow of air and blood through the lungs. These growths are also known as neuroendocrine lung tumors, pulmonary carcinoids, and lung carcinoids.

Description

These cancers account for 1% to 3% of all lung tumors. Most lung carcinoids measure between slightly less than 1/4" (0.63 cm) and slightly more than 3/4" (1.9 cm). These tumors usually develop in the right lung.

Doctors classify lung carcinoids according to what tumor cells look like under a microscope, and where in the lung the tumor is located. Typical lung carcinoids occur about nine times as often as atypical tumors. They grow slowly and rarely spread beyond the lungs. Atypical lung carcinoids grow somewhat faster than typical tumors and are more likely to spread to other organs. In their most invasive form, atypical lung carcinoids look and behave like small-cell lung cancers.

About 80% of lung carcinoids are central carcinoids. Located in the walls of the large airways in the center of the lungs, where the neuroendocrine cells that form them are most concentrated, these tumors are almost always typical tumors. Carcinoids that develop in the narrower airways, close to the edges of the lungs, are called peripheral carcinoids. Most are typical tumors.

Demographics

Lung carcinoids usually develop between the ages of 45 and 55. These tumors are equally common in men and women and rarely affect children.

Causes and symptoms

Lung carcinoids are not caused by smoking or by exposure to chemicals at work or in the environment.

Doctors believe that central carcinoids develop from glands beneath the surface of the large air passages. Lung biopsies performed to diagnose or treat other conditions sometimes reveal microscopic clusters of neuroendocrine cells. These carcinoid tumorlets look like tiny peripheral carcinoids. They are most common when disease has caused scar tissue to form in the lungs, and may grow to be carcinoid tumors.

Patients who have peripheral or small central carcinoids don't usually show symptoms, but some patients who have central carcinoids cough, wheeze, or cough up blood (**hemoptysis**).

A large carcinoid that blocks part or all of an airway can cause post-obstructive **pneumonia**. Doctors may not consider the possibility of a carcinoid until **antibiotics** fail to cure this lung infection.

About 10% to 20% of lung carcinoids produce hormone-like substances that release into the bloodstream. These substances can cause symptoms such as **Cushing's syndrome**, acromegaly, or **hypercalcemia**. They may also cause carcinoid syndrome, which is a constellation of symptoms including facial flushing, abdominal cramps, **diarrhea**, and breathlessness, among others.

Diagnosis

A thorough physical examination will detect symptoms of syndrome health problems associated with these tumors. If a patient has one or more symptoms that suggest the presence of a lung carcinoid, the doctor will inquire about:

- chest pain
- cough
- blood-tinged sputum
- asthma
- wheezing
- pneumonia not cured by antibiotics
- recent weight gain
- facial flushing
- diarrhea

The doctor will use one or more methods to determine whether the patient has a lung tumor. Lung carcinoids that do not cause symptoms usually show up on chest x rays taken during a routine physical or as a result of other health problems.

Chest x rays cannot detect tumors that are very small or hidden by other organs in the chest. A doctor who suspects a lung carcinoid may order additional **imaging studies** in order to make a more detailed search.

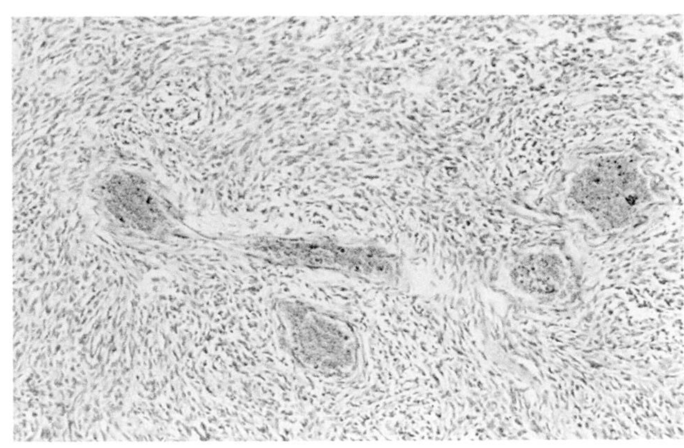

Lung carcinoid, spindle cell form. *(© Parviz M. Pour, Science Source/Photo Researchers, Inc. Photo reproduced by permission.)*

About 75% of lung carcinoids can be seen through a long, lighted tube called a bronchoscope. Doctors also use CT scans, octreoscans, or MIBG (metaiodobenzyl-guanidine) scans to locate lung carcinoids and determine how far they have spread. CT scans provide a detailed view of the lungs. Octreoscans and MIBG scans trace the path of radioactive substances that are attracted to lung carcinoids.

Also called indium-111-labeled DTPA-octreotide scintigraphy, octreoscan involves injecting a small amount of a radioactive hormone-like substance into the patient's vein. Carcinoid tumors attract this substance, and a special camera locates tumors by pinpointing the area where the radioactive material accumulates.

Doctors perform MIBG scans by attaching radioactive iodine to a chemical absorbed by carcinoid tumors. This compound is injected into the patient's bloodstream, drawn to carcinoid tumor cells, and tracked by a special scanner.

Although diagnostic procedures can indicate that a patient might have a lung carcinoid, **biopsy** is the only way to confirm the diagnosis. Doctors use several different techniques to remove samples of these tumors.

BRONCHOSCOPIC BIOPSY. To obtain a sample of a tumor in one of the large airways, the doctor uses a bronchoscope to examine the lining of these organs. When a tumor is located, the doctor manipulates pincers or tongs (biopsy forceps) through the bronchoscope to remove a small sample of tissue. The patient leaves the hospital a few hours after undergoing this outpatient procedure. If serious bleeding occurs, the doctor narrows or seals the blood vessels by injecting drugs or aiming a laser beam.

BRUSHING SAMPLE. A doctor who performs a bronchoscopic biopsy may also wipe a tiny brush over the surface of the tumor. Tumor cells extracted in this way (brushing sample) are examined under a microscope. A

KEY TERMS

Acromegaly—Hormonal disorder causing progressive enlargement of hands and feet and elongation of the face, headache, muscle pain, and visual and emotional disturbances in middle-aged men and women.

Carcinoid syndrome—Rare malignant disease characterized by facial flushing, abdominal cramps, diarrhea, breathlessness, and other symptoms. Affects fewer than 10% of patients with carcinoid tumor.

Cushing's syndrome—Hormonal disorder characterized by a round face, mental or emotional instability, high blood pressure, weight gain, or abnormal growth of facial and body hair in women.

Emphysema—Abnormal lung condition characterized by breathing problems, cough, rapid heartbeat. Later stages are characterized by restlessness, weakness, confusion, increased breathlessness, and may cause fluid to collect around the lungs (pulmonary edema) and congestive heart failure.

Hypercalcemia—Abnormally high levels of calcium in the blood, causing muscle pain and weakness and loss of appetite. Severe cases can result in kidney failure.

brushing sample can add useful information to the results of bronchoscopic biopsy.

NEEDLE BIOPSY. Doctors often use needle biopsy to obtain samples of tumors that are not close to the large airways. Guided by a **computed tomography** scan (CT scan) image, a long needle is passed between the ribs and into the lung to remove a small piece of the tumor. Because carcinoid tumors are usually small, localization using a needle biopsy may be difficult or impossible.

THORACOTOMY. If neither bronchoscopic biopsy nor needle biopsy yields enough tissue to identify the tumor type, the doctor may open the patient's chest (**thoracotomy**) to remove a tissue sample. A doctor who feels certain that a tumor is a carcinoid may perform a thoracotomy and remove the entire tumor without having taken a biopsy sample.

Treatment team

Lung carcinoids are treated by thoracic and cardiothoracic surgeons.

Clinical staging, treatments, and prognosis

Staging

Once lung carcinoids have been diagnosed, more tests are done to find out if the cancer has spread from the lung to other parts of the body (staging). A doctor needs to know the stage to plan treatment. Doctors stage lung carcinoids the same way they stage non-small cell lung cancers:

- Stage 0: Cancer is only found in a local area and only in a few layers of cells. It has not grown through the top lining of the lung.
- Stage I: The cancer is only in the lung, and normal tissue is around it.
- Stage II: Cancer has spread to nearby lymph nodes.
- Stage III: Cancer has spread to the chest wall or diaphragm near the lung; or the cancer has spread to the lymph nodes in the area that separates the two lungs (mediastinum); or to the lymph nodes on the other side of the chest or in the neck. Stage III is further divided into stage IIIA (usually can be operated on) and stage IIIB (usually cannot be operated on).
- Stage IV: Cancer has spread to other parts of the body.

Treatment of lung carcinoids

Doctors consider tumor size and location, and whether the patient has additional lung problems or serious disease affecting any other organ, in order to determine the most appropriate treatment for lung carcinoids.

SURGERY. Removing the tumor (surgical resection) is the treatment of choice for these cancers because most lung carcinoids:

- can be cured by surgery alone
- do not respond to **chemotherapy** or radiation
- must be removed in order to prevent airway obstruction and other complications of tumor growth

If the tumor is located in a large airway, the surgeon may remove the tumor and normal tissue above and below it, then sew together the remaining lung tissue. This procedure is a sleeve resection.

If tumor size or location makes sleeve resection impossible, the surgeon removes the affected lobe of the lung (**lobectomy**). In rare cases, the surgeon removes the entire right or left lung (**pneumonectomy**).

Surgeons use lobectomy to remove peripheral carcinoids located at the edges of the lungs farthest from the large airways. If the tumor is very small, the surgeon may remove it and a wedge-shaped piece of lung tissue surrounding it (wedge resection).

Surgeons who remove lung carcinoids usually remove some of the lymph nodes near the lungs because:

- About 10% of typical carcinoids and 30% to 50% of atypical carcinoids have spread to lymph nodes by the time the disease is diagnosed.
- Not removing lymph nodes might increase the risk of cancer spreading to other organs.
- Surgery alone cannot cure lung carcinoids that have spread to other organs.
- Examining lymph nodes can indicate the likelihood that cancer will recur.

Surgeons who remove lung carcinoids try to preserve the patient's lung function by removing the smallest possible amount of normal lung tissue.

PALLIATIVE TREATMENT. A patient who has severe emphysema, chronic bronchitis, heart disease, or other medical problems may not be able to withstand the stress of surgery to cure lung carcinoids or to cope with breathing difficulties resulting from removal of normal lung tissue.

Doctors use a bronchoscope and a laser to burn away (vaporize) most of the tumor in a patient who is too ill to withstand surgery. These palliative treatments can relieve most symptoms associated with lung carcinoids, but cannot cure the disease. They are often supplemented by radiation administered externally or directly into the air passages (intrabronchial radiation).

MEDICAL TREATMENTS. Guidelines issued in 2001 by the National Comprehensive Cancer Network recommend the use of radiation following surgery to remove carcinoid lung tumors, and chemotherapy and radiation following surgery to remove atypical lung carcinoids.

Injected into a vein or taken by mouth, chemotherapy drugs are also used to treat lung carcinoids that have spread to other organs, are causing severe symptoms, or have not responded to other medications. Doctors may combine two or more chemotherapy drugs or add them to other medications to relieve symptoms of lung carcinoids that have spread to other organs.

Octreotide controls wheezing, flushing, and other symptoms of carcinoid syndrome. This medication may temporarily shrink lung carcinoids but does not cure them.

Alpha-interferon can shrink some lung carcinoids that have spread to other parts of the body and relieve symptoms of carcinoid syndrome. Doctors can prescribe other medications to relieve specific symptoms.

Radiation may be an option for patients who are too frail or ill to undergo surgery but is not a very effective treatment for lung carcinoids. High doses of radiation can damage lung tissue, create scar tissue, cause breathing problems, and make the patient more susceptible to infection.

QUESTIONS TO ASK THE DOCTOR

- What kind of lung carcinoid do I have?
- What treatment do you recommend?
- Will this treatment cure me?
- What can I do to make this treatment more successful?

PROGNOSIS. Five-year survival rates for patients with lung carcinoids are 90% to 100% for typical tumors, and 40% to 76% for atypical tumors. Ten-year survival rates are about 10% lower than five-year rates for both types of tumors. The prognosis is worse for lung carcinoids that measure 1 1/4" (3.2 cm) or larger or have spread to lymph nodes.

Some patients who have had lung carcinoids must continue to have regular x rays and blood tests to help doctors detect recurrent disease in its earliest stages. Any patient who has had a lung carcinoid should notify the doctor whenever new symptoms develop. These symptoms could be side effects of treatment or signs that the disease has recurred. A patient who has recovered from surgery should ask the doctor about an exercise routine to restore energy and reduce shortness of breath.

Clinical trials

Researchers are currently investigating whether:

- new methods of delivering radiation can shrink lung carcinoids that have not responded to treatment
- inhaling chemotherapy drugs can shrink advanced lung carcinoids
- biological therapy can starve lung carcinoids by cutting off the flow of blood that nourishes them and stimulate patients' white blood cells to kill cancer cells
- new methods of delivering chemotherapy can kill cancer cells without harming normal cells
- new combinations of chemotherapy drugs can prevent cancer cells from multiplying
- chemotherapy drugs combined with radioactive substances can locate and kill cancer cells without harming normal cells

Moore, Katen, and Libby Schmais. *Living Well with Cancer: A Nurse Tells You Everything You Need to Know About Managing the Side Effects of Your Treatment.* New York: Putnam Publishing Group, 2001.

PERIODICALS

Ginsburg, A.D. "Doxorubicin-induced Cardiomyopathy."*New England Journal of Medicine* 340, no. 8 (February, 1999): 654.

OTHER

Heart Center Online Home Page. 6 June 2001 <http://www.heartcenteronline.com/> This website serves cardiologists and their patients and has sections on pericardiocentesis, pericarditis and tamponade.

Marianne Vahey, M.D.

Carmustine

Definition

Carmustine is an antineoplastic drug, meaning that it inhibits the growth of cancer. It does this by disrupting DNA and synthesis, which leads to cell death. Carmustine is often referred to as BCNU, and along with other chemically similar drugs (**lomustine**, **semustine**, and **streptozocin**) is classified as a nitrosourea. Brand names for carmustine in the U.S. include BiCNU and Gliadel Wafers.

Purpose

Because it readily crosses the blood-brain barrier, carmustine is used to treat several types of brain tumors, including **astrocytoma**, **ependymoma**, glioblastoma, brainstem glioma, **medulloblastoma**. It is usually given intravenously, but it is also available as a wafer that is implanted in the brain during surgery. Carmustine is also used in the treatment of **multiple myeloma** and **melanoma**, usually in combination with other agents. It is also used in high does for patients undergoing bone marrow or stem cell transplants. Patients with non-Hodgkin's or Hodgkin's lymphoma whose disease has either relapsed or not responded to initial therapy, may be treated with carmustine used in combination with other drugs.

Description

Carmustine was approved for use by the U.S. Food and Drug Administration (FDA) in 1977. Carmustine comes in vial, in a powder form, and is reconstituted with sterile water according to the manufacturer's instructions. It may be used as a single agent, meaning it is administered alone; or it may be used with other drugs. It is further diluted in a larger volume of fluid and given slowly into a vein over a one- to two-hour period. Faster administration may cause a burning sensation in the vein, as well as facial flushing. The wafer is implanted surgically.

Carmustine is excreted by the kidneys during urination, and the lungs during expiration. Studies have shown that within four days, up to 70% of the drug is excreted in the urine, while an additional 10% is excreted in exhaled carbon dioxide. No one is certain what happens to the remaining 20% of the drug.

Recommended dosage

Because carmustine can have delayed toxic effects on the bone marrow, doses should be given at least four to six weeks apart. If carmustine is given in conjunction with other drugs that also suppress the bone marrow, dosages may be reduced. Blood tests are performed frequently during and after treatment, and their results may require dosage adjustments. Currently, there is no known remedy for a carmustine overdose.

Chemotherapy dosages are based on a person's body surface area (BSA), which is calculated in square meters using height and weight measurements. Drug dosages are ordered in milligrams per square meter (mg/m^2). Carmustine doses vary, but common doses include 75–250 mg/m^2 every four to six weeks, and 80 mg/m^2 daily for three days every six weeks. Higher doses are used for patients undergoing bone marrow or stem cell transplants. The specific dose should be verified for each patient. Continued doses after the first course of carmustine depend on the patient's response and on toxicity. Sometimes doses are adjusted because of toxicity or low blood counts.

Precautions

Carmustine may be damaging to an unborn fetus. Women of child-bearing potential should take measures to prevent pregnancy and women receiving carmustine should not breast-feed.

Side effects

Carmustine should be used after careful consideration of the risks and benefits involved, as there can be serious adverse side effects.

Myelosuppression

Effects on the bone marrow can lead to reduced numbers of platelets and white blood cells, which can have potentially life-threatening results, including bleeding and infection. These effects are first seen from four to six weeks after treatment is started, are cumulative, and are related to the amount of the drug given. A patient taking carmustine who develops a **fever** or notices an increased tendency to bleed or bruise may have dangerously low blood counts, and should be evaluated by a physician.

Pulmonary damage

Patients taking carmustine are at risk for damage to the lungs marked by pulmonary fibrosis. The main symptom of pulmonary fibrosis is shortness of breath. Pulmonary fibrosis can lead to heart failure. It is most likely to develop in patients with total cumulative doses greater than 1400 mg/m^2, although lower doses may also cause damage.

Individuals with underlying lung disease, such as chronic obstructive pulmonary disease, may be more likely to develop carmustine-associated pulmonary injury. Prior to initiating treatment with carmustine, a doctor will usually evaluate how well the lungs function by performing pulmonary function tests (PFTs). Patients are more likely to develop lung damage if portions of these tests are abnormal. PFTs may be repeated during treatment to monitor for adverse effects of carmustine. If carmustine is used in conjunction with other drugs that have toxic effects on pulmonary function, there may be a greater risk of lung damage.

Nausea and vomiting

Like many antineoplastic drugs, carmustine can cause **nausea and vomiting**. Before carmustine is administered, medications called **antiemetics** should be given to prevent or minimize nausea. Patients who experience severe nausea, or nausea that is uncontrolled with antiemetics, should notify their doctor.

Organ damage

Carmustine may cause damage to the kidneys. With careful monitoring and frequent blood tests, this damage can be prevented or reversed. Kidney damage is more likely to occur in individuals who have received prolonged therapy with large cumulative doses. Blood tests to evaluate renal function should be performed routinely. Carmustine may be discontinued or reduced depending on these results.

Secondary malignancies

Although carmustine is used to treat cancer, it may also cause secondary malignancies when used long-term.

KEY TERMS

Antiemetic—A drug that prevents or alleviates nausea and vomiting.

Body surface area—A measurement based on height and weight that is expressed in square meters. It is used to determine chemotherapy dosages.

Myelosuppression—Suppression of bone marrow function that results in decreased platelets, red blood cells, and white blood cells.

Carmustine wafers

Intracranial implantation of carmustine wafers has been associated with abnormal wound healing after surgery, brain edema or accumulation of fluid, infection, and the formation of cysts near the site of implantation.

Interactions

Patients should tell their doctor about medications they are taking in addition to their cancer treatment, as these medications may interact with carmustine. For example, cimetidine, a drug used to treat heartburn and ulcers, may increase the toxic effects of carmustine on the bone marrow. Carmustine, on the other hand, may decrease blood levels of **phenytoin**, a drug used in the treatment of patients with seizures. If blood levels are too low, seizures may not be prevented.

Patients undergoing treatment for cancer with carmustine should talk to their doctor prior to taking any **vaccines**. Live vaccines, in particular, can increase the likelihood of complications.

Aspirin and ibuprofen, which are found in many over-the-counter products, should be avoided. These drugs can increase the potential for bleeding in people who may already have decreased platelet counts due to carmustine therapy.

Tamara Brown, R.N.

CAT scan *see* **Computed tomography**

Cefepime *see* **Antibiotics**

Ceftazidime *see* **Antibiotics**

Ceftriaxone *see* **Antibiotics**

Celecoxib *see* **Cyclooxygenase 2 inhibitors**

Cellcept *see* **Mycophenolate mofetil**

Central nervous system carcinoma

Definition

A central nervous system **carcinoma** is a malignant tumor arising in the cells of the brain or spinal cord.

Description

The central nervous system (CNS) is comprised of the brain and spinal cord. The CNS takes its name from the crucial role it plays in maintaining physical and mental well-being (homeostasis). The brain controls and monitors the body's activity; the spinal cord conveys information to the body from the brain, and vice versa. Consequently, a tumor in the CNS disrupts motor (e.g., standing, walking, writing) and sensory (e.g., seeing, tasting, hearing) activities.

The two major components of brain tissue are neurons (nerve cells) and glial cells. About half of all malignant CNS tumor growth starts in glial cells. Long thought to be mere space-holders, glial cells have been found to be extremely important. These cells actually protect and nourish the neurons, and may also help them transmit information. There are many different types of glial carcinomas, or gliomas.

The three layers of tissue, meninges, that cover the brain and spinal cord; and the pituitary and pineal parts of the brain, are also common sites for tumor growth. About 40% of benign (noncancerous) CNS tumors occur in the meninges, and the pituitary and pineal glands.

Some cancers that originate in organs, such as the kidneys, spread (metastasize) to the brain and spinal cord. These metastases differ from CNS carcinomas, however.

Demographics

About 35,000 cases of CNS carcinoma are diagnosed each year. The Central Brain Tumor Registry of the United States (CBTRUS) puts the incidence of CNS tumors at 12.8 per 100,000 person-years. The rate is slightly higher in males and slightly lower in females. Over a lifetime the chance a man will be diagnosed with and die from a CNS tumor is 1 in 200 and for a woman that rate is 1 in 263.

The older a person is the more likely he or she is to be diagnosed with CNS carcinoma. According to CBTRUS, the pediatric (individuals ages 0-19 years) incidence of CNS tumors is significantly lower, or about 3.8 per 100,000 person-years. People under the age of 20 years also have a higher survival rate. They are five times more likely to live at least five years with a CNS tumor than are people between the ages of 45 and 64 years.

In addition to the diagnoses of primary CNS tumors (those that originate in the brain and spinal cord) is the diagnoses of metastatic cancer. Metastatic cancers are those that have spread from other primary sites, such as the breast, prostate, lungs, and colon. For every person diagnosed with a primary CNS tumor, at least four other individuals will be diagnosed with cancer that has metastasized to the brain and spinal cord. Occasionally, the identification of a metastatic brain cancer leads a physician to discover a cancer in another organ, or the **primary site**.

Causes and symptoms

The cause of CNS carcinoma is unknown. Important factors might include heredity, genetic make-up, and exposure to radiation and chemicals. Head injury might lead to meningiomas (carcinoma of the meninges). Extra or missing chromosomes or other genetic abnormalities are linked to the development of some CNS tumors. In one study a group of researchers led by T. Ballard showed pilots and flight attendants are at greater risk for CNS carcinoma, perhaps because of their frequent exposure to high levels of cosmic radiation.

Many individuals display no symptoms of CNS carcinoma until the tumor has grown large enough to exert pressure on part of the CNS. Because the skull covers the brain and the vertebral column protects the spinal cord, a growing tumor soon pushes up against a barrier of bone. The bone limits the expansion of the tumor and the cancerous and adjacent parts of the CNS become distorted. The meninges then swell in response to the distortion, producing symptoms.

Symptoms include:

- headache
- muscle weakness
- exhaustion
- **nausea and vomiting**
- changes in vision
- seizures

When a tumor is in the spinal cord, symptoms include back pain and **incontinence** (inability to control defecation and urination). Paralysis on one side of the body (hemiparesis), which often indicates a stroke in an elderly person, sometimes occurs because of a brain tumor.

Diagnosis

Seizures and difficulties with walking, speech, sight, or other day-to-day activities usually cause patients with CNS carcinoma to consult a physician. The techniques a physician uses to diagnose CNS carcinoma begins with an examination and medical history. Some combination of blood tests, **x ray**, **computed tomography** (CT), and **magnetic resonance imaging** (MRI) is used. If a tumor is detected with a CT or MRI scan a **biopsy** is usually done to determine the type of tumor.

Treatment team

A CNS carcinoma requires attention from several different types of physician specialists. A neurologist, a physician specializing in the nervous system, does the initial assessment. A radiologist interprets x rays, CT and MRI images. A hematologist or oncologist evaluates the results of blood tests. A pathologist studies the tissue from a biopsy. The surgery team that removes the tumor typically includes a neurosurgeon and an orthopedic surgeon. The orthopedic surgeon takes part because it is necessary to cut through bone to reach the brain and maneuver around vertebrae to reach the spinal cord. At premier cancer centers teams of physicians work collaboratively with one person, usually an oncologist, taking the lead. Physical and occupational therapists who help with rehabilitation following treatment and surgery, and registered nurses who administer **chemotherapy**, are also part of the team.

Clinical staging, treatments, and prognosis

By studying tissue from the tumor and surrounding cells the oncologist determines whether the tumor is growing and, if so, how fast. There is an elaborate system for assigning grades to the tumors that depends on things such as which part of the brain was served by the glial cell(s) in which the tumor began.

A plan for treatment is based on the location, size, and rate of growth of the tumor. Surgical removal of the tumor, radiation, and chemotherapy are all used. Method of treatment depends on the type of CNS carcinoma. In some cases the treatment is strictly palliative (provides comfort) and is not expected to halt the course of the cancer. Drugs, such as steroids, are often given to reduce swelling and, correspondingly, reduce pain and other symptoms.

About three-quarters of all individuals diagnosed with CNS carcinoma die before attaining a five-year survival rate.

Alternative and complementary therapies

Relaxation techniques may help to relieve pain from swelling.

Coping with cancer treatment

Being an active participant in the treatment team, something that specialized cancer centers encourage, is one way to cope. Joining a support group also may help.

KEY TERMS

Biopsy—Tissue sample taken from body for microscopic examination.

Carcinoma—A cancer that originates in cells that developed from epithelial tissue, a tissue that forms layers and often specializes to cover and protect organs.

Computed tomography (CT)—X rays aimed at sections of the body (by rotating equipment) and images appear as slices. Results are assembled with a computer to give a three-dimensional image.

Homeostasis—Self-regulating mechanisms are working, body is in equilibrium, no uncontrolled cell growth.

Magnetic resonance imaging (MRI)—Magnetic fields and radio frequency waves are used to make images of the inside of the body.

Meninges—The three layers of tissue that cover the brain and spinal cord.

Pineal—A very small gland in the center of the brain that is sensitive to light.

Pituitary—A gland at the base of the brain that produces hormones.

Clinical trials

The National Cancer Institute at the National Institutes of Health operates an information service that provides the most up-to-date information about **clinical trials**. The number is (800) 4-CANCER ([800] 422-6237).

Prevention

Limiting exposure to cosmic radiation and chemicals might lower the risk. However, experts have no specific recommendations for prevention.

Special concerns

Psychological changes as simple as mood swings and as severe as major changes in personality are possible. Sensory impairment is also possible. **Advance directives**, or written instructions for the care a person wants at each juncture of treatment, should be prepared and legalized as early in the therapeutic process as possible. Such directives make the patient's choices clear should he or she become unable to express them as the cancer progresses. Doing so relieves loved ones of the

QUESTIONS TO ASK THE DOCTOR

- Which type of CNS carcinoma do I have?
- With this type of carcinoma, what is the five-year survival rate for a person of my age and gender?
- What is the one-year survival rate?
- Is there a center that specializes in treating this type of cancer?
- Are there any clinical trials in which I might be eligible to participate?
- Does this health care institution have a support group for individuals with my type of carcinoma?
- What is your approach to relieving pain? (Do we agree?)

responsibility for making those decisions, which can become extremely difficult.

See Also Brain and central nervous system tumors

Resources

BOOKS

Schold, S. Clifford Jr. et al. *Primary Tumors of the Brain and Spinal Cord.* Boston: Butterworth-Heinemann, 1997.

PERIODICALS

Ballard, T. et al. "Cancer Incidence and Mortality Among Flight Personnel: A Meta-Analysis" *Aviation, Space, and Environmental Medicine.* 71 (March 2000): 216-24.

Black, P. M. "Brain Tumors" (part two) *New England Journal of Medicine* 324 (May 31,1991): 1555-1564.

Huncharek, M. et al. "Chemotherapy Response Rates in Recurrent/Progressive Pediatric Glioma; Results of a Systematic Review" *Anticancer Research* 19 (July-Aug. 1999): 3569-74.

ORGANIZATIONS

American Brain Tumor Association. 2720 River Road, Des Plaines, IL 60018 (800) 886-2282 <http://www.abta.org>

The Brain Tumor Society. 124 Watertown Street, Suite 3-H, Watertown, MA 02472. (617) 924-9997 <http://www.tbts. org>

OTHER

"Year 2000 Standard Report" *Central Brain Tumor Registry of the United States* 28 March 2001 6 July 2001 <http://www.cbtrus.org/2000/y2kstats_report.htm>

"Facts and Statistics from the American Brain Tumor Association" *CancerWise.org* 28 March 2001. 6 July 2001 <http://www.cancerwise.org/archive/august/facts_figures/ff_brain.html>

Diane M. Calabrese

Central nervous system lymphoma

Definition

Central nervous system (CNS) lymphoma is a malignant growth, or neoplasm, that originates in the white blood cells of the lymphatic fluid in the brain and spinal cord.

Description

CNS lymphoma affects the brain and the spinal cord, the two components of the CNS. The brain and spinal cord work together to control, monitor, and interpret all the physical and mental processes of the body. They make possible the activities a person takes for granted, such as walking, talking, thinking and remembering. A malignancy, or neoplasm, in the brain or spinal cord interferes with the normal functions of the body.

An uncontrolled growth of cells called lymphocytes causes lymphoma. Lymphocytes are the white blood cells in the lymphatic system. Under normal conditions they help the body resist invasion by foreign substances and organisms. In other words, they assist with **immune response** or defense.

When the uncontrolled growth of lymphocytes originates in the brain or spinal cord, it is called primary CNS lymphoma, or simply, CNS lymphoma. The specific place of origin of CNS lymphoma is probably in cells known as B cells. Other kinds of lymphoma begin elsewhere in the lymphatic system. They may also eventually affect the brain and spinal cord, but they are not called CNS lymphoma.

In most cases, CNS lymphoma does not produce a defined and specific site of growth, or a tumor. Generally, the cancer cells spread throughout the brain and spinal cord. The spread gives way to lesions, which are places where tissue breaks down.

Demographics

Although the number of cases is on the increase, CNS lymphoma is rare. Between 1 and 2% of all uncontrolled growths in the brain result from CNS lymphoma. The most common age of diagnosis in the general population is between 52 and 55 years. However, in patients that have experienced immune system problems, age at diagnosis is much younger, at about 34 years.

Events and conditions that affect the immune system put a person at greater risk for CNS lymphoma. For example, someone who has had an organ transplant is more vulnerable to the disease. Part of the reason is that transplant patients are given drugs to suppress, or reduce, the action of the immune system so their bodies will accept an organ from a donor. Individuals with acquired immunodeficiency syndrome (AIDS) are also at higher risk for CNS lymphoma.

Causes and symptoms

The cause of CNS lymphoma is not known. It is more common in individuals with suppressed immune systems, and individuals with some conditions linked to the X chromosome, one of the two sex chromosomes, seem to be at higher risk. Studies indicate that exposure to certain herbicides also increases risk.

One role of the lymphatic system is to collect fluid that builds up outside cells and to return it to blood vessels. CNS lymphoma obstructs this process. Fluid builds up in the body and puts particular pressure on the cranial nerves, the nerves that carry information directly from the brain to organs such as the eyes and ears. Consequently, symptoms of CNS lymphoma often occur in the organs of the head and in the face.

Symptoms include:

- change in personality
- headache
- **nausea and vomiting**
- seizures
- weakness
- numbness, particularly in the face
- sensory problems (cannot hear, see)
- difficulty swallowing

Diagnosis

Symptoms cause a person to consult a physician. The initial assessment is made using **computed tomography** (CT) or **magnetic resonance imaging** (MRI). To confirm a diagnosis a physician does a variety of tests. They include a physical examination of lymph nodes, chest **x ray**, blood and urine tests, eye exam, bone marrow **biopsy**, and—in males—an ultrasound of the testes. Some of the tests are done to rule out other kinds of lymphoma.

Treatment team

CNS lymphoma requires attention from several different types of physician specialists. A neurologist—a physician specializing in the nervous system—does the initial assessment. A radiologist interprets x rays, CT scans, and MRI images. A hematologist or oncologist evaluates the results of blood tests. A pathologist studies the tissue from a biopsy. If there is surgery, and in many cases there is not, the surgery team that removes the tumor typically includes a neurosurgeon and an orthopedic surgeon. The orthopedic surgeon takes part because it is necessary to cut through bone to reach the brain, and maneuver around vertebrae to reach the spinal cord. At premier cancer centers, teams of physicians work collaboratively, with one person (usually an oncologist) taking the lead. Physical and occupational therapists who help with rehabilitation following treatment and surgery, and registered nurses who administer **chemotherapy**, are also part of the team.

KEY TERMS

B lymphocyte—Cell in the lymph system that produces antibodies, which protect against foreign substances.

Biopsy—Tissue sample taken from the body for microscopic examination.

Computed tomography (CT)—X rays are aimed at sections of the body (by rotating equipment) and images appear as slices. Results are assembled with a computer to give a three-dimensional picture of a structure within the body.

Herbicide—A chemical compound used to kill plants.

Lymphatic system—The nodes of tissue and the fluid that moves among them. This system works to protect the body from invading substances and organisms, and to return fluid that collects outside cells to the blood vessels.

Magnetic resonance imaging (MRI)—Magnetic fields and radio frequency waves take pictures (images) of the inside of the body.

Ultrasound—Sound waves are bounced off structures in the body to produce an image of those structures.

Clinical staging, treatments, and prognosis

All treatment is palliative (designed to provide relief from symptoms and make a patient comfortable). Surgery is sometimes used to eliminate well-defined masses that are causing pressure in the brain and spinal cord. This pressure causes the symptoms, such as headache and numbness, because it contributes to swelling and dislocation. However, because CNS lym-

QUESTIONS TO ASK THE DOCTOR

- Will my quality of life be better with or without radiation treatment? How much of the time that I gain from radiation treatment will be time that I can function and do some of the things I enjoy?
- Is there a clinical trial in which I could participate?
- Is there a support group for CNS lymphoma at this institution or in this town?

phoma generally spreads throughout the brain and spinal cord, surgery is usually not a treatment choice.

Medication in the form of steroids and radiation treatment both give good results over the short term by causing clusters of malignant cells to shrink briefly. However, neither treatment is effective for much more than six months. A great deal of interest surrounds research aimed at finding chemotherapy that works effectively for this type of cancer. Chemotherapy for CNS lymphoma is sometimes given by putting drugs directly into the brain or spinal cord.

The prognosis (outlook for recovery) for a patient with CNS lymphoma is poor. Untreated, the disease usually results in death in just a few weeks. If it is treated, life can be extended by perhaps six months to one year, and occasionally longer.

Ulrich Herrlinger, M.D., and colleagues in Tuebingen, Germany, have reported that the combination of **radiation therapy** and chemotherapy gives patients a much better chance of extended survival, prolonging life for more than six years in one individual. Eleven of the 21 patients in their study lived for 33 months or longer.

Alternative and complementary therapies

Any relaxation program, such as biofeedback or yoga, often help a patient deal with the poor prognosis, pain, and symptoms of CNS lymphoma.

Coping with cancer treatment

Radiation therapy, particularly of the entire brain that is required to treat most CNS lymphoma, can greatly alter memory and thought processes. Being prepared for the effects of radiation before the treatment begins is important. For example, a patient can write out a daily schedule of things to do—the essentials of an ordinary day such as brushing teeth and combing hair. This schedule can then be used as a memory aid after treatment.

Having a patient taking an active part in planning the course of treatment can be helpful, such as participating in meetings with the treatment team. Premier cancer treatment centers encourage patients to be an integral member of the team. Because some individuals beat the odds and live much longer than expected, an optimistic attitude is important.

Clinical trials

The National Cancer Institute at the National Institutes of Health, Bethesda, MD, offers a Cancer Information Service that can connect people with **clinical trials**. The toll free number for the Service is 1-800-4-CANCER (1-800-422-6237).

Prevention

No prevention is known; however, any effort that reduces the number of people infected with the virus that causes AIDS will indirectly reduce the number of people with CNS lymphoma. Three percent of all AIDS patients exhibit CNS lymphoma.

Special concerns

Because CNS lymphoma is a fatal disease, patients must make decisions about end-of-life care. How will it be arranged: at home, in a hospice, in some other setting? Who will make decisions if the patient is no longer able to state his or her desires? **Advance directives**, or written instructions for how a person wishes the medical team to respond at each juncture of the illness, should be completed as soon as possible after a diagnosis is made.

Resources

BOOKS

Canellos, George P., et al.*The Lymphomas.* Philadelphia: W.B. Saunders Co., 1997.

PERIODICALS

Herrlinger, Ulrich, et al. "Primary Central Nervous System Lymphoma"*Cancer* 91 (Jan.1, 2001): 131-135.

OTHER

Lymphoma Information Network. Mike Barela, host. 1 July 2001 <http://www.lymphomainfo.net>

Diane M. Calabrese

Central nervous system tumors *see* **Brain and Central nervous system tumors**

Cerebrospinal fluid analysis, *see* **Lumbar puncture**

Cervical cancer

Definition

Cervical cancer is a disease in which the cells of the cervix become abnormal and start to grow uncontrollably, forming tumors.

Description

In the United States, cervical cancer is the fifth most common cancer among women aged 35-54, and the third most common cancer of the female reproductive tract. In some developing countries, it is the most common type of cancer. It generally begins as an abnormality in the cells on the outside of the cervix. The cervix is the lower part or neck of the uterus (womb). It connects the body of the uterus to the vagina (birth canal).

Approximately 90% of cervical cancers are squamous cell carcinomas. This type of cancer originates in the thin, flat, squamous cells on the surface of the ectocervix, the part of the cervix that is next to the vagina. (Squamous cells are the thin, flat cells of the surfaces of the skin and cervix and linings of various organs.) Another 10% of cervical cancers are of the adenocarcinoma type. This cancer originates in the mucus-producing cells of the inner or endocervix, near the body of the uterus. Occasionally, the cancer may have characteristics of both types and is called adenosquamous **carcinoma** or mixed carcinoma.

The initial changes that may occur in some cervical cells are not cancerous. However, these precancerous cells form a lesion called dysplasia or a squamous intraepithelial lesion (SIL), since it occurs within the epithelial or outer layer of cells. These abnormal cells can also be described as cervical intraepithelial neoplasia (CIN). Moderate to severe dysplasia may be called carcinoma in situ or non-invasive cervical cancer.

Dysplasia is a common condition and the abnormal cells often disappear without treatment. However, these precancerous cells can become cancerous. This may take years, although it can happen in less than a year. Eventually, the abnormal cells start to grow uncontrollably into the deeper layers of the cervix, becoming an invasive cervical cancer.

Although cervical cancer used to be one of the most common causes of cancer death among American women, in the past 40 years there has been a 75% decrease in mortality. This is primarily due to routine screening with Pap tests (Pap smear), to identify precancerous and early-invasive stages of cervical cancer. With treatment, these conditions have a cure rate of nearly 100%.

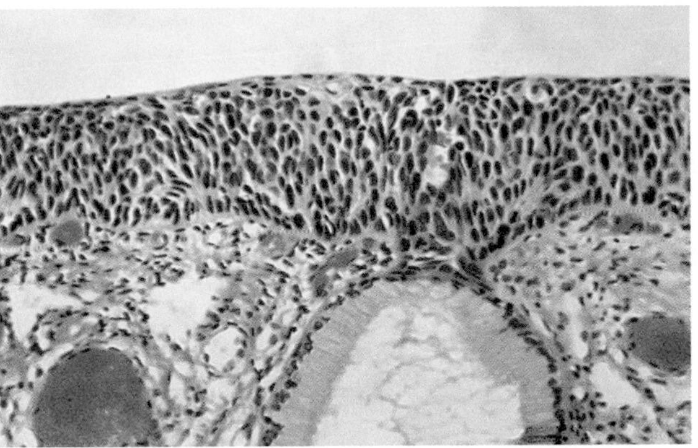

A biopsied section of the cervix indicating a carcinoma in situ. *(Custom Medical Stock Photo. Reproduced with permission.)*

Demographics

Worldwide, there are more than 400,000 new cases of cervical cancer diagnosed each year. The American Cancer Society (ACS) estimates that there will be 12,900 new cases of invasive cervical cancer diagnosed in the United States in 2001. More than one million women will be diagnosed with a precancerous lesion or non-invasive cancer of the cervix.

Older women are at the highest risk for cervical cancer. Although girls under the age of 15 rarely develop this cancer, the risk factor begins to increase in the late teens. Rates for carcinoma in situ peak between the ages of 20 and 30. In the United States, the incidence of invasive cervical cancer increases rapidly with age for African-American women over the age of 25. The incidence rises more slowly for Caucasian women. However women over age 65 account for more than 25% of all cases of invasive cervical cancer.

The incidence of cervical cancer is highest among poor women and among women in developing countries. In the United States, the death rates from cervical cancer are higher among Hispanic, Native American, and African American women than among Caucasian women. These groups of women are much less likely to receive regular Pap tests. Therefore, their cervical cancers usually are diagnosed at a much later stage, after the cancer has spread to other parts of the body.

Causes and symptoms

Human papilloma virus

Infection with the common **human papilloma virus** (HPV) is a cause of approximately 90% of all cervical cancers. There are more than 80 types of HPV. About 30 of these types can be transmitted sexually, including those that cause genital warts (papillomas). About half of the sexually transmitted HPVs are associated with cervical cancer. These "high-risk" HPVs produce a protein that can cause cervical epithelial cells to grow uncontrollably. The virus makes a second protein that interferes with tumor suppressors that are produced by the human immune system. The HPV-16 strain is thought to be a cause of about 50% of cervical cancers.

More than six million women in the United States have persistent HPV infections, for which there is no cure. Nevertheless, most women with HPV do not develop cervical cancer.

Symptoms of invasive cervical cancer

Most women do not have symptoms of cervical cancer until it has become invasive. At that point, the symptoms may include:

- unusual vaginal discharge
- light vaginal bleeding or spots of blood outside of normal menstruation
- pain or vaginal bleeding with sexual intercourse
- post-menopausal vaginal bleeding

Once the cancer has invaded the tissue surrounding the cervix, a woman may experience pain in the pelvic region and heavy bleeding from the vagina.

Diagnosis

The Pap test

Most often, cervical cancer is first detected with a **Pap test** that is performed as part of a regular pelvic examination. The vagina is spread with a metal or plastic instrument called a speculum. A swab is used to remove mucus and cells from the cervix. This sample is sent to a laboratory for microscopic examination.

The Pap test is a screening tool rather than a diagnostic tool. It is very efficient at detecting cervical abnormalities. The Bethesda System commonly is used to report Pap test results. A negative test means that no abnormalities are present in the cervical tissue. A positive Pap test describes abnormal cervical cells as low-grade or high-grade SIL, depending on the extent of dysplasia. About 5-10% of Pap tests show at least mild abnormalities. However, a number of factors other than cervical cancer can cause abnormalities, including inflammation from bacteria or yeast infections. A few months after the infection is treated, the Pap test is repeated.

Biopsy

Following an abnormal Pap test, a colposcopy is usually performed. The physician uses a magnifying scope to view the surface of the cervix. The cervix may be coated with an iodine solution that causes normal cells to turn brown and abnormal cells to turn white or yellow. This is called a Schiller test. If any abnormal areas are observed, a colposcopic **biopsy** may be performed. A biopsy is the removal of a small piece of tissue for microscopic examination by a pathologist.

Other types of cervical biopsies may be performed. An endocervical curettage is a biopsy in which a narrow instrument called a curette is used to scrape tissue from inside the opening of the cervix. A cone biopsy, or conization, is used to remove a cone-shaped piece of tissue from the cervix. In a cold knife cone biopsy, a surgical scalpel or laser is used to remove the tissue. A loop electrosurgical excision procedure (LEEP) is a cone biopsy using a wire that is heated by an electrical current. Cone biopsies can be used to determine whether abnormal cells have invaded below the surface of the cervix. They also can be used to treat many precancers and very early cancers. Biopsies may be performed with a local or general anesthetic. They may cause cramping and bleeding.

Diagnosing the stage

Following a diagnosis of cervical cancer, various procedures may be used to stage the disease (determine how far the cancer has spread). For example, additional pelvic exams may be performed under anesthesia.

There are several procedures for determining if cervical cancer has invaded the urinary tract. With **cystoscopy**, a lighted tube with a lens is inserted through the urethra (the urine tube from the bladder to the exterior) and into the bladder to examine these organs for cancerous cells. Tissue samples may be removed for microscopic examination by a pathologist. **Intravenous urography** (intravenous pyelogram or IVP) is an **x ray** of the urinary system, following the injection of special dye. The kidneys remove the dye from the bloodstream and the dye passes into the ureters (the tubes from the kidneys to the bladder) and bladder. IVP can detect a blocked ureter, caused by the spread of cancer to the pelvic lymph nodes (small glands that are part of the immune system).

A procedure called proctoscopy or **sigmoidoscopy** is similar to cystoscopy. It is used to determine whether the cancer has spread to the rectum or lower large intestine.

Computed tomography (CT or CAT) scans, ultrasound, or other imaging techniques may be used to determine the spread of cancer to various parts of the body. With a CT scan, an x-ray beam rotates around the body, taking images from various angles. It is used to determine if the cancer has spread to the lymph nodes. **Magnetic resonance imaging** (MRI), which uses a magnetic field to image the body, sometimes is used for evaluating the spread of cervical cancer. Chest x rays may be used to detect cervical cancer that has spread to the lungs.

Treatment team

Pap smears usually are performed by a women's health specialist, a nurse practitioner, a family practice physician, or a gynecologist. These practitioners may treat precancerous conditions. Procedures for diagnosing cervical cancer are performed by a gynecologist. A pathologist examines the biopsied tissue for cancer cells. Following diagnosis, a specialist in cancers of the female reproductive system, a gynecological oncologist, as well as a radiation oncologist and a surgeon may join the team.

Clinical staging, treatments, and prognosis

Following a diagnosis of cervical cancer, the physician takes a medical history and performs a complete physical examination. This includes an evaluation of symptoms and risk factors for cervical cancer. The lymph nodes are examined for evidence that the cancer has spread from the cervix. The choice of treatment depends on the clinical stage of the disease.

The FIGO system of staging

The International Federation of Gynecologists and Obstetricians (FIGO) system usually is used to stage cervical cancer:

- Stage 0: Carcinoma in situ; non-invasive cancer that is confined to the layer of cells lining the cervix.
- Stage I: Cancer that has spread into the connective tissue of the cervix but is confined to the uterus.
- Stage IA: Very small cancerous area that is visible only with a microscope.
- Stage IA1: Invasion area is less than 3 mm (0.13 in) deep and 7 mm (0.33 in) wide.
- Stage IA2: Invasion area is 3–5 mm (0.13-0.2 in) deep and less than 7 mm (0.33 in) wide.
- Stage IB: Cancer can be seen without a microscope or is deeper than 5 mm (0.2 in) or wider than 7 mm (0.33 in).
- Stage IB1: Cancer is no larger than 4 cm (1.6 in).
- Stage IB2: Stage IB cancer is larger than 4 cm (1.6 in).
- Stage II: Cancer has spread from the cervix but is confined to the pelvic region.
- Stage IIA: Cancer has spread to the upper region of the vagina, but not to the lower one-third of the vagina.
- Stage IIB: Cancer has spread to the parametrial tissue adjacent to the cervix.
- Stage III: Cancer has spread to the lower one-third of the vagina or to the wall of the pelvis and may be blocking the ureters.
- Stage IIIA: Cancer has spread to the lower vagina but not to the pelvic wall.
- Stage IIIB: Cancer has spread to the pelvic wall and/or is blocking the flow of urine through the ureters to the bladder.
- Stage IV: Cancer has spread to other parts of the body.
- Stage IVA: Cancer has spread to the bladder or rectum.
- Stage IVB: Cancer has spread to distant organs such as the lungs.
- Recurrent: Following treatment, cancer has returned to the cervix or some other part of the body.

In addition to the stage of the cancer, factors such as a woman's age, general health, and preferences may influence the choice of treatment. The exact location of the cancer within the cervix and the type of cervical cancer also are important considerations.

Treatment of precancer and carcinoma in situ

Most low-grade SILs that are detected with Pap tests revert to normal without treatment. Most high-grade SILs require treatment. Treatments to remove precancerous cells include:

- cold knife cone biopsy
- LEEP
- cryosurgery (freezing the cells with a metal probe)
- cauterization or diathermy (burning off the cells)
- laser surgery (burning off the cells with a laser beam)

These methods also may be used to treat cancer that is confined to the surface of the cervix (stage 0) and other early-stage cervical cancers in women who may want to become pregnant. They may be used in conjunction with other treatments. These procedures may cause bleeding or cramping. All of these treatments require close follow-up to detect any recurrence of the cancer.

Surgery

A simple hysterectomy is used to treat some stages O and IA cervical cancers. Usually only the uterus is removed, although occasionally the fallopian tubes and ovaries are removed as well. The tissues adjoining the uterus, including the vagina, remain intact. The uterus may be removed either through the abdomen or the vagina.

In a radical hysterectomy, the uterus and adjoining tissues, including the ovaries, the upper region (1 in) of the vagina near the cervix, and the pelvic lymph nodes,

KEY TERMS

Adenocarcinoma—Cervical cancer that originates in the mucus-producing cells of the inner or endocervix.

Biopsy—Removal of a small sample of tissue for examination under a microscope; used for the diagnosis and treatment of cervical cancer and precancerous conditions.

Carcinoma in situ—Cancer that is confined to the cells in which it originated and has not spread to other tissues.

Cervical intraepithelial neoplasia (CIN)—Abnormal cell growth on the surface of the cervix.

Cervix—Narrow, lower end of the uterus forming the opening to the vagina.

Colposcopy—Diagnostic procedure using a hollow, lighted tube (colposcope) to look inside the cervix and uterus.

Conization—Cone biopsy; removal of a cone-shaped section of tissue from the cervix for diagnosis or treatment.

Dysplasia—Abnormal cellular changes that may become cancerous.

Endocervical curettage—Biopsy performed with a curette to scrape the mucous membrane of the cervical canal.

Human papilloma virus (HPV)—Virus that causes abnormal cell growth (warts or papillomas); some types can cause cervical cancer.

Hysterectomy—Removal of the uterus.

Interferon—Potent immune-defense protein produced by viral-infected cells; used as an anti-cancer and anti-viral drug.

Laparoscopy—Laparoscopic pelvic lymph node dissection; insertion of a tube through a very small surgical incision to remove lymph nodes.

Loop electrosurgical excision procedure (LEEP)—Cone biopsy performed with a wire that is heated by electrical current.

Lymph nodes—Small round glands, located throughout the body, that filter the lymphatic fluid; part of the body's immune defense.

Pap test—Pap smear; removal of cervical cells to screen for cancer.

Pelvic exenteration—Extensive surgery to remove the uterus, ovaries, pelvic lymph nodes, part or all of the vagina, and the bladder, rectum, and/or part of the colon.

Squamous cells—Thin, flat cells of the surfaces of the skin and cervix and linings of various organs.

Squamous intraepithelial lesion (SIL)—Abnormal growth of squamous cells on the surface of the cervix.

Vaginal stenosis—Narrowing of the vagina due to a build-up of scar tissue.

are all removed. A radical hysterectomy usually involves abdominal surgery. However it can be performed vaginally, in combination with a laparoscopic pelvic **lymph node dissection**. With **laparoscopy**, a tube is inserted through a very small surgical incision for the removal of the lymph nodes. These operations are used to treat stages IA2, IB, and IIA cervical cancers, particularly in young women. Following a hysterectomy, the tissue is examined to see if the cancer has spread and requires additional radiation treatment. Women who have had hysterectomies cannot become pregnant, but complications from a hysterectomy are rare.

If cervical cancer recurs following treatment, a pelvic **exenteration** (extensive surgery) may be performed. This includes a radical hysterectomy, with the additional removal of the bladder, rectum, part of the colon, and/or all of the vagina. Such operations require the creation of new openings for the urine and feces. A new vagina may be created surgically. Often the clitoris and other outer genitals are left intact.

Recovery from a pelvic exenteration may take 6 months to 2 years. This treatment is successful with 40-50% of recurrent cervical cancers that are confined to the pelvis. If the recurrent cancer has spread to other organs, radiation or **chemotherapy** may be used to alleviate some of the symptoms.

Radiation

Radiation therapy, which involves the use of high-dosage x rays or other high-energy waves to kill cancer cells, often is used for treating stages IB, IIA, and IIB cervical cancers, or in combination with surgery. With external-beam radiation therapy, the rays are focused on the pelvic area from a source outside the body. With implant or internal radiation therapy, a pellet of radioactive material is placed internally, near the tumor. Alternatively, thin needles may be used to insert the radioactive material directly into the tumor.

Radiation therapy to the pelvic region can have many side effects:

- skin reaction in the area of treatment
- **fatigue**
- upset stomach and loose bowels
- vaginal stenosis (narrowing of the vagina due to build-up of scar tissue) leading to painful sexual intercourse
- premature menopause in young women
- problems with urination

Chemotherapy

Chemotherapy, the use of one or more drugs to kill cancer cells, is used to treat disease that has spread beyond the cervix. Most often it is used following surgery or radiation treatment. Stages IIB, III, IV, and recurrent cervical cancers usually are treated with a combination of external and internal radiation and chemotherapy. The common drugs used for cervical cancer are **cisplatin**, **ifosfamide**, and **fluorouracil**. These may be injected or taken by mouth. The National Cancer Institute recommends that chemotherapy with cisplatin be considered for all women receiving radiation therapy for cervical cancer.

The side effects of chemotherapy depend on a number of factors, including the type of drug, the dosage, and the length of the treatment. Side effects may include:

- **nausea and vomiting**
- fatigue
- changes in appetite
- hair loss (**alopecia**)
- mouth or vaginal sores
- infections
- menstrual cycle changes
- premature menopause
- infertility
- bleeding or **anemia** (low red blood cell count)

With the exception of menopause and infertility, most of the side effects are temporary.

Alternative and complementary therapies

Biological therapy sometimes is used to treat cervical cancer, either alone or in combination with chemotherapy. Treatment with the immune-system protein interferon is used to boost the **immune response**. Biological therapy can cause temporary flu-like symptoms and other side effects.

Some research suggests that vitamin A (carotene) may help to prevent or stop cancerous changes in cells such as those on the surface of the cervix. Other studies suggest that **vitamins** C and E may reduce the risk of cervical cancer.

Prognosis

For cervical cancers that are diagnosed in the pre-invasive stage, the 5-year-survival rate is almost 100%. When cervical cancer is detected in the early invasive stages, approximately 91% of women survive 5 years or more. Stage IVB cervical cancer is not considered to be curable. The 5-year-survival rate for all cervical cancers combined is about 70%. The death rate from cervical cancer continues to decline by about 2% each year. Women over age 65 account for 40-50% of all deaths from cervical cancer.

Coping with cancer treatment

Medications can alleviate some of the side effects of radiation and chemotherapy, such as nausea and menopausal symptoms. Premature menopause may require estrogen-replacement therapy. Vaginal dilators and lubricants can relieve the effects of vaginal stenosis. A nutritious diet, rest, and a strong emotional support system help with recovery from treatment.

Following treatment for cervical cancer, additional tests are conducted to check for recurrence. These tests include frequent Pap smears, biopsies, and blood tests. X rays, CT or MRI scans, or other **imaging studies** such as ultrasound also may be used.

Clinical trials

There are many **clinical trials**, ongoing throughout the United States, for the treatment of most stages of cervical cancer. These include the testing of new chemotherapy drugs, new methods of radiation therapy, and new combinations of surgery and radiation or chemotherapy. New methods for performing Pap tests also are being studied.

A new test for HPV, called the Hybrid Capture HPV test, is being studied. Results suggest that this test may be useful for determining which women with abnormal Pap test results should have colposcopy. Clinical trials also are examining whether an HPV test can replace a Pap test as a routine screen for cervical cancer. Various types of HPV **vaccines** are being tested. These include vaccines that prevent HPV infection, vaccines for women

QUESTIONS TO ASK THE DOCTOR

- What type of biopsy will I have? What type of anesthetic will be used? What are the after-effects?
- What type of cervical cancer do I have?
- What is the stage of my cancer?
- What are my treatment choices?
- Which treatment do you recommend and why?
- What should I do to prepare for treatment?
- What are the side effects of this treatment and how can I alleviate them?
- What is the recovery period for this treatment?
- Will I be able to get pregnant after this treatment?
- Are there clinical trials that may be appropriate for me?
- What is my prognosis?

infected with HPV, and vaccines for women with advanced cervical cancer.

Prevention

Viral infections

Most cervical cancers are preventable. More than 90% of women with cervical cancer are infected with HPV. HPV infection is the single most important risk factor. This is particularly true for young women because the cells lining the cervix do not fully mature until age 18. These immature cells are more susceptible to cancer-causing agents and viruses.

Since HPV is a sexually-transmitted infection, sexual behaviors can put women at risk for HPV infection and cervical cancer. These behaviors include:

- sexual intercourse at age 16 or younger
- partners who began having intercourse at a young age
- multiple sexual partners
- sexual partners who have had multiple partners ("high-risk males")
- A partner who has had a previous sexual partner with cervical cancer

HPV infection may not produce any symptoms, so sexual partners may not know that they are infected. However, Pap tests can detect the infection. Condoms do not necessarily prevent HPV infection.

Infection with the human immunodeficiency virus (HIV) that causes acquired immunodeficiency syndrome (AIDS) is a risk factor for cervical cancer. Women who test positive for HIV may have impaired immune systems that cannot correct precancerous conditions. Furthermore, sexual behavior that puts women at risk for HIV infection, also puts them at risk for HPV infection. There is some evidence suggesting that another sexually-transmitted virus, the genital herpes virus, also may be involved in cervical cancer.

Smoking

Smoking may double the risk of cervical cancer. Chemicals produced by tobacco smoke can damage the DNA of cervical cells. The risk increases with the number of years a woman smokes and the amount she smokes.

Diet and drugs

Diets that are low in fruits and vegetables increase the risk of cervical cancer. Women also have an increased risk of cervical cancer if their mothers took the drug diethylstilbestrol (DES) while they were pregnant. This drug was given to women between 1940 and 1971 to prevent miscarriages. Some statistical studies have suggested that the long-term use of oral contraceptives may slightly increase the risk of cervical cancer.

Pap tests

Most cases of cervical cancers are preventable, since they start with easily-detectable precancerous changes. Therefore, the best prevention for cervical cancer is a regular Pap test. When precancerous changes are detected, appropriate treatment can prevent the development of invasive cancer. The ACS recommends that women have annual Pap tests beginning when they first start having sex or at age 18. Women who are past menopause or some women with hysterectomies continue to require Pap tests.

The National Breast and Cervical Cancer Early Detection Program provides free or low-cost Pap tests and treatment for women without **health insurance**, for older women, and for members of racial and ethnic minorities. The program is administered through individual states, under the direction of the Centers for Disease Control and Prevention.

Special concerns

If a woman is diagnosed with very early-stage (IA) cervical cancer while pregnant, the physician usually will recommend a hysterectomy after the baby is born. For later-stage cancers, the pregnancy is terminated or the baby is removed by cesarean section as soon as it can survive outside the womb. This is followed by a hysterectomy and/or radiation treatment. For the most advanced stages of cervical cancer, treatment is initiated despite the pregnancy.

Many women with cervical cancer have hysterectomies, which are major surgeries. Although normal activities, including sexual intercourse, can be resumed in 4-8 weeks, a woman may have emotional problems following a hysterectomy. A strong support system can help with these difficulties.

See Also Gynecologic cancers

Resources

BOOKS

Falco, Kristine. *Reclaiming Our Lives After Breast and Gynecologic Cancer.* Northvale, NJ: Jason Aronson, Inc., 1998.

Holland, Jimmie C. and Sheldon Lewis. *The Human Side of Cancer: Living with Hope, Coping with Uncertainty.* New York: HarperCollins, 2000.

Runowicz, Carolyn D., Jeanne A. Petrek, and Ted S. Gansler. *Women and Cancer: A Thorough and Compassionate Resource for Patients and their Families.* New York: Villard Books, 1999.

Sweeney, Julia. *God Said "Ha!"* New York: Bantam Books, 1997.

ORGANIZATIONS

American Cancer Society. 1599 Clifton Road, N.E., Atlanta, GA 30329. (800) ACS-2345. <http://www.cancer.org>. Information, funds for cancer research, prevention programs, and patient services, including educational and support programs for patients and families and temporary accommodations for patients.

Centers for Disease Control and Prevention. National Center for Chronic Disease Prevention and Health Promotion. Mail Stop K-64. 4770 Buford Highway NE, Atlanta, GA 30341-3717. (770) 488-4751. (888) 842-6355. <http://www.cdc.gov/cancer>. Research and public education and outreach for disease prevention under the U.S. Department of Health and Human Services.

EyesOnThePrize.Org. 446 S. Anaheim Hills Road, #108, Anaheim Hills, CA 92807. <http://www.eyesontheprize.org>. On-line information and emotional support for women with gynecologic cancer.

Gynecologic Cancer Foundation. 401 North Michigan Avenue, Chicago, IL 60611. (800) 444-4441. (312) 644-6610. <http://www.wcn.org/gcf/>. Research, education, and philanthropy for women with gynecologic cancer.

National Cancer Institute. Public Inquiries Office, Building 31, Room 10A31, 31 Center Drive, MSC 2580, Bethesda, MD 20892-2580. (800)-4-CANCER. <http://www.nci.nih.gov/>. <http://cancernet.nci.nih.gov>. Research, information, and clinical trials.

National Cervical Cancer Coalition. 16501 Sherman Way, Suite #110, Van Nuys, CA 91406. (800) 685-5531. (818) 909-3849. <http://www.nccc-online.org/>. Information, education, access to screening and treatment, and support services; sponsors the Cervical Cancer Quilt Project.

OTHER

"Cancer of the Cervix." *CancerNet.* 12 Dec. 2000. National Cancer Institute. NIH Publication No. 95-2047. 3 Apr. 2001. > http://cancernet.nci.nih.gov/wyntk_pubs/cervix.htm#2>.

"Cervical Cancer." *Cancer Resource Center.* American Cancer Society. 16 Mar. 2000. 3 Apr. 2001. <http://www3.cancer.org/cancerinfo/load_cont.asp?ct=8&doc=25&Language=English>.

"Cervical Cancer." *National Institutes of Health Consensus Development Conference Statement.* 1-3 Apr. 1996. 3 Apr. 2001. <http://text.nlm.nih.gov/nih/cdc/www/102txt.html>.

"Cervical Cytology: Evaluation and Management of Abnormalities." *American College of Obstetricians and Gynecologists (ACOG) Techincal Bulletin.* Number 183 (August 1993).

Lata Cherath, Ph.D.
Margaret Alic, Ph.D.

Chemoembolization

Definition

Utilized to treat tumors in the liver, chemoembolization is the process of injecting **chemotherapy** directly into the blood vessels which feed the tumor.

Purpose

Chemoembolization is a treatment that can be focused on cancerous cells that have spread to the liver but does not expose the rest of the body to the effects of chemotherapy. It is not a cure but does offer relief (palliative) and preserves the quality of life. The technique is minimally invasive and approximately 70% of patients will experience improvement in liver function and survival time.

Precautions

The referring physician will probably recommend several tests prior to the procedure, such as, liver function blood tests and a CAT scan or an MRI of the liver. These tests insure there is no blockage of the portal vein in the liver; there is no cirrhosis of the liver; and there is no blockage of the bile ducts. Any of these complications may prevent the procedure from being performed.

KEY TERMS

CAT—Computerized axial tomography, also called computed tomography.

Chemotherapy—The treatment of illness by chemical means, by medications.

Liver function tests—Laboratory procedures that measure some aspect of liver functions and involves a wide range of tests.

MRI—Magnetic resonance imaging

cirrhosis—A liver disease characterized by the loss of normal microscopic structures within the liver that are replaced by fibrous tissue that cause the organ to constrict and divide into irregular nodules.

Palliative—Any treatment that offers relief but does not cure.

Description

A radiologist performs this procedure in a hospital under x-ray guidance by inserting a small catheter (tiny tube) through a hollow needle into the femoral artery, located in the groin. It is then threaded up through the aorta and into the artery in the liver that feeds the tumor. During chemoemolization, three chemotherapy drugs are injected directly into this artery and it is then "embolized" or blocked off with a mixture of oil and tiny particles. Since the drugs are injected directly into the tumor, the dosage is 20-200 times greater than that received with standard treatment via a vein in the arm. Since the tumor is blocked off, the drugs stay in it for a much longer time. Also, with the blood supply blocked, the tumor is deprived of oxygen and nutrients, which serves to hasten its destruction. The liver has two blood supplies, a hepatic artery and a large portal vein so it can still function with one blocked off.

The procedure takes approximately three hours to perform, occurs while the patient is under conscious sedation, and usually involves an overnight stay in the hospital. It is usually performed on a monthly basis with three sessions being the average treatment regimen.

Preparation

The evening before the procedure nothing may be taken by mouth after dinner. Generally, a patient must arrive at the hospital early in the morning to permit the infusion of large amounts of fluids by an intravenous (IV) line placed in the arm. These fluids contain **antibiotics** and other medications needed prior to the procedure. The patient is then taken to the Department of Radiology for the treatment.

Aftercare

Immediately following the injection of the chemotherapy mixture, the patient is returned to a hospital room and must lie flat in bed for at least six hours. More IV fluids are provided during this time as well as overnight. Most patients are discharged the next day. It is important to spend as much time as possible in bed 1-2 days following the procedure in order to improve blood flow to the liver.

Risks

Serious complications are extremely rare from this procedure. Some statistics have quoted that in less than 3% of the procedures, the liver tumor that was destroyed became infected and abscessed. Others have noted approximately one fatality per 100 procedures due to liver failure.

Normal results

The patient may experience varying degrees of pain, **fever** and nausea following the treatment, which may last any where from a few hours to a few days. Pain or high fevers the first few days following the treatment are a result of the tumor breaking down and is normal. Frequently, one of the **laxatives** called Lactulose is given to help the body rid itself of metabolic waste usually eliminated by the liver. This may cause loose stools for several days. Extreme **fatigue** is a common problem for 3-4 weeks after the procedure. With the tumor now blocked, liver function should improve and thus, the quality of life.

Follow-up scans may be performed in order to determine any changes in the tumor and to look for the appearance of any new tumors. Chemoembolization can be repeated many times over a period of many years depending on the status of the patient.

Abnormal results

A sudden change in the degree of pain and/or fever that persists after the first week should be reported to a physician. Any unusual changes should be communicated immediately.

Resources

BOOKS

American Cancer Society's Consumer's Guide to Cancer Drugs. Published by Jones and Bartlett, 2000.

QUESTIONS TO ASK THE DOCTOR

- Am I a good candidate for this procedure?
- Do I have any contraindications that should be considered before having the procedure?
- Will I experience any improvement in my quality of life?
- What are the advantages and disadvantages of the procedure?
- Does the physician performing the procedure do this often or just once in awhile?

ORGANIZATIONS

American Society of Clinical Oncology,1900 Duke Street, Suite 200, Alexandria, VA 22314. Phone: 703-299-0150. <http://www.asco.org>.

American Cancer Society, P.O. Box 102454, Atlanta, GA 30368-2454. <http://www.ca.cancer.org>.

OTHER

Montgomery, Sue. *Chemotherapy Delivered Directly to Liver Tumors Doubles Life Expectancy.* University of Pennsylvania Cancer Center, April 13, 2001.

Linda K. Bennington, C.N.S., M.S.N.

Chemoprevention

Definition

Chemoprevention is the attempt to prevent cancer from developing by using substances that interfere in the process of **carcinogenesis**.

Purpose

Clinical trials are currently investigating chemoprevention for people at high risk of certain cancers. For instance, to prevent **breast cancer** in the second breast of women who have already been treated for breast cancer, or women who have never had breast cancer but are determined to be at high risk; or to prevent **colon cancer** in people with a genetic predisposition for that cancer. Individuals not at a particularly high risk can use behavioral and dietary modifications for chemoprevention. Since the 1980s, the National Cancer Institute has identified more than 1,000 natural and synthetic chemicals with some degree of cancer preventive activity. Currently, over 400 potential agents are under investigation for their ability to prevent cancer and at least 40 compounds or combinations are undergoing human clinical trials.

Chemopreventive agents have been identified that interact with all stages of carcinogenesis; initiation, promotion and progression. They work by inactivating carcinogens (cancer-causing agents), inducing enzymes, or as **antioxidants**. Later in the process they may inhibit tumor growth by acting as suppressors or stimulating apoptosis.

Description

Chemoprevention differs from **chemotherapy** in that it is used long before cancer develops to prevent cancer or to inhibit pre-cancer, possibly in at-risk individuals. Chemotherapy on the other hand seeks to kill cells that have already become cancerous. Chemoprevention uses natural products from foods or synthetic preparations. Because chemoprevention is used long-term, it must be non-toxic, effective, easy to administer and inexpensive. Few specific agents are currently advised for widespread clinical use since clinical trials that last up to 15 years are still ongoing.

Dietary factors and lifestyle changes are important areas in chemoprevention. It is estimated that through dietary improvements there could be a 50% reduction in colon and rectal cancers, 25% reduction in breast cancer and a 15% reductions each in prostate, endometrial and gallbladder cancers. Cancers of the stomach, esophagus, pancreas, ovaries, liver, lung and bladder may also be affected by dietary factors. Agents of importance in chemoprevention include **vitamins** A, C and E as well as nonnutrient compounds from plants called phytochemicals.

Phytochemicals from food are a source of many chemopreventive agents. Garlic alone contains 30 cancer preventing compounds including selenium. Broccoli contains indole-3-carbinol as well as phenethylisothiocyanate, a sulfur-containing compound. Soy products contain phytoestrogens such as genistein. Tea, both black and green, contains an abundance of polyphenols such as the catechins that have antioxidant and anti-cancer activity. Compounds in tea also have anti-estrogen activity and can modulate detoxification enzymes. Curcumin from the spice turmeric is gaining attention as a chemopreventive agent. It is both an anti-inflammatory agent and an antioxidant. In laboratory animals curcumin has shown inhibition towards colon, breast, and **stomach cancer**.

Chemoprevention of breast cancer

Anti-estrogens can counteract the growth effect estrogen has on some breast cancers. Two **antiestrogens**,

KEY TERMS

apoptosis—A process of cell death performed by a damaged cell.

anti-inflammatory—An agent that reduces inflammation. The most common example is aspirin.

phytochemical—A non-nutrient compound from plants.

tamoxifen and **raloxifene**, have been shown in clinical trials to prevent breast cancer in women at high risk for the disease. As a result of these trials, Tamoxifen has been approved by the FDA as a preventative as well as a treatment. Other anti-estrogens including soy isoflavones are still under investigation. The synthetic retinoid, fenretinide, also shows promise in preventing breast cancer. Decreasing the amount of fat in the diet is also under investigation to prevent breast cancer. Also under investigation are indole-3-carbinol from broccoli.

Chemoprevention of colon cancer

Because there are more identifiable **tumor markers** known for colon cancer, the evaluation of chemopreventive agents can be a shorter process. The recurrence of polyps rather than the development of malignant cancer can be used as an endpoint. Inflammation has been linked to cancer for some time and the anti-inflammatory agents sulindac and sulindac sulfone as well as specific **Cyclooxygenase-2 inhibitors** are proving useful in preventing colon cancer. A combination of beta-carotene, vitamin C and vitamin E are also under investigation as well as high-fiber wheat cereal supplements. Adding fruits and vegetables to the diet also appears from epidemiological studies to have a protective effect on colon cancer.

Chemoprevention of prostate cancer

Anti-androgens and anti-estrogens are both important in preventing **prostate cancer**. Finasteride is under investigation as an anti-estrogen to prevent prostate cancer in at-risk men. Finasteride is a drug that can reduce the levels of dihydrotestosterone, which is associated with prostate enlargement and possibly cancer. It has been used to treat enlarged prostate and is currently being investigated to prevent prostate cancer in men over the age of 55 years. Men at an increased risk for prostate cancer include those with a history of prostate cancer, those with a high-fat diet, increasing age, and those of African-American descent. Soy products and indole-3-carbinol may also be effective for this reason. Lycopene, a vitamin A-like compound found in tomatoes and other red fruits and vegetables is associated with a decreased risk of prostate cancer. Both selenium and tea may also have chemopreventive effects on prostate cancer.

Chemoprevention of skin cancer

The incidence of skin cancer has dramatically increased in recent years, probably due to the popularity of sun tanning. Compounds under investigation for the prevention of skin cancer include compounds from tea, silymarin from milk thistle, vitamin A and coumarins found in a number of plants.

Recommendations

Changes in lifestyle can significantly affect an individual's risk for cancer. It is estimated that 32% of colon cancers are related to physical inactivity, which may also play a part in other cancers. Tobacco accounts for 30% of all cancers and not just lung cancer. **Alcohol consumption** is related to cancers of the oral cavity, pharynx, larynx, esophagus and liver and possibly colorectal and breast cancers. The combination of alcohol and tobacco is especially dangerous. The main cause of skin cancers is exposure to UV radiation. Fair skinned individuals are at an increased risk. Obesity puts an individual at an increased risk of death from uterus, gallbladder, kidney, stomach, colon, breast, colon, and prostrate cancers. Obese women are at a 55% greater risk of mortality from cancer than women of normal weight, while obese men are at a 33% greater risk of mortality from cancer.

The lifestyle recommendations from the American Cancer Society for preventing cancer include:

- Maintain a desirable body weight.
- Eat a variety of foods.
- Include both fruits and vegetables in the daily diet.
- Eat more high-fiber foods.
- Cut down on total fat intake.
- Limit consumption of alcoholic beverages.
- Limit consumption of salt-cured, smoked and nitrite preserved foods.

Risks

Because chemopreventive agents can be administered in high doses and for long periods of time, the risk of side effects is increased. During the 1980's the CARET study found that beta-carotene actually increased the risk of lung cancer in male smokers. Studies of tamoxifen to prevent breast cancer can increase the risks of uterine cancer, cataracts and blood-clot formation. Long-term use of **non-steroidal anti-inflammato-**

ry drugs to prevent colon cancer can result in gastrointestinal problems and liver toxicity. Current recommendations are to increase consumption of fruits, vegetables and fiber in the diet rather than taking supplements.

Resources

BOOKS

Bal, Dileep G. Daniel W. Nixon, Susan B. Foerster, and Ross C. Brownson, "Cancer Prevention" In *Clinical Oncology*, edited by Murphy, Gerald P., Walter Lawrence, and Raymond E. Atlanta, GA: The American Cancer Society, 1995.

Kelloff, Gary J, James A. Crowell, Vernon E. Steele, Ronald A. Lubet, et. al. "Progress in Cancer Chemoprevention" In *Cancer Prevention: Novel Nutrient and Pharmaceutical Developments,* Annals of The New York Academy of Sciences, edited by Bradlow, H. Leon, Jack Fishman, and Michael P. Osborne. New York: The New York Academy of Sciences, 1999, vol 889.

American Institute for Cancer Research *Stopping Cancer Before it Starts*, New York: Golden Books, 1999.

PERIODICALS

Greenwald, Peter, "Chemoprevention of Cancer" *Scientific American* (September 1996).

Osborne, Michael, Peter Boyle, Peter and Martin Lipkin, "Cancer Prevention" *Lancet* 1997;349:SII27–30.

Rao, Chinthalapally V. Abraham Rivenson, Barbara Simi, and Bandaru S. "Chemoprevention of Colon Cancer by Dietary Curcumin" In *Annals New York Academy of Sciences* 1995; 768:201–204.

OTHER

Dresbach, Sereana Howard and Amy Rossi. "Chemoprevention—The Answer to Cancer?" *Ohio State University Extension Fact Sheet, Family and Consumer Sciences* <http://www.ag.ohio-state.edu/~ohioline/hyg-fact/5000/5051.html.> 4 July 2001.

Greenwald, Peter and Sharon S. McDonald. "Cancer Prevention: The Roles of Diet and Chemoprevention."*Cancer Control Journal* <http://www.moffitt.usf.edu/providers/ccj/v4n2/article2.html> 4 July 2001.

Cindy L. A. Jones, Ph.D.

Chemotherapy

Definition

Chemotherapy is the systemic (whole body) treatment of cancer with anticancer drugs.

Purpose

The main purpose of chemotherapy is to kill cancer cells. It can be used as the primary form of treatment or as a supplement to other treatments. Chemotherapy is often used to treat patients with cancer that has spread from the place in the body where it started (metastasized), but it may also be used the keep cancer from coming back (adjuvant therapy). Chemotherapy destroys cancer cells anywhere in the body. It even kills cells that have broken off from the main tumor and traveled through the blood or lymph systems to other parts of the body.

Chemotherapy can cure some types of cancer. In some cases, it is used to slow the growth of cancer cells or to keep the cancer from spreading to other parts of the body. When a cancer has been removed by surgery, chemotherapy may be used to keep the cancer from coming back (adjuvant therapy). It is also helpful in reducing the tumor size prior to surgery (primary [neoadjuvant] chemotherapy). Chemotherapy can ease the symptoms of cancer (palliate), helping some patients have a better quality of life.

Types of chemotherapy

Chemotherapy may be used as the first line of treatment or it may be started after a tumor is removed. A variety of factors, including the type and stage of cancer, will determine the type of chemotherapy used.

Adjuvant chemotherapy

Adjuvant chemotherapy refers to giving patients anticancer drugs after the primary tumor has been removed and there is no evidence that cancer remains in the body. It was first studied in the 1950s. This form of treatment initially gained popularity because it showed promise in improving the survival for patients with certain cancers. The theory was that adjuvant chemotherapy would attack microscopic cancer cells that remained after tumor removal. Adjuvant chemotherapy may be effective in some types of cancers, including **breast cancer**, colorectal cancer, osteogenic sarcoma, and **Wilms' tumor**.

A patient's response to adjuvant therapy is determined by a variety of factors, including drug dosage, schedule of drug therapy, and **drug resistance**. Toxic side effects and cost-effectiveness are other important issues. This area is undergoing further investigation.

Primary (neoadjuvant) chemotherapy

Primary chemotherapy, also sometimes called neoadjuvant chemotherapy or induction chemotherapy, is the use of anticancer drugs as the main form of treatment. Chemotherapy can be the primary treatment with cancers such as these: certain lymphomas, childhood and some adult forms of **Hodgkin's disease**, Wilms' tumor, embryonal **rhabdomyosarcoma**, and small cell lung cancer.

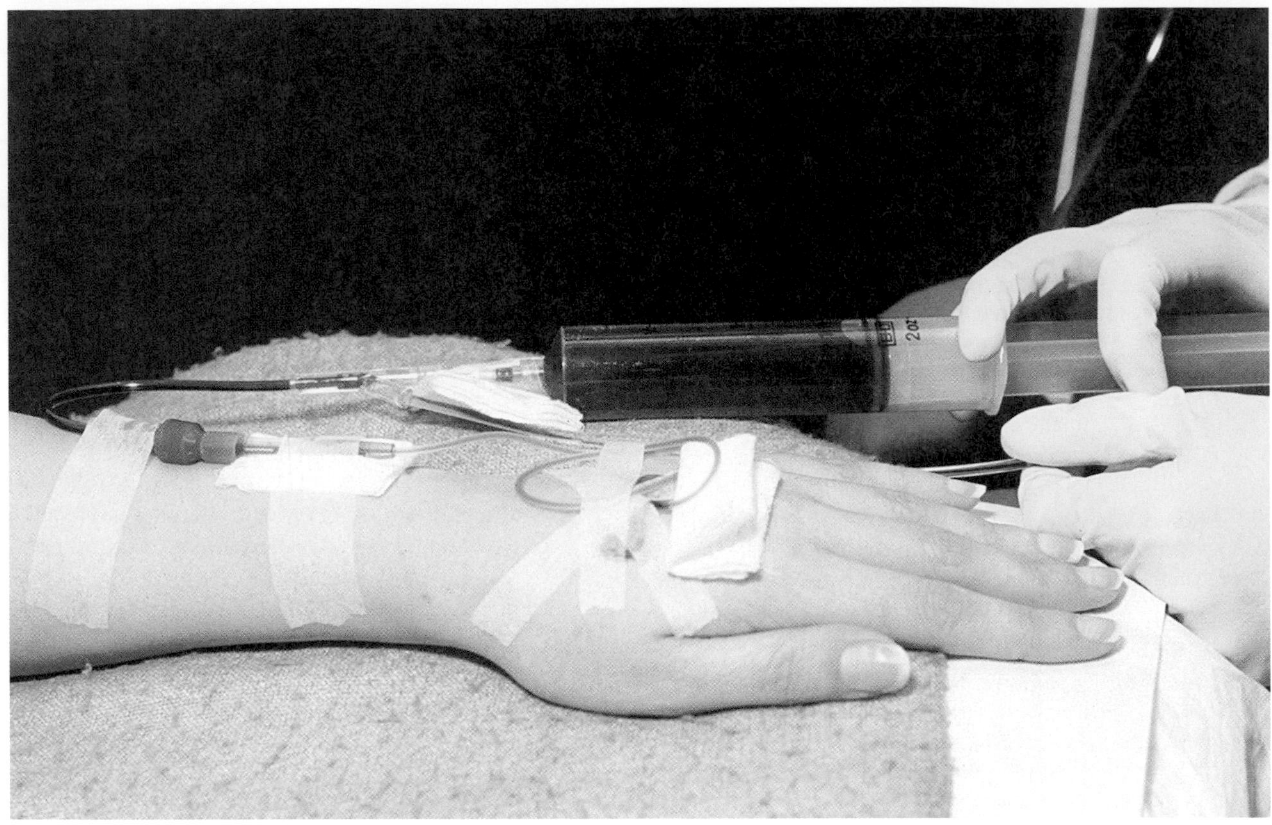

A woman receiving Adriamycin (doxorubicin) chemotherapy. *(Custom Medical Stock Photo. Reproduced by permission.)*

Primary chemotherapy can also be used to treat tumors prior to surgery or radiation. In some cases, the tumor may be so large that surgery to remove it would destroy major organs or would be quite disfiguring. Primary neoadjuvant chemotherapy may reduce the tumor size, making it possible for a surgeon to perform a less traumatic operation. Examples of cancers in which primary chemotherapy may be followed-up with less extensive surgeries include: **anal cancer**, **bladder cancer**, breast cancer, **esophageal cancer**, **laryngeal cancer**, osteogenic sarcoma, and soft tissue sarcoma.

An advantage of primary chemotherapy is that the blood vessels are intact since they have not been exposed to surgery or radiation. Therefore, drugs can easily travel through the bloodstream toward the tumor. In fact, the therapy can improve the tumor's blood flow, making it more receptive to the impact of radiation. In addition, the use of chemotherapy before surgical removal of cancer allows the physician to assess the responsiveness of the tumor to the drug(s) used. Since not all chemotherapy regimens are equally effective, knowing how a particular tumor responds to the chemotherapy regimen prescribed can be an advantage in treating the disease.

Primary chemotherapy does have drawbacks. Some cancer cells may be drug-resistant, making the therapy ineffective. (Although discovering that the drug is ineffective minimizes the number of cycles of the drug that the patient must undergo.) The drug may not significantly reduce tumor size, or the tumor may continue to grow despite treatment. Furthermore, the initial use of a drug may lead to higher toxicity when chemotherapy is given later in the course of treatment.

Primary chemotherapy is becoming the norm in treating some patients with certain cancers, such as specific types of lymphomas, some small cell lung cancers, **childhood cancers**, **head and neck cancers**, and locally advanced breast cancer. Additional research using this type of chemotherapy is underway.

Combination chemotherapy

In most cases, single anticancer drugs cannot cure cancer alone. The use of two or more drugs together is often a more effective alternative. This approach is called combination chemotherapy. Scientific studies of different drug combinations help doctors learn which combinations work best for various types of cancers.

Combination chemotherapy provides a higher chance of destroying cancerous cells. An oncologist decides which chemotherapy drug or combination of drugs will work best for each patient. Different drugs attack cancer cells at varying stages of their growth cycles, making the combination a stronger weapon against cancerous cells. Furthermore, using a combination of drugs may reduce the chance of drug resistance.

When selecting the combination of drugs, a variety of factors are examined. It is important for each drug to be effective against the particular tumor being targeted. Toxicity must also be studied to be sure that each different drug used in a combination is not toxic for the same organ. For example, if two drugs are each toxic to the liver, the combination could be more damaging to that organ.

How chemotherapy is given

Chemotherapy medications enter a person's body in different ways, depending on the drugs to be given and the type of cancer.

The goal is for the chemotherapy drug to reach the tumor. Some areas of the body are less accessible for anticancer drugs, and this is considered when the doctor determines the route of administration. For example, the blood-brain barrier refers to the inability of some anticancer drugs to travel through the bloodstream and enter the brain or the fluid surround the brain. Areas of the body that are inaccessible to a particular drug create a phenomenon called the sanctuary effect. In other words, the tumor is safe because the chemotherapy cannot reach it. To overcome a problem such as this one, the doctor must consider the route that will most effectively deliver the drug to the cancerous cells. Chemotherapy may be given by one or more of the following methods:

- oral (by mouth)
- injection (intramuscular or subcutaneous)
- intravenous (IV)
- intra-arterial (into the arteries)
- intralesional (directly into the tumor)
- intraperitoneal (into the peritoneal cavity)
- intrathecal (into the spinal fluid)
- topically (applied to the skin)

Orally

Oral chemotherapy is given by mouth in the form a pill, capsule, or liquid. This is the easiest method and can usually be done at home.

Injection

Intramuscular (IM) chemotherapy is injected into a muscle. Chemotherapy given by intramuscular injection is absorbed into the blood more slowly than IV chemotherapy. Because of this, the effects of IM chemotherapy may last longer than chemotherapy given intravenously. Chemotherapy may also be injected subcutaneously (SQ or SC), which means under the skin.

Intravenous

Intravenous (IV) chemotherapy is the most common way to deliver anticancer drugs into a person's body. The drug is injected directly into a vein. A small needle is inserted into a vein on the hand or lower arm.

Chemotherapy may also be given by a catheter or port inserted into a central vein or body cavity, where it can remain for an extended period of time. A port is a small reservoir or container that is placed in a vein or under the skin in the area where the drug will be given. These methods eliminate the need for repeated injections and may allow patients to spend less time in the hospital while receiving chemotherapy. A common location for a permanent catheter is the external jugular vein in the neck. Catheters and ports require meticulous care and cleaning to avoid complications, such as blood clots or infection. They may be inserted using a surgical procedure.

Chemotherapy given by the IV method may be administered intermittently or continuously. The main reasons for a continuous flow are to increase effectiveness against the tumor or to lower toxicity. Some drugs perform more effectively when exposed to the cancer over a period of time, making a continuous flow more desirable. A drug that is commonly used to treat colorectal cancer in continuous infusions is **fluorouracil**, also known as 5-FU. A drug that has less toxicity to the heart with continued infusion is **doxorubicin**, also known as Adriamycin. In some cases, toxicity occurs when the drug reaches a peak level. Offering a continuous infusion prevents the drug from reaching this level, thus lowering the chance of toxic side effects.

Intra-arterial

Cancerous tumors require a supply of blood and oxygen so that they can grow. They get these essentials from the arteries that supply organs with their blood and oxygen. Putting chemotherapy drugs into the arteries provides good access to the cancerous tumor. Intra-arterial chemotherapy is not designed for all patients. The tumor must be confined to one specific organ and the blood supply to the tumor must be accessible. The liver is

Types of chemotherapy

Type	Definition
Adjuvant	Given to improve survival when cancer is no longer evident
Primary (formerly called neo-adjuvant)	Use of chemotherapy drugs as main treatment, or as a treatment prior to surgery or radiation
Induction	Initiation of chemotherapy with plans for further treatments
Combination	Use of two or more chemotherapy drugs together

the most common organ targeted in this type of chemotherapy, although it is also effective in certain brain cancers. Its use in head and neck cancers remains controversial. Further use of this type of chemotherapy is being investigated.

A catheter is inserted using radiologic techniques or surgery. Surgical insertion is the most common. Although it is less costly and less stressful, radiologic insertion results in a catheter that cannot stay in place as long as one inserted surgically. A radiologically inserted catheter stays in place for weeks compared to surgically inserted catheters designed to stay in place from weeks to years. In the long run, the surgically implanted arterial catheter has fewer complications, such as thrombosis or infection, and is more highly acceptable to the patient.

The radiologically placed catheter is initially inserted into an artery in the person's arm or leg, and then it is guided to its final destination near the tumor, where it can remain for an extended period.

The catheters require meticulous care to keep them clean and securely in place, which lessen the chance of complications. Problems associated with catheters include movement of the tip, blood clots and infection.

Pumps may be used to move the drug through the artery and into the tumor. A pump may be external or internally planted. External pumps range from large machines found in hospitals to portable wallet-sized devices. Implanted pumps give patients greater freedom, and are safe and effective. Some internal pumps deliver a constant flow of drugs, while others are programmed to deliver intermittent doses.

Drugs used for intra-arterial chemotherapy include FUDR (**floxuridine**), FU (fluorouracil), mitomycin, **cisplatin**, and streptomycin. Less frequently, doxorubicin has been used intra-arterially for treating certain cancers of the breast, bladder, stomach, and other areas.

Intralesional

Intralesional chemotherapy is the injection of anticancer drugs directly into a tumor that is in the skin, under the skin, or in an organ inside the body. Some examples involving the use of intralesional chemotherapy include **melanoma** and **Kaposi's sarcoma**. This type of chemotherapy shows promise for other malignancies such as laryngeal cancers, and further uses are under investigation.

Intraperitoneal

Intraperitoneal (IP) chemotherapy is administered into the abdominal cavity through a catheter or port that is put into place by surgery.

Ovarian cancer is sometimes treated with IP chemotherapy because this type of cancer usually stays within a confined area. This type of therapy is only suitable for some patients. Ovarian cancer patients whose tumors have a diameter greater than two centimeters may not receive this therapy because the anticancer drug does not reach very far into the tumor. Also, patients whose cancers are resistant to certain drugs may not undergo IP therapy. Patients with smaller tumors, or those who show response to chemotherapy are better candidates.

Drugs used in IP chemotherapy include cisplatin, **paclitaxel**, floxuridine, 5-FU, **mitoxantrone**, **carboplatin**, and alfa-interferon.

Intrathecal

Intrathecal chemotherapy is the injection of anticancer drugs into the spinal fluid. This method is used primarily in treating **acute lymphocytic leukemia**. It is effective in placing the anticancer drug directly into the cerebrospinal fluid that surrounds the spinal cord and the brain. A spinal tap, also called **lumbar puncture**, is the procedure usually used to gain access to the spinal fluid. If many treatments are needed, a device called an **Ommaya reservoir** may be used. This device is inserted under the scalp and allows injection of anticancer drugs throughout the spinal fluid via the reservoir. Patients can go home with the Ommaya reservoir in place. Common drugs used intrathecally include **methotrexate** and **cytarabine**, which are usually given by a doctor with a nurse's assistance. Some leukemia patients receive IV treatments at the same time they are having intrathecal treatments.

Topical chemotherapy

Topical chemotherapy is given as a cream or ointment applied directly to the cancer. This method is more common in the treatment of certain types of skin cancer. An example is fluorouracil, also known as 5-FU, which is a topical anticancer cream.

Chemotherapy drugs

More than 50 chemotherapy drugs are currently available to treat cancer and many more are being tested for their ability to destroy cancer cells. About 30% of anticancer drugs come from or are derived from natural sources. Most chemotherapy drugs interfere with the cell's ability to grow or multiply. Although these drugs affect all cells in the body, many useful treatments are most effective against rapidly growing cells. Cancer cells grow more quickly than most other body cells. Other cells that grow fast are cells of the bone marrow that produce blood cells, cells in the stomach and intestines, and cells of the hair follicles. Therefore, the most common side effects of chemotherapy are linked to their effects on other fast growing cells. Some tumor cells are resistant to drugs, making them more difficult to target.

Alkylating agents

Alkylating drugs kill cancer cells by directly attacking DNA, the genetic material of the genes. By attacking the DNA, the drug prevents the cell from forming new cells. Nitrogen mustards, which were the first nonhormonal chemicals with anticancer abilities, are alkylating drugs. **Cyclophosphamide** and Mustargen are two alkylating agents. Cyclophosphamide, the most common alkylating agent, is often used in combination with other drugs to treat breast cancer, lymphomas, and other tumors in both children and adults. Mustargen is part of the treatment for Hodgkin's disease.

Platinum drugs

Drugs containing platinum are useful in treating a number of malignant tumors. Examples of these drugs include cisplatin, carboplatin, and **oxaliplatin**. Cisplatin is more toxic than the other two, and it is subject to resistance by the cancerous tumors. In fact, it was cisplatin's high toxicity that prompted the discovery of the other two platinum drugs, which are less toxic and more effective. Carboplatin has been shown to cause less **nausea and vomiting** than cisplatin, and it has replaced cisplatin in many treatment regimes. New platinum drugs are being investigated.

Antimetabolites

Antimetabolites interfere with the production of DNA and keep cells from growing and multiplying. They are used to treat a variety of cancers including breast cancer, leukemia, **lymphoma**, colorectal cancer, head and neck cancer, osteogenic sarcoma, choriocarcinoma (a rare uterine cancer), and urothelial cancer. Some drug resistance has occurred with these types of drugs. Examples of antimetabolites are 5-fluorouracil (5-FU), Tegafur, and Uracil.

Chemotherapy

Routes of delivering chemotherapy	Some common drugs used
Oral	Capecitabine
Intravenous	Fluorouracil (5–FU) Doxorubicin
Intra-arterial (into the arteries)	Floxuridine Fluorouracil BUDR FCNU Doxorubicin Mitomycin-C Cisplatin Streptomycin
Intralesional (directly into the tumor)	Vinblastine Vincristine
Intraperitoneal (into the cavity surrounding the abdominal organs)	Cisplatin Paclitaxel Floxuridine Fluorouracil Mitoxantrone Carboplatin Alpha interferon
Intrathecal (into the spinal fluid)	Methotrexate Cytarabine
Topical (applied to skin)	Fluorouracil

Antitumor antibiotics

Antitumor **antibiotics** are made from natural substances such as fungi in the soil. They interfere with important cell functions, including production of DNA and cell proteins. Doxorubicin, **daunorubicin**, **idarubicin**, **epirubicin**, **dactinomycin**, and **bleomycin** belong to this group of chemotherapy drugs.

Topoisomerase inhibitors

Topoisomerase inhibitors are effective in treating a number of cancers. Topoisomerase is an enzyme necessary for the replication of DNA within the cell. The topoisomerase inhibitors act on this enzyme, and the cell eventually dies. Drugs in this class include **etoposide** and **teniposide**.

Camptothecin analogues are also classed as topoisomerase inhibitors. Specific drugs are **topotecan** and **irinotecan**.

Anthracyclines are topoisomerase inhibitors such as daunorubicin, doxorubicin, epirubicin, and idarubicin. A drawback of the anthracyclines is their toxicity to the heart. Because of this, there have been efforts to develop synthetic drugs similar to the anthracyclines. Mitoxantrone and losoxantrone are two examples of synthetics.

Dactinomycin is another drug acting on the DNA of the cell. It is an effective drug for treating a variety of cancers including **Ewing's sarcoma**, Wilms' tumor, embryonal rhabdomyosarcoma, and gestational choriocarcinoma (rare uterine cancer). It has also been used to treat cancer of the testicles, lymphoma, and Kaposi's sarcoma.

Antimicrotubule Agents

A microtubule is an important part of a cell, and is the target of a class of anticancer drugs.

Vinca alkaloids, which attack the cell's microtubules, are found in very small amounts in the periwinkle plant. Three types of vinca alkaloids are **vincristine**, **vinblastine** and **vinorelbine**. Vincristine is used more frequently in treating childhood, rather than adult, cancers. It is used in combination chemotherapy for the treatment of acute lymphocytic leukemia and Hodgkin's and non-Hodgkin's lymphoma, as well as other cancers. Vinblastine is used in combination chemotherapy for Kaposi's sarcoma, as well as cancers of the bladder, brain and breast. It is also used in the treatment of advanced cases of lymphoma and germ cell cancers.

The taxanes are another group of antimicrotubule agents. They are from the Pacific yew tree, and were first isolated in 1963. In 1971, **paclitaxel** was found to be an active ingredient in the bark of this tree. Paclitaxel has shown promising results in people with cancers of the ovaries or breasts. It is also used for AIDS patients who have Kaposi's sarcoma, and in combination with cisplatin in the treatment of non-small cell lung cancer. Paclitaxel is also part of the chemotherapy treatment in breast cancer patients whose cancer has spread to the lymph nodes. A related drug, **docetaxel** is used for treating advanced cases of breast cancer as well as certain non-small cell lung cancers.

Estramustine phosphate is related to nitrogen mustard. This drug acts on the microtubule of the cell, and has been effective in treating certain prostate cancers.

Hormones

Steroid hormones slow the growth of some cancers that depend on hormones. For example, **tamoxifen** is used to treat breast cancers that depend on the hormone estrogen for growth. Additionally, androgen suppression therapy is used in the treatment of **prostate cancer**. The goal of this therapy is to lower the levels of male hormones (androgens), especially **testosterone**, that can cause prostate cancer cells to grow. Lutenizing hormone-releasing hormone (LHRH) analogs lower testosterone levels by decreasing the androgens produced by the testicles. Two LHRH analogs available in the U.S. in 2001 are **leuprolide acetate** and **goserelin**.

Treatment location and schedule

Patients may take chemotherapy at home, in the doctor's office, or as an inpatient or outpatient at the hospital. Most patients stay in the hospital when first beginning chemotherapy, so their doctor can check for any side effects and change the dose if needed. A very important part of chemotherapy is determining the appropriate dose. To do this, the doctor must consider the person's size as well as any toxic side effects the drug may have.

How often and how long chemotherapy is given depends on the type of cancer, how patients respond to the drugs, patients' health and ability to tolerate the drugs, and on the types of drugs given. Chemotherapy administration may take only a few minutes or may last as long as several hours. Chemotherapy may be given daily, weekly, or monthly. A rest period may follow a course of treatment before the next course begins. In combination chemotherapy, more than one drug may be given at a time, or they may be given alternately, one following the other.

Precautions

There are many different types of chemotherapy drugs. Oncologists, doctors who specialize in treating cancer, determine which drugs are best suited for each patient. This decision is based on the type of cancer, the patient's age and health, and other drugs the patient is taking. Some patients should not be treated with certain chemotherapy drugs. Age and other conditions may affect the drugs with which a person may be treated. Heart disease, kidney disease, and diabetes are conditions that may limit the choice of treatment drugs. Pregnancy is another precaution because of the anticancer drug's impact on fetal development.

Preparation

A number of medical tests are done before chemotherapy is started. The oncologist will determine how much the cancer has spread from the results of x rays and other imaging tests and from samples of the tumor taken during surgery.

A patient's complete medical history will be taken, including any past chemotherapy. The patient will be asked to sign a consent form, and will be told about the drugs and procedures involved with chemotherapy. It is essential that the patient understand both the risks and benefits of treatment.

The nurse explains what will take place during the treatment, and what side effects to expect. In addition to the physical side effects, the stress of chemotherapy will be discussed. Patients who are better prepared tend to have fewer side effects and a higher emotional ability to handle the chemotherapy treatments.

Blood tests give the doctor important information about the function of the blood cells and levels of chemicals in the blood. A complete blood count (CBC) is commonly done before and regularly during treatment. The CBC shows the numbers of white blood cells, red blood cells, and platelets in the blood. Because chemotherapy affects the bone marrow, where blood cells are made, levels of these cells often drop during chemotherapy. The white blood cells and platelets are most likely to be affected by chemotherapy. A drop in the white blood cell count means that the immune system cannot function properly. Low levels of platelets can cause a patient to bleed easily from a cut or other wound. A low red blood cell count can lead to **anemia** (deficiency of red blood cells) and **fatigue**.

When a chemotherapy treatment takes a long time, the patient may prepare for it by wearing comfortable clothes. Bringing a book to read or a tape to listen to may help pass the time and ease the stress of receiving chemotherapy. Some patients bring a friend or family member to provide company and support during treatment.

Sometimes, patients taking chemotherapy drugs known to cause nausea are given medications called **antiemetics** before chemotherapy is administered. Anti-emetic drugs help to lessen feelings of nausea. Two anti-nausea medications that may be used are Kytril and Zofran.

Other ways to prepare for chemotherapy and help lessen nausea are:

- Regularly eat nutritious foods and drink lots of fluids.
- Eat and drink normally until about two hours before chemotherapy.
- Eat high carbohydrate, low-fat foods and avoid spicy foods.

Aftercare

To control side effects after chemotherapy, patients should:

- Follow any instructions given by the doctor or nurse.
- Take all prescribed medications.
- Eat small amounts of bland foods.
- Drink lots of fluids.
- Get plenty of rest.

Some patients find it helps to breathe fresh air or get mild exercise, such as taking a walk.

Risks

Chemotherapy drugs are toxic to normal cells as well as cancer cells. A dose that will destroy cancer cells will probably cause damage to some normal cells. Doctors adjust doses to do the least amount of harm possible to normal cells. Some patients feel few or no side effects, and others may have more serious side effects. In some cases, a dose adjustment is all that is needed to reduce or stop a side effect.

A person may experience a side effect right away or the reaction may be delayed. Side effects are classified as follows:

- acute, develops within 24 hours of treatment
- delayed, develops after 24 hours but within six to eight weeks of treatment
- short-term, combination of acute and delayed
- late/long-term, develops months or years after treatment, or lasts for an extended period of time
- expected, a side effect that develops in three quarters of patients

KEY TERMS

Adjuvant therapy—Treatment given after surgery or radiation therapy when there is no further evidence of cancer to prevent the cancer from coming back.

Alkaloid—A type of chemical commonly found in plants and often having medicinal properties.

Alykylating drug—A drug that kills cells by directly damaging DNA.

Antiemetic—A medicine that helps control nausea; also called an anti-nausea drug.

Antimetabolite—A drug that interferes with a cell's growth or ability to multiply.

Combination chemotherapy—The use of two or more anticancer drugs over the same course of treatment.

Lumbar puncture—A procedure in which a person lies on his or her side and a doctor inserts a needle into the spinal column. It can be used to withdraw spinal fluid or to deliver chemotherapy into the spinal fluid.

Peritoneal cavity—The space between the two layers of the peritoneum, the membrane that covers the abdominal wall of the body.

Platelets—Blood cells that function in blood clotting.

Primary chemotherapy—Chemotherapy that is the primary form of treatment. It may be used to shrink a tumor prior to surgically removing it.

- common, occurs in 25–75% of patients
- uncommon/occasional, occurs in less than a quarter of patients
- rare, occurs in 5% of patients
- very rare, occurs in less than 1% of patients

Certain chemotherapy drugs have more side effects than others. While some drugs have immediate effects, other effects are delayed. Patients are encouraged to discuss the potential for side effects with their doctor. They must seek immediate medical attention if they are experiencing any unusual symptoms. Some of the most common side effects are discussed in this section.

Nausea and vomiting/loss of appetite

Nausea and vomiting are common, but can usually be controlled by taking antinausea drugs, drinking enough fluids, and avoiding spicy foods. Loss of appetite (**anorexia**) may be due to nausea or the stress of undergoing cancer treatment. Drugs that have a high likelihood of causing nausea or vomiting include cisplatin, **mechlorethamine**, **streptozocin**, **dacarbazine**, **carmustine**, and dactinomycin. Those with moderate nausea-inducing potential include cyclophosphamide, doxorubicin, carboplatin, mitomycin, and L-**asparaginase**. Anticancer drugs with a low chance of causing nausea or vomiting include fluorouracil, methotrexate, etoposide, vincristine, and bleomycin.

Hair loss

Some chemotherapy drugs cause hair loss (**alopecia**), but it is almost always temporary. Hair re-growth may not begin until several weeks have passed since the final treatment. This is the most common impact that chemotherapy has on the outer surfaces of the body. In some patients, an ice wrap, called an ice turban, can reduce hair loss. The effectiveness will depend on factors such as the type of drug, dose, and treatment schedule. This preventive treatment must be avoided by patients with leukemia, lymphoma, **mycosis fungoides** or by those with scalp tumors. People should use with caution if they have conditions such as vasculitis, cryoglobulinemia or a history of radiation to the head. Patients should discuss the ice turban treatment with their doctor before trying it.

Anemia and fatigue

Low blood cell counts caused by the effect of chemotherapy on the bone marrow can lead to **anemia**, infections, and easy bleeding and bruising. Patients with anemia have too few red blood cells to deliver oxygen and nutrients to the body's tissues. Anemic patients feel tired and weak. If red blood cell levels fall too low, a blood transfusion may be given.

Infections

Patients receiving chemotherapy are more likely to get infections. This happens because their infection-fighting white blood cells are reduced. The level of reduction can vary depending on the dose and schedule of treatments, and whether the drug is used alone or in combination with other anticancer agents.

It is important for chemotherapy patients to avoid infection. When the white blood cell count drops too low, the doctor may prescribe medications called colony stimulating factors that help white blood cells grow. Neupogen and Leukine are two colony stimulants used as treatments to help fight infection.

Easy bleeding and bruising

Platelets are blood cells that make the blood clot. When patients do not have enough platelets, they may bleed or bruise easily, even from small injuries. Patients with low blood platelets should take precautions to avoid injuries. Medicines such as aspirin and other pain relievers can affect platelets and slow down the clotting process.

Sores in the mouth

Chemotherapy can cause irritation and dryness in the mouth and throat. An inflammation in the mouth is called **stomatitis**. Painful sores may form that can bleed and become infected. Precautions to avoid this side effect include getting dental care before chemotherapy begins, brushing the teeth and gums regularly with a soft brush, and avoiding mouth washes that contain salt or alcohol. Good oral hygiene is important. It is helpful for some patients to chew on ice chips for half an hour during chemotherapy treatments, but this should be discussed with the doctor before it is done.

Neuropathy and other damage to the nervous system

Cancer patients may develop neurological problems due to the cancer or the anticancer drugs. A variety of problems can develop, including altered mental alertness, changes in taste and smell, seizures, and peripheral **neuropathy** (tingling and burning sensations and/or weakness or numbness in the hands and/or feet). Different drugs can lead to different types of neurological disorders. Patients should discuss neurological symptoms with the doctor.

Heart damage

Some anticancer drugs are damaging to the heart. In these cases, the dosage is closely monitored in an attempt to avoid heart damage. Specific drugs that may be toxic to the heart include doxorubicin, daunorubicin, high doses of cyclophosphamide, and, in some cases, 5-FU. Patients experiencing chest pain or any cardiac symptoms should seek immediate medical help.

Kidney damage

A number of anticancer drugs can damage the kidney. Examples include high doses of methotrexate or 6-MP, as well as regular doses of L-asparaginase, cisplatin, mithramycin, streptozocin, and mitomycin C. Some kidney problems can be lessened by taking in adequate amounts of fluids. A secondary danger of kidney damage is that a less functional kidney can be more susceptible to further toxicity caused by other anticancer drugs that the patient is taking.

Respiratory problems

Cancer patients who have had radiation in the chest area are more susceptible to respiratory complications. Nitrosourea or bleomycin cause the most common type of respiratory toxicity, called pulmonary fibrosis. Patients should get immediate medical assistance if they have difficulty breathing.

Sexual function

Some drugs can lead to impaired sexual function. Alkylating agents and **procarbazine** may result in the absence of sperm in a man and the lack of menstruation in a woman. Patients of child-bearing age are usually told to refrain from conceiving while undergoing chemotherapy because of the defects it can cause in the fetus.

Vision problems

Some anticancer drugs can impact a person's vision. High doses of cyclophosphamide can cause blurred vision in children, while some alkylating agents can cause cataracts. Tamoxifen may be damaging to the retina, and cisplatin can damage the optic nerve. Conjunctivitis, commonly called pinkeye, is a treatable problem that occurs with many anticancer drugs.

Results

The main goal of chemotherapy is to cure cancer. Many cancers are cured by chemotherapy. The chemotherapy treatment may be used in combination with surgery to keep a cancer from spreading to other parts of the body. Some widespread, fast-growing cancers are more difficult to treat. In these cases, chemotherapy may slow the growth of the cancer cells.

Doctors can tell if the chemotherapy is working by the results of medical tests. Physical examination, blood tests, and x rays are all used to check the effects of treatment on the cancer.

The possible outcomes of chemotherapy are:

- Complete remission or response. The cancer completely disappears for at least one month. The course of chemotherapy is completed and the patient is tested regularly for a recurrence.
- Partial response. The cancer shrinks in size by at least 30–50%, the reduction in size is maintained for at least one month, and no new lesions are found during treatment. The same chemotherapy may be continued or a different combination of drugs may be used.
- Minor response. The cancer shrinks 1–29%.
- Stabilization. The cancer does not grow or shrink. Other therapy options may be explored. A tumor may stay stabilized for many years.
- Progressive disease. The cancer continues to increase in size by at least 25%, or new lesions are noted. Other therapy options may be explored.
- A secondary malignancy may develop from the one being treated, and that second cancer may need additional chemotherapy or other treatment.

See Also Cancer biology; Clinical trials; Complementary cancer therapies; Fatigue; Fertility issues; Infection and sepsis; Memory change; Metastasis; Nutritional support; Pregnancy and cancer; Radiation therapy; Second cancers; Sexuality; Taste alteration; Vascular access

Resources

BOOKS

DeVita, Vincent T. et al, eds. *Cancer: Principles and Practice of Oncology.* 6th ed. Philadelphia, PA: Lippincott, Williams & Wilkins, 2001.

Dollinger, Malin, Ernest H. Rosenbaum, and Greg Cable. *Everyone's Guide to Cancer Therapy.* Rev. 3rd ed. Kansas City, MO: Andrews McMeel Publishing, 1997.

Drum, David. *Making the Chemotherapy Decision.* Los Angeles, CA: Lowell House, 1996.

Haskell, Charles M. *Cancer Treatment,* 5th ed. Philadelphia, PA: W.B.Saunders Company, 2001.

McKay, Judith, and Nancee Hirano. *The Chemotherapy Survival Guide.* Oakland, CA: New Harbinger Publications, 1993.

Perry, Michael C. *The Chemotherapy Source Book.* 2nd ed. Baltimore, MD: Williams & Wilkins, 1996.

ORGANIZATION

American Cancer Society. 1599 Clifton Road, N.E., Atlanta, GA 30329. 1-800-ACS-2345.

Cancer Information Service of the National Cancer Institute. 1-800-4-CANCER.

QUESTIONS TO ASK THE DOCTOR

- What type of anticancer drugs will be used?
- Why were these drugs selected?
- How will the drugs be administered?
- Where will the chemotherapy take place?
- What preparation is necessary before treatment?
- What are the side effects?
- How can side effects be lessened?
- What are the symptoms of dangerous side effects?
- Who will give the chemotherapy?
- How often will the chemotherapy be given?
- How often are blood tests needed between treatments?
- What special care is needed while undergoing this type of treatment?
- When will the treatments be completed?
- What is the expected result?

OTHER

American Cancer Society. "How Will the Chemotherapy Be Administered?" 28 May 2001. <http://www3.cancer.org>.

American Cancer Society. Laryngeal and Hypopharyngeal Cancer Resource Center. "How Are Laryngeal and Hypopharyngeal Cancers Treated?" 28 May 2001. <http://www3.cancer.org>.

Cuesta-Romero, Carlos, and Grado-Pena, Jesus de. "Intralesional Methotrexate in Solitary Keratoacanthoma." *Archives of Dermatology,* April, 1998. 28 May 2001. <http://archderm.ama-assn.org/issues/v134n4/ffull/dlt0498-6.html>.

National Cancer Institute. National Institutes of Health. "Chemotherapy and You: A Guide to Self-Help During Treatment." <http://www.cancernet.nci.nih.gov/chemotherapy/chemoint.html>.

OncoLink. "What is Chemotherapy?" University of Pennsylvania Cancer Center, September, 1997. <http://www.oncolink.upenn.edu/specialty/chemo/general/whatis_chemo.html>.

OncoLink. "Introduction to Chemotherapy." University of Pennsylvania Cancer Center, 1998. <http://www.oncolink.upenn.edu/specialty/chemo/general/chemo_intro.html>.

Toni Rizzo
Rhonda Cloos, R.N.

Chest x ray *see* **X ray**

Childhood cancers

Definition

Childhood cancers are malignant diseases that affect children under the age of 18 years.

Description

Cancer in children (pediatric cancers) differs from cancer in adults in several important ways. The most important difference is that children have generally better prognoses than do adults. Two-thirds of children with cancer are cured of the disease. Still, despite enormous progress in the treatment of childhood cancer since the 1960s, it is the second-most common cause of death in children older than one year, with accidents being the first.

One difference between pediatric and adult cancer is found in the cells in which the cancers originate. Many adult cancers begin in specific organs, such as a lung, the breast, or the colon. Childhood cancer, except for leukemias and brain tumors, often arise in connective tissues such as bone and muscle.

Childhood cancer is often more aggressive than adult cancers. It grows faster and is frequently metastatic (has moved to other parts of the body or to the major organs) by the time of diagnosis. Thus, surgery alone is less likely to cure a child. Nevertheless, the cancers children develop tend to be more responsive to **chemotherapy** and radiation than those of adults.

The median age for children at the time of a cancer diagnosis is six years; for adults it is 67 years. Most children with cancer are otherwise healthy; many adults have conditions, such as heart disease, that make their treatment and recovery more difficult. Another important difference is that screening tests are available for some adult cancers, such as mammograms for **breast cancer** and Pap smears for **cervical cancer**. There are no useful screening tests for childhood cancers. Not infrequently, the diagnosis is made at a routine pediatric visit.

An extremely important factor in the improved prognosis of children with cancer has been the enrollment of the majority of children with cancer in research trials. Although only 2% of all cancers diagnosed in the United States occur in children, more than 70 percent of those children are enrolled in formal research protocols. By contrast, although adults have 98% of all cancers diagnosed in the United States, only 3% enroll in trials. Research protocols permit rapid collection of data on the effectiveness of treatment; they recognize adverse effects quickly, and foster valuable communication and collaboration among pediatric oncologists throughout the country and the world. In 1998, the four major pediatric research consortia in the United States joined forces. The Pediatric Oncology Group, the Children's Cancer Group, the Intergroup **Rhabdomyosarcoma** Study Group, and the National **Wilms' Tumor** Study Group, combined to form the Children's Oncology Group—to the great benefit of children with cancer.

Demographics

About 8,700 cases of cancer are diagnosed in children under the age of 15 years in the United States each year. Another 2,000-3,000 are diagnosed in teenagers over 15 years of age, but these are often recorded with adult diagnoses. The number of cases of childhood cancer has remained steady for a number of years. Researchers estimate that 1 of every 333 children will be diagnosed with cancer before the age of 20 years.

Leukemia accounts for 31% of the cancers in children, with about three-quarters of those being acute lymphoblastic leukemia and the other one-fourth mostly **acute myelocytic leukemia**. Central nervous system (CNS) cancers, commonly lumped together as brain tumors, are the next largest group, constituting another 17%. **Lymphoma**, both Hodgkin's and non-Hodgkin's, accounts for 15 percent of childhood cancers. The rest of the diagnoses are divided among what are referred to as solid tumors, such as **neuroblastoma**, **retinoblastoma**, Wilms' tumor, rhabdomyosarcoma, and bone cancers.

These statistics are similar in other parts of the developed world. In Africa, the most common form of childhood cancer is **Burkitt's lymphoma**, which is associated with the Epstein-Barr viral infection.

The survival rate for children with cancer is approaching 80% in the United States.

Causes

The causes of most childhood cancers are unknown, but some associations are recognized. The risk of childhood leukemia is increased in children with Down syndrome, in boys, in whites, and in those of higher socioeconomic status. Exposure to radiation *in utero* increases the risk as well. Central nervous system cancers are also more common in boys, in whites, and in those who have received radiation treatments for other cancers.

A number of inherited and developmental conditions are associated with an increased risk of childhood cancer. These include neurofibromatosis, Bloom's syndrome, ataxia-telangiectasia, and tuberous sclerosis. A family history of **Hodgkin's disease** increases its likelihood, and a family history of retinoblastoma in both eyes confers a 50% chance of an offspring carrying the gene. Ninety percent of children carrying the gene will develop the disease.

Special concerns

Family

Few situations test a family or a marriage like a diagnosis of cancer in a child. One day, parents have a healthy child with unlimited potential and a bright future; the next day, they have a child with a possibly fatal disease.

With a diagnosis of cancer in a child, parents must begin to negotiate complicated medical, social, family, and financial issues. Because children are generally best treated in centers that have pediatric oncologists, and because such centers can be far from a family's home, whole families can be uprooted, parents forced to spend weeks apart, and siblings left home with other relatives for long stretches of time.

Guilt can consume parents. They often assume they are responsible for their child's illness, they feel guilty if finances or insurance coverage issues force both to remain employed during their child's illness, and they worry that they are neglecting their other children.

One of the most difficult aspects of dealing with a diagnosis of cancer in a child is deciding what to tell that child and when. For infants and toddlers, this is not a concern, but older children need to know that they are ill, that they need these painful and unpleasant treatments, and—importantly—that they are not being punished for some misdeed, which is a common fear.

School

More than 80% of children with cancer miss at least some school during their treatments. Some children must miss school for prolonged periods. Federal law requires all states to provide education to handicapped children, and children with cancer are considered handicapped under the law. An individual education plan must be developed and an education provided, even for those who are homebound due to illness. Hospital social workers can be good resources for parents to explore their children's rights under their state's laws.

Completion of treatment

One of the surprisingly difficult aspects of cancer treatment comes when the treatment itself is completed. Parents, and certainly older children, can find the loss of the routine of regular treatment and the comfort of knowing that something active is being done to keep the cancer at bay can be quite frightening. Some parents and children become excessively focused on minor symptoms, fearful of recurrence. Occasionally, children who survive cancer become risk-takers as they grow, engaging in dangerous sports or hobbies.

Death

Though the survival rates for children with cancer continue to improve, the tragic truth is that some children will die of their disease. For parents, the day they learn that no further treatment is available is even harder than the day they learned their child's diagnosis. No decision is more difficult than stopping futile treatment and turning to care that is palliative (aimed solely at making the child comfortable).

Hospice care can be a valuable part of the end-of-life treatment for a child with cancer. Though not all inpatient hospice facilities accept children, they do provide home hospice care. Most families find that bringing their terminally ill child home, letting the child die in familiar surroundings with their loved ones at their side, offers them the only comfort to be had in a time of great sadness.

Grief for the death of a parent or spouse can last for months or even years, but most adults eventually come to accept those losses. Grief for the death of a child is life long. One of the hardest tasks for a parent in mourning can be offering the necessary support and love to their other surviving children. Some parents who lose a child to cancer can find some solace from support groups. Such groups are available through hospitals, hospices, churches, counseling, and cancer organizations. Other parents prefer solitude and time to face their loss.

Treatments

The treatment of childhood cancer depends on the specific disease, what tissues are affected, and how extensively it has spread at the time of diagnosis.

Acute lymphocytic leukemia and acute myelocytic leukemia

Acute lymphocytic leukemia (ALL) is the most common form of cancer in children, occurring about three times as often as **acute myelocytic leukemia** (AML). Leukemia of either type causes symptoms such as fevers, pallor, **fatigue**, bleeding or bruising, swollen glands, and bone pain—which can manifest itself as a limp or refusal to walk.

The diagnosis is made based on blood tests and bone marrow studies. The treatment is similar for both types. ALL has a very good prognosis, with a cure rate of about 80%; AML has a poorer prognosis, with different studies citing cure rates of 35-55%.

Treatment for ALL requires prolonged chemotherapy, consisting of remission induction, consolidation or intensification therapy, and maintenance. An essential component of the successful treatment of ALL is prophylactic (preventative) treatment to the CNS, a common site of relapse. In the past, children received radiation to the CNS, but this carried a risk of later brain tumors and significant neurologic and psychiatric deficits. Only the highest-risk children now receive CNS radiation; the rest receive intrathecal chemotherapy, which means that the medications are introduced directly into the spinal fluid during spinal taps.

Similar strategies are used in children with AML, but since far more of these patients relapse, **bone marrow transplantation** becomes an important option.

Non-Hodgkin's lymphoma

Non-Hodgkin's lymphoma constitutes about 60% of the lymphomas in children, and 10% of all childhood cancers. It is a cancer of the lymphatic system, which includes the spleen and lymph nodes. It is more common in boys than in girls, and other risks for the development of **non-Hodgkin's lymphomas** include conditions that depress the immune system, such as AIDS or immune suppressive treatment after organ or bone marrow transplant. Many such cases are Burkitt's lymphomas, and are associated with the presence of **Epstein-Barr virus**. These often manifest as masses in the jaw.

Non-Hodgkin's lymphoma has survival rates of 60-90%, depending upon the stage at which it is diagnosed. Lymphoma might be found at a routine examination, with nothing but swollen lymph nodes or an enlarged spleen as early signs. Some children do experience fevers or drenching **night sweats**, while others complain of persistent **itching**. Like adults, some teenagers will experience unexplained abdominal pain with alcohol ingestion, but might never report this symptom to parents for fear of consequences for underage drinking.

Non-Hodgkin's lymphoma is treated with chemotherapy, with radiation generally reserved for emergency treatment of bulky tumors that threaten other organs.

Hodgkin's disease

Hodgkin's disease is rare in young children but becomes more common in the teen years. Early Hodgkin's disease is one of the most curable of all cancers, with a cure rate as high as 95%. Early disease is often treated with chemotherapy alone, while more advanced disease is often treated with both chemotherapy and radiation.

Central nervous system cancers

CNS tumors account for about 17% of all childhood cancers. Several major categories of brain cancers are found in children.

KEY TERMS

Ataxia-telangiectasia—An inherited disorder of abnormal gait, skin lesions, and respiratory infections associated with a greater-than-average risk of developing childhood cancer.

Bloom's syndrome—An inherited disorder featuring skin abnormalities with a higher-than-average risk of childhood cancers.

Connective tissues—Those parts of the body that give it structure and form, including bones, joints, muscles, tendons, and ligaments.

Familial polyposis—An inherited disorder featuring multiple polyps in the colon with a very high likelihood of developing colon cancer by age 40; also associated with a greater-than-average risk of developing childhood cancer.

Fetal alcohol syndrome—A variety of birth defects that occur in children of mothers who abuse alcohol while pregnant, including mental retardation and facial abnormalities. Children with this syndrome have a higher than average risk of developing liver cancer.

Neurofibromatosis—An inherited disorder characterized by skin lesions, including brown spots called café au lait spots, small to large skin tumors, and neurofibromas, tumors within nerves. This carries a higher than average risk of developing childhood cancer.

Pituitary gland—The gland that produces multiple hormones that in turn affect other glands. The pituitary influences the nerves, the thyroid gland, the adrenal glands, and the ovaries and testes.

Tuberous sclerosis—An inherited disorder that includes skin abnormalities, mental retardation, and seizures, and carries a higher-than-average risk of childhood cancer.

Ureterosigmoidostomy—A surgical procedure that reroutes the ureters, the tubes that carry urine from the kidneys to the bladder, by implanting them instead into the sigmoid colon.

Ventricles—Spaces within the body. In the brain, these are spaces filled with cerebrospinal fluid. In the heart, these are the largest pumping chambers.

MEDULLOBLASTOMA. This is the most common brain tumor found in children. Its symptoms can appear as headaches, **nausea and vomiting**, and it can also cause gait disturbances and damage to the cranial nerves (those nerves that control such functions as eye movement and facial muscle control). **Medulloblastoma** is treated by surgical removal of the tumor and postoperative radiation. Chemotherapy appears to improve survival rates in those children with the most advanced disease at the time of diagnosis.

GLIOMA. These arise most often in the brainstem, at the base of the brain. Those that arise in the segment of the brain known as the pons have the poorest prognosis. Many gliomas produce gait abnormalities and cranial nerve problems such as double vision, and swallowing and speech disorders. Their location makes them difficult to reach surgically, so the primary treatment is **radiation therapy**. Most trials of chemotherapy have not shown benefit, but newer agents are being explored.

High-grade malignant gliomas include astrocytomas and glioblastomas. They are treated by surgical removal when possible, radiation therapy, and sometimes chemotherapy.

EPENDYMOMA. These cancers arise in the cells that line spaces within the brain—known as the ventricles—or the spinal column. In addition to nausea, vomiting, and headache, an **ependymoma** can cause head tilting and hearing loss. Treatment consists of surgery to remove the tumor followed by radiation. Chemotherapy does have benefit in children under three years of age but has less value in older children.

Neuroblastoma

Neuroblastoma, which accounts for about 8% of all childhood cancers, is far more common in infants than in older children. It originates in the sympathetic nervous system, a complicated system involving nerves and the adrenal glands, which produce hormones such as epinephrine and norepinephrine (also called adrenaline and noradrenaline). Most neuroblastomas arise in the adrenal glands, and are noticed as a mass in the abdomen. However, they can arise anywhere in the sympathetic nervous system, appearing as masses in the neck, the chest, or the pelvis.

Symptoms are usually related to whatever organs are compressed by the growing tumors. Thus, abdominal masses produce discomfort, vomiting or loss of appetite.

Neck masses can press on certain nerves and cause an eyelid to droop, the pupil to constrict, and the eye to stop producing tears. Masses in the pelvis can cause constipation or urinary retention. Because these cancers arise in tissues that produce epinephrine and similar substances, symptoms may be related to high levels of those substances. Children might be noted to sweat, flush, become pale, complain of palpitations or a rapid heartbeat, or develop high blood pressure.

Neuroblastomas are staged based on the age at diagnosis, location of the tumor, and degree of spread. Children considered at low or intermediate risk have the best prognoses, with up to 90% achieving long-term survival. Those at the highest risk have traditionally had a poor prognosis, with only about 15% surviving. The use of more intensive chemotherapy had improved the survival rate to 30% 1995.

Treatment consists of surgery to remove as much tumor as possible, chemotherapy, and often radiation therapy.

Wilms' tumor

Wilms' tumor, or nephroblastoma, is a cancer that arises in the kidney. It accounts for 5% of all cancers in children. Signs and symptoms of Wilms' tumors include abdominal masses, abdominal pain or swelling, high blood pressure, and blood in the urine—either visible or in microscopic examination. Treatment consists of removal of the kidney along with the tumor. Many children also receive radiation or chemotherapy, depending upon the extent of the original disease and the specific cell types involved. Wilms' tumors diagnosed at the very earliest stages have extremely favorable prognoses, with as high as a 98% cure rate.

Sarcomas

Soft tissue **sarcomas** are broadly divided into rhabdomyosarcoma and nonrhabdomyosarcoma soft tissue sarcomas. These are cancers of connective tissue. Rhabdomyosarcomas constitute about half of these types of cases. It is the fourth most common solid tumor in children, after brain tumors, neuroblastoma, and Wilms' tumor. It begins most commonly in sites in the head and neck, but can also arise in the urinary tract and the extremities. Symptoms can vary depending on the site of origin but, most often, rhabdomyosarcoma develops as a painless mass.

The nonrhabdomyosarcomas arise in a variety of different cell types. Among those cell types are the cells of the linings of peripheral nerves, the linings of joints, and other fibrous tissue. The most common sites of origin are the limbs, the trunk, the abdomen, and the pelvis.

The prognosis of both types of sarcomas varies with the extent of spread at the time of diagnosis and the type of cell from which the cancer arose. About 90% of children with early stage sarcomas can be cured, while only 20% of those with the most advanced disease at the time of diagnosis can be cured. Treatment consists of surgery and chemotherapy.

Osteogenic sarcoma

This is a form of bone cancer. In the past, all such cancers were treated with **amputation**. Now, **limb salvage** surgery can be performed in a number of cases. Chemotherapy and surgery combined have improved the prognosis for this disease to a 60% long-term survival rate.

Ewing's sarcoma

Ewing's sarcoma is a rare bone cancer that usually occurs in teenagers. It is more common in girls than in boys, and often starts in the femur (thighbone). Between 50 and 60% of children with Ewing's sarcoma will survive up to five years.

Retinoblastoma

Retinoblastoma is a cancer that arises in the cells of the retinas of the eyes. It is a disease of young children and has been diagnosed at birth. It can occur in both eyes in an inherited syndrome, and siblings of children with retinoblastoma in both eyes need to be screened. First symptoms include a sudden onset of squinting or crossed eyes. Radiation therapy will cure the disease in about 90% of children and, although most will suffer some visual changes, few lose their eyesight.

Germ cell cancers

These include teratomas, choriocarcinomas, embryonal carcinomas, and germinomas. These are all cancers of stem cells—cells that represent the earliest, or embryonal, stages of cell development and which have the potential to develop into mature cells. Some **germ cell tumors** are benign; others are malignant. They arise in the ovaries, testes, or sites along the midline of the interior of the body. Symptoms vary with the site of origin. Testicular masses are usually painless; ovarian masses can be accompanied by abdominal pain and swelling. Midline germ cell cancers can cause constipation or urinary retention as they grow and block internal organs. They are treated with surgery, radiation, and chemotherapy, and long-term survival rates are as high as 80% percent.

Hepatic cancers

Hepatic (liver) cancers are rare but not unheard of in children. There are two types of liver cancer in children.

Hepatoblastoma, which accounts for about two-thirds of these, is associated with familial polyposis, an inherited disease of multiple polyps in the colon. It has also been associated with fetal alcohol syndrome. Its incidence has risen since the 1970s.

The second type is hepatocellular **carcinoma**, which accounts for about one-third of the cases of liver cancer in children, and its incidence has been falling. Hepatocellular carcinoma has been associated with hepatitis B and C, exposure to anabolic steroids, aflatoxins (food contaminants), pesticides, and vinyl chloride.

Treatment of both of these cancers includes surgical removal of the cancer and chemotherapy, although hepatoblastoma is more responsive to chemotherapy than is hepatocellular carcinoma.

Alternative and complementary therapies

Alternative and complementary treatments have not been studied extensively in children, and some have been proven harmful. Herbal remedies can be particularly dangerous, in that children have very different metabolisms from adults and relatively benign treatments for adults can be fatal in children. For example, *jin bu hua*, a traditional Chinese medicine, can produce heart problems or difficulty breathing. Life root or comfrey might cause fatal liver damage in children.

Techniques such as guided imagery can be adapted for children. Providing favorite toys or videotapes can serve as focal points for children to distract them from painful or frightening procedures.

Late effects of treatment

The high cure rates for children with cancer have not come without a price. While chemotherapeutic drugs and radiation are highly toxic to cancer cells, they are highly toxic to healthy cells and organs, as well. Most organ systems can be affected by cancer treatment, and children who have been cured of cancer frequently face lifelong consequences of those treatments.

Organ systems

CENTRAL NERVOUS SYSTEM. Children who receive radiation therapy to their brains often experience a decline in scores on cognitive tests. More than one-half of the children who receive high-dose brain radiation have IQ scores below 90. Children with **acute leukemia** who are given chemotherapeutic agents directly into their spinal fluid are also at risk for developing learning disabilities and other neurologic effects.

EYES AND VISION. Both radiation to the brain and chemotherapy can cause damage to vision. If the eyes are included in a radiation field, the child can develop radiation cataracts. The long-term use of steroids, which are part of most chemotherapeutic regimens and used after bone marrow transplant, can also cause cataracts.

HEARING. Both radiation and the drug, **cisplatin**, can cause hearing loss.

TEETH AND SALIVARY GLANDS. Radiation therapy to the head and neck can damage permanent teeth and salivary glands. The chemotherapy administered to very young children with acute lymphoblastic leukemia can also cause damage to the teeth.

HEART. Heart damage can occur from the toxic effects of radiation therapy and from certain chemotherapeutic drugs. That damage can be centered in the heart muscle, the pericardium (lining) of the heart, or the coronary arteries. The drugs most noted for causing heart damage are **daunorubicin** and **doxorubicin**. They do particular damage to the left ventricle, the main pumping chamber of the heart. This can lead to congestive heart failure, in which the heart fails to pump blood effectively throughout the body. This might not appear until later life, precipitated by such stressors as vigorous exercise or pregnancy. Some survivors of childhood (and adult) cancers eventually come to require heart transplant.

LUNGS. **Bleomycin** and **carmustine**, two chemotherapeutic drugs, can cause inflammation of the lungs with later scarring and decrease in lung function. Radiation treatment of the chest can also impair lung function.

KIDNEYS. The kidneys can be damaged by radiation therapy to the abdomen or by a number of chemotherapeutic drugs. Some of those drugs are cisplatin, BCNU, **ifosfamide**, **methotrexate**, **vinblastine**, and bleomycin. Children treated for Wilms' tumors can develop kidney disease in the unaffected kidney years after treatment.

BLADDER. Radiation to the pelvis combined with the drug **cyclophosphamide** can produce a cystitis or bladder inflammation.

LIVER. Liver damage can occur with radiation or with chemotherapy. The agents used to treat leukemias are particularly known for their liver toxicity. BCNU is another agent with known liver toxicity.

Because so many children receive transfusions of blood products, they are at risk for developing transfusion-related hepatitis, which can progress to cirrhosis in a few cases. Blood products are now screened for the presence of hepatitis B and C viruses, but many older surviving children received transfusions before the screening tests were available.

SMALL INTESTINE. Radiation can cause an acute inflammation of the intestines with vomiting and **diarrhea**. Some children go on to develop scarring of the intestines that can lead to blockages requiting surgical repair.

MUSCULOSKELETAL SYSTEM. Radiation to the spine, sometimes used for children with Hodgkin's disease or medulloblastoma, can produce curvature of the spine, in the form of kyphosis, or hunchback, or scoliosis, an S-shaped curve of the spine. Radiation to the hips can cause damage to the hipbones. The two most common forms of that damage are slipped capital femoral epiphysis and avascular necrosis, both of which involve damage to the end of the thighbone where it meets the pelvic bones.

Loss of the necessary minerals within the bones can be seen in children who have been treated for brain cancers, acute lymphoblastic leukemia, lymphoma and some solid tumors. Long-term use of steroids or methotrexate is a common cause of this. These children are at risk of fractures.

ENDOCRINE SYSTEM. The endocrine system is the group of glands responsible for the production of hormones. Almost any gland can be affected.

Pituitary gland: Brain radiation can cause growth hormone deficiency. Even when normal levels of growth hormone are found, children who have undergone brain radiation are often obese and fail to achieve their expected height. Those whose levels are low will grow when growth hormone injections are administered.

Thyroid gland: The thyroid gland can be damaged by radiation treatment that involves the neck, typically becoming underactive. This might not occur until several years after treatment, and is treated with oral thyroid hormone.

Reproductive function: Radiation therapy and chemotherapy can both damage the ovaries, causing loss of hormones, lack of periods and infertility. The testes are less easily damaged and adult male survivors often have normal hormonal levels and sexual function, but might be sterile. Adolescents might be offered the opportunity to bank sperm before treatment to ensure that they might have future children through artificial insemination. Those who have had surgery to remove internal nodes involved in **testicular cancer** might be impotent as adults due to damage to the nerves that control sexual function.

Concerns have been raised that since chemotherapeutic agents can cause genetic mutations, those survivors whose fertility has been preserved might be at risk of giving birth to children with birth defects. This has not been observed yet, but children of women treated for Wilms' tumors often have low birth weights.

Second cancers

The most serious late effect of successful treatment for childhood cancer is a second cancer. **Second Cancers** are a different type and are related to either inherited factors or far more often to late effects of treatments.

GENETIC CAUSES. About fifty percent of those who have been treated for the hereditary form of retinoblastoma develop a second cancer at some point in their lives.

SURGICAL TREATMENT. Children with cancers that obstruct the flow of urine sometimes require a procedure called ureterosigmoidostomy. In this, the ureter, which carries urine from the kidney to the bladder, is attached instead to the sigmoid colon. Such children have a significant risk of developing adenocarcinoma of the colon at the site of the connection in adulthood.

RADIATION THERAPY. Radiation to the neck can cause later **thyroid cancer**. Radiation to the brain can cause later brain tumors, such as meningiomas or gliomas. This was once fairly common in children treated for leukemia and given prophylactic radiation therapy to prevent central nervous system relapse. Bone sarcomas are possible after radiation treatment of retinoblastomas or Ewing's sarcoma. The risk of later breast cancer is increased in those who were treated with radiation for Hodgkin's disease in childhood.

CHEMOTHERAPY. **Etoposide** and **teniposide**, chemotherapeutic drugs known as epipodophyllins, are associated with a risk of developing acute myelogenous leukemia in the years after initial treatment for cancer. These are used in treatment of some germ cell tumors, ALL, and non-Hodgkin's lymphoma.

IMMUNE SUPPRESSION. To prevent rejection, children who undergo bone marrow transplant receive drugs to suppress their immune systems. Long-term use of these medications is associated with a risk of developing cancer that originates in the white blood cells known as B cells.

See Also Cancer genetics; Extragonadal germ cell tumor; Osteosarcoma

Resources

BOOKS

Fromer, Margaret Joan. *Surviving Childhood Cancer: A Guide for Families.* Oakland: New Harbinger Publications, 1998.

Janes-Hodder, Honna, and Nancy Keene. *Childhood Cancer: A Parent's Guide to Solid Tumor Cancers.* Sebastopol: O'Reilly & Associates, 1999.

Keene, Nancy, Kathy Ruccione, and Wendy L. Hobbie. *Childhood Cancer Survivors: A Practical Guide to Your Future.* Sebastopol: O'Reilly & Associates, 2000.

Keene, Nancy, and Linda Lamb. *Childhood Leukemia: A Guide for Families, Friends & Caregivers.* Sebastopol: O'Reilly & Associates, 1999.

Laszlo, John. *The Cure of Childhood Leukemia: Into the Age of Miracles.* New Brunswick: Rutgers University Press, 1995.

PERIODICALS

Dixon-Woods, M., M. Findlay, B. Young, H. Cox, and D. Henry. "Parents' Accounts of Obtaining a Diagnosis of Childhood Cancer." *Lancet* 357, no. 9257 (March 3, 2001): 670-4.

Gaynon P. S., M. E. Trigg, N. A. Heerema, M. G. Sensel, H. N. Sather, G. D. Hammond, and W. A. Bleyer. "Children's Cancer Group Trials in Childhood Acute Lymphoblastic Leukemia: 1983-1995." *Leukemia* 14, no. 12 (December 2000): 2223-33.

Green, D. M., A. Hyland, M. P. Barcos, J. A. Reynolds, R. J. Lee, B. C. Hall, and M. A. Zevon. "Second Malignant Neoplasms after Treatment for Hodgkin's Disease in Childhood or Adolescence." *Journal of Clinical Oncology* 18, no. 7 (April 2000): 1492-9.

Hasle, H., I. H. Clemmenson, M. Mikkelsen. "Risks of Leukaemia and Solid Tumours in Individuals with Down's Syndrome." *Lancet* 355, no. 9199 (January 15, 2000): 165-9.

Pui, C. H. "Acute Lymphoblastic Leukemia in Children." *Current Opinions in Oncology* 12, no. 1 (January 2000): 3-12.

ORGANIZATIONS

Candlelighters Childhood Cancer Foundation. 7910 Woodmont Avenue, Suite 460, Bethesda, MD 20814. (800)366-CCCF. <http://www.candlelighters.org>

National Childhood Cancer Foundation. 440 E. Huntington Drive, P.O. Box 60012, Arcadia, CA 91066-6012. (626)447-1674. <http://www.nccf.org>

Childhood Cancer Ombudsman Program. P.O. Box 595, Burgess, VA 22432. Fax: (804)580-2502

American Cancer Society. 1599 Clifton Road, Atlanta, GA, 30329. (800)ACS-2345. <http://www.cancer.org>

The Leukemia and Lymphoma Society of America (formerly The Leukemia Society of America). 1311 Mamaroneck Avenue, White Plains, NY 10605. (914)949-5213. <http://www.leukemia-lymphoma.org/>

The National Cancer Institute. Cancer Information Service. Building 31, Room 10A31, 31 Center Drive, MSC 2580, Bethesda, MD 20892-2580. (301)435-3848. <http://www.nci.nih.gov/>

Cancer Care, Inc. 1180 Avenue of the Americas, New York, NY 10036. (212)302-2400 or (800)813-4673. <http://www.cancercare.org>

National Marrow Donor Program. Suite 500, 3001 Broadway Street NE, Minneapolis, MN 55413-1753. (800)MARROW2 (800-627-7692). <http://www.marrow.org/>

OTHER

National Children's Cancer Society. 1 July 2001 <http://www.children-cancer.com>

Why, Charlie Brown, Why? Videotape. Topper Books, 1990.

PDQ (Physician Data Query). (800)4-CANCER. 1 July 2001 <http://cancernet.nci.nih.gov>

QUESTIONS TO ASK THE DOCTOR

- What type of cancer does my child have?
- What characteristics of my child's illness are favorable? Which are unfavorable?
- What course of therapy do you recommend?
- What medications will you use and what side effect should we anticipate?
- Will my child require surgery?
- Will my child need radiation therapy?
- Will my child need to be hospitalized for treatments?
- Should my child be enrolled in a clinical trial?
- Should my child be treated at a pediatric oncology center?
- Can my child continue to go to school?
- Can I stay with my child for procedures; for hospitalizations?
- How and what should we tell our child about the illness?
- What should we tell our other children?
- What should we expect after treatment is finished?

GrannyBarb and Art's Leukemia Links. 1 July 2001 <http://www.acor.org/diseases/hematology/Leukemia/leukmain.html>

Patient-centered Guides. 1 July 2001 <http://www.patientcenters.com/leukemia/>

CancerNet clinical trials listings. 1 July 2001 <http://www.cancernet.nci.nih.gov/trialsrch.shtml>

Veritas A service of Harvard Medical School, listing clinical trials throughout the U.S. 1 July 2001 <http://www.veritasmedicine.com/leukemia>

International clinical trials listings. 1 July 2001 <http://www.graylab.ac.uk/cancerweb/trials.html>

Marianne Vahey, M.D.

Chlorambucil

Definition

Chlorambucil (marketed under the brand name Leukeran) is a **chemotherapy** medicine used to treat cancer by interfering with the growth of cancer cells.

KEY TERMS

Anemia—A reduction in the normal number of red blood cells in the blood.

Chemotherapy—Specific drugs that are used to treat cancer.

Cystitis—An irritation of the bladder lining.

DNA—Deoxyribonucleic acid; genetic material inside of cells.

Food and Drug Administration—A government agency that oversees public safety in relation to drugs and medical devices. The FDA gives the approval to pharmaceutical companies for commercial marketing of their products.

Intravenous—Entering the body through a vein.

Leukopenia—A reduction in the normal number of white blood cells in the blood.

Metastatic—Cancer that has spread to one or more parts of the body.

Purpose

Chlorambucil is approved by the Food and Drug Administration (FDA) to treat **chronic lymphocytic leukemia** and malignant lymphomas. It has also been less commonly used for other types of cancer including **breast cancer**, **ovarian cancer**, and choriocarcinoma. Chlorambucil is not used with the intent to cure the cancer but to improve symptoms of the disease.

Description

Chlorambucil is a member of the group of chemotherapy drugs known as alkylating agents. Alkylating agents interfere with the genetic material (deoxyribonucleic acid, or DNA) inside the cancer cells and prevent them from further dividing and growing more cancer cells. Chlorambucil is a tablet that is taken orally.

Recommended dosage

Chlorambucil can be taken according to several different dosing schedules, depending on the disease to be treated. Chlorambucil is a 2mg oral tablet, and patients may need to take more than one tablet at a time depending on the dose. The dose is based on a patient's weight in kilograms. Patients with leukemia take chlorambucil daily for three to six weeks at a dose of 0.1 to 0.2 mg/kg/day (milligram per kilogram of body weight per day).

Precautions

Patients who have received a full course of **radiation therapy** or chemotherapy generally should not receive chlorambucil until four weeks after the radiation or chemotherapy has been completed. Heath care providers should be notified if patients have had any previous allergic reactions to chemotherapy treatment. Patients should also increase the amount of fluids that they drink while on this medicine.

Blood counts will be monitored regularly while on chlorambucil therapy. During a certain time period after receiving chlorambucil there may be an increased risk of getting infections. Caution should be taken to avoid unnecessary exposure to infectious agents. Patients should check with their doctors before receiving live virus **vaccines** while on chemotherapy.

Patients who may be pregnant or trying to become pregnant should tell their doctor before receiving chlorambucil. Men and women undergoing chemotherapy are at risk of becoming sterile.

Side effects

The most common side effect from taking chlorambucil is **myelosuppression**, a suppression of bone marrow activity resulting in a low blood cell count. Myelosuppression is usually the goal when treating leukemia with chlorambucil. When the white blood cell count is lower than normal (leukopenia), patients are at an increased risk of developing a **fever** and infections.

The platelet count can also be decreased due to chlorambucil administration. Platelets are blood cells normally found in large numbers that aid in clot formation. When the platelet count is low, patients are at an increased risk for bruising and bleeding. If the platelet count remains too low, a platelet blood transfusion is an option for treatment. More rarely, chlorambucil causes a condition called **anemia** in which the number of circulating red blood cells drops, resulting in dizziness and/or **fatigue**. **Erythropoietin** is a drug that can be used to increase the red blood cell count.

Less common side effects from chlorambucil include nausea, vomiting, loss of appetite, mouth sores, skin rashes, and **diarrhea**. **Antiemetics** may be given to patients before taking chlorambucil to help prevent or reduce **nausea and vomiting**. Liver problems may occur due to chlorambucil administration, but they are typically mild and resolve when the drug is stopped.

Damage to nerves and nervous system tissues is uncommon with chlorambucil therapy. Some reports do exist of nerve damage that has resulted in seizures, muscle twitching, muscle shaking, confusion, visual hallucinations, irritability, and loss of muscle control. Other rare reactions to chlorambucil include hair loss (**alopecia**), **itching**, fever, lung problems, eye problems, tingling of the hands and feet, cystitis (bladder infection), and the development of another type of cancer or leukemia.

Interactions

There are no significant drug interactions associated with taking chlorambucil.

Nancy J. Beaulieu, RPh.,BCOP

Cholangiocarcinoma *see* **Bile duct cancer**

Chondrosarcoma

Definition

Chondrosarcoma is a malignant tumor that arises from cells that produce cartilage, the rubbery tissue around joints. Therefore, it is a type of sarcoma that is predominantly found in the area around bones.

Description

Sarcomas of the bone are rare and represent about 0.2% of all new cancer cases each year. The two most common forms of bone cancer are **osteosarcoma** and **Ewing's sarcoma**. Among the less common are chondrosarcoma, **fibrosarcoma**, and **malignant fibrous histiocytoma**, all of which arise from spindle cell neoplasms.

Chondrosarcomas arise from chondroblasts, cells that form cartilage. Cartilage is the matrix found at the tip of the nose and ears. However, cancer that develops from chondroblasts is usually observed on the surface of the pelvis, in the femur of the upper leg, around the shoulder, in the humerus of the upper arm, and in the ribs.

Depending on the type and location of the chondrosarcoma, the tumor can either be high grade and aggressive or low grade and not as invasive. There are two different categories of chondrosarcomas—classic chondrosarcomas and variant chondrosarcomas. Together they have five main types.

Central chondrosarcoma and peripheral chondrosarcoma are both classic chondrosarcomas. Central chondrosarcoma occurs within a bone, and peripheral chondrosarcoma develops on the surface of a bone. Both can develop as a primary tumor or as a secondary tumor to an existing tumor elsewhere in the body. Most, however, are primary tumors. Seventy-six percent of primary chondrosarcomas occur centrally within a bone.

There are three variant chondrosarcomas: clear cell chondrosarcoma, mesenchymal chondrosarcoma, and dedifferentiated chondrosarcoma. Clear cell chondrosarcoma is the most rare form of chondrosarcoma. It is a low grade, slow growing tumor that typically occurs locally in the epiphysis, or end part, of long tubular bones such as the femur and humerus, meaning that it does not normally invade into surrounding soft tissue. As the name implies, cells biopsied from this type of chondrosarcoma appear clear with many large vacuoles.

Mesenchymal chondrosarcoma is another rare variant. However, as opposed to clear cell chondrosarcoma, it is highly malignant and frequently metastasizes, commonly to the lungs, lymph nodes and other bones. This variant has a tendency to develop in flat bones such as vertebra, the pelvis, or the skull, as opposed to long tubular bones. Under a microscope, the cells appear round and contain spindle cell elements and neoplastic cartilage formation.

Dedifferentiated chondrosarcoma is also rare and is the most malignant form of chondrosarcoma. It is characterized by the presence of a mix of low-grade chondrosarcoma and has undergone malignant degeneration, producing a fully malignant soft tissue mass that is no longer identifiable as cartilage. These cancers occur most commonly in the flat bones of individuals over the age of sixty. Despite varied treatments, they are almost always fatal.

Due to the location of chondrosarcoma tumors, the result is often a decrease in the range of motion of limbs, especially tumors occurring on the epiphysis of bones such as those seen in clear cell chondrosarcoma.

Demographics

Although there are exceptions, chondrosarcomas occur mainly in older adults forty to sixty years old and typically occur more in men than in women. Chondrosarcomas are rarely seen in infants and children. Dedifferentiated chondrosarcomas predominantly arise in the elderly over the age of sixty, equally between males and females. Mesenchymal chondrosarcoma develops in the young adult population between the ages of twenty and forty years old, and it is slightly more common in females. Classic chondrosarcomas usually develop in people over the age of forty. However, when they occur in younger age groups, they have a propensity to be highly malignant, capable of **metastasis**.

Causes and symptoms

As of 2001, there is little known about what causes chondrosarcomas. However, researchers have discovered

KEY TERMS

Carcinogen—An agent that is capable of causing cancer.

Epiphysis—The end of long tubular bones such as femur in the leg and the humerus in the arm. Initially separated from the main bone by a layer of cartilage that eventually allows the parts to fuse.

Spindle cells—Spindle-shaped cells typically found in connective tissue.

that chondrosarcomas are sometimes associated with underlying benign bone tumors. They can also result as a side effect from previous **radiation therapy** for unrelated primary cancer treatment. Individuals with other bone diseases such as Maffucci's syndrome and Ollier's disease are at a higher risk for developing chondrosarcomas.

There are many symptoms associated with the onset of chondrosarcomas. They tend to develop slowly in most cases, except when the cancer is aggressive. The following is a list of the main symptoms that may present:

- pain
- swelling
- firm lump
- broken bone
- impeded normal range of motion
- urinary frequency (seen in pelvic chondrosarcomas)
- urinary obstruction (seen in pelvic chondrosarcomas)

The above symptoms are not always indicators of the presence of chondrosarcoma. Any one of these symptoms could be related to another, less serious condition. A doctor should be seen to diagnose the problem properly.

Diagnosis

In order to diagnose bone cancer, a doctor will take the patient's history and conduct a thorough physical exam. Blood tests will be performed to rule out other conditions and identify cancer markers.

The most revealing initial exam is an **x ray**. It can show the location, size, and shape of the tumor. If a malignant tumor is present, the x ray will expose a soft tissue mass with ill-defined edges. This procedure takes less than an hour and can be performed in the doctor's office. Depending on the medical facilities, the results can be returned the same day after being interpreted by a physician, and perhaps a consulting oncologist and radiologist.

Once there is evidence of a tumor, one or more of several other procedures may be performed, including CT scans, MRI (**magnetic resonance imaging**), angiograms, and **biopsy**.

Treatment team

If the patient is seeing a primary care provider, the provider may perform the initial diagnostic tests. However, in order to comprehensively diagnose and treat chondrosarcomas, the primary care provider will refer the patient to an orthopaedic oncologist (bone cancer specialist). Radiologists, pathologists and orthopaedic surgeons will also be involved to read x rays, examine tissue samples, and remove the tumor if necessary.

Many other individuals will be involved with the treatment of chondrosarcoma. For example, nurses and dieticians are available to explain side effects of treatment and offer suggestions on eating healthy meals to help fight the side effects. If a limb is totally or partially removed, a physical therapist or vocational therapist will assist the patient in learning how to use a prosthetic limb.

Clinical staging, treatments, and prognosis

After the physician makes the diagnosis, it is important to determine the stage of the cancer. This will help reveal how far the cancer has progressed and how much tissue has been affected.

A new system of staging was adopted in 1980 by the Musculoskeletal Tumor Society. It is based on the fact that differing tissue types associated with the bone behave similarly when cancerous. This classification system uses grade (G), location (T), and lymph node involvement and metastasis (M).

Surgical grade (G) refers to how aggressive the cancer is. For example, G0 represents a benign tumor and G2 represents a highly aggressive tumor. The anatomical location (T) establishes whether or not the tumor is inside the bone (T1) or outside the bone (T2). If metastases are present, then the tumor is classified as M0; and if metastases are not present, the tumor is classified as M1. The following is a list of stages and their indications:

- Stage IA (G1, T1, M0): low grade within the bone, without metastasis
- Stage IB (G1, T2, M0): low grade outside the bone, without metastasis
- Stage IIA (G2, T1, M0): high grade within the bone, without metastasis

- Stage IIB (G2, T2, M0): high grade outside the bone, without metastasis
- Stage IIIA (G1 or G2, T1, M1): inside the bone, with metastasis
- Stage IIIB (G1 or G2, T2, M1): outside the bone, with metastasis

Physicians can employ several courses of treatment to remove chondrosarcomas. The most effective treatment is surgical removal. When performing the surgery, the doctor will remove the tumor and some healthy tissue or bone around it to ensure that the tumor does not recur near the original site. The physician may replace the removed bone with a metal device. In children, the metal device can be lengthened as the child grows, but this will require further surgeries. The fact that most chondrosarcomas tend to be low grade and slow-progressing makes this procedure one that does not necessitate entire limb removal except in extreme cases when the tumor is large.

Even individuals with low-grade chondrosarcoma that have undergone surgery experience a moderate risk of local recurrence. To combat recurrence, **chemotherapy** (the use of one or more cancer killing drugs) and radiation therapy (the use of high energy rays) have also been used to complement surgery. Employing chemotherapy or radiation therapy individually (without surgery) is much less effective. In fact, chondrosarcomas are generally resistant to chemotherapy alone.

Low stage chondrosarcomas (Stages IA and IB) have greater one and five-year survival rates than the high stages (Stages IIIA and IIIB). High-grade tumors are more aggressive and highly metastatic than lower grade tumors, and therefore they have a lower survival rate. Not only is the grade of the tumor (the estimate of its aggressiveness) important in determining prognosis, but the age of the patient is also crucial. Generally, chondrosarcomas that occur in childhood and infancy have a higher mortality rate than those that occur in adults.

Metastases appear later in the development of chondrosarcomas. The lungs are the sites of primary metastasis. Once metastasis to the lungs has occurred, survival rate decreases.

Coping with cancer treatment

Chemotherapy often results in several side effects, depending on the drug used and the patient's individual tolerance. Patients may have to deal with nausea, vomiting, loss of appetite, and hair loss. Often, chemotherapy and radiation therapy are better handled if the patient is eating well. Nurses and dieticians can aid in choosing healthful foods to incorporate into the patient's diet.

If the chondrosarcoma necessitates limb **amputation**, the patient will need to learn how to cope with a prosthetic device. Both physical and vocational therapists can help the patient adjust and learn to use prosthetic devices to perform daily activities in new ways.

Clinical trials

Since chondrosarcomas are rare forms of cancer, there is still much to be learned. Clearly, surgery is the most effective treatment. New techniques in cryosurgery are being developed in various institutions across the country.

Chemotherapy trials have shown improved results with more intense regimens. Such drugs that are under study include **methotrexate**, **leucovorin**, **vincristine**, **bacillus Calmette-Guérin**, **doxorubicin**, or a combination of two or three of these.

Patients should consult with their physicians or contact the American Cancer Society to learn what procedures are currently in **clinical trials**. In some cases, insurance companies will not cover clinical trial procedures. Patients should talk with their doctor and insurance company to determine which procedures are covered.

Prevention

Since little is known about what causes chondrosarcomas, there is also little known about how to prevent them. In general, the prevention of cancer can be assisted by avoiding known chemical carcinogens such as alpha-naphthylamine, carbon tetrachloride, and benzene. Another way to avoid developing cancer—especially bone cancer—is to minimize exposure to penetrating radiation such as x rays and radioactive elements. Medical x rays revolutionized the field of medicine and are used to detect and treat many diseases. In most cases, the benefits of medical x rays outweigh the risks.

Special concerns

Cancer treatments, especially surgical amputation, can take a physical and psychological toll on cancer patients and their families. To deal with the psychological impact, many different support groups and psychotherapists are available to help. Some therapists will consider amputation a post-traumatic stress disorder and treat it accordingly. Faith practices are also beneficial for cancer patients in dealing with their condition. Patients should discuss all options with their physician to determine what is available to them.

Once the cancer has been treated, patients should make sure to schedule follow-up appointments with their

QUESTIONS TO ASK THE DOCTOR

- What diagnostic procedures are best for the location and type of tumor suspected?
- What treatments are best for the location and type of tumor suspected?
- What kinds of side effects will this course of treatment result?
- Are there support services available?
- What treatments are currently in clinical trials?
- What treatments will my health care insurance cover?

physicians. Physicians will want to monitor the patient for side effects or possible recurrence that may develop years after treatment.

See Also Tumor staging; Tumor grading; Limb Salvage

Resources

BOOKS

Malawer, Martin M. "Sarcomas of Bone." In *Cancer Principles and Practice of Oncology,* edited by Vincent T. DeVita, Jr., M.D., et al. New York: Lippincott-Raven Publishers, 1997, pp.1789-852.

Rosen, Gerald, M.D. "Neoplasms of the Bone and Soft Tissue." In *Cancer Medicine,* edited by Robert C. Bast, Jr., M.D., et al. London: BC Decker, Inc., 2000, pp.1870-95.

PERIODICALS

Lee, Francis, M.D., et al. "Chondrosarcoma of Bone: An Assessment of Outcome."*The Journal of Bone and Joint Surgery* (March 1999): 326-38.

Mitchell, A.D., et al. "Experience in the treatment of dedifferentiated chondrosarcoma"*The Journal of Bone and Joint Surgery* (January 2000): 55-61.

ORGANIZATIONS

American Cancer Society. <http://www.cancer.org>.

National Cancer Institute. <http://cancernet.nci.nih.gov>.

Sally C. McFarlane-Parrott

Chordoma

Definition

Chordomas are rare tumors of the central nervous system (brain and spinal cord).

Description

Chordomas are slow-growing tumors that invade bone and tissue surrounding the spinal column. They rarely spread to other parts of the body, but they can cause considerable damage or death because they destroy bone and soft tissue and often grow along the roots of nerves, putting pressure on the nerves and disrupting their function.

Chordomas appear at the base of the skull about 60% of the time and in the sacrum, located at the base of the spine, about 30% of the time. The other 10% of chordomas can occur anywhere else along the spinal column.

Demographics

Chordomas are very rare, accounting for between 1–4% of tumors of the brain and spinal column. Chordomas that occur at the base of the skull are most common in adults between 30 and 40 years of age. Those tumors that arise at the sacrum, located at the base of the spine, most commonly appear in older adults between the ages of 50 and 70. Chordomas are about twice as common in men as they are in women.

Causes and symptoms

During the fourth through sixth week of fetal development, a group of cells come together to form a structure called the notochord. The notochord defines the vertical mid-line of the body, and the spinal column develops around it. Normally, as development progresses, the notochord degenerates and disappears, except for small bits that become part of the disks between the spinal vertebrae. Chordomas are believed to develop from pieces of notochord that, for some reason, do not break down as they should. Over many years, these harmless bits of notochord transform and become malignant, forming chordomas.

Symptoms of chordoma depend on where the tumor is located. They are often vague and similar to symptoms of other tumors or even other conditions. Tumors located at the base of the skull may cause headaches, difficulty swallowing, or seizures depending on how much they have invaded the bones of the skull. Tumors located on the sacrum can cause general low back pain or difficulty with bowel and bladder control.

Diagnosis

Diagnosis has two parts: first, determining that the patient has a central nervous system tumor and where it is located, and second, determining what type of tumor it is. It is not easy to diagnose either of these.

A battery of tests is used to diagnose chordomas. A basic neurological examination tests the patient's reflexes, vision, hearing, senses of touch and smell, mental

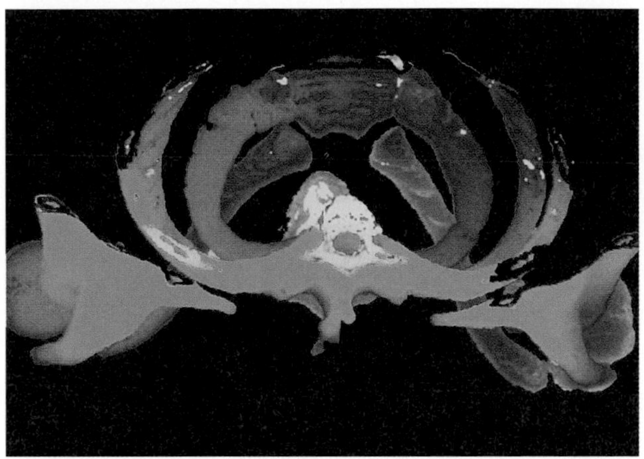

Colored 3-D computed tomography (CT) scan of the spine and ribcage of a male patient, showing cancer of the spine. The front of the body is at top, and at bottom left and right are the shoulder blades. The vertebral bone of the spine appears yellow and to the left of the vertebra is the cancerous tumor. *(© Simon Fraser, Science Source/Photo Researchers, Inc. Reproduced by permission.)*

acuity, orientation, memory, and head and neck movements. If the results of the test indicate central nervous system dysfunction, the patient is usually referred to a neurologist (specialist in the central nervous system).

Several different scans are done to locate the tumor. Two of the most common are the **computed tomography** (CT or CAT) scan and **magnetic resonance imaging** (MRI). A CT scan uses x-ray images taken from many angles and computer reconstruction to show parts of the body in cross section. This helps to locate and estimate the size the tumor, and provides information on whether it can be surgically removed. MRI uses magnets and radio waves to create more detailed cross-sectional scans than computed tomography. There are many variations on these two scans that use dyes or radioactive materials to provide information about blood flow around the tumor and help determine whether the tumor can be surgically removed.

Treatment team

A neurosurgeon (a surgeon that specializes in the nervous system) will most likely lead the treatment team. A radiologist that specializes in nervous system radiology will interpret CT and MRI scans. Depending on the treatment plan, other members of the team may include a radiation oncologist (a specialist in **radiation therapy**), radiation technicians, and nurses with special training in assisting cancer patients.

Clinical staging, treatments, and prognosis

Staging of chordomas is less important in developing a treatment plan than it is for some other cancers, since chordomas rarely spread from their original location. If the tumor is in a location where it can safely be removed without damaging other nerves or structures, surgery is the preferred treatment.

But chordomas can be difficult to treat because the location of the tumor often makes it inoperable or impossible to remove completely. This is especially true of chordomas located at the base of the skull. When the tumor is inoperable, radiation therapy is the preferred treatment. Proton therapy, also called charged particle therapy, is a type of radiation treatment that spares the tissues around the tumor. For this reason, it is sometimes recommended for chordoma around the skull. One drawback of proton therapy is that the procedure is only offered at a few sites around in the United States. It is always appropriate to get a second opinion before agreeing to any treatment plan. Some insurers require second opinions before surgery.

The success of the treatment plan depends almost entirely on the location of the tumor. Chordomas can recur after either surgery or radiation therapy. They rarely spread (metastasize) to other parts of the body.

Alternative and complementary therapies

Alternative and complementary therapies range from herbal remedies, vitamin supplements, and special diets to spiritual practices, acupuncture, massage, and similar treatments. When these therapies are used in addition to conventional medicine, they are called complementary therapies. When they are used instead of conventional medicine, they are called alternative therapies.

No specific alternative therapies have been directed toward chordoma. However, good nutrition and activities, such as yoga, meditation, and massage, that reduce stress and promote a positive view of life have no unwanted side effects and appear to be beneficial. Alternative and experimental treatments are normally not covered by insurance.

Coping with cancer treatment

Cancer treatment, even when successful, has many unwanted side effects. Radiation therapy may cause

KEY TERMS

Sacrum—The last five vertebrae (bones) of the spinal column, which are fused into a single mass commonly called the tail bone.

QUESTIONS TO ASK THE DOCTOR

- What kinds of tests will you do?
- What will these tests tell you about my cancer?
- What are my treatment options?
- How will my treatment affect my daily life?
- Since chordoma is a rare tumor, how much experience do you have with it?
- Are there hospitals that specialize in the treatment of chordoma where I might receive treatment unavailable here?

fatigue, and **nausea and vomiting**. Bladder control and sexual function may be impaired after surgery on sacral chordomas. Mental functions may be impaired because of inoperable chordomas near the brain.

Discovering one has cancer is a traumatic event. Not only is one's health affected, one's whole life suddenly revolves around trips to the doctor for cancer treatment and adjusting to the side effects of these treatments. As this is a stressful time for both the cancer patient and family members, support groups and psychological counseling may be helpful. Many national organizations that support cancer education can provide information either in person or through on-line support and education groups.

Clinical trials

Chordoma is a rare tumor. In 2001, there were no **clinical trials** related to its diagnosis or treatment. However, the selection of clinical trials underway changes frequently. Current information on what clinical trials are available and where they are being held can be found by entering the search term "chordoma" at the following websites:

- National Cancer Institute <http://cancertrials.nci.nih.gov> or (800) 4-CANCER.
- National Institutes of Health Clinical Trials <http://clinicaltrials.gov>.
- Center Watch: A Clinical Trials Listing <http://www.centerwatch.com>.

Prevention

There is no way to prevent chordoma. There appear to be no environmental factors that affect the development of this tumor.

Resources

ORGANIZATIONS

American Brain Tumor Association. 2720 River Road, Des Plaines, IL 60018. (847) 827-9910. Patient line (800) 886-2282. <http://www.abta.org>.

Tish Davidson, A.M.

Choriocarcinoma *see* **Gestational trophoblastic tumors**

Choroid plexus tumors

Definition

Choroid plexus tumors (CPTs) are rare abnormal growths on a part of the brain called the choroid plexus. The choroid plexus is the structure in the brain that produces the cerebrospinal fluid that coats the brain and spinal cord.

Description

There are two types of CPT: choroid plexus papilloma (CPP) and choroid plexus **carcinoma** (CPC). CPPs account for the majority of all CPTs.

A CPP is a benign, slow-growing, wart-like tumor that tends to grow on the surface of the choroid plexus. CPPs can spread by growing and by multiplying, just like warts, but they do not spread (metastasize) to organs that are not directly attached to the brain. A CPC is a malignant slow-growing tumor that tends to invade healthy brain tissue. CPCs can metastasize to distant parts of the body.

A primary brain tumor is a tumor that begins in the brain, as opposed to a secondary (or metastatic) brain tumor, which begins in another organ and metastasized to the brain. CPPs make up approximately 1% of primary brain tumors in adults and 3% of primary brain tumors in children.

Demographics

CPTs occur in approximately two of every one million people. CPTs can occur in people of any age, but greater than 70% of all CPTs occur in children younger than two years of age. When CPPs occur in children, they tend to be located in the uppermost portion of the spinal fluid pathway (the lateral ventricles). When they occur in adults, they tend to be located in the lower portion of the spinal fluid pathway in the brain (the fourth ventricle).

CPCs occur almost exclusively in children, most under the age of two years, and are almost always located in the lateral ventricles.

CPTs occur with equal frequency in members of all races and ethnic groups. There does not appear to be any relationship of CPTs to any geographic region. Males and females are affected in equal numbers by CPTs.

Causes and symptoms

The cause, or causes, of CPTs are not known. In early 2001, ongoing investigations attempted to determine if environmental factors, genetic factors, viruses, or other factors caused primary brain tumors. Primary brain tumors are not contagious.

The symptoms of CPTs are the result of increased pressure in the fluid within the skull (intracranial hypertension). These symptoms include:

- nausea
- vomiting
- irritability
- headache
- vision disturbances
- enlargement of the head
- seizures

CPCs may also be accompanied by:

- bleeding (hemorrhage) at the site of the tumor
- weakness or paralysis on the side of the body opposite to the side of the brain where the tumor is located.

Diagnosis

The diagnosis of CPTs begins in the doctor's office. After taking a complete medical history, the doctor will perform a basic neurological examination. This examination involves:

- testing eye reflexes, eye movement, and pupil reactions
- testing hearing with a tuning fork or ticking watch
- reflex tests with a rubber hammer
- balance and coordination tests
- pin-prick and cotton ball tests for sense of touch
- sense of smell tests with various odors
- facial muscle tests: smiling, frowning, etc.
- tongue movement and gag reflex tests
- head movement tests
- mental status tests: asking what year it is, who the president is, etc.
- abstract thinking tests: asking for the meaning of a common saying, such as "every cloud has a silver lining."
- memory tests: asking to have a list of objects repeated, asking for details of what a patient ate for dinner last night, etc.

If the doctor suspects a brain tumor may be present, further diagnostic tests will be ordered. These tests are performed by a neurological specialist. Imaging tests that may be ordered include:

- **computed tomography** (CT scan)
- **magnetic resonance imaging** (MRI)

Other tests may include:

- a **lumbar puncture**, or spinal tap, to examine the cerebrospinal fluid
- an electroencephalogram (EEG), which measures the electrical activity of the brain

Treatment team

Treatment of any primary brain tumor, including the CPTs, is different from treating tumors in other parts of the body. Brain surgery requires much more precision than most other surgeries. Also, many medicinal drugs cannot cross the blood-brain barrier. Therefore, the therapies that are used to treat CPTs, and the side effects of these therapies, are quite complex.

The most up-to-date treatment opportunities are available from experienced, multidisciplinary medical professional teams made up of doctors, nurses, and technologists

KEY TERMS

Choroid plexus—Tissues of the brain that produce the fluid that coats the brain and spinal cord.

Choroid plexus carcinoma (CPC)—A malignant tumor of the choroid plexus that often invades the underlying brain tissues and can spread to other parts of the body.

Choroid plexus papilloma (CPP)—A benign tumor of the choroid plexus that does not invade the underlying brain tissues and does not spread to other parts of the body.

Intracranial hypertension—A higher than normal pressure of the fluid in the skull.

Spinal fluid shunt—A small tube that is surgically implanted to allow excess spinal fluid to drain directly into the abdominal cavity.

QUESTIONS TO ASK THE DOCTOR

- Which type of CPT do I have?
- Is my tumor operable?
- What is the likelihood of my type of CPT coming back?
- How often should I seek follow-up examinations?

who specialize in cancer (oncology), neurology, medical imaging, drug or **radiation therapy**, and anesthesiology.

Clinical staging, treatments, and prognosis

CPTs and other primary brain tumors are diagnosed, or staged, in grades of severity from I to IV. Grade I tumors have cells that are not malignant and are nearly normal in appearance. Grade II tumors have cells that appear to be slightly abnormal. Grade III tumors have cells that are malignant and clearly abnormal. Grade IV, the most severe type of brain tumor, contains fast-spreading and abnormal cells. The standard treatment for all grades of CPTs is surgery to completely remove the tumor or tumors. This surgery is generally aided by an image guidance system that allows the surgeon to determine the most efficient route to take to the location of the tumor.

Approximately one-half of CPT patients gain relief of the increased intracranial pressure after complete removal of their tumors. The other half require a spinal fluid shunt to allow drainage of the excess fluid.

In some instances of CPC, the tumor is inoperable. Patients with inoperable CPCs are generally treated with radiation therapies. CPPs are highly resistant to radiation treatment, so these therapies are not used for CPPs.

As of 1999, 8.6% of patients who had surgery to remove CPTs died within five years of the surgery. One-half of these patients (4.3%) died during the surgery itself.

Alternative and complementary therapies

There are no effective alternative treatments for CPTs other than surgery and radiation therapies in the case of inoperable CPCs.

Coping with cancer treatment

Most patients who undergo brain surgery to remove their tumors can resume their normal activities within a few days of the operation.

Clinical trials

There were 19 **clinical trials** underway in early 2001 aimed at the treatment of CPTs. More information on these trials, including contact information, may be found by conducting a clinical trial search at the Web site of the National Cancer Institute, CancerNet (http://cancernet.nci.nih.gov/trialsrch.shtml).

Prevention

Because the causes of CPTs are not known, there are no known preventions.

Special concerns

Repeat surgery may be necessary for CPTs because these tumors sometimes redevelop. Careful monitoring by the medical team will be required.

Resources

BOOKS

Scott, R. Michael, and John Knighty. "Choroid Plexus Papilloma." In *Brain Tumors: An Encyclopedic Approach*, edited by Andreeo H. Kaye. New York: Churchill Livingstone, 1995, pp.505-524.

ORGANIZATIONS

National Brain Tumor Foundation. 785 Market Street, Suite 1600, San Francisco, CA 94103. Telephone (415)284-0208. <http://www.braintumor.org>

The Brain Tumor Society. 124 Watertown Street, Suite 3-H. Watertown, MA 02472. Telephone (617)924-9997. Fax (617)924-9998. <http://www.tbts.org>.

OTHER

Tavares, Marcio P.*Choroid Plexus Tumors—MEDSTUDENTS—Neurosurgery.* (25 March 2001) 1 July 2001 <http://www.medstudents.com.br/neuroc/neuroc5.htm>

Paul A. Johnson, Ed.M.

Chromic phosphate P32 *see* **Radiopharmaceuticals**

Chromosome rearrangements

Definition

A chromosome rearrangement is a structural change in a chromosome such as a deletion, translocation, inversion, or gene amplification. Chromosome rearrangements can contribute to the transformation of a normal cell into a cancerous cell and are therefore found in many cancer cells.

Description

Chromosomes and genes

A chromosome is a microscopic structure which is composed of proteins and DNA and is found in every cell of the body. Each cell of the body, except for the egg and the sperm cells, contains 23 pairs of chromosomes and 46 chromosomes in total. All cells of the body except for the egg and sperm cells are called the somatic cells. The egg and sperm cells each contain 23 chromosomes. Both males and females have 22 pairs of chromosomes, called the autosomes, that are numbered one to twenty-two in order of decreasing size. The final pair of chromosomes, called the sex chromosomes, determine the sex of the individual. Women possess two identical chromosomes called the X chromosomes while men possess one X chromosome and one Y chromosome.

Each type of chromosome contains different genes that are found at specific locations along the chromosome. Men and women possess two of each type of autosomal gene since they inherit one of each type from each parent. Each gene contains the instructions for the production of a particular protein. The proteins produced by genes have many functions and work together to create the traits of the human body, such as hair and eye color, and are involved in controlling the body's basic functions. Some genes produce proteins that are involved in controlling the growth cycle of the cell and are therefore involved in preventing the development of cancer.

Types of chromosome rearrangements

Sometimes a spontaneous break or breaks occur in a chromosome or chromosomes in a particular cell and can result in a deletion, inversion, or translocation. If the break or breaks result in the loss of a piece of chromosome, it is called a deletion. An inversion results when a segment of chromosome breaks off, is reversed (inverted), and is reinserted into its original location. When a piece of one chromosome is exchanged with a piece from another chromosome it is called a translocation.

Sometimes a small segment of chromosome is amplified, which results in the presence of multiple copies of that section of the chromosome. In most cases the segment of the chromosome that is duplicated contains only one gene, although it is possible for more than one gene to be amplified. Sometimes amplified genes form a separate and unique chromosome and sometimes they are located within an otherwise normal chromosome.

KEY TERMS

Chromosome—A microscopic structure, made of a complex of proteins and DNA, that is found within each cell of the body.

Deletion—A piece missing from a chromosome.

Gene—A building block of inheritance, made up of a compound called DNA (deoxyribonucleic acid) and containing the instructions for the production of a particular protein. Each gene is found on a specific location on a chromosome.

Gene amplification—When multiple copies of a small segment of chromosome containing one or more genes are present as a separate chromosome or as part of an otherwise normal chromosome.

Inversion—A piece of a chromosome that was removed from the chromosome, inverted, and reinserted into the same location on the chromosome.

Leukemia—Cancer of the blood-forming organs which results in an overproduction of white blood cells.

Lymphoma—Cancer involving cells of the immune system.

Oncogene—A changed proto-oncogene that promotes uncontrolled cell division and growth.

Protein—A substance produced by a gene that is involved in creating the traits of the human body such as hair and eye color or is involved in controlling the basic functions of the human body.

Proto-oncogene—A gene involved in stimulating the normal growth and division of cells in a controlled manner.

Somatic cells—All the cells of the body except for the egg and sperm cells.

Translocation—An exchange of a piece of one chromosome with a piece from another chromosome.

Tumor-suppressor gene—Gene involved in controlling normal cell growth and preventing cancer.

Chromosome rearrangements and cancer

A chromosome rearrangement can delete or disrupt the functioning of genes that are located on the chromo-

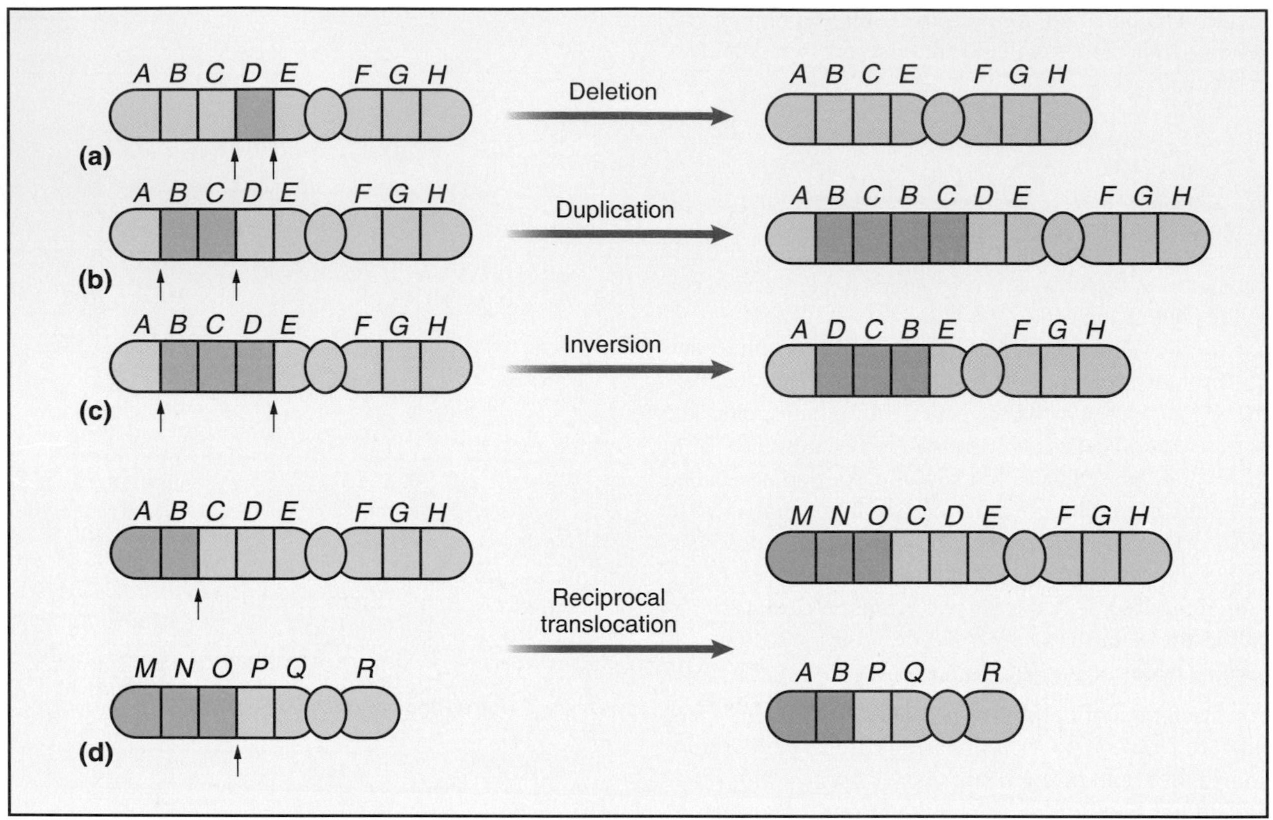

Four kinds of chromosome rearrangements. Arrows indicate where chromosomes break, and dark green indicates the genes affected. (a) A deletion removes a chromosome segment. (b) Duplication repeats a segment. (c) Inversion reverses the order of a segment. (d) A translocation moves a segment from one chromosome to another. Each chromosome contains genes found at specific locations along the chromosome, and each gene contains the instructions for the production of a protein. If a gene produces proteins involved in controlling the cell's growth cycle, and this gene is affected by a chromosome rearrangement, uncontrolled cell growth (cancer) could result. *(Illustration by Argosy Publishing.)*

somal pieces involved. Chromosome rearrangements that delete or disrupt genes that regulate the cell cycle can contribute to the transformation of a normal cell into a cancerous cell. That is why chromosomal rearrangements are found in many cancers.

THE TRANSFORMATION OF A NORMAL CELL INTO A CANCEROUS CELL. The process by which a normal cell is transformed into a cancerous cell is a complex, multistep process involving a breakdown in the normal cell cycle. Normally a somatic cell goes through a growth cycle during which it produces new cells. The process of cell division is necessary for the growth of tissues and organs of the body and for the replacement of damaged cells.

Cell division is tightly regulated by genes. Normal cells have a limited lifespan and only go through the cell cycle a certain number of times. Genes regulate the cell cycle by producing regulatory proteins. Different types of regulatory proteins regulate cell growth and division in different types of cells. For example, a skin cell may be regulated by a different combination of proteins than a breast cell or a liver cell.

A cell that loses control of its cell cycle and replicates out of control is called a cancer cell. Cancer cells undergo many cell divisions, often at a quicker rate than normal cells, and do not have a limited lifespan. They also have loss of apoptosis, or cell death, which is characteristic of a normal cell. This allows them to eventually overwhelm the body with a large number of abnormal cells and hurt the functioning of the normal cells.

A cell becomes cancerous only after changes or deletions occur in a number of genes that are involved in the regulation of its cell cycle. However, a change or deletion of one regulatory gene can result in the change or deletion of other regulatory genes.

Proto-oncogenes and tumor-suppressor genes are the two most common types of genes involved in regulating the cell cycle. We inherit two of each type of proto-oncogene and two of each type of tumor-suppressor gene. Tumor-suppressor genes produce proteins that are involved in helping to prevent uncontrolled cell growth and division. Only one normal copy of a tumor-suppressor gene needs to be present to maintain its normal role in the regulation of the cell cycle. If both copies of a tumor-suppressor gene are changed, however, then not enough normal tumor-suppressor protein will be produced and the cell is more likely to become cancerous.

Proto-oncogenes produce proteins that are largely involved in stimulating the growth and division of cells in a controlled manner. A change in a proto-oncogene can convert it into an oncogene. An oncogene produces an abnormal protein, which is involved in stimulating uncontrolled cell growth. Only one proto-oncogene of a pair needs to be changed into an oncogene for it to promote the transformation of a normal cell into a cancerous cell.

A chromosome rearrangement involving a tumor-suppressor gene or proto-oncogene can contribute to the transformation of a normal cell into a cancerous cell. Certain types of chromosome rearrangements are found more commonly in cancers of certain types of cells. This is because these chromosome rearrangements involve genes that regulate the cell cycle in those specific cells. More than one chromosome rearrangement is usually present in a particular cancer cell since it is necessary for more than one regulatory gene to be altered during the transformation of a normal cell into a cancerous cell. Different types of chromosome rearrangements contribute to the formation of cancer cells in different ways. Researchers don't always know how a chromosome rearrangement contributes to the development of cancer.

How specific types of rearrangements contribute to the development of cancer

Deletions

A deletion of a piece of chromosome that contains a tumor suppressor gene can contribute to the transformation of a normal cell into a cancerous cell. If both copies of a tumor suppressor gene are deleted or changed then little or no tumor suppressor protein is produced. This in turn can impact the regulation of the cell cycle and contribute to the transformation of the normal cell.

A deletion of a segment of chromosome 13, for example, can result in the loss of a tumor-suppressor gene that helps to prevent an eye cancer called

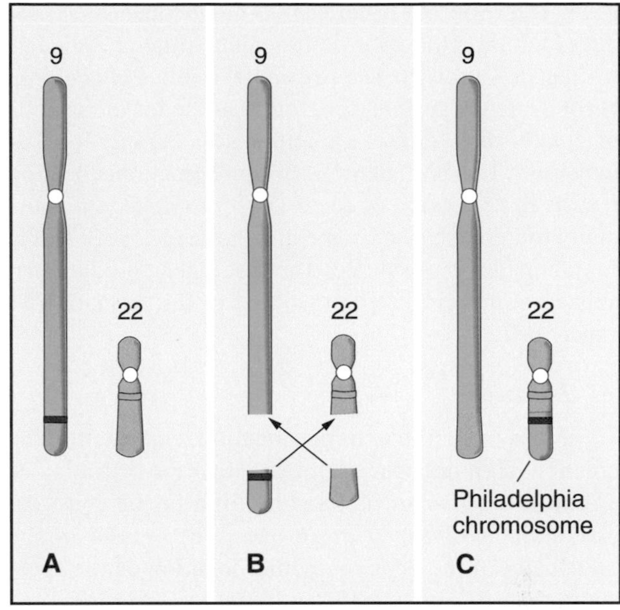

A. Normal chromosomes. B. Breakage occurs near a proto-oncogene on chromosome 9. C. Translocation chromosomes. This translocation, called the Philadelphia chromosome, can result in chronic myelocytic leukemia. *(Illustration by Argosy Publishing.)*

retinoblastoma. If both retinoblastoma tumor-suppressor genes are deleted or changed in one of the cells of the eye then that cell can become cancerous.

Translocations

A translocation involving a proto-oncogene can result in its conversion into an oncogene which can contribute to the development of cancer. A translocation involving a proto-oncogene results in the transfer of the proto-oncogene from its normal location on a chromosome to a different location on another chromosome. Sometimes this results in the transfer of a proto-oncogene next to an activating gene. This activating gene abnormally activates the proto-oncogene and converts it into an oncogene. When this oncogene is present in a cell, it contributes to uncontrolled cell growth and the development of cancer.

For example, the translocation of the c-myc proto-oncogene from its normal location on chromosome eight to a location on chromosome 14 results in the abnormal activation of c-myc. This type of translocation is involved in the development of a type of cancer called **Burkitt's lymphoma**. The translocated c-myc proto-oncogene is found in the cancer cells of approximately 85% of people with Burkitt's lymphoma.

A translocation involving a proto-oncogene can also result in the fusion of the proto-oncogene with another gene. The resulting fused gene is an oncogene that produces an unregulated protein which stimulates uncontrolled cell growth. One example is the Philadelphia chromosome translocation, found in the leukemia cells of greater than 95% of patients with a chronic form of leukemia. The Philadelphia chromosome translocation results in the fusion of the c-abl proto-oncogene, normally found on chromosome nine, to the bcr gene that is found on chromosome 22. The fused gene produces an abnormal protein that is involved in the formation of cancer cells.

Inversions

An inversion, like a translocation, can result in the creation of an oncogene through either the activation of a proto-oncogene or the creation of a fusion gene. An inversion involving a proto-oncogene results in the movement of the gene to another location on the same chromosome. For example, an inversion of chromosome ten can move a proto-oncogene called RET and cause it to fuse with a gene called ELEI or a gene called H4. The fusion of RET with either of these genes creates an oncogene. When the RET oncogene is present in a thyroid cell it promotes the transformation of that cell into a cancerous cell.

Gene amplification

Gene amplification can also contribute to the development of cancer. Amplification of a segment of chromosome that contains a proto-oncogene can result in the formation of many copies of a proto-oncogene. Each copy of the proto-oncogene produces protein that is involved in stimulating cell growth. This can result in a significant increase in the amount of protein produced, which can promote uncontrolled cell growth. Multiple copies of proto-oncogenes are found in many tumors.

See Also Cancer genetics

Resources

BOOKS

Vogelstein, Bert and Kenneth Kinzler, eds. *The Genetic Basis of Human Cancer* New York, NY: McGraw-Hill, 1998.

OTHER

"Chromosome Rearrangements" *University of Wisconsin–Madison Department of Genetics* 3 July 2001 <http://www1.genetics.wisc.edu/466/Fall98/lect08/index.html>.

"The Genetics of Cancer—an Overview" *Robert H. Lurie Comprehensive Cancer Center of Northwestern University*. 17 Feb. 1999. 29 June 2001 <http://www.cancergenetics.org/gncavrvu.htm>.

Lisa Andres, M.S., CGC

Chronic leukemia

Definition

A slowly progressing cancer that starts in blood-forming cells of the bone marrow. Leukemias are the result of an abnormal development of leukocytes (white blood cells) and their precursors. Leukemia cells look different than normal cells and do not function properly.

Description

There are four main types of leukemia, which can be further divided into subtypes. When classifying the type of leukemia, the first steps are to determine whether the cancer is lymphocytic or myelogenous (cancer can occur in either the lymphoid or myeloid white blood cells) and whether it is acute or chronic (rapidly or slowly progressing).

Chronic leukemia cells live much longer than normal white blood cells, resulting in an accumulation of too many mature granulocytes or lymphocytes. Chronic leukemia progresses slowly but can develop into an acute form. Major types include **chronic lymphocytic leukemia** (CLL) and **chronic myelocytic leukemia** (CML).

Kate Kretschmann

Chronic lymphocytic leukemia

Definition

Chronic lymphocytic leukemia (CLL) is a cancer of white blood cells. In CLL, mature white blood cells of certain types called lymphocytes function abnormally and cause disease.

Description

Chronic leukemia is a cancer that starts in the blood cells made in the bone marrow. The bone marrow is the spongy tissue found in the large bones of the body. The bone marrow makes precursor cells called "blasts" or "stem cells" that mature into different types of blood cells. Unlike acute leukemias, in which the process of maturation of the blast cells is interrupted, in chronic leukemias, most of the cells do mature and only a few remain as immature cells. However, even though the cells appear normal, they do not function as normal cells.

The different types of cells produced in the bone marrow are red blood cells (RBCs), which carry oxygen and other materials to all tissues of the body, and white blood cells (WBCs), which fight infection. Platelets play a part in the clotting of the blood. The white blood cells can be further subdivided into three main types: the granulocytes, monocytes, and the lymphocytes.

The granulocytes, as their name suggests, contain granules (particles). These granules contain special proteins (enzymes) and several other substances that can break down chemicals and destroy microorganisms such as bacteria. Monocytes are the second type of white blood cell. They also are important in defending the body against pathogens.

The lymphocytes form the third type of white blood cell. There are two main types of lymphocytes: T lymphocytes and B lymphocytes. They have different functions within the immune system. The B cells protect the body by making "antibodies." Antibodies are proteins that can attach to the surfaces of bacteria and viruses. The occurrence of this attachment sends signals to many other cell types to travel through the blood and destroy the antibody-coated organism. The T cell protects the body against viruses. When a virus enters a cell, it produces certain proteins that are projected onto the surface of the infected cell. T cells recognize these proteins and produce certain chemicals (cytokines) capable of destroying the virus-infected cells. In addition, T cells destroy some types of cancer cells.

Chronic leukemias develop very gradually. The abnormal lymphocytes multiply slowly, and in a poorly regulated manner. These lymphocytes live much longer than normal lymphocytes and, thus, their numbers build up in the body. In CLL, lymphocytes accumulate. The enlarged lymphocyte population congregates in the blood, bone marrow, lymph nodes, spleen, and liver. The two types of chronic leukemias can be easily distinguished under the microscope. Chronic lymphocytic leukemia (CLL) involves the T or B lymphocytes. B-cell abnormalities are more common than T-cell abnormalities. T cells are affected in only 5% of the patients.

Demographics

Ninety percent of CLL cases are seen in people who are 50 years or older, with the average age at diagnosis being 65. Rarely is CLL diagnosed in a patient who is less than 35 years of age. The incidence of the disease increases with age. It is almost never seen in children. According to the estimates of the American Cancer Society (ACS), approximately 8,100 new cases of CLL were diagnosed in 2000, 4,600 in men and 3,500 in women.

CLL affects both sexes. Among patients younger than 65, the disease is slightly more common in men.

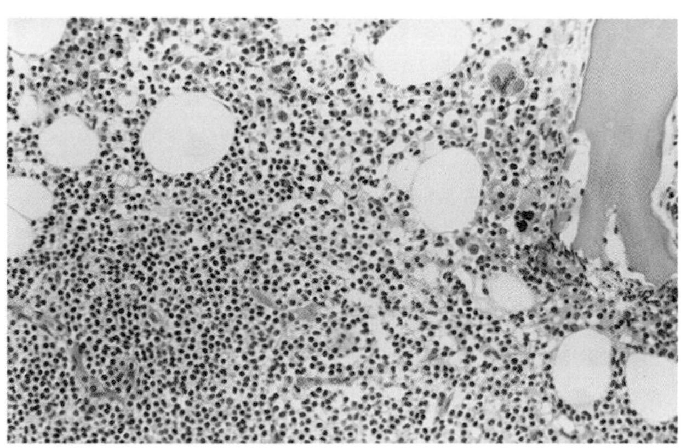

Bone marrow in chronic lymphocytic leukemia. In this disease, bone marrow is replaced by small, mature lymphoid cells. *(© Biophoto Associates, Science Source/Photo Researchers, Inc. Reproduced by permission.)*

However, among patients older than 75 years of age, CLL appears almost equally in men and women. Within the United States, CLL affects African-Americans as frequently as it does Caucasians. However, CLL appears more frequently among Americans than among people living in Asia, Latin America, and Africa.

In the United States and Europe, CLL accounts for more than one-quarter of all diagnosed leukemias. Over the past 50 years, the rate at which CLL has been appearing has increased significantly. However, many doctors think that this increase is not necessarily due to the disease actually being more common than in the past, but instead due to the fact that the disease is now more likely to be diagnosed when it does appear. Fifty years ago, only one out of ten CLL patients was diagnosed during the early stages of the disease. Now, half of all CLL patients are diagnosed during this early stage.

Causes and symptoms

The cause of CLL is unknown. It is certain, however, that CLL is linked to genetic abnormalities and environmental factors. For example, close family members of patients with CLL are twice as likely to seven times as likely to be diagnosed with CLL as people in the general population. For another example, exposure to certain chemicals used in farming and other agricultural occupations may increase the risk that a person will develop CLL. In contrast, CLL is not associated with exposure to radiation known to cause other cancers. As of 2001, doctors were unsure whether people who have had certain virus infections are more likely to develop CLL than are people in the general population. If there does turn out to be such an association, it would not be with all viruses but with two human retroviruses (HTLV-I and HTLV-II) or with **Epstein-Barr virus** (EBV).

The symptoms of CLL are generally vague and nonspecific. One out of five patients with CLL has no symptoms at all, and the disease is discovered only through a routine blood test. A patient may experience all or some of the following symptoms:

- chronic **fatigue**
- weakness
- a general feeling of malaise or of things being not quite right
- swollen lymph nodes
- an enlarged spleen, which could make the patient complain of abdominal fullness
- a general feeling of ill health
- **fever**
- frequent bacterial or viral infections.
- unusually severe response to insect bites
- **night sweats**
- **weight loss** not due to dieting or exercise

Diagnosis

There is no **screening test** for CLL. If the doctor has reason to suspect leukemia, he or she will conduct a very thorough physical examination to look for enlarged lymph nodes in the neck, underarm, and pelvic region. In addition, the doctor will look to see whether the liver and spleen are enlarged. Urine and blood tests may be ordered to check for microscopic amounts of blood in the urine and to obtain a complete differential blood count. This count will give the numbers and percentages of the different cells found in the blood. An abnormal blood test might suggest leukemia. Some authorities state that CLL may be diagnosed if the number of lymphocytes in the blood exceeds a certain level.

The doctor may perform a **bone marrow aspiration and biopsy** to confirm the diagnosis of leukemia. During the bone marrow biopsy, a cylindrical piece of bone and marrow is removed. The tissue is generally taken out of the hipbone. These samples are sent to the laboratory for examination. In many CLL patients, more than one-fourth of the bone marrow is made up of mature lymphocytes. In addition to diagnosis, bone marrow biopsy is also conducted during the treatment phase of the disease to see if the leukemia is responding to therapy.

Some CLL patients have a condition called hypogammaglobulinemia. Immunoglobulins are normal parts of the body's immune system, the system used to fight off infection. Patients with hypogammaglobulinemia have very low levels of all of the various types of immunoglobulins.

The doctor may also conduct immunophenotyping. This involves taking a sample of the blood and looking at what types of cells of the immune system are being affected by the CLL. Approximately 19 out of 20 CLL patients have the B-cell type of CLL. Far more rare is the T-cell type of CLL. In addition, the doctor may look for abnormalities in the chromosomes of the affected cells. Chromosomes are a unit of genetic material within cells. Patients exhibiting no chromosomal abnormalities have a better prognosis than those who do have such abnormalities. If the abnormalities become more complex over time, the patient's prognosis may worsen.

Standard imaging tests such as x rays, **computed tomography** scans (CT scans), and **magnetic resonance imaging** (MRI) may be used to check whether the leukemic cells have invaded other organs of the body, such as the bones, chest, kidneys, abdomen, or brain.

Clinical staging, treatments, and prognosis

Staging

Usually one of two systems are used to stage CLL. One of these is the Binet system and the other the Rai system. According to the Rai system, patients at low risk have no enlargement of lymph nodes, spleen or liver. The occurrence of these marks entry into the intermediate stage, according to Rai. High risk patients have, in addition, **anemia** and a significant decrease in the number of blood platelets in their blood. Blood platelets help blood to clot. According to the Binet system, a patient's stage depends upon how much hemoglobin (part of red blood cells that carry oxygen) and how many platelets are in the blood, as well as how many other areas the disease has affected. According to both systems, patients at low risk usually survive more than ten years. Patients at intermediate risk usually survive about six years. Patients at high risk usually survive about 2 years. Other factors with important implications for prognosis include the pattern at which bone marrow is being affected by the CLL and the amount of time it takes for the number of lymphocytes to double.

Treatment

Because the long-term prognosis for many patients with CLL is excellent, many patients receive no treatment at all at first. Many patients go for years before developing aggressive disease that requires treatment. Treatment for early stage CLL should be started only when one of the following conditions appears:

- Symptoms of the disease are growing worse, for example, there is a greater degree of fever, weight loss, night sweats, and so forth.

- The spleen is enlarging or enlargement of the spleen has become painful.
- Disease of the lymph nodes has become more severe.
- The condition of the bone marrow has deteriorated and there is anemia and a marked reduction in the number of blood platelets.
- There is anemia or reduction in the number of blood platelets for reasons not specifically related to the condition of the bone marrow.
- The population of lymphocytes is rapidly growing.
- The patient is experiencing numerous infections caused by bacteria.

Therapy for CLL usually starts with **chemotherapy**. Depending on the stage of the disease, single or multiple drugs may be given. Drugs commonly prescribed include **fludarabine**, **cladribine**, **chlorambucil** and **cyclophosphamide**. Studies have also provided evidence that a combination of fludarabine and cyclophosphamide is effective. However, this combination has not yet been evaluated over periods of ten years or more. Another combination now being studied involves fludarabine and **mitoxantrone** (Novantrone). Yet another involves fludarabine and anthracyclines. Low-dose **radiation therapy** may be given to the whole body, or it may be used to alleviate the symptoms and discomfort due to an enlarged spleen and lymph nodes. The spleen may be removed in a procedure called a **splenectomy**.

Bone marrow transplantation (BMT) has produced some positive outcomes in patients with CLL, although it has not been the subject of sufficient systematic study to permit doctors to know how effective it is. In BMT, the patient's diseased bone marrow is replaced with healthy marrow. There are two ways of performing a bone marrow transplant. In an allogeneic bone marrow transplant, healthy marrow is taken from another person (donor) whose tissue is either the same or very closely resembles the patient's tissues. The donor may be a twin, a sibling, or a person who is not related at all. First, the patient's bone marrow is destroyed with very high doses of chemotherapy and radiation therapy. To replace the destroyed marrow, healthy marrow from the donor is given to the patient through a needle in the vein.

In the second type of bone marrow transplant, called an autologous bone marrow transplant, some of the patient's own marrow is taken out and treated with a combination of anticancer drugs to kill all the abnormal cells. This marrow is then frozen to save it. The marrow remaining in the patient's body is then destroyed with high-dose chemotherapy and radiation therapy. Following that, the patient's own frozen marrow is thawed and given back to the patient through a needle in the vein. The use of this mode of bone marrow transplant for the treatment of CLL is currently being investigated in **clinical trials**.

KEY TERMS

Antibodies—Proteins made by the B lymphocytes in response to the presence of infectious agents, such as bacteria or viruses, in the body.

Biopsy—The surgical removal and microscopic examination of living tissue for diagnostic purposes.

Chemotherapy—Treatment with drugs that act against cancer.

Chromosome —Part of the cell that carries genetic material.

Cytokines—Chemicals made by the cells that act on other cells to stimulate or inhibit their function. Cytokines that stimulate growth are called "growth factors."

Immunotherapy—Treatment of cancer by stimulating the body's immune defense system.

Maturation—The process by which stem cells transform from immature cells without a specific function into a particular type of blood cell with defined functions.

Radiation therapy—Treatment using high-energy radiation from x-ray machines, cobalt, radium, or other sources.

Remission—A disappearance of a disease as a result of treatment. Complete remission means that all disease is gone. Partial remission means that the disease is significantly improved by treatment, but residual traces of the disease are still present.

Allogeneic BMT has been successfully used with younger patients with CLL who have not responded positively to chemotherapy. Autologous BMT has produced some positive results in older CLL patients. However, BMT is generally not considered an option in treating most patients with CLL because they are too old to be considered good candidates for the procedure.

Other CLL therapies that are being investigated include monoclonal antibody-targeted therapy and **interferons**. **Monoclonal antibodies** (MoAbs) are laboratory-manufactured chemicals that closely resemble parts of the body's natural immune system. Studies of MoAbs-targeted therapies have shown some positive results in CLL, although definitive studies have not been performed at the time of this writing in 2001. Interferon is a chemical normally made in the cells of the body. It helps protect the body against viruses and also seems to have some effect against certain cancers. The interferon used as medicine is a laboratory-manufactured copy of the interferon produced by the body. As of this writing in 2001, interferon therapy has produced some response in CLL patients. However, interferon therapy has not as yet been shown to be associated with prolongation of remission.

Radiation therapy is very effective for approximately one in three of those CLL patients for whom it is considered appropriate.

Because leukemia cells can spread to all the organs via the blood stream and the lymph vessels, surgery is not considered an option for treating leukemias.

Treatment of CLL and its complications

During therapy for CLL, complications frequently appear. Many patients develop infectious illnesses. Sometimes, two or more infectious diseases attack a patient at the same time. These infections should be treated with great care. Most people whose death has been directly attributed to CLL have actually died from bacterial infections. The patient should be involved in identifying symptoms of infection and reporting these to the doctor without delay. Doing so may save the patient's life.

Many patients develop anemia, which is treated with the drug prednisone. Patients who do not respond to prednisone therapy may have their spleen removed and may receive therapy with immunoglobulin, a component of the blood.

Treatment after transformation of CLL

Between three and ten out of every hundred patients with CLL experiences transformation of the disease into large-cell lymphoma (LCL). When this happens it is called Richter's transformation. Its occurrence is often marked by fever, weight loss, and night sweats. Treatments for LCL are being studied, although outcomes have not been very good. Very infrequently, CLL may transform into another disease, called prolymphocytic leukemia. Attempts to develop adequate therapies for this disease are ongoing.

Prognosis

For many CLL patients, the prognosis is excellent. Using the Binet and Rai staging systems, patients at low risk usually survive more than ten years. Patients at intermediate risk usually survive about six years. Patients at high risk usually survive about two years. The average patient survives approximately nine years following diagnosis. Factors with important implications for prognosis that are not included in the Binet or Rai systems are the pattern at which bone marrow is being affected by the CLL and the amount of time it takes for the number of lymphocytes in the blood to double. It is uncertain whether BMT may prolong the lifespan of CLL patients. Many of the chemotherapy agents used to treat disease do effectively control the leukemia and its effects but, as yet, the more established chemotherapy agents have not been shown to increase the life span of patients.

Coping with cancer treatment

Since many CLL patients die from infection, it is essential that patient be very alert to the signs of infection. If patients perform this role and seek medical attention as soon as symptoms of infection appear, then treatment can be started early. This may save a life.

It is very difficult for some patients to be not only informed that they have leukemia but then to also be told that they do not need treatment. This may be very confusing, unless the patient realizes that treatment may be necessary at some future time and that starting therapies too soon may be counterproductive.

Because nutritional alteration, weight loss, and psychosocial problems may accompany CLL, it may be prudent for patients to consult with a registered dietitian.

Cancer patients need supportive care to help them come through the treatment period with physical and emotional strength in tact. Many patients experience feelings of **depression**, anxiety, and fatigue, and many experience **nausea and vomiting** during treatment. Studies have shown that these can be managed effectively if discussed with the attending physician.

Prevention

Although some cancers are related to known risk factors, such as smoking, in leukemias, there are no known risk factors. Therefore, at the present time, there is no way known to prevent the leukemias from developing. Everyone should undergo periodic medical checkups.

Resources

BOOKS

Braunwald, Eugene, et al. *Harrison's Principles of Internal Medicine* 15th ed. New York: McGraw-Hill, 2001.

deWitt, Susan C. *Essentials of Medical-Surgical Nursing* 4th ed. Philadelphia: W. B. Saunders, 1998.

Herfindal, Eric T., Dick R. Gourley. *Textbook of Therapeutics: Drug and Disease Management,* 7th ed. Philadelphia: Lippincott Williams & Wilkins, 2000.

Humes, H. David, et al.*Kelley's Textbook of Internal Medicine* 4th ed. Philadelphia: Lippincott Williams & Wilkins, 2000.

Pazdur, Richard, et al. *Cancer Management: A Multidisciplinary Approach: Medical, Surgical, & Radiation Oncology* 4th ed. Melville, NY: PRR, 2000.

Souhami, Robert, Jeffrey Tobias. *Cancer and Its Management* 3rd ed. London: Blackwell Science, 1998.

PERIODICALS

Mauro, F. R., et al. "Clinical characteristics and outcome of young chronic lymphocytic leukemia patients: A single institution study of 204 cases." *Blood* 1999; 94: 448-454.

ORGANIZATIONS

The National Cancer Institute publishes useful texts available through the internet or by mail, and answers questions by telephone. Some titles include: *What You Need to Know about Leukemia*, and *PDQ - Treatment - Patients: Chronic Lymphocytic Leukemia.* Call 1-800-4CANCER or visit on the Internet at <www.nci.nih.gov/>.

The American Cancer Society publishes useful texts, such as *Adult Chronic Leukemia - Overview,Leukemia - Adult Chronic: Treatment,Leukemia - Adult Chronic: Detection and Symptoms,Leukemia: Adult Chronic FAQ [Frequently Asked Questions],* and *Leukemia - Adult Chronic: Prevention & Risk.* Call 1-800-ACS-2345 or on the Internet at <www.cancer.org/>

The Leukemia & Lymphoma Society (Formerly Leukemia Society of America) publishes useful texts available through the Internet or by mail, including *Chronic Lymphocytic Leukemia (CLL),Making Intelligent Choices About Therapy,Understanding Blood Counts,Patient Aid Program,Family Support Group,* and *Information Resource Center.* Call 1-800-955-4572 or visit on the Internet at <www.leukemia-lymphoma.org/>.

National Coalition for Cancer Survivorship. 1010 Wayne Avenue, 7th Floor, Silver Spring, MD 20910-5600. Telephone: (301) 650-9127 and (877) NCCS-YES [877-622-7937). Web site: <www.cansearch.org>.

Lata Cherath, Ph.D.
Bob Kirsch

Chronic myelocytic leukemia

Definition

Chronic myelocytic leukemia (CML) is a cancer of white blood cells in which too many white blood cells are made in the bone marrow. Chronic myelogenous leukemia and chronic myeloid leukemia are other names for CML and refer to the identical disease. In CML, there is an increased proliferation of white blood cells called granulocytes.

Description

Chronic leukemia is a cancer that starts in the blood cells made in the bone marrow. The bone marrow is the spongy tissue found in the large bones of the body. The bone marrow makes precursor cells called "blasts" or "stem cells" that mature into different types of blood cells. Unlike acute leukemias, in which the process of maturation of the blast cells is interrupted, in chronic leukemias, the cells do mature and only a few remain as immature cells. However, even though the cells appear normal, they do not function as normal cells.

The different types of cells produced in the bone marrow are red blood cells (RBCs), which carry oxygen and other materials to all tissues of the body; white blood cells (WBCs), which fight infection; and platelets, which play a part in the clotting of the blood. The white blood cells can be further subdivided into three main types: the granulocytes, monocytes, and the lymphocytes.

The granulocytes, as their name suggests, have granules (particles) inside them. These granules contain special proteins (enzymes) and several other substances that can break down chemicals and destroy microorganisms such as bacteria. Monocytes are also important in defending the body against pathogens.

The lymphocytes form the third type of white blood cell. There are two main types of lymphocytes: T lymphocytes and B lymphocytes. They have different functions within the immune system. The B cells protect the body by making antibodies. Antibodies are proteins that can attach to the surfaces of bacteria and viruses. This attachment sends signals to many other cell types to come and destroy the antibody-coated organism. The T cell protects the body against viruses. When a virus enters a cell, it produces certain proteins that are projected onto the surface of the infected cell. The T cells can recognize these proteins and produce certain chemicals (cytokines) that are capable of destroying the virus-infected cells. In addition, the T cells can destroy some types of cancer cells.

Chronic leukemias develop very gradually. The abnormal lymphocytes multiply slowly, but in a poorly regulated manner. They live much longer than normal cells and thus their numbers build up in the body. The two types of chronic leukemias can be easily distinguished under the microscope. Chronic lymphocytic leukemia (CLL) involves the T or B lymphocytes. In chronic myelocytic leukemia (CML), the cells affected are the granulocytes. In addition, CML involves abnormalities of both the blood platelets, structures that help blood to clot, and the red blood cells, the blood cells that carry oxygen.

Very rarely will CML appear in children. Juvenile CML is a distinct disease of children younger than 14

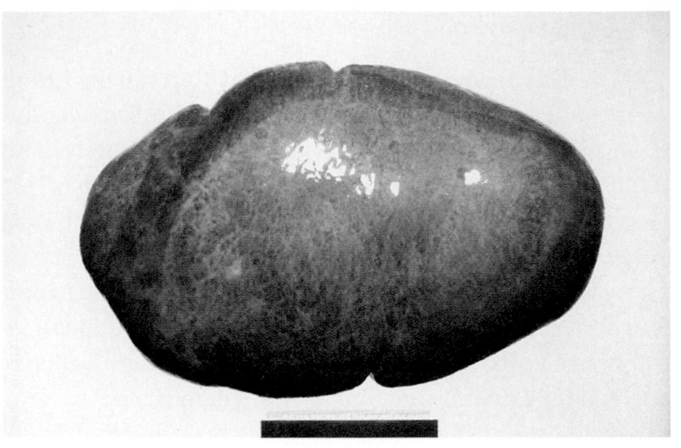

This spleen was removed from a patient with chronic myelocytic leukemia.The spleen has many functions—it removes old red blood cells, stores blood, and produces lymphocytes and plasma cells. Many blood disorders and cancers (including leukemias and lymphomas) can cause the spleen to enlarge. *(Custom Medical Stock Photo. Reproduced by permission.)*

years of age. There is a decrease in the number of blood platelets, substances that help the blood to clot. And there is an increase in certain white blood cells.

Demographics

Slightly more men than women are affected by CML. The average patient is between 50 and 60 years of age. However, CML can affect people of any age. Chronic leukemias account for 1.2% of all cancers. Chronic myelocytic leukemia is generally seen in people in their mid-40s. According to the estimates of the American Cancer Society (ACS), approximately 4,400 new cases of leukemia were diagnosed in the year 2000, 2,600 in men and 1,800 in women. Between 1973 and 1991, the rate at which CML appeared in the United States decreased slightly.

Causes and symptoms

People exposed to nuclear and other radiation are at increased risk for CML. Thus, people who have had higher exposure to radiation for medical reasons are at increased risk of developing this cancer. Parents with CML do not have children who are more than normally likely to develop CML. However, it is possible that people whose immune system exhibits certain characteristics are at increased risk for the disease.

CML develops in a two- or three-stage progression. First, the chronic phase appears. Between 60 and 80 percent of patients next exhibit the symptoms of what is called the accelerated phase. The final stage of CML is the terminal blastic phase.

Symptoms of chronic phase CML appear in 60%–85% of patients. This means 15% to 40% of all the people diagnosed with CML have no symptoms at all and are diagnosed with the disease only because of the results of a routine blood test. Patients who do have symptoms most frequently find themselves to have **fatigue**, **weight loss**, or pain. Some patients have a mass of tissue or an enlarged liver that the doctor is able to feel. Some patients experience strokes, visual problems, a lowering of alertness or responsiveness, priapism, and ringing in the ear. Many patients in accelerated phase CML have no specific symptoms. However, **fever**, weight loss, and **night sweats** may appear.

Patients with terminal, blastic phase CML often experience symptoms. There may be fever, weight loss, night sweats, and **bone pain**. Many patients develop infections. Many have **anemia** (low counts of red blood cells) and many bleed easily.

Diagnosis

There are no screening tests available for chronic leukemias. The detection of these diseases may occur by chance during a routine physical examination.

People who have CML have an unusually high number of white blood cells. Somewhat less than half of these people also have high numbers of blood platelets. Most patients have mild anemia. The composition of the bone marrow in CML patients also differs from that of a healthy person. The marrow is described as being hypercellular. This means that the number of cells present in the bone marrow is unusually great.

If the doctor has reason to suspect leukemia, he or she will conduct a very thorough physical examination to look for enlarged lymph nodes in the neck, underarm, and pelvic region. Swollen gums, an enlarged liver or spleen, bruises, or pinpoint red rashes all over the body are among the signs of leukemia. Urine and blood tests may be ordered to check for microscopic amounts of blood in the urine and to obtain a complete differential blood count. This count will give the numbers and percentages of the different cells found in the blood.

Standard imaging tests such as x rays, **computed tomography** scans (CT scans), and **magnetic resonance imaging** (MRI) may be used to check whether the leukemic cells have invaded other organs of the body, such as the bones, chest, kidneys, abdomen, or brain.

Many doctors consider the presence of the Philadelphia (Ph) chromosome to be a crucial factor in the diagnosis of CML. The Ph chromosome is formed if some of the genetic material in two specific parts of two specific genetic units, called chromosomes, have exchanged some content in a particular way and created an arrangement of genetic material characteristic of CML patients.

Laboratory findings indicate when a patient enters the accelerated phase of CML. There may be more than 15% blasts (immature cells) in the blood. Alternately, the accelerated phase has started when more than 30% of the blood may be composed of a combination of blasts and promyelocytes. Promyelocytes are immature granulocytes. Another marker for the start of the accelerated phase is when the blood contains more than 20% of another white blood cell, called a basophil. Finally, the accelerated phase may be heralded by there being more than 100,000,000,000 platelets per liter of blood. The terminal, blastic phase of CML is heralded by measurements of 30% or more of blasts in either the bone marrow or the blood.

Clinical staging, treatments, and prognosis

Staging

Several different staging systems are in use. Most of these make use of the fact that a number of factors relevant to patients with CML say something about the patient's prognosis. Among these factors are the patient's age, the white blood cell count, the platelet count, the percentage of blast cells and basophil cells in either the blood or the bone marrow, the size of the liver, the size of the spleen, population of red blood cells that have a central portion called a nucleus, and the evolution of certain cell clones.

Treatment

It is very fortunate that several years ago the American Society of Hematology convened an Expert Panel on Chronic Myeloid Leukemia. This panel reviewed available therapies and published its findings in 1999. The findings were rigorously based upon evidence provided by the best research. The panel, comprised of top doctors from around the world, carefully sifted through all of the studies on treatment for CML and put aside all those studies performed with questionable methodology. This is a most important document relevant to CML therapy.

Since the publication of the findings of the expert panel, however, a new medicine has demonstrated great success in studies. This new medicine is known as STI571, **Imatinib mesylate**, or Gleevec. Since Gleevec was such a new drug in 2001, few studies have been conducted to evaluate its long-term effects. Furthermore, researchers have not had an opportunity to view the effects of imatinib mesylate over a period of five, 10, or 20 years.

In terms of CML therapy, the situation in 2001 was the following: physicians have the reliable report of the Expert Panel and a little bit of new information about a new medication. How the Expert Panel's findings and this new information should be integrated with the results of recent studies of imatinib mesylate is an issue that cancer doctors are currently resolving.

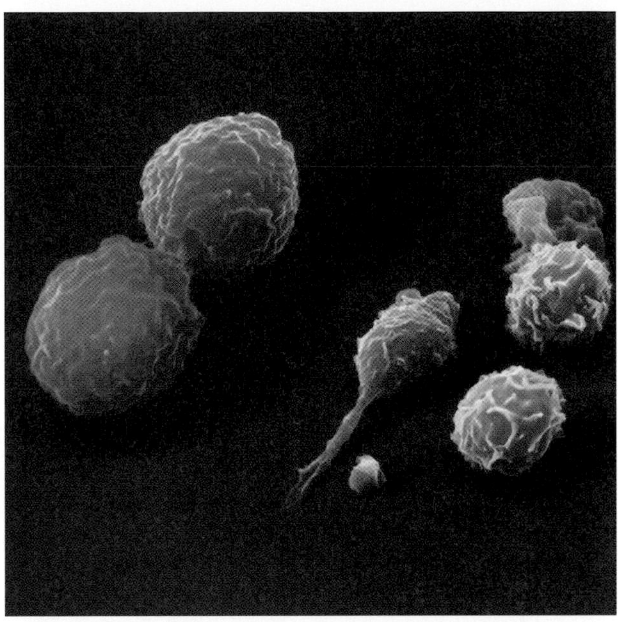

Color-enhanced scanning electron microscope image of leukemia cells. Leukemia cells (left) are compared to healthy bone marrow cells. The leukemia cells are larger and have a higher metabolism than the normal cells. *(© Meckes/Ottawa, Science Source/Photo Researchers, Inc. Reproduced by permission.)*

The Expert Panel looked at treatment of the chronic phase of CML. One therapy examined by the panel is **busulfan** (BUS). Another is **hydroxyurea** (HU). Both BUS and HU are **chemotherapy** medications. Studies have demonstrated that CML patients in chronic phase given HU live longer than patients given BUS.

Another therapy examined by the expert panel is interferon-alpha. Interferon is a chemical normally made in the cells of the body. It helps protect the body against viruses and also seems to have some effect against certain cancers. The interferon used as medicine is a laboratory-manufactured copy of the interferon produced by the body. The Expert Panel concluded that patients in chronic phase CML who have received interferon live longer than those given HU or BUS. This conclusion applies, in particular, to patients who have had little prior treatment for CML, who start interferon treatment soon after diagnosis, and who have certain other characteristics. However, side effects of interferon therapy are greater than those of therapy with HU or BUS. Patients who develop the side effects of interferon may feel like they have the flu. Patients receiving interferon seem to do

KEY TERMS

Accelerated phase—The middle one of the three-phase course of CML. However, between 20 and 40 percent of patients never enter the accelerated phase but, rather, go directly from the chronic to the terminal blastic phase.

Basophil—A type of white blood cell

Blast—An immature cell

Bone marrow—Spongy tissue found in the large bones of the body

Chemotherapy—Treatment with drugs that act against cancer.

Chronic phase—The initial phase of CML.

Hypercellular—Bone marrow is described as being hypercellular if the number of cells present in the bone marrow is unusually great.

Leukapheresis —A procedure to remove or extract excessive white blood cells from the blood.

Philadelphia (Ph) chromosome —The Philadelphia (Ph) chromosome is present if some of the genetic material in two specific parts of two specific genetic units, called chromosomes, have exchanged some content in a particular way.

Remission—Remission of a disease is achieved if the disease becomes diminished for a period.

Terminal blastic phase—The final stage of CML.

better if they also receive chemotherapy with either HU or a medicine called Ara-C, or **cytarabine**.

Bone marrow transplantation (BMT) is an effective treatment for CML. In BMT, the patient's diseased bone marrow is replaced with healthy marrow. There are two ways of doing a bone marrow transplant. In an allogeneic bone marrow transplant, healthy marrow is taken from another person (donor) whose tissue is either the same or very closely resembles the patient's tissues. The donor may be a twin, a sibling, or a person who is not related at all. First, the patient's bone marrow is destroyed with very high doses of chemotherapy and **radiation therapy**. To replace the destroyed marrow, healthy marrow from the donor is given to the patient.

In the second type of bone marrow transplant, called an autologous bone marrow transplant, some of the patient's own marrow is taken out and treated with a combination of anticancer drugs to kill all the abnormal cells. This marrow is then frozen to save it. The marrow remaining in the patient's body is then destroyed with high dose chemotherapy and radiation therapy. Following that, the patient's own marrow that was frozen is thawed and given back to the patient.

Allogeneic BMT may be used soon after diagnosis or after a patient has been treated with interferon or chemotherapy. The Expert Panel found that carefully designed, well-controlled, randomized studies have not been conducted on BMT therapy for CML. In the studies that do exist, scientists performed BMT on a group of patients and then observed the results. These studies show that BMT may lead to long-term remission. Remission is achieved if the disease becomes diminished for a period. Patients appear to live longer if they received chemotherapy followed by BMT. But the Expert Panel cautions that the results of these observational studies cannot be relied upon. One problem with them might be, for example, that the patients chosen to receive BMT might have started out being healthier than patients who did not receive BMT. The side effects of BMT may be severe, and a large number of CML patients receiving BMT die as a direct result of the BMT.

Therefore, one important consideration when BMT is being considered is whether the conditions under which the individual patient might receive BMT are favorable. In other words, is a very suitable marrow donor available? Is the patient within two years of CML diagnosis? It is important that patients understand clearly the ptential benefits and risks of BMT. One comment made by the Expert Panel is that younger patients who hope to live a very long time after CML diagnosis are more likely to benefit from allogeneic BMT. Autologous BMT has not achieved superior long-term results.

The recent studies of imatinib mesylate found it very effective in two groups of CML patients. One group was made up of patients who had unsuccessful results with interferon alfa therapy. The other group of CML patients studied were in the blast phase of the disease. Both studies found the medication to be effective and well tolerated. However, studies reporting on the effectiveness of imatinib mesylate over periods of five years or longer were not yet available in 2001.

Because leukemia cells can spread to all the organs via the blood stream and the lymph vessels, surgery is not considered an option for treating the leukemias.

The Expert Panel was careful to state that patient preferences should be taken into account as a treatment plan is developed. No approach to CML therapy is perfect. Each provides some benefit and is accompanied by certain side effects and risks. Which therapy or therapies is best for each individual patient depends upon on certain facts, such as the age of the patient and whether the patient is suffering from illnesses other than CML. In addition, the Expert Panel explains that the personal preferences of each patient are an important consideration. For example, some patients would rather avoid potential severe side effects and would be willing to give up the potential of living another few months or years. Other patients would be entirely unwilling to accept this way of looking at risks and benefits. It is important that health care professionals educate patients as to what treatment options are available and the perfections and imperfections associated with each. The opinions of each patient should be an important factor in deciding which treatment is best for that patient.

In the accelerated and blastic phase of CML, aggressive chemotherapy may be given. Combination chemotherapy, in which multiple drugs are used, is more effective than using a single drug for the treatment. Interferon and BMT may be used, although results are not as good as for patients in the chronic phase of CML.

It should be mentioned that during treatment the doctor may order a procedure called leukapheresis. This lowers the numbers of white blood cells circulating in the patient's body. Also, either before or after therapy, it may be necessary to provide the patient with a transfusion of blood platelets. In addition, **antibiotics** are often used to help prevent infection in leukemia patients.

Prognosis

The most important factor in determining the likelihood that a patient receiving interferon therapy will achieve long-term survival is whether there is a positive response to interferon-alfa. Although experience with imatinib mesylate is being gathered in studies, this drug remains so new that doctors do not know what effect it will have on the prognosis of CML patients. Once the threat of transplantation-related complications has passed, patients receiving BMT may achieve longer survival than patients receiving interferon therapy.

Before the discovery of modern therapies, patients often spent between three-and-a-half and five years in the chronic phase. Then some patients entered an accelerated phase, from which most died within 18 months. Once patients were in the terminal, blastic phase most died within six months. However, all of this has changed with the arrival of newer therapeutic techniques. Just as many patients used to die from heart attack while similar patients may now live for decades, so cancer patients are achieving longer lives.

Coping with cancer treatment

Cancer patients need supportive care to help them come through the treatment period with physical and emotional strength in tact. Many patients experience feelings of **depression**, anxiety, and fatigue, and many experience **nausea and vomiting** during treatment. Studies have shown that these can be managed effectively if discussed with the doctor.

QUESTIONS TO ASK THE DOCTOR

- How can I obtain supportive care so I come through this not only alive but with my family and emotional life intact?
- What sort of benefit and what sort of side effects might each of the available treatment options bring?
- Would you please inform me about the treatment options and let me tell you about the priorities in my life so I can participate in forming a treatment plan?
- What is my prognosis?
- Are blasts present?
- Has complete remission or partial remission been achieved?
- What can I do to lower my risk of infection during chemotherapy?

Prevention

Although some cancers are related to known risk factors, such as smoking, in leukemias, there are no definitive risk factors. Therefore, at the present time, there is no way known to prevent the leukemias from developing. People who are at an increased risk for developing leukemia because of proven exposure to ionizing radiation, the organic liquid benzene, or people who have a history of other cancers of the lymphoid system (Hodgkin's lymphoma) should undergo periodic medical checkups.

See Also Chromosome rearrangements

Resources

BOOKS

Braunwald, Eugene, et al. *Harrison's Principles of Internal Medicine,* 15th ed. New York: McGraw-Hill, 2001.

deWitt, Susan C. *Essentials of Medical-Surgical Nursing,* 4th ed. Philadelphia: W. B. Saunders, 1998.

Humes, H. David, et al. *Kelley's Textbook of Internal Medicine,* 4th ed. Philadelphia: Lippincott Williams & Wilkins, 2000.

Pazdur, Richard, et al. *Cancer Management: A Multidisciplinary Approach: Medical, Surgical, & Radiation Oncology,* 4th ed. Melville, NY: PRR, 2000.

Souhami, Robert, Jeffrey Tobias. *Cancer and Its Management,* 3rd ed. London: Blackwell Science, 1998.

PERIODICALS

Drucker, B. J., et al. "Efficacy and safety of a specific inhibitor of the BCR-ABL tyrosine kinase in chronic myeloid leukemia." *New England Journal of Medicine,* 344 (2001): 1031-1037.

Drucker B. J., et al. "Activity of a specific inhibitor of the BCR-ABL tyrosine kinase in the blast crisis of chronic myeloid leukemia and acute lymphoblastic leukemia with the Philadelphia chromosome." *New England Journal of Medicine,* 344 (2001): 1038-1042.

Silver, Richard T., et al. "An evidence-based analysis of the effect of busulfan, hydroxyurea, interferon, and allogeneic bone marrow transplantation in treating the chronic phase of chronic myeloid leukemia: developed for the American Society of Hematology." *Blood,* 94 (1999): 1517-1536.

ORGANIZATIONS

The National Cancer Institute publishes useful texts available through the Internet or by mail, and answers questions by telephone. Some publications include: *Leukemia,What You Need to Know About Leukemia,PDQ - Treatment - Patients: Chronic Myelogenous Leukemia,* and *Complementary & Alternative Therapies for Leukemia, Lymphoma, Hodgkin's Disease, & Myeloma.* Telephone: 1-800-4CANCER. Web site: <www.nci.nih.gov/>.

The Leukemia & Lymphoma Society (Formerly Leukemia Society of America) publishes useful texts available through the Internet or by mail. Some publications include: *Chronic Myelogenous Leukemia (CML),Choosing a Specialist. Choosing a Treatment Facility,Making Intelligent Choices About Therapy,Understanding Blood Counts,Patient Aid Program,* and *Family Support Group.* Telephone:1-800-955-4572. Web site: <www.leukemia-lymphoma.org/>.

The American Cancer Society publishes useful texts, which include: *Adult Chronic Leukemia - Overview, Leukemia - Adult Chronic: Treatment, Leukemia - Adult Chronic: Detection and Symptoms,Leukemia: Adult Chronic FAQ [Frequently Asked Questions],* and *Leukemia - Adult Chronic: Prevention & Risk.* Telephone:1-800-ACS-2345. Web site: <www.cancer.org/>.

National Coalition for Cancer Survivorship. 1010 Wayne Avenue, 7th Floor, Silver Spring, MD 20910-5600. Telephone: (301) 650-9127 and (877)NCCS-YES [877-622-7937). Web site: <www.cansearch.org>.

Lata Cherath, Ph.D.
Bob Kirsch

Chronic myelogenous leukemia *see* **Chronic myelocytic leukemia**

Cigarettes

Description

Farmers were harvesting tobacco crops eight thousand years ago. Its uses since that time have ranged from weather forecasting, appetite suppression, and pain relief, to the ceremonial smoking of the peace pipe and recreational use. Although tobacco was smoked and chewed in the United States back in the days of Columbus, it was not until the 1880s that smoking cigarettes became a widespread custom. At its peak in 1965, 52% of all adult men and 32% of all adult women in the United States routinely smoked. By the year 2001, smoking rates in the United States had decreased to 25.5% in men, and 21.3% in women.

The potential adverse health effects of smoking were suspected as far back as 1859. It was then that an evaluation of 68 patients with oral cavity cancer linked 66 of them with the practice of smoking tobacco through short-stemmed clay pipes. Epidemiological evidence of the potentially harmful effects of cigarette smoking continued to mount over the following years. Finally, in 1962, the Royal College of Physicians of London officially deemed smoking a serious threat to health; in 1964 the U.S. Surgeon General followed suit.

Health risks of cigarette smoking

By 2001, an estimated 450,000 Americans died annually from diseases related to cigarette smoking. According to the American Cancer Society, 3,000 non-smoking adults die each year of lung cancer from the effects of secondhand smoke. Pregnant women who smoke are more likely to give birth to low-weight babies, and smokers have increased rates of heart disease and respiratory problems.

In addition to those health risks, smokers are at a higher risk for the development of many types of cancer. In fact, 38% of all cancer deaths in men and 23% of all cancer deaths in women are believed to be attributed to cigarette smoking. As cigarette smoking becomes more prevalent in developing countries, the incidence of particular diseases, such as lung cancer, has also increased.

Cancers associated specifically with tobacco use include:

- Lung cancer: Smoking is now the primary modifiable risk factor for lung cancer. Tobacco was first linked to lung cancer in 1898, when it was theorized to be the cause for several cases of lung cancers in tobacco workers. Since then, studies have continued to document the relationship between smoking and lung cancer. Lung cancer incidence—the number of new cases diagnosed per year—closely follows smoking trends. As more and more women began to smoke, for example, the incidence of lung cancer in women also increased. By the late 1900s, 90% of lung cancer cases in men and 79% in women were believed to be related to smoking.

- Head and neck cancer: Smoking increases the risk of **head and neck cancers**. When tobacco is used in conjunction with alcohol, there is believed to be an even higher risk of these types of diagnoses. The precise mechanism of this relationship, known as a "synergistic effect," is not yet well understood.
- **Esophageal cancer**: Smokers, particularly women smokers, are at an increased risk for developing esophageal cancer—a risk that increases with the quantity of cigarettes smoked per day.
- Pancreatic cancer: An estimated 22,000 people die from pancreatic cancer each year, and an alarming 30% of these deaths are related to cigarette smoking.
- Colorectal cancer: Individuals who smoke cigarettes are more likely to develop polyps in the colon, which in turn increases the risk of **colon cancer**. There is also evidence that the risk of colon and/or **rectal cancer** increases with pack years for smokers. (Pack years are calculated by multiplying the number of packs of cigarettes smoked a day by the number of years smoked.)
- **Stomach cancer**: Although some studies have found no existing relationship between smoking and stomach cancer, others have shown an increased risk for smokers over the age of 50 years and a relationship between the disease and pack-years of smoking. More conclusive research is necessary to better understand the role that smoking plays in the development of stomach, or gastric, cancer.
- **Bladder cancer**: Smoking is believed to be related to 30-40% of all bladder cancers, most of which are of the transitional cell type. The risk of developing bladder cancer is believed to be related to the duration of smoking and inversely related to the age at which smoking began (that is, the younger a person is when he or she starts smoking, the higher the chances of developing bladder cancer).
- **Cervical cancer**: There appears to be a relationship between smoking and cervical cancer—the higher the "dose," or amount smoked, the higher the likelihood of developing cervical cancer. Smoking is also associated with **human papilloma virus** infection, or HPV. Certain types of HPV can cause warts to develop in the genital area and cervix. These types of infections are a major cause of cervical cancer. Because of these overlapping relationships, the exact effect of smoking in cervical cancer needs further study.
- **Breast cancer**: Smoking is not yet a well-established risk factor for breast cancer: some studies indicate an increased risk among smokers, and others report a decreased risk among smokers. Genetic susceptibility to certain components of tobacco may explain the varying results, but more research is needed to better understand the relationship.

Although cancer is not always preventable, avoiding known risk factors, such as smoking, is an important part of prevention. The best approach to prevent disease is not to start smoking at all. However, even individuals who have smoked for years can decrease their risk of cancer and improve their health and well being by breaking the habit. Shortly after quitting smoking, a person will notice an improvement in their sense of taste and smell. After a smoke-free ten years, lung cancer risk declines by up to 50%. After 15 smoke-free years, an ex-smoker has the same risk of early death than a person who never smoked at all. Although quitting smoking does reduce the likelihood of cancer development, the risk depends upon the amount smoked, the number of years smoked, and whether or not a person is ill at the time of **smoking cessation**.

Resources

BOOKS

Varricchoi, C., ed. *A Cancer Source Book for Nurses,* 7th ed. Sudbury, MA: Jones and Bartlett Publishers, 1997.

PERIODICALS

Christiani, D., "Smoking and Pulmonary and Cardiovascular Diseases." *Clinics in Chest Medicine* 21 (March 2000): 87-93.

Johnson, B., "Tobacco and Lung Cancer." *Primary Care: Clinics in Office Practice* 25 (June 1998): 279-91.

Leistikow, B., "Smoking and Pulmonary and Cardiovascular Diseases." *Clinics in Chest Medicine* 21 (March 2000): 189-97.

Mitchell, B. et al., "Tobacco Use and Cessation: The Adverse Health Effects of Tobacco and Tobacco-Related Products." *Clinics in Office Practice* 26 (September 1999): 463-98.

Smith, R., "Epidemiology of Lung Cancer." *Radiologic Clinics of North America* 38 (May 2000): 453-460.

Tanoue, L., "Cigarette Smoking and Women's Respiratory Health." *Clinics in Chest Medicine* 21 (March 2000): 47-65.

Tamara L. Brown, R.N.

Cimetidine *see* **Histamine 2 antagonists**

Ciprofloxacin *see* **Antibiotics**

Cisplatin

Definition

Cisplatin, also known by the brand name Platinol-AQ, Cis-platinum, CDDP, or DDP, is a **chemotherapy** medicine used to treat certain types of cancer by destroying cancerous cells.

Purpose

Cisplatin is approved by the Food and Drug Administration (FDA) to treat metastatic **testicular cancer** and metastatic **ovarian cancer**. It is also approved for late-stage **bladder cancer** and has been used to treat other types of cancer including head and neck cancer, **esophageal cancer**, **stomach cancer**, lung cancer, skin cancer, **prostate cancer**, **lymphoma** and others (breast, **neuroblastoma**, sarcoma, bladder, cervical, **myeloma**, **mesothelioma**, **osteosarcoma**).

Description

Cisplatin is a member of the group of chemotherapy drugs known as heavy metal alkylating-like agents. These drugs interfere with the genetic material (DNA) inside the cancer cells and prevent them from further dividing and growing more cancer cells.

Cisplatin has been used to treat cancer for more than 30 years. It can be used alone or in combination with other chemotherapies, including bleomycin-etoposide, **ifosfamide**, **gemcitabine**, **paclitaxel**, fluorouracil-leucovorin, **vinorelbine**, methotrexate-vinblastine-doxorubicin. Cisplatin may also be given with **radiation therapy**.

Recommended dosage

A cisplatin dose can be determined using a mathematical calculation that measures body surface area (BSA), which depends on a person's overall size. Body surface area is measured in the units known as square meter (m^2). The body surface area is calculated and then multiplied by the drug dosage in milligrams per m^2 (mg/m^2), which gives the proper dosage.

Cisplatin is a clear, colorless solution administered by an infusion into a vein. Infusions can be given once every three to four weeks over a 30 minutes up to two hours. It can also be given continuously over 24 hours a day for several days in a row. One cycle of cisplatin should not be given more frequently than once every three to four weeks. Dosages depend on the cancer being treated.

To treat metastatic testicular cancer

Dosages are 20 mg/m^2 per day administered into a vein every day for five days in a row. This regimen is used in combination with other chemotherapy drugs, mainly **bleomycin** and **etoposide** or **vinblastine**.

To treat metastatic ovarian cancer

Dosages are 50 mg/m^2 to 100 mg/m^2 administered into a vein once every four weeks. This regimen can be combined with the chemotherapy drug **cyclophosphamide** or **doxorubicin**.

To treat advanced bladder cancer

Cisplatin doses range from 50 mg/m^2 to 70 mg/m^2 administered into a vein once every 3 to 4 weeks. Cisplatin is usually given alone for bladder cancer.

Before receiving cisplatin large volumes of intravenous fluids are given to keep the kidneys flushed with water. If patients have severe kidney problems the physician will either not use cisplatin or decrease the dose being used.

Normal metal ions found in the body, called electrolytes, can be lost due to administration of cisplatin. These may be added to these intravenous fluids for replacement.

Precautions

When receiving cisplatin, it is important to drink a lot of fluids to help flush the kidneys and prevent kidney damage. Patients also receive additional fluids through their veins before, during, and after receiving cisplatin.

Blood counts will be monitored regularly while on cisplatin therapy. During a certain time period after receiving cisplatin, there is an increased risk of getting infections. Caution should be taken to avoid unnecessary exposure to crowds and people with infections.

Patients with a known previous allergic reaction to chemotherapy drugs or any other medications should tell their doctor.

Patients who may be pregnant or trying to become pregnant should also tell their doctor before receiving cisplatin.

Chemotherapy can cause men and women to be sterile (not able to have children).

Patients should check with their doctors before receiving live virus **vaccines** while on chemotherapy.

Side effects

Common side effects include **nausea and vomiting**, which can begin from 1 hour after receiving the drug and last as long as a week. Patients are given medicines known as **antiemetics**, before and after receiving cis-

KEY TERMS

Anemia—A red blood cell count that is lower than normal.

Chemotherapy—Specific drugs used to treat cancer.

DNA—Genetic material inside of cells that carries information to make proteins that are necessary to run the cells and keep the body functioning properly.

Electrolytes—Refers to the elements normally found in the body (sodium, potassium, calcium, magnesium, phosphorus, chloride, and acetate) that are important to maintain the many cellular functions and growth.

Food and Drug Administration—A government agency that oversees public safety in relation to drugs and medical devices. The FDA gives approval to pharmaceutical companies for commercial marketing of their products.

Intravenous—To enter the body through a vein

Metastatic—Cancer that has spread to one or more parts of the body.

Neutropenia—a white blood cell count that is lower than normal.

Radiation therapy—The use of high-energy beams focused to treat cancerous tumors.

platin to help prevent or decrease this side effect. **Diarrhea** has also been known to occur.

A serious common side effect related to the total dose of cisplatin received is kidney damage, which can occur in up to one-third of patients. Taking fluids before, during and after receiving cisplatin help prevent this from occurring.

Hearing damage can also occur in up to one-third of patients. Patients may experience ringing in the ears and hearing loss of high-pitched frequency. Hearing tests may be requested before and/or after cisplatin therapy.

Low blood counts, referred to as **myelosuppression**, are expected due to cisplatin administration. When the white blood cell count is low this is called **neutropenia** and patients are at an increased risk of developing a **fever** and infections. Platelets are blood cells in the body that allow for the formation of clots. When the platelet count is low, patients are at an increased risk for bruising and bleeding. Low red blood cell counts, referred to as **anemia**, may also occur due to cisplatin administration. Low red counts make people feel tired.

Cisplatin can also cause damage to nerves and nervous system tissues. Patients may feel tingling, numbness and sometimes burning of the fingers and toes. This side effect is common and can be severe.

Less common side effects include change of taste sensation, loss of appetite, dizziness, seizures, confusion, muscle cramps and uncontrolled muscle contractions. Other side effects include, hair loss (**alopecia**), hiccups, rash, allergic reactions with difficulty breathing, swelling and a fast heart rate.

Cisplatin may cause the body to waste normal electrolytes that circulate in the body (potassium, magnesium, phosphate, sodium, calcium) resulting in low levels of these electrolytes. These will be monitored by the doctor and replacement drugs will be given if necessary.

All side effects should be reported to the doctor or nurse.

Interactions

Patients should avoid other drugs that may cause damage to the kidneys.

Certain water pills and cisplatin given together may increase the risk of hearing damage. Before starting any medications, patients should notify their doctors.

Cisplatin may make medications that control seizures less effective.

Nancy J. Beaulieu, RPh., BCOP

Cladribine

Definition

Cladribine, also known by the brand name Leustatin, is a **chemotherapy** medicine used to treat certain types of cancer by destroying cancerous cells.

Purpose

Cladribine is approved by the Food and Drug Administration (FDA) to treat active **hairy cell leukemia**. It has also been used to treat other types of leukemias and lymphomas.

Description

A member of the group of chemotherapy drugs known as a purine nucleoside analog, cladribine may also

KEY TERMS

Anemia—A red blood cell count that is lower than normal.

Complete response—No sign of leukemia in the blood or bone marrow.

Chemotherapy—Specific drugs used to treat cancer.

DNA—Genetic material inside of cells that that carry information to make proteins that are necessary for proper cell functioning.

Food and Drug Administration—A government agency that oversees public safety in relation to drugs and medical devices. The FDA gives approval to pharmaceutical companies for commercial marketing of their products

Intravenous—To enter the body through a vein.

Neutropenia—White blood cell count that is lower than normal.

be referred to as 2-CdA, chlorodeoxyadenosine, and 2-chlorodeoxyadenosine. The purine nucleosides interfere with the genetic material (DNA) inside the cancer cells, cause DNA strand breaks, and block RNA synthesis. These traits help prevent cancer cells from further dividing and growing and also may cause the cancer cells to die.

Recommended dosage

Cladribine is a clear solution that is administered through a vein. The dose of cladribine is based on a patient's weight in kilograms. The approved dose for hairy cell leukemia is 0.09 mg per kilogram of body weight administered each day as a continuous intravenous infusion administered over 24 hours each day for seven continuous days. Some patients may receive this treatment in more than one cycle.

Other doses include 0.1 to 0.3 mg per kilogram of body weight per day for seven days administered as a continuous infusion. Patients may also receive cladribine as a two-hour infusion daily for five days in a row.

Precautions

Blood counts will be monitored regularly while on cladribine therapy. During a certain time period after receiving cladribine, there is an increased risk of getting infections. Caution should be taken to avoid unnecessary exposure to crowds and people with infection.

Patients with a known previous allergic reaction to chemotherapy drugs should tell their doctor.

Patients who may be pregnant or are trying to become pregnant should tell their doctors before receiving cladribine.

Although chemotherapy can cause men and women to be sterile (not able to have children), it is unknown if cladribine has this effect on humans.

Patients should check with their doctors before receiving live virus **vaccines** while on chemotherapy.

Side effects

The most common side effect from taking cladribine is low blood counts, referred to as **myelosuppression**. When the white blood cell count is lower than normal, referred to as **neutropenia**, patients are at an increased risk of developing a **fever** and infections. The platelet blood count can also be decreased due to cladribine administration, but generally returns back to normal within two weeks after the end of the infusion. Platelets are blood cells in the body that cause clots to form these clots stop bleeding. When the platelet count is low, patients are at an increased risk for bruising and bleeding. Cladribine causes low red blood cell counts, which is referred to as **anemia**. Low red counts make people feel tired and dizzy.

Other common side effects of cladribine include skin rashes or reactions, pain, redness, or swelling at the injection site. Half of patients with hairy cell leukemia experience a rash.

Patients may experience infections, chills, and fever when being treated with cladribine. This may result in treatment with **antibiotics**.

Nausea,vomiting, loss of appetite, abdominal pain, constipation and **diarrhea** are mild side effects from cladribine. If **nausea and vomiting** are a problem, patients can be given medicines known as **antiemetics** before receiving cladribine to help prevent or decrease these side effects.

Damage to the kidneys and nervous system tissues is uncommon with cladribine, unless given in high doses for bone marrow transplant patients. At high doses, kidney problems and nerve damage have resulted in weakness of the arms and legs.

Less common side effects of cladribine are hair loss, **itching**, a fever from taking the drug, lung problems, cough, inability to sleep, headache, dizziness, fast heart rate, muscle and joint aches, and **fatigue**.

Interactions

Patients should notify their doctors of any medications they are taking. In the case of cladribine, medications to make special note of include antithyroid agents, **azathioprine**, chloramphenicol, flucytosine, ganciclovir, interferon, **plicamycin**, zidovudine, probenecid, sulfinpyrazone.

Patients should tell their doctors if they have a known allergic reaction to **amifostine** or any other medications or substances, such as foods and preservatives. Before taking any new medications, including nonprescription medications, **vitamins**, and herbal medications, the patients should notify their doctors.

Nancy J. Beaulieu, RPh.,BCOP

KEY TERMS

Leukemia—Cancer of the blood and bone marrow.

Maximum tolerated dose (MTD)—The highest dose of an investigational drug that patients can tolerate without life-threatening or fatal side effects.

Oncology—The study of cancer.

Osteosarcoma—A tumor of the bone. The most common childhood cancer.

Placebo—A preparation without medication.

Protocol—A written, scientific guideline used for treatment planning in clinical trials.

Wilms' tumor—A malignant tumor of the kidney; occurs most frequently in children.

Clinical trials

Definition

A clinical trial is a research study designed to answer specific medical questions regarding cancer care.

Description

The clinical trial is a scientific study that follows a written guideline (protocol) or recipe for treatment. It is the only scientific mechanism designed to test the effectiveness of new and promising therapies. The clinical trial provides intensive testing of new or updated treatment regimens. Almost all standard treatments in the field of oncology (cancer) originated from clinical trials. These trials are conducted by medical, surgical and radiation oncologists (cancer specialists).

Cancer clinical trials are the key to preventing, diagnosing and treating all types of cancer. It is estimated that 60% of all cancer patients in the United States are being cured. Yet, fewer than 3% of adult cancer patients participate in clinical trials. In contrast, about 71% of children enter clinical trials. This has led to major advancements in treatment and high cure rates for many **childhood cancers** such as **Wilms' tumor** (malignant neoplasm of the kidney), **osteosarcoma** (tumor of the bone), and childhood leukemia (cancer of the blood).

Types of clinical trials

Clinical trials that involve new drugs or devices for humans must first be tested in animals. When a new or **investigational drug** has been discovered that shows anti-tumor activity in laboratory animals, it is tested on a small number of patients with different types of cancer, usually in a university setting. These are called Phase I trials and are designed to test the maximum tolerated dose (MTD) and side effects or toxicities of a new drug. This phase also helps determine how a new drug should be given (by mouth or by injection). The patients being tested are those with advanced cancer who have exhausted other treatment options. These patients may not personally benefit from participation in the trial.

If the investigational agent or drug continues to show anti-tumor activity and if the side effects are tolerable and not life-threatening, the drug is moved into a Phase II trial for further testing. In a Phase II trial, the drug is offered to a specific group of patients having the same tumor type. The drug is being tested to determine if it regresses tumor growth. Additional information on side effects of the treatment is also evaluated in this phase.

If the drug continues to show response to the patient's cancer, it is moved into a Phase III trial. At this phase, the investigational treatment is compared to the standard cancer therapy. This is to ensure that no one in a study is left without any treatment when standard treatment is available. If there is no standard therapy, a placebo (a pill that looks like the drug being studied but contains no active medication) may be used for comparison. However, researchers must inform potential patients of this possibility before patients decide whether to participate. Patients are usually assigned their treatment by a process called randomization, which is similar to the toss of a coin. Comparison or randomized trials help

QUESTIONS TO ASK THE DOCTOR

- Am I eligible for a clinical trial?
- Where can I get more information?

researchers find the most effective treatment for a specific type of cancer.

The objectives of Phase III trials include tumor response to treatment, survival, and quality of life during therapy. This phase can involve 400-1000 patients. Antitumor response by a significant proportion of the involved patients indicates that the investigational drug or treatment is ready to be submitted to the Food and Drug Administration (FDA) for approval. If approved, the drug is released from investigational status and made available for commercial use in patients with the specifically tested type of cancer.

What to expect as part of a clinical trial

Taking part in a clinical trial does not mean that patients are seen as or treated like "guinea pigs," or that they will receive substandard care. Cancer patients who enroll in clinical trials may be the first to receive a new technique or drug that becomes the standard of care. Clinical trials, however, have risks, as well. The treatment or drug being tested is new, and the side effects may be unknown. The cancer patient, his or her loved ones, and the patient's physician must weigh the risks and benefits when deciding whether or not to enroll in a clinical trial.

When patients participate in a clinical trial, they receive treatment in a cancer center, hospital, clinic, and/or doctor's office. Doctors, nurses, social workers, and other health professionals may be part of the treatment team, and will closely monitor progress. Cancer clinical trial patients:

- are, as stated above, under close scrutiny
- are seen frequently by the members of the treatment team
- are tested often
- follow the treatment plan their doctor prescribes and as according to the study's protocol
- and may also have other responsibilities, such as keeping a log or filling out health forms.

Some studies continue to check on patients after their treatment is completed.

Resources

BOOKS

Klimaszewski, Angela D., Jennifer L. Aikin, Monica A. Bacon, Susan A. DiStasio, Heidi E. Ehrenberger, Bertie A. Ford, Ed. *Manual for Clinical Trials Nursing.* Pittsburgh: Oncology Nursing Press, Inc., 2000.

Murphy, Gerald P., Walter Lawrence, Jr., and Raymond E. Lenhard, Jr., Ed. *American Cancer Society Textbook of Clinical Oncology.* Atlanta: American Cancer Society, 1995.

Varricchio, Claudette, Ed.*A Cancer Source Book for Nurses.* Atlanta: Jones and Barlett Publishers, 1997: pp. 69-79.

OTHER

National Cancer Institute. *An Introduction to Clinical Trials.* January 2000 National Cancer Institute. 8 July 2001. <http://cancertrials.nci.nih.gov>.

National Cancer Institute. *Cancer Trials.* 8 July 2001. <http://cancertrials.nci.nih.gov/>

Phyllis M. Stein, B.S., CCRP

Codeine *see* **Opioids**

Cold sore *see* **Herpes simplex**

Colectomy

Definition

Colectomy is the surgical removal of all or part of the colon, the first part of the large intestine.

Purpose

Doctors perform colectomy to remove large Stage I **colon cancer** lesions or to cure colon cancer that: has spread beyond the mucous membrane, has infiltrated or spread beyond the intestinal wall, or is likely to recur.

Doctors also perform this procedure to improve patients' quality of life by relieving pain and preventing bleeding and other symptoms that occur when colon cancer invades organs near the bowel, and also, when nonsurgical methods are unsuccessful, to treat diverticulitis, ulcerative colitis, and benign colon polyps.

Precautions

This surgery can significantly diminish bowel control and sexual function.

Description

Colectomy is the preferred therapy for colon cancers that can be cured. Performed in a hospital, under general

Before

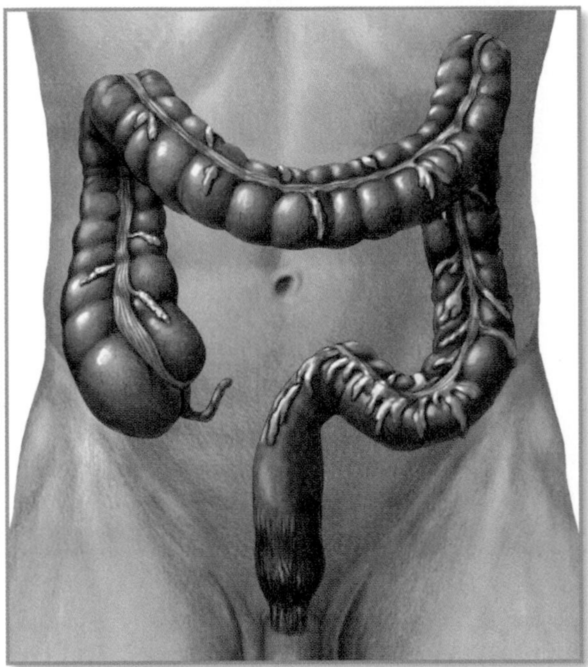

After

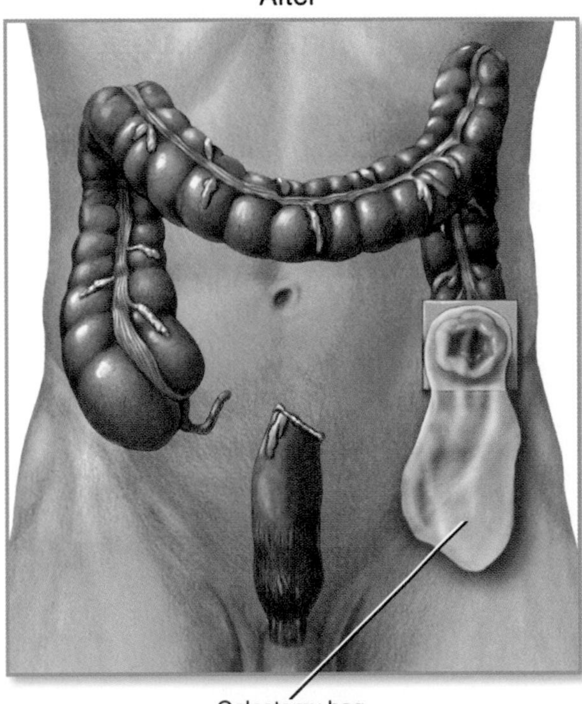

Above, diseased colon before colectomy. After the diseased portion is removed, the parts of the remaining colon are reattached. If reattachment is not possible, a colostomy is performed (below). *(Copyright 2001 adam.com, Inc. Reproduced by permission.)*

KEY TERMS

Diverticulitis—Inflammation or infection in pockets/ pouches that primarily develops in the wall of the large or small intestine.

Hemicolectomy—Surgical removal of half of the large intestine.

Hepatic—Of the liver.

Ulcerative colitis—Chronic inflammation of the large intestine and rectum.

anesthesia, this procedure involves removing the cancerous part of the colon, a margin of normal bowel, and any tissue or lymph nodes affected by the disease, and reconnecting the healthy segments of the colon (anastomosis). If infection or obstruction make it impossible to reconnect the colon, the surgeon creates an opening (stoma) in the abdominal wall (**colostomy**) through which feces passes from the body into a disposable collection bag.

Colostomy may be:

- temporary, with the ends of the intestines being reconnected at a later time, or
- permanent in patients whose cancer cannot be completely removed.

Open and laparoscopic procedures

Traditional, or open, colectomy is an invasive procedure requiring a wide surgical incision. This surgery allows the surgeon to view the internal organs very clearly.

Laparoscopic colectomy requires only a few small incisions, enables doctors to view the internal organs, and results in a shorter hospital stay and fewer side effects. Studies suggest that laparoscopic colectomy may be safer than open surgery for elderly patients. A clinical trial funded by the National Institutes of Health (NIH) is comparing survival rates for the two procedures.

Types of colectomy

LEFT RADICAL HEMICOLECTOMY. Doctors perform left radical hemicolectomy to remove cancer and other abnormal tissue in the:

- descending colon, which extends from the pelvis to the spleen,
- and splenic flexure, the place where the descending colon joins the part of the large intestine that extends across the middle of the abdomen (transverse colon).

When cancer is found in the splenic flexure, the surgeon removes the splenic flexure, the first half of the descending colon, and about one-third of the transverse colon.

RIGHT RADICAL HEMICOLECTOMY. Doctors perform this procedure to remove tumors and other abnormalities of the:

- section of large intestine nearest the appendix (cecum)
- portion of the large intestine that extends along the right side of the body from the small intestine to the transverse colon (ascending colon).

This procedure involves removing the cecum, descending colon, the hepatic flexure where the ascending colon joins the transverse colon, and the first one-third of the transverse colon. These procedures are considered radical because they involve removing nerves, blood vessels, and lymph nodes near the tumor.

TRANSVERSE COLECTOMY. Performed to remove disease in the transverse colon, this procedure includes removing the:

- transverse colon,
- and hepatic and splenic flexures.

SIGMOID RESECTION. Used to remove cancer in the part of the colon (sigmoid) between the descending colon and rectum, this procedure involves removing the:

- sigmoid colon
- bottom two-thirds of the descending colon

RECTOSIGMOID RESECTION. Used to remove tumors in the part of the colon (rectosigmoid) just above the rectum (sigmoid flexure), this procedure removes:

- the sigmoid colon
- most of the rectum and surrounding rectal tissue (mesorectum)

Because tumors in this part of the colon usually involve the bladder, uterus, or other organs, the surgeon may insert drainage tubes or a catheter to draw urine from the bladder.

ABDOMINOPERINEAL RESECTION (APR). This extensive procedure, which may be performed in two parts or by two surgical teams operating at the same time, involves removing the:

- lower sigmoid colon
- rectum
- anus
- nearby lymph nodes, blood vessels, and nerves

Sphincter-saving APR is designed to minimize loss of bowel control by:

- removing only the tumor
- preserving nerves and blood vessels near the tumor.

These specialized procedures involve repositioning the tumor while removing it, can cause shedding of tumor cells, and may not be available in all hospitals.

After completing any of these procedures, the surgeon uses:

- sutures
- clips
- heat and electrical current (electrothermal bipolar vessel sealer)

to tie off the ends of blood vessels before closing the incision.

Preparation

The day before the operation, the patient may consume only clear liquids, and may take nothing by mouth after midnight.

To reduce the possibility of infection, **antibiotics** are given to the patient the night before the operation.

Aftercare

A patient who has had an open colectomy will spend at least a week in the hospital and experience significant postoperative pain.

A patient who has had a laparoscopic colectomy will spend 4–5 days in the hospital, experience less pain, and resume normal activities within two weeks.

A patient who has had a colostomy must learn to care for the collection bag and keep the area clean. Patients who have had colostomies often worry about:

- not being able to care for themselves
- odors, gas, and leakage from the collection bag
- health problems
- recurrence of cancer

A patient who is depressed about sexual dysfunction, bowel problems, or other aspects of treatment may benefit from professional counseling or from joining a support group.

Risks

Side effects of colectomy include bladder complications, **diarrhea**, bowel irregularities, urinary urgency, and sexual dysfunction.

Normal results

Most patients experience postoperative pain. Patients who have laparoscopic surgery have less pain than patients who have open colectomy. Some patients require temporary colostomy until normal bowel function returns.

Most of these procedures do not affect sexual function, but rectosigmoid resection can make it difficult for a man to achieve erection during intercourse.

QUESTIONS TO ASK THE DOCTOR

- Which type of colectomy should I have?
- How will I feel and look after the operation?
- If I have to have a colostomy, will people be able to tell I'm wearing a bag?

Abnormal results

Extensive surgery can cause:

- infection
- severe pain
- fecal incontinence
- prolonged recovery

Resources

OTHER

Colectomy. <http://www.medterms.com/script/main/art.asp?article key=12529>. 20 May 2001.

Colorectal Cancer Treatments. <http://www.cancerfacts.com> 20 May2001

Laparoscopic Colorectal Surgery 20 January 2000. 21 May 2001 <http://www.lapsurgery.com/colectom.htm>.

Surgery & Colon Cancer 5 May 2001<http://www.colorectal-cancer.net/surgerycoloncancer> <http://www.colorectal-cancer.net/surgerycoloncancer.htm> 20 May 2001

What Are the Latest Treatments of Colon and Rectal Cancers? June 1999. 20 May 2001. <http://content.health.msn.com/content/dmk/dmk_article_5462002 7gt; 20 May 2001

Maureen Haggerty

Colon cancer

Definition

Cancer of the colon is the disease characterized by the development of malignant cells in the lining or epithelium of the first and longest portion of the large intestine. Malignant cells have lost normal control mechanisms governing growth. These cells may invade surrounding local tissue or they may spread throughout the body and invade other organ systems.

Synonyms for the colon include the large bowel or the large intestine. The rectum is the continuation of the large intestine into the pelvis that terminates in the anus.

Description

The colon is a tubular organ beginning in the right lower aspect of the abdomen. Anatomically, it ascends on the right side of the abdomen, traverses from right to left in the upper abdomen, descends vertically down the left side, takes an S-shaped curve in the lower left abdomen, and then flows into the rectum as it leaves the abdomen for the pelvis. These portions of the colon are named separately though they are part of the same organ.

- cecum, the beginning of the colon
- ascending colon, the right vertical ascent of the colon
- transverse colon, the portion traversing from right to left
- descending colon, the left vertical descent of the colon
- sigmoid colon, the s-shaped segment of colon above the pelvis

These portions of the colon are recognized anatomically based on the arterial blood supply and venous and lymphatic drainage of these segments of the colon. Lymph, a protein-rich fluid that bathes the cells of the body, is transported in small channels known as lymphatics that run alongside the veins of the colon. Lymph nodes are small filters through which the lymph travels on its way back to the blood stream. Cancer can spread elsewhere in the body by invading the lymph and vascular systems. Therefore, these anatomic considerations become very important in the treatment of colon cancer.

The small intestine is the continuation of the upper gastrointestinal tract responsible for the transport of ingested nutrients into the body. The waste left after the small intestine has completed absorption of nutrients amounts to a few liters, (about the same as quart), of material per day and is directly delivered to the colon, (at the cecum), for processing. Physiologically, the colon is responsible for the preservation of fluid and electrolytes as it propels the increasingly solid waste towards the rectum and anus for excretion.

When cells lining the colon become malignant, they first grow locally and may invade partially or totally through the wall of the bowel and even into adjacent structures and organs. In the process, the tumor can penetrate and invade the lymphatics or the capillaries locally and it gains access to the circulation. As the malignant cells work their way to other areas of the body, they again become locally invasive in the new area to which they have spread. These tumor deposits, originating from the colon primary tumor, are then known as metastases. If metastases are found in the regional lymph nodes from the primary, they are known as regional metastases, or regional nodal metastases. If they are distant from the primary tumor, they are known as distant metastases. The patient with distant metastases has systemic disease. Thus the cancer originating in the colon begins locally and, given time, can become systemic in its extent.

By the time the primary tumor is originally detected it is usually larger than one cm, (about 3/8 inches), in size and has over a million cells. This amount of growth itself is estimated to take about three–seven years. Each time the cells double in number, the size of the tumor quadruples. Thus like most cancers, the part that is identified clinically is later in the progression than would be desired and screening becomes a very important endeavor to aid in earlier detection of this disease.

Demographics

There are about 94,000 cases of colon cancer diagnosed per year in the United States. Together, colon and rectal cancers account for 10% of cancers in men and 11% of cancers in women. It is the second most common site-specific cancer affecting both men and women. (Lung cancer is the first affecting both men and women, breast is the leader in women and prostate the leader in men). Nearly 48,000 people died from colon cancer in the United States in 2000. In recent years the incidence of this disease is decreasing very slightly, as has the mortality rate. It is difficult to tell if the decrease in mortality reflects earlier diagnosis, less death related to the actual treatment of the disease, or a combination of both factors.

Cancer of the colon is thought to arise sporadically in about 80% of those who develop the disease. 20% of cases are thought to have genetic predisposition that ranges from familial syndromes affecting 50% of the offspring of a mutation carrier, to a risk of 6% when there is just a family history of colon cancer occurring in a first degree relative. Development of colon cancer at an early age, or at multiple sites, or recurrent colon cancer suggests a genetically transmitted form of the disease as opposed to the sporadic form.

Causes and symptoms

Causes

Causes of colon cancer are probably environmental in the sporadic cases, (80%), and genetic in the heredity predisposed cases (20%). Since malignant cells have a changed genetic makeup, this means that in 80% of cases, the environment spontaneously induces change, whereas in those born with a genetic predisposition, they are either destined to get the cancer or it will take less environmental exposure to induce the cancer. Exposure to agents in the environment that may induce mutation is the process of **carcinogenesis** and is caused by agents known as carcinogens (cancer-causing agents). Specific carcinogens have been difficult to identify; however, dietary factors seem to be involved.

Colon cancer is more common in industrialized nations and diets high in fat, red meat, total calories, and alcohol seem to predispose. Diets high in fiber are associated with a decreased risk. The mechanism for protection by high-fiber diets may be related to less exposure of the colon lining to carcinogens from the environment, as the transit time through the bowel is faster with a high-fiber diet than it is with a low fiber diet.

Age plays a definite role in the predisposition to colon cancer. Colon cancer is uncommon before age 40. This incidence increases substantially after age 50 and doubles with each succeeding decade.

There is also a slight increase risk for colon cancer in the individual who smokes.

Patients who suffer from inflammatory diseases of the colon known as ulcerative colitis and Crohn's colitis are also at increased risk.

As for genetic predisposition, on chromosome 5, there is a gene called the APC gene associated with the familial adenomatous polyposis syndrome. There are multiple different mutations that occur at this site, yet they all cause a defect in tumor suppression that results in early and frequent development of colon cancer. This genetic aberration is transmitted to 50% of offspring and each of those affected will develop colon cancer, usually at an early age. There is another syndrome, hereditary non-polyposis colon cancer (also known as Lynch syndrome), related to mutations in any of four genes responsible for DNA mismatch repair. In patients with colon cancer, the p53 gene is mutated 70% of the time. When the p53 gene is mutated and ineffective, cells with damaged DNA escape repair or destruction. This allows for the damaged cell to perpetuate itself, and continued replication of the damaged DNA may lead to tumor development. Though these syndromes have a very high incidence of colon cancer, family history without the syndrome is also a substantial risk factor. When considering first-degree relatives, history of one with colon cancer raises the baseline risk of 2% to 6%. (Most physicians think that this baseline is about 4%.) The presence of a second raises the risk to 17%.

The development of polyps of the colon almost always precedes the development of colon cancer by five or more years. Polyps are benign growths of the colon lining. They can be unrelated to cancer, precancerous, or malignant. Polyps, when identified, are removed for diagnosis. If the polyps are benign, the patient should undergo careful surveillance for the development of more polyps or the development of colon cancer.

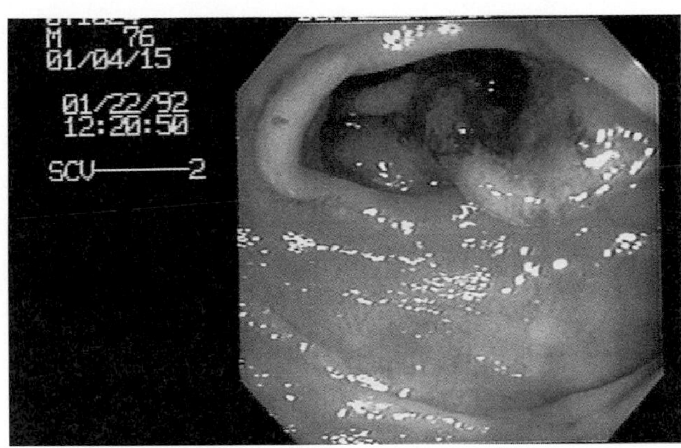

An endoscopic view of a colorectal tumor. *(Custom Medical Stock Photo. Reproduced by permission.)*

Symptoms

Colon cancer causes symptoms related to its local presence in the large bowel or by its effect on other organs if it has spread. These symptoms may occur alone or in combination:

- a change in bowel habit
- blood in the stool
- bloating, persistent abdominal distention
- constipation
- a feeling of fullness even after having a bowel movement
- narrowing of the stool—so-called ribbon stools
- persistent, chronic **fatigue**
- abdominal discomfort
- unexplained **weight loss**
- and, very rarely, **nausea and vomiting**

Most of these symptoms are caused by the physical presence of the tumor mass in the colon. Similar symptoms can be caused by other processes; these are not absolutely specific to colon cancer. The key is recognizing that the persistence of these types of symptoms without ready explanation should prompt the individual to seek medical evaluation.

Many of the symptoms are understood by remembering that the colon is a tubular conduit. If a tumor

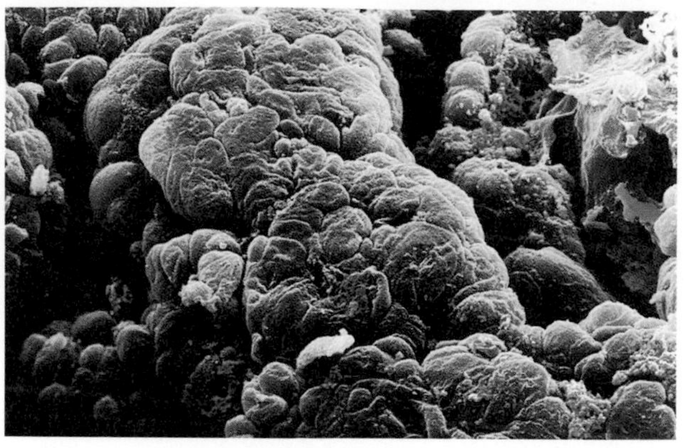

Scanning electron micrograph (SEM) image of the inner surface of the human colon diseased with cancer. *(© Oliver Meckes, Science Source/Photo Researchers, Inc. Reproduced by permission.)*

develops, as it reaches a certain size it will begin to cause symptoms related to the obstruction of that conduit. In addition, the tumor commonly oozes blood that is lost in the stool. (Often, this blood is not visible.) This phenomenon results in **anemia** and chronic fatigue. Weight loss is a late symptom, often implying substantial obstruction or the presence of systemic disease.

Diagnosis

Screening

Of all of the major cancers, only colorectal cancer can be prevented by screening. In all other cancers (breast and prostate, for example), screening tests look for small, malignant lesions. Screening for colorectal cancers, however, is the search for pre-malignant, benign polyps. This screening can be close to 100% effective in preventing cancer development, not just in detecting small cancers.

Screening involves physical exam, simple laboratory tests, and the visualization of the lining of the colon. The ways to visualize the colon epithelium are with x rays (indirect visualization), and endoscopy (direct visualization).

The physical examination involves the performance of a digital rectal exam (DRE). The DRE includes manual examination of the rectum, anus and the prostate. During this examination, the physician examines the anus and the surrounding skin for hemorrhoids, abscesses, and other irregularities. After lubricating the gloved finger and anus, the examiner gently slides the finger into the anus and follows the contours of the rectum. The examiner notes the tone of the anus and feels the walls and the edges for texture, tenderness and masses as far as the examining finger can reach. At the time of this exam, the physician checks the stool on the examining glove with a chemical to see if any occult (invisible), blood is present. At home, after having a bowel movement, the patient is asked to swipe a sample of stool obtained with a small stick on a card. After 3 such specimens are on the card, the card is then easily chemically tested for occult blood also. (The stool analysis mentioned here is known as a **fecal occult blood test**, or FOBT, and, while it can be helpful, it is not 100% accurate—only about 50% of cancers are FOBT-positive.) These exams are accomplished as an easy part of a routine yearly physical exam.

Proteins are sometimes produced by cancers and these may be elevated in the patient's blood. When this occurs, the protein produced is known as a tumor marker. There is a tumor marker for some cancers of the colon; it is known as carcinoembryonic antigen, or CEA. Unfortunately, this protein may be made by other adenocarcinomas as well, or it may not be produced by a particular colon cancer. Therefore, screening by chemical analysis for CEA has not been helpful. CEA has been helpful when used in a follow-up role for patients treated for colon cancer if their tumor makes the protein.

Indirect visualization of the colon may be accomplished by placing barium through the rectum and filling the colon with this compound. Barium produces a white contrast image of the lining of the colon on **x ray** and thus the contour of the lining of the colon may be seen. Detail can be increased if the barium utilized is thinned and air also introduced. These studies are known as the **barium enema** (BE), and the double contrast barium enema (DCBE).

Direct visualization of the lining of the colon is accomplished using a scope or endoscope. The physician introduces the instrument through the rectum and passes it proximally, visualizing the colon epithelium in the process. Older, shorter scopes were rigid. Today, utilizing fiberoptic technology, the scopes are flexible and can reach much farther. If the left colon only is visualized, it is called flexible **sigmoidoscopy**. When the entire colon is visualized, the procedure is known as **colonoscopy**.

Unlike the indirect visualizations of the colon (the BE and the DCBE), the endoscopic screeenings allow the physician to remove polyps and **biopsy** suspicious tissue. (A biopsy is a removal of tissue for examination by a pathologist.) For this reason, many physicians prefer endoscopic screening. All of the visualizations, the BE, DCBE, and each type of endoscopy require pre-procedure preparation (evacuation) of the colon.

The American Cancer Society has recommended the following screening protocol for those of normal risk over 50 years of age:

- yearly DRE with occult blood in stool testing

KEY TERMS

Adenocarcinoma—Type of cancer beginning in glandular epithelium.

Adjuvant therapy—Treatment involving radiation, chemotherapy (drug treatment), or hormone therapy, or a combination of all three given after the primary treatment for the possibility of residual microscopic disease.

Anastomosis—surgical reconnection of the ends of the bowel after removal of a portion of the bowel.

Anemia—The condition caused by too few circulating red blood cells, often manifested in part by fatigue.

Carcinogens—Substances in the environment that cause cancer, presumably by inducing mutations, with prolonged exposure.

Electolytes—Salts, such as sodium and chloride.

Epithelium—Cells composing the lining of an organ.

Lymphatics—Channels that are conduits for lymph.

Lymph nodes—cellular filters through which lymphatics flow.

Malignant—Cells that have been altered such that they have lost normal control mechanisms and are capable of local invasion and spread to other areas of the body.

Metastasis—Site of invasive tumor growth that originated from a malignancy elsewhere in the body.

Mutation—A change in the genetic make up of a cell that may occur spontaneously or be environmentally induced.

Occult blood—Presence of blood that cannot be seen with the naked eye.

Polyps—Localized growths of the epithelium that can be benign, precancerous, or harbor malignancy.

Radical resection—Surgical resection that takes the blood supply and lymph system supplying the organ along with the organ.

Resect—to remove surgically.

Sacrum—Posterior bony wall of the pelvis.

Systemic—Throughout the body.

- flexible sigmoidoscopy at age 50
- flexible sigmoidoscopy repeated every 5 years

Many physicians, however, recommend full colonoscopy every five to seven years. Screening evaluations should start sooner for patients who have predisposing factors, such as family history, history of polyps, or a familial syndrome.

Evaluation of patients with symptoms

For those whose symptoms prompt them to visit their physician, and if their symptoms could possibly be related to colon cancer, the entire colon will be inspected. The combination of a flexible sigmoidoscopy and double contrast barium enema may be performed but the preferred evaluation of the entire colon and rectum is that of complete colonoscopy. Colonoscopy allows direct visualization, photography, as well as the opportunity to obtain a biopsy of any abnormality visualized. If, for technical reasons, the entire colon is not visualized endoscopically, a double contrast barium enema should complement the colonoscopy.

The diagnosis of colon cancer is actually made by the performance of a biopsy of any abnormal lesion in the colon. When a tumor growth is identified, it could be either a benign polyp (or lesion) or a cancer; the biopsy resolves the issue. The endoscopist may take many samples so as to exclude any sampling errors.

If the patient presents with advanced disease, or has advanced disease at the time of diagnosis, areas where the tumor has spread (such as the liver) may be amenable to biopsy. Such biopsies are usually obtained using a special needle under local anesthesia.

Once a diagnosis of colon cancer has been established by biopsy, in addition to the physical exam, studies will be performed to assess the extent of the disease. Blood studies include a complete blood count, liver function tests, and a CEA. **Imaging studies** will include a chest x ray and a CAT scan (**computed tomography** scan) of the abdomen. The chest x ray will determine if there is spread to the lung, the CAT scan will evaluate potential spread to the liver as well as any local invasive characteristics of the primary tumor. If the patient has any neurologic symptoms, a CAT scan of the brain will be performed, and if the patient is experiencing **bone pain**, a bone scan will also be performed.

Treatment team

The surgeon and the medical oncologist each have a role in therapy that is dictated by the degree of progression of the disease. A radiation oncologist may also play a role on the team; however, radiation treatment is rare in colon cancer.

Clinical staging, treatments, and prognosis

Clinical staging

Once the diagnosis has been confirmed by biopsy, the clinical stage of the cancer is assigned. Using the characteristics of the primary tumor, its depth of penetration through the bowel, and the presence or absence of regional or distant metastases, stage is derived. Often, the depth of penetration through the bowel or the presence of regional lymph nodes can't be assigned before surgery.

Colon cancer is assigned stages I through IV, based on the following general criteria:

- Stage I: the tumor is confined to the epithelium or has not penetrated through the first layer of muscle in the bowel wall.
- Stage II: the tumor has penetrated through to the outer wall of the colon or has gone through it, possibly invading other local tissue.
- Stage III: Any depth or size of tumor associated with regional lymph node involvement.
- Stage IV: any of previous criteria associated with distant **metastasis**.

With many cancers other than colon cancer, staging plays an important pre-treatment role to best determine treatment options. In colon cancer, almost all colon cancers are treated with surgery first, regardless of stage. Colon cancers through Stage III, and even some Stage IV colon cancers, are treated with surgery first, before any other treatments are considered.

Treatments

SURGERY. Surgical removal of the involved anatomic segment of colon (**colectomy**) along with its blood supply and regional lymph nodes is the primary therapy for colon cancer. Usually, on the basis of the blood supply, the partial colectomies are separated into right, left, transverse, or sigmoid. The removal of the blood supply at its origin along with the regional lymph nodes that accompany it assures an adequate margin of normal colon on either side of the primary tumor. When the cancer lies in a position such that the blood supply and lymph drainage lies between two of the major vessels, both vessels are taken to assure complete radical resection, or removal (extended radical right or left colectomy). If the primary tumor penetrates through the bowel wall, any tissue adjacent to the tumor extension is also taken if feasible.

Surgery is used as primary therapy for stages I through III colon cancer unless there are signs that local invasion will not permit complete removal of the tumor, as may occur in advanced stage III tumors. However, this circumstance is very rare, and occurs in less than 2% of all colon cancer cases.

After the resection is completed, the ends of the remaining colon are reconstructed; the hook-up is called an anastomosis. Once healing has occurred, there may be a slight increase in the frequency of bowel movements. This effect usually lasts only for several weeks. Most patients go on to develop completely normal bowel function.

Occasionally, the anastomosis would be risky and cannot be performed. (Most commonly, this occurs when the bowel could not be adequately evacuated in an emergency circumstance due to bowel obstruction.) When the anastomosis cannot be performed, a **colostomy** is performed instead. A colostomy is performed by bringing the end of the colon through the abdominal wall and sewing it to the skin. The patient will have to wear an appliance (a bag) to manage the stool. The colostomy may be temporary and the patient may undergo a hook-up at a later, safer date, or the colostomy may be permanent. In most cases, emergent colostomies are not reversed and are permanent.

RADIATION. **Radiation therapy** is used as an adjunct to surgery if there is concern about potential for local recurrence post-operatively and the area of concern will tolerate the radiation. For instance, if the tumor invaded muscle of the abdominal wall but was not completely removed, this area would be considered for radiation. Radiation has significant dose limits when residual bowel is exposed to it because the small and large intestine do not tolerate radiation well.

Radiation is also used in the treatment of patients who present with or progress to having metastatic disease. It is particularly useful in shrinking metastatic colon cancer to the brain.

CHEMOTHERAPY. **Chemotherapy** is useful for patients who have had all identifiable tumor removed and are at risk for recurrence (adjuvant chemotherapy). Chemotherapy may also be used when the cancer is stage IV and is beyond the scope of regional therapy, but this use is rare.

Adjuvant therapy is considered in stage II disease with deep penetration or in stage III patients. Standard therapy is treatment with **fluorouracil**, (5FU) combined with **leucovorin** for a period of 6 to 12 months. 5FU is an antimetabolite and leukovorin improves the response rate. (A response is a temporary regression of the cancer in response to the chemotherapy.) Another agent, **levamisole**, (which seems to stimulate the immune system), may be substituted for leucovorin. These protocols reduce rate of recurrence by about 15% and reduce mortality by about 10%. The regimens do have some toxicity but usually are tolerated fairly well.

Similar chemotherapy may be administered for stage IV disease or if a patient progresses and develops metastases. Results show response rates of about 20%. Unfortunately, these patients eventually succumb to the disease, and this chemotherapy may not prolong survival or improve quality of life in Stage IV patients. **Clinical trials** have now shown that the results can be improved with the addition of another agent to this regimen. **Irinotecan** does not seem to increase toxicity but it improved response rates to 39%, added 2-3 months to disease-free survival, and prolonged overall survival by a little over two months.

Prognosis

Prognosis is the long-term outlook or survival after therapy. Overall, about 50% of patients treated for colon cancer survive the disease. As expected, the survival rates are dependent upon the stage of the cancer at the time of diagnosis, making early detection a very worthwhile endeavor.

About 15% of patients present with stage I disease and 85-90% survive. Stage II represents 20-30% of cases and 65-75% survive. 30-40% comprise the stage III presentation of which 55% survive. The remaining 20-25% present with stage IV disease and are very rarely cured.

Alternative and complementary therapies

Alternative therapies have not been studied in a large-scale, scientific way. Large doses of **vitamins**, fiber, and green tea are among therapies tried. Avoiding **cigarettes** and alcohol may be helpful. Before initiating any alternative therapies, the patient is wise to consult his/her physician to be sure that these therapies do not complicate or interfere with the established therapy.

Coping with cancer treatment

For those with familial syndromes causing colon cancer, genetic counseling may be appropriate. Psychological counseling may be appropriate for anyone having trouble coping with a potentially fatal disease. Local cancer support groups may be helpful and are often identified by contacting local hospitals or the American Cancer Society.

The Colon Cancer Alliance offers internet online support at the following web page: <http://www.ccalliance.org/connect/support.html>.

Clinical trials

Clinical trials are scientific studies in which new therapies are compared to current standards in an effort to identify therapies that give better results.

Agents being tested for efficacy in patients with advanced disease include **oxaliplatin** and CPT-11. Please see reference below for current information available from the National Cancer Institute regarding these clinical trials.

Prevention

There is not an absolute way of preventing colon cancer. Still, there are steps an individual can take to dramatically lessen the risk or to identify the precursors of colon cancer so that it does not manifest itself. The patient with a familial history can enter screening and surveillance programs earlier than the general population. High-fiber diets and vitamins, avoiding obesity, and staying active lessen the risk. Avoiding cigarettes and alcohol may be helpful. By controlling these environmental factors, an individual can lessen risk and to this degree prevent the disease.

By undergoing appropriate screening when uncontrollable genetic risk factors have been identified, an individual may be rewarded by the identification of benign polyps that can be treated as opposed to having these growths degenerate into a malignancy.

Special concerns

Polyps are growths of the epithelium of the colon. They may be completely benign, premalignant or cancerous. The association of colon cancers in patients with certain types of polyps is such that it is thought that many polyps begin as a benign growth and later acquire malignant characteristics. There are two types of polyps, pedunculated and sessile. This terminology comes from their appearance; those that are pedunculated are on a stalk like a mushroom, and the sessile polyps are broad based and have no stalk. Unless a pedunculated polyp gets large, malignant potential is very small. This type may also be easily removed at colonoscopy, by a snaring technique. (A snare is like a lasso introduced through the endoscope to encircle the polyp at its base and amputate it.) The sessile polyp is also known as a villous **adenoma** and as many as 1/3 of these harbor a malignancy. Therefore, the villous adenoma is considered premalignant. Sessile polyps may or may not be able to be managed with the colonoscope and may need surgical removal because of their pre-malignant nature.

Polyps commonly present with occult blood in the stool. Since they are associated with the development of cancer, patients who have developed polyps need to enter a program of careful surveillance.

There is an occasional patient who develops a pattern of metastatic disease that is isolated to either the liver or the lung and the deposit appears to be solitary. When patients have this type of pattern of metastatic disease, especially if there has been a long interval between the primary management and the development of metastasis, they may be considered for surgical resection of the isolated metastasis to effect a cure. In carefully selected patients, long-term survival approaching 20% has been achieved.

When a patient has developed metastatic cancer in the liver alone, a technique of administering chemotherapy directly to the liver is sometimes considered. This is called **hepatic arterial infusion** and requires the placement of a special device into the artery supplying the liver. This method of utilizing chemotherapy has been helpful in carefully selected patients only, and currently is not used as a cure.

Resources

BOOKS

Abelhoff, Martin, MD, James O. Armitage MD, Allen S. Lichter MD, and John E. Niederhuber MD.*Clinical Oncology Library.* Philadelphia: Churchill Livingstone, 1999.

Jorde, Lynn B., Ph.D., John C. Carey MD, Michael J. Bamshad MD, and Raymond L. White, Ph.D. *Medical Genetics,* Second Edition. St. Louis: Mosby, 1999.

Kirkwood,John M., MD, Michael T. Lotze MD, Joyce M. Yasko Ph.D. *Current Cancer Therapeutics,* Third Edition. Philadelphia: Churchill Livingstone, 1998

PERIODICALS

Greenlee, Robert T., Ph.D., MPH, Mary Beth Hill-Harmon, MSPH, Taylor Murray, and Michael Thun, MD, MS. "Cancer Statistics 2001." *CA: A Cancer Journal for Clinicians,* Volume 51 No. 1 (Jan/Feb 2001).

Saltz, Leonard, et al. "Irinotecan plus Fluorouracil and Leucovorin for Metastatic Colorectal Cancer." *The New England Journal of Medicine* Volume 343, No. 13 (September 28, 2000).

ORGANIZATIONS

American Cancer Society. (800) ACS-2345. <http://www.cancer.org>.

Cancer Information Service of the NCI. (1-800-4-CANCER). <http://wwwicic.nci.nih.gov>.

Colon Cancer Alliance. <http://www.ccalliance.org>.

National Cancer Institute Cancer Trials. <http://cancertrials.nci.nih.gov/system>. <http://www.cancertrials.com>.

Richard A. McCartney, M.D.

Colonoscopy

Definition

Colonoscopy is a medical procedure during which a long, flexible, tubular instrument called the colonoscope is used to view the entire inner lining of the colon (large intestine) and the rectum.

Purpose

A colonoscopy is generally recommended when the patient complains of rectal bleeding or has a change in bowel habits or other unexplained abdominal symptoms. The test is frequently used to test for colorectal cancer, especially when polyps or tumor-like growths have been detected using the **barium enema** and other diagnostic tests. Polyps can be removed through the colonoscope and samples of tissue (biopsies) can be taken to test for the presence of cancerous cells.

The test also enables the physician to check for bowel diseases such as ulcerative colitis and Crohn's disease. It is a necessary tool in monitoring patients who have a past history of polyps or **colon cancer**. It may also be used as a screening tool for people at high risk of developing colon cancer, such as those with a strong family history of the disease.

Precautions

Patients who are pregnant or have a history of heart and lung disease and those with blood-clotting problems should tell the doctor about their health history before the procedure. Special precautions may be needed. For instance, a patient with artificial heart valves or a history of infection of the lining of the heart may need to take **antibiotics** to prevent infection. Patients also should tell the doctor about all medications they are taking. The doctor may want the patient to stop taking some drugs, such as aspirin, for a period of time before the procedure. Patients with some intestinal conditions should not have a colonoscopy. Examples of these conditions include acute diverticulitis, acute inflamatory bowel disease, a suspected perforation or break in the intestines, and recent abdominal surgery. Patients must be able to cooperate during the procedure.

Description

The procedure can be done either in the doctor's office or in a special procedure room of a local hospital. An intravenous (IV) line will be started in a vein in the arm. Through the IV line, the patient generally receives a sedative and a pain-killer if needed.

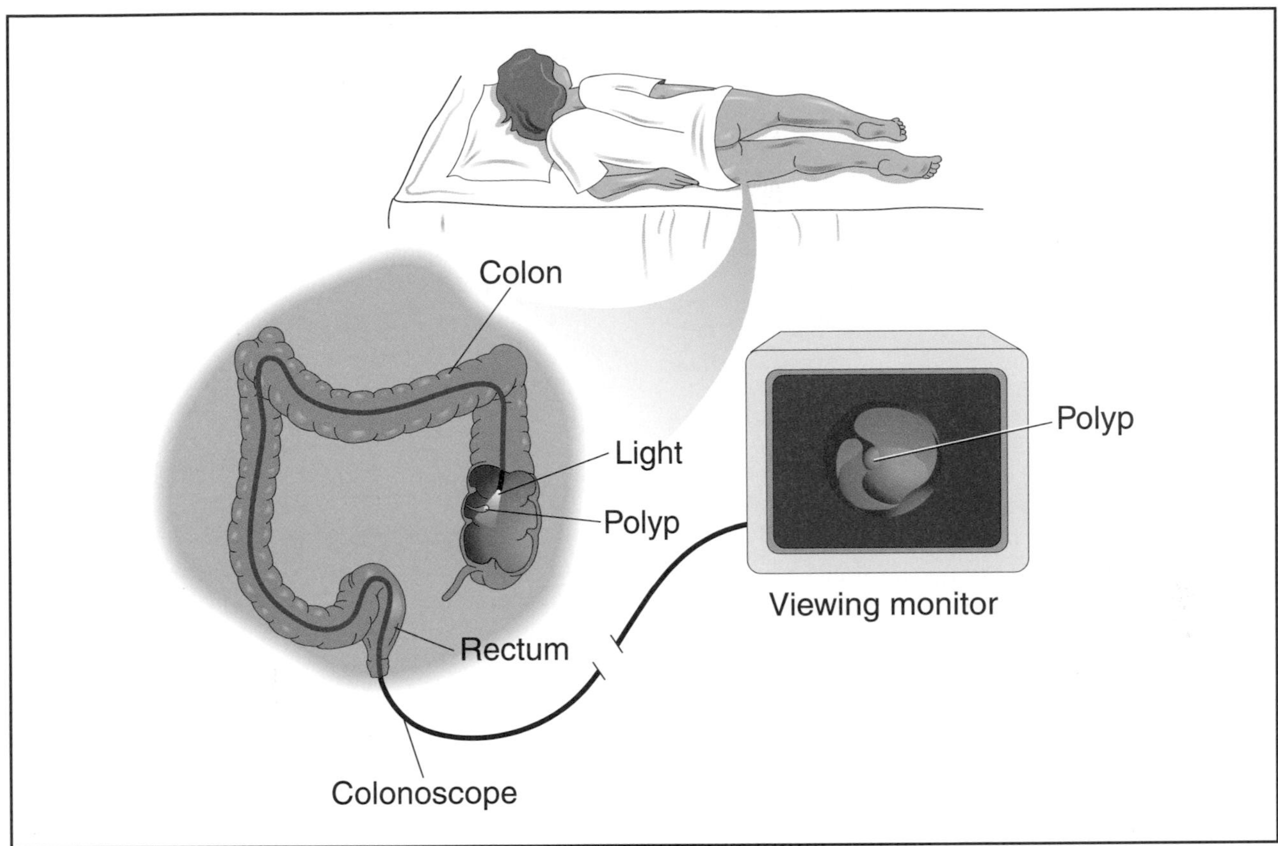

Colonoscopy is a procedure in which a long, flexible, tubular instrument called a colonoscope is inserted into the patient's anus in order to view the lining of the colon and rectum. It is performed to test for colorectal cancer and other bowel diseases and it enables the physician to collect tissue samples for laboratory analysis. *(Illustration by Electronic Illustrators Group.)*

During the colonoscopy, the patient will be asked to lie on his/her left side with his/her knees drawn up toward the abdomen. The doctor begins the procedure by inserting a lubricated, gloved finger into the anus to check for any abnormal masses or blockage. A thin, well-lubricated colonoscope will then be inserted into the anus and it will be gently advanced through the colon. The lining of the intestine will be examined through the scope. Air is pumped through the colonoscope to help clear the path or make it easier to view the lining of the colon. If there are excessive secretions, stool or blood that obstruct the viewing, they will be suctioned out through the scope. The doctor may press on the abdomen or ask the patient to change his/her position in order to advance the scope through the colon.

The entire length of the large intestine can be examined in this manner. If suspicious growths are observed, tiny biopsy forceps or brushes can be inserted through the colonoscope and tissue samples can be obtained. Small polyps can also be removed through the colonoscope. Biopsies and the removal of polyps through the colonoscope are both painless procedures. After the procedure, the colonoscope is slowly withdrawn and the instilled air is allowed to escape. The anal area is then cleansed with tissues.

The procedure may take anywhere from 30 minutes to one hour, depending on how easy it is to advance the scope through the colon.

The bowel cleaning preparation may be tiring and often produces **diarrhea** and cramping. During the colonoscopy, the sedative will keep the patient drowsy and relaxed. Most patients complain of minor discomfort, such as cramping or a feeling of fullness. However, the procedure is not painful.

Preparation

The doctor should be notified if the patient has allergies to any medications or anesthetics, has any bleeding problems, or if a female patient is pregnant. The doctor should also be informed of all the medications that the patient is currently taking and if he or she has had a barium x-ray examination recently. The doctor may instruct the patient not to take certain medications, like aspirin

KEY TERMS

Barium enema—An x-ray test of the bowel after giving the patient an enema of a white chalky substance that outlines the colon and the rectum.

Biopsy—Removal of a tissue sample for examination under the microscope to check for cancer cells.

Colonoscope—A thin, flexible, hollow, lighted tube that in inserted through the rectum into the colon to enable the doctor to view the entire lining of the colon.

Crohn's disease—A chronic inflammatory disease resulting from the immune system attacking one's own body. The disease generally affects the gastrointestinal tract and may cause the formation of deep ulcers.

Diverticulosis—A pouchlike section that bulges through the large intestine's muscular walls but is not inflamed. It may cause bleeding, stomach distress and excess gas.

Pathologist—A doctor who specializes in the diagnosis of disease by studying cells and tissues under a microscope.

Polyps—An abnormal growth that develops on the inside of a hollow organ such as the colon.

Ulcerative colitis—A chronic condition where recurrent ulcers are found in the colon. It is manifested clinically by abdominal cramping, and rectal bleeding.

and anti-inflammatory drugs that interfere with clotting, for a period of time prior to the procedure. If the patient has had heart valves replaced or a history of an inflammation of the inside lining of the heart, the doctor should be informed, so that appropriate antibiotics can be administered to prevent any chance of infection. The risks of the procedure will be explained to the patient before performing the procedure and the patient will be asked to sign a consent form.

It is important that the colon be thoroughly cleaned before performing the examination. Hence, before the examination, considerable preparation is necessary to clear the colon of all stool. The patient will be asked to refrain from eating any solid food for 24–48 hours before the test. Only clear liquids such as juices, broth, and gelatin are recommended. The patient is advised to drink plenty of water to avoid dehydration.

The day before the test, the patient will have to drink a special cleansing solution or take a strong laxative that the doctor has prescribed. The patient will also be given specific instructions as to how to use an enema, as a warm water enema may be necessary the next morning.

On the morning of the examination, one or two enemas of warm tap water may have to be taken. Generally, the procedure has to be repeated until the return from the enema is clear of stool particles. The patient is instructed not to eat or drink anything. The preparatory procedures are extremely important because the colon must be thoroughly clean for the exam to be performed.

Aftercare

After the procedure, the patient is kept under observation until the effects of the medications wear off. The patient will not be able to drive immediately after the procedure and can generally resume a normal diet and usual activities unless otherwise instructed. The patient will be advised to drink lots of fluids to replace those lost by **laxatives** and fasting.

For a few hours after the procedure, the patient may feel groggy. There may be some abdominal cramping and a considerable amount of gas may be passed. If a biopsy was performed or a polyp was removed, there may be small amounts of blood in the stool for a few days. If the patient experiences severe abdominal pain or has persistent and heavy bleeding, it should be brought to the doctor's attention immediately.

Risks

The procedure is considered safe. Very rarely (2 in 1,000 cases) there may be a perforation (a hole) in the intestinal wall. Heavy bleeding due to the removal of the polyp or from the biopsy site occurs very infrequently (1 in 1,000 cases). Infections due to a colonoscopy are also extremely rare. Patients with artificial or abnormal heart valves are usually given antibiotics before and after the procedure to prevent an infection.

Normal results

The results are said to be normal if the lining of the colon is a pale reddish pink and there are no abnormal looking masses that are found in the lining of the colon.

Abnormal results

Abnormal results would imply that polyps or other suspicious-looking masses were detected in the lining of the intestine. Polyps can be removed during the procedure

QUESTIONS TO ASK THE DOCTOR

- Did you see any abnormalities?
- How soon will you know the results of the biopsy (if one was done)?
- When can I resume any medications that were stopped?
- What future care will I need?

and tissue samples can be biopsied. If cancerous cells are detected in the tissue samples, then a diagnosis of colon cancer is made. The pathologist analyzes the tumor cells further to estimate the aggressiveness of the tumor and the extent of spread of the disease.

Abnormal findings also could be due to inflammatory bowel diseases such as ulcerative colitis or Crohn's disease. A condition called diverticulosis, in which many small fingerlike pouches protrude from the colon wall, may also be identified.

Resources

BOOKS

Berkow, Robert et al., eds. *Merck Manual of Diagnosis and Therapy, 17th edition.* Rahway, NJ: Merck Publishing Group, 1999.

Fauci, Anthony S. "Gastrointestinal Endoscopy." In *Harrison's Principles of Internal Medicine,14th edition.* New York, NY: The McGraw-Hill Companies, 2000.

Pfenninger, John L.*Procedures for Primary Care Physicians, 2nd edition.* St. Louis: Mosby, Inc. 2000.

Stauffer, Joseph and Joseph C. Segen. *The Patient's Guide to Medical Tests.* New York: Facts On File, 1997.

ORGANIZATIONS

American Cancer Society (National Headquarters). 1599 Clifton Road, N.E. Atlanta, Georgia 30329. (800) 227-2345. <http://www.cancer.org>

American Gastroenterological Association. 7910 Woodmont Ave., Seventh Floor, Bethesda, MD 20814. Phone: (301) 654-2055. www.gastro.org.

Cancer Research Institute (National Headquarters). 681 Fifth Avenue, New York, N.Y. 10022. (800) 992-2623. <http://www.cancerresearch.org>

National Cancer Institute. 9000 Rockville Pike, Building 31, Room 10A31, Bethesda, Maryland, 20892. (800) 422-6237. <http://www.icic.nci.nih.gov>

Society of American Gastrointestinal Endoscopic Surgeons (SAGES). 2716 Ocean Park Boulevard, Suite 3000, Santa Monica, CA 90405. (310) 314-2404. <http://www.sages.org>

United Ostomy Association, Inc. (UOA). 19772 MacArthur Blvd., Suite 200, Irvine, CA 92612. (800) 826 0826. <http://www.uoa.org.>

Lata Cherath, Ph.D.

Colorectal cancer *see* **Colon cancer; Rectal cancer**

Colostomy

Definition

Ostomy is a surgical procedure used to create an opening for urine or feces to be released from the body. Colostomy refers to a surgical procedure in which a portion of the large intestine is brought through the abdominal wall to carry stool out of the body.

Purpose

A colostomy is created as a result of treatment for various disorders of the large intestine, including cancer, obstruction, inflammatory bowel disease, ruptured diverticulum, ischemia (compromised blood supply), or traumatic injury. Temporary colostomies are created to divert stool from injured or diseased portions of the large intestine, allowing rest and healing. These temporary colostomies are removed at a later date, with restoration of normal bowel function. Permanent colostomies are performed when the distal bowel (bowel at the farthest distance) must be removed or is blocked and inoperable. Although colorectal cancer is the most common indication for a permanent colostomy, only about 10–15% of patients with this diagnosis require a colostomy.

Description

Surgery will result in one of three types of colostomies:

- End colostomy. The functioning end of the intestine (the section of bowel that remains connected to the upper gastrointestinal tract) is brought out to the surface of the abdomen, forming the stoma by cuffing the intestine back on itself and suturing the end to the skin. A stoma is an artificial opening created to the surface of the body. The surface of the stoma is actually the lining of the intestine, usually appearing moist and pink, and it has no pain sensation. The distal portion of bowel (now connected only to the rectum) may be removed, or sutured closed and left in the abdomen. An end

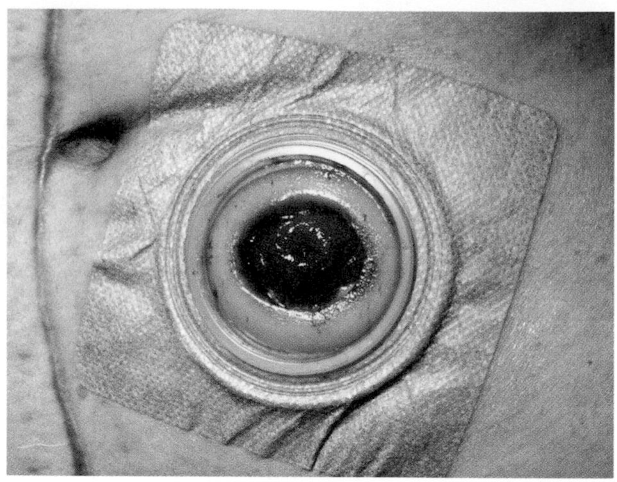

Colostomy stoma with ring for stoma bag. *(Custom Medical Stock Photo. Reproduced by permission.)*

colostomy is usually a permanent ostomy, resulting from trauma, cancer or another pathological condition.

- Double–barrel colostomy. This colostomy involves the creation of two separate stomas on the abdominal wall. The proximal (nearest) stoma is the functional end that is connected to the upper gastrointestinal tract and will drain stool. The distal stoma, connected to the rectum and also called a mucous fistula, drains small amounts of mucus material. This is most often a temporary colostomy performed to rest an area of bowel, and to be later closed.
- Loop colostomy. This colostomy is created by bringing a loop of bowel through an incision in the abdominal wall. An incision is made in the bowel to allow the passage of stool through the loop colostomy. In the past, a plastic rod was used to hold the loop in place, and this supporting rod was removed approximately 7-10 days after surgery, when healing had occurred. The use of the plastic supporting rod is becoming less common. A loop colostomy is most often performed for creation of a temporary stoma to divert stool away from an area of intestine that has been blocked or ruptured.

Preparation

As with any surgical procedure, the patient will be required to sign a consent form after the procedure is explained thoroughly. Blood and urine studies, along with various x rays and an electrocardiograph (ECG) may be ordered as the doctor deems necessary. If possible, the patient should visit an enterostomal therapist, who will mark an appropriate place on the abdomen for the stoma, and offer pre-operative education on ostomy management.

In order to empty and cleanse the bowel, the patient may be placed on a low-residue diet for several days prior to surgery. A liquid diet may be ordered for at least the day before surgery, with nothing by mouth after midnight. A series of enemas and/or oral preparations (GoLytely or Colyte) may be ordered to empty the bowel of stool. Oral **antibiotics** (neomycin, erythromycin, or kanamycin sulfate) may be given to decrease bacteria in the intestine and help prevent post-operative infection. A nasogastric tube may be inserted from the nose to the stomach on the day of surgery or during surgery to remove gastric secretions and prevent **nausea and vomiting**. A urinary catheter (a thin plastic tube) may also be inserted to keep the bladder empty during surgery, giving more space in the surgical field and decreasing chances of accidental injury.

Aftercare

Post-operative care for the patient with a new colostomy involves monitoring of blood pressure, pulse, respiration, and temperature. Breathing tends to be shallow because of the effect of anesthesia and the patient's reluctance to breathe deeply and experience pain caused by the abdominal incision. The patient is instructed how to support the operative site during deep breathing and coughing, and given pain medication as necessary. Fluid intake and output is measured, and the operative site is observed for color and amount of wound drainage.

Two to three days after the operation, the patient will be able to resume eating. For both open and laparoscopic resections, most patients are discharged from the hospital in five to seven days. Healing may take one to two months.

A colostomy pouch will generally have been placed on the patient's abdomen, around the stoma during surgery. During the hospital stay, the patient and caregivers will be educated about how to care for the colostomy. Determination of appropriate pouching supplies and a schedule of how often to change the pouch should be established. Regular assessment and meticulous care of the skin surrounding the stoma is important to maintain an adequate surface on which to apply the pouch. Some patients with colostomies are able to routinely irrigate the stoma, resulting in regulation of bowel function; rather than needing to wear a pouch, these patients may need only a dressing or cap over their stoma. Often, an enterostomal therapist will visit the patient at home after discharge to help the patient resume normal daily activities.

Risks

Potential complications of colostomy surgery include:

- excessive bleeding

- surgical wound infection
- thrombophlebitis (inflammation and blood clot to veins in the legs)
- pneumonia
- pulmonary embolism (blood clot or air bubble in the lungs' blood supply)

Normal results

Complete healing is expected without complications. The period of time required for recovery from the surgery varies depending on the patient's overall health prior to surgery. The colostomy patient without other medical complications should be able to resume all daily activities once recovered from the surgery.

Abnormal results

The doctor should be made aware of any of the following problems after surgery:

- increased pain, swelling, redness, drainage or bleeding in the surgical area
- headache, muscle aches, dizziness or **fever**
- increased abdominal pain or swelling, constipation, nausea or vomiting or black, tarry stools

Stomal complications to be monitored include:

- Death (necrosis) of stomal tissue. Caused by inadequate blood supply, this complication is usually visible 12–24 hours after the operation and may require additional surgery.
- Retraction (stoma is flush with the abdomen surface or has moved below it). Caused by insufficient stomal length, this complication may be managed by use of special pouching supplies. Elective revision of the stoma is also an option.
- Prolapse (stoma increases length above the surface of the abdomen). Most often results from an overly large opening in the abdominal wall or inadequate fixation of the bowel to the abdominal wall. Surgical correction is required when blood supply is compromised.
- Stenosis (narrowing at the opening of the stoma). Often associated with infection around the stoma or scarring. Mild stenosis can be removed under local anesthesia. Severe stenosis may require surgery for reshaping the stoma.
- Parastomal hernia (bowel causing bulge in the abdominal wall next to the stoma). Usually due to placement of the stoma where the abdominal wall is weak or creation of an overly large opening in the abdominal wall. The use of an ostomy support belt and special pouching supplies may be adequate. If severe, the defect in the abdominal wall should be repaired and the stoma moved to another location.

KEY TERMS

Diverticulum—Pouches that project off the wall of the intestine, visible as opaque on an x ray after the patient has swallowed a contrast (dye) substance.

Embolism—Blockage of a blood vessel by any small piece of material traveling in the blood. The emboli may be caused by germs, air, blood clots, or fat.

Enema—Insertion of a tube into the rectum to infuse fluid into the bowel and encourage a bowel movement. Ordinary enemas contain tap water, mixtures of soap and water, glycerin and water, or other materials.

Intestine—Commonly called the bowels, divided into the small and large intestine. They extend from the stomach to the anus. The small intestine is about 20 ft (6 m) long. The large intestine is about 5 ft (1.5 m) long.

Ischemia—A compromise in blood supply delivered to body tissues that causes tissue damage or death.

Ostomy—A surgically created opening in the abdomen for elimination of waste products (urine or stool).

Resources

BOOKS

Doughty, Dorothy. *Urinary and Fecal Incontinence.* St. Louis: Mosby-Year Book, Inc., 1991.

Hampton, Beverly and Ruth Bryant. *Ostomies and Continent Diversions.* St. Louis: Mosby-Year Book, Inc., 1992.

Monahan, Frances. *Medical-Surgical Nursing.* Philadelphia: W. B. Saunders Company, 1998.

Murphy, Gerald P. et al. *American Cancer Society Textbook of Clinical Oncology.* Atlanta, Georgia: American Cancer Society, 1995, pp.72-73.

Suddarth, Doris. *The Lippincott Manual of Nursing.* Philadelphia: J. B. Lippincott, 1991.

PERIODICALS

Edwards, D. P. et al. "Stoma -related complications are more frequent after transverse colostomy than loop ileostomy: a prospective randomized clinical trial." *British Journal of Surgery.* March 2001 88:3, pp. 360-363.

Whitehead, William E. et al. "Treatment options for Fecal Incontinence." *Diseases of the Colon and Rectum.* January 2001 44:1, pp. 131-144.

ORGANIZATIONS

The United Ostomy Association, a self-help organization, provides useful information. 36 Executive Park, Suite 120, Irvine, CA 92714. Phone: (800) 826-0826 or (714) 660-8624. uoa@deltanet.com. <http://www.uoa.org.>

Wound Ostomy and Continence Nurses Society. 2755 Bristol Street, Suite 110, Costa Mesa, CA 92626. (714) 476-0268. <http://www.wocn.org>.

Kathleen Dredge Wright

Complementary cancer therapies

Definition

Alternative and complementary therapies refer to treatments outside the mainstream of Western scientific medicine. They cover a wide variety of approaches, ranging from the medical systems of other cultures to special diets or medications, spiritual practices, herbal remedies, and external energy sources. As a general rule, *complementary* is used to refer to treatments that are offered alongside mainstream methods of cancer therapy to relieve the patient's discomfort or contribute to his or her overall sense of well-being. Other terms that are sometimes used for complementary therapies are *adjunctive*, which means helping or assisting, and *supportive*. Complementary or supportive treatments are not considered cures for cancer. When they are given together with mainstream cancer treatments, the combination is called *integrative* therapy.

The word *alternative* refers to treatments used instead of mainstream cancer treatments in an attempt to cure cancer. Some alternative treatments have not yet been tested by scientific researchers while others have been tested and shown not to work. If alternative remedies are used instead of proven cancer treatments, they may harm the patient by allowing the cancer to grow and reducing the chances of curing it by standard therapies. Treatments that are still being tested on animals or humans are called research or investigational therapies. In the United States, medications or other methods of treatment must be approved by the Food and Drug Administration (FDA) before they can be considered standard treatments for cancer. In 1991, Congress established the Office of Alternative Medicine as part of the National Institutes of Health. It includes the National Center for Complementary and Alternative Medicine, or NCCAM. As of October 2000, NCCAM supports 15 specialized research centers that study the safety and effectiveness of various complementary and alternative medicine (CAM) treatments for cancer.

Description

Today there are over two hundred complementary/alternative substances and treatment methods that have been given to cancer patients. They can be grouped for purposes of discussion into ten major categories.

Biologic

Biologic treatments are drugs or other medical products that are derived naturally from plants, animals, or the human body itself. They are thought to help the body fight cancer by restoring its biochemical balance.

Many biologic treatments have already been tested by researchers. They vary widely in their effectiveness:

- Antineoplaston therapy. Antineoplastons, which are extracted from blood serum and urine, are short-chain amino acids that supposedly reprogram the DNA of cancer cells so that the cells reproduce normally instead of uncontrollably. The FDA and National Cancer Institute (NCI) have permitted **clinical trials** of antineoplastons in cancer patients. However, the clinical trials were closed in 1995 because of small enrollment numbers in the trials and lack of consensus about how to recruit more patients for the trials. Because of the small numbers in the trials, the NCI draws no conclusions about the effectiveness of antineoplastons. Antineoplaston therapy can be used with standard **chemotherapy**.
- 714X. 714X is a treatment consisting of three 21-day rounds of injections of camphor and organic salts directly into the lymphatic system. It is based on a theory that cancer cells use up large amounts of nitrogen and secrete a poisonous K-cofactor that paralyzes the immune system so that nitrogen can be drawn from healthy cells. Since the camphor in 714X contains nitrogen, the cancer cells do not have to secrete the K-cofactor, which in turn allows the immune system to recover.
- Cancell/Entelev. Cancell/Entelev is a liquid marketed as a treatment for cancer as well as AIDS, epilepsy, lupus, and other diseases. It is also sold as Cantron, Sheridan's Formula, Jim's Juice, and Crocinic Acid. Cancell is a mixture of 12 common chemicals—including nitric acid and sulfuric acid—none of which are known to be effective against cancer. The NCI tested Cancell four times between 1978 and 1991; no benefit to this therapy could be demonstrated, and the NCI decided not to study it further.

- Hydrazine sulfate. Hydrazine sulfate is a chemical that has been used to treat the loss of appetite (**anorexia**) and wasting away of body tissue (cachexia) that occur in late-stage cancer; it has not been promoted as a cure for cancer. It is available in the United States as a dietary supplement. Hydrazine sulfate has been studied by the Russian government as well as the NCI, but test results are not conclusive. As of 2001, no clinical trials of hydrazine sulfate are being conducted in the United States.
- Laetrile. Laetrile, which is also known as amygdalin or vitamin B_{17}, is a chemical found in fruit pits, lima beans, sorghum, and clover; it contains sugar and produces cyanide. The cyanide is considered to be the primary anti-cancer agent in laetrile. Laetrile has been used by itself to treat cancer and as part of metabolic therapy, but it has not shown any anti-cancer effectiveness in NCI clinical trials. It is not approved for use in the United States but is available in Mexico. When taken by mouth, laetrile can produce side effects resembling the symptoms of cyanide poisoning.
- Hydrogen peroxide therapy. Hydrogen peroxide has been used in the United States and Japan since the 1960s as an adjunctive treatment to **radiation therapy**. The hydrogen peroxide is diluted in water and injected directly into the patient's arteries. Some researchers think that hydrogen peroxide helps to shrink tumors by making them more sensitive to radiation.

Metabolic therapies

Metabolic therapies combine enzyme treatments, diets, and nutritional supplements with herbal medicines or special formulas. They are based on the belief that cancer results from many factors acting together, and that it should be treated by strengthening the entire body, not just by removing the tumor.

Most of these therapies are considered questionable by mainstream physicians:

- Kelley/Gonzalez therapy. Kelley/Gonzalez therapy focuses on cancer of the pancreas. Its practitioners regard cancer as resulting from inadequate levels of pancreatic enzymes, which help the body to digest protein. Kelley/Gonzalez therapy includes a diet tailored to each individual, nutritional supplements, digestive aids, enzyme supplements, and colonic irrigation. It is the most promising of the metabolic therapies. As of 2001, the NCI is conducting clinical trials of Kelley/Gonzalez therapy at Columbia University.
- Gerson therapy. Gerson therapy combines a low-salt vegan diet with large quantities of fruit and vegetable juices, as well as three or four coffee enemas each day to detoxify the body. It is based on the notion that cancer patients have too much sodium in their bodies and not enough potassium. Gerson therapy is not recommended as an alternative to conventional treatment for cancer.
- Issel's whole-body therapy. This form of metabolic therapy originated in Germany. It includes psychotherapy, oxygen therapy, and the removal of amalgam dental fillings (which contain small amounts of mercury) as well as a special diet.
- Revici therapy. Revici therapy is based on the belief that cancer is associated with imbalances in the body's tissue-building and tissue-breakdown processes. These imbalances are treated with intravenous injections of lipids (fatty or waxy organic substances) containing oxygen, copper, calcium, and selenium.

Immune enhancement therapies

Immune enhancement therapies are based on the theory that cancers in humans result from a weakened immune system.

Therapies in this category are not recommended as alternatives to conventional cancer treatment:

- Immuno-augmentative therapy (IAT). IAT is based on the theory that cancer results from an imbalance among four blood protein components, called the tumor antibody, the tumor complement, the blocking protein, and the deblocking protein. Treatment consists of injecting various amounts of these components to restore the proper balance.
- Livingston therapy. Livingston therapy uses a raw-food vegetarian diet combined with nutritional supplements and **vaccines** to restore the patient's immune system. It is based on a theory that cancer is caused by a bacterium called progenitor cryptocides, found in eggs, milk, poultry, and beef products.

Bodywork/movement therapies

Doctors often recommend bodywork and movement therapies as adjunctive treatments for cancer because they benefit patients emotionally as well as physically. The exercise involved in dance therapy, yoga, and t'ai chi helps to preserve muscle tone and joint flexibility. Therapeutic massage can relieve muscle soreness resulting from emotional stress.

Some common forms of body work and movement therapy include:

- Acupuncture and acupressure. Acupuncture is a basic form of treatment in traditional Chinese medicine. It involves the insertion of very thin steel needles into points on the body associated with the flow of vital energy. In acupressure, the energy points are stimulated by finger pressure. These forms of treatment are often combined with massage.

- Chiropractic. A chiropractor treats the patient's nervous system by manipulating or adjusting the segments of the spinal column. Some people find that chiropractic relieves back pain. As of 2001, one of the NCCAM's 15 research centers is specializing in studies of chiropractic.
- Yoga. Yoga is a good form of low-impact exercise for releasing stress and tension. Its stretches and poses can be modified to fit the needs or limitations of individual patients. Cancer patients who have had surgery should consult their doctor before starting a yoga program.
- T'ai chi. T'ai chi is a Chinese system of meditative exercise that involves a series of slow circular or stretching movements. Many patients find it relaxing and calming. In clinical settings, control groups practicing t'ai chi showed improvements in symptoms and signs such as strength, appetite, weight gain, stamina, and bowel function, hence increasing the ability for self-cure. In addition, t'ai chi and related practices are simple to learn and produce no side effects.
- Therapeutic massage. Therapeutic massage is often recommended as a complementary treatment to mainstream cancer therapy, but should not be given near the area of any recent surgery.
- Dance therapy. Dance therapy allows patients to release strong emotions as well as exercising their joints and muscles.

Diets and digestive treatments

These forms of treatment are based on the belief that the human digestive tract stores or produces toxic substances and should be cleansed periodically by special foods, fasting, or washing out the lower bowel.

Dietary therapies vary in their usefulness as complementary cancer treatments:

- Vegan diets. Vegan diets are vegetarian diets that omit eggs and dairy products as well as meat. They are thought to offer some protection against cancer, because the milk as well as the tissues of animals raised for meat may contain carcinogenic (cancer-causing) chemicals. In addition, the high fiber content of vegan diets appears to lower the risk of colon cancer.
- Fasting and juice therapies. These therapies are a major part of naturopathic treatment. Naturopaths maintain that the body can devote more of its energy to healing itself when it does not have to digest high-fat, high-calorie foods. In addition, they regard fasting as a way to help the body rid itself of toxic wastes.
- Macrobiotics. Macrobiotic diets originated in Japan, and classify foods according to the Eastern distinction between yin and yang rather than Western nutritional categories. These diets emphasize brown rice, fruits and vegetables eaten in season, and cooking over a flame rather than using electricity. Although macrobiotic diets have been credited with preventing or curing cancer, no scientific studies have verified these claims.
- Colonic irrigation. This is a treatment method that circulates warm water through the patient's large intestine to remove feces and toxic substances from the walls of the colon. It has been recommended by some alternative therapists for AIDS-related cancers.

Herbal therapies and food supplements

Herbal treatments are historically important because of their role in the development of a number of standard medications. Complementary herbal treatments are presently used to relieve the side effects of mainstream cancer therapy, such as peppermint tea for nausea or ginger for **diarrhea**. Patients should, however, consult a health professional before taking any herbal preparation by mouth to make sure that the herb(s) will not interact with prescription medications. Fragrant herbs (rosemary, lemongrass, mint, etc.) can be added to massage oils or bath water for aromatherapy.

Other herbal therapies and dietary supplements have been advertised as cures for cancer:

- Hoxsey formulas. The Hoxsey formulas are herbal remedies for external as well as internal use. The external Hoxsey formula contains bloodroot, which was used by some Native Americans to treat cancer. The internal formula is a mixture of red clover, buckthorn, burdock, licorice root, and several other herbs. The American Cancer Society placed the Hoxsey formulas on its list of unproven methods in 1968.
- Cartilage. Both bovine (cow) and shark cartilage are available in the United States as dietary supplements. Shark cartilage is presently being studied as a cancer treatment in clinical trials approved by the FDA. It appears to slow down or stop the formation of new blood vessels (angiogenesis) in tumors in animals. As of 2001, however, it is not clear that shark cartilage is an effective anti-cancer treatment in humans.
- Coenzyme Q_{10}. Coenzyme Q_{10}, also known as vitamin Q_{10}, ubiquinone, or ubidecarenone, is a compound that occurs naturally in the human body. It appears to help cells produce energy and to stimulate the immune system. Coenzyme Q_{10} has not been investigated widely as a treatment for cancer in humans as of 2001, but it has been reported to lengthen the survival of cancer

patients. It is sold in the United States as a dietary supplement.

- Mistletoe. Mistletoe (*Viscum album*) is a parasitic plant that has been shown to kill cancer cells in laboratory tests and stimulate the immune system. Although the leaves and berries are toxic to humans, mistletoe extracts are available over the counter in Europe and Asia. There is no clinical evidence that mistletoe is an effective treatment for human cancer, and mistletoe extracts have not been approved for sale in the United States.
- Pau d'arco. Pau d'arco comes from a tree in the South American rainforest. The bark is dried and used to brew a medicinal tea. Pau d'arco was investigated by the NCI for possible anti-tumor effectiveness, but the study concluded in 1974 that a dose strong enough to shrink tumors in humans would have toxic side effects. In small doses, however, pau d'arco tea does appear to stimulate the immune system. It can be purchased in the United States in health food stores.
- Essiac tea. Essiac is a mixture of herbs including burdock, slippery elm inner bark, sheep sorrel, Turkish rhubarb, watercress, red clover, and kelp. Promoters of Essiac claim that the tea strengthens the immune system, relieves pain, increases appetite, reduces tumor size, and extends survival. Some also claim that it cleanses the blood, promotes cell repair, restores energy levels, and detoxifies the body. Despite testimonials, there is no scientific evidence to support the use of this mixture for cancer treatment. NCI studies of Essiac in 1983 found no anticancer activity. However, serious side effects from these herbs are rare, and patients may benefit psychologically from the treatment.

External energy therapies

Treatments in this category are based on the belief that there are forms of energy in the universe that can be tapped for purposes of human healing. These energies, which are sometimes called "subtle energies," are thought to be present in mineral formations, plants, the earth's magnetic field, the spectrum of visible light, interpersonal contact, and certain structures or energy fields within the human body itself. Most practitioners of external energy therapies do not ask cancer patients to avoid or give up conventional treatment methods.

The most common forms of external energy therapies include:

- Crystal/gemstone healing. Crystal or gemstone healing is based on the theory that the human body is surrounded by an invisible energy field, or aura, and that the color or crystal structure of a gemstone or mineral can transmit healing energy to the body through the aura.
- Shamanism. Shamanism is the belief that certain persons (shamans) have unusual spiritual powers that can be used for healing. The shaman (who may be a woman in some traditions) acts as an intermediary between the patient and supernatural beings or powers. Native American healers are one type of shaman.
- Bach flower remedies. The 38 Bach flower remedies are tinctures of wildflowers discovered by an English homeopath in the 1920s. They are said to assist physical healing by clearing up negative emotional states or conditions.
- Light/color therapy. Light or color treatment combines the physical effects of the different wavelengths in visible light with the psychological or symbolic meanings attached to specific colors. The practitioner may suggest wearing or visualizing certain colors, or shine colored lights on specific energy points on the patient's body.
- Reiki. Reiki is a holistic approach based on Eastern concepts of universal life energy in which the practitioner holds her or his hands in symbolic patterns over the affected part of the patient's body. It is not a form of massage. Reiki can be used for self-healing as well as treating someone else.
- Therapeutic touch. Therapeutic touch resembles Reiki in that the practitioner is thought to transmit universal energy or "life force" to the patient. Instead of touching the patient directly, however, the practitioner passes his or her hands over the patient's energy field, two to four inches above the body.

Mind- and spirituality-based approaches

Mind-based or spirituality-based approaches draw on the mental and spiritual dimensions of human beings to treat the physical side effects of cancer treatment. They are related to the belief that all dimensions of a person's being should be involved in cancer treatment, and that the mind and spirit can affect or influence physical processes.

These approaches are frequently recommended by health professionals as complementary treatments that allow patients to regain a sense of personal effectiveness and active participation in their lives:

- Prayer. Prayer has been shown in over a hundred reputable double-blind clinical studies to have positive effects on anxiety, high blood pressure, headaches, heart disease, and wounds. As of 2001, NCCAM is conducting a study of the effects of prayer on **breast cancer** in African-American women.
- Meditation. Meditation is helpful in relieving stress, pain, and other side effects of cancer treatment. There are several different approaches to meditation, such as using a mantra (a sacred word or phrase), chanting, focusing on a visual image, or focusing on one's breath.

KEY TERMS

Adjunctive—Any form of therapy that is considered to help or assist a patient's primary treatment.

Alternative—A form of treatment outside mainstream medicine that is used as a cure instead of standard treatments.

Angiogenesis—The formation of blood vessels. Shark cartilage is undergoing tests on its effects on angiogenesis in tumors.

Anorexia—Loss of appetite. Anorexia is a common side effect of chemotherapy.

Aura—The field of subtle energy that surrounds the human body, according to external energy therapists.

Biologics—Drugs or other medical products made from biological sources.

Cachexia—The wasting away of body tissue.

Complementary—Any form of treatment outside the mainstream that is not considered a cure but is given to ease symptoms or contribute to general well-being.

Detoxification—Ridding the body of digestive wastes considered toxic through fasting, drinking large quantities of juice, or colonic irrigation.

Holistic—Any approach to health care that emphasizes the patient's total well-being, including psychological and spiritual as well as physical aspects.

Integrative—An approach to cancer treatment that combines mainstream therapies with one or more complementary therapies.

Investigational—A drug or therapy that is approved for use in clinical trials but not for regular treatment of patients.

Mantra—A sacred word or phrase, used in some forms of meditation to deepen the meditative state.

Quackery—A fraudulent form of treatment or therapy.

Vegan—A vegetarian who omits all animal products, including eggs and milk, from their diet.

- Biofeedback. Biofeedback is a method of learning to modify certain body functions (temperature, heart rate, etc.) related to relaxation with the help of electronic monitors. Eventually, the patient can learn to control his or her relaxation responses without feedback from the machine.
- Hypnosis. Hypnosis is often recommended to lower anxiety and relieve pain. Patients can be hypnotized by a therapist or taught to hypnotize themselves. Hypnosis and biofeedback have both been shown to ease chemotherapy-related nausea and anticipatory nausea (queasiness caused by psychological triggers, such as the sight of the chemotherapy room or smell of treatment chemicals).
- Imagery and visualization. Patients are asked to picture or create an inner image that symbolizes their resistance to cancer. They might visualize their medications as a fire burning up their cancer cells, or their white blood cells as soldiers fighting the enemy.

Sensory-based therapies

Treatments in this category are often used in integrative treatment plans. They are given to help cancer patients cope with the side effects of radiation or chemotherapy, to provide positive sensory experiences, and to improve overall quality of life.

Sensory-based treatments include:

- Aromatherapy. Aromatherapy is the use of fragrances—usually the essential oils of flowers and other plant parts—to relax cancer patients or lift their spirits. The fragrant oils are used to scent oil for massage or added to bath water.
- Art therapy. Art therapy allows cancer patients to express their feelings through their creations and to find satisfaction in learning new skills or techniques. Art therapy may include painting, sculpture, making pottery, quilting, metalwork, print making, photography, or other activities.
- Journaling. Keeping a journal can aid a patient's psychological well being by providing an emotional and creative outlet. Journaling also offers an arena in which patients can sort out thoughts and concerns about their disease.
- Music therapy. Music therapy can be used to help patients relax, release feelings of sadness or anger, or participate in a group activity. It can involve making music as well as listening to it.
- Pet therapy. Pet therapy is the use of trained animals (usually cats, small dogs, birds, or rabbits) in hospital

settings to provide comfort and companionship to cancer patients. Petting and talking to the animals has been shown to benefit patients psychologically and physically.

Traditional approaches

Some of the therapies in this category developed outside the European medical tradition, while the last two developed in the West during the eighteenth and nineteenth centuries:

- Native American medicine. Specific beliefs about the causes of disease vary among the five hundred tribes of Native Americans. In general, however, Native American medicine emphasizes the importance of people living in beauty, harmony, and peace with one another and with their environment. Native American healing rituals are most often used as complementary treatments within integrative treatment plans.
- Ayurveda. Ayurveda is the traditional medical system of India. It emphasizes identifying a person's physical and psychological constitution as part of the healing process. Treatments include dietary recommendations and herbal or mineral remedies.
- Traditional Chinese medicine (TCM). TCM includes five major forms of treatment: diet, exercise, acupuncture, massage, and traditional herbal remedies. It regards human health as resulting from balancing the various vital energies within the human body and keeping the body in harmony with its external environment. As of 2001, the Center for Cancer Complementary Medicine at Johns Hopkins is conducting two studies of Chinese herbal remedies.
- Homeopathy. Homeopathy is a system of treating disease with extremely small doses of substances that would produce symptoms in a healthy person similar to those of the disease being treated. For example, a homeopathic practitioner might give a feverish patient belladonna, which can cause **fever** in a healthy person.
- Naturopathy. Naturopathy is an approach to healing that rejects surgery and synthetic drugs. Naturopaths recommend vitamin supplements, natural herbal remedies, diets, and fasting to assist the body's natural healing processes.

Special concerns

Because complementary and alternative therapies vary so widely in their underlying assumptions, their claims to effectiveness, their licensing standards for practitioners, and the materials and equipment involved in their use, patients should talk to their doctor before beginning any complementary or alternative form of treatment. Patients should also investigate said treatments and the practitioner's level of experience in this area.

Surgery

Cancer patients who have had recent surgery should consult their doctor before starting yoga, t'ai chi, or any other form of movement therapy. In addition, Swedish massage and certain forms of deep tissue massage are not suitable for patients who have not fully recovered from surgery.

Clinical trials

Patients who are interested in a specific complementary or alternative therapy may wish to participate in a study of that treatment. Information about CAM trials can be obtained from the NCI's CancerNet at <http://www.cancernet.nci.nih.gov/cam>.

Fraudulent treatments

False claims about a treatment, such as stating that it cures or prevents cancer when it is known to be useless, are sometimes referred to as "quackery." Several groups and organizations can help patients evaluate questionable therapies.

Treatment decisions

Patients considering CAM therapies should ask their doctor:

- What does the treatment claim to do? Cure cancer? Increase the effectiveness of standard treatments? Or relieve symptoms or side effects?
- How is the practitioner licensed or credentialed? For example, there are licensing boards in most states for massage therapists, acupuncturists, practitioners of Chinese medicine, yoga instructors, and homeopaths.
- Is the treatment based on specific theories about the causes of cancer? How are these theories regarded by mainstream health professionals?
- Is the treatment associated with specific types of cancer, such as cancers of the digestive tract or the nervous system?
- Does the treatment have any restrictions or side effects of its own?
- Is the treatment recommended for other diseases or conditions, or only for cancer?
- How is the treatment advertised or promoted? In medical journals, mainstream health publications, the mass media, or only in "New Age" or special-interest magazines?

Patients should look for "red flags" that may indicate that a treatment is fraudulent:

- The treatment is unusually expensive.

- It is based on unproven or discredited theories.
- It claims to be a "secret" offered by only a few providers.
- Patients must go outside the United States or Canada for the treatment.
- Patients are told not to use standard cancer treatments.
- The treatment lacks any connection to reputable licensing bodies, medical schools, research institutions, or cancer organizations.

Resources

BOOKS

Altman, Nathaniel. *Oxygen Healing Therapies for Optimum Health and Vitality.* Rochester, VT: Healing Arts Press, 1995.

American Cancer Society. *The American Cancer Society's Guide to Complementary and Alternative Cancer Methods.* New York: American Cancer Society, 2000.

Borysenko, Joan, Ph.D.. *Minding the Body, Mending the Mind.* Reading, MA: Addison-Wesley Publishing Co., Inc., 1987. Dr. Borysenko has worked as a cancer researcher at Tufts Medical School as well as Director of the Mind/Body Clinic at Harvard University.

The Burton Goldberg Group. *Alternative Medicine: The Definitive Guide.* Fife, WA: Future Medicine Publishing, Inc., 1995.

Cassileth, Barrie R., Ph.D.. "Questionable and Unproven Cancer Therapies." In *Cancer Therapy.* Dollinger, Malin, MD, Ernest H. Rosenbaum, MD, and Greg Cable, eds. Kansas City, MO: Andrews and McMeel, 1994.

Chiazzari, Suzy. "Healing with Color." In *The Complete Book of Color: Using Color for Lifestyle, Health, and Well-Being.* Boston: Element Books Ltd., 1998.

Collinge, William, Ph.D.. *Subtle Energy: Awakening to the Unseen Forces in Our Lives.* New York: Warner Books, 1998.

Dass, Ram. *Journey of Awakening: A Meditator's Guidebook.* New York: Bantam Books, 1978. An excellent brief guide to the different methods of meditation in all the major religious traditions, as well as an introduction to the practice itself.

Dossey, Larry, MD. *Healing Words: The Power of Prayer and the Practice of Medicine.* New York: HarperCollins, 1993. Dr. Dossey is affiliated with the NIH's Office of Alternative Medicine.

Feuerstein, Georg, and Stephan Bodian. *Living Yoga: A Comprehensive Guide for Daily Life.* New York: Jeremy P. Tarcher/Perigee Books, 1993.

Kabat-Zinn, Jon. *Full Catastrophe Living: Using the Wisdom of Your Body and Mind to Face Stress, Pain, and Illness.* New York: Dell Publishing, 1990. The author is the director of the Stress Reduction Clinic at the University of Massachusetts Medical Center.

Mehl-Madrona, Lewis, M.D.*Coyote Medicine: Lessons from Native American Healing.* New York: Fireside, 1997.

Melody. *Love Is in the Earth—A Kaleidoscope of Crystals,* 2nd ed. Wheat Ridge, CO: Earth-Love Publishing House, 1997.

Murray, Michael, ND, and Joseph Pizzorno, ND. *Encyclopedia of Natural Medicine.* Rocklin, CA: Prima Publishing, 1991. Parts I and II explain the theories and principles of naturopathy.

National Cancer Institute of the National Institutes of Health. *Chemotherapy and You: A Guide to Self-Help During Cancer Treatment.* NIH Publication #99-1136. Can be downloaded from <http://cancernet.nci.nih.gov>.

Price, Shirley. *Practical Aromatherapy.* London: Thorsons, 1994.

Reid, Daniel P. *Chinese Herbal Medicine.* Boston: Shambhala, 1993.

Stein, Diane. *Essential Reiki: A Complete Guide to an Ancient Healing Art.* Freedom, CA: The Crossing Press Inc., 1997.

Stein, Diane. *All Women Are Healers: A Comprehensive Guide to Natural Healing.* Freedom, CA: The Crossing Press Inc., 1996. Includes chapters on the Bach flower remedies, acupressure, homeopathy, gemstone therapy, herbal treatments, and vitamin therapy.

Svoboda, Robert, and Arnie Lade. *Tao and Dharma: Chinese Medicine and Ayurveda.* Twin Lakes, WI: Lotus Press, 1995.

Vithoulkas, George. *Homeopathy: Medicine of the New Man.* New York: Simon & Schuster, 1992.

ORGANIZATIONS

American Academy of Medical Acupuncture. (800) 521-2262.

American Association of Naturopathic Physicians. 601 Valley St., Suite 105, Seattle, WA 98109. (206) 298-0126. Fax: (206) 298-0129. <http://www.naturopathic.org>.

American Botanical Council. <http://www.herbalgram.org>.

American Cancer Society (ACS). 1599 Clifton Road, NE, Atlanta, GA 30329. (404) 320-3333 or (800) ACS-2345. Fax: (404) 329-7530. <http://www.cancer.org>.

American Foundation of Traditional Chinese Medicine (AFTCM). 505 Beach Street, San Francisco, CA 94133. (415) 776-0502. Fax: (415) 392-7003. E-mail: aftcm@earthlink.net.

American Herbal Products Association. 8484 Georgia Ave., Suite 370, Silver Spring, MD 20910. (301) 588-1174. <http://www.ahpa.org>.

American Indian Science and Engineering Society (AISES). 5661 Airport Blvd., Boulder, CO 80301-2339. (303) 939-0023. Fax: (303) 939-8150. E-mail: aisehq@spot.colorado.edu. <http://www.colorado.edu/aises>.

Consumer Reports Health Letter. P.O. Box 52145, Boulder, CO 80321.

Delta Society (pet therapy). <http://www.deltasociety.org>.

National Cancer Institute, Office of Cancer Communications. 31 Center Drive, MSC 2580, Bethesda, MD 20892-2580. (800) 4-CANCER. TTY: (800) 332-8615. Email: cancermail@cips.nci.nih.gov. <http://www.nci.nih.gov>.

National Center for Homeopathy (NCH). 801 North Fairfax St., Suite 306, Alexandria, VA 22314. (703) 548-7790. Fax: (703) 548-7792.

National Certification Board for Therapeutic Massage and Bodywork. 8201 Greensboro Drive, Suite 300, McLean, VA 22102. (703) 610-9015.

National Council Against Health Fraud. P.O. Box 1276, Loma Linda, CA 92354.

NIH National Center for Complementary and Alternative Medicine (NCCAM) Clearinghouse. P. O. Box 8218, Silver Spring, MD 20907-8218. TTY/TDY: (888) 644-6226. Fax: (301) 495-4957. <http://www.nccam.nih.gov>.

NIH Office of Dietary Supplements. Building 31, Room 1B25, 31 Center Drive, MSC 2086, Bethesda, MD 20892-2086. (301) 435-2920. Fax: (301) 480-1845. Web site: http://odp.od.nih.gov/ods.

Office of Cancer Complementary & Alternative Medicine of the National Cancer Institute (OCCAM). Email: ncioccam1-r@mail.nih.gov. <http://www.occam.nci.nih.gov>.

Quackwatch. <http://www.quackwatch.com>.

OTHER

Cancer Supportive Care Programs. 21 June 2001 <http://www.cancersupportivecare.com>. Provides information about pain control, nutrition, and other aspects of supportive care for cancer patients.

The Wellness Community. 21 June 2001 <http://www.wellness-community.org>. Offers support groups, stress reduction workshops, exercise programs, social events, and nutritional counseling for cancer patients and their families.

Rebecca J. Frey, Ph.D.

Computed tomography

Definition

Computed tomography (CT) scanning is a valuable diagnostic tool that provides physicians with views of internal body structures. During a CT scan, multiple x rays are passed through the body, producing cross-sectional images, or "slices," on a cathode-ray tube (CRT), a device resembling a television screen. These images can then be preserved on film for examination.

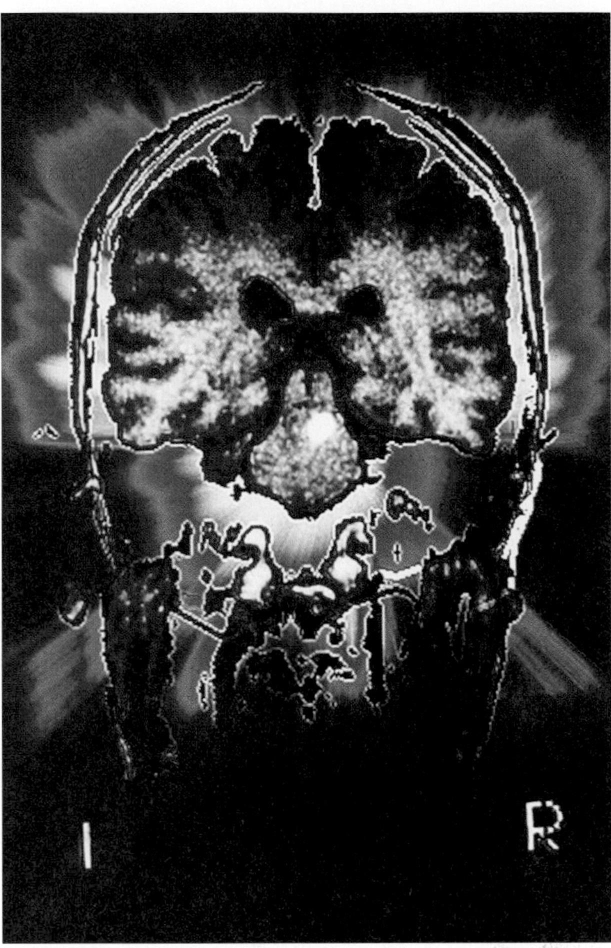

A computed tomography (CT) scan, colorized, of the human brain. *(Custom Medical Stock Photo. Reproduced by permission.)*

Purpose

CT scans are used to image bone, soft tissues, and air. Since the 1990s, CT equipment has become more affordable and available. CT scans have become the imaging exam of choice for the diagnoses of most solid tumors. Because the computerized image is sharp, focused, and three-dimensional, many structures can be better differentiated than on standard x rays.

Common indications for CT scans include:

- Sinus studies. The CT scan can show details of sinusitis, bone fractures, and the presence of bony tumor involvement. Physicians may order a CT scan of the sinuses to provide an accurate map for surgery.
- Brain studies. Brain CT scans can detect hematomas, tumors, strokes, aneurysms, and degenerative or infected brain tissue. The introduction of CT scanning, especially spiral CT, has helped reduce the need for more invasive procedures such as cerebral angiography.
- Body scans. CT scans of the chest, abdomen, spine, and extremities can detect the presence of tumors, enlarged lymph nodes, abnormal collection of fluid, and vertebral disc disease. These scans can also be helpful in evaluating the extent of bone breakdown in osteoporosis.
- Heart and aorta scans. CT scans can focus on the thoracic or abdominal aorta to locate aneurysms and other possible aortic diseases. A newer type of CT scan, called electron beam CT, can be used to detect calcium buildup in arteries. Because it is a new technology, it is not yet widely used and its indications are not yet well-defined.
- Chest scans. CT scans of the chest are useful in distinguishing tumors and in detailing accumulation of fluid in chest infections.

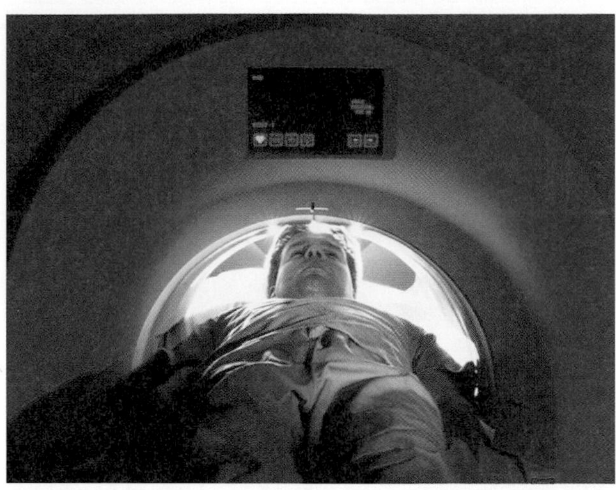

Patient passes into a CT (computed tomography or CAT) scanner. *(© Volker Steger/Science Photo Library, Science Source/Photo Researchers, Inc. Reproduced by permission.)*

Precautions

Pregnant women or those who could possibly be pregnant should not have a CT scan, particularly a full body or abdominal scan, unless the diagnostic benefits outweigh the risks. If the exam is necessary for obstetric purposes, technologists are instructed not to repeat films if there are errors. Pregnant patients receiving a CT scan or any **x ray** exam away from the abdominal area may be protected by a lead apron; most radiation, known as scatter, travels through the body, however, and is not blocked by the apron.

Contrast agents are often used in CT exams, though some types of tumors are better seen without it. Patients should discuss the use of contrast agents with their doctor, and should be asked to sign a consent form prior to the administration of contrast. One of the common contrast agents, iodine, can cause allergic reactions. Patients who are known to be allergic to iodine or shellfish should inform the physician prior to the CT scan; a combination of medications can be given to such patients before the scan to prevent or minimize the reaction. Contrast agents may also put patients with diabetes at risk of kidney failure, particularly those taking the medication glucophage.

Description

Computed tomography, also called CT scan, CAT scan, or computerized axial tomography, is a combination of focused x-ray beams and the computerized production of an image. Introduced in the early 1970s, this radiologic procedure has advanced rapidly and is now widely used, sometimes in the place of standard x rays.

CT equipment

A CT scan may be performed in a hospital or outpatient imaging center. Although the equipment looks large and intimidating, it is very sophisticated and fairly comfortable. The patient is asked to lie on a gantry, or narrow table, that slides into the center of the scanner. The scanner looks like a doughnut and is round in the middle, which allows the x-ray beam to rotate around the patient. The scanner section may also be tilted slightly to allow for certain cross-sectional angles.

CT procedure

The gantry moves very slightly as the precise adjustments for each sectional image are made. A technologist watches the procedure from a window and views the images on a computer screen. Generally, patients are alone during the procedure, though exceptions are sometimes made for pediatric patients. Communication is possible via an intercom system.

It is essential that the patient lie very still during the procedure to prevent motion blurring. In some studies, such as chest CTs, the patient will be asked to hold his or her breath during image capture.

Following the procedure, films of the images are usually printed for the radiologist and referring physician to review. A radiologist can also interpret CT exams on the computer screen. The procedure time will vary in length depending on the area being imaged. Average study times are from 30 to 60 minutes. Some patients may be concerned about claustrophobia but the width of the "doughnut" portion of the scanner is such that many patients can be reassured of openness. Doctors may consider giving sedatives to patients who have severe claustrophobia or difficulty lying still.

The CT image

While traditional x-ray machines image organs in two dimensions, often resulting in organs in the front of the body being superimposed over those in the back, CT scans allow for a more three-dimensional effect. CT images can be likened to slices in a loaf of bread. Precise sections of the body can be located and imaged as cross-sectional views. The screen before the technologist shows a computer's analysis of each section detected by the x-ray beam. Thus, various densities of tissue can be easily distinguished.

Contrast agents

Contrast agents are often used in CT exams and in other radiology procedures to illuminate certain details of anatomy more clearly. Some contrasts are natural, such as air or water. A water-based contrast agent is sometimes administered for specific diagnostic purposes. Barium sulfate is commonly used in gastroenterology procedures. The patient may drink this contrast or receive it in an enema. Oral or rectal contrast is usually given when examining the abdomen or cells, but not when scanning the brain or chest. Iodine is the most widely used intravenous contrast agent and is given through an intravenous needle.

If contrast agents are used in the CT exam, these will be administered several minutes before the study begins. Patients undergoing abdominal CT may be asked to drink a contrast medium. Some patients may experience a salty taste, flushing of the face, warmth or slight nausea, or hives from an intravenous contrast injection. Technologists and radiologists have the equipment and training to help patients through these minor reactions and to handle more severe reactions. Severe reactions to contrast are rare, but do occur.

Newer types of CT scans

The spiral CT scan, also called a helical CT, is a newer version of CT. This type of scan is continuous in motion and allows for the continuous re-creation of images. For example, traditional CT allows the technologist to take slices at very small and precise intervals one after the other. Spiral CT allows for a continuous flow of images, without stopping the scanner to move to the next image slice. A major advantage of spiral CT is the ability to reconstruct images anywhere along the length of the study area. Because the procedure is faster, patients are required to lie still for shorter periods of time. The ability to image contrast more rapidly after it is injected, when it is at its highest level, is another advantage of spiral CT's high speed.

Electron beam CT scans are another newer type of CT technology that can be used to detect calcium buildup in arteries. These calcium deposits are potential risk factors for coronary artery disease. Electron beam CT scans take pictures much more quickly than conventional CTs, and are therefore better able to produce clear images of the heart as it pumps blood. Because it is a newer and expensive test, electron beam CT scanning is not widely used.

Some facilities will have spiral, electron, and conventional CT available. Although spiral is more advantageous for many applications, conventional CT is still a superior and precise method for imaging many tissues and structures. The physician will evaluate which type of CT works best for the specific exam purpose.

Preparation

If a contrast medium is administered, the patient may be asked to fast for about four to six hours prior to the procedure. Patients will usually be given a gown (like a typical hospital gown) to be worn during the procedure. All metal and jewelry should be removed to avoid artifacts on the film. Depending on the type of study, patients may also be required to remove dentures.

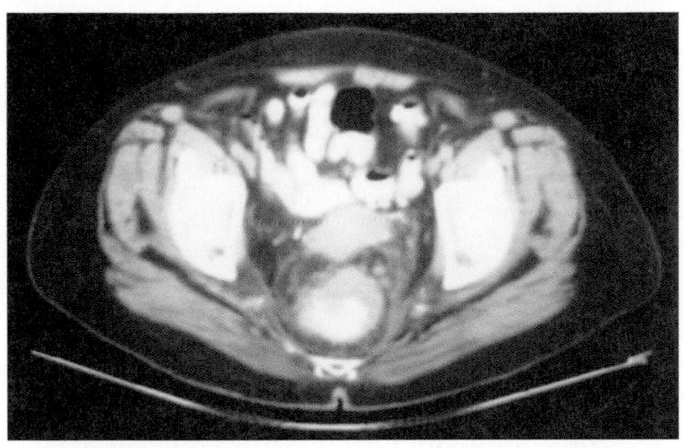

CT scan (without color added) of cancer of the rectum. *(Custom Medical Stock Photo. Reproduced by permission.)*

Aftercare

Generally, no aftercare is required following a CT scan. Immediately following the exam, the technologist will continue to watch the patient for possible adverse contrast reactions. Patients are instructed to advise the technologist of any symptoms, particularly respiratory difficulty. The site of contrast injection will be bandaged and may feel tender following the exam.

Risks

Radiation exposure from a CT scan is similar to, though higher than, that of a conventional x ray. Although this is a risk to pregnant women, the risk for other adults is minimal and should produce no effects. Severe contrast reactions are rare, but they are a risk of many CT procedures.

Normal results

Normal findings on a CT exam show bone, the most dense tissue, as white areas. Tissues and fat will show as various shades of gray, and fluids will be gray or black. Air will also look black. Intravenous, oral, and rectal contrast appear as white areas. The radiologist can determine if tissues and organs appear normal by the sensitivity of the gray shadows.

Abnormal results

Abnormal results may show different characteristics of tissues within organs. Accumulations of blood or other

KEY TERMS

Aneurysm—The bulging of the blood vessel wall. Aortic aneurysms are the most dangerous. Aneurysms can break and cause bleeding.

Contrast (agent, medium)—A substance injected into the body that illuminates certain structures that would otherwise be hard to see on the radiograph (film).

Gantry—A name for the couch or table used in a CT scan. The patient lies on the gantry while it slides into the x-ray scanner.

Hematoma—A collection of blood that has escaped from the vessels. It may clot and harden, causing pain to the patient.

Metastasis—Secondary cancer, or cancer that has spread from one body organ or tissue to another.

Radiologist—A medical doctor specially trained in radiology (x ray) interpretation and its use in the diagnosis of disease and injury.

Spiral CT—Also referred to as helical CT, this method allows for continuous 360-degree x-ray image capture.

Thoracic—Refers to the chest area. The thorax runs between the abdomen and neck and is encased in the ribs.

fluids where they do not belong may be detected. Radiologists can differentiate among types of tumors throughout the body by viewing details of their makeup.

Sinus studies

The increasing availability and lowered cost of CT scanning has lead to its increased use in sinus studies, either as a replacement for a sinus x ray or as a follow-up to an abnormal sinus radiograph. The sensitivity of CT allows for the location of areas of sinus infection, particularly chronic infection. Sinus tumors will show as shades of gray indicating the difference in their density from that of normal tissues in the area.

Brain studies

The precise differences in density allowed by CT scan can clearly show tumors, strokes, or lesions in the brain area as altered densities. These lighter or darker areas on the image may indicate a tumor or hematoma within the brain and skull area. Different types of tumors can be identified by the presence of edema, by the tissue's density, or by studying blood vessel location and activity. The speed and convenience of CT often allows for detection of hemorrhage before symptoms even occur.

QUESTIONS TO ASK THE DOCTOR

- Why is a CT scan recommended in my case?
- What are the benefits associated with this procedure?
- What are the risks associated with this procedure?
- How do I prepare for the CT scan?
- When will I know the results?

Body scans

The body CT scan can identify abnormal body structures and organs. A CT scan may indicate tumors or cysts, enlarged lymph nodes, abnormal collections of fluids, blood or fat, or cancer **metastasis**. Tumors resulting from metastasis are different in makeup than primary (original) tumors.

Chest scans

In addition to those findings which may indicate aortic aneurysms, chest CT studies can show other problems in the heart and lungs, and distinguish between an aortic aneurysm and a tumor adjacent to the aorta. CT will not only show differences between air, water, tissues and bone, but will also assign numerical values to the various densities. Coin-sized lesions in the lungs may be indicative of tuberculosis or tumors. CT will help distinguish among the two. Enlarged lymph nodes in the chest area may indicate **Hodgkin's disease**.

Teresa G. Norris

Resources

BOOKS

Abeloff, M. *Clinical Oncology, 2nd Ed.* Orlando, Florida: Churchill Livingstone, Inc., 2000.

Springhouse Corporation. *Illustrated Guide to Diagnostic Tests.* Springhouse, PA: Springhouse Corporation, 1998.

PERIODICALS

Holbert, J. M. "Role of Spiral Computed Tomography in the Diagnosis of Pulmonary Embolism in the Emergency

Department." *Annals of Emergency Medicine* (May 1999): 520-28.

ORGANIZATION

American College of Radiology. 1891 Preston White Drive, Reston, VA 22091. (800) ACR-LINE. <http://www.acr. org>.

Computerized axial tomography *see* **Computed tomography**

Corticosteroids

Definition

Corticosteroids are a group of related drugs used in cancer treatment to reduce the growth of tumors, stimulate the appetite, and treat skin rashes, **nausea and vomiting**, allergic reactions, inflammation, accumulation of fluid in the brain, and autoimmune disease.

KEY TERMS

Autoimmune disease—An illness occurring when the body's tissues are attacked by its own immune system

Intravenous injection—Injection directly into the vein

Purpose

Corticosteroids have broad use in cancer treatment. Some are used to treat adult leukemias, adult lymphomas, acute childhood leukemia, **multiple myeloma**, and advanced **prostate cancer**. Others are used in creams to treat skin rashes from **radiation therapy**. Corticosteroids are also used to reduce swelling, especially in the brain and spinal column, reduce nausea and vomiting, and improve appetite.

Description

Corticosteroids occur naturally in the body. They are produced by the cortex of the adrenal glands, a small, pea-sized pair of glands that are located in the lower back, just above the kidney. Some corticosteroids regulate fluid balance in the body. Others influence fat and sugar (glucose) usage. Corticosteroids are chemically related to the sex hormones estrogen and **testosterone**.

Many different corticosteroids are produced artificially to use as drugs. They are administered as creams, tablets, liquids, or intravenously (or injection directly into a vein). Many people are already familiar with hydrocortisone, a corticosteroid found in low doses in over-the-counter creams.

The most common corticosteroids used in cancer treatment are:

- dexamethasone (Decadron)
- hydrocortisone
- methylprednisolone (Medrol)
- prednisone
- cortisone
- betamethasone
- prednisolone

There are many trade names for drugs containing these corticosteroids.

Recommended dosage

Corticosteroids come in tablets, liquids, intravenous solutions, and creams. Because of their wide variety of uses and forms, there is no standard recommended dose. Dosage is individualized, and depends on the type of cancer, the patient's body weight and general health, the goal of the treatment, the other drugs being given, and the way a patient's cancer responds to the drug. Corticosteroids should be stored away from heat.

Precautions

People taking corticosteroids may want to go on a low-salt, high-potassium diet in order to reduce water retention. They may also want to watch their calorie intake unless corticosteroids are being given to improve appetite. Patients taking large doses of corticosteroids are more susceptible to infection and should try to avoid contact with crowds or any individuals that may have an infection. Patients should seek immediate medical advice if they are exposed to chicken pox or measles.

Side effects

Corticosteroids have several side effects. Not every side effect is seen in every patient. The most serious, although rare, side effect is an allergic reaction to corticosteroids when given intravenously (IV). Other side effects can include:

- salt and water retention
- excessive potassium loss

- high blood pressure
- other fluid and electrolyte imbalances
- loss of muscle tissue
- loss of bone strength (osteoporosis)
- easily fractured bones
- heartburn and ulcers
- thin, fragile skin
- slow wound healing
- skin rashes
- masking of infection
- convulsions
- headache
- dizziness
- reproductive irregularities
- strong mood changes
- changes in the functioning of the adrenal gland
- increased pressure in the eye
- glaucoma, cataracts, and blindness (rare)
- nausea
- **fatigue**
- increased appetite
- weight gain
- increased urination

Interactions

Many drugs interact with nonprescription (over-the-counter) drugs and herbal remedies. Patients should always tell their health care providers about these remedies, as well as any prescription drugs they are taking. Patients should also notify their physician if they are on a special diet.

Corticosteroids can also interact with anticoagulants (blood thinners such as Coumadin), **cyclosporine**, phenobarbitol, and antidepressants.

Tish Davidson, A.M.

Coughing up blood *see* **Hemoptysis**

Craniopharyngioma

Definition

Craniopharyngioma is a cancer which arises in the pituitary gland, in tissue originally found in the embryo. One of the most common childhood brain cancers, it is also sometimes called a Rathke's pouch tumor or a suprasellar cyst.

Description

Craniopharyngioma is the second most common type of childhood brain tumor, accounting for almost 10% of all brain tumors in children. This cancer has very little tendency to spread to other parts of the body. It readily invades local tissues, however, and since it occurs deep within the brain, invasion of local tissues alone can result in serious illness or even death.

The pituitary gland produces many hormones that play critical roles in the development and regulation of the body. Because this cancer arises in the pituitary gland, it often results in deficiencies of the various hormones that the pituitary gland produces. The tumor can be either solid or cystic or mixed, and most (up to 90%) of craniopharyngiomas contain calcium deposits, an indication of diseased tissue readily observable on x rays.

Demographics

The large majority of craniopharyngiomas are childhood tumors. The median age at diagnosis is eight years; peak incidence is between the ages of six and eleven. Almost 70% of all craniopharyngiomas occur before the age of 20, although a small peak occurs after the age of 50. Diagnosis before the age of two is very rare. Girls and boys and all races are affected equally.

Causes and symptoms

The cause of craniopharyngioma is not really understood, although it is believed to be primarily a congenital illness. Nests of embryonic cells exist in a part of the pituitary gland known as Rathke's pouch. In craniopharyngioma, these nests appear to contain cancerous cells which, over time, multiply and become a tumor.

The symptoms of craniopharyngioma can be divided into two categories. Some are nonspecific symptoms which occur because of increased pressure within the skull; some result from deficiencies of the hormones that the pituitary gland normally produces. Any individual patient may have various combinations of symptoms and both the number of symptoms and the severity of the symptoms typically increase over time. Nonspecific symptoms of increased intracranial pressure include:

- headache
- visual disturbances
- irritability
- personality changes
- mental disturbances

Symptoms that can result from hormone deficiencies include:

- diabetes
- growth retardation
- sexual dysfunction (in adults)

Diagnosis

Most patients seek medical attention because of headaches or visual disturbances, failure to match normal growth patterns (due to a deficiency of growth hormone), or symptoms of diabetes. If (after other causes of symptoms are ruled out) a craniopharyngioma is suspected, usually some kind of imaging technique is performed. Traditional x rays reveal an enlargement of the space at the base of the skull where the tumor is typically found, and will also show calcification of cancerous cells. **Computed tomography** (CT scan or CAT scan) may show calcification that does not show up on x rays and also shows whether the tumor is cystic or solid in nature. **Magnetic resonance imaging** (MRI) can show how much the tumor has invaded the surrounding tissues.

Often the amounts of pituitary hormones in the blood are measured as well. Measurements may be made of gonadatropins (hormones which regulate reproduction), thyrotropin (a hormone that regulates the thyroid gland), growth hormones (regulates growth), corticotropin (a hormone that regulates carbohydrate metabolism, vasopressin (a hormone that regulates water retention), or prolactin (a hormone that regulates milk production in mothers of infants).

Treatment team

As the understanding of cancer grows and new treatment approaches are developed, the complexity of cancer treatment also increases. Today, a multidisciplinary approach to cancer treatment is considered necessary for effective patient care. Since craniopharyngioma is a neuroendocrine tumor that occurs deep in the brain and mainly in children, optimal treatment requires a particularly complex and sophisticated team of health professionals. The types of people who may be involved in treating or caring for a patient with craniopharyngioma and their family typically include oncologists (pediatric), pathologists (neuropathologists), radiation oncologists, radiation technicians, psychiatrists, oncology social workers, nutritionists, home health care providers, endocrinologists, rehabilitative specialists, and neurosurgeons. The surgeon, specifically, should be a pediatric neurosurgeon, as these specialists have been shown to provide better long-term outcomes than general neurosurgeons.

Clinical staging, treatments, and prognosis

Standard treatment for craniopharyngioma consists of surgical removal of as much of the tumor as is readily accessible, followed by **radiation therapy**. Although total removal of the tumor yields the best odds of survival, the location in which this cancer occurs (and the fact that these tumors are typically covered by a thick membrane that adheres tightly to surrounding tissues) can make total removal difficult. Attempts to remove the tumor completely, therefore, often result in significant and unacceptable side effects. A better quality of life, and therefore better overall outcome, is obtained through partial removal of the tumor followed by radiation therapy. This is now generally accepted as the best treatment approach.

Chemotherapy is not routinely used for treatment of craniopharyngioma, although some medications are commonly used to treat symptoms. Drugs that decrease inflammation and reduce the probability of convulsions may be given preoperatively to make surgical removal of the tumor safer. Hormone replacement therapy may be necessary if the cancer, occurring in the pituitary gland, causes serious hormone deficiency problems.

Therapies that are not routinely used but have shown some promise include internal placement of radioactive material and improvements in surgical techniques, including stereotactic surgery, which utilizes a radioactive "gamma knife" for excision of the tumor.

Since this type of cancer does not demonstrate a tendency to spread to remote areas of the body, staging or grading systems are not usually used. Factors that improve survival are complete removal of the tumor (although this often results in greatly decreased quality of life), the size of the tumor at diagnosis, a cystic rather than solid nature of the tumor, and an age of at least five years old at diagnosis. Unfortunately, most patients who survive have significant remaining illness, and predicting how much function may be lost is as important in this cancer as prognosis of survival. It is important to remember, especially with regards to extent of functional capacity to be expected, that the physician's prognosis is only an educated guess, and that positive thinking can contribute significantly to a better quality of life.

Alternative and complementary therapies

Alternative and complementary therapies are treatments which are not traditional, first-line therapies like surgery, chemotherapy and radiation. Complementary therapies are those that are meant to supplement traditional therapies and usually have the objective of relieving symptoms or helping cancer patients cope with the disease or traditional treatments. Alternative therapies are nontraditional treatments which are chosen instead of

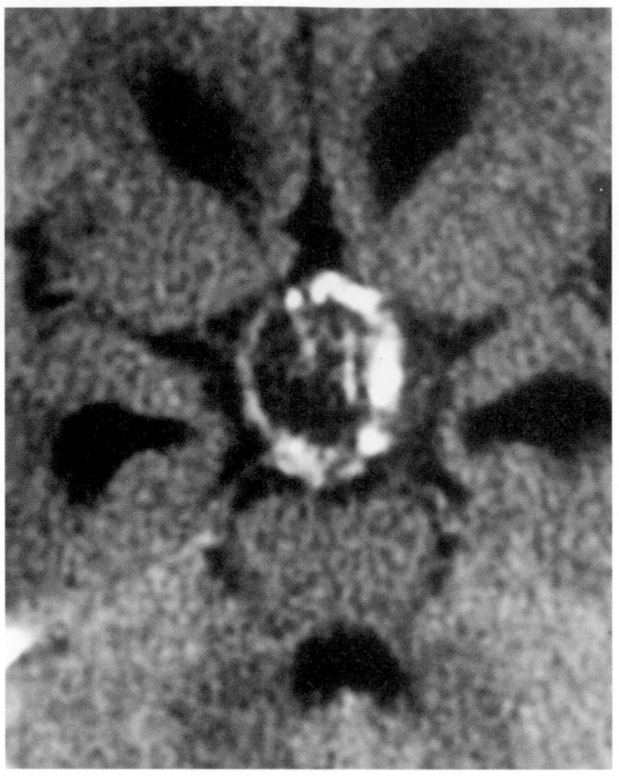

Magnetic resonance image (MRI) of a craniopharyngioma brain tumor. *(Custom Medical Stock Photo. Reproduced by permission.)*

traditional treatments in an attempt to cure the disease. Alternative therapies have typically not been proven to be effective in the same way that traditional drugs are evaluated, in studies called **clinical trials**, and are usually not recommended for use with children.

Common complementary therapies that may be employed by cancer patients include aromatherapy, art therapy, massage, meditation, music therapy, prayer, t'ai chi, and yoga or other forms of exercise, which reduce anxiety and can increase a patient's feeling of well-being. Many patients also take high doses of **vitamins** and other nutritional supplements, especially A, C, E, and selenium, which are thought to act as **antioxidants**. Any physical activities or nutritional supplements (especially when treating a child) should be discussed with then patient's physician.

Numerous alternative therapies exist in cancer treatment. Special caution must be used, however, when considering alternative therapies for children's cancers. Although alternative treatments, by definition, have not been proven effective by scientific methods, some brain tumor patients believe that the use of alternative therapies has been beneficial. Some alternate therapies include:

- Laetrile, a product of apricot seeds, contains a form of cyanide that proponents believe may be released by tumor enzymes and act to kill cancerous cells. Laetrile is not approved by the Food and Drug Administration for use in the United States. The National Cancer Institute sponsored two studies of laetrile in the late 1970s and early 1980s, but concluded after the second study that no additional research was necessary.
- Vitamin E, melatonin, aloe vera, and a compound called beta-1,3-glucan are reported to stimulate the immune system. Some practitioners believe that natural substances like garlic, ginger, and shark cartilage shrink tumors, although how they are supposed to work is not really defined.
- Antineoplastons are believed by some to be another alternative approach to a cancer cure. Antineoplastons are small proteins which may act as molecular messengers and which may be absent from the urine and blood of many cancer patients. The therapy is based on the idea that replacing these proteins may have beneficial effects. However, the National Cancer Institute proposed phase II clinical trials, and protocols were developed, but the trials never got underway on a large scale because of lack of patient participation. The National Cancer Institute draws no definitive conclusions about the treatment's effectiveness due to lack of clinical trials.

Coping with cancer treatment

Children have special needs when coping with treatment, depending on their age. Some comprehensive resources are available about how families can cope with cancer diagnoses, but some coping strategies are summarized here. Very young children need affection, soothing, time to play, reassurances, while toddlers have these same needs, but also may need to be taught how to express their anger or frustration, and simple explanations about what is happening. School-age children may enjoy a little more involvement in their treatment plan, and will need empathy about missing school and activities. They may benefit from drawing or keeping a journal, communicating with friends, and, if possible, a little physical activity each day. Adolescents have similar needs, but also may want to keep some thoughts and feelings private, and also may have more complex spiritual concerns along with feelings of anger and frustration. The siblings and parents of the child with cancer will have needs and concerns and will need to adopt coping strategies as well. The patient's treatment team can help point the family to helpful resources.

Treatment of craniopharyngioma commonly includes surgery and radiation therapy. Although the use of radiation therapy in addition to surgery has improved the quality of life for craniopharyngioma patients, treatments unavoidably result in damage to some healthy tissues and other undesirable side effects.

Fatigue is a very common side effect of radiation therapy. Patients should expect to be very sleepy and therefore to cut back on activities, allowing plenty of time for resting and letting the body heal. It is also important to try maintain a well-balanced,nutritious diet. Patients should avoid as much extra stress as possible and should limit visitors, if needed, to avoid being overtired.

Another problem for those undergoing radiation therapy is dry, sore skin in the area being treated. (Radiation does not hurt during treatment and does not make the person radioactive.) Skin in the treatment area is essentially "burned" and may blister and peel, becoming painful. Patients with fair skin or those who have undergone previous chemotherapy have a greater risk of more serious reactions. Dry, itchy or sore skin is temporary, but skin in the treatment area may remain more sensitive to sun exposure, so a good sunscreen should be used whenever affected skin is exposed to sunlight.

Radiation therapy requires a substantial level of commitment from the patient in terms of time and emotional energy. Fear and anxiety are major factors in coping with cancer in general and these cancer treatments specifically. The feelings are completely normal. Some patients find that concentrating on restful, pleasurable activities like hobbies, prayer, or meditation is helpful in decreasing negative emotions. It is also very important that patients have people to whom they can express their fears and other negative emotions. If friends or family members are unable to provide this to patients, support groups may help to provide an environment where fears can be freely expressed and understood.

Clinical trials

Although numerous clinical trials are in progress which evaluate treatments for childhood brain tumors, few of these are specifically concerned with craniopharyngioma. Most clinical trials for childhood brain tumors are evaluating new medications or new chemotherapy combinations. Although some of these may prove effective against craniopharyngiomas, chemotherapy at this time is not considered an appropriate approach to treatment of this disease. Some new therapies with potential value for cranipharyngioma patients include new forms of drug delivery, including liposomes, and immune-based therapies like **monoclonal antibodies**. In addition, new refinements of surgical techniques, including MRI-assisted surgery and stereotactic surgery, including the bloodless "gamma knife" surgery, are being evaluated. A clinical trial evaluating a pharmaceutical therapy for a common side effect of surgical treatment of craniopharygioma, hypothalmic obesity, is ongoing.

KEY TERMS

Congenital—Existing at birth.

Cystic tumor—A tumor that consists of a sac filled with fluid.

Solid tumor—A tumor that consists of tissue.

Neuroendocrine—Relating to nerves and glands that produce hormones.

Stereotactic surgery—Surgery that used sophisticated methods of imaging internal organs in order to make the most precise surgical incisions.

Monoclonal antibodies—Antibodies produced in bulk that act against a single target.

Liposomes—An artificially produced, microscopic sphere, consisting of a drug surrounded by cell membrane, used to help drugs get into target cells.

Prevention

Craniopharyngioma is believed to be a congenital disease, and there is no known way to prevent this cancer.

Special concerns

This tumor is characterized by various diseases related to hormone deficiencies which may arise as the result of the tumor itself or as the result of either surgical or radiation therapy. The tumor may cause problems related to hormone deficiencies, especially diabetes or growth retardation, and these are often the reason that medical attention is first sought. Craniopharyngioma patients may also experience sleep disorders, changes in personality, and mental disturbances. In addition, treatment for craniopharyngioma can create a condition called hypothalmic obesity, in which a patient steadily gains weight although eating patterns may not have changed. Although many of these problems may significantly improve with time, care of a family member with a brain tumor is a significantly stressful experience for caregivers, which creates a huge strain on normal family life.

As mentioned, **childhood cancers** create unique concerns for the children diagnosed and their families. Parents and siblings, as well as the cancer patient, all have emotional issues to address, in addition to everyday

QUESTIONS TO ASK THE DOCTOR

- Can you explain what kind of cancer I have?
- Can you show me where my tumor is located?
- How was this cancer diagnosed?
- What is my prognosis? What limitations will I have?
- What treatments are we going to pursue? What goals will these treatments have? What happens if these don't work?
- Are there any alternatives to these treatments?
- Do you have experience in treating this type of cancer?
- Is there anything I can do to optimize treatment? Are there any particular side effects I should expect?
- Are there complementary therapies that you would recommend?

concerns, such as social development, friends, and school. Hospital staff and social workers can help direct a family to useful resources for support. Support groups for craniopharyngioma patients and for parents of craniopharyngioma patients offer patients and parents a place to discuss their fears and concerns with other people who have been impacted by this disease.

Resources

BOOKS

Abeloff, ed. *Clinical Oncology.* New York: Churchill Livingstone.

Bracken, Jeanne Munn. *Children with Cancer: A Comprehensive Reference Guide for Parents.* New York:Oxford University Press, 1986.

Buckman, R. *What You Really Need to Know About Cancer.* Baltimore: Johns Hopkins University Press, 1999.

Cook, Allan R., ed. *The New Cancer Sourcebook.* New York: Omnigraphics, Inc.,1996.

Fromer, Margot Joan. *Surviving Childhood Cancer: A Guide for Families.* Washington D.C.: American Psychiatric Press, 1998.

Ganz, Pam. *Life Isn't Always A Day at the Beach: A Book for All Children Whose Lives Are Affected by Cancer.* Lincoln, Nebraska: High-Five Publishing, 1996.

Pizzo and Poplack, eds. *Principles and Practice of Pediatric Oncology.* Baltimore, MD: Lippincott-Raven Publishers, 1997.

PERIODICALS

Lafferty, A. R. "Pituitary Tumors in Children and Adolescents." *Journal of Clinical Endocrinology and Metabolism* 84 (December 1999):4317-4322.

ORGANIZATIONS

American Cancer Society, 1599 Clifton Road, NE, Atlanta, GA 30329-4251. (800)586-4872 <http://www.cancer.org>

National Cancer Institute, 9000 Rockville Pike, Bethesda, Maryland, 20892. (800)422-6237. <http:..www.nci.nih.gov>

The Wellness Community, 10921 Reed Harman Highway, Cincinnati, Ohio, 45242 (888)793-9355.

Childhood Brain Tumor Foundation, 20312 Watkins Meadow Drive, Germantown, MD 20867. (301)515-2900. <http://www.childhoodbraintumor.org>

Candlelighter Childhood Cancer Foundation, 3910 Warner St., Kensington, MD 20895. 1-800-366-2223.<http://www.candlelighters.org>

National Children's Cancer Society, Suite 600, 1015 Locust St. St. Louis, MO 63101. 1-800-532-6459. <http://www.children-cancer.com>

Wendy Wippel, M.Sc.

Craniotomy

Definition

A craniotomy is the surgical removal of part of the skull to expose the brain.

Purpose

A craniotomy is the most commonly performed surgery to remove a brain tumor. It may also be done to remove a blood clot and control hemorrhage, to inspect the brain, to perform a **biopsy**, or to relieve pressure inside the skull.

Precautions

The outcome of surgery will depend on the type and location of the tumor. **Radiation therapy** or **chemotherapy** are sometimes given before surgery to shrink the tumor.

Description

There are two basic ways to open the skull. A curving incision may be made from behind the hairline, in front of the ear, to arch above the eye, or at the nape of the neck around the occipital lobe. The surgeon marks with a felt tip pen a large square flap on the scalp that

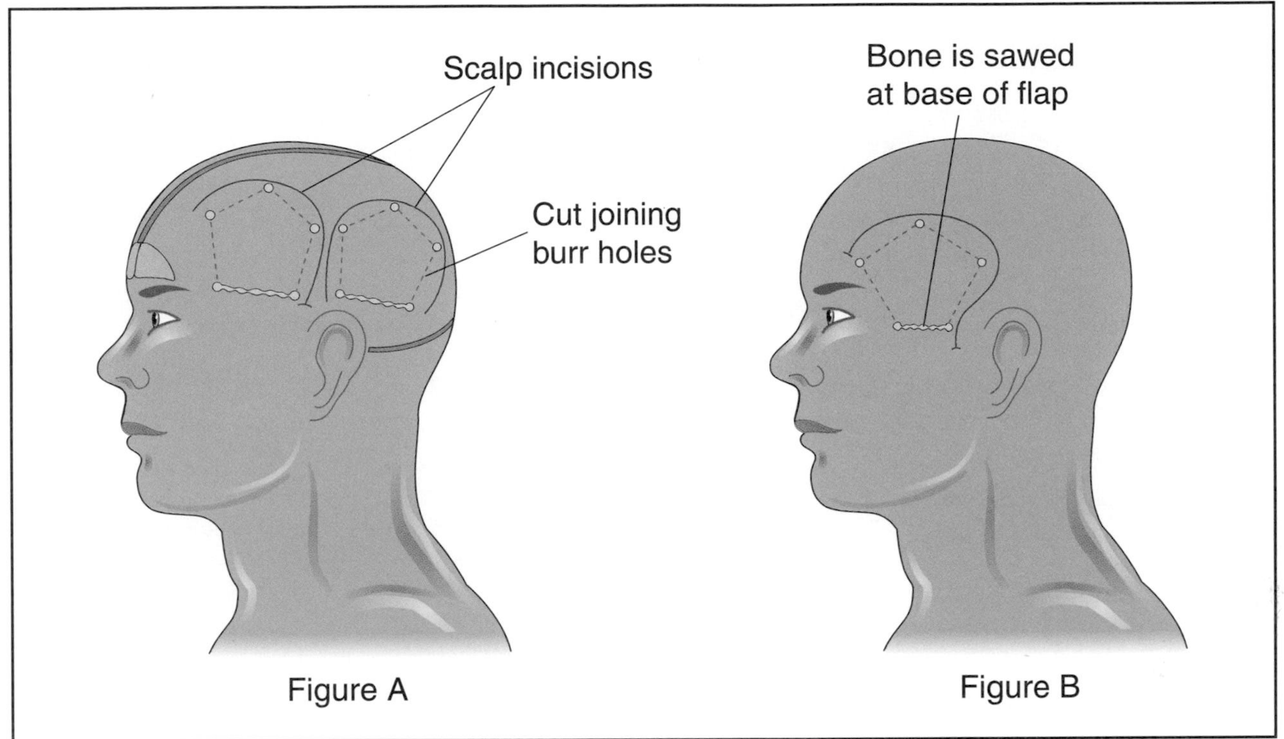

A craniotomy is the most commonly performed brain surgery for brain tumor removal. There are two basic ways to open the skull: a curving incision from behind the hairline in front of the ear and at the nape of the neck (figure A). To reach the brain, the surgeon uses a hand drill to make holes in the skull, pushing a soft metal guide under the bone. The bone is sawed through until the bone flap can be removed to expose the brain (figure B). *(Illustration by Electronic Illustrators Group.)*

covers the surgical area. Following this mark, the surgeon makes an incision into the skin as far as the thin membrane covering the skull bone. Because the scalp is well supplied with blood, the surgeon will have to seal many small arteries. The surgeon then folds back a skin flap to expose the bone.

Using a high speed hand drill or an automatic craniotome, the surgeon makes a circle of holes in the skull and pushes a soft metal guide under the bone from one hole to the next. A fine wire saw is then moved along the guide channel under the bone between adjacent holes. The surgeon saws through the bone until the bone flap can be removed to expose the brain.

After the surgery for the underlying cause is completed, the piece of skull is replaced and secured with pieces of fine, soft wire. Finally, the surgeon sutures the membrane, muscle, and skin of the scalp.

Recent advances in computer-assisted technology have enhanced this operation. Image-guided craniotomy uses information from magnetic resonance imagining scans (MRIs) or **computed tomography** (CT) scans to produce three-dimensional images of the brain for the surgeon before the operation is begun. This makes it possible for the surgeon to remove less skin and bone, to tell exactly where the tumor stops and the healthy brain begins, and to remove tumors that were previously too deep for surgery.

Preparation

Before the operation, the patient undergoes diagnostic procedures such as CT and MRI scans to determine the underlying problem that requires the craniotomy and to get a better look at the brain's structure. Cerebral **angiography** is a diagnostic procedure that may be used to study the blood supply to the tumor, aneurysm, or other brain lesion.

Before the surgery, patients are given drugs to ease anxiety, and other medications to reduce the risk of swelling, seizures, and infection after the operation. Fluids may be restricted, and a diuretic (water pill) may be given before and during surgery if the patient has a tendency to retain water. A urinary catheter is inserted before the patient goes to the operating room. The scalp is shaved in the operating room immediately before surgery; this is done so that any small nicks in the skin won't have a chance to become infected before the operation.

KEY TERMS

Craniotome—A type of surgical drill used to operate on the skull. It has a self-controlled system that stops the drill when the bone is penetrated.

Computed tomography (CT or CAT) scan—Using x rays taken from many angles and computer modeling, CT scans help locate and size tumors and provide information on whether they can be surgically removed.

Magnetic resonance imaging (MRI)—MRI uses magnets and radio waves to create detailed cross-sectional pictures of the interior of the body.

Aftercare

Oxygen, painkillers, and drugs to control swelling and seizures are given after the operation. Codeine may be given to relieve potential headaches caused by the stretching or irritation of the nerves of the scalp. Some type of drainage from the head may be in place, depending on the reason for the surgery.

Patients are usually out of bed within a day and out of the hospital within a week. Headache and pain from the scalp wound can be controlled with medications. Some patients will receive radiation therapy or chemotherapy after surgery.

The bandage on the skull should be changed regularly. Sutures closing the scalp will be removed, but soft wires used to reattach the skull are permanent and require no further attention. The patient should avoid getting the scalp wet until all the sutures have been removed. A clean cap or scarf can be worn until the hair grows back.

Risks

Accessing the area of the brain that needs repair may damage other brain tissue. Therefore, the procedure carries with it risk of brain damage that could leave the patient with some loss of brain function. The surgeon performing the operation can give the patient an assessment of the risk of his or her particular procedure based on the location of the tumor.

Normal results

While every patient's experience is different depending on the reason for the surgery, age, and overall health, recovery from a successful surgery is usually rapid because of the good supply of blood to the area.

Abnormal results

Possible complications after craniotomy include:

- swelling of the brain
- excessive intracranial pressure
- infection
- seizures

See Also Brain and central nervous system tumors; Computed tomography; Magnetic resonance imaging

Resources

ORGANIZATIONS

American Cancer Society. 1599 Clifton Road NE, Atlanta, GA 30329. 800 (ACS)-2345). <http://www.cancer.org>.

Cancer Information Service, National Cancer Institute. Building 31, Room 10A19, 9000 Rockville Pike, Bethesda, MD 20892. (800) 4-CANCER. <http://www.nci.nih.gov/cancerinfo/index.html>.

Carol A.Turkington

Cryotherapy

Definition

Cryotherapy is a technique that uses an extremely cold liquid or instruments to freeze and destroy abnormal or cancerous skin cells that require removal. The technique has been in use since the turn of the century, but modern techniques have made it widely available to dermatologists and primary care doctors. Recent advances have also lead to more use of cryotherapy in treating internal cancer. The technique is also called cryosurgery.

Purpose

Cryotherapy can be employed to destroy a variety of benign skin growths, such as warts, precancerous lesions (such as actinic keratoses), and malignant lesions (such as basal cell and squamous cell cancers). It has also found new use in treating internal cancers, such as cancers of the prostate gland and the breast. The goal of cryotherapy is to freeze and destroy targeted skin growths or cancers while preserving the surrounding tissue from injury.

Precautions

Cryotherapy is not recommended for certain areas of the body because of the danger of destruction of normal tissue or unacceptable scarring. These areas include: skin that overlies nerves, the corners of the eyes, the fold of skin between the nose and lip, the skin surrounding the nostrils, and the border between the lips and the rest of the face. Lesions that are suspected or known to be malignant **melanoma**, an aggressive form of skin cancer, should not be treated with cryotherapy, but should instead be removed surgically. Similarly, basal cell or squamous cell skin cancers that have reappeared at the site of a previously treated tumor should also be removed surgically.

If it remains unclear whether a growth is benign or malignant, a sample of tissue should be removed for analysis (**biopsy**) by a pathologist before any attempts to destroy the lesion with cryotherapy. Care should be taken in people with diabetes or certain circulation problems when cryotherapy is considered for growths located on their lower legs, ankles, and feet. In these patients, healing can be poor and the risk of infection can be high.

Description

There are three main techniques used to perform cryotherapy. In the simplest technique, usually reserved for warts and other benign skin growths, the physician will dip a cotton swab or other applicator into a cup containing a "cryogen," such as liquid nitrogen, and apply it directly to the skin growth to freeze it. At a temperature of −320°F (–196°C), liquid nitrogen is the coldest cryogen available. The goal is to freeze the skin growth as quickly as possible, and then let it thaw slowly to cause maximum destruction of the skin cells. A second application may be necessary depending on the size of the growth.

In another cryotherapy technique, a device is used to direct a small spray of liquid nitrogen or other cryogen directly onto the skin growth. Freezing may last from 20–30 seconds, depending on the size of the lesion. A second freeze-thaw cycle may be required. In a third option, liquid nitrogen or another cryogen is circulated through a probe to cool it to low temperatures. The probe is then brought into direct contact with the lesion, either on the skin or in the case of internal cancers, inside the patient. The freeze time can take two to three times longer than with the spray technique.

Preparation

Extensive preparation prior to cryotherapy is not required for external lesions. The area to be treated should be clean and dry, but sterile preparation is not necessary. Patients should know that they will experience some pain at the time of the freezing, but local anesthesia is usually not required. The physician may want to

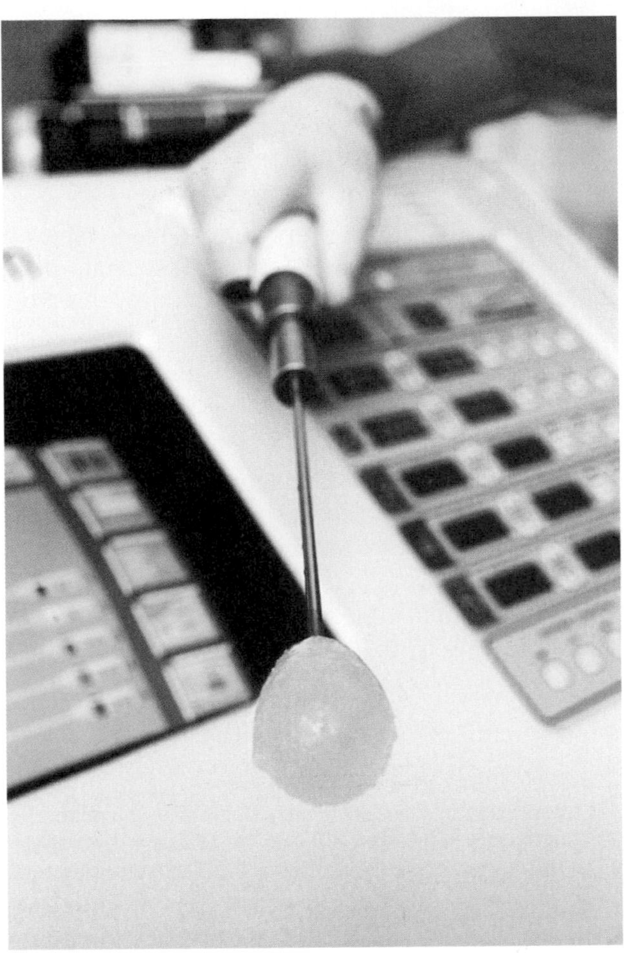

Metal cryoprobe used to treat prostate cancer. *(© Hank Morgan, Science Source/Photo Researchers, Inc. Reproduced by permission.)*

reduce the size of certain growths, such as warts, prior to the cryotherapy procedure, and may have patients apply salicylic acid preparations to the growth over several weeks. Sometimes, the physician will pare away some of the tissue using a device called a curette or a scalpel.

Preparation for treating cancers inside the body, such as **prostate cancer**, is slightly more complicated. The areas that are to be cooled are precisely mapped using ultrasound imaging or a specialized x-ray machine known as a computed axial tomography (CAT) scan. Temperature sensors are then placed inside and around the tumor to monitor the temperature. Lastly, cooling probes are then placed in and around the tumor.

Risks

Cryotherapy poses little risk and can be well tolerated by elderly and other patients who are not good candidates for other surgical procedures. As with other surgical procedures, there is some risk of scarring, infection, and dam-

KEY TERMS

Actinic keratosis—A crusty, scaly precancerous skin lesion caused by damage from the sun. Frequently treated with cryotherapy.

Basal cell cancer—The most common form of skin cancer; it usually appears as one or several nodules having a central depression. It rarely spreads (metastasizes) but is locally invasive.

Cryogen—A substance with a very low boiling point, such as liquid nitrogen, used in cryotherapy treatment.

Melanoma—The most dangerous form of skin cancer. It should not be treated with cryotherapy but should be removed surgically instead.

Squamous cell cancer—A form of skin cancer that usually originates in sun-damaged areas or preexisting lesions; at first local and superficial, it may later spread to other areas of the body.

age to underlying skin and tissue. These risks are generally minimal in the hands of experienced users of cryotherapy.

Normal results

Some redness, swelling, blistering, and oozing of fluid are all common results of cryotherapy. Healing time can vary by the site treated and the cryotherapy technique used. When cryogen is applied directly to the growth, healing may occur in three weeks. Growths treated on the head and neck with the spray technique may take four to six weeks to heal; growths treated on other areas of the body may take considerably longer. Cryotherapy boasts high success rates in permanently removing skin growths; even for malignant lesions such as squamous cell and basal cell cancers, studies have shown a cure rate of up to 98%. For certain types of growths, such as some forms of warts, repeat treatments over several weeks are necessary to prevent the growth's return.

In the case of internal tumors, such as cancers of the prostate, cryotherapy has been shown to be at least as effective as other means, such as **radiation therapy**, with fewer side effects and faster recovery time.

Abnormal results

Although cryotherapy is a relatively low risk procedure, some side effects may occur as a result of the treatment. They include:

- Infection. Though uncommon, infection is more likely on the lower legs where healing can take several months.
- Pigmentary changes. Both hypopigmentation (lightening of the skin) and hyperpigmentation (darkening of the skin) are possible after cryotherapy. Both generally last a few months, but can be longer lasting.
- Nerve damage. Though rare, damage to nerves is possible. Reports suggest this will disappear within several months.

Resources

BOOKS

Abeloff, Martin D., James O. Armitage, Allen S. Lichter, and John E. Niederhuber. *Clinical Oncology.* New York: Churchill Livingstone, 2000.

PERIODICALS

Baust, John, et al. "Minimally Invasive Cryosurgery-Technological Advances."*Cryobiology* 34 (1997): 373-384.

Fintor, Lou. "Cancer Cryosurgery Potentially "Hot" For Patients, New Markets."*Journal of the National Cancer Institute* 92 (September 2000): 1464-1466.

ORGANIZATIONS

American Academy of Dermatology. 930 N. Meacham Road, P.O. Box 4014, Schaumburg, IL 60168-4014. (847)330-0230. <http://www.aad.org>.

OTHER

National Cancer Institute. <http://cis.nci.nih.gov>.

Edward R. Rosick, D.O., M.P.H.

CT scan *see* **Computed tomography**

CT-guided biopsy

Definition

A CT-guided **biopsy** is a procedure by which the physician uses a very thin needle and a syringe to withdraw a tissue or fluid specimen from an organ or suspected tumor mass. The needle is guided while being viewed by the physician on a **computed tomography** (CT) scan.

Purpose

A definite diagnosis of cancer is almost always based on the histological examination of cell or tissue samples. The procedure used to obtain a specimen for this testing is called a biopsy. Biopsies can be performed by surgical removal of the specimen if the suspicious area is located near the surface of the body or during surgery. If, however, the suspected tumor is located deep inside the body and cannot be seen or felt by the physician, he may decide to perform a CT-guided biopsy. The main advantage of a CT-guided biopsy is that it does not require an incision, but the disadvantage is that in some cases, the needle may not be able to remove enough tissue for analysis.

Precautions

CT-guided biopsy can be performed on almost all organs of the body, for example on the lungs, liver, kidneys, adrenal glands, pancreas, and pelvis. The procedure is not indicated for the spleen because there is a high risk of severe post-biopsy hemorrhage. CT-guided biopsy is not indicated for patients with bleeding disorders such as hemophilia, or who are at risk for bleeding as a result of cancer treatments (chemo-radiation) or the cancer itself, as when a patient develops **thrombocytopenia**.

Description

The development of CT technology provided a powerful means to visualize the inner features of the human body which previously could only be seen during surgery or autopsy. Before CT, if a patient had a tumor located in the chest, abdomen, or pelvis, biopsies could only be performed with a surgical procedure. If the patient needed surgery so as to treat the tumor, then biopsy specimens were also collected at the same time for analysis. However, there was no way to obtain samples from patients whose tumors could not be treated with surgery, such as patients with metastatic cancer or with general conditions not allowing surgery. CT-guided needle biopsy has become a welcome alternative to surgical exploration and biopsy.

Preparation

The technique will vary depending on the site of specimen collection and the patient's general condition. In most procedures, the patient lies on the CT table on his back, or on either side, depending on where the needle is to be inserted. Some patients may require intravenous injection of pain killers. A CT scan is first performed, to locate the best site for needle insertion. The skin is then disinfected and anesthetized with its underlying tissue. The needle is inserted through the skin into the body. Another CT scan is perfomed to confirm that the tip of the needle lies at the desired location. When the tip of the needle is seen to be in the proper position, the biopsy specimen is withdrawn through the needle.

Aftercare

After the procedure, the patient is monitored in the hospital or clinic department or in an observation unit for a few hours, and then sent home.

KEY TERMS

Anesthesia—Loss of normal sensation or feeling. Insensitivity to pain.

Autopsy—Postmortem surgical procedure performed to examine body tissues and determine the cause of death.

Hemorrhage—Escape of blood from blood vessels; bleeding.

Histology—The study of tissue with a microscope.

Incision—Cutting through the skin.

Metastasis—The transfer of cancer from one organ to another one not directly connected to it.

Pelvis—Bassin-shaped body cavity containing and protecting the bladder, the rectum and the reproductive organs.

Pneumothorax—A collapse of the lung due to a sudden change of pressure within the chest cavity.

Sterile—Procedures carried out with instruments that have been sterilized, meaning that they are completely free from microorganisms (germs) that could cause infection.

Risks

CT-guided biopsy is a fairly safe procedure. The risks are certainly less than the risks involved with the alternative method, surgical biopsy. In any case, recovering from CT-guided biopsy takes considerably less time than it would if the biopsy were surgically performed.

The risks associated with CT-guided biopsy depend on the site where the biopsy specimen is collected. They include:

- Bleeding: Most patients have had their blood evaluated before the procedure. Although rare, bleeding can occur and may require surgery to control.
- Infection: An infection is possible whenever an object, —such as the needle used in CT-guided biopsy—, pierces the skin, —even if sterile procedures are always followed during the procedure. This is a very rare complication.
- Pneumothorax: Partial or total collapse of a lung is a reported complication in approximately 25% of lung biopsies. It is also a risk during CT-guided biopsies of the liver and adrenal glands.

QUESTIONS TO ASK THE DOCTOR

- Will the CT-guided biopsy procedure be painful?
- How many times will I need to have one?
- What is the normal success rate in obtaining enough tissue to make a diagnosis?
- What kind of complications may I experience at the biopsy site?
- When will I know the results?

Normal results

A preliminary evaluation of the CT-guided biopsy specimen is often performed by the physician. If enough tissue has been obtained for the required tests, the procedure is terminated and the specimen is sent to the histology lab for analysis.

Abnormal results

If the CT-guided biopsy has not been successful, it may be repeated or another biopsy procedure may be selected. Abnormal results indicate that a malignancy or other abnormality is present.

See Also Imaging studies; Biopsy

Resources

BOOKS

Seeram, E. *Computed Tomography: Physical Principles, Clinical Applications and Quality Control.* W. Saunders & Co., 2001

Webb, R. et al.*Fundamentals of Body CT.* W. Saunders & Co., 1998.

PERIODICALS

Ben-Yehuda, D., Polliack, A., Okon, E., Sherman, Y., Fields, S., Lebenshart, P., Lotan, H., and E. Libson. "Image-guided core-needle biopsy in malignant lymphoma: experience with 100 patients that suggests the technique is reliable." *Journal of Clinical Oncology* 14 (September 1996):2431-34.

Golder, W. A., Borchert, M., and K.J. Wolf. "Outcomes and benefits of CT-guided biopsy." *Academy of Radiology* 5 (September 1998)Suppl.2:S317-20.

Nashed, Z., Klein, J. S., and M.A. Zarka. "Special techniques in CT-guided transthoracic needle biopsy."*American Journal of Roentgenology* 171 (December 1998):1665-68.

Sklair-Levy, M., Polliack, A., Shaham, D., Applbaum, Y. H., Gillis, S., Ben-Yehuda, D., Sherman, Y., and E. Libson. "CT-guided core-needle biopsy in the diagnosis of mediastinal lymphoma."*European Radiology* 10 (2000):714-8.

Monique Laberge, Ph.D.

CT scan *see* **Computed tomography**

CUP *see* **Carcinoma of unknown primary**

Cushing's syndrome

Definition

Cushing's syndrome is a relatively rare endocrine (hormonal) disorder resulting from excessive exposure to the hormone cortisol. The disorder, which leads to a variety of symptoms and physical abnormalities, is most commonly caused by taking medications containing the hormone over a long period of time. A more rare form of the disorder occurs when the body itself produces an excessive amount of cortisol.

Description

The adrenals are two glands, each of which is perched on the upper part of the two kidneys. The outer part of the gland is known as the cortex; the inner part is known as the medulla. Each of these parts of the adrenal gland is responsible for producing different types of hormones. Regulation of hormone production and release from the adrenal cortex involves the pituitary gland, a small gland located at the base of the brain. After the hypothalamus (the part of the brain containing secretions important to metabolic activities) sends "releasing hormones" to the pituitary gland, the pituitary secretes a hormone called adrenocorticotropic hormone (ACTH). The ACTH then travels through the bloodstream to the adrenal cortex, where it encourages the production and release of cortisol (sometimes called the "stress" hormone) and other adrenocortical hormones.

Cortisol, a very potent glucocorticoid—a group of adrenocortical hormones that protects the body from stress and affect protein and carbohydrate metabolism—is involved in regulating the functioning of nearly every type of organ and tissue in the body, and is considered to be one of the few hormones absolutely necessary for life. Cortisol is involved in:

- complex processing and utilization of many nutrients, including sugars (carbohydrates), fats, and proteins
- normal functioning of the circulatory system and the heart
- functioning of muscles
- normal kidney function
- production of blood cells
- normal processes involved in maintaining the skeletal system

- proper functioning of the brain and nerves
- normal responses of the immune system

Cushing's syndrome, also called hypercortisolism, has an adverse effect on all of the processes described above. The syndrome occurs in approximately 10 to 15 out of every onc million people per year, usually striking adults between the ages of 20 and 50.

Causes and symptoms

The most common cause of Cushing's syndrome is the long-term use of glucocorticoid hormones in medications. Medications such as prednisone are used in a number of inflammatory conditions. Such conditions include rheumatoid arthritis, asthma, vasculitis, lupus, and a variety of other autoimmune disorders in which the body's immune cells accidentally attack some part of the body itself. In these disorders, the glucocorticoids are used to dampen the **immune response**, thereby decreasing damage to the body.

Cushing's syndrome can also be caused by three different categories of disease:

- a pituitary tumor producing abnormally large quantities of ACTH
- the abnormal production of ACTH by some source other than the pituitary
- a tumor within the adrenal gland overproducing cortisol

Although it is rare, about two-thirds of endogenous (occurring within the body rather than from a source outside the body, like a medication) Cushing's syndrome is a result of Cushing's disease. The term "Cushing's disease" refers to Cushing's syndrome, which is caused by excessive secretion of ACTH by a pituitary tumor, usually an **adenoma** (noncancerous tumor). The pituitary tumor causes increased growth of the adrenal cortex (hyperplasia) and increased cortisol production. Cushing's disease affects women more often than men.

Tumors in locations other than the pituitary can also produce ACTH. This is called ectopic ACTH syndrome ("ectopic" refers to something existing out of its normal place). Tumors in the lung account for more than half of all cases of ectopic ACTH syndrome. Other types of tumors which may produce ACTH include tumors of the thymus, the pancreas, the thyroid, and the adrenal gland. In each case, the secreting part of the tumor may be in the primary tumor, part of the primary tumor, or may be a small, difficult-to-find, metastatic lesion(s). Nearly all adrenal gland tumors are benign (noncancerous), although in rare instances a tumor may actually be cancerous.

Symptoms of cortisol excess (resulting from medication or from the body's excess production of the hormone) include:

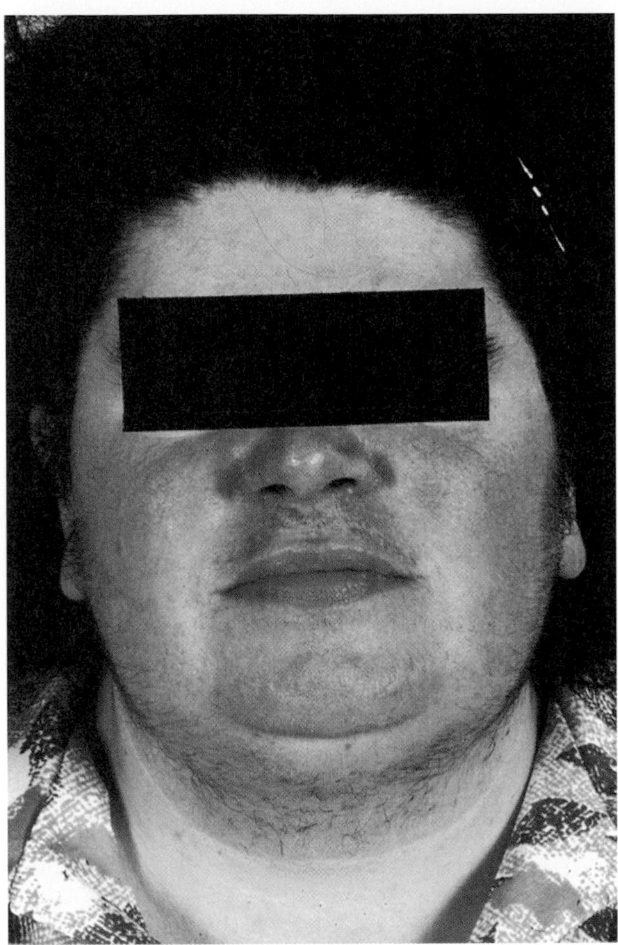

Woman exhibiting symptoms of Cushing's syndrome. *(© John Radcliff Hospital/Science Source/Photo Researchers, Inc. Reproduced by permission.)*

- weight gain
- an abnormal accumulation of fatty pads in the face (creating the distinctive "moon face" of Cushing's syndrome); in the trunk (termed "truncal obesity"); and over the upper back and the back of the neck (giving the individual what has been called a "buffalo hump")
- purple and pink stretch marks across the abdomen and flanks
- high blood pressure
- weak, thinning bones (osteoporosis)
- weak muscles
- low energy
- thin, fragile skin, with a tendency toward both bruising and slow healing
- abnormalities in the processing of sugars (glucose), with occasional development of actual diabetes
- kidney stones
- increased risk of infections

KEY TERMS

Adenoma—A type of noncancerous (benign) tumor that often involves the overgrowth of certain cells of the type normally found within glands.

Adrenocorticotropic hormone (ACTH)—A pituitary hormone that stimulates the cortex of the adrenal glands to produce adrenal cortical hormones.

Cortisol—A hormone secreted by the cortex of the adrenal gland. Cortisol regulates the function of nearly every organ and tissue in the body.

Ectopic—In an abnormal position.

Endocrine—Pertaining to a gland that secretes directly into the bloodstream.

Gland—A collection of cells whose function is to release certain chemicals (hormones) that are important to the functioning of other, sometimes distantly located, organs or body systems.

Glucocorticoids—General class of adrenal cortical hormones that are mainly active in protecting against stress and in protein and carbohydrate metabolism.

Hormone—A chemical produced in one part of the body, which travels to another part of the body in order to exert its effect.

Hypothalamus—the part of the brain containing secretions important to metabolic activities.

Pituitary—A gland located at the base of the brain, the pituitary produces a number of hormones, including hormones which regulate growth and reproductive function.

- emotional disturbances, including mood swings, **depression**, irritability, confusion, or even a complete break with reality (psychosis)
- irregular menstrual periods in women
- decreased sex drive in men and difficulty maintaining an erection
- abormal hair growth in women (in a male pattern, such as in the beard and mustache area), as well as loss of hair from the head (receding hair line).

Diagnosis

Diagnosing Cushing's syndrome can be complex. Diagnosis must not only identify the cortisol excess but also locate its source. Many of the symptoms listed above can be attributed to numerous other diseases. Although a number of these symptoms seen together would certainly suggest Cushing's syndrome, the symptoms are still not specific to Cushing's syndrome. Following a review of the patient's medical history, physical examination, and routine blood tests, a series of more sophisticated tests is available to achieve a diagnosis.

24-hour free cortisol test

This is the most specific diagnostic test for identifying Cushing's syndrome. It involves measuring the amount of cortisol present in the urine over a 24-hour period. When excess cortisol is present in the bloodstream, it is processed by the kidneys and removed as waste in the urine. This 24-hour free cortisol test requires that an individual collect exactly 24-hours' worth of urine in a single container. The urine is then analyzed in a laboratory to determine the quantity of cortisol present. This technique can also be paired with the administration of **dexamethasone**, which in a normal individual would cause urine cortisol to be very low. Once a diagnosis has been made using the 24-hour free cortisol test, other tests are used to find the exact location of the abnormality causing excess cortisol production.

Dexamethasone suppression test

This test is useful in distinguishing individuals with excess ACTH production due to a pituitary adenoma from those with ectopic ACTH-producing tumors. Patients are given dexamethasone (a synthetic glucocorticoid) orally every six hours for four days. Low doses of dexamethasone are given during the first two days; for the last two days, higher doses are administered. Before dexamethasone is administered, as well as on each day of the test, 24-hour urine collections are obtained.

Because cortisol and other glucocorticoids signal the pituitary to decrease ACTH, the normal response after taking dexamethasone is a drop in blood and urine cortisol levels. Thus, the cortisol response to dexamethasone differs depending on whether the cause of Cushing's syndrome is a pituitary adenoma or an ectopic ACTH-producing tumor.

However, the dexamethasone suppression test may produce false-positive results in patients with conditions such as depression, alcohol abuse, high estrogen levels, acute illness, and stress. On the other hand, drugs such as **phenytoin** and phenobarbital may produce false-negative results. Thus, patients are usually advised to stop taking these drugs at least one week prior to the test.

Corticotropin-releasing hormone (CRH) stimulation test

The CRH stimulation test is given to help distinguish between patients with pituitary adenomas and those with either ectopic ACTH syndrome or cortisol-secreting **adrenal tumors**. In this test, patients are given an injection of CRH, the corticotropin-releasing hormone that causes the pituitary to secrete ACTH. In patients with pituitary adenomas, blood levels of ACTH and cortisol usually rise. However, in patients with ectopic ACTH syndrome, this rise is rarely seen. In patients with cortisol-secreting adrenal tumors, this rise almost never occurs.

Petrosal sinus sampling

Although this test is not always necessary, it may be used to distinguish between a pituitary adenoma and an ectopic source of ACTH. Petrosal sinus sampling involves drawing blood directly from veins that drain the pituitary. This test, which is usually performed with local anesthesia and mild sedation, requires inserting tiny, flexible tubes (catheters) through a vein in the upper thigh or groin area. The catheters are then threaded up slowly until they reach veins in an area of the skull known as the petrosal sinuses. X rays are typically used to confirm the correct position of the catheters. Often CRH is also given during the test to increase the accuracy of results.

When blood tested from the petrosal sinuses reveals a higher ACTH level than blood drawn from a vein in the forearm, the likely diagnosis is a pituitary adenoma. When the two samples show similar levels of ACTH, the diagnosis indicates ectopic ACTH syndrome.

Radiologic imaging tests

Imaging tests such as **computed tomography** scans (CT) and **magnetic resonance imaging** (MRI) are only used to look at the pituitary and adrenal glands after a firm diagnosis has already been made. The presence of a pituitary or adrenal tumor does not necessarily guarantee that it is the source of increased ACTH production. Many healthy people with no symptoms or disease whatsoever have noncancerous tumors in the pituitary and adrenal glands. Thus, CT and MRI is often used to image the pituitary and adrenal glands in preparation for surgery.

Treatment

The choice of a specific treatment depends on the type of problem causing the cortisol excess. Pituitary and adrenal adenomas are usually removed surgically. Malignant adrenal tumors always require surgical removal.

Treatment of ectopic ACTH syndrome also involves removing all of the cancerous cells which are producing ACTH. This may be done through surgery, **chemotherapy** (using combinations of cancer-killing drugs), or **radiation therapy** (using x rays to kill cancer cells), depending on the type of cancer and how far it has spread. Radiation therapy may also be used on the pituitary (with or without surgery), for patients who cannot undergo surgery, or for patients whose surgery did not successfully decrease pituitary release of ACTH.

There are a number of drugs that are effective in decreasing adrenal production of cortisol. These medications include **mitotane**, ketoconazole, metyrapone, trilostane, **aminoglutethimide**, and mifepristone. These drugs are sometimes given prior to surgery in an effort to reverse the problems brought on by cortisol excess. However, the drugs may also need to be administered after surgery (sometimes along with radiation treatments) in patients who continue to have excess pituitary production of ACTH.

Because pituitary surgery can cause ACTH levels to drop too low, some patients require short-term treatment with a cortisol-like medication after surgery. Patients who need adrenal surgery may also require glucocorticoid replacement. If the entire adrenal gland has been removed, the patient must take oral glucocorticoids for the rest of his or her life.

Prognosis

Prognosis depends on the source of the problem. When pituitary adenomas are identified as the source of increased ACTH leading to cortisol excess, about 80% of patients are cured by surgery. When cortisol excess is due to some other form of cancer, the prognosis depends on the type of cancer and the extent of its spread.

Resources

BOOKS

Brickner, Colleen. *Inside Out: An Autobiography.* Spokane, WA: A.H. Clark Co., 1992.

DeGroot, Leslie J., ed., et al. "Cushing's syndrome." In *Endocrinology, Vol. 2.* Philadelphia: W.B. Saunders Co., 1995, 1741-69.

Williams, Gordon H., and Robert G. Dluhy. "Hyperfunction of the Adrenal Cortex." In *Harrison's Principles of Internal Medicine,* edited by Anthony S. Fauci, et al. New York: McGraw-Hill, 1998.

PERIODICALS

Boscaro, Marco, Luisa Barzon, Francesco Fallo, and Nicoletta Sonino. "Cushing's Syndrome."*Lancet* 357 (2001): 783-91.

Boscaro, Marco, Luisa Barzon, and Nicoletta Sonino. "The Diagnosis of Cushing's Syndrome: Atypical Presentations and Laboratory Shortcomings."*Archives of Internal Medicine* 160 (2000): 3045-53.

Findlay, C.A., J.F. Macdonald, A.M. Wallace, N. Geddes, and M.D.C. Donaldson. "Childhood Cushing's Syndrome Induced by Betamethasone Nose Drops, and Repeat Prescriptions."*British Medical Journal* 3, no.17 (12 September, 1998): 739-40.

Kirk, Lawrence F., Robert B. Hash, Harold P. Katner, and Tom Jones. "Cushing's Disease: Clinical Manifestations and Diagnostic Evaluation."*American Family Physician* 62, no.5 (1 September, 2001): 1119-27.

Newell-Price J., and A. Grossman. "Diagnosis and Management of Cushing's Syndrome." *Lancet* 353 (1999): 2087-88.

Orth, David N. "Cushing's Syndrome."*The New England Journal of Medicine* 332, no. 12 (23 March, 1995): 791-803.

Utiger, Robert D. "Treatment, and Retreatment, of Cushing's Disease."*The New England Journal of Medicine* 336, no.3 (16 January, 1997): 215-17.

ORGANIZATION

Cushing's Support and Research Foundation, Inc. 65 East India Row, Suite 22B, Boston, MA 02110. (617) 723-3674. <http://www.world.std.com>.

National Adrenal Disease Foundation. 505 Northern Boulevard, Suite 200, Great Neck, NY 11021. (516) 487-4992. <http://www.medhelp.org>.

National Institute of Neurological Disorders and Stroke (NINDS). National Institutes of Health, Bethesda, MD 20892-2560. <http://www.ninds.nih.gov>.

Pituitary Network Association. 16350 Ventura Boulevard, #231, Encino, CA 91436. (805)499-9973. <http://www.pituitary.org>.

Rosalyn Carson-DeWitt, M.D.

Cutaneous T-cell lymphoma

Definition

Cutaneous T-cell lymphoma (CTCL) is a malignancy of the T helper (CD4+) cells of the immune system.

Description

CTCL is a cancer of the white blood cells that primarily affects the skin and only secondarily affects other sites. The disease usually develops slowly, advancing from itchy dark patches on the skin to mushroom shaped tumors, a condition known as **mycosis fungoides**. This disease involves the uncontrollable proliferation of T-lymphocytes known as T helper cells, so named because of their role in the **immune response**. T-helper cells are characterized by the presence of a protein receptor on their surface called CD4. Accordingly, T-helper cells are said to be CD4+.

The proliferation of T-helper cells results in the penetration, or infiltration, of these abnormal cells into the epidermal layer of the skin. The skin reacts with slightly scaling lesions that itch, although the sites of greatest infiltration do not necessarily correspond to the sites of the lesions. The lesions are most often located on the trunk, but can be present on any part of the body. In the most common course of the disease, the patchy lesions progress to palpable plaques that are deeper red and have more defined edges. As the disease worsens, skin tumors develop that are often mushroom-shaped, hence the name mycosis fungoides (the name was not meant to imply that a fungus is involved in the disease). Finally, the cancer progresses to extracutanous involvement, often in the lymph nodes or the viscera.

The progression of the disease is often not linear, although the probability of spread to the viscera (internal organs in the abdomen) is directly related to the amount of skin involvement. Visceral involvement is almost never seen with minimal skin involvement. About 8% of those with generalized plaques have extracutaneous spread, while 30% with tumors have viscera involved. Overall, visceral involvement occurs with only 15 to 20% of all patients diagnosed with the disease.

Some patients present with an overall redness of the skin, with or without overlying plaques or tumors. The skin can be atrophic (shrunken) or lichenified (having small, firm bumps, close together), with cold intolerance and intense **itching**. These patients have swollen lymph nodes and large numbers of abnormal cells circulating the blood. This particular manifestation of CTCL is known as Séary syndrome.

Demographics

CTCL is a rare disease, with an annual incidence of about.29 cases per 100,000 persons in the United States. It is about half as common in Eastern Europe. However, this discrepancy may be attributed to a differing physician awareness of the disease rather than a true difference in occurrence. In the U.S., there are about 500 to 600 new cases a year and about 100 to 200 deaths. Usually seen in older adults, CTCL strikes twice as many men as women and the median age at diagnosis is 55 to 60 years.

Causes and symptoms

The cause of CTCL is unknown. Exposure to chemicals or pesticides has been suggested but the most recent study on the subject failed to show a connection between exposure and development of the disease. The ability to isolate various viruses from cell lines grown from cells of CTCL patients raises the question of a viral cause, but studies have been unable to confirm these suspicions.

The symptoms of CTCL are seen primarily in the skin, with itchy red patches or plaques and, usually over time, mushroom-shaped skin tumors. Any part of the skin can be involved and the extent and distribution of the rash or tumors vary greatly from patient to patient. The only universal symptom of the disease is the itch and this symptom is usually what brings the patient to the doctor for treatment. If the disease spreads outside of the skin, the symptoms include swelling of the lymph nodes, usually most severe in those draining the areas with skin involvement. Spread to the viscera is most often manifested as disorders of the lungs, upper digestive tract, central nervous system, or liver but virtually any organ can be shown to be involved at autopsy.

Diagnosis

Diagnosis of CTCL is often difficult in the early stages because of its slow progression and ability to mimic many other benign skin conditions. The early patches of CTCL resemble closely the rashes of eczema, psoriasis, and contact dermatitis. In a further complication, the early manifestations of the disease can respond favorably to the topical corticosteroid treatments prescribed for these skin disorders. This has the unfortunate result of the disease being missed and the patient remaining untreated for years. CTCL is most likely discovered when a physician maintains a suspicion about the disease, performs multiple skin biopsies, and provides close follow-up after the initial presentation.

Skin biopsies showing penetration of abnormal cells into the epidermal tissue are necessary to make a firm diagnosis of CTCL. Several molecular studies can also help support the diagnosis. The first looks at the cellular proteins seen on the surface of the abnormal cells. Many cases of CTCL show the retention of the CD4+ protein, but the loss of other proteins usually seen on the surface of mature CD4+ cells, such as Leu-8 or Leu-9. The abnormal cells also show unusual rearrangements at the genetic level for the gene that encodes the T-cell receptors. These rearrangements can be identified using Southern blot analysis. The information from the molecular tests, combined with the presence of abnormal cells in the epidermis, strongly supports the CTCL diagnosis.

Treatment team

This disease is treated by a dermatologist, a medical oncologist, and, if **radiation therapy** is used, a radiation oncologist.

Clinical staging, treatments, and prognosis

The current staging of this disease was first presented at the International Consensus Conference on CTCL in 1997. This staging attempts to show the complex interac-

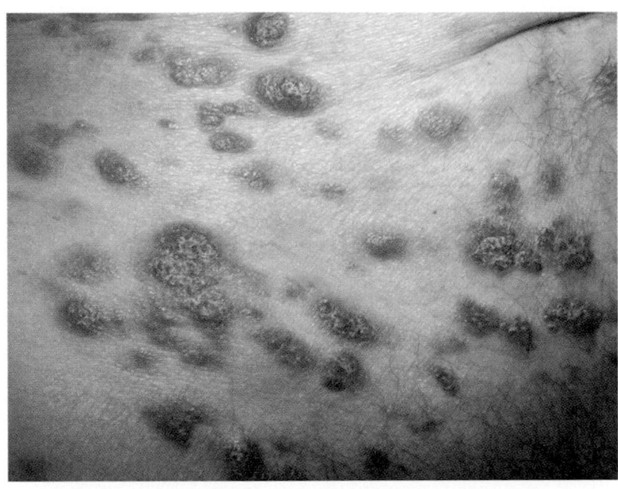

Itchy, crusted plaque on the skin of a patient with cutaneous T-cell lymphoma. *(Custom Medical Stock Photo. Reproduced by permission.)*

tion between the various outward symptoms of the disease and prognosis. The system has seven clinical stages based on skin involvement (tumor = T), lymph node involvement (LN), and presence of visceral metastases (M).

The first stage, IA, is characterized by plaques covering less than 10 percent of the body (T1) and no visceral involvement (M0). Lymph node condition at this stage can be uninvolved, reactive to the skin disease, or dermatopathic (biopsies showing CTCL involvement) but not enlarged (LN0-2). The shorthand expression of this stage is therefore T1, LN0-2, M0. Prognosis is very good if the disease has only progressed this far, with an average survival of 20 or more years. Most deaths occurring to persons in this group are unrelated to CTCL.

The next stage, IB, differs from IA in that greater than 10 percent of the body is covered by plaques (T2, LN0-2, M0). Stage IIA occurs with any amount of plaques in addition to the ability to palpate the lymph node and the lymph uninvolved, reactive, or dermatopathic (T1-2, LN0-2, M0). Average survival for patients in stages IB and IIA is about 12 years.

Treatments applied to the skin are preferred for patients having these preliminary stages of the disease. These commonly include topical **chemotherapy** with **mechlorethamine** hydrochloride (nitrogen mustard) or phototherapy of psoralen plus ultraviolet A (PUVA). Topical chemotherapy involves application to the skin of nitrogen mustard, an alkylating agent, in a concentration of 10 to 20 mg/dL in an aqueous or ointment base. Treatment of affected skin is suggested at a minimum and application over the entire skin surface is often recommended. Care needs to be taken that coverage of involved skin is adequate, as patients who self-apply the

KEY TERMS

Alkylating agent—A chemical that alters the composition of the genetic material of rapidly dividing cells, such as cancer cells, causing selective cell death; used as a topical chemotherapeutic agent to treat CTCL.

Erythroderma—An abnormal reddening of the entire skin surface.

Mycosis fungoides—A well-defined subset of CTCL in which mushroom shaped tumors form on the skin.

Séary Syndrome—A variant of CTCL that is characterized by circulating abnormal T-cells and erythroderma.

T-helper cells—A cellular component of the immune system that plays a major role in ridding the body of bacteria and viruses, characterized by the presence of the CD4 protein on its surface; the type of cell that divides uncontrollable with CTCL.

Total-skin Electron Beam Therapy—A method of radiation therapy used to treat CTCL that involves bombarding the entire body surface with high energy electrons.

drug often cannot reach all affected areas. The most common side effect is skin hypersensitivity to the drug. Nearly all patients respond favorably to this treatment, with a 32 to 61% complete response rate, based on amount of skin involvement. Unfortunately, only 10 to 15% of patients maintain a complete response rate after discontinuing the treatment.

Phototherapy involves treatment with an orally administered drug, 8-methyloxypsoralen, that renders the skin sensitive to long-wave ultraviolet light (UVA), followed by controlled exposure to the radiation. During the initial treatment period, which may last as long as 6 months, patients are treated two to three times weekly. This is reduced to about once monthly after initial clearing of the lesions. Redness of the skin and blistering are the most common side effects of the treatment and are much more common in patients presenting with overall skin redness, or erythroderma, so lower intensities of light are usually used in this case. About 50% of all patients experience complete clearance with this treatment. Some patients with very fair skin and limited skin involvement can successfully treat themselves at home with special lamps and no psoralen.

The next stage, IIB, involves one or more cutaneous tumors, in combination with absent or present palpable lymph nodes, lymph uninvolved, reactive, or dermatopathic, and no visceral involvement (T3, LN0-2, M0). Stage III is characterized by erythroderma, an abnormal redness over widespread areas of the skin (T4, LN0-2, M0). The disease in both of these stages involves intermediate risk to the patient.

For more extensive disease, radiation therapy is an effective treatment option. It is generally used after the topical treatments have proven ineffective. Individual plaques or tumors can be treated using electrons, orthovoltage x rays, or megavoltage photons with exposure in the range of 15 to 25 Gy. Photon therapy has proven particularly useful once the lymph nodes are involved. Another possibility is total-skin electron beam therapy (TSEB), although the availability of this treatment method is limited. It involves irradiation of the entire body with energized electrons. Side effects of this treatment include loss of finger and toe nails, acute redness of the skin, and inability to sweat for about 6 to 12 months after therapy. Almost all patients respond favorably to radiation treatment and any reoccurrence is usually much less severe.

Combinations of different types of treatments is a very common approach to the management of CTCL. Topical nitrogen mustard or PUVA is often used after completion of radiation treatment to prolong the effects. The addition of genetically engineered interferon to PUVA therapy significantly increases the percentage of patients showing a complete response. Furthermore, although treatments using chemotherapy drugs alone, such as deoxycofomycin or etretinate, have been disappointing for CTCL, combining these drugs with interferon has shown promising results. Interferon has also been combined with retinoid treatments, although the mechanism of action of retinoids (Vitamin A analogues) against CTCL is unknown.

The final two stages of the disease are IVA and IVB. IVA presents as any amount of skin involvement, absent or present palpable lymph nodes, no visceral involvement, and lymph that contains large clusters of convoluted cells or obliterated nodes (T1-4, LN3-4). Patients in stage III and IVA have an average life expectancy of about five years. IVB differs in the addition of palpable lymph nodes and visceral involvement (T1-4, LN3-4, M1). At these stages the disease is high risk, with most deaths occurring by infection, due to the depleted immune system of the later stage patient. Once a patient has reached stage IVB, the average life expectancy is one year. All of the treatment methods described above are appropriate for the final two stages of the disease.

Alternative and complementary therapies

Itching of the skin is one of the most troublesome symptoms of CTCL. One alternative treatment for itchiness is the application of a brewed solution of chickweed that is applied to the skin using cloth compresses. Another suggested topical application is a mixture of vitamin E, vitamin A, unflavored yogurt, honey, and zinc oxide. Evening primrose oil applied topically may also reduce itch and promote healing.

Coping with cancer treatment

Topical chemotherapy and radiation treatment of the skin require special care of the areas being exposed to the drug or emission. Use of mild soap and special sensitive formulas for moisturizer and other skin products is suggested. Tight clothing in the area should be avoided. It is important that the treated area is not exposed to the sun during the treatment course. In general, special care to not irritate the area that is being treated will help ease the treatment course.

Clinical trials

Recent **clinical trials** for CTCL have focused on testing molecular treatment approaches. Anti-T-cell **monoclonal antibodies**, that would theoretically target the abnormal T-cells for destruction by the patient's own immune system, have been tried. Unfortunately, the responses to this treatment have been brief and limited by the development of an immune reaction against the antibodies themselves (which are made in mouse cells and therefore seen as foreign by the patient's immune system). Studies continue using newly developed, more specific antibodies and radiolabeled antibodies (to target radiation therapy to the T-helper cells).

Genetically engineered fusion proteins that link diphtheria toxin (a protein that kills cells) with interleukin-2 (a protein that binds to T-helper cells through a receptor on its surface) have also been administered intravenously to CTCL patients. The toxin was taken into the abnormal cells and did kill them. Three out of five patients in a phase I trial achieved significant tumor response to this novel therapy.

Prevention

Studies have been unable to link CTCL to any environmental or genetic factors, so prevention at this time is not possible.

Special concerns

Because the initial diagnosis of CTCL can be difficult, any dermatitis-like or ecuzema-like rash that does not respond to treatment or recurs after running the full course of topical **corticosteroids** should be brought to the attention of a doctor. This is particularly important given the good prognosis with early diagnosis and treatment of CTCL but rapidly worsening prognosis with progression of the disease.

QUESTIONS TO ASK THE DOCTOR

- What is the stage of the disease at this point and what is the prognosis?
- What are the treatment options and what side effects can be expected?
- Is total-skin electron beam therapy (TSEB) available and is this a treatment that should be considered?
- What are the chances of complete clearance of the disease?

See Also Non-Hodgkin's lymphoma

Resources

BOOKS

Hoppe, Richard, T. "Mycosis Fungoides and Other Cutanous Lymphomas." In *The Lymphomas*, edited by Canellos, George P. et al. Philadephia: W.B. Saunders Co., 1999, pp. 495–406.

Wilson, Lynn D., et al. "Cutaneous T-Cell Lymphomas" In *Cancer Principles & Practice of Oncology*, edited by DeVita, Vincent T. et al. Philadelphia: Lippincott Williams & Wilkins, 2001, pp. 2316–2329.

PERIODICALS

Elmer, Kathleen B., and Rita M. George. "Cutaneous T-Cell Lymphoma Presenting as Benign Dermatoses."*American Family Physician* 59(May 1999): 2809–2815.

ORGANIZATIONS

National Cancer Institute. Building 31 Room 10A31 31 Center Drive MSC 2580 Bethesda, MD 20892-2580. (800)4-CANCER. <http://cancernet.nci.nih.gov>

Michelle Johnson, M.S., J.D.

Cyclooxygenase 2 inhibitors

Definition

Cyclooxygenase 2 inhibitors, also known as COX-2 inhibitors, are useful as pain and antiflammatory medica-

KEY TERMS

Cyclooxygenase—A chemical important for the normal functioning of the human body. The body produces cyclooxygenase 1 (COX 1) and cyclooxygenase 2 (COX 2).

Cyclooxygenase 1 (COX 1) —The cyclooxygenase that helps the stomach, kidneys, and blood function well.

Cyclooxygenase 2 (COX 2)—The cyclooxygenase that helps mediate inflammation and that helps the brain feel pain and regulate fever.

tions for cancer patients. COX-2 inhibitors are not better at stopping pain and inflammation than other **nonsteroidal anti-inflammatory drugs** (NSAIDs), but are less likely to cause stomach ulcers and bleeding.

Purpose

Nonsteroidal anti-inflammatory drugs (NSAIDs) used to treat pain and inflammation are relatively effective in controlling these symptoms but can cause serious side effects. These side effects include stomach ulcers, kidney problems, and increased likelihood of bleeding. Aspirin is the most serious offender, although other pain medications in the NSAID class of medication present similar problems. COX-2 inhibitors were developed as a type of pain medication less likely to cause stomach and bleeding problems than existing NSAID pain medications.

Description

Cyclooxygenase is a chemical important for the normal functioning of the human body. Cyclooxygenase helps the stomach and kidneys to function normally, the platelets in the blood to function normally, and the brain to regulate body temperature and feel pain. Scientists have discovered that there are two distinct types of cyclooxygenase (abbreviated COX). These two types of COX are known as COX-1 and COX-2. COX-1 is needed to maintain the normal body functions of platelet aggregation, the regulation of blood flow in the kidney and stomach, and the regulation of gastric acid secretion in the stomach.

COX-2 is produced only when the body's tissues have been injured. COX-2 mediates inflammation, helps the nerves feel pain, and helps the brain regulate **fever**. A medication that inhibits COX-2 can suppress inflammation, relieve pain, and reduce fever. Inhibition of COX-1, on the other hand, results in bleeding and kidney and stomach toxicity.

The problem with many older pain medications is that they affect both COX-1 and COX-2, even though they provid benefit only through how they affect COX-2. That is why their long-term use may be associated with such side effects as stomach ulcers, decreased kidney function, and a tendency for excessive bleeding. COX-2 inhibitors inhibit COX-2 while exerting less effect on COX-1.

As of 2001, two COX-2 inhibitors are available by prescription in the United States. Celecoxib (brand name Celebrex) was the first to be available, followed by rofecoxib (brand name Vioxx).

Recommended dosage

Celecoxib comes in 100 mg and 200 mg capsules that are taken orally either once or twice a day.

Rofecoxib comes in 12.5, 25, and 50 mg tablets for oral use. In addition, it comes in 12.5 mg per 5 milliliter and 25 mg per 5 milliliter liquid doses. Both tablets and liquid are taken orally once a day.

Precautions

Celecoxib should not be taken by patients with sulfonamide allergy. This medication should not be taken during the last few months of pregnancy.

Rofecoxib is safe for patients who are allergic to sulfonamides. It should not be taken during the last few months of pregnancy.

Side effects

Celecoxib has few side effects. A small number of patients report stomach upset and even fewer report abdominal pain. Other effects reported rarely with celecoxib include kidney problems, fluid retention, and retention of water in the tissues. The occurrence of ulcers in patients taking celecoxib is less frequent than for many other pain medications. However, the long-term safety of celecoxib has not been well-researched.

Rofecoxib may cause **diarrhea**, dyspepsia, and abdominal pain. More rarely, headache, kidney problems, high blood pressure, **anemia**, respiratory infections, and retention of water in the legs is seen. The occurrence of ulcers in patients taking rofecoxib is less frequent than for many other pain medications. However, the long-term safety of rofecoxib has not been well-researched.

Interactions

Celecoxib may affect the activities of **warfarin**, a medication that limits the ability of blood to clot. Celecoxib may also be involved in interactions with: furosemide, a diuretic; angiotensin-converting enzyme inhibitors (ACE inhibitors), medicines used for high blood pressure and some heart problems; lithium, a medication for bipolar disorder; and fluconazole, an antifungal medication. Celecoxib may be taken with any of the medicines mentioned above—however, the doctor should closely monitor these drug combinations. Because celecoxib is a relatively new medication, more remains to be learned about its potential to interact with other drugs.

Rofecoxib may interact with the anti-tuberculosis medication rifampin. It may also be involved in interactions with lithium, ACE inhibitors, warfarin, and **methotrexate**, a medication used for cancer and arthritis. Rofecoxib may be taken with any of the medicines mentioned above—again, however, the doctor should closely monitor these drug combinations. Because rofecoxib is a relatively new medication, more remains to be learned about its potential to interact with other drugs.

Bob Kirsch

Cyclophosphamide

Definition

Cyclophosphamide is an anticancer (antineoplastic) agent. It also acts as a suppressor of the immune system. It is available under the brand names Cytoxan and Neosar.

Purpose

Cyclophosphamide is approved by the Food and Drug Administration (FDA) to treat several forms of cancer. These include:

- **breast cancer**
- leukemia
- malignant lymphoma
- **multiple myeloma**
- **ovarian cancer**
- soft tissue sarcoma
- **mycosis fungoides**
- nephrotic syndrome
- **neuroblastoma**
- **Wilms' tumor**
- **retinoblastoma**

Cyclophosphamide has activity against a wide variety of other cancers and conditions not specifically approved by the FDA, and patients should be aware that it may be commonly prescribed for these other disease states:

- bone cancer
- **cervical cancer**
- **endometrial cancer**
- **germ cell tumors**
- **gestational trophoblastic tumors**
- **histiocytosis X**
- lung cancer
- **prostate cancer**
- **testicular cancer**
- Wilms' tumor

Description

Cyclophosphamide chemically interferes with the synthesis of the genetic material (DNA and RNA) of cancer cells by cross-linking DNA strands, preventing these cells from being able to reproduce and continue the growth of the cancer.

Recommended dosage

Cyclophosphamide may be taken either orally (in pill form) or as an injection into the vein. The dosage prescribed may vary widely depending on the patient, the cancer being treated, and whether or not other medications are also being taken.

A typical oral dosage for adults is 1 to 5 mg per kg of body weight per day for initial and maintenance dose, or 400 to 1000 milligrams per squared meter of body surface area for four to five days every three to four weeks. A typical dosage by injection is 40 to 50 mg per kg, divided in several smaller doses, for two to five days. The dose for patients receiving bone marrow transplant may be as high as 60 mg per kg per day for two days.

Precautions

Cyclophosphamide should be taken on an empty stomach. If stomach irritation occurs, it should be taken with small amounts of food or milk. Cyclophosphamide should always be taken with plenty of fluids.

Cyclophosphamide can cause an allergic reaction in some people. Patients with a prior allergic reaction to cyclophosphamide should not receive this drug.

Cyclophosphamide can cause serious birth defects if either the man or the woman is taking this drug at the time of conception or if the woman is taking this drug during pregnancy. Contraceptive measures should be

KEY TERMS

Antineoplastic—A drug that prevents the growth of a neoplasm by interfering with the maturation or proliferation of the cells of the neoplasm.

Neoplasm—New abnormal growth of tissue.

taken by both men and women while on this drug. Sterility is a common side effect of cyclophosphamide. This sterility is dependent upon the dose, duration of therapy, and state of function of the ovary or testicle at the time of administration of the drug. The sterility may be irreversible in some patients.

Because cyclophosphamide is easily passed from mother to child through breast milk, breast feeding is not recommended while under treatment.

Cyclophosphamide suppresses the immune system and interferes with the normal functioning of certain organs and tissues, and its excretion from the body is dependent on a normal functioning kidney and liver. For these reasons, it is important that the prescribing physician is aware of any of the following pre-existing medical conditions:

- a current case of, or recent exposure to, chicken pox
- herpes zoster (shingles)
- all current infections
- kidney disease
- liver disease
- a prior removal of one, or both, adrenal gland(s)

Also, because cyclophosphamide is such a potent immunosuppressant, patients taking this drug must exercise extreme caution to avoid contracting any new infections.

Side effects

Inflammation and irritation of the bladder, causing blood in the urine, is a common and severe side effect of cyclophosphamide. However, this side effect can be prevented and controlled with the administration of vigorous hydration with intravenous fluids before, during, and after **chemotherapy**. Patients should urinate frequently (at least every 2 hours) to enhance removal of the drug from the body, drink 3 to 4 liters of fluids a day while taking the drug by mouth and for 2 to 3 days after discontinuation of the drug unless otherwise instructed by the physician. Patients who are taking cyclophosphamide orally should avoid taking the drug at night so that they can go to the bathroom frequently during the day. The bladder-protectant drug **mesna** is usually administered if the patient is receiving more than 2,000 mg per square meter of body surface area of the cyclophosphamide. Another common side effect of cyclophosphamide is increased susceptibility to infection due to decreased production of cells that fight infection. Increased risk of bleeding can occur due to decrease of platelets, which are involved with the clotting process. Decreased production of red blood cells can cause **anemia** and patients may experience **fatigue**, and shortness of breath.

Nausea and vomiting can occur, usually at the higher doses. Taking the appropriate **antiemetics** prescribed by the physician can prevent this side effect. Temporary hair loss (**alopecia**) usually begins 3-6 weeks after the start of therapy, but hair will regrow (although it may be a different color and/or texture). Sterility can occur in both men and women, and some women may also experience stoppage of menstruation. **Diarrhea** and ulcers of the mouth are also possible side effects of cyclophosphamide treatment.

Less common side effects include:

- nasal stuffiness
- runny eyes
- runny nose
- sinus congestion
- dizziness
- darkening of skin or fingernails
- skin rash
- sneezing (if the drug is given too rapidly by injection into the vein
- facial flushing

Some patients may also develop a second cancer years later with cyclophosphamide therapy alone or in combination with other anti cancer drugs. Patients should discuss this side effect with their physicians and determine the risks versus the benefits of this drug for treatment of the immediate cancer.

A doctor should be consulted immediately if the patient experiences any of the following:

- painful or difficult urination
- increase in frequency or feeling of urgency to urinate
- blood in the urine
- shortness of breath
- signs of infection such as cough, sore throat, **fever** and chills
- pain in the lower back or sides

- unusual bleeding or bruising
- blood in the stool
- tiny red dots on the skin
- delayed healing of any wounds
- skin rash
- yellowing of the skin or eyes

Interactions

Cyclophosphamide should not be taken in combination with any prescription drug, over-the-counter drug, or herbal remedy without prior consultation with a physician.

Paul A. Johnson, Ed.M.

KEY TERMS

Intravenous line—A tube that is inserted directly into a vein to carry medicine directly to the bloodstream, bypassing the stomach and other digestive organs that might alter the medicine.

Lymphatic system—The system that collects and returns fluid in tissues to the blood vessels and produces defensive agents for fighting infection and invasion by foreign bodies.

Kilogram (kg)—Metric measure that equals 2.2 pounds.

Milligram (mg)—One-thousandth of a gram. A gram is the metric measure that equals about 0.035 ounces.

Cyclosporine

Definition

Cylosporine is an immunosuppressant drug used to prevent rejection of kidney, liver, and heart transplants, to prevent graft-versus-host disease in patients receiving allogeneic bone marrow transplants, and for severe autoimmune diseases that are resistant to **corticosteroids** and other therapy. Cyclosporine, also spelled as cyclosporin and ciclosporin, takes several brand names in the United States, including Neoral, Sandimmun, Sandimmune, and Sang Cya. It is also known in slight variant forms, such as cyclosporin A, CsA, and CyA. The Neoral and Sang Cya brand name products are interchangeable, but the Sandimmune brand name product can not be used interchangeably for those other two products.

Purpose

Cyclosporine is best known as a drug used to prevent the rejection of organ transplants and bone grafts.

Description

Discovered in 1972, cyclosporine was first isolated from a fungus. It suppresses (prevents the activity of) the cells in the lymphatic system, known as T cells, that would otherwise mount an **immune response**. This suppression makes cyclosporine useful in conjunction with organ transplants. (In a transplant, the patient receiving a donated organ can react to the organ as though it were a foreign substance, rejecting it.) Cyclosporine is also used to treat severe rheumatoid arthritis, and is being used investigationally as a drug that may help to temper multidrug resistance in cancer patients.

The drug is available in several forms, including an intravenous (I.V.) solution, an oral solution, and an oral capsule. Cyclosporine is broken down in the liver.

Recommended dosage

The dosage varies, depending on the reason for use and the patient, and the dosage is also often adjusted by the physician. The dosage is based on the patient's ideal body weight, and the oral dose is approximately three times higher than the intravenous dose. I.V. use is only reserved for patients who cannot take the oral dose, and it is recommended that patients who can be switched to the oral form be switched as soon as possible.

The usual initial oral dose is 14–18 mg/kg per day, beginning four–twelve hours before organ transplantation. After the transplantation, the dose is decreased, and then usually tapered to 3–10 mg/kg per day.

Precautions

Cyclosporine can cause infection and possibly **lymphoma**, and is toxic to the kidneys. The use of this drug along with other drugs that are toxic to the kidneys must be closely monitored. It should be ingested and swallowed in its capsule without breaking the capsule. The liquid solution should only be mixed in a glass container. Pregnant or nursing women should not take this drug, and patients taking this drug will be more susceptible to infection. Therefore, crowds of people should be avoided, and no live **vaccines** should be adminstered to the patient without consulting the patient's doctor. Patients should inform their doctor of any hypersensitivities or drug allergies they have before taking this drug. (Cyclosporine in both liquid and capsule form has some castor oil components in it, which could cause an allergic reaction for some.) Some allergic reactions to the I. V. solution may be severe. This drug has not been specifically studied for use with the elderly.

Side effects

More than 10% of patients taking this drug experience the following:

- high blood pressure
- unusual hair growth
- kidney toxicity
- tremors
- thickening of the gums

Other, less common side effects include: seizures, headache, acne, abdominal pain, **nausea and vomiting**, leg cramps, and some endocrine/metabolic conditions known as hypomagnesia, hypokalemia, hyperkalemia, and hyperlipidemia.

Interactions

Cyclosporine interacts with a long list of other drugs. A physician should be informed about each and every drug a person eligible for treatment with cyclosporine is taking. Drugs that may make cyclosporine less effective include: **carbamazepine**, phenobarbital, **phenytoin**, and others. Drugs that may increase cyclopsporine's toxicity include: acyclovir, amphotericin B, corticosteroids, erythromycin, certain **antibiotics**, and some antifungals including fluconazole, itraconazole, and ketaconazole. Cyclosporine should not be taken with grapefruit or related juices because the combination can make it more toxic. Vaccinations should not be given while a person is taking cyclosporine.

Diane M. Calabrese

Cystoscopy

Definition

Cystoscopy (cystourethroscopy) is a diagnostic procedure that is used to look at the bladder (lower urinary tract), collect urine samples, and examine the prostate gland. Performed with an optic instrument known as a cystoscope (urethroscope), this instrument uses a lighted tip for guidance to aid in diagnosing urinary tract disease and prostate disease. Performed by a urologist, this surgical test also enables biopsies to be taken or small stones to be removed by way of a hollow channel in the cystoscope.

Purpose

Categorized as an endoscopic procedure, cystoscopy is used by urologists to examine the entire bladder lining and take biopsies of any areas that look questionable. This test is not used on a routine basis but may benefit the urologist who needs further information about a patient who displays the following symptoms or diagnosis:

- blood in the urine (also known as hematuria)
- incontinence, or the inability to control urination
- a urinary tract infection
- a urinary tract that display signs of congenital abnormalities
- tumors located in the bladder
- the presence of bladder or kidney stones
- a stiffness or strained feeling of the urethra or ureters
- symptoms of an enlarged prostate

Blood and urine studies, in addition to x rays of the kidneys, ureters, and bladder may all occur before a cystoscopy. At the time of the procedure, a retrograde pyelogram may also be performed. Additional blood studies may be needed immediately following cystoscopy.

Precautions

While the cystoscopy procedure is commonly relied on to gather additional diagnostic information, it is an invasive surgical technique that may involve risks for certain patients. Those who are extremely overweight (obese), smoke, are recovering from a recent illness, or are treating a chronic condition may face additional risks from surgery.

Surgical risk also increases in patients who are currently using certain drugs including antihypertensives; muscle relaxants; tranquilizers; sleep inducers; insulin; sedatives; beta blockers; or cortisone. Those who use mind-altering drugs also put themselves at increased risk of complications during surgery. The following mind-altering drugs should be avoided: narcotics, psychedelics, hallucinogens, **marijuana**, sedatives, hypnotics, or cocaine.

Description

Depending on the type of information needed from a cystoscopy, the procedure typically takes 10–40 minutes to complete. The patient will be asked to urinate before the procedure, which allows an accurate measurement of the remaining urine in the bladder. A well-lubricated cystoscope is inserted through the urethra into the bladder, where a urine sample is taken. Fluid is then pushed in to inflate the bladder and allow the urologist to examine the entire bladder wall.

During an examination, the urologist may take the following steps: remove either bladder or kidney stones; gather tissue samples; and treat any suspicious lesions. In order to perform the x-ray studies known as a retrograde pyelogram, a harmless dye is injected into the ureters by way of a catheter that is passed through the previously placed cystoscope. After completion of all needed tests, the cystoscope is removed.

Preparation

A cystoscopic procedure can be completed in a hospital, a doctor's office, or an outpatient surgical facility. An injection of spinal or general anesthetic may be used prior to a cystoscopy. Although this test is typically performed on an outpatient basis, a patient may require up to three days' recovery in the hospital.

Aftercare

Patients who have undergone a cystoscopy will be instructed to follow these steps to ensure a quick recovery:

- Because of soreness or discomfort that may occur in the urethra, especially while urinating, several warm baths a day are recommended to relieve any pain.
- Allow four days for recovery.
- Be aware that blood may appear in the urine. This is common and soon clears up in one to two days following the procedure.
- Avoid strenuous exercise for a minimum of two weeks following cystoscopy.
- Sexual relations may continue when the urologist determines that healing is complete.
- Wait at least two days after surgery before driving.

Patients may also be prescribed pain relievers and **antibiotics** following surgery. Minor pain may also be treated with over-the-counter, nonprescription drugs such as acetaminophen.

Risks

As with any surgical procedure, there are some risks involved with a cystoscopy. Complications may include profuse bleeding, a damaged urethra, a perforated bladder, a urinary tract infection, or an injured penis.

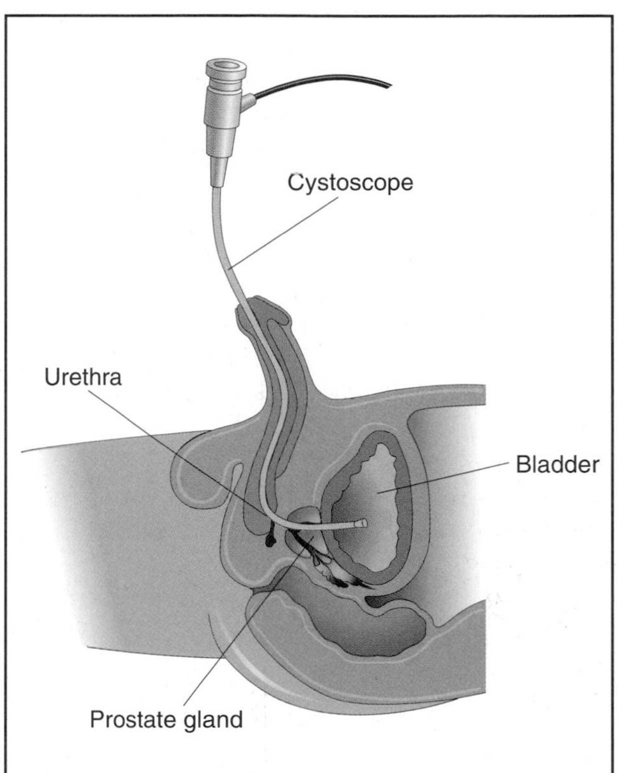

Cystoscopy is a diagnostic procedure which is used to view the bladder, collect urine samples, and examine the prostate gland. This procedure also enables biopsies to be taken. The primary instrument used in cystoscopy is the cystoscope, a tube which is inserted through the penis, into the urethra, and ultimately into the bladder. *(Illustration by Electronic Illustrators Group.)*

Patients should also contact their physician if they experience any of the following symptoms following surgery: pain at or redness or swelling around the surgical site; drainage or bleeding from the surgical site; signs of infection, which may include headache, muscle aches, dizziness, an overall ill feeling, and **fever**; nausea or vomiting; strenuous or painful urination; or symptoms that may result as side effects from the medication.

Normal results

A successful cystoscopy includes a thorough examination of the bladder and collection of urine samples for cultures. If no abnormalities are seen, the results are indicated as normal.

Abnormal results

Cystoscopy allows the urologist to detect inflammation of the bladder lining, prostatic enlargement, or tumors. If these are seen, further evaluation or biopsies may be needed, in addition to the removal of some tumors.

KEY TERMS

Cystoscopy with bladder distention (hydrodistention)—Under anesthesia, the bladder is stretched to capacity (distended) with either liquid or gas and then examined with a cystoscope. The examination will detect bladder wall inflammation; thick, stiff bladder wall; Hunner's ulcers; and glomerulations.

Endoscopy—Examination of body organs or cavities through the use of an endoscope (a lighted optical instrument used to see inside body cavities), such as a cystoscope used to complete a cystoscopy.

Glomerulation—Pinpoint bleeding caused by recurrent irritation that can appear on the bladder wall.

Retrograde pyelogram—A pyelography or x-ray technique in which radiopaque dye is injected into the kidneys from below, by way of the ureters, allowing further examination of the kidneys.

Ureter—The tube that carries urine from the kidney to the bladder, with each kidney having one ureter.

Urethra—A passageway from the bladder to the outside for the discharge of urine. In the female this canal lies between the vagina and the clitoris; in the male the urethra travels through the penis, opening at the tip.

QUESTIONS TO ASK THE DOCTOR

- Why do I need a cystoscopic examination?
- How long will a cystoscopic procedure take?
- How long is recovery from a cystoscopic procedure?

Resources

BOOKS

Segen, Joseph C., and Joseph Stauffer. "Cystoscopy." In *The Patient's Guide to Medical Tests: Everything you Need to Know about the Tests Your Doctor Prescribes.* New York: Facts on File, 1998.

PERIODICALS

Chew, Lisa, and Stephan D. Fihn. "Recurrent cystitis in non-pregnant women."*Western Journal of Medicine* (May 1999)170: 274-277.

Gilmour, D.T., P.L. Dwyer, M.P. Carey. "Lower urinary tract injury during gynecologic surgery and its detection by intraoperative cystoscopy"*Obstetrics and Gynecology*(1999)5(2):883-889.

Neumayer, Leigh, A., Mary K. Mastin, and Douglas M. Hinson. "Performance Standards: Piece of Cake or Pie in the sky?"*Journal of Surgical Research* (2000)88:47-50.

Weinberger, M.W. "Cytosurethroscopy for the Practicing Gynecologist."*Clinical Obstetrics and Gynecology* (September 1998)41(2): 764-776.

ORGANIZATIONS

American Cancer Society. 1599 Clifton Road, NE, Atlanta, GA 30329-4251. (800)ACS-2345. http://www.cancer.org/. The American Cancer Society (ACS) is a nationwide community-based voluntary health organization dedicated to eliminating cancer as a major health problem and is the largest source of private, nonprofit cancer funds. The ACS hopes to prevent cancer, save lives, and diminish suffering from cancer through research, education, advocacy, and service.

Interstitial Cystitis Association (ICA), 51 Monroe Street, Suite 1402, Rockville, MD 20850, 1-800-HELP-ICA, http://www.ichelp.org. Founded in 1984, the ICA is a not-for-profit health organization dedicated to providing patient and physician educational information and programs, patient support, public awareness, and research funding.

National Institute of Diabetes & Digestive & Kidney Disease, Office of Communications and Public Liaison, NIDDK, NIH, 31 Center Drive, MSC 2560, Bethesda, MD 20892-2560, NIDDK_Inquiries@nih.gov. http://www.niddk.nih.gov. Mission to understand, treat, and prevent diseases, such as diabetes and obesity, digestive diseases such as hepatitis and inflammatory bowel disease, kidney and urologic diseases such as kidney failure and prostate enlargement, and blood diseases such as the anemias.

National Kidney and Urologic Diseases Information Clearinghouse, 3 Information Way, Bethesda, MD 20892-3580, 1-800-891-5390, nkudic@info.niddk.nih.gov, http://www.niddk.nih.gov/health/kidney/nkudic.htm. Knowledge and understanding about diseases of the kidneys and urologic system among people with these conditions and their families, health care professionals, and the general public.

Beth A. Kapes

Cytarabine

Definition

Cytarabine (also known as ARA-C, and by the brand name Cytosar) is an anticancer agent that kills cancer cells. It is very frequently used with other anticancer drugs in the treatment of **acute myelocytic leukemia** (AML), lymphomas, and for leukemia and **lymphoma** affecting the surrounding membranes of the brain and spinal cord (meninges).

Purpose

There are two formulations of this drug: cytarabine, and cytarabine liposomal, where the drug is encapsulated in a molecule of lipid. Cytarabine is used to treat acute myelogenous leukemia, **acute lymphocytic leukemia** (ALL), **chronic myelocytic leukemia** (CML), central nervous system (CNS) leukemia affecting the membrane surrounding the brain and spinal cord, and Hodgkin's and non-Hodgkin's lymphoma (NHL). Cytarabine liposomal (brand name Depocyt) is primarily used to treat lymphoma involving the meninges (the membrane covering the brain and spinal cord).

Description

Cytarabine is a cytotoxic drug. This means that its task is to kill cancer cells. Cytarabine kills cells by interfering with the production of DNA.

Recommended dosage

The dose for cytarabine may be different depending on the protocol used by the physician. An example dose of cytarabine is 100 to 200 mg per square meter of body surface area per day for seven days as an intravenous (IV) medication.

High-dose cytarabine may be 2 to 3 grams per square meter of body surface area twice a day for three days. Cytarabine is also administered directly into the cerebral spinal fluid for lymphoma or leukemia involving the meninges. The dose is 5 to 75 mg per square meter of body surface area every two to seven days. The dose for cytarabine liposomal in the cerebral spinal fluid is usually 50 mg.

Precautions

Liposomal cytarabine not be given to patients with infections of the meninges, allergic reaction to cytarabine, or if the patient is pregnant.

Side effects

Side effects include **fever** in greater than 80% of patients, hair loss (**alopecia**), **nausea and vomiting**, **diarrhea**, ulcers of the mouth, decreased white blood cells (responsible for fighting infections), decreased platelets (responsible for blood clotting), decreased red blood cells (responsible for oxygenation of tissues), and decrease in liver function. Abdominal pain, loss of appetite, and a metallic taste in the mouth may develop, as may an allergic reaction. Tearing, eye pain, foreign body sensation in the eye, blurred vision, and sensitivity of the eyes to light occurs with high-dose cytarabine and may be prevented or relieved with corticosteroid eyedrops. Patients receiving high-dose cytarabine may also experience skin sloughing, redness and pain of the palms of the hand and soles of the feet, dizziness, headaches, drowsiness, confusion, personality changes, abnormal movements of the eye, loss of coordination, and in severe cases, loss of consciousness.

Although it is uncommon, one of the most serious side effects of cytarabine may involve sudden respiratory distress involving abnormal, shallow, and rapid breathing, which may progress to **pneumonia**.

High doses of cytarabine may trigger what is known as cytarabine syndrome, which consists of fever, muscle ache, **bone pain**, occasional chest pain, rash, inflammation of the membrane that covers the outer surface of the eye. This syndrome occurs six to 12 hours after the drug is given. **Corticosteroids** can treat this syndrome or prevent it from occurring.

Interactions

Drugs that decrease the function of the kidneys may increase the toxic side effects of cytarabine. Cytarabine may decrease the effect of digoxin and the **antibiotics** gentamicin and flucytosine. Prior to starting any new medications or herbal remedies, patients should consult with their physician, nurse, or pharmacist to prevent any drug interactions.

Bob Kirsch

KEY TERMS

Cytotoxic drug—A medicine that kills (cancer) cells.

DNA—An acid found in all living cells that contains tiny bits of genetic information.

Lipids—Substances including fats, waxes, and related compounds that (with proteins and carbohydrates) constitute the principal structural components of living cells.

Cytogenetic analysis

Definition

Cytogenetics is the analysis of blood or bone marrow cells that reveals the organization of chromosomes. Chromosomes are the physical structures that contain the genetic material, DNA.

Purpose

Cytogenetic analyses are essential to the diagnosis and treatment of different forms of cancer, especially leukemia, cancers of the blood cell-forming system. The results of cytogenetic tests can help to confirm the diagnosis of a particular form of leukemia, and permit the best treatment to be selected for each patient.

Precautions

This test is performed on tissue or cells that have been removed during the initial surgery or diagnostic procedure used to determine the precise nature of the leukemia or other cancer. It usually does not require any new surgery or blood draw on the patient and, so, does not entail any additional precautions for the patient.

Description

The development of leukemia and other cancers involves alterations, or mutations, in the cellular genetic material. The types of changes seen differ among various forms of cancer, but include changes in the specific sequence of DNA substituent units (termed nucleotides), as well as more dramatic alterations. Some of these more dramatic alterations include loss or duplication of large stretches of DNA sequence, or chromosomal rearrangements that correspond to the movement of genetic sequences from one chromosome to another. These rearrangements can lead to the production of novel, and often characteristic, molecules that are believed to play essential parts in the development of particular cancers.

Cytogenetic analysis focuses upon chromosomal rearrangements. In essence, this type of testing is a hybrid approach that combines genetics, analysis of mutations, with examination of cells. The cells to be tested, usually obtained from circulating blood or bone marrow, are treated in such a way that the chromosomes are made visible. Cells that are about to divide and which have condensed and organized their chromosomes into pairs are most suitable for this type of analysis. Often cells will be treated in the laboratory to increase the frequency of such cells, in which the chromosomes are visible as what are called mitotic figures. Cells containing such mitotic figures are then chemically stained in a way that makes it possible to identify specific chromosomes. When such stained chromosomes are visualized and enumerated, the resulting pattern is termed the karyotype of that cell.

The karyotypes of many cells are usually scrutinized to establish whether some fraction of cells display a reproducible genetic alteration that can be associated with a specific cancer. Historically, the first such abnormality recognized was the Philadelphia chromosome, which is associated with chronic myelogenous leukemia (also called **chronic myelocytic leukemia**, or CML). In virtually all cases of CML, cytogenetic analyses will reveal a Philadelphia chromosome. The presence of this marker can be used to monitor response to treatment. There are a variety of other genetic abnormalities that are associated with specific forms of cancer. Most of these have been recognized using cytogenetics, and to varying degrees have become useful in diagnosis of leukemia and solid tumors, or in predicting treatment outcome.

Cytogenetics examines microscopically visible chromosomal changes. More recently developed molecular approaches can recognize the same sorts of genetic rearrangements as seen in abnormal karyotypes. In addition, these molecular tests can recognize smaller, more subtle alterations affecting just one or a few of the nucleotide units within a cancer-related gene. These techniques can, in some cases, be more sensitive than cytogenetic approaches, and along with the large body of information derived from the human genome project, hold the promise or providing more accurate tests for diagnosis and treatment of cancer.

KEY TERMS

Chromosome—The self-replicating genetic the structures in cells that containing the cellular DNA, the hereditary material, that includes the genes in a particular order.

DNA sequence—The relative order of nucleotides, the chemical subunits of a DNA molecule.

Gene rearrangement—A change in the structure of a chromosome that changes the order of genes.

Karyotype—A complete set of chromosomes that are examined to look for genetic abnormalities

QUESTIONS TO ASK THE DOCTOR

- Are the cytogenetic results what you would expect based upon other diagnostic tests and examinations I have undergone?
- Will you want to repeat this test? At what point in my treatment will you want to do so?
- Do these test results tell you anything about my prospects for a disease-free survival?

Preparation and Aftercare

The only preparation and aftercare would be the preparation and aftercare required for the sample collection—a blood draw or a **bone marrow aspiration and biopsy**. The cytogenetic analysis itself requires no additional preparation or aftercare on the part of the patient.

Risks

This test is performed on tissue or cells that have been removed during the initial surgery or diagnostic procedure used to determine the precise nature of the leukemia or other cancer. It usually does not require any new surgery or blood draw on the patient and, so, does not entail any additional risk to the patient.

Results

Human body cells, exclusive of reproductive cells, have 23 pairs of chromosomes. Any deviation from this is considered abnormal. Cytogenetic analysis directed toward leukemia or other cancer cells is considered to have an abnormal result when a specific, distinctive genetic alteration is seen in the configuration of these chromosomes. The absence of a cytogenetic alteration is not, by any means, a basis to conclude there is an absence of a particular disease or that the prognosis is better than if a genetic abnormality was observed. For example, in **acute lymphocytic leukemia** (ALL) there are several different genetic rearrangements that are each associated with a different outcome. The patients who do the best are not those without any cytogenetic abnormality, but rather those with one specific chromosomal rearrangement. Therefore the potential use of cytogenetics, and similar molecular analyses, is to enable doctors to more accurately determine the diagnosis, treatment, and follow-up of patients with leukemia and other forms of cancer.

See Also Chromosome rearrangements

Resources

PERIODICALS

Nowell P.C., J. D. Rowley, A. D. Knudson, Jr. "Cancer genetics, cytogenetics: defining the enemy within." *Nature Medicine* 4(October 1998):1107-11.

Warren Maltzman, Ph.D.

Cytology

Definition

Cytology is the examination of individual cells and small clusters of cells, and may be used for the diagnosis and screening of diseases, including cancers. Cytology can also be referred to as cytopathology.

Purpose

Diagnostic tests are used to detect a disease in individuals who have signs, symptoms, or some other abnormality that is indicative of disease. A **screening test** identifies those who might have a certain disease, sometimes before they develop any symptoms, but does not absolutely prove that disease is present. If a screening test is positive, a diagnostic test can be used as follow-up to verify the diagnosis.

Precautions

Procedures to gather cells for cytology are often less invasive than other forms of **biopsy**, and therefore may

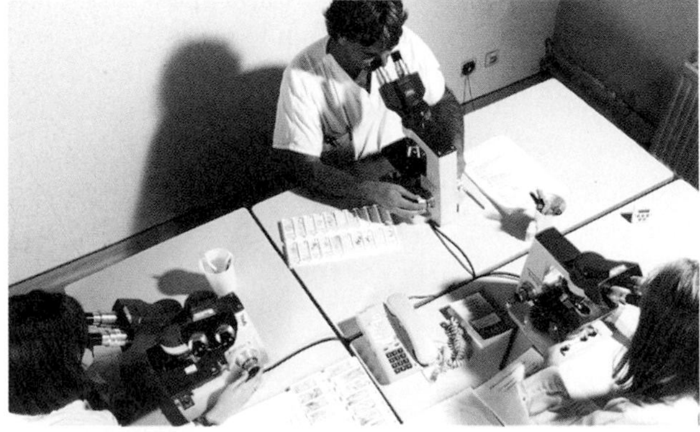

Researchers at binocular light microscopes analyze biological samples in a laboratory. The samples have been prepared on glass slides in trays and have been stained with dyes to highlight certain types of cells or tissues. *(© CC Studio Science Source/Photo Researchers, Inc. Reproduced by permission.)*

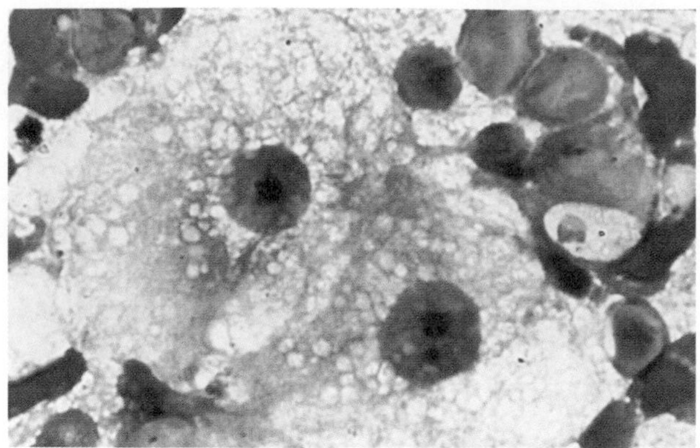

Kidney cancer cells for examination by a pathologist. *(© Parviz M. Pour, Science Source/Photo Researchers, Inc. Reproduced by permission.)*

cause less discomfort, be less likely to result in serious complications, and cost less to perform. In some situations, however, where a piece of tissue is removed rather than individual cells, a different type of biopsy may be required to confirm the cytologic diagnosis.

Description

Samples for cytology can be obtained in more than one way. Fine needle aspiration (FNA) is a type of biopsy in which tumor samples are taken through thin needles.

Scrape or brush cytology is another technique in which cells are scraped or brushed from the organ or tissue being tested. Samples from the esophagus, stomach, bronchi (breathing tubes that lead to the lungs), and mouth can be obtained using this procedure.

How a cytology sample is processed depends on what type of sample it is. A doctor can smear a sample directly on a glass microscope slide. The slide is then stained and viewed by a cytopathologist. In other cases, the fluid is concentrated before being smeared and stained on a slide. This is especially useful for dilute samples such those from body cavities.

Most routine cytology results are available one or two days after the sample is received in the laboratory. There are many reasons why some results take longer to return, such as if special stains are required to confirm a diagnosis.

Preparation, Aftercare, and Risks

Because this analysis is performed on cells that had been already gathered during initial diagnostic procedures, there is no additional preparation, aftercare, or risks for the patient. The only procedure, aftercare, or risks to note would be those associated with the sample collection itself.

KEY TERMS

Biopsy—Removing tissue from living patients for a diagnostic examination.

Cytology/cytopathology—The study of cells or cell types.

Fine needle aspiration—Removal of tissue or suspensions of cells using a small needle.

Pap smear—A common cytology test used to screen for malignant and premalignant changes of the cervix.

QUESTIONS TO ASK THE DOCTOR

- What is a cytology test?
- How accurate is a cytology test?
- How long will it take to get cytology test results?

Normal results

A cytopathologist examines and identifies the normal and abnormal cells on the slide using a microscope.

Abnormal results

A pathologist reviews the cells identified as abnormal to decide on a diagnosis.

See Also Biopsy; Pap test

Resources

PERIODICALS

Dahlstrom, Jane E., Gillian M. Langdale-Smith, and Daniel T. James. "Fine Needle Aspiration Cytology of Pulmonary Lesions: A Reliable Diagnostic Test" *Pathology* 33 (2001): 13-16.

ORGANIZATIONS

American Cancer Society. 1599 Clifton Road NE, Atlanta, GA 30329. (404) 320-3333. <http://www.cancer.org>.

American Society for Clinical Pathologists (ASCP). 2100 West Harrison Street, Chicago, IL 60612. (312) 738-1336. <http://www.ascp.org.>.

American Society for Cytopathology (ASC). 400 West 9th Street, Suite 201, Wilmington, DE 19801. (302) 429-8802. <http://www.cytopathology.org.>.

College of American Pathologists (CAP). 325 Waukegan Road, Northfield, IL 60093. (800) 323-4040. <http://www.cap.org>.

International Academy of Cytology (IAC). 1640 East 50th Street, Ste. 20C, Chicago, IL 60615-3161. (773) 955-1406. <http://www.cytology-iac.org>.

Laura Ruth, Ph.D.

Cytopenias *see* **Neutropenia and Thrombocytopenia**

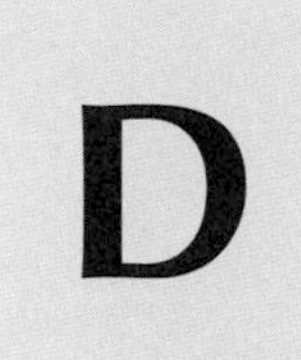

D & C *see* **Dilatation and Curettage**

Dacarbazine

Definition

Dacarbazine, also known as DTIC-Dome or DTIC, is an anticancer agent best known for its long-time use in treating metastatic malignant **melanoma**.

Purpose

Dacarbazine has been approved by the Federal Drug Administration (FDA) for use in the treatment of metastatic malignant melanoma and Hodgkin's lymphoma, as well as other neoplasms.

Metastatic malignant melanoma

Dacarbazine used alone produces a response in up to 25% of patients with **metastasis** to the surrounding skin and lymph nodes. Though it has been studied in combination with other drugs, and some three-drug combinations have shown promise, evidence thus far does not indicate a clear advantage over traditional single-agent treatment with dacarbazine.

Hodgkin's disease

In **Hodgkin's disease**, dacarbazine is indicated as a second-line therapy, meaning it is used after initial therapies have failed or if the patient's disease recurs. It is usually used in conjunction with other drugs, most commonly in a regimen called "ABVD," which is comprised of the drugs **doxorubicin** (Adriamycin), **bleomycin**, **vinblastine** and dacarbazine. ABVD has produced complete remission in up to 70% of cases.

Other neoplasms

Dacarbazine has other, unlabeled uses. It has been used to treat soft tissue **sarcomas** and malignant metastatic pheochromocytomas. When used with other **chemotherapy** agents, it has also shown to have some activity in the treatment of non-small cell lung cancer.

Description

Dacarbazine is a non-classical alkylating agent that causes DNA mispairing and strand breakage, leading to cell death (necrosis). Its exact mechanism is not completely understood. It is a cell cycle nonspecific drug, meaning that it causes cell damage and death throughout the life cycle of a cell, and not at any one particular time. When a patient is treated with dacarbazine 50% of the drug is metabolized by the liver, and 50% excreted in urine.

Recommended dosage

Dacarbazine comes in a vial, and must be mixed with sterile water according to manufacturer instructions prior to administration. It may be given directly into a vein, slowly, or by infusion over a time period of 15 minutes to an hour. Safety and effectiveness of this drug have not yet been established in children.

Chemotherapy dosages are usually based on a person's body surface area (BSA), which is calculated in square meters using height and weight measurements. Drug dosages are ordered in milligrams per square meter (mg/m^2). In some cases, chemotherapy may be ordered in milligrams per kilogram body weight. (One kilogram equals 2.2046 pounds.)

There are three regimens that may be considered when prescribing dacarbazine for metastatic malignant melanoma: the ten-day, five-day, and one-day regimen. The dosages recommended are as follows: 2-4.5mg/kg/day for ten days, repeated every four weeks; 250mg/square meter/day every five days, and repeated every three weeks; and 850-1000mg/square meters for one day, repeated every three weeks. Because of recently developed drugs called 5HT3 **antiemetics** that treat **nausea and vomiting**, the one-day regimen is currently the most

KEY TERMS

Antiemetic—A drug that prevents or alleviates nausea and vomiting.

Body surface area—A measurement based on height and weight that is calculated in square meters. It is used to determine chemotherapy dosages.

Carcinogenic—A substance capable of causing cancer.

Extravasation—To pass from a blood vessel into the surrounding tissue.

Hematopoietic—Referring to proteins that cause growth and maturity in blood cells.

Myelosuppression—Suppression of bone marrow function that results in decreased platelets, red blood cells, and white blood cells.

commonly used. To date, no studies have indicated that schedule or daily dose affects response rates.

Dacarbazine is usually given in combination with other drugs in the treatment of Hodgkin's lymphoma. The recommended dosage is 150mg/square meter, given once a day for five days. Treatment is repeated every four weeks. Alternatively, the drug may be given on only the first day of treatment, and every 15 days thereafter. For this regimen, the recommended dose is 375mg/square meter.

Precautions

Anaphylaxis is rarely associated with dacarbazine. Dacarbazine should not be used in patients who have demonstrated previous sensitivity to it.

Dacarbazine is classified as both an irritant, meaning that the drug has the potential to cause pain and inflammation at the site if it seeps out of the vein and into the surrounding tissue. Should this event, called extravasation, occur, hot packs should be applied. Rarely, extravasation of dacarbazine results in tissue damage or death.

Animal studies have indicated that dacarbazine may be carcinogenic and damaging to an unborn fetus It should be used only when the need outweighs the risks There have not been adequate studies to determine whether it does pass to the milk. To be safe, women undergoing treatment with dacarbazine should not breast-feed.

Side effects

Hematopoietic

The most common side effect of dacarbazine is moderate bone marrow suppression. White blood cells and platelets are most affected, though red blood cells may also be decreased. These effects are potentially life threatening, requiring frequent blood level monitoring, and potentially a decrease or complete cessation of the drug. These effects may be delayed from two to four weeks after the drug is administered. Patients should be monitored for symptoms of low white blood cell count. Symptoms may include sore throat, burning during urination, **diarrhea**, or **fever**. Symptoms of low platelet count may include bleeding, increased bleeding with menstruation, and unexplained bruising. Symptoms of **anemia** may include dizziness, **fatigue**, and/or pallor.

Gastrointestinal

Dacarbazine is a highly emetogenic drug, meaning it frequently causes nausea and/or vomiting. Symptoms begin after one to six hours of administration, and can last up to five days. However, with appropriate supportive care, dacarbazine is usually well tolerated. Preventing nausea and vomiting can usually be accomplished by administering antiemetic medications before dacarbazine is administered, and even up to several days afterwards. There are several regimens available. In addition, restricting food intake for several hours prior to the administration of the drug can help reduce adverse gastrointestinal effects.

Cardiovascular

Dacarbazine has been associated with episodes of low blood pressure that resolve when the drug is stopped. Dacarbazine is prepared in vials with citric acid and the drug mannitol. There is some consideration that these hypotensive episodes may be related to the citric acid, and not the dacarbazine itself.

Dermatological

Although photosensitivity (sensitivity to sunlight) is rare, patients should be instructed to avoid sun exposure after treatment. When outdoors, patients should wear sunscreen and protective clothing. Reactions may include redness, swelling and/or **itching** of the skin. In more serious cases, blisters may develop.

Dacarbazine may also affect the skin in other ways. For example, it may cause hyperpigmentation of the nails. When used in conjunction with the drugs doxorubicin, bleomycin, and vinblastine, dacarbazine can cause brown streaks to form over the sites of infusion. Dacarbazine may also cause flushing, a temporary redness of the face, neck and chest area. Dacarbazine can also cause hair loss, although uncommon. Once treatment stops, hair growth nearly always recurs.

Other

Dacarbazine is sometimes associated with a flu-like syndrome that causes fatigue, muscle aches, and sometimes an increased temperature. Reportedly, symptoms begin about a week after therapy, and resolve within one to three weeks. Rarely, dacarbazine causes liver toxicity, symptoms of which may include yellowing of the whites of the eyes or skin, abdominal pain and nausea.

Interactions

Dacarbazine is best administered in Dextrose 5% water or normal saline. It should not be given with the following medications, as they are chemically incompatible: **allopurinol** sodium, cefepime HCl, **Heparin** sodium, or piperacillin sodium. Patients should let their doctors know what medications they are taking, as there may be some adverse reactions. Patients at risk for bone marrow suppression, such as those taking dacarbazine, should avoid aspirin-containing medicines as they may increase the risk of bleeding.

Tamara Brown, R.N.

Daclizumab

Definition

Daclizumab is a humanized monoclonal antibody of the IgG1 type produced by recombinant DNA technology that binds to a specific interleukin-2 (IL-2) receptor known as CD25 or Tac. This receptor is expressed on the surface of cancerous lymphocytes in a number of blood malignancies. Daclizumab has also been known as dacliximab and is marketed in the United States under the Zenapax brand name.

Purpose

When used against cancer, this drug is intended to stop the growth of blood cell (hematologic) cancers that express the CD25 protein on the surface of the cancerous cells. Some representative cancers include adult T-cell leukemia/lymphoma (ATL), **hairy cell leukemia** (HCL), **cutaneous T-cell lymphoma** (CTCL), chronic lymphocytic lymphoma (CLL), **Hodgkin's disease**, non-Hodgkin's lymphoma (NHL), and other peripheral T-cell or lymphoid leukemias or lymphomas.

KEY TERMS

Antibody—A protective protein made by the immune system in response to an antigen, also called an immunoglobulin.

Exotoxin—A protein produced by a bacteria that is both toxic and produced an immune response by the host.

IgG—Immunoglobulin type gamma, the most common type found in the blood and tissue fluids.

Interleukin-2—A cytokine responsible for the activation of B and T-cells of the immune system that induces growth and maturation.

Humanization—Fusing the constant and variable framework region of one or more human immunoglobulins with the binding region of an animal immunoglobulin, done to reduce human reaction against the fusion antibody.

Monoclonal—Genetically engineered antibodies specific for one antigen.

Based on the antibody's known ability to block IL-2 binding experimentally, this drug would be expected to work most effectively at the times that the cancerous cells require IL-2 for growth. Generally, this is in the early stages of the disease. However, limited clinical evidence and some experimental evidence support an as of yet uncharacterized alternative method of action that may work during the later, IL-2 independent stages of the cancers.

Description

Daclizumab is a genetically engineered monoclonal antibody that was approved by the FDA in late 1997 as an immunosuppressive drug for use in kidney transplantation. The use of this drug in transplantation is based on the known interaction of activated lymphocytes with IL-2 during the rejection of transplanted tissue. It has not yet been approved for use as a cancer therapy. As of mid-2001 there were at least three active **clinical trials** to test the ability of daclizumab to treat hematologic cancers. The drug has also been used experimentally to treat IL-2-mediated autoimmune diseases such as uveitis and tropical spastic paraparesis.

Monoclonal antibodies are proteins of the immune system that bind specifically to a particular antigen.

Daclizumab was constructed to bind specifically to the alpha subunit of the IL-2 high affinity receptor, a protein also known as CD25 or Tac. By binding to the IL-2 receptor, it is theorized that daclizumab will block the action of IL-2 on the cell, whether it be uncontrolled growth or an uncontrolled immune reaction.

Fusion antibodies related to daclizumab have been developed and are being studied in clinical trials. One fusion antibody links the antibody with radioactive yttrium (Y 90), effectively bringing **radiation therapy** directly to the cancer cells. Another called LMB-2 fuses the antibody binding site with a bacterial exotoxin that is toxic to the cancer cells. This drug is the first recombinant immunotoxin to induce major responses in cancer during a clinical trial.

Most of the daclizumab sequence is derived from human sequences, while about 10% are from mouse sequences. The human sequences were derived from the constant domains of human IgG1 (called "constant" because it is essentially the same for all IgG antibodies) and the variable framework regions of a human antibody against an antigen seen on the surface of **myeloma** cells. These areas do not bind to the IL-2 receptor. Using human sequences in this part of the antibody helps to reduce patient **immune response** to the antibody itself and is called humanization. The actual binding site of daclizumab to the IL-2 receptor is from a mouse anti-Tac antibody.

Recommended dosage

Clinical trials are currently ongoing to determine the most effective dosage and treatment cycles for daclizumab against hematologic cancers.

Precautions

Daclizumab therapy on an outpatient basis requires regular visits to the doctor to check progress. Laboratory tests are needed to make sure daclizumab is working properly and not overly compromising immune function. Because of the possible suppression of the immune system by this drug it is important to maintain good dental hygiene and see a dentist regularly. Also, because the drug would cross the placenta and the effects on an unborn child is unknown, effective contraception is necessary for women of childbearing age while receiving this medicine.

Side effects

Some uncommon side effects of daclizumab needing medical attention include chest pain; coughing; dizziness; **fever**; nausea; rapid heart rate; red, tender, oozing skin; shortness of breath; swelling of the feet or lower legs; trembling or shaking of the hands or feet; vomiting; weakness and, rarely, frequent urination.

Some also uncommon and less serious side effects include constipation; **diarrhea**; headache; heartburn; joint pain; muscle pain; slow wound healing and trouble in sleeping.

Interactions

The following medications have been administered in clinical trials with daclizumab with no increase in adverse reactions: **cyclosporine**, **mycophenolate mofetil**, ganciclovir, acyclovir, **azathioprine**, and **corticosteroids**. Daclizumab has also been used by small numbers of patients without reaction with other immune suppressive drugs such as **tacrolimus**, **muromonab-CD3**, antithymocyte globulin, and antilymphocyte globulin.

See Also Monoclonal antibodies

Michelle Johnson, M.S., J.D.

Dactinomycin

Definition

Dactinomycin is a chemotherapeutic agent belonging to a family of medicines known as antineoplastic drugs. Alternative trade names or brand names for dactinomycin include Actinomycin-D and Cosmegen.

Description

Dactinomycin is one of the older **chemotherapy** drugs, having gained approval from the Food and Drug Administration (FDA) in 1982. This highly potent and effective cytotoxic agent is a mixture of substances produced by the bacteria *Streptomyces parvullus*. Its toxic properties prevent its use as an antibiotic.

Dactinomycin interferes with the growth of cancer cells by complexing with a cell's genetic material (deoxyribonucleic acid, or DNA). This prevents the cell from producing the proteins necessary to function and grow, thereby killing it. Dactinomycin may be used as a single chemotherapeutic agent or in conjunction with other antineoplastics (such as **vincristine** and **cyclophosphamide**) for greater efficacy.

Purpose

Dactinomycin is used in the treatment of **Ewing's sarcoma**, **Wilms' tumor**, **rhabdomyosarcoma**, **gestational trophoblastic tumors**, **Kaposi's sarcoma**, and soft tissue **sarcomas**. It is less commonly used for cancers of the uterus and testis.

Recommended dosage

The exact schedule and method of dactinomycin administration will be prescribed by an oncologist based on the type and stage of the cancer. An appropriate starting treatment regimen for adult patients is 500 mg/day for five consecutive days at two to four week intervals if the drug is tolerated. For children the dose is 15 mg/day over the same time course as prescribed for adults. Dactinomycin is not recommended for children less than one year of age; little clinical data is available on the use of dactinomycin in the elderly. Administration may be by intravenous (IV) injection, through a running IV infusion, or through a central line inserted under the skin into a vein near the collarbone.

Precautions

To maximize treatment effects, patients receiving dactinomycin should observe the following guidelines, as well as any modifications given by the oncologist:

- The area surrounding the injection site should be monitored.
- Patients should have regular laboratory testing for white blood cell count and kidney, liver, and bone marrow function.
- In order to reduce the possibility of immunosuppression, immunizations not approved or prescribed by the oncologist should be avoided.
- Patients should avoid contact with individuals taking or that have recently taken the oral polio vaccine, or individuals that have an active infection. When necessary a protective facemask should be worn.
- Oral hygiene procedures should be followed to reduce the risk of gum abrasion.
- Patients should not touch eye and nasal areas unless hands have been properly washed immediately prior to contact.
- To reduce bleeding and bruising complications, patients should exercise extreme caution when handling sharp instruments and decline participation in contact sports.
- Prior to treatment, the patient's medical history should be thoroughly reviewed to avoid complications that might arise from previous conditions such as gout, kidney stones, liver disease, chickenpox, shingles, or a history of allergic reactions to various drugs.
- The oncologist should be made aware if the patient is pregnant or if there is the possibility the patient might be pregnant, or if the patient is a breast-feeding mother.
- Only prescribed medications or over the counter (OTC) drugs approved by the oncologist should be taken by a patient receiving dactinomycin.

KEY TERMS

Antineoplastics—Agents that inhibit or prevent the maturation and proliferation of malignant cells.

Cytotoxic—Toxic to cells.

Ewing's sarcoma—A highly malignant primary bone tumor most often found in young adults under the age of 30.

Gestational trophoblastic cancer—A pregnancy associated cancer in which a grape-like mole develops in the uterus instead of a fetus.

Kaposi's sarcoma—A type of cancer associated with the skin and mucous membranes.

Myeloma—A malignant tumor composed of plasma cells normally found in the bone marrow.

Oncologist—A doctor who specializes in the diagnosis and treatment of patients with cancer.

Rhabdomyosarcoma—A malignant tumor derived from striated muscle.

Wilms' tumor—A cancerous tumor found in the kidneys of children.

Side effects

Possible side effects of treatment with dactinomycin should be discussed with the patient prior to initiation of treatment. The patient should be instructed to notify the oncologist of any side effects. Side effects that may not be life threatening but give the patient cause for concern include hair loss (**alopecia**), intermittent **diarrhea**, **nausea and vomiting**, loss of appetite, difficulty swallowing, mouth sores or ulcers, and a general rash or change in skin tone. Side effects that should be reported immediately to the oncologist include unusual bleeding or bruising, black tarry stools, blood in the urine or stool, development of a cough, wheezing or hoarseness, **fever** or chills, lower back or side pain, painful or difficult urination, pinpoint red spots on the skin, and pain at the site of the injection. The oncologist will decide what type of intervention is best suited to control or extinguish the presented side effects, including changing the dosage, changing the treatment schedule, or discontinuing dactinomycin treatment.

Interactions

Certain medications should never be used together, but there are cases in which multiple drug treatment may be advisable even when drug interaction is well documented. Dactinomycin may be used in conjunction with other antineoplastic drugs or **radiation therapy** for increased efficacy of treatment. Under such conditions the oncologist will balance dosage and treatment schedules to maximize the positive effects of all drugs given and minimize any negative interactions.

It is essential that the oncologist be aware of any drugs that the patient is presently taking or has recently taken, or if the patient has recently received radiation therapy. A careful review of drugs that may interact with dactinomycin to lower its efficiency should be covered with the patient prior to treatment. These may include, but are not limited to, amphotericin B, antithyroid agents, **azathioprine**, chloramphenicol, flucytosine, ganciclovir, interferon, **plicamycin**, zidovudine, probenecid, and sulfinpyrazone.

See Also Antineoplastic agents

Jane Taylor-Jones, Research Associate, M.S.

Dalteparin *see* **Low molecular weight Heparin**

Danazol

Definition

Danazol is a synthetic androgen hormone that the Federal Drug Administration (FDA) approved in 1976. It is also known by its trade name, Danocrine.

Purpose

Danazol is approved for use in the treatment of endometriosis, fibrocystic breast changes, and in the prevention of hereditary angioedema. In addition, it has shown promise in the treatment of certain cytopenias.

Endometriosis

Endometriosis is a condition in which endometrial tissue, normally found in the uterus, implants itself in other areas of the body. The tissue continues to respond to hormones estrogen and progesterone during menstruation as it does in the uterus, but because the tissue cannot exit the body through the vagina during menstruation, it builds up, causing pain and inflammation. Danazol does not cure endometriosis, but renders the endometrial tissue located outside the uterus inactive. In most cases that are amenable to hormonal treatment, the endometrial lesions completely resolve, but can return within six months of stopping treatment.

Fibrocystic breast changes

Many women experience benign lumps or cystic changes in the breast. Most often, supportive bras and over-the-counter pain medication relieves symptoms. However, in some women, pain and discomfort may be so great that medical treatment is warranted. Danazol is the only drug approved by the FDA for fibrocystic breast disease, and in this patient population usually results in complete resolution of nodularity and pain. However, symptoms usually return when medication is stopped.

Hereditary angioedema

Hereditary angioedema is a condition in which parts of the body, most dangerously the airway, develop episodic swelling. Danazol is used to prevent these rare, but potentially fatal, attacks.

Other

In addition to the aforementioned indications, there are other, unlabeled uses for danazol. The drug may be used to treat precocious puberty (premature sexual development), menorrhagia (excessively long menstrual periods), and gynecomastia (excess breast development in males).

Because it stimulates erythropoiesis (the production of red blood cells), it is sometimes administered to treat certain types of **anemia**. However, the use of danazol to combat anemia has declined since the recent developments in the synthetic production of **erythropoietin**, a hormone naturally produced by the kidney that promotes the formation of red blood cells in bone marrow. In cancer patients, danazol may be used for its ability to stimulate erythropoiesis in individuals with types of **thrombocytopenia** (decreased platelets), often associated with HIV, or anemia. Danazol has shown promise in the management of autoimmune **hemolytic anemia**, a group of conditions in which the body produces antibodies that attack red blood cells. Myelodysplastic syndrome (MDS), a term that describes a group of hematologic cancers that often develop into **acute leukemia**, has shown some response to danazol treatment. However, more research is needed to better evaluate its potential in these patient populations.

Description

The pituitary gland produces hormones necessary for reproduction—follicle stimulating hormone (FSH) and luteinizing hormone (LH). Danazol suppresses the production of these and other hormones (estrogen and progesterone), inhibiting ovulation as a result. The effects are usually reversible. Approximately 60 to 90 days after treatment is stopped, ovulation and cyclic bleeding usually return.

Recommended dosage

The lowest therapeutic dose possible should be administered to minimize side effects. In some cases, doctors may periodically stop treatment or decrease dosages. In women, danazol should be started during menstruation or after tests to ensure the woman is not pregnant. Patients should be careful not to miss a dose, and if they do, should not take a double dose.

Endometriosis

Severe cases of endometriosis are initially treated with 800 milligrams (mg) of danazol, given in two divided doses. Gradually, the amount of medication is reduced to a level that is sufficient to suppress menstruation. Mild cases of endometriosis respond to lower doses of danazol. Typically, a doctor will first prescribe 200 to 400 mg a day, in two divided doses. Treatment should continue for three to six months, but in some cases, may last up to nine months.

Fibrocystic breast changes

Treatment for fibrocystic breast changes ranges from 100 to 400 mg given in two divided doses. Up to six months of danazol treatment may be needed to reduce breast nodularity and pain. However, in half of women treated with danazol, symptoms recur within a year. In these cases, treatment can be restarted.

Hereditary angiodema

Treatment for hereditary angioedema usually starts with a 200 mg dose given two or three times a day. Further adjustments are made based on the patient's response. If episodes are prevented, the amount may be decreased by half. If an attack occurs, the dose can be increased by up to 200 mg.

Other

Treatment of anemia in myelodysplastic syndrome usually begins with a dose of 200 mg three times a day.

Precautions

The use of danazol requires that liver and kidney function be routinely tested, as it can cause damage to these organs. In fact, with long-term use, there have been reported incidents of cancerous tumors in the liver.

KEY TERMS

Androgen—A steroid that produces masculine characteristics.

Cytopenia—Deficiencies of certain elements in blood, such as red blood cells, white blood cells and/or platelets.

Menorrhagia —Excessive menstrual bleeding.

Breast cancer should be ruled out prior to starting treatment. This may be difficult when there are multiple nodules in the breast. Any lumps that persist once danazol has started warrant consideration for breast cancer. Although danazol is effective in managing dysfunctional uterine bleeding, it should not be used in cases where **endometrial cancer** has not been ruled out.

Danazol should be used cautiously in people with high cholesterol. Danazol may cause a decrease in high-density lipoproteins (HDL; "good cholesterol"), which in, high levels, remove cholesterol from the arteries. At the same time, danazol can cause an increase in the low density lipoproteins (LDL; "bad cholesterol"), which act to move cholesterol into the arteries.

Danazol can cause androgenic effects on the fetus, and should not be used during pregnancy. Effects on a female fetus can include genital abnormalities such as clitoral enlargement, labia fusion, or vaginal closure. Treatment should not be initiated until pregnancy is ruled out. Throughout therapy, non-hormonal methods of birth control should be used to prevent pregnancy. If pregnancy does occur, the drug should be stopped and a doctor notified immediately.

Danazol is rarely associated with a condition called benign intracranial hypertension, symptoms of which include headache, nausea, vomiting, and visual disturbances. Should these symptoms occur, patients should stop taking the drug and see a neurologist.

When men, particularly adolescent men, take danazol, semen should be tested for volume, viscosity, sperm-count, and sperm motility every three to four months. Any changes may indicate a need to stop treatment.

Conditions that are worsened by swelling, a possible side effect of danazol, should be carefully monitored. This is particularly relevant in patients with epilepsy or cardiac problems.

Side effects

Long-term effects of danazol are unknown. Androgenic side effects may result, and may be an effect of decreased estrogen. These symptoms may include acne, swelling, abnormal hair growth, decreased breast size, deepening of voice, oily skin or hair, weight gain, enlargement of the clitoris, or reduction in the size of the testicles. Flushing, sweating, vaginitis, nervousness or emotional lability (instability) may also develop. Danazol may cause liver damage. In addition to routine lab testing, patients should be monitored for yellowing of the skin or whites of the eyes due to jaundice.

Interactions

The effects of oral anticoagulants, such as coumadin, may be increased in patients taking danazol, and should be used with caution. Individuals taking insulin for diabetes should carefully monitor their blood sugars. Taken in conjunction with danazol, insulin's effects are reduced. Danazol is also known to increase effects of the medications **carbamazepine** and **cyclosporine**.

Tamara Brown, R.N.

Daunorubicin

Definition

Daunorubicin is an anti-cancer drug that kills cancer cells. The brand names are DaunoXome for the liposomal formulation and Cerubidine for the daunorubicin hydrochloride formulation.

Purpose

Daunorubicin is available in two different formulations, the daunorubicin hydrochloride and daunorubicin citrate liposome. The liposomal daunorubicin formulation places the drug in lipid molecules. This formulation is able to penetrate cancer cells more effectively because of its smaller size, and it remains in the body longer when compared to the daunorubicin hydrochloride formulation. The daunorubicin hydrochloride is approved by the Food and Drug Administration (FDA) to treat **acute myelocytic leukemia** (AML) and **acute lymphocytic leukemia** (ALL). It is also sometimes used to treat chronic myelogenous leukemia (CML), non-Hodgkin's **lymphoma**, and psoriasis. The liposomal formulation of daunorubicin is used to treat advanced HIV-associated **Kaposi's sarcoma**.

Description

Daunorubicin interferes with the cells' production of DNA and RNA by inserting itself between the molecules that make up DNA and RNA. It also works by inhibiting the enzyme responsible for repairing of DNA (topoisomerase II enzyme). The structure of daunorubicin is very similar to that of **doxorubicin**, and both drugs function in the same way.

Recommended dosage

In the treatment of acute myelocytic leukemia (AML), the dose is 30 to 60 mg of daunorubicin per square meter of body surface area given for three to five days, and the dose is repeated every three to four weeks.

In acute lymphocytic leukemia (ALL), 25 to 45 mg per square meter of body surface area of daunorubicin may be given on day one every week for four cycles, or alternatively may be given at a dose of 30 to 45 mg per square meter of body surface area for three days. The dose for patients receiving daunorubicin citrate liposome is 20 to 40 mg per square meter of body surface area every two weeks, or 100 mg per square meter of body surface area every three weeks.

Patients with decreased liver or kidney function may receive lower doses of the medication than other patients. This medication is usually administered directly into the vein (intravenous, or IV) over the course of three to five minutes. It may also be diluted in a solution to be given over fifteen minutes to one hour.

Precautions

A major problem with the use of daunorubicin is that it may cause a serious heart problem known as heart failure. Some authorities suggest that giving any individual patient more than 900 to 1000 mg of daunorubicin per square meter over the course of their entire life may increase risk of heart injury. Other authorities recommend that the total lifetime cumulative dose not exceed 550 milligrams per square meter. The patient's baseline heart function is obtained prior to starting therapy and is monitored every few cycles of **chemotherapy**. If the heart function is significantly decreased from baseline, the drug is discontinued.

Side effects

There is a risk that heart rhythm problems will occur during daunorubicin therapy. Later, patients may develop heart failure. However, patients receiving daunorubicin are, in fact, less likely to develop such problems than are patients receiving doxorubicin.

In addition, the activity of the bone marrow in producing white blood cells to fight infections, platelets to control bleeding, and red blood cells for oxygenation

KEY TERMS

DNA—A molecule found in all living cells that contains tiny bits of genetic information

RNA—A molecule that interacts with the genetic information contained in cells.

may be impaired by the drug. This and the development of heart problems are the major side effects that may cause doctors to lower the dose of daunorubicin.

Other side effects associated with daunorubicin therapy are nausea, vomiting, ulcerations of the mouth, **diarrhea**, and hair loss. In addition, the medication has a harmless side effect about which patients should be forewarned; urine and tears may take on a red color.

Patients receiving daunorubicin in conjunction with certain other anticancer drugs may (very rarely) develop a certain type of leukemia. The drug is also an irritant to the skin and tissues of the body. Patients who notice burning or pain with infusion of the drug should notify the nurse immediately to assess if the drug has leaked from the vein into the surrounding tissue. If this occurs, the drug infusion is stopped immediately and appropriate actions are taken to minimize side effects due to tissue damage.

Bob Kirsch

Demeclocycline

Definition

Demeclocycline, more accurately demeclocycline hydrochloride, is a broad-spectrum antibiotic of the tetracycline family. Demeclocycline is marketed under the trade name Declomycin.

Purpose

Demeclocycline is used to treat cancer patients who have developed a condition known as **syndrome of inappropriate antidiuretic hormone** (SIADH). A wide variety of malignacies, especially small-cell lung cancer, as well as various other non-cancer conditions, give rise to SIADH, which is caused by overproduction of antidiuretic hormone (ADH). SIADH can also develop as a side effect of the anticancer drugs **vincristine**, **vinblastine**, **cisplatin**, **melphalan**, and **cyclophosphamide**. The increased ADH levels lead to insufficient elimination of water from the kidneys, and the retained water leads to dilution of the serum sodium concentration, a condition called hyponatremia. Symptoms of hyponatremia include weight gain in spite of appetite loss, **fatigue**, headache, and confusion. When the condition is severe or the onset sudden, the symptoms may develop into seizures or coma. Although treating the underlying cancer is the ideal approach, the metabolic imbalances may be alleviated in other ways. The tetracycline derivative demeclocycline has been found to be effective in treating SIADH.

Description

This tetracycline derivative is isolated from a mutant strain of the bacterium *streptomyces aureofaciens*.

Demeclocycline was first investigated as a treatment for SIADH in 1976, and had become established as the treatment regimen of choice by 1986. The drug acts to interfere with the response of the kidneys to ADH and has consistently been found to be effective in treating SIADH with relatively few side effects.

Recommended dosage

Demeclocycline hydrochloride is taken orally. It is supplied as 150 and 300 mg tablets and 150 mg capsules. The usual dosage of demeclocycline for SIADH is from 600 to 1200 mg/day, and should not exceed 2400 mg/day. Within five days of beginning the drug, the diuretic action begins, and it generally lasts for two to six days after the drug is discontinued.

Precautions

Absorption of demeclocycline is reduced when taken with food or dairy products, and thus should be given one hour before or two hours after a meal or ingestion of dairy products. The dose should be taken with 8 oz (240 mL) of water, and the last dose of the day should be taken at least one hour before bedtime.

Antacids containing aluminum, calcium, or magnesium interfere with absorption of orally administered tetracyclines and should not used by patients taking demeclocycline.

Photosensitivity reactions are more frequent and more severe with demeclocycline than with other tetracyclines. Patients should be advised that this reaction can occur and be cautioned to avoid exposure to direct sunlight or ultraviolet light.

KEY TERMS

Anaphylactoid purpura—A short-term allergic condition of blood vessels, found chiefly in children, that is characterized by wet sores on the skin of the buttocks, legs, and lower abdomen. Joint pain, stomach bleeding, and blood in the urine are also common findings. The disease, also called Henoch-Schonlein (Schonlein-Henoch) purpura, usually lasts for about 6 weeks and has no long-term effects unless kidney involvement is severe.

Anaphylaxis—A severe allergic reaction to a foreign substance (antigen) that a patient has had previous contact with, characterized by redness and swelling, itching, water build-up, and, in severe cases, extremely low blood pressure, lung spasms, and shock.

Angioedema—A sudden, painless, swelling of short duration that can affect the face, neck, lips, throat, hands, feet, genitals, or abdominal organs; also called angioneurotic edema.

Antidiuretic hormone—A peptide hormone, also called vasopressin, synthesized in the hypothalamus and released by the posterior pituitary gland in response to decreased blood volume, that stimulates capillary muscles and concentrates and reduces the elimination of urine.

Benign intracranial hypertension—Also called pseudotumor cerebri or meningeal hydrops, a condition of swelling of the optic nerve and mild paralysis of the cranial nerves, with headache, nausea, and vomiting.

Dysphagia—Difficulty in swallowing.

Hyponatremia—A condition in which the serum sodium concentration falls to less than 135 milliequivalents per liter (mEq/L), caused by too little excretion of water or by too much water in the bloodstream; in severe cases, hyponatremia leads to water intoxication, characterized by confusion, lethargy, muscle spasms, convulsions, and coma.

Lupus erythematosus—A long-term disease that affects women four times more often than men, characterized by severe swelling of the blood vessels giving rise to arthritis, kidney disorders, red rash over the nose and cheeks, weakness, fatigue, weight loss, photosensitivity, fever, and skin sores that may spread to the mucous membranes and other tissues of the body; also called systemic or disseminated lupus erythematosus.

Nephrogenic diabetes insipidus—A condition in which the kidneys do not retain urine, resulting in excess urination and thirst, and very watered-down urine.

Pancreatitis—An inflammation of the pancreas diagnosed on the basis of severe pain that begins in the abdomen and moves to the back, fever, loss of appetite, nausea, vomiting, and jaundice.

Pericarditis—An inflammation of the pericardium, the membrane covering the heart, marked by pain that begins in the chest and moves to the shoulder or neck, fever, difficulty breathing, and a dry cough.

Photosensitivity—An abnormal sensitivity of the skin to ultraviolet light, often resulting from use of an oral or topical drug, that leads to accelerated and severe burning and blistering of the skin.

Prothrombin—A plasma protein, produced by the liver and converted to thrombin by activation factors in the plasma, involved in blood coagulation; also called factor II.

Superinfection—An overgrowth, during antimicrobial treatment for another infection, of a microorganism not affected by the treatment.

Tetracycline—A broad-spectrum antibiotic.

Tinnitus—A sensation of ringing or other similar sound in the ears.

With renal impairment, even usual doses of demeclocycline may lead to accumulation of the drug and the possibility of liver toxicity. Serum level determinations of the drug may be advisable under such conditions, and the dosage should be lower than usual.

Tetracyclines can cross the placenta and can have toxic effects on the developing fetus, and the drug is found in the milk of lactating women taking tetracyclines. Tetracyclines form a complex with calcium and act to decrease the rate of bone growth in any bone-forming tissue while the drug is being administered.

Side effects

Dermatological

Skin reactions, including redness, swelling, rashes, and flaking or peeling of the skin can result from demeclocycline administration. Demeclocycline should be discontinued if the skin becomes swollen and reddened.

Patients taking demeclocycline are likely to be photosensitive. Phototoxic reactions occur with moderate to large doses and are characterized by severe skin burns resulting from direct exposure to sunlight.

Gastrointestinal

Demeclocycline can cause loss of appetite, nausea, vomiting, and **diarrhea**. Inflammations of the upper GI tract have also been reported as side effects, involving the tongue and esophagus, with resultant dysphagia, but many of these patients were found to have taken the medication immediately before going to bed. Inflammation of the small and large intestines has also been reported, and, as with all antibiotic therapy, overgrowth in the lower GI tract of other organisms, especially of the *candida* genus of yeast-like fungi, can lead to inflammatory lesions in the anogenital area.

Central nervous system

Dizziness, tinnitus, benign intracranial hypertension (pseudotumor cerebri), and visual disturbances have been reported. More rarely, myasthenic (Eaton-Lambert) syndrome and muscle weakness have been reported.

Immune system

Possible allergic reactions to demeclocycline include hives, angioedema, anaphylaxis, anaphylactoid purpura, pericarditis, and worsening of systemic lupus erythematosus.

Other

Superinfection due to overgrowth of nonsusceptible organisms is a common side effect of demeclocycline administration. Renal toxicity has been reported. Acute pancreatitis and nephrogenic diabetes insipidus are possible side effects of demeclocycline treatment. Increases in liver enzymes and hepatic toxicity have been rarely observed. Blood conditions such as **hemolytic anemia**, **thrombocytopenia**, **neutropenia**, and eosinophilia have also been reported. Individuals still undergoing tooth development (infants and children up to 8 years old, and in the fetus during the last half of pregnancy) may develop permanent yellowish-grayish-brown discoloration of the teeth and poor enamel development.

Interactions

Tetracyclines such as demeclocycline can interfere with the bactericidal action of penicillins, and should not be administered together with penicillin. Tetracyclines coadministered with oral contraceptives can render oral contraceptives less effective. The activity of plasma prothrombin can be depressed by tetracyclines, thus patients on anticoagulant therapy may be required to decrease their anticoagulant dosage.

Patricia L.Bounds, Ph.D.

Denileukin

Definition

Denileukin (denileukin difitox) is a fusion protein, or a protein made from two different proteins, that is used to treat recurrent **cutaneous T-cell lymphoma**.

Purpose

Cutaneous T-cell lymphoma (CTCL)is a form of non-Hodgkin's lymphoma, or an uncontrolled growth of cells in the lymph system that begins in the skin. It may spread to other organs.

Denileukin is known by the full name denileukin difitox, and also by the brand name Ontak. It causes the death of T cells or lymphocytes that are being made in enormous numbers by tricking the troublesome cells into binding with it, and then killing them.

Description

Denileukin is a genetically engineered protein, created by fusing a piece of the toxin that causes diphtheria with interleukin-2 (also known as IL-2 or **aldesleukin**). Because of the presence of IL-2 in the fusion protein denileukin, cells that have IL-2 receptors bind with it. Thus, the cells are fooled into binding with a protein they recognize, only to be killed by the toxin that is fused with it.

Not all malignant T cells and lymphocytes have IL-2 receptors. If the cells do not have the receptors, denileukin is not useful.

Recommended dosage

Denileukin is given through intravenous line. The best therapy course has not yet been determined. But the standard dose is either 9 or 18 micrograms per kilogram of body weight per day for five consecutive days, every three weeks.

Precautions

Because the use of the treatment can contribute to an environment that encourages infections, largely because

KEY TERMS

Genetically engineered—An organism that has been modified by the intervention of humans, usually by the addition of DNA, or hereditary material, from one species to the DNA of another species.

Intravenous line—A tube that is inserted directly into a vein to carry medicine directly to the blood stream, bypassing the stomach and other digestive organs that might alter the medicine.

Kilogram—Metric measure that equals 2.2 pounds.

Lymphatic system—The system that collects and returns fluid in tissues to the blood vessels and produces defensive agents for fighting infection and invasion by foreign bodies.

Lymphocyte—One of the specialized white blood cells in the lymphatic system.

Microgram—One-thousandth of a milligram, and one-millionth of a gram.

Milligram—One-thousandth of a gram. There are one thousand grams in a kilogram. A gram is the metric measure that equals about 0.035 ounces.

Receptor—A part of a cell that is a structural and functional fit for a compound to which the cell is exposed.

Recurrent—Returns, or keeps coming back.

T cell—A cell in the lymphatic system that contributes to immunity by attacking foreign bodies, such as bacteria and viruses, directly.

of the fluid that accumulates around cells, patients must be monitored closely for infection.

Oncologists using the treatment must first test the cells of the patient for receptivity to IL-2. The treatment should not be used in patients that do not have the specific receptors for IL-2 that tricks the cells into binding with denileukin. The receptors of the cells that will bind all have a component known as CD25.

About 60% of patients diagnosed with CTCL have the receptors for IL-2. The Food and Drug Administration (FDA) has approved denileukin for use in patients that have not responded to other treatments.

Side effects

Vascular leak, or the seepage of fluid from blood vessels, accumulates and causes swelling (edema) and may contribute to infection. Infection is an important and dangerous side effect. It causes some patients to discontinue treatment. Flu symptoms are common, and include pain, headache, and **nausea and vomiting**. Low blood pressure, skin eruptions, and liver toxicity (poisoning) are also side effects. Fast heart rate and numbness are possible side effects.

Interactions

Denileukin was so recently approved for use that drug interaction studies are not available. As with all drugs, the physician in charge of the care plan must be told about all drugs a patient is taking that might interfere with the activity of the denileukin.

Diane M. Calabrese

Depression

Description

Everybody feels sad sometimes, but to be clinically depressed is not just a matter of feeling sad. A patient with cancer is diagnosed as having major depression only if certain symptoms, such as loss of pleasure or thoughts of death, are present for at least two weeks. Only a healthcare professional can accurately determine whether a patient is depressed or is simply upset because of the disease.

A note on depression and children with cancer

Few children with cancer experience depression. For many children survivors of cancer, the experience of having had cancer makes them deeper, more understanding human beings later in adulthood and old age. However, some children with cancer do experience depression, sleep problems, and relationship problems. Depression appearing in a child who has cancer should be treated by a healthcare professional.

The symptoms of depression in children are somewhat different from those in adults. The physician should be notified of a sad mood (or, in children less than six years of age, a facial expression that appears to express sadness) that continues for at least two weeks and is accompanied by at least four of the following: (a) appetite changes, (b) sleep problems or excessive sleep, (c) excessive activity or inactivity, (d) loss of pleasure, (e) not caring about anything, (f) fatigue, (g) being overly critical of himself or herself, (h) feeling worthless or guilty for no apparent reason, (i) inability to concentrate, and (j) thoughts of death.

Are most people who have cancer depressed?

Most people who have cancer are not depressed. Depression is found in cancer patients about as frequently as in patients hospitalized for major, noncancer illnesses such as heart disease. However, depression is more often present in people who have cancer than in the general population. Approximately one out of eight people with cancer are depressed. Among hospitalized people with cancer, roughly one in four is depressed.

Depression and embarrassment

Doctors and nurses can do a great deal to help a depressed person feel better. Being embarrassed can get in the way of the patient's getting help. While depression is a disease that happens to a minority of cancer patients, it does appear in a sizable number of these patients. Doctors and nurses are trained to deal with depression in cancer patients. If one out of eight people with cancer are depressed, it is no surprise to healthcare professionals that some patients require treatment for depression. It is not "bothering" a good health care professional to let them know that the patient is experiencing some symptoms that may signal depression. Competent doctors and nurses will not think less of a patient who is depressed. Rather, they will respect the patient who acknowledges the willingness to seek and accept treatment for depression. Cooperative patients are not those who hide depression but those who deal with depression when it appears. Dealing honestly and with the aid of doctors and allied healthcare professionals is the right way to address any cancer-related symptom.

How does depression affect someone who has cancer?

Depression is not something that can be pointed to, as one would point to a runny nose or an earache. That does not mean it is not real, nor does it mean the depression does not have a major effect on the cancer patient. The fact is that depression may not only affect what patients can do and how they feel, depression may also affect how well they function and how long they live.

A study of patients with **acute leukemia** who were receiving **bone marrow transplantation** found that those who were not depressed lived longer. A study of **breast cancer** patients showed that depression can be treated successfully and life extended. In this study, women with metastatic breast cancer who joined a support group lived twice as long as matched patients who did not join a support group. In light of these types of studies it would be incorrect to assume that depressed cancer patients who work with their doctors and nurses to treat their depression do not live as long as patients without depression.

Untreated depression or inadequately treated depression may slow recovery time. A study of depressed colorectal cancer patients found they were not able to function as well six months after surgery as patients who were not depressed. Another study found that breast cancer patients who were more anxious and depressed felt more pain than those who were not. Other studies have also shown that depression affects how people function and cope with illness.

Causes

It is certainly understandable that someone with a serious illness feels sad. Many cancer patients are confronted with difficulties. These may include having to take medications, dealing with the side effects of these medications, undergoing operations, submitting to other medical procedures, and generally taking time away from other things they would prefer to do. In addition, many patients feel a sense of loss. They may feel a loss of good health; there may be a loss of part of the body, such as a segment of a breast; there may be a loss of the ability to do certain tasks. There may also be financial strains. Any such things are difficult for most people to deal with. It takes time and effort, and sometimes medical intervention, for people to deal with such loss and gradually get their lives back on track.

If patients are in pain it is extremely important that the pain be adequately treated. Pain is often under-treated. When pain is not treated appropriately, patients may be more likely to develop depression.

Patients with cancer of the pancreas are particularly likely to become depressed. In addition, patients with breast, colon, gynecologic, oropharyngeal, and **stomach cancer** are more likely to experience depression than patients with other types of cancers. No one knows why depression is more likely to be associated with these cancers.

Approximately one out of every four patients with depression associated with cancer already was depressed at the time of diagnosis. In contrast, approximately three out of four develop the depression after the diagnosis has been made.

Risk factors for depression among cancer patients

Anyone can become depressed, and this includes people with cancer and people who are perfectly healthy.

Often, there is no way of predicting who will develop major depression. However, some groups of cancer patients are more likely to develop depression than are others. This include patients who:

- are younger
- have a personal or family history of depression or other mental health problems
- have a personal or family history of substance abuse
- have **body image** problems
- are hospitalized
- are experiencing unrelieved cancer-related symptoms, such as pain
- have advanced or relapsed cancer, or have experienced a treatment failure
- have been diagnosed with stroke or with Parkinson's disease

In addition, some patients are receiving medicines that may cause depression as a side effect. Among these medicines are certain anticancer drugs, antihistamines, blood pressure medicines, anti-Parkinson's disease medicines, medications for convulsions, sedatives, steroids, stimulants, and tranquilizers.

Signs and symptoms

A patient with cancer is diagnosed as having major depression only if certain symptoms are present for at least two weeks. Among these symptoms are:(a) loss of pleasure or interest in activities, (b) major **weight loss** or weight gain not associated with dieting, (c) serious sleep problems, (d) loss of energy, (e) **fatigue**, (f) feeling worthless, (g) feeling guilty without adequate reason, (h) problems concentrating, (i) indecisiveness, (j) thoughts of death or suicide. Symptoms such as sleep problems, fatigue, and weight loss may, however, affect cancer patients who are not depressed in the slightest. So, the diagnosis must be made by a healthcare professional.

Often depression appears gradually. At first, the patient seems no more than sad. At times, the person who is in a very early stage of depression brightens up. For many people things never get worse than this and true depression never touches them. However, other people progress to where negative thoughts have a grip upon them.

Gradually, some of the neurotransmitters in the nervous system may stop working in the most healthy way. Neurotransmitters are the chemicals released by nerves to communicate with other nerves. Once a patient's neurotransmitters are affected, the depression is definitely not simply happening in the patient's mind. The way the body uses actual chemicals is being altered by the depressive disease.

Precisely how the depression shows itself may differ from patient to patient. For example, some patients start to respond to little setbacks as though these are catastrophes. Other patients start making big assumptions, usually in negative directions; for example, they may assume their current therapy will not help them, even although there is good medical evidence that it probably will. For yet another example, they may blame themselves for having cancer, or irrationally see the cancer as a punishment visited upon them for something they have done. Patients may try to be too perfect and repeatedly fail. They may think other people have negative feelings about them, or they may focus upon the negative portions of situations. One danger is that the looming depression may encourage patients to push away and alienate those health professionals, friends, and family members who are trying to be helpful. For a final example, a depressed patient may deny the seriousness of the cancer, saying something like, "The tumor is small so I don't really need to be careful about taking my medicines."

Some patients experience a milder form of depression, called dysthymia. Symptoms of dysthymia include annoyance, feelings of sadness, irritability, loss of pleasure, and self-criticism. The patient with dysthymia may develop aches and pains, express excessive guilt, and distance themselves from loved ones. Dysthymia may be almost unnoticeable; however, many patients with dysthymia are unable to function quite as well as they can when they are healthy.

Depression screens

The attending doctor or nurse may request that the patient complete a depression screen. This screen is nothing more than a page or two of questions about how the patient is feeling. The patient's responses give healthcare professionals a picture of whether or not depression may be present.

Prevention

It is important for patients to have an idea of the psychological and social stressors they may have to address because of the cancer. Knowing in advance that something may be a problem is a good way of making sure that it is not quite as stressful once it does appear as it otherwise would be. Patients, their families, and close friends should be able to recognize the most important signs and symptoms of depression and should know which healthcare professional to call should depression appear. However, no one except a professional is capable of accurately diagnosing depression. It is a good idea to try to develop an honest relationship with a healthcare professional you trust. Parents of a child who has cancer may find a parent support group helpful, as there is a great deal to learn from other parents who have been through a similar situation.

Treatments

Most important is that study after study has shown that depression in cancer patients can be successfully treated. It is important to understand that this problem probably can get better. Several different approaches to treatment can be taken, and several of these approaches can be effectively combined with one another

If the patient has a doctor or nurse capable of providing sustained emotional support, that can be helpful. On the other hand, it is important for patients to realize that doctors and nurses are usually extremely busy and that it may be necessary to find someone else to provide sustained emotional support. This other person may be a trained professional, such as a social worker, a psychiatric nurse, a psychologist, or a psychiatrist. The persons who provide support may also be family members or friends. A support group may be helpful. During periods of crisis, it is beneficial to have several people who can provide support. The family member or friend who is trying to provide such support should try to listen well and sympathetically.

Cognitive interventions

Cognitive interventions are also known as cognitive-behavioral treatment (CBT). CBT helps patients' view in a realistic way what is happening to them, where they are, and what they should or should not be doing. This type of intervention can be useful in helping patients give up negative perspectives and replace them with views that rely more upon the facts about what is going on. CBT may be practiced with a healthcare provider, or in a group with other patients and one or more providers.

Among the techniques CBT makes use of are:

- Cognitive distraction: This is the phrase used for techniques that shift the mind-frame of the patient from negative things to more positive thoughts. Music is one of the basic tools of cognitive distraction. Patients should be encouraged to listen to the type of music they like best. Headphones may be helpful if brought to diagnostic and treatment sessions and occasions when waiting is necessary. Imagery is another technique important for cognitive distraction. Imagery can help the mind shift from negative thoughts and difficult situations to helpful images. Each patient should select those images that feel right and good. For one patient this may be swimming at the beach; for another, visiting special friends; for another, walking through the forest.

KEY TERMS

Cognitive-behavioral therapy—One of several effective ways of treating depression in cancer patients. CBT helps patients view what is happening to them in a realistic way. It may make use of music, imagery, and providing accurate information.

Depression screen—A questionnaire on how the patient is feeling used to help healthcare professionals diagnose depression.

Dysthymia—A milder form of depression.

- Psychoeducation: This CBT technique involves providing information to patients so patients can feel that what is going on is not entirely beyond their control. People often find it difficult to deal with the unknown, and psychoeducation attempts to remove some of what is unknown. Another important psychoeducation technique is having patients make lists of questions to ask their nurse or doctor.
- Image rehearsal: This CBT technique involves working with a healthcare professional. The patient may use image rehearsal to rehearse some activity she or he finds to be stressful. For example, image rehearsal may be used if the patient finds MRI scans or radiation treatments to be stressful.

Other CBT techniques involve relaxation techniques and the conscious decision to participate in activities the patient likes doing.

Psychotherapy

Talking to a psychologist, social worker, psychiatric nurse, psychiatrist, or other health care professional can be helpful. In addition to the cancer and problems associated with therapy, this talk therapy can help the patient address unresolved matters that were already bothersome before cancer was diagnosed.

Group therapy

Studies have shown group therapy to be an effective approach for patients with cancer-related depression. Various approaches to group therapy may be taken. In all, however, it involves communication not only between patient and healthcare professional, but also among and between patients. Group therapy can also be helpful for loved ones of cancer patients.

Important to note is that studies have shown that cancer patients may tend to isolate themselves from friends and family. In other words, the amount of contact and communication between friends and family may be less than it had been before cancer was diagnosed. This is not a helpful trend. Research suggests that social support can have beneficial effects on a person's physical health. Group therapy can provide this type of social support to patients. In addition, group therapy may furnish a place where patients are able to learn about how to maintain contact with family and friends. It can also provide a way for patients to identify which family members and friends are not supportive.

Medication

A variety of antidepressant medications are available. Among those most frequently prescribed are psychostimulants, tricyclic antidepressants (TCAs), selective serotonin reuptake inhibitors (SSRIs), and monoamine oxidase inhibitors (MAOIs). These medications help return the neurotransmitters to a normal, balanced function. There are at least three different psychostimulants, six different TCAs, three different SSRIs, and three different MAOIs that doctors may choose among. In addition, there are various other medications that have proven to be effective as treatment for depression. All of these drugs have been shown to work well in general; however, while one specific type of drug may be appropriate for one patient, another patient may require a completely different type of drug. Use of some of these drugs may be accompanied by side effects. Just as there are different antidepressant drugs, so are there different side effects that may appear. However, many patients have no side effects from antidepressant medications or, at most, exhibit only minor side effects. Other patients find that, although they had side effects from one drug, they experienced no side effects after they switched to another medication. Many patients find they are able to successfully combine medications and other treatment approaches, but honest communication with the physician is essential.

The suicidal patient

If a patient is suicidal it is extremely important to immediately contact a healthcare professional capable of dealing with such a crisis.

Resources

BOOKS

Spiegel, David, and Catherine Classen. *Group Therapy for Cancer Patients: A Research-Based Handbook of Psychosocial Care.* New York: Basic Books, 2000.

Waller, Alexander, and Nancy L. Caroline. *Handbook of Palliative Care in Cancer* 2nd ed. Boston: Butterworth Heinemann, 2000.

Yarboro, Connie H., Margaret H. Frogge, and Michelle Goodman. *Cancer Symptom Management.* 2nd ed. Boston: Jones and Bartlett Publishers, 1999.

PERIODICALS

Lovejoy, Nancy C., Derek Tabor, Margherite Matteis, and Patricia Lillis. "Cancer-related Depression: Part I—Neurologic Alterations and Cognitive-Behavioral Therapy." *Oncology Nursing Forum* 27 (2000): 667-677.

Sheard, T., and P. Maguire. "The Effect of Psychological Interventions on Anxiety and Depression in Cancer Patients: Results of Two Meta-Analyses." *British Journal of Cancer* 80 (1999): 1770-1780.

ORGANIZATION

The National Cancer Institute.(800)4-CANCER. <http://www.nci.nih.gov>

The American Cancer Society. (800)ACS-2345. <http://www.cancer.org>

National Coalition for Cancer Survivorship. 1010 Wayne Avenue, 7th Floor, Silver Spring, MD 20910-5600. (301) 650-9127 and (877)NCCS-YES [(877)622-7937]. <http://www.cansearch.org>

Bob Kirsch

Dexamethasone

Definition

Dexamethasone is a synthetic glucocorticoid. Its naturally occuring counterparts are hydrocortisone and cortisone. Although the drug is used in a variety of ways, in general, it reduces inflammation and depresses the immune system. Dexamethasone may also be called by its brand name, Decadron, and is one of the **corticosteroids**.

Purpose

Dexamethasone is used in the treatment of many disorders. For example, it may be used:

- as replacement therapy in the treatment of Addison's disease
- in the management of various inflammatory disorders, such as rheumatoid arthritis
- in managing allergic disorders, such as asthma

Patients with ulcerative colitis may benefit from dexamethasone therapy, as might those with exacerbations of multiple sclerosis. Blood disorders, such as thrombocytopenic purpura or erythroblastopenia, may also be managed with dexamethasone.

Dexamethasone is often prescribed to patients with cancer. In some cases, the drug is part of the drug treatment for the disease, and in other cases it is used to manage side effects caused by the treatment or the cancer itself.

Dexamethasone may be used to decrease abnormally high levels of potassium that develop in association with cancer. In some cases, it may be used as palliation in leukemia or **lymphoma**. Because of its antiinflammatory properties, dexamethasone may help reduce swelling in the brain caused by a brain tumor. It may also help prevent hypersensitivity reactions associated with drugs like **paclitaxel**. Dexamethasone is also commonly used to treat nausea associated with **chemotherapy**. It is particularly useful with the drug **cisplatin**, which frequently causes **nausea and vomiting**.

In non-Hodgkin's lymphoma (NHL), dexamethasone is part of a drug regimen known as "DHAP." Here, dexamethasone is given with chemotherapy drugs called cisplatin and **cytarabine**. Also in treating NHL, dexamethasone may be used in a regimen caled "m-BACOD," which also includes the administration of **methotrexate**, **leucovorin**, **bleomycin**, **doxorubicin**, **cyclophosphamide**, and **vincristine**. Dexamethasone may also be helpful in patients with **multiple myeloma**. In the "EDAP" regimen, dexamethasone is given with **etoposide**, cytosine arabinoside (cytarabine), and cisplatin; in VAD, it is given with vincristine and doxorubicin.

KEY TERMS

Addison's disease—A potentially life-threatening condition that results when adrenocortical function fails. Hypoadrenalism.

Glucocorticoid—An adrenocortical steroid hormone that is stimulated by the anterior pituitary. The three naturally-occuring types are hydrocortisone, corticosterone, and cortisone.

Hyperglycemia—An abnormally increased level of glucose (sugar) in the blood.

Palliation—Therapy aimed at relieving symptoms and promoting comfort, but not producing a cure.

Description

Patients should not stop taking dexamethasone without first consulting their physician. When dexamethasone treatment stops, it must be gradually reduced over time before it can be completely discontinued. Sudden withdrawal of glucocorticoids may result in adrenal insufficiency.

When possible, the drug should be taken before nine A.M. to imitate the time that the body's corticosteroid levels are typically at their highest. A child taking dexamethasone will be carefully monitored to ensure the drug is not affecting his or her growth. Patients taking large doses of dexamethasone should try to take the drug with meals. Antacids may be recommended between meals to reduce gastrointestinal effects and to prevent peptic ulcer.

Recommended dosage

Dexamethasone is available in oral, intravenous (IV), topical, ophthalmic, or inhaled form. In cancer patients, the oral and IV routes are used most frequently. The pill is available in several color-coded dosages [0.25 milligrams (mg), 0.5mg, 0.75mg, 1.5mg, 4mg, and 6mg]. Dexamethasone should be given very slowly by the IV route.

Dosages to treat disease are highly individualized, but generally start at 0.75 to 9.0 mg per day. The lowest therapeutic dose should be given, though amounts given may need to be increased during times of stress. Dosages of medications may be changed based on factors specific to the individual. The following dosages are general guidelines for dexamethasone when it is used in conjunction with chemotherapy agents:

- DHAP. Forty milligrams of dexamethasone is given in pill or IV form per day for the first four days of treatment, followed by cisplatin and cytarabine.
- M-BACOD. Six milligrams per meter square (mg/m2) of dexamethasone is given as a pill on the first five days of treatment.
- EDAP. Forty milligrams of dexamethasone is given in pill form on the first four days of treatment. It is given again on days 9-12, and 17-20.

When used to prevent or manage nausea or vomiting associated with chemotherapy, dexamethasone is given in the following dosages: 4–20 mg IV every 4–6 hours. Alternatively, a one-time dose of 10–20 mg may be given IV. When pills are preferred, 4–8 mg of dexamethasone may be given four times, every four hours. When used to prevent hypersensitivity reactions in paclitaxel treatment, 20mg should be given orally twelve and six hours before treatment begins.

Precautions

Dexamethasone should be used cautiously in patients with kidney or liver problems, hypothyroidism, high blood pressure, or a history of heart attack. Patients with diabetes mellitus should monitor blood sugar levels carefully, as hyperglycemia may result. If changes occur, patients should notify their doctors immediately. Sudden cessation of dexamethasone therapy is dangerous for patients on therapy for longer than two weeks. The drug should be gradually withdrawn under a physician's guidance.

Side effects

Adverse effects vary widely, and depend on the dosage and route of the drug. Certain drugs may result in decreased blood levels, and therefore render dexamethasone less effective. Patients taking the following drugs should be carefully monitored for decreased levels of dexamethasone: **phenytoin**, phenobarbitol, ephedrine, and rifampin. Conversely, some drugs, such as troleandomycin, may increase blood levels of dexamethasone.

Because of its immunosuppressive properties, dexamethasone may decrease the signs and symptoms of infection. Depending on the amount of drug being administered, patients may consider taking measure to prevent infection by avoiding crowded areas and washing their hands frequently. Patients should inform their doctor if they notice a **fever**, sore throat, or cuts or abrasions that don't heal. Laboratory tests may also be affected—false negative results may occur in the nitroblu-tetrazolium test for bacterial infections.

Glucocorticoids, such as hydrocortisone, tend to make the body retain salt. Although dexamethasone's salt-retaining properties are not as severe as hydrocortisone's, salt retention may result in fluid and electrolyte imbalances. Patients at risk may experience high blood pressure or even congestive heart failure. Weight gain or swelling may indicate salt and fluid retention.

Other adverse effects may include headache, dizziness, insomnia, increased appetite, mood swings, menstrual changes, muscle weakness, acne and/or sweating. **Depression** may be worsened with dexamethasone use. Some men experience changes in the motility and number of their sperm with steroid treatment. Patients should talk to their doctors about any unusual symptoms they experience. In cancer patients, increased appetite may actually be beneficial.

Dexamethasone crosses the placenta and is excreted in breast milk. If a pregnant woman is taking large doses of the drug, her newborn should be monitored for evidence of hypoadrenalism. Optimally, breast-feeding should be avoided. There is some concern that dexamethasone, in large quantities, suppresses growth or disrupts the baby's normal corticosteroid production.

Interactions

Patients should discuss all their medications, prescription and non-prescription, with their doctor. If dexamethasone is administered in amounts that suppress the immune system, live **vaccines**, such as small pox, should not be administered. Dexamethasone may alter the effect of anticoagulant drugs. Frequent laboratory tests should be performed to monitor blood levels. If dexamethasone is given with diuretics, potassium levels may be abnormally low, and should be frequently monotired. Doctors may recommend that patients on long-term therapy follow a potassium-rich diet.

Tamara Brown, R.N.

Dexrazoxane

Definition

Dexrazoxane, known by the brand name Zinecard or may be referred to as ADR-529, is a medicine that protects the heart from damage caused by the **chemotherapy** drug **doxorubicin**.

Purpose

Dexrazoxane is approved by the Food and Drug Administration (FDA) as a protectant medicine given to women with metastatic **breast cancer** who are being treated with the chemotherapy drug doxorubicin. In most cases these women already will have received greater than 300 mg per square meter (mg/m^2) of the chemotherapy drug doxorubicin before dexrazoxane is added. Dexrazoxane is given in combination with doxorubicin. Doxorubicin can cause damage to heart muscle and the risk of this damage increases as the total dose increases. The addition of dexrazoxane at the appropriate time in therapy can decrease the extent of damage to the heart muscle.

Description

Dexrazoxane is a clear, colorless solution. It is administered intravenously, into a vein, over a 15-30 minute period. Dexrazoxane is given within 30 minutes prior to receiving the doxorubicin. When doxorubicin gets into cells, it combines with iron to form toxic substances that destroy heart muscle. Dexrazoxane interferes with the doxorubicin binding to the iron compound so that the toxic substance is not formed and the heart muscle is protected.

Recommended dosage

Dexrazoxane doses can be determined using a mathematical calculation that measures a person's body surface area (BSA). This number is dependent upon a patient's height and weight. The larger the person, the greater the body surface area. Body surface area is measured in units known as meters squared (m^2). The body surface area is calculated and then multiplied by the drug dosage in mg/m^2. This calculates the actual dose a patient is to receive.

Dexrazoxane is dosed in mg/m^2 as a 10:1 ratio of the doxorubicin dose. For example, if a patient is to receive doxorubicin 50 mg/m^2, then the patient would receive dexrazoxane 500 mg/m^2. Once the dose is determined, the drug is administered either directly into the vein over a few minutes as an intravenous push, or as a quick infusion from an infusion bag. This is then followed by the doxorubicin intravenously.

Precautions

Blood counts will be monitored regularly while on dexrazoxane therapy. During a certain time period after receiving chemotherapy, there is an increased risk of getting infections. Caution should be taken to avoid unnecessary exposure to crowds and people with infections.

Patients should not expect their doctor to use dexrazoxane the first time they receive chemotherapy. It is thought that dexrazoxane may interfere with the chemotherapy drug's ability to destroy cancer cells. Dexrazoxane is therefore only used when absolutely necessary.

Patients who may be pregnant or are trying to become pregnant should tell their doctor before receiving dexrazoxane.

Chemotherapy can cause men and women to be sterile (not able to have children). It is unknown if dexrazoxane causes sterility.

Patients should check with their doctors before receiving live virus **vaccines** while on chemotherapy along with dexrazoxane.

Side effects

The most common side effect from receiving the dexrazoxane is pain at the injection site. Another common side effect when dexrazoxane is given with chemotherapy is that the blood counts fall lower than with just chemotherapy alone. However, the time it takes for the blood counts to return to normal is the same with or without the dexrazoxane.

Low blood counts, referred to as **myelosuppression**, are expected due to chemotherapy with dexrazoxane administration. A low white blood cell count is called **neutropenia**, and patients are at an increased risk of developing a **fever** and infections. Platelets are blood cells in the body that allow for the formation of clots. When the platelet count is low, patients are at an increased risk for bruising and bleeding. Low red blood cell counts, referred to as **anemia**, may also occur due to chemotherapy administration. Low red counts cause **fatigue**.

Most other side effects occur due to the administration of the chemotherapy agents that accompany dexrazoxane. Common side effects include **nausea and vomiting**. Patients are given medicines before receiving chemotherapy that can help prevent or decrease these side effects from happening. Other common side effects are hair loss (**alopecia**), fatigue, loss of appetite, mouth sores, fevers, infections, **diarrhea**, and changes in liver function.

Less common side effects are nerve damage, swelling and inflammation of the veins where the chemotherapy is administered, difficulty swallowing, bleeding, **itching**, and skin reactions in areas of previous radiation.

All side effects a patient experiences should be reported to his or her doctor.

KEY TERMS

Anemia—A lower than normal red blood cell count.

Anthracyclines—a group of chemotherapy medicines that are used to treat cancer. They have similar characteristics and are known for their ability to cause heart damage. The drugs included as anthracyclines are doxorubicin, daunorubicin, idarubicin, and epirubicin.

Antineoplastics—Medicines used to treat cancers.

Chemotherapy—A specific drug used to treat cancer.

Food and Drug Administration—A government agency that oversees public safety in relation to drugs and medical devices. The FDA gives approval to pharmaceutical companies for commercial marketing of their products

Intravenous—To enter the body through a vein.

Metastatic—Cancer that has spread to one or more parts of the body.

Neutropenia—A lower than normal white blood cell count.

Radiation therapy—The use of high-energy beams focused to treat cancerous tumors.

Sterility—Inability to have children.

Toxic—Poisonous.

Interactions

Dexrazoxane should only be used with chemotherapy combinations that contain doxorubicin or other agents in the anthracycline class of antineoplastics.

Patients should tell their doctors if they have a known allergic reaction to dexrazoxane or any other medications or substances, such as foods and preservatives. Before taking any new medications, including nonprescription medications, **vitamins**, and herbal medications, the patients should notify their doctors.

Nancy J. Beaulieu, RPh.,BCOP

Diarrhea

Description

Diarrhea is the abnormal increase of liquid in stool and increase in the frequency of passing stool (defecation). The person with diarrhea has watery or loose stool more than three times a day. Other symptoms include cramping, pain, feeling the urge to defecate, irritation of the skin around the anus (perianal), and inability to control defecation (fecal **incontinence**). Approximately 10% of the patients with advanced cancer suffer from diarrhea. Diarrhea lasting fewer than two weeks is called "acute diarrhea," and diarrhea lasting for longer than two months is called "chronic diarrhea."

Diarrhea is a debilitating condition that can significantly affect quality of life. Diarrhea can prevent patients from participating in social activities and going to work. Persons with diarrhea fear soiling their clothing or bed linens, a fear that prevents them from leaving home. Loss of sleep due to nighttime diarrhea can cause fatigue, which ultimately affects the patient's ability to function normally. Uncontrolled diarrhea can lead to chemical imbalances, loss of fluids (dehydration), and even death.

Causes

Although there are many causes of diarrhea, only those associated with cancer will be discussed. The most common cause of diarrhea in cancer patients is related to constipation or its treatment. Cancer patients may experience diarrhea as a result of their treatment, or it can be due to dietary changes, infections, hormone imbalances, digestion disorders, or inflammation. Treatment-related diarrhea can be caused by **chemotherapy**, hormone therapy, **radiation therapy**, biological response modifiers (drugs that improve the patient's immune system), or surgery. In addition, cancer patients may develop temporary lactose intolerance, which causes diarrhea.

Chemotherapy drugs kill the rapidly growing cancer cells. However, certain normal cells of the body are rapidly growing and they too are affected. Rapidly growing cells are found in the intestines, as well as other parts of the body. Diarrhea occurs as a result of injury to the cells of the intestine. These effects are temporary. Chemotherapy drugs, hormones, and biological response modifiers that frequently cause diarrhea include:

- **Dactinomycin**
- **Daunorubicin**
- **Diethylstilbestrol diphosphate**
- **Doxorubicin**
- **Fluorouracil**
- Flutamide
- **Hydroxyurea**
- Interferon
- Interleukin-2 (**Aldesleukin**)
- **Irinotecan**
- **Methotrexate**
- Nitrosoureas
- Thioguanine

Radiation therapy can cause diarrhea if the intestines are in the treatment field. Diarrhea results from the injury and destruction of the cells lining the intestines, which leads to a decrease in the uptake (absorption) of fluids and an increase in the speed with which stool moves through the intestines. Radiation therapy can cause diarrhea, and other intestinal problems, many months or years after treatment has been completed.

Diarrhea usually develops within one week following pretreatment (chemotherapy and irradiation) for **bone marrow transplantation**. This diarrhea usually disappears within two weeks. Also, bone marrow transplant patients with **graft-versus-host disease** develop severe diarrhea.

Treatments

Prevention

There are some measures that can prevent diarrhea. Patients who are receiving abdominal radiation therapy can be put into certain positions to minimize exposure of healthy intestines to radiation. Diarrhea caused by chemotherapy cannot be prevented; however, the administration of atropine during treatment with irinotecan may prevent diarrhea. Patients should stop taking dietary supplements, as these can cause diarrhea.

There are many dietary changes that can be made to prevent or reduce diarrhea. Foods to avoid include:

- whole grain breads and cereals
- fresh or frozen fruits (except banana)
- dried fruits
- fruit juices with pulp and prune juice
- raw vegetables
- canned onions, corn, olives, pickles, and Brussels sprouts
- fatty foods
- dried beans
- rich desserts
- milk and milk products
- alcohol and caffeinated coffee and tea
- spicy foods
- fried foods

Management

Of the utmost importance in the treatment of diarrhea is the replacement of fluids lost by frequent, watery stools. The patient should drink six to eight glasses of fluid daily, including clear broth, ginger ale (without the fizz), water, weak tea, and commercial formulas that contain sugars and minerals (electrolytes). Patients with severe diarrhea may need intravenous fluid replacement either at home or in the hospital.

Diarrhea can cause the perianal skin to become irritated and painful; therefore, it needs to be cleaned thoroughly after each bout of diarrhea. Baby wipes or a mild soap with water can be used to clean the irritated skin. The area should be patted dry and occasionally exposed to air. Taking a sitz bath (sitting in a bathtub of shallow water) with lukewarm water may relieve the discomfort. Petroleum jelly or other type of barrier cream may be used.

The patient should eat small, frequent meals. Foods and drinks should be taken at room temperature. Foods that can help control diarrhea include:

- bananas
- applesauce
- boiled white rice
- tapioca
- white bread
- plain pasta
- creamed cereals
- eggs
- potatoes (without skin; mashed or baked)
- fish
- chicken or turkey (without skin)

There are some medications that can slow down the movement of stool through the intestines and increase intestinal water absorption. The patient may need a combination of drugs and/or dose adjustments to achieve relief. A physician should be consulted before any over-the-counter antidiarrheal medications are taken. Antidiarrheal medications include:

- Atropine sulfate with diphenoxylate HCl (Lomotil)
- Codeine phosphate
- Loperimide HCl (Imodium-AD)
- Octreotide phosphate (Sandostatin)

These medications should not be used if infection as the cause of diarrhea has not been eliminated.

Patients who are experiencing diarrhea due to graft-versus-host disease will continue to take their immunosuppressant drugs. They may also be treated with **corticosteroids** and antidiarrheal medications.

Alternative and complementary therapies

Peppermint tea, chamomile tea, valerian capsules, or aloe vera juice may reduce cramping and intestinal spasms. An Ayurvedic physician may recommend taking equal parts of yogurt and water with fresh ginger, or a powder of beleric myrobalan fruit. Ginger capsules may relieve intestinal spasms and pain. Glutamine supplements may speed up the healing process and relieve irritated intestines.

Resources

BOOKS

Lenhard, Raymond E, Robert T. Osteen, and Ted Gansler. *Clinical Oncology.* American Cancer Society, 2000.

Maleskey, Gale. *Nature's Medicines: from Asthma to Weight Gain, from Colds to High Cholesterol—The Most Powerful All-Natural Cures.* Emmaus, PA: Rodale Press, Inc., 1999.

Somerville, Robert, ed. *The Medical Advisor.* Alexandria, VA: Time-Life Books, 1997.

Yarbro, Connie Henke, Michelle Goodman, Margaret Hansen Frogge, and Susan L. Groenwald, eds. *Cancer Nursing, Principles and Practice, 5th ed.* Sudbury, MA: Jones and Bartlett Publishers, 2000.

Yarbro, Connie Henke, Margaret Hansen Frogge, and Michelle Goodman, eds. *Cancer Symptom Management, 2nd ed.* Sudbury, MA: Jones and Bartlett Publishers, 1999.

PERIODICALS

Kornblau, Steven, Al B. Benson III, Robert Catalano, Richard E. Champlin, Constance Engelking, et al. "Management

KEY TERMS

Defecation—The passage of stool from the body.

Dehydration—The condition caused by excessive loss of water from the body.

Electrolytes—Molecules, such as sodium and potassium, that are necessary for normal body functioning. Diarrhea can cause electrolytes to become lost and/or unbalanced.

Perianal—The skin surrounding the anal opening.

of Cancer Treatment—Related Diarrhea: Issues and therapeutic Strategies." *Journal of Pain and Symptom Management* 19, no. 2 (February 2000): 118-127.

Wadler, Scott, Al B. Benson III, Constance Engelking, Robert Catalano, Michael Field, et al. "Recommended Guidelihnes for the Treatment of Chemotherapy-Induced Diarrhea." *Journal of Clinical Oncololgy* 16, no. 9 (September 1998): 3169-3178.

OTHER

"What About Diarrhea?" *American Cancer Society, Inc.* 2000. 1 July 2001 <http://www3.cancer.org/cancerinfo>

Belinda Rowland, Ph.D.

Diethylstilbestrol diphosphate

Definition

Diethylstilbestrol diphosphate is a synthetic (manufactured) form of the female hormone estrogen. Brand names for diethylstilbestrol include Stilphostrol, and is also referred to as Stilbestrol and DES.

Purpose

Diethylstilbestrol is used to relieve symptoms of advanced **breast cancer** that has metastasized, or spread, from the breast to other parts of the body. It is used to treat breast cancer in men and in postmenopausal women. Diethylstilbestrol also has been used to relieve symptoms of advanced cancer of the prostate in men.

Description

Diethylstilbestrol was the first form of estrogen made in the laboratory. It was prescribed to millions of women in the 1950s and 1960s to prevent miscarriage and premature birth. This use was discontinued in the 1970s, when abnormalities of the reproductive systems were found in some children of women who took the drug during pregnancy. Furthermore, daughters of women who took this drug during pregnancy are at an increased risk for developing certain types of cervical and vaginal cancers.

Diethylstilbestrol is used to relieve some symptoms of advanced breast cancer in certain men and women. The drug can interfere with the spread of cancer cells that require estrogen to grow and divide.

Diethylstilbestrol sometimes is used to relieve symptoms of advanced **prostate cancer** in men. This drug can lower the levels of the male hormone **testosterone**, which is required for the growth and division of these cancer cells. However, diethylstilbestrol can cause severe side effects in men, including breast enlargement and increased risk of heart disease and blood clots. Thus, it is no longer widely used for the treatment of prostate cancer.

Recommended dosage

Diethylstilbestrol usually is given as a pill, which should be taken at the same time each day. The dosage varies depending on body weight and the type of cancer that is being treated. For breast cancer, the dose is 15 mg per day.

For inoperable prostate cancer, the dose is 50 mg three times a day and can be increased up to 200 mg or more three times a day. Maximum dose is 1 gram a day. For the treatment of prostate cancer, diethylstilbestrol can also be injected slowly into a vein. The dosage may be as high as 1 gram per day for five or more days. The dosage then may be lowered to 250-500 mg once or twice per week.

Precautions

Diethylstilbestrol can cause serious birth defects in humans. Children of women who take diethylstilbestrol (DES) during pregnancy may develop reproductive system abnormalities at puberty, and daughters are at an increased risk for developing **vaginal cancer**. Therefore, this drug should not be taken by pregnant women, or by either the man or the woman at the time of conception. Women should not breast-feed infants while taking this drug, since estrogens pass into the breast milk.

Diethylstilbestrol may not be indicated, or should be used with caution, for individuals whose medical histories include any of the following:

- heart, kidney, or liver damage

- disease of the gallbladder or gallstones
- inflammation of the pancreas
- bone or uterine cancer
- fibroid tumors of the uterus
- unusual vaginal bleeding
- endometriosis (uterine cells in the ovaries or other pelvic organs)
- high cholesterol
- blood clots or circulatory problems in males

Side effects

Diethylstilbestrol affects normal cells as well as cancer cells, so side effects can occur with this medicine. The side effects associated with diethylstilbestrol usually are mild and temporary. Common side effects include:

- enlargement of the breasts
- breast tenderness
- decreased sexual desire
- voice changes
- swelling of the feet and lower legs
- fluid retention
- weight gain

Less common side effects of diethylstilbestrol include:

- **nausea and vomiting** during the first few weeks of treatment
- changes in vaginal bleeding
- loss of bladder control
- lumps or discharge from the breasts
- stomach, side, or abdominal pain
- yellow skin or eyes

Taking the medicine with food may reduce or prevent nausea.

Rarely, diethylstilbestrol results in the formation of blood clots in the legs or in the lungs. This primarily affects men who are receiving high-dosage treatment for breast or prostate cancers. Symptoms of blood clots include:

- pain, redness, or swelling in the calf
- weakness or tingling in an arm or leg
- faintness
- sudden severe headache
- vision changes
- shortness of breath
- chest pain
- coughing up blood (**hemoptysis**)

KEY TERMS

Estrogen—Female sex hormone.

Hormone—Substance produced by the body to regulate the activity of a tissue or organ.

Metastasis—Spread of cancer from its point of origin to other parts of the body.

Prostate—Gland in males that surrounds the urine tube (urethra) at the base of the bladder.

Testosterone—Principal male sex hormone.

Interactions

Medicines that may adversely affect the liver when taken along with diethylstilbestrol include:

- acetaminophen (as in Tylenol; long-term or high-dose usage)
- amiodarone (Cordarone)
- anabolic steroids (such as nandrolone, oxandrolone, oxymetholone, stanozolol)
- androgens (male hormones)
- antithyroid drugs that are used to treat an overactive thyroid
- birth control pills containing estrogen
- **carbamazepine** (Tegretol)
- **carmustine** (BiCNU)
- chloroquine (Aralen)
- dantrolene (Dantrium)
- **daunorubicin** (Cerubidine)
- disulfiram (Antabuse)
- divalproex (Depakote)
- etretinate (Tegison)
- gold salts to treat arthritis
- hydroxychloroquine (Plaquenil)
- isoniazid
- medicines to treat infections
- **mercaptopurine** (Purinethol)
- **methotrexate** (Mexate)
- methyldopa (Aldomet)

- naltrexone (Trexan; long-term or high-dose usage))
- phenothiazines
- **phenytoin** (Dilantin)
- **plicamycin** (Mithracin)
- valproic acid (Depakene)

In addition, diethylstilbestrol and other estrogens can prevent **cyclosporine** (Sandimmune) from being removed from the body, leading to possible kidney or liver problems. Protease inhibitors such as ritonavir (Norvir) may reduce the activity of diethylstilbestrol.

Margaret Alic, Ph.D.

Digital rectal examination

Definition

The digital rectal examination (DRE) is a routine part of the physical examination and includes manual examination of the rectum, anus and, in men, the prostate.

Purpose

The purpose of the digital rectal examination is to identify lesions within the rectum and the prostate. It is the most widely used and oldest technique for the detection of **prostate cancer** and is used in screening for **colon cancer** and for the detection of rectal polyps.

Description

Usually the patient is positioned on the left side with the knees close to the chest. Sometimes the patient is asked to stand up and lean over the examination table. For women, sometimes this examination is part of the routine gynecological exam, and it may be done in a different manner than described here.

During the examination, the health care practitioner examines the anus and the surrounding skin for hemorrhoids, tags, fissures and abscesses. After lubricating the gloved finger and anus, the examiner gently slides the finger into the anus and follows the contours of the rectum. The examiner notes the tone of the anus and feels the walls and the edges for texture, tenderness and masses as far as the examining finger can reach. The examiner evaluates the prostate for nodules and tenderness. Stool on the finger should be examined for blood, color, texture and tested for fecal occult blood.

The examination takes less than two minutes and can be uncomfortable when the patient is not relaxed or is anxious. Occasionally, when the DRE is performed on a man the penis may become erect. A gentle reminder and reassurance helps to relieve the embarrassment associated with the unexpected erection.

KEY TERMS

Fissure—Any cleft or groove, normal or otherwise, especially a deep fold in the anus.

Lesion—Any pathological or traumatic discontinuity of tissues or loss of function of a part.

Palpation—A simple technique in which a doctor presses lightly on the surface of the body to feel the organs or tissues underneath.

Peritonitis—Inflammation of the peritoneum. It may be accompanied by abdominal pain and tenderness, constipation, vomiting and moderate fever.

Polyp—Growth, usually benign, protruding from a mucous membrane.

Rectal prolapse—Protrusion of the rectal mucous membrane through the anus.

Skin tag—A small outgrowth of skin tissue that may be smooth or irregular, flesh-colored and benign.

Preparation

The patient must be carefully positioned and the doctor should take care to explain the examination to the patient and to explain to the patient what to expect. The digital rectal examination may be uncomfortable and embarrassing. Much of the discomfort can be reduced by an understanding, unhurried and gentle examiner.

Precautions

When there are infections of the anus and of the rectum, the digital rectal examination should not be performed. Manipulation of the anal and rectal tissues increases the risk of infection and of bleeding.

Results

In the normal anus and rectum, there are no hemorrhoids or bleeding about the anus. The anal tone is not loose. The rectum is smooth and non-tender. No masses should be palpated, or felt.

The digital rectal examination is helpful in identifying areas of peritonitis or tender areas that can be felt through the wall of the rectum. It is used to identify perineal disease or deformity, abnormal location of the anus, rectal prolapse and atrophy of the gluteal muscle. Digital examination can detect a stenosis (or narrowing) of the anal canal, assess the tone and strength of the anal muscles or detect the presence of a rectal mass or fecal impaction.

Any masses, including hard stool, blood or tenderness is considered abnormal. Cancer masses may be flattened, nodular, cauliflower-like or ring-shaped. Polyps can be felt, but must be visualized using **anoscopy** or flexible **sigmoidoscopy** to be distinguished from other lesions, such as internal hemorrhoids or malignant growths. Hard masses of feces may be felt and may be removed.

Aftercare

Aftercare of the digital rectal examination is minimal. It requires removal of the lubricating jelly residue from around the anus. The lubricating jelly dissolves easily in water and may be washed off in bathing after the examination. It can be removed with toilet paper immediately after the examination.

See Also Rectal cancer

Resources

BOOKS

DeGowin, R. and D. D. Brown. *DeGowin's Diagnostic Examination Seventh Edition.* New York, New York: McGraw-Hill, 2000.

Yamada, Tadatake, ed. *Textbook of Gastroenterology Volumes One and Two, 3rd Edition.* Philadelphia: Lippincott, Williams & Wilkins, 1999.

Cheryl L. Branche, M. D.

DiGuglielmo syndrome *see* **Acute erythroblastic leukemia**

Dilatation and curettage

Definition

Dilatation and curettage (D&C) is a gynecological procedure in which the lining of the uterus (endometrium) is scraped away.

Purpose

D&C is commonly used to obtain tissue for microscopic evaluation to rule out cancer. The procedure may also be used to diagnose and treat heavy menstrual bleeding and to diagnose endometrial polyps and uterine fibroids. D&C can be used to remove pregnancy tissue after a miscarriage, incomplete abortion, or childbirth, or as an early abortion technique up to 16 weeks. Endometrial polyps may be removed, and sometimes benign uterine tumors (fibroids) may be scraped away.

Description

D&C is usually performed under general anesthesia, although local or epidural anesthesia can also be used. Using local anesthesia reduces risk and costs, but the patient will feel cramping during the procedure. The type of anesthesia used often depends upon the reason for the D&C.

To begin the procedure (which takes only minutes to perform), the doctor inserts an instrument to hold open the vaginal walls, and then stretches the opening of the uterus to the vagina (the cervix). This is done by inserting a series of tapering rods, each thicker than the previous one, or by using other specialized instruments. The process of opening the cervix is called dilation.

Once the cervix is dilated, the physician inserts a spoon-shaped surgical device called a curette into the uterus. The curette is used to scrape away the uterine lining. One or more small tissue samples from the lining of the uterus or the cervical canal are sent for analysis by microscope to check for abnormal cells.

Although simpler, less expensive techniques such as a vacuum aspiration are quickly replacing the D&C as a diag-

KEY TERMS

Endomerial hyperplasia—Thickening of the uterine lining. The types of hyperplasia include: simple, complex, and atypical.

Endometrial polyps—A growth in the lining of the uterus (endometrium) that may cause bleeding and can develop into cancer.

Epidural anesthesia—A type of anesthesia that is injected into the epidural space of the spinal cord to numb the nerves leading to the lower half of the body.

Hysteroscopy—A procedure in which the doctor can see the uterine lining with a tube and viewing system. This is sometimes done with a D&C.

Uterine fibroid—A noncancerous tumor of the uterus that can range from the size of a pea to the size of a grapefruit. Small fibroids require no treatment, but those causing serious symptoms may need to be removed.

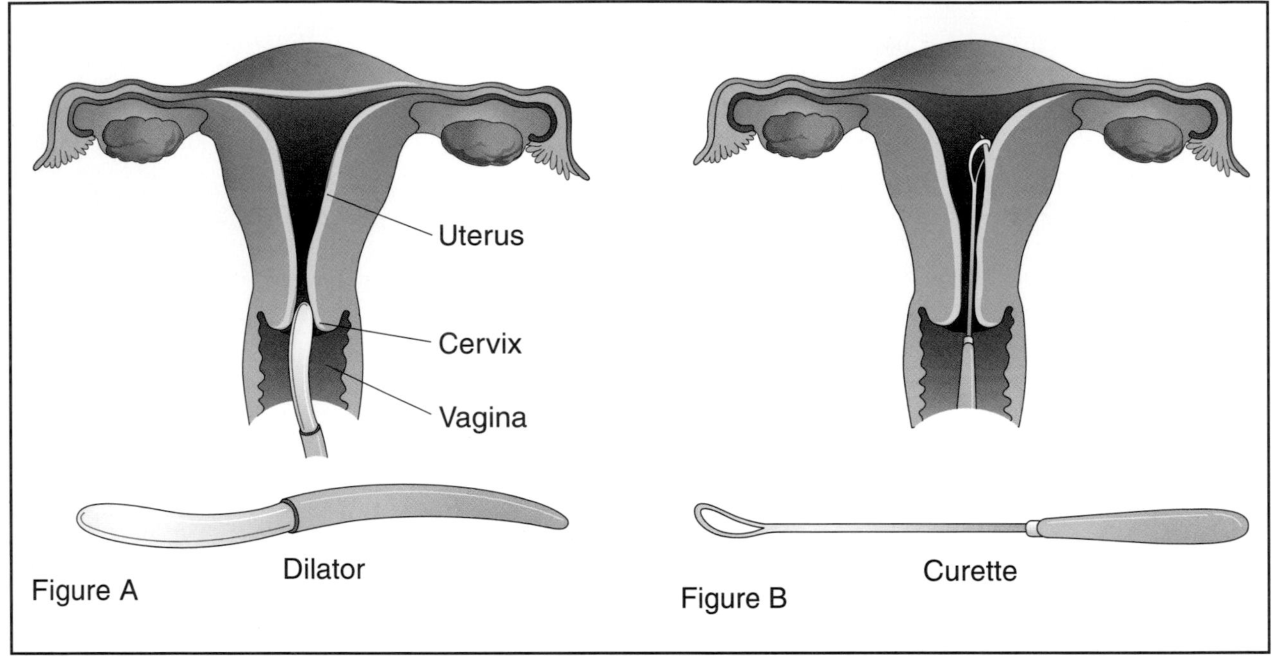

Dilatation and curettage (D & C) is used primarily to diagnose and treat heavy menstrual bleeding and to diagnose endometrial polyps, uterine fibroids, uterine cancer and cervical cancer. When performing a D & C, the physician inserts a speculum to separate and hold the vaginal walls, then stretches open the cervix with a dilator. Once the cervix is dilated, the physician will insert a curette into the uterus and scrape away small portions of the uterine lining for laboratory analysis. *(Illustration by Electronic Illustrators Group.)*

nostic method, it is still often used to diagnose and treat a number of conditions, especially when cancer is suspected.

Preparation

Because opening the cervix can be painful, sedatives may be given before the procedure begins. Deep breathing and other relaxation techniques may help ease cramping during cervical dilation.

Aftercare

A woman who has had a D&C performed in a hospital can usually go home the same day or the next day. Many women experience backache and mild cramps after the procedure, and may pass small blood clots for a day or so. Vaginal staining or bleeding may continue for several weeks.

Most women can resume normal activities almost immediately. Patients should avoid sexual intercourse, douching, and tampon use for at least two weeks to prevent infection while the cervix is closing and to allow the endometrium to heal completely.

Risks

The primary risk after the procedure is infection. Signs of infection include:

- **fever**
- heavy bleeding
- severe cramps
- foul-smelling vaginal discharge

A woman should report any of these symptoms to her doctor, who can treat the infection with **antibiotics** before it becomes serious.

D&C is a surgical operation, which carries certain risks associated with general anesthesia. Rare complications include puncture of the uterus (which usually heals on its own) or puncture of the bowel or bladder (which requires further surgery to repair).

Normal results

Results are considered normal if no unusual thickening, growths, or cancers are found. Removal of the uterine lining causes no side effects, and may be beneficial if the lining has thickened so much that it causes heavy periods. The uterine lining soon grows again normally, as part of the menstrual cycle.

Abnormal results

Some types of uterine thickening, called hyperplasia, are considered abnormal. Simple hyperplasia is a benign

QUESTIONS TO ASK THE DOCTOR

- What are you looking for in the D&C?
- Do you recommend any special preparation before the procedure?
- How long will the procedure take?
- What is the risk of finding cancer in my case?
- What action will be taken if cancer is found?
- Will a repeat D& C be necessary?

condition in which the uterine lining becomes thicker and with more endometrial glands. In complex hyperplasia, another condition where the uterine lining has thickened, the endometrial glands are crowded together. In 80% of cases these conditions will improve, and there is little risk of cancer. Only 1% of simple hyperplasia and 3% of complex hyperplasia will become cancerous.

Atypical hyperplasia is a more serious finding. In this type of endometrial thickening, the cells are abnormal. Twenty-nine percent of women with atypical hyperplasia develop cancer. In fact, in 17% to 25% of women with atypical hyperplasia who have a hysterectomy within one month of diagnosis, a **carcinoma** is found elsewhere in the endometrium.

A D&C is not a fool-proof procedure because only a portion of the uterine lining is sampled. Therefore, it is possible for a cancer to be missed. Because of this, patients with atypical hyperplasia must have another D&C in three or four months. Combining a hysteroscopy (a procedure where a physician can see the lining of the uterus using a special tool) with D&C may increase the accuracy of the diagnosis in some cases. However, this combination is not recommended when endometrial carcinoma is suspected because of the possibility that the hysteroscopy itself can aid in the spread of cancer through the fallopian tubes.

See Also Biopsy; Endometrial cancer; Gynecologic cancers

Resources

BOOKS

Berman, Michael L. and Michael T. McHale. "Uterus." In *Cancer Treatment, 5th ed.*, edited by Charles M. Haskell. Philadelphia: W.B. Saunders, 2001, pp. 951-55.

Byers, Lowell J. et al. "Uterus." In *Clinical Oncology, 2nd ed.*, edited by Abeloff, Martin D. et al. Philadelphia: Churchill Livingstone, 2000, pp. 1987-97.

Carlson, Karen J., Stephanie A. Eisenstat, and Terra Ziporyn. *The Harvard Guide to Women's Health.* Cambridge: Harvard University Press, 1996.

ORGANIZATIONS

American College of Obstetricians and Gynecologists. 409 12th St. SW, PO Box 96920, Washington, DC 20090-6920. <http://www.acog.org>.

Carol A.Turkington

Diphenhydramine

Definition

Diphenhydramine is an antihistamine, used to treat allergies, motion sickness, allergic reactions, insomnia, cough, nausea, and phenothiazine drug-induced abnormal muscle movement.

Purpose

Diphenhydramine is frequently ordered for cancer patients to aid in controlling nausea and **itching**. It may be given after a blood transfusion to limit allergic reactions to blood products. Because of its sedating properties, diphenhydramine is often used to assist in inducing sleep. It is also used to control nausea, treat the stiffness and tremor of Parkinson's disease, and control symptoms of extrapyramidal neurologic movement disorders (tremors and abnormal involuntary movements of the muscles) caused by some drugs used to treat psychosis or **nausea and vomiting**). The drug may also be formulated as a syrup and used to relieve a cough caused by minor throat irritation due to a cold or hay fever.

Description

Diphenhydramine is an antihistamine that dries, sedates, and is distributed throughout the body. It is readily absorbed when taken by mouth, with peak action occurring about one hour after ingestion. The effects last from four to six hours. This type of drug seems to compete with histamine for receptor sites after exposure to an allergen. By blocking histamine from attaching to the receptor site, the drug decreases itchiness, a runny nose, hives, and other symptoms of an allergic reaction.

Recommended dosage

The dose should be adjusted depending on the needs of the patient and their response to the medication. Adults generally take from 25 mg to 50 mg, three to four times daily. For sleep, 50 mg at bedtime is the usual

KEY TERMS

Allergen—Something that triggers an allergic reaction

Antihistamine—Agent that blocks or counteracts the action of histamine

Extrapyramidal movement disorders—Involuntary movements that occur as a side effect of psychiatric medications

Histamine—Substance released during allergic reaction

dose. Injectable diphenhydramine, 10 mg to 50 mg, may be administered through a vein or injected deep within a muscle. Some patients may require 100 mg injections. The daily dose should not exceed 400 mg. Patients should not double up on doses if one is missed.

Children weighing more than 20 pounds may take from 12.5 mg to 25 mg, three to four times daily. Children should not consume more than 300 mg in one day. The doctor may calculate a recommended dosage based on the child's weight. Parents should not double up on doses if one is missed.

Lotions or creams with diphenhydramine may be applied to the skin to relieve itching in adults and children older than two. The creams contain 1% or 2% diphenhydramine and may be used on the affected area three to four times per day. Topical diphenhydramine should not be applied to large areas of the body, blistered or oozing skin, sunburn, or lesions caused by poison ivy or chickenpox. Patients should not use topical diphenhydramine with other antihistamine-containing lotions or creams.

Precautions

Patients with angle closure glaucoma, peptic ulcer disease, bowel obstructions, an enlarged prostate, or difficulty urinating due to a blockage in the bladder should not use this medication without a doctor's order and monitoring. This drug should be used with caution in patients with asthma, heart disease, high blood pressure, or an overactive thyroid. Prior to taking this medication, patients with these conditions should discuss this medication with their doctor. Patients should not take diphenhydramine for several days prior to an allergy test. It will interfere with obtaining accurate results.

Elderly patients are prone to diphenhydramine's sedating effects. The drug may also cause dizziness and lower blood pressure in this population group. Patients should slowly change position from sitting or lying to standing when taking this medication.

Children also may experience drowsiness. In young children, this drug may produce the opposite effect. Pregnant women and those breast feeding should discuss the use of this and other drugs with their physician prior to use.

Side effects

Drowsiness commonly occurs after taking diphenhydramine. This effect may be more pronounced if alcohol or another central nervous system depressant, such as a tranquilizer or pain medication, is also ingested. Those taking the drug should refrain from driving or operating machinery or appliances until the medication has worn off. It also may cause dizziness, coordination difficulties, confusion, restlessness, nervousness, difficulty sleeping, blurry or double vision, ringing in the ears, headache, or convulsions.

Stomach distress also is common with diphenhydramine. Patients may develop a poor appetite, **nausea and vomiting**, **diarrhea** or constipation. Patients also may experience low blood pressure, palpitations, a rapid or irregular heart beat, an early onset of menstruation, frequent urination, or difficulty urinating, with urine retained in the bladder.

Diphenhydramine may also cause hives, a rash, sensitivity to the sun, and a dry mouth and nose. Thickened lung secretions are common.

Interactions

Alcohol, pain medications, sleeping pills, tranquilizers and antidepressants may make the drowsiness associated with diphenhydramine more severe.

Diphenhydramine's drying effects may be stronger and last longer when taken with an antidepressant called an MAO inhibitor.

Debra Wood, RN

Diphenoxylate *see* **Antidiarrheal agents**

Disseminated intravascular coagulation (DIC)

Description

This condition is a bleeding disorder resulting from the widespread overstimulation of the body's clotting and anticlotting mechanisms in response to illness, stress, or both. Disseminated intravascular coagulation (DIC) occurs mainly within the capillaries or the microcirculation. It is a secondary complication of a diverse group of disorders that activate, in some way, the coagulation system.

Causes

Disseminated intravascular coagulation occurs when the body's clotting mechanisms are activated throughout the body in response to an injury or a disorder, instead of being isolated to the area of initial onset. Platelets circulating throughout the body form small blood clots (thrombi) primarily in the area of the capillaries. This eventually causes the clotting factors to be used up, and none are left to form clots at the site of the injury. The presence of numerous small clots precipitates the release of clot-dissolving mechanisms, and the end result is generalized bleeding throughout the body. It is, in essence, a paradoxical situation—numerous microthrombi are being formed in the capillaries and the body reacts to dissolve these clots. It is sometimes called consumptive coagulopathy to indicate this paradox because the intravascular clotting rapidly consumes the products necessary for clotting: fibrinogen, platelets, prothrombin, and clotting factors V, VIII, and X.

Disseminated intravascular coagulation should be suspected in any individual who has an unexplained tendency toward bleeding and has experienced any clinical condition that introduces coagulation-promoting factors into the circulation. These conditions include placental abruption; retained dead fetus; amniotic fluid embolism; metastatic cancer of the pancreas, lung, stomach, or prostate; and **acute leukemia**. Any condition that also causes decreased blood flow, such as hypotension, can stimulate DIC. Widespread injury to the tissues throughout the body, as in severe burns, trauma, heat stroke, surgery, various types of infections by bacteria and fungus, snake bites, and fat embolism, can precipitate the cascade of factors to produce DIC. Excessive bleeding can appear suddenly and progress rapidly to severe or fatal hemorrhage. Signs and symptoms that appear gradually are prolonged bleeding from a venipuncture site, bleeding gums, nosebleeds, and bruising easily as well as the presence of minute, pinpoint red spots caused by bleeding under the layer of the skin.

Treatments

The objective of treatment is to determine the underlying cause of DIC and treat it, because this underlying cause predicts the probable outcome. The presence of inadequate blood components can be overcome with fresh frozen plasma and blood transfusions. Fibrinogen replacement can also occur by transfusion of blood products. When the primary disease cannot be treated, intravenous injections of **heparin**, a medication used to prevent thrombosis, are sometimes used in combination with replacement therapy. The use of heparin is, however, very controversial because it can cause bleeding itself.

Alternative and complementary therapies

Disseminated intravascular coagulation is an extremely serious condition precipitated by extraordinary events. Because it is an immediate, life-threatening situation, alternative and complementary therapies are not recommended during this phase. As an individual improves, it is important to utilize relaxation, visualization and imagery as well as vitamin and mineral supplements to promote healing.

Linda K. Bennington, C.N.S., M.S.N.

KEY TERMS

Cryoprecipitate—A preparation of antihemophilic factor used in the management of hemophilia.

Embolism—The sudden blocking of an artery by a clot of foreign material (fat, air bubble, tissue, clump of bacteria, blood clot). This foreign material is referred to as the embolus.

Polycythemia—An increase in the total red cell mass of the blood.

Thrombus—Blood clot: an accumulation of blood factors, primarily platelets and fibrin with entrapment of cellular elements, which frequently cause an obstruction in the circulation of blood. Microthrombi are very small blood clots.

Venipuncture—Surgical puncture of a vein.

DNA *see* **Cancer genetics**

DNA flow cytometry

Definition

DNA **flow cytometry** is a method of measuring the amount of deoxyribonucleic acid (DNA, genetic materi-

KEY TERMS

Aneuploid—A cell that has an irregular number of chromosomes.

Cell cycle—The events that take place during the time in which a cell replicates itself.

Diploid—A cell that has two sets (the normal number in humans) of chromosomes.

Mitosis—The process of cell division.

al) in tumor cells and the percentage of cells actively replicating.

Purpose

DNA flow cytometric analysis is sometimes done to assess a patient's prognosis. It is used to help the physician determine how the tumor cells are likely to behave. It may also be used to monitor a patient if the tumor is expected to recur.

Description

DNA flow cytometric analysis may be performed on tissue from a **biopsy** or it may require a sample of blood or body fluid from the patient. If a blood sample is used, it will be separated into its different components and the red blood cells will be removed. If material from a biopsy is used, cells from the solid tissue will be separated from each other. The cells to be analyzed will then be mixed with a dye called propidium iodide that binds tightly to DNA. This dye gives off fluorescent light as the cells pass through the laser beam of the cytometer. The cytometer can also measure other information about the cells, such as their size.

By analyzing the amount of fluorescence that the cells emit, the pathologist can evaluate the DNA content; this is also sometimes referred to as the DNA index or **ploidy analysis**. It can also determined whether or not the cancer cells are dividing; this is called S-phase analysis. The physician sometimes uses this information to determine the patient's prognosis and choose the most effective treatment.

Preparation

If a biopsy is required, the patient should be prepared for the biopsy as suggested by the physician. Alternatively, a routine blood or body fluid sample may be required. Other special preparations are not usually necessary.

Risks

The risks associated with DNA flow cytometry are limited to those associated with blood or biopsy sample collection.

Normal results

Most cells are normally in a resting, or non-proliferating, phase of the cell cycle. During this time the cells are diploid, meaning they have two copies of each chromosome. Cells duplicate their DNA during what is called S-phase so that they can reproduce, resulting in four copies of each chromosome. The cells rest again until a period called mitosis, when they begin to divide.

Normal DNA flow cytometry results will show that most of the cells are resting and have only two copies of each chromosome. Less than 10% of the cells will be in S-phase. DNA flow cytometry results are usually presented in graphical form for easier analysis. A normal graph will show one large peak of resting cells, followed by a flat area and another smaller peak of cells about to divide.

Abnormal results

Abnormal results will show as several peaks of differing sizes. This means that some of the cells in the sample have extra DNA or an irregular number of chromosomes. An increased percentage of cells may be in S-phase replicating their DNA. An abnormal result does not necessarily mean malignancy; DNA flow cytometry results must be combined with other tests to diagnose malignancy. Interpretation of results is also dependent on the type of tumor being examined. In most types of cancers the presence of cells with irregular amounts of DNA is associated with a poor prognosis, but in some types of cancers, it may indicate a good prognosis.

See Also Tumor grading

Resources

BOOKS

Javois, Lorette C., ed. *Immunocytochemical Methods and Protocols.* Totowa, NJ: Humana Press, 1999.

PERIODICALS

Chassevent, A., et al. "S-phase Fraction and DNA Ploidy in 633 t1t2 Breast Cancers: A Standardized Flow Cytometric Study." *Clinical Cancer Research* 7 (April 2001): 909-17.

Rosen, Shara. "Flow Cytometry: An Underexploited Diagnostic Power." *Medical Laboratory Observer* 30 (March 1998): 52-8.

OTHER

"FACS Laboratory." *Imperial Cancer Research Fund* 3 July 2001 <http://www.icnet.uk/axp/facs/davies/flow.html>.

QUESTIONS TO ASK THE DOCTOR

- What type of information do you expect to learn from this test?
- Are there any alternatives to doing this test?
- Is it possible that the test may give unclear or inaccurate results?
- Are there any risks or complications that could take place?

"Flow Cytometry Core Educational Links." *University of Florida* 3 July 2001 <http://www.biotech.ufl.edu/~fccl/flow_edu.html>.

Racquel Baert, M.Sc.

Docetaxel

Definition

Docetaxel is a drug used to treat certain types of cancer. Docetaxel is available under the trade name Taxotere.

Purpose

Docetaxel is an antineoplastic agent used to treat **breast cancer** and non-small cell lung **carcinoma**.

Description

Docetaxel was approved by the Food and Drug Administration (FDA) in 1996.

Docetaxel is a synthetic derivative of the naturally occurring compound **paclitaxel**. Docetaxel is synthesized from the naturally occurring compound, 10-deacetyl baccatin III, which is extracted from the needles of yew plants. Docetaxel belongs to a group of chemicals called taxoids. The chemical structure and biological action of docetaxel is similar to that of paclitaxel.

Docetaxel promotes the formation of microtubules that do not function properly. One of the roles of normal microtubules is to aid in the replication of cells. By disrupting this function, docetaxel inhibits cell replication.

Docetaxel is used in patients who have breast cancer that has recurred or progressed following treatment with other drugs. It is also used to treat non-small cell lung carcinoma alone, or in combination with platinum-containing drugs such as **cisplatin**. Statistically significant increases in survival times have been observed in patients treated with regiments that include docetaxel compared to control populations.

Recommended dosage

There is no known antidote for docetaxel overdose, so patients should be carefully monitored during treatment for toxicity.

Docetaxel is administered intravenously, in a dose that ranges from 60–100 mg/m^2, over one hour, once every three weeks. The initial dose may be adjusted downward depending on patient tolerance to the toxic side effects of the drug. Also, blood tests may be necessary to ensure that the bone marrow is functioning adequately to continue treatment at the recommended interval.

All patients should be pretreated with **corticosteroids** such as **dexamethasone** prior to docetaxel administration, to help prevent adverse side effects. These side effects include severe hypersensitivity to docetaxel treatment and fluid retention. Premedication should start one day prior to docetaxel treatment and continue for three to five days.

Precautions

Docetaxel should only be used under the supervision of a physician experienced in the use of cancer chemotherapeutic agents. Special caution should be taken to monitor the toxic effects of docetaxel, especially suppression of bone marrow function and hypersensitivity reactions. Premedication to prevent hypersensitivity reactions is recommended. Minor to severe hypersensitivity reactions may occur within a few minutes of the start of treatment. Severe hypersensitivity requires treatment to stop. Docetaxel has a low therapeutic index at its maximum recommended dosage. Certain complications will only be possible to manage if the necessary diagnostic and treatment resources are readily available.

Because docetaxel is administered intravenously, the site of infusion should be monitored for signs of inflammation.

Adverse effects of docetaxel treatment in patients with significant liver dysfunction are more likely. High doses of treatment may also increase the likelihood and severity of adverse side effects.

Docetaxel should not be administered to patients who are known to have severe hypersensitivity to

KEY TERMS

10-deacetyl baccatin III—A naturally occuring compound that can be converted to docetaxel.

Hypersensitivity—An abnormally sensitive reaction to a stimulus. Similar to an allergic reaction.

Microtubles—A tubular structure located in cells that help them to replicate.

Taxoids—A complex molecule that is chemically similar to paclitaxel.

Therapeutic index—A ratio of the maximum tolerated dose of a drug divided by the dose used in treatment.

polysorbate 80, which is a component of the treatment that helps dissolve the drug.

The safety of docetaxel in children under 16 years of age has not been established.

Docetaxel can cause harm to a fetus when administered to pregnant women. Only in life-threatening situations, should this treatment be used during pregnancy. Women of child bearing age are advised not to become pregnant during treatment. Women should stop nursing before beginning treatment, due to the potential for serious adverse side effects in the nursing infants.

Side effects

Suppression of bone marrow function is the principal adverse side effect associated with docetaxel treatment. Blood tests will allow a doctor to determine if there is adequate bone marrow function to begin or continue treatment. Hypersensitivity and fluid retention may also occur during treatment. Corticosteroids are administered prior to treatment to help alleviate these side effects. Ulceration of the mouth and surrounding areas is possible. Additional side effects, including **fever**, decrease in blood pressure, **nausea and vomiting**, **diarrhea**, pain, abnormal liver function, skin rash, nerve damage, and hair loss (**alopecia**) may occur.

Interactions

As of 2001, no formal studies have explored the interactions between docetaxel and other medications. Drugs that may alter the metabolism of docetaxel such as **cyclosporine**, terfenadine, ketoconazole, erythomycin and troleandomycin should be used with caution due to the potential for interactions.

Marc Scanio

Docusate *see* **Laxatives**

Dolasetron *see* **Antiemetics**

Double contrast barium enema *see* **Barium enema**

Doxorubicin

Definition

Doxorubicin, which kills cancer cells, is among the most widely used **chemotherapy** drugs. It is also known by its trade name, Adriamycin.

Purpose

This anticancer drug may be used to fight several different cancers: **breast cancer**, **ovarian cancer**, gastric (stomach) cancer, **thyroid cancer**, lung cancer, **testicular cancer**, and **endometrial cancer**. In addition it may be used against Hodgkin's and non-Hodgkin's **lymphoma**, acute lymphoblastic leukemia (ALL), acute myeloblastic leukemia (AML), **sarcomas** of the soft tissue, sarcomas of the bone (osteosarcomas), **neuroblastoma**, **Wilms' tumor**, small cell lung cancer (SCLC), and non-small cell lung cancer (NSCLC).

Because doxorubicin is used to treat so many different cancers, a complete description of how it may be combined with other medications in the treatment of each of the cancers cannot be given here. A few examples follow: In the treatment of Hodgkin's disease, for instance, one widely used chemotherapy regimen is the so-called ABVD, which consists of doxorubicin, **bleomycin**, **vinblastine**, and **dacarbazine**. Another is the so-called MOPP/ABV, which consists of **mechlorethamine**, **vincristine** (Oncovin), prednisone, **procarbazine**, doxorubicin, bleomycin, and vinblastine. Yet another is the so-called EVA: **etoposide**, vinblastine, and doxorubicin. Still another is the so-called EPOCH, which consists of etoposide, vincristine, doxorubicin, **cyclophosphamide**, and prednisone.

Doctors may treat stage III and IV non-Hodgkin's lymphoma with the so-called m-BACOD chemotherapy regimen, which consists of **methotrexate**, bleomycin, doxorubicin, cyclophosphamide, vincristine, and **dexamethasone**. Yet another regimen called the ProMACE-CytaBOM, which consists of cyclophosphamide, doxorubicin, etoposide, prednisone, **cytarabine**, bleomycin, vincristine, methotrexate, and **leucovorin**.

Complete remission (CR) is the total elimination of all diseased cells detectable following therapy. Continuous complete remission is CR that continues indefinitely. In the treatment of **acute lymphocytic leukemia** (ALL), it has been found that the likelihood that continuous complete remission will be achieved is increased if the patient receives at least three drugs. Two of these are usually prednisone and vincristine. The third may be doxorubicin.

Description

Doxorubicin is a DNA-binding anticancer drug and belongs to an anthracycline antibiotic, although doctors do not use this drug to attack microbial infections.

Recommended dosage

Between 60 and 90 milligrams per square meter of doxorubicin are administered via a single intravenous (IV) injection every 21 days. Alternately, between 20 and 30 milligrams per square meter per day may be given via IV for three days every three to four weeks. Alternately, 20 milligrams per square meter may be given via IV weekly. The dose of doxorubicin used depends upon which regimen for cancer is being followed.

For example, in the treatment of **acute myelocytic leukemia** (AML), 30 milligrams per square meter may be given over a period of three days. When the medication is used in the treatment of breast cancer, one chemotherapy regimen is the so-called AC, which consists of doxorubicin plus cyclophosphamide. A total of 60 milligrams of doxorubicin per square meter are given per day. AC is then repeated every 21 days.

Another chemotherapy regimen used for breast cancer is known as either FAC or CAF: **fluorouracil**, doxorubicin, and cyclophosphamide. In this regimen, 50 milligrams of doxorubicin are given per square meter per day.

Doxorubicin is not given by mouth, as an insufficient amount of the medication would be transported through the stomach wall if this were done. Rather this medication is usually administered through an intravenous (IV) procedure. Patients with liver problems may be given a reduced dose of doxorubicin.

Precautions

Doxorubicin may cause serious heart problems. To prevent these, doctors may limit the amount of doxorubicin given to each patient so that the total amount of doxorubicin a patient receives over her or his entire lifetime is 550 milligrams per square meter, or less. An encouraging recent development is that medication is now available that appears to help protect the patient's heat from the effects of doxorubicin. This new medication is called **dexrazoxane** (Zinecard).

Side effects

Patients may develop problems with heart rhythms while doxorubicin is being taken. In addition, a serious heart illness known as heart failure may develop later. Some patients develop heart failure more than 20 after having received doxorubicin.

Studies have shown that the use of the new medication dexrazoxane (Zinecard) helps protect the patient's heart from the harmful effects of doxorubicin. However, dexrazoxane itself has side effects. For example, it may intensify the reduction of blood cells that may occur with doxorubicin therapy. In addition, it may make doxorubicin less effective in attacking cancer. Dexrazoxane is used only in patients being treated for breast cancer and only in patients who have already been given more than half of the total lifetime amount of doxorubicin they should ever receive.

The activity of the bone marrow in producing blood cells may be harmed by doxorubicin. Side effects affecting the heart and bone marrow may cause doctors to lower the dose of doxorubicin. Other side effects associated with doxorubicin are **nausea and vomiting**, stomach problems, eye problems, loss of appetite (**anorexia**), and hair loss (**alopecia**). Blistering may result if bleeding occurs. In addition, the medication has a harmless side effect about which patients should be forewarned: the urine and tears may have a red color.

Patients receiving doxorubicin in conjunction with certain other anticancer drugs may, very rarely, develop a type of leukemia.

Bob Kirsch

Dronabinol *see* **Antiemetics**

Droperidol *see* **Antiemetics**

Drug resistance

Definition

Drug resistance refers to the ability of an organism, such as the HIV virus, the tuberculosis bacillus (TB), or cancer, to overcome the effects of a drug prescribed to destroy it. Well-known examples are the resistance of the HIV virus to AZT, or that of TB to **antibiotics**. Resistance has been observed to occur with every anti-HIV drug prescribed. According to the Mayo Clinic in Rochester, Minnesota, drug resistance may have played a role in the 58% rise in infectious disease deaths observed in the United States between 1980 and 1992.

Due to the immunocompromised state of cancer patients caused by the cancer treatment effect, infections with viruses and bacteria are commonplace and infectious disease treatment is paramount.

Causes

A virus like HIV becomes resistant to drugs because it has the ability to mutate. This happens because a typical virus creates billions of new viruses in the body every day—viruses that are replicas of itself. However, these replicas are not always perfect. In this daily production of billions of viruses, several small differences can occur in some of the new viruses. These differences are called *mutations*. When such mutations occur on that part of the virus that the drug is designed to chemically attach to, the drug's action is effectively stopped because it cannot attach. When a drug no longer works against its target, this is called drug resistance and the virus that the drug can no longer destroy is said to be resistant to the drug.

An example of drug resistance is a patient with AIDS. The patient may have a few HIV viruses that mutate in such a way that prevents AZT from working on those mutated viruses. The drug will still work against the HIV that has not mutated, eventually destroying it. However, reproduction of the mutated virus is then unchecked, and the infection keeps spreading as the mutated virus makes more copies of itself, which are also resistant to AZT. After some time, this mutated AZT-resistant HIV will be the only type of HIV left, and AZT will no longer work for that patient.

A similar scenario may occur with cancer drug resistance. Since the early 1970s, multiple drug resistance (MDR) has also been known to exist in several types of cancer cells. It now appears that certain cancers have the capacity to resist the cytotoxic (toxic to cells) effects of cancer **chemotherapy**, probably due to genetic abnormalities in the cancer cells. Normal tissues never develop resistance to chemotherapy. Initially, sensitive cancer cells are destroyed by chemotherapy but since mutated cancer cells are allowed to replicate (unlike normal cells that are destroyed when defective) these mutated cancer cells are no longer sensitive to some chemotherapy.

Resistance of cytomegalovirus (CMV) against antiviral drugs is another example showing that drug resistance is becoming an increasingly serious medical problem.

Like viruses, bacteria can also become drug resistant. Every time a patient takes an antibiotic, such as penicillin, to fight a bacterial infection, the antibiotic destroys most of the bacteria. However, a few tough germs may survive—either by mutating like viruses or by obtaining resistance genes from other bacteria. These survivors can then reproduce quickly, creating new drug-resistant bacteria. As is the case with mutated viruses, the presence of these resistant bacterial strains usually means that the next infection will not be cured by the first-choice antibiotic prescribed by the doctor.

Some bacteria that have already become resistant to antibiotic attack include:

- Staphylococcus aureus: This bacterium causes the majority of infections in patients in U.S. hospitals. It spreads and infects cuts, burns, skin, as well as surgical wounds. Since 1996, at least four patients have been reported to be infected with a strain that was partially resistant to normal doses of the most powerful antibiotic available, vancomycin.
- Streptococcus pneumoniae: This bacterium causes **pneumonia**, meningitis, and ear infections. According to the Mayo Clinic, it has also become partially resistant to antibiotics of the penicillin family.
- Enterococcus: This bacterium can cause everything from urinary tract to heart valve infections and it is also becoming increasingly antibiotic-resistant, including vancomycin-resistant.

If a virus or bacteria mutates at a specific location that represents the target for the drug to attach to, then modifying the drug so as to have it attach at a different place will succeed in overcoming the drug resistance. In the case of HIV, compiled databases of mutations in HIV genes that confer resistance to anti-HIV drugs are available to assist researchers in the design and production of new drugs.

Treatments

The strategies used to overcome drug resistance depend upon the nature of the organism causing the infection but generally involve the following steps:

- Accurate and rapid diagnosis: Swift identification and treatment—the sooner the infectious organism is detected and correctly identified, the higher the chances that it will not become drug resistant since it will have less time to mutate.
- Drug combination: New combinations of drugs can be very effective. Given a mixture of mutated and unmutated pathogens, a drug "cocktail" is likely to contain a drug that may be effective against a new mutated form

KEY TERMS

AIDS (Acquired Immunodeficiency Syndrome)—A state of severe immune suppression caused by the HIV virus. A diagnosis of AIDS is given to a patient infected with HIV and who also experiences at least one condition from a list compiled by the Center for Disease Control and Prevention (CDC), as for example an infection with cytomegalovirus (CMV) or a cancer such as Kaposi's sarcoma.

Antibiotic—A drug that slows bacterial growth or kills bacteria.

Antiviral drug—A drug that slows viral growth or kills viruses.

AZT (Retrovir, zidovudine, ZDV)—The first drug licensed to treat HIV. It is almost always used in combination with other anti-HIV drugs. AZT is also used to prevent transmission of HIV from mother to fetus.

Bacterium—A tiny microorganism that reproduces by cell division. It can be shaped like a rod, sphere, or spiral and is found virtually everywhere. Many types of bacteria cause infection and disease.

CMV (Cytomegalovirus)—A virus that belongs to the herpes virus family and is present as a silent infection in almost everyone. CMV often becomes activated in people with AIDS.

Cytoxic—A substance toxic (poisonous) to cells.

Gene—The part of DNA responsible for determining a person's characteristics. It also transfers information from old cells to new cells.

Gene therapy—The use of genes to treat cancer and other diseases.

Immune system—The system within the body, consisting of many organs and cells, that recognizes and fights foreign cells and disease.

Pathogen—Anything capable of causing disease, usually a virus or bacterium, but it also refers to chemical substances, such as asbestos.

Tuberculosis—An infectious disease of the lungs caused by a type of bacterium called amycobacterium. Symptoms include weight loss, fever, and cough, often with blood-streaked mucus. Tuberculosis is highly contagious.

of the virus, thus preventing it from making billions of new copies every day. The less virus created, the less chance of further mutations occurring.

- New drugs: There is a problem facing all the strategies used to overcome drug resistance and it is that drugs have to be given at high—and sometimes toxic—doses, and also in combinations that have become quite expensive. Increasingly, they also must be taken on schedules that are difficult to follow by patients. Even then, new varieties of resistant strains still appear. There is, therefore, an urgent need to understand how drug resistance develops at the molecular level, and to use this understanding to develop more effective drugs.

See Also AIDS-related cancers

Resources

BOOKS

Huemer R. P., and J. Challem. *The Natural Health Guide to Beating the Supergerms: and Other Infections, Including Colds, Flus, Ear Infections and Even HIV* New York: Pocket Books, 1997.

Kaspers, G. J. L., R. Pieters, and A. J. P. Veerman, eds.*Drug Resistance in Leukemia and Lymphoma III (Advances in Experimental Medicine and Biology)* 457 New York: Plenum Press, 1999.

Kellen, J. A.*Alternative Mechanisms of Multidrug Resistance in Cancer* New York: Springer Verlag, 1995.

Levy, S. B. *The Antibiotic Paradox: How Miracle Drugs Are Destroying the Miracle* Boulder, CO: Perseus Press, 1992.

PERIODICALS

Brenner, B. G., and M. A. Wainberg. "The role of Antiretrovirals and Drug Resistance in Vertical Transmission of HIV-1 Infection." *Annals of the New York Acadademy of Sciences* 918(November 2000): 9-15.

Broxterman, H. J., and N. Georgopapadakou. "Cancer Research 2000: Drug Resistance, New Targets and Drugs In Development." *Drug Resistance Updates* 3 (June 2000): 133-138.

Clavel, F., E. Race, and F. Mammano. "HIV Drug Resistance and Viral Fitness." *Advances in Pharmacology* 49 (2000):41-66.

Durant, J., P. Clevenbergh, P. Halfon, P. Delgiudice, S. Porsin, et al. "Drug-Resistance Genotyping in HIV-1 Therapy." *Lancet* 353 (June 1999): 2195-2199.

Emery, V. C. "Cytomegalovirus Drug Resistance." *Antiviral Therapy* 3 (1998): 239-242.

Norgaard, J. M., and P. Hokland "Biology of Multiple Drug Resistance in Acute Leukemia." *International Journal of Hematology* 72 (October 2000): 290-297.

Teicher, B. A. "Molecular Targets and Cancer Therapeutics: Discovery, Development and Clinical Validation." *Drug Resistance Updates* 3 (April 2000):67-73.

ORGANIZATIONS

National Cancer Institute, HIV Drug Resistance Program. NCI-Frederick, Building 535, Room 109, P.O. Box B, Frederick, MD 21702-1201. Phone:(301)846-1168. <http://www.ncifcrf.gov/hivdrp>

U. S. Food and Drug Administration. 5600 Fishers Lane, Rockville, MD 20857. Phone:(888)INFO-FDA [(888)463-6332] <http://www.fda.gov/default.htm>

HIV Drug Resistance Database. <http://204.121.6.64:581/Resist_DB/default.htm>

OTHER

The AIDS Treatment Data Network. Factsheet: Understanding Drug Resistance. 1 July 2001 <http://www.aidsinfonyc.org/network/simple/resistance.html>

The AIDS Treatment Data Network. Factsheet: Trials of drugs for treating HIV. 1 July 2001 <http://www.aidsinfonyc.org/network/trials/hiv.html>

Monique Laberge, Ph.D.

Dryness of the mouth, *see* **Xerostomia**

Ductogram

Definition

A ductogram, also called a galactogram, is a special type of mammogram used for imaging the breast ducts. It can aid in diagnosing the cause of abnormal nipple discharges.

Purpose

The purpose of a ductogram is to locate the origin of an abnormal discharge from the nipple of the breast.

Precautions

Women who are pregnant should not undergo a ductogram without adequate protection of the abdomen from the x rays that are used in this test.

Description

A ductogram is performed by first cleansing the nipple and areola with an antiseptic. The radiologist performing the test then presses gently on the nipple to determine which duct is leaking fluid. Once the leaking duct has been identified, a small needle (cannula) is inserted into that duct. A dye is then injected into the leaking duct and an **x ray** similar to a mammogram is performed.

This test is performed in a **mammography** or breast imaging facility, either in a hospital department or an outpatient x-ray center. During this procedure, the patient is in a sitting, standing, or horizontal position depending on the x-ray equipment available at the testing center where the ductogram is to be performed. The x-ray camera may change position during the study, but the patient is usually stationary. The procedure typically takes 30 to 60 minutes. It is important for the patient not to move except when directed to do so by the technologist.

Preparation

There is usually little or no preparation required of the patient for a ductogram. Prior to the test, the patient should not attempt to express a discharge from the affected nipple or nipples. Jewelry or metallic objects that may interfere with the x-ray image should be removed for the duration of the ductogram. No deodorant or powder should be used as this can interfere with the test.

If the nipple drainage suddenly stops on the day of the ductogram, the patient should notify her health care provider prior to undergoing this test.

Aftercare

No special care is required after the test. Fluids are encouraged after the procedure to aid in the excretion of the dye from the body.

Risks

The risks of a ductogram are very low. Most ductograms use the same amount of radiation as a conventional x ray. Side effects or negative reactions are very rare. Possible side effects include pain, infection, and bleeding from the nipple where the cannula was inserted.

KEY TERMS

Cannula—A small tube or hollow needle designed for insertion into a duct.

Ductogram—A special type of mammogram used diagnosing the cause of abnormal nipple discharges.

Pathologic—Diseased or abnormal.

QUESTIONS TO ASK THE DOCTOR

- Were any abnormalities detected?
- What future care is necessary?
- What are the risks and precautions of any further procedures?

Normal results

A normal ductogram shows the expected distribution of the dye material within the ducts of the breast and no unusual shape or size of the scanned tissue.

Abnormal results

An abnormal ductogram shows an abnormality within the ducts of the breast that may be causing the pathologic discharge of fluid from that breast. If an abnormality is identified, additional procedures, including surgery, may be necessary.

Resources

BOOKS

Cardeonsa, Gilda. *Ductography.* New York: Creative Education Options, LLC, 1996.

ORGANIZATIONS

American Cancer Society. (800) ACS-2345. <http://www.cancer.org>.

National Alliance of Breast Cancer Organizations (NABCO). 9 East 37th St., 10th Floor, New York, NY 10016. (888) 806-2226. <http://www.nabco.org>.

OTHER

Breast Cancer Overview. 25 May 2001. <http://cancer.mps-group.com/breast_cancer.htm>.

Paul A. Johnson, Ed.M.

Duplex ultrasound *see* **Ultrasonography**

Dysplastic nevus syndrome *see* **Melanoma**

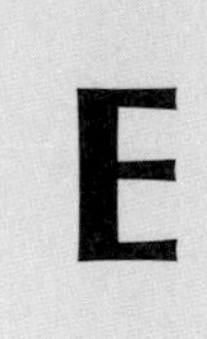

Eaton-Lambert syndrome

Description

Eaton-Lambert syndrome, also called Lambert-Eaton myasthenic syndrome (LEMS), is a rare disorder affecting the muscles and nerves. LEMS is known to be associated with small cell lung cancer. It may also be associated with cancers such as **lymphoma**, non-Hodgkin's lymphoma, T-cell leukemia, non-small cell lung cancer, **prostate cancer**, and **thymoma**.

The primary symptom of LEMS is muscular weakness or paralysis that varies in intensity and location throughout the body. Other symptoms of LEMS include tingling sensations on the skin, double vision, difficulty maintaining a steady gaze, and dry mouth or difficulty in swallowing.

The first signs of LEMS tend to be:

- changes in vision
- decreased posture and muscle tone
- difficulty in chewing or swallowing
- difficulty in climbing stairs
- difficulty in lifting simple objects
- speech impairment
- a drooping head
- fatigue
- and/or a need to use hands to get up from a sitting or lying position

LEMS is often misdiagnosed as **myasthenia gravis** because of the similarities between the symptoms of these two disorders.

Causes

The symptoms of LEMS are the result of an insufficient release of neurotransmitter by nerve cells. Neurotransmitter is a chemical which passes signals from the nerve cells to the muscles in order for the muscles to move. The decreased level of neurotransmitter causes a muscle reaction to the nerve signal that is lower than normal. The underlying cause of the lower-than-normal neurotransmitter release seen in LEMS patients is believed to be related to a malfunction of the patient's own immune system (an autoimmune reaction).

This autoimmune reaction is caused by antibodies that a patient produces in response to small cell lung cancer, or one of the other cancers associated with LEMS.

Since continued use of the muscles may lead to a build-up of the neurotransmitter to normal levels, symptoms of LEMS can often be lessened or alleviated by use of the affected muscles. Myasthenia gravis, another disorder that has symptoms similar to LEMS, is caused by a blockage of neurotransmitters by antibodies. Symptoms of myasthenia gravis do not improve with continued muscle use. The improvement in symptoms that is observable in LEMS patients often helps to differentiate LEMS from myasthenia gravis.

LEMS is aggravated by neuromuscular blocking agents used during surgery; certain **antibiotics**, such as aminoglycoside and fluoroquinolone; magnesium; calcium channel blockers; and iodinated intravenous contrast agents used for medical imaging.

Treatments

The goal of treatment for LEMS patients is to improve muscle strength while also treating the cancer or other underlying disorder that is causing LEMS.

When possible, patients affected with LEMS should undergo a physical therapy program that is tailored to their health status and abilities. This may include stretching and flexibility manuevers as well as light strength and cardiovascular exercises. Symptoms of LEMS tend to be aggravated by prolonged exercise, so any physical therapy undertaken should be relatively short in duration.

KEY TERMS

Autoimmune reaction—An immune reaction in which the body attacks healthy tissue, mistaking it for a foreign antigen.

Neurotransmitter—A chemical that is released at the end of a nerve to transmit a signal to another nerve or to a muscle.

Plasmapheresis—Also called plasma replacement, this technique is used to replace a patient's blood plasma, usually with donated plasma.

Some LEMS patients are not able to undergo physical therapy because of their current state of health. In these cases, plasmapheresis (also called plasma exchange), a procedure in which blood plasma is removed from the patient and replaced, may be recommended. This procedure can be effective in a majority of LEMS patients.

Medications that suppress the **immune response** or that suppress the antibodies responsible for the weakness have also been shown to improve LEMS symptoms in some patients.

Alternative and complementary therapies

Yoga and other stretching exercises may be effective treatments for alleviating the physical symptoms of LEMS patients. Some LEMS patients also report improvement of symptoms after deep body massage or hydrotherapy.

Resources

BOOKS

Lisak, Robert P., ed. *Handbook of Myasthenia Gravis and Myasthenic Syndromes.* Detroit: Wayne State University, 1994.

ORGANIZATIONS

Muscular Dystrophy Association. 3300 E. Sunrise Dr., Tucson, AZ 85718. (800) 572-1717. <http://www.mdausa.org/>.

Myasthenia Gravis Foundation of America, Inc. 5841 Cedar Lake Road, Suite 204, Minneapolis, MN 55416. (800) 541-5454. <http://www.myasthenia.org/>.

OTHER

"Calcium Channel Autoantibodies in the Diagnosis of the Lambert-Eaton Syndrome." *Diagnostika GMBH* June 2001. 28 June 2001 <http://dld-diagnostika.de/>.

"Eaton Lambert Syndrome." *Reader's Digest Health* 29 March 2001. 28 June 2001 <http://www.rd.com/comma/nav/index.jhtml?articleld= 8612775>.

"Lambert-Eaton Syndrome." *HealthCentral* June 2001. 28 June 2001 <http://www.healthcentral.com/mhc/top/000710.cfm>.

"Myasthenia Gravis Support and Community Forum." *MGFriends.com* 15 April 2001. 28 June 2001 <http://www.mgfriends.com/>.

"Myasthenic Syndrome (Lambert-Eaton; LEMS): Autoimmune." *Neuromuscular Disease Center* June 2001. 28 June 2001 <http://www.neuro.wustl.edu/neuromuscular/synmg.html#lems>.

Paul A. Johnson, Ed.M.

Edatrexate

Definition

Edatrexate is an investigational (experimental) medicine similar to **methotrexate** used to stop growth of cancer and formation of new cancer cells.

Purpose

Edatrexate has been shown to have anticancer activity in research studies in patients with lung cancer, head and neck cancer, **breast cancer**, and non-Hodgkins lymphoma.

Description

Edatrexate is an anticancer drug that belongs to a family of drugs called antimetabolites. It is an antagonist of **folic acid** closely related to methotrexate in its structure and antitumor activity. However, edatrexate has several potential advantages over methotrexate, including better transport across cancer cell membranes (walls surrounding cancer cells), increased selectivity for tumor cells, and greater antitumor effect. Edatrexate inhibits formation of genetic material and reproduction of cancer cells by inhibiting a certain enzyme needed to make folic acid. Without folic acid, formation of protein and new genetic material in cancer cells cannot occur. Unlike methotrexate, edatrexate has additive activity when used with **cisplatin** (a **chemotherapy** agent often used to treat non-small cell lung cancer) in animal studies. It also showed additive anticancer effects with **cyclophosphamide**, **paclitaxel** and **docetaxel**.

Edatrexate has been used in combination with paclitaxel, cisplatin, clyclophosphamide, mitomycin, or **vinblastine** in research studies. **Leucovorin** has been shown to be effective in reducing edatrexate side effects, but it may also decrease its antitumor effectiveness.

Recommended Dosage

Adults

SOLID TUMORS (LUNG, BREAST, HEAD AND NECK CANCER). Doses vary between different chemotherapy protocols. The most commonly used dose in research studies was 40-80 mg per square meter of body surface area given as intravenous infusion once a week. Maximum tolerated dose when edatrexate was used in combination with paclitaxel was 120 mg per meter square per week.

Children

There is no data available on dosing and use of edatrexate in children.

Precautions

To maximize treatment effects, patients receiving edatrexate should observe certain guidelines. Including any modifications given by the oncologist, these guidelines should include regular visits with the oncologist and laboratory testing for white blood cell count, kidney, liver, and bone marrow function. Patients should: avoid any immunizations not approved or prescribed by the oncologist; avoid contact with individuals taking or who have recently taken oral polio vaccine, or individuals who have an active infection; wear a protective facemask when necessary; avoid prolonged or direct exposure to sunlight, as some patients experience an increased sensitivity; ask for specific instructions on oral hygiene procedures to reduce the risk of gum abrasion, and avoid touching the eye and nasal areas unless hands have been properly washed immediately prior to contact. To reduce bleeding and bruising complications, patients should exercise extreme caution when handling sharp instruments and decline participation in contact sports. Prior to treatment, the patient's medical history should be thoroughly reviewed to avoid complications that might arise from previous conditions such as gout, kidney stones or kidney disease, liver disease, chickenpox, shingles, intestinal blockage, colitis, suppressed immune system, stomach ulcers, mouth sores, or a history of allergic reactions to various drugs.

The oncologist should also be made aware if the patient is pregnant or if there is the possibility the patient might be pregnant, or if the patient is a breast-feeding mother. Only prescribed medications or over the counter (OTC) drugs approved by the oncologist should be taken by a patient receiving edatrexate.

Side effects

The side effect profile of edatrexate is similar to that of methotrexate, with mouth ulcers as the dose-limiting toxicity. Other side effects include bone marrow suppression and decreased formation of all blood elements, **diarrhea**, skin rash, nausea, vomiting, inflammation of the lungs (pneumonitis) and mild increase in liver function tests.

KEY TERMS

Bone marrow—The tissue filling the cavities of bones.

Non-Hodgkin's lymphoma—Lymphomas are some of the most treatable cancers with cure rates around 50% in 1990's. Non-Hodgkin's lymphoma mainly affects people over 50 years of age and has been more difficult to treat than the Hodgkin's type. There has been an increase in non-Hodgkin's lymphoma cases in the last two decades in patients with HIV.

Interactions

There is no published information available at this point about any potential drug or food interactions with edatrexate. As a general rule, **vaccines** should be avoided due to the immunosuppressive action of edatrexate, and alcohol should be avoided to reduce the risk of liver complications.

Olga Bessmertny, Pharm.D.

Endocrine system tumors

Definition

The group of tumors that are associated with the hormone-secreting (endocrine) glands of the body.

Description

The glands in the body that make and secrete hormones comprise the endocrine system. All endocrine glands secrete hormones directly into the bloodstream, where they travel to a target organ or cell to trigger a specific reaction. These glands are primarily involved in controlling many of the slow and long-term activities in the body, such as growth, sexual development, and regulation of blood levels for many important proteins and essential chemical elements.

Endocrine glands are found in the head and neck region, the abdominal region, and the pelvic area (the region where the reproductive organs are located). The following are the main endocrine glands of the body:

- Pituitary gland. Found at the base of the brain, this small gland is important because it secretes several hormones that control the activity of other endocrine glands.

- Thyroid gland. Situated in the front of the neck, in the region of the Adam's apple, this gland secretes hormones that regulate body temperature, heart rate, and metabolism.
- Parathyroid glands. These four glands, with a pair on either side of the thyroid gland in the neck region, produce parathyroid hormone, which helps control the level of calcium in the blood.
- Pancreas. Found close to the stomach in the abdominal region, the pancreas contains two groups of cells. One group functions as an exocrine gland, secreting digestive enzymes into the intestines through a duct. The other, known as islets of Langerhans (or islet cells), functions as an endocrine gland and secretes hormones that control blood sugar levels and aid digestion.
- Adrenal glands. These two glands, one located above each kidney, secrete hormones that prevent inflammation and help regulate blood pressure, blood sugar levels, and metabolism.
- Ovary. A woman has two small ovaries in the pelvic area. They contain the egg cells and secrete the hormones progesterone and estrogen. These hormones have many functions, including controlling the onset of puberty, the timing of menstruation, and the changes associated with pregnancy.
- Testis (also called testicle). Men typically have two testes located outside the body in the lower pelvic area. They produce sperm and the hormone **testosterone**, which signals the onset of puberty, maintains the expression of male characteristics, such as facial hair, and stimulates sperm production.

Endocrine system tumors are rare. Although certain types are likely to be diagnosed as malignant (cancerous), endocrine tumors are often noncancerous (benign). Each year endocrine system cancers account for only around 4% of all new cancer cases in the United States. In 2001, it is expected that 53,460 Americans will develop an endocrine system cancer, resulting in an estimated 16,600 deaths.

The most common cancers of the endocrine system are **ovarian cancer** and **thyroid cancer**. Ovarian cancer represents about 44% of all endocrine system cancers and affects eight out of every 100,000 American women. New cases of ovarian cancer in 2001 will likely reach over 23,000, and nearly 13,000 will die from the disease. Roughly six out of every 100,000 Americans develop thyroid cancer, which accounts for 36% of all endocrine system cancers. It is estimated that 19,000 new cases will be diagnosed in 2001 and result in 1,300 deaths. Other malignant endocrine tumors are much rarer. **Testicular cancer** affects about two out of every 100,000 American men, while the remaining cancer types combined affect roughly one out of every 100,000 Americans.

Endocrine system tumors

Pituitary tumors
Thyroid tumors
Parathyroid tumors
Endocrine pancreatic tumors, including gastrinoma, insulinoma, and glucagonoma
Adrenal tumors, including pheochromocytoma and adrenocortical carcinoma
Ovarian tumors
Testicular tumors
Multiple endocrine gland tumors (tumors on several endocrine glands at once)

Many benign and malignant endocrine tumors are treatable with a combination of surgery and medication, and the survival rates for many endocrine cancers is good. Two exceptions are ovarian cancer and **adrenocortical carcinoma**, a tumor of the adrenal gland. About 50% of ovarian cancer patients and 40% of those diagnosed with an adrenocortical carcinoma will survive five years or more after the initial diagnosis. These cancers have poor survival rates because they are usually first diagnosed after they have spread or reached an advanced stage. Among the different cancers, thyroid cancer and testicular cancer have some of the better 5-year survival rates; both approach 95%.

Symptoms of many endocrine tumors are associated with the excessive secretion of hormones. Hormone-producing tumors are called functional tumors, while those that do not secrete hormones are called nonfunctional tumors. Both types are potentially malignant.

Types of cancers

Proceeding from the head region to the pelvic area, endocrine system tumors include:

- Pituitary tumors. These tumors are classified by the type of hormone they secrete. They are rarely malignant but can cause heath problems, including visual complications. One type of tumor results in **Cushing's syndrome**.
- Thyroid tumors. Only 5% of the tumors found on the thyroid are malignant. A malignant tumor can indicate one of the four types of thyroid cancer.
- Parathyroid tumors. Around 5% are malignant and result in a diagnosis of **parathyroid cancer**. Overproduction of parathyroid hormone, a condition known as hyperparathyroidism, is a common condition associated with both benign and malignant tumors. Untreated, hyperparathyroidism can result in osteoporosis (bones become brittle and fracture easily), kidney stones, peptic ulcers, and nervous system problems.
- Endocrine pancreatic tumors. Benign and malignant tumors are often treatable with surgery. Malignant

KEY TERMS

Endocrine gland—Any gland that makes hormones and secretes them directly into the bloodstream.

Exocrine gland—Any gland that secretes substances outward through a duct into a body cavity or onto a body surface (e.g., sweat glands and salivary glands).

Germ cell—Any cell in the body that eventually produces either a mature egg cell (female) or a mature sperm cell (male).

Inherited disorder—A disease that has a tendency to occur within a family. A disorder may be acquired due to a gene or genes that are passed from parent to child.

tumors are rare. The most common types of tumors are a gastrinoma, which is associated with **Zollinger-Ellison syndrome**, insulinoma, and glucagonoma.

- Adrenal tumors. One type of tumor, a **pheochromocytoma**, is found on the inner part of the adrenal gland (the adrenal medulla). About 10% are malignant. An adrenocortical carcinoma is a malignant tumor on the outer part of the gland (adrenal cortex), and a common symptom is the occurrence of Cushing's syndrome. Both tumors are very rare.
- Ovarian tumors. Tumors can develop in the egg cells inside the ovary (**germ cell tumors**), but most occur in the cells lining the outside of the ovary, and most of these tumors are benign.
- Testicular tumors. Tumors can occur in one or both of the testes. Over 90% develop in the germ cells and only 4% involve the endocrine cells of the testes.
- Multiple endocrine gland tumors. Some disorders result in the simultaneous occurrence of tumors on several endocrine glands. Many of these are inherited disorders, including **multiple endocrine neoplasia syndromes**, **Von Hippel-Lindau syndrome**, and **Von Recklinghausen's neurofibromatosis**.

See Also Adenoma; Craniopharyngioma; Neuroendocrine carcinomas; Pancreatic cancer, exocrine

Resources

BOOKS

Greenspan, Francis S., and Gordon J. Strewler.*Basic and Clinical Endocrinology.* Stamford, Conn: Appleton & Lange, 1997.

Wilson, Jean D., Charles Cameron, Daniel W. Foster, Donald W. Seldin, Henry M. Kronenberg, and P. Reed Larsen.*Williams Textbook of Endocrinology.* Philadelphia: W. B. Saunders, 1998.

PERIODICALS

Monson, J. C."The Epidemiology of Endocrine Tumours."*Endocrine-Related Cancer* 7 (2000): 29–36.

ORGANIZATIONS

American Association of Clinical Endocrinologists. 1000 Riverside Ave., Suite 205, Jacksonville, FL 32204. (904) 353-7878. <http://www.aace.com>.

OTHER

EndocrineWeb.com 3 July 2001 <http://www.endocrineweb.com>.

Monica McGee, M.S.

Endometrial cancer

Definition

Endometrial cancer develops when the cells that make up the inner lining of the uterus (the endometrium) become abnormal and grow uncontrollably.

Description

Endometrial cancer (also called uterine cancer) is the fourth most common type of cancer among women and the most common gynecologic cancer. Approximately 34,000 women are diagnosed with endometrial cancer each year. In 1998, approximately 6,300 women died from this cancer. Although endometrial cancer generally occurs in women who have gone through menopause and are 45 years of age or older, 30% of the women with endometrial cancer are younger than 40 years of age. The average age at diagnosis is 60 years old.

The uterus, or womb, is the hollow female organ that supports the development of the unborn baby during pregnancy. The uterus has a thick muscular wall and an inner lining called the endometrium. The endometrium is very sensitive to hormones and it changes daily during the menstrual cycle. The endometrium is designed to provide an ideal environment for the fertilized egg to implant and begin to grow. If pregnancy does not occur, the endometrium is shed causing the menstrual period.

More than 95% of uterine cancers arise in the endometrium. The most common type of uterine cancer is adenocarcinoma. It arises from an abnormal multiplication of endometrial cells (atypical adenomatous hyperplasia) and is made up of mature, specialized cells (well-differentiated). Less commonly, endometrial cancer arises without a preceding hyperplasia and is made up of poorly differentiated cells. The more common of these types are the papillary serous and clear cell carcinomas. Poorly differentiated endometrial cancers are often associated with a less promising prognosis.

Demographics

The highest incidence of endometrial cancer in the United States is in Caucasians, Hawaiians, Japanese, and African Americans. American Indians, Koreans, and Vietnamese have the lowest incidence. African–American and Hawaiian women are more likely to be diagnosed with advanced cancer and, therefore, have a higher risk of dying from the disease.

Causes and symptoms

Although the exact cause of endometrial cancer is unknown, it is clear that high levels of estrogen, when not balanced by progesterone, can lead to abnormal growth of the endometrium. Factors that increase a woman's risk of developing endometrial cancer are:

- Age. The risk is considerably higher in women who are over the age of 50 and have gone through menopause.
- Obesity. Being overweight is a very strong risk factor for this cancer. Fatty tissue can change other normal body chemicals into estrogen, which can promote endometrial cancer.
- Estrogen replacement therapy. Women receiving estrogen supplements after menopause have a 12 times higher risk of getting endometrial cancer if progesterone is not taken simultaneously.
- Diabetes. Diabetics have twice the risk of getting this cancer as nondiabetic women. It is not clear if this risk is due to the fact that many diabetics are also obese and hypertensive. One 1998 study found that women who were obese and diabetic were three times more likely to develop endometrial cancer than women who were obese but nondiabetic. This study also found that nonobese diabetics were not at risk of developing endometrial cancer.
- Hypertension. High blood pressure (or hypertension) is also considered a risk factor for uterine cancer.
- Irregular menstrual periods. During the menstrual cycle, there is interaction between the hormones estrogen and progesterone. Women who do not ovulate regularly are exposed to high estrogen levels for longer periods of time. If a woman does not ovulate regularly, this delicate balance is upset and may increase her chances of getting uterine cancer.
- Early first menstruation or late menopause. Having the first period at a young age (a 1997 *Pediatrics* article identified the mean age of menses as 12.16 years in African-American girls and 12.88 years in white girls) or going through menopause at a late age (over age 51 according to a 2001 *Prevention* article) seem to put women at a slightly higher risk for developing endometrial cancer.
- **Tamoxifen**. This drug, which is used to treat or prevent **breast cancer**, increases a woman's chance of developing endometrial cancer. Tamoxifen users tend to have more advanced endometrial cancer with an associated poorer survival rate than those who do not take the drug. In many cases, however, the value of tamoxifen for treating breast cancer and for preventing the cancer from spreading far outweighs the small risk of getting endometrial cancer.
- Family history. Some studies suggest that endometrial cancer runs in certain families. Women with inherited mutations in the BRCA1 and BRCA2 genes are at a higher risk of developing breast, ovarian, and other **gynecologic cancers**. Those with the hereditary nonpolyposis colorectal cancer gene have a higher risk of developing endometrial cancer.
- Breast, ovarian, or **colon cancer**. Women who have a history of these other types of cancer are at an increased risk of developing endometrial cancer.
- Low parity or nulliparity. Endometrial cancer is more common in women who have born few (low parity) or no (nulliparity) children. The high levels of progesterone produced during pregnancy has a protective effect against endometrial cancer. The results of one study suggest that nulliparity is associated with a lower survival rate.
- Infertility. Risk is increased due to nulliparity or the use of fertility drugs.
- Polycystic ovary syndrome. The increased level of estrogen associated with this abnormality raises the risk of cancers of the breast and endometrium.

The most common symptom of endometrial cancer is unusual vaginal spotting, bleeding or discharge. In women who are near menopause (perimenopausal), symptoms of endometrial cancer could include bleeding between periods (intermenstrual bleeding), heavy bleeding that lasts for more than seven days, or short menstrual cycles (fewer than 21 days). For women who have gone through menopause, any vaginal bleeding or abnormal discharge is suspect. Pain in the pelvic region and the presence of a lump (mass) are symptoms that occur late in the disease.

Diagnosis

If endometrial cancer is suspected, a series of tests will be conducted to confirm the diagnosis. The first step will involve taking a complete personal and family medical history. A physical examination, which will include a thorough pelvic examination, will also be done.

The doctor may order an endometrial **biopsy**. This is generally performed in the doctor's office and does not require anesthesia. A thin, flexible tube is inserted through the cervix and into the uterus. A small piece of endometrial tissue is removed. The patient may experience some discomfort, which can be minimized by taking an anti-inflammatory medication (like Advil or Motrin) an hour before the procedure.

If an adequate amount of tissue was not obtained by the endometrial biopsy, or if the biopsy tissue looks abnormal but confirmation is needed, the doctor may perform a **dilatation and curettage** (D & C). This procedure is done in the outpatient surgery department of a hospital and takes about an hour. The patient may be given general anesthesia. The doctor dilates the cervix and uses a special instrument to scrape tissue from inside the uterus.

The tissue that is obtained from the biopsy or the D & C is sent to a laboratory for examination. If cancer is found, then the type of cancer will be determined. The treatment and prognosis depends on the type and stage of the cancer.

Transvaginal ultrasound may be used to measure the thickness of the endometrium. For this painless procedure, a wand-like ultrasound transducer is inserted into the vagina to enable visualization and measurement of the uterus, the thickness of the uterine lining, and other pelvic organs.

Other possible diagnostic procedures include sonohysterography and hysteroscopy. For sonohysteroscopy, a small tube is passed through the cervix and into the uterus. A small amount of a salt water (saline) solution is injected through the tube to open the space within the uterus and allow ultrasound visualization of the endometrium. For hysteroscopy, a wand-like camera is passed through the cervix to allow direct visualization of the endometrium. Both of these procedures cause discomfort, which may be reduced by taking an anti-inflammatory medication prior to the procedure.

Treatment team

The treatment team for endometrial cancer may include a gynecologist, gynecologic oncologist, surgeon, radiation oncologist, gynecologic nurse oncologist, sexual therapist, psychiatrist, psychological counselor, and social worker.

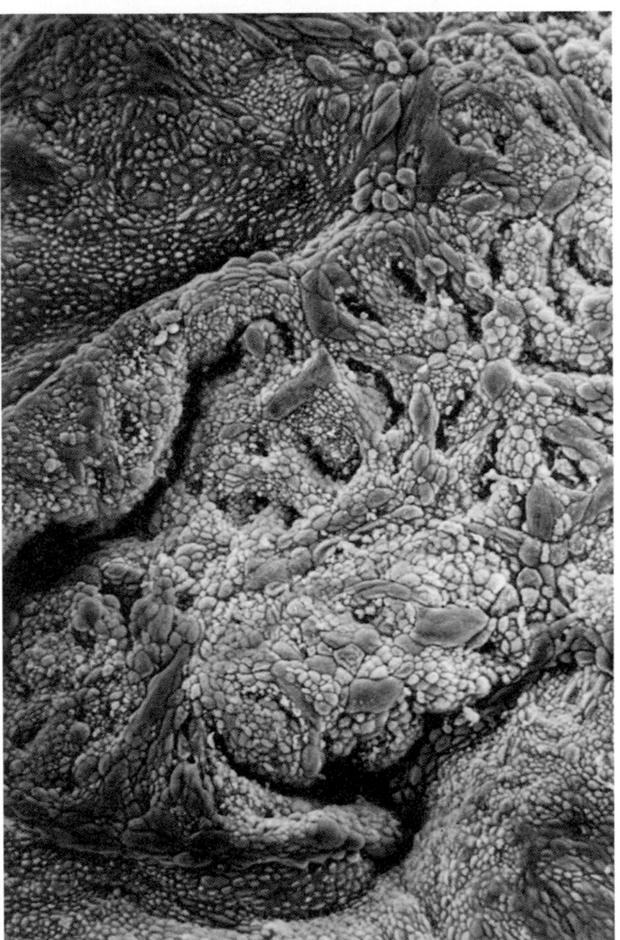

Colored scanning electron micrograph of adenocarcinoma cancer in the endometrium. Surface epithelial cells are seen (yellow), with cavities forming the openings of glands. Adenocarcinoma cells are large (green) and proliferative, invading the surface and glands. *(© Professors P.M. Motta and S. Makabe, Science Source/Photo Researchers, Inc. Photo reproduced by permission.)*

Clinical staging, treatments, and prognosis

Clinical staging

The International Federation of Gynecology and Obstetrics (FIGO) has adopted a staging system for endometrial cancer. The stage of cancer is determined after surgery. Endometrial cancer is categorized into four stages (I, II, III, and IV) which are subdivided (A, B, and possibly C) based on the depth or spread of cancerous tissue. Seventy percent of all uterine cancers are stage I, 10% to 15% are stage II, and the remainder are stages III and IV. The cancer is also graded (G1, G2, and G3) based upon microscopic analysis of the aggressiveness of the cancer cells.

KEY TERMS

Adjuvant therapy—A treatment done when there is no evidence of residual cancer in order to aid the primary treatment. Adjuvant treatments for endometrial cancer are radiation therapy, chemotherapy, and hormone therapy.

Atypical adenomatous hyperplasia—The overgrowth of the endometrium. This precancerous condition is estimated to progress to cancer in one third of the cases.

Dilation and curettage (D & C)—A procedure in which the doctor opens the cervix and uses a special instrument to scrape tissue from the inside of the uterus.

Endometrial biopsy—A procedure in which a sample of the endometrium is removed and examined under a microscope.

Endometrium—The mucosal layer lining the inner cavity of the uterus. The endometrium's structure changes with age and with the menstrual cycle.

Estrogen—A female hormone responsible for stimulating the development and maintenance of female secondary sexual characteristics.

Estrogen replacement therapy (ERT)—A treatment in which estrogen is used therapeutically during menopause to alleviate certain symptoms such as hot flashes. ERT has also been shown to reduce the risk of osteoporosis and heart disease in women.

Progesterone—A female hormone that acts on the inner lining of the uterus and prepares it for implantation of the fertilized egg.

Progestins—A female hormone, like progesterone, that acts on the inner lining of the uterus.

The FIGO stages for endometrial cancer are:

- Stage I. Cancer is limited to the uterus.
- Stage II. Cancer involves the uterus and cervix.
- Stage III. Cancer has spread out of the uterus but is restricted to the pelvic region.
- Stage IV. Cancer has spread to the bladder, bowel, or other distant locations.

Treatments

The mainstay of treatment for most stages of endometrial cancer is surgery. **Radiation therapy**, hormonal therapy, and **chemotherapy** are additional treatments (called adjuvant therapy). The necessity of adjuvant therapy is a controversial topic which should be discussed with the patient's treatment team.

SURGERY. Most women with endometrial cancer, except those with stage IV disease, are treated with hysterectomy. A simple hysterectomy involves the removal of the uterus. In a bilateral salpingo-oophorectomy with total hysterectomy, the ovaries, fallopian tubes, and uterus are removed. This may be necessary because endometrial cancer often spreads to the ovaries first. The lymph nodes in the pelvic region may also be biopsied or removed to check for **metastasis**. Hysterectomy is traditionally performed through an incision in the abdomen (laparotomy), however, endoscopic surgery (**laparoscopy**) with vaginal hysterectomy is also being used. Women with stage I disease may require no further treatment. However, those with higher grade disease will receive adjuvant therapy.

RADIATION THERAPY. The decision to use radiation therapy depends on the stage of the disease. Radiation therapy may be used before surgery (preoperatively) and/or after surgery (postoperatively). Radiation given from a machine that is outside the body is called external radiation therapy. Sometimes applicators containing radioactive compounds are placed inside the vagina or uterus. This is called internal radiation therapy or brachytherapy and requires hospitalization.

Side effects are common with radiation therapy. The skin in the treated area may become red and dry. **Fatigue**, upset stomach, **diarrhea**, and nausea are also common complaints. Radiation therapy in the pelvic area may cause the vagina to become narrow (vaginal stenosis), making intercourse painful. Premature menopause and some problems with urination may also occur.

CHEMOTHERAPY. Chemotherapy is usually reserved for women with stage IV or recurrent disease because this therapy is not a very effective treatment for endometrial cancer. The anticancer drugs are given by mouth or intravenously. Side effects include stomach upset, vomiting, appetite loss (**anorexia**), hair loss (**alopecia**), mouth or vaginal sores, fatigue, menstrual cycle changes, and premature menopause. There is also an increased chance of infections.

HORMONAL THERAPY. Hormonal therapy uses drugs like progesterone to slow the growth of endometrial cells. These drugs are usually available as pills. This therapy is usually reserved for women with advanced or recurrent disease. Side effects include fatigue, fluid retention, and appetite and weight changes.

Prognosis

Because it is possible to detect endometrial cancer early, the chances of curing it are excellent. The five year survival rates for endometrial cancer by stage are: 90%, stage I; 60%, stage II; 40%, stage III; and 5%, stage IV. Endometrial cancer most often spreads to the lungs, liver, bones, brain, vagina, and certain lymph nodes.

Alternative and complementary therapies

Although alternative and complementary therapies are used by many cancer patients, very few controlled studies on the effectiveness of such therapies exist. Mind-body techniques such as prayer, biofeedback, visualization, meditation, and yoga, have not shown any effect in reducing cancer but they can reduce stress and lessen some of the side effects of cancer treatments. Clinical studies of hydrazine sulfate found that it had no effect on cancer and even worsened the health and well-being of the study subjects. One clinical study of the drug amygdalin (Laetrile) found that it had no effect on cancer. Laetrile can be toxic and has caused deaths. Shark cartilage, although highly touted as an effective cancer treatment, is an improbable therapy that has not been the subject of clinical study.

The American Cancer Society has found that the "metabolic diets" pose serious risk to the patient. The effectiveness of the macrobiotic, Gerson, and Kelley diets and the Manner metabolic therapy has not been scientifically proven. The FDA was unable to substantiate the anti-cancer claims made about the popular Cancell treatment.

There is no evidence for the effectiveness of most over-the-counter herbal cancer remedies. Some herbals have shown an anticancer effect. As shown in clinical studies, Polysaccharide krestin, from the mushroom *Coriolus versicolor*, has significant effectiveness against cancer. In a small study, the green alga *Chlorella pyrenoidosa* has been shown to have anticancer activity. In a few small studies, evening primrose oil has shown some benefit in the treatment of cancer.

For more comprehensive information, the patient should consult the book on complementary and alternative medicine published by the American Cancer Society listed in the Resources section.

Coping with cancer treatment

The patient should consult her treatment team regarding any side effects or complications of treatment. Vaginal stenosis can be prevented and treated by vaginal dilators, gentle douching, and sexual intercourse. A water-soluble lubricant may be used to make sexual intercourse more comfortable. Many of the side effects of chemotherapy can be relieved by medications. Women should consult a psychotherapist and/or join a support group to deal with the emotional consequences of cancer and hysterectomy.

Clinical trials

Because endometrial cancer is a common type of cancer there are many studies underway to optimize its treatment. Women should consult with their treatment team to determine if they are candidates for any ongoing studies.

QUESTIONS TO ASK THE DOCTOR

- What type of cancer do I have?
- What stage of cancer do I have?
- What is the 5-year survival rate for women with this type of cancer?
- Has the cancer spread? What tests will be used to determine this?
- What are my treatment options?
- Is adjuvant therapy really necessary in my case?
- What are the risks and side effects of these treatments?
- What medications can I take to relieve treatment side effects?
- Are there any clinical studies underway that would be appropriate for me?
- What effective alternative or complementary treatments are available for this type of cancer?
- How debilitating is the treatment? Will I be able to continue working?
- How will the treatment affect my sexuality?
- Are there any restrictions regarding sexual activity?
- Are there any local support groups for endometrial cancer patients?
- What is the chance that the cancer will recur?
- Is there anything I can do to prevent recurrence?
- How often will I have follow-up examinations?

Prevention

Women (especially postmenopausal women) should report any abnormal vaginal bleeding or discharge to the doctor. Controlling obesity, blood pressure, and diabetes can help to reduce the risk of this disease. Women on estrogen replacement therapy have a substantially reduced risk of endometrial cancer if progestins are taken simultaneously. Long-term use of birth control pills has been shown to reduce the risk of this cancer. Women who have irregular periods may be prescribed birth control pills to help prevent endometrial cancer. Women who are taking tamoxifen and those who carry the hereditary non-polyposis colorectal cancer gene should be screened regularly, receiving annual pelvic examinations.

Special concerns

Of special concern to the young woman with endometrial cancer is the impact that a hysterectomy will have on her fertility, **sexuality**, and **body image**. **Depression** is common. Symptoms caused by the sudden onset of menopause, due to removal of the ovaries, can be more severe than with natural menopause. Estrogen replacement therapy is not commonly used due to the potential risk of cancer recurrence. Without estrogen replacement, osteoporosis becomes a concern and calcium supplements should be considered. Weight bearing exercise and alendronate (Fosamax) will also decrease the development rate of osteoporosis. Vaginal stenosis following radiation treatment is a concern.

Resources

BOOKS

Bruss, Katherine, Christina Salter, and Esmeralda Galan, eds. *American Cancer Society's Guide to Complementary and Alternative Cancer Methods.* Atlanta: American Cancer Society, 2000.

Burke, Thomas, Patricia Eifel, and Muggia Franco. "Cancers of the Uterine Body." In *Cancer: Principles & Practice of Oncology*, ed. Vincent DeVita, Samuel Hellman, and Steven Rosenberg. Philadelphia: Lippincott Williams & Wilkins, 2001, pp.1573– 86.

Long, Harry. "Carcinoma of the Endometrium." In *Current Therapy in Cancer*, ed. John Foley, Julie Vose, and James Armitage. Philadelphia: W. B. Saunders Company, 1999, pp.162–66.

Primack, Aron. "Complementary/Alternative Therapies in the Prevention and Treatment of Cancer." In *Complementary/Alternative Medicine: An Evidence-Based Approach*, ed. John Spencer and Joseph Jacobs. St. Louis: Mosby, 1999, pp.123–69.

PERIODICALS

Bristow, Robert. "Endometrial Cancer."*Current Opinion in Oncology* 11 (September 1999): 388– 393.

Canavan, Timothy and Nipa Doshi. "Endometrial Cancer." *American Family Physician* 59 (June 1999): 3069–3077.

Elit, Laurie. "Endometrial Cancer: Prevention, Detection, Management, and Follow up." *Canadian Family Physician* 46 (April 2000): 887–892.

Hogberg, Thomas, Margareta Fredstorp, and Anuja Jhingran. "Indications for Adjuvant Radiotherapy in Endometrial Carcinoma."*Hematology/Oncology Clinics of North America: Current Therapeutic Issues in Gynecologic Cancer* 13 (February 1999): 189– 209.

ORGANIZATIONS

American Cancer Society, National Headquarters. 1599 Clifton Rd. NE, Atlanta, GA 30329. (800) 227-2345. <http://www.cancer.org/>.

Cancer Research Institute, National Headquarters. 681 Fifth Ave., New York, NY 10022. (800) 992-2623. <http://www.cancerresearch.org>.

Gynecologic Cancer Foundation. 401 North Michigan Ave., Chicago, IL 60611. (800) 444-4441. <http://www.wcn.org>.

National Cancer Institute, National Institutes of Health. 9000 Rockville Pike, Bethesda, MD 20892. (800) 422-6237. <http://cancernet.nci.nih.gov/>.

OTHER

"Cancer of the Uterus."*Cancernet.* Dec. 2000. 13 Mar. 2001 <http://cancernet.nci.nih.gov/wyntk_pubs/uterus.htm>.

Lata Cherath, Ph.D.
Belinda Rowland, Ph.D.

Endorectal ultrasound

Definition

Ultrasound is a type of imaging technique that painlessly uses sound waves to produce an image of internal structures, organs, and masses. Endorectal ultrasound, also called transrectal ultrasound, is a special ultrasound technique in which the transducer is directly inserted through the anus and into the patient's rectum. The sound wave echoes detected by the transducer are converted by a computer into an image.

Purpose

Ultrasound technology has been used in medicine since World War II and is recognized as a non-invasive, non-radiative, real-time and inexpensive imaging capacity. It has become standard medical practice to produce fetal images and to identify and assess various anatomical features of the body.

Endorectal ultrasound is a specialized ultrasound application and it represents one of the most useful diagnostic tools for diseases of the anal and rectal regions of the body, especially for rectal, anal, and prostrate cancer screening and staging.

For **rectal cancer**, endorectal ultrasound is the most preferred method for staging both depth of tumor penetration and local lymph node metastatic status. Endorectal ultrasound:

- differentiates areas of invasion within large rectal adenomas that seem benign
- determines the depth of tumor penetration into the rectal wall
- determines the extent of regional lymph node invasion
- can be combined with other tests (chest x rays and **computed tomography** scans, or CT scans) to determine the extent of cancer spread to distant organs, such as the lungs or liver

The resulting rectal cancer staging allows physicians to determine the need for—and order of—radiation, surgery, and **chemotherapy**.

For patients diagnosed with **anal cancer**, endorectal ultrasound may help to stage the lesion and may be used as follow-up care to check for recurrence of cancer after treatment.

In the diagnosis of prostrate cancer, endorectal ultrasound has become a companion technique to **digital rectal examination** (DRE). It is also the most frequent method used to guide **biopsy** needle insertion. If surgery is indicated, endorectal ultrasound can also assist the preoperative evaluation of the depth of cancer penetration and of the presence of metastases, as required to design appropriate surgical procedures.

Endorectal ultrasounds can also be used to check the overall treatment results.

KEY TERMS

Anal—Pertaining to the anus, which is the terminal orifice of the digestive—or alimentary—canal.

Anatomy—Structure of the body and of the relationship between its parts.

Biopsy—Procedure that involves obtaining a tissue specimen for microscope analysis to establish a precise diagnosis.

Cancer screening—Examination of people to detect early stages in the development of cancer even though they have no symptoms.

Colon—Large intestine.

Digital rectal examination (DRE)—Examination performed by a physician to detect rectal cancer. The physician inserts a gloved, lubricated finger into the rectum of the patient and feels for abnormal areas.

Endorectal probe—Instrument which sends sound waves through the prostrate. Sound echoes are then recorded as an image.

Enema—Injection of a liquid into the rectum.

Metastasis—The transfer of cancer from one part of the body to another not directly connected with it.

Rectal—Pertaining to the rectum, which is the last portion of the large intestine.

Sonogram —A computer picture of areas inside the body created by bouncing sound waves off organs and other tissues. Also called ultrasonogram or ultrasound.

Precautions

This is a very easy procedure. Unlike other imaging techniques, it uses no radiation and thus requires no special precautions.

Description

The instrumentation used for endorectal ultrasound consists of a hand-held probe, the transrectal transducer, a scanner, and an imaging screen. During the procedure, high-frequency acoustical (sound) waves are sent out by the small microphone-like transducer, which is inserted into the rectum. The waves bounce off the organ being examined and produce echoes sent by the transducer to a computer so as to generate a picture called a sonogram. Doctors examine the sonogram for echoes that may represent abnormal areas.

Usually, the patient lies on his side during the test. An endorectal probe is covered with a protective covering and inserted into the patient. The probe looks like a small enema tip and there is a minimal amount of discomfort associated with the procedure itself. Once inserted, the sonographer or radiologist gently moves the probe forward and backward to best evaluate the organ being examined. An endorectal ultrasound generally takes five to ten minutes. After the procedure, the radiologist interprets the results and sends a report to the referring physician.

Preparation

The patient requires no anesthetic or sedation, but needs an enema about two hours before the test in order to provide a clean rectal wall through which to scan. The

> **QUESTIONS TO ASK THE DOCTOR**
>
> - How many endorectal ultrasounds will I have to undergo?
> - Are any other imaging tests indicated?
> - How will this test help you diagnose my cancer?

evening before the procedure, it is recommended that the patient eat a small dinner, drinking only clear liquids and avoiding coffee, tea, or soft drinks after dinner.

Aftercare

The patient should enjoy a good meal and remember to keep a follow-up appointment if scheduled. In some cases, there may be some bleeding from the rectum, though this usually settles within a few days. **Antibiotics** may be prescribed in some cases.

Risks

Multiple studies have shown that the sound waves used with ultrasound imaging are harmless and may be directed at patients with complete safety. However, some patients may develop infections following the procedure, which could require further treatment. These may cause shivering and **fever**. Any manifestation of such symptoms should be immediately reported to the treating physician. Generally speaking, the entire procedure is well tolerated and there is usually minimal bleeding afterwards.

Normal results

Normal sonograms produce images that have the correct shape of the organ or tissue examined by the procedure, meaning that it corresponds to the true anatomy.

Abnormal results

Abnormal sonograms produce images which highlight abnormal features of the organ being scanned. In a tumor is present, it will show up as a distinct contrast feature on the sonogram.

See Also Imaging studies

Resources

BOOKS

Bankman, I. *Handbook of Medical Imaging.* Academic Press, 2000

Bushong, S. C. *Diagnostic Ultrasound.* New York: McGraw-Hill & Co., 1999.

Edelstein, Peter, M.D. *Colon and Rectal Cancer.* New York: Wiley-Liss, 2000.

PERIODICALS

Gavioli, M., A. Bagni, I. Piccagli, S. Fundaro, G. Natalini. "Usefulness of endorectal ultrasound after preoperative radiotherapy in rectal cancer: comparison between sonographic and histopathologic changes." *Diseases of the Colon and Rectum* 43 (August 2000):1075-83.

Hsieh, J.-S., C.-J. Huang, J.-Y. Wang, T.-J. Huang. "Benefits of Endorectal Ultrasound for Management of Smooth-Muscle Tumor of the Rectum." *Diseases of the Colon and Rectum* 42 (August 1999):322-8

Ott, D. J. "EUS and rectal cancer staging." *American Journal of Gastroenterology* 93 (April 1998):659-60.

Saclarides, T. J. "Endorectal ultrasound." *Surgical Clinics of North America* 78 (April 1998):237-49.

Sudhanshu, G. et al. "Staging of prostate cancer using 3-dimensional transrectal ultrasound images: a pilot study." *Journal of Urology* 162 (1999):1318-1321.

van den Berg, J. C., J. P. van Heesewijk, H. W. van Es. "Malignant stromal tumour of the rectum: findings at endorectal ultrasound and MRI." *British Journal of Radiology* 73 (September 2000):1010-12.

Monique Laberge, Ph.D.

Endoscopic retrograde cholangiopancreatography

Definition

Endoscopic retrograde cholangiopancreatography (ERCP) is a technique in which a hollow tube called an endoscope is passed through the mouth and stomach to the duodenum (the first part of the small intestine). This procedure was developed to examine abnormalities of the bile ducts, pancreas, and gallbladder. It was developed during the late 1960s and is used today to diagnose and treat blockages of the bile and pancreatic ducts.

The term has three parts to its definition:

- "Endoscopic" refers to the use of an endoscope.
- "Retrograde" refers to the injection of dye up into the bile ducts in a direction opposing, or against, the normal flow of bile down the ducts.
- Cholangiopancreatography means visualization of the bile ducts (cholangio) and pancreas (pancreato).

Purpose

Until the 1970s, methods to visualize the bile ducts produced images that were of relatively poor quality and often misleading; in addition, the pancreatic duct could not be examined at all. Patients with symptoms related to the bile ducts or pancreatic ducts frequently needed surgery to diagnose and treat their conditions.

Using ERCP, physicians can obtain high-quality x rays of these structures and identify areas of narrowing (strictures), cancers, and gallstones. This procedure can help determine whether bile or pancreatic ducts are blocked; it also identifies where they are blocked along with the cause of the blockage. ERCP may then be used to relieve the blockage. For patients requiring surgery or additional procedures for treatment, ERCP outlines the anatomical changes for the surgeon.

Precautions

The most important precaution is that the examination should be performed by an experienced physician. The procedure is much more technically difficult than many other gastrointestinal endoscopic studies. Patients should seek physicians with experience performing ERCP. Patients should inform the physician about any allergies (including allergies to contrast dyes, iodine, or shellfish), medication use, and medical problems. Occasionally, patients may need to be admitted to the hospital after the procedure.

Description

After sedation, a specially adapted endoscope is passed through the mouth, through the stomach, then into the duodenum. The opening to ducts that empty from the liver and pancreas is identified, and a plastic tube or catheter is placed into the orifice (opening). Contrast dye is then injected into the ducts, and with the assistance of a radiologist, pictures are taken.

Preparation

The upper intestinal tract must be empty for the procedure, so patients should NOT eat or drink for at least 6 to 12 hours before the exam. Patients should ask the physician about taking their medications before the procedure.

Aftercare

Someone should be available to take the person home after the procedure and stay with them for a while; patients will not be able to drive themselves because they undergo sedation during this test. Pain or any other unusual symptoms should be reported to the physician.

Risks

ERCP-related complications can be broken down into those related to medications used during the procedure, the diagnostic part of the procedure, and those related to endoscopic therapy. The overall complication rate is 5% to 10%; most of those occur when diagnostic ERCP is combined with a therapeutic procedure. During the exam, the endoscopist can cut or stretch structures (such as the muscle leading to the bile duct) to treat the cause of the patient's symptoms. Although the use of sedatives carries a risk of decreasing cardiac and respiratory function, it is very difficult to perform these procedures without these drugs.

The major complications related to diagnostic ERCP are pancreatitis (inflammation of the pancreas) and cholangitis (inflammation of the bile ducts). Bacteremia (the passage of bacteria into the blood stream) and perforation (hole in the intestinal tract) are additional risks.

Normal results

Because certain standards have been set for the normal diameter or width of the pancreatic duct and bile ducts, measurements using x rays are taken to determine if the ducts are too large (dilated) or too narrow (strictured). The ducts and gallbladder should be free of stones or tumors.

Abnormal results

When areas in the pancreatic or bile ducts (including those in the liver) are too wide or too narrow compared with the standard, the test is considered abnormal. Once these findings are demonstrated using ERCP, symptoms are usually present; they generally do not change without

KEY TERMS

Endoscope, endoscopy—An endoscope used in the field of gastroenterology is a hollow, thin, flexible tube that uses a lens or miniature camera to view various areas of the gastrointestinal tract. When the procedure is performed to examine the bile ducts or pancreas, the organs are not viewed directly, but rather indirectly through the injection of contrast. The performance of an exam using an endoscope is referred to as endoscopy. Diagnosis through biopsies or other means and therapeutic procedures can also be done using these instruments.

Visualization—The process of making an internal organ visible. A radiopaque substance is introduced into the body, then an x-ray picture of the desired area is taken.

QUESTIONS TO ASK THE DOCTOR

- How soon will you know the results?
- Did you see any abnormalities?
- When can I resume any medications that were stopped?
- When can I resume normal activities?
- What future care will I need?

treatment. Stones, identified as opaque or solid structures within the ducts, are also considered abnormal. Masses or tumors may also be seen, but sometimes the diagnosis is made not by direct visualization of the tumor, but by indirect signs, such as a single narrowing of one of the ducts. Overall, ERCP has an excellent record in diagnosing these abnormalities.

Resources

BOOKS

Ostroff, James W., and Jeanne M. LaBerge. "Endoscopic and Radiologic Treatment of Biliary Disease." In *Sleisenger & Fordtran's Gastrointestinal and Liver Disease.* Edited by Mark Feldman, et al. Philadelphia: W.B. Saunders Company, 1997.

PERIODICALS

Aliperti, Giuseppe. "Complications Related to Diagnostic and Therapeutic Endoscopic Retrograde Cholangiopancreatography"*Gastrointestinal Endoscopy Clinics of North America* (April 1996): 379–407.

Baillie, John. "Treatment of Acute Biliary Pancreatitis."*New England Journal of Medicine* 336, no. 4 (1997): 286.

"Guidelines—The role of ERCP in diseases of the biliary tract and pancreas." *Gastrointestinal Endoscopy* 50, no. 6 (1999): 915-920.

OTHER

Endoscopic Retrograde Cholangiopancreatography. 21 June 2001 <http://www.asge.org>.

Measuring Procedural Skills. 21 June 2001 <http://www.acponline.org/journals/annals/15dec96/procskil.htm>.

Treatment of Acute Biliary Pancreatitis. 21 June 2001 <http://content.nejm.org>.

David S. Kaminstein

Endoscopic ultrasound *see* **Ultrasonography**

Enoxaparin *see* **Low molecular weight Heparin**

Enteritis

Description

Enteritis is an inflammation of the intestine; the term applies chiefly to the small intestine. In the context of cancer, enteritis is a functional disorder of the large and small bowel that occurs as a result of **radiation therapy** applied to the abdomen, pelvis, or rectum. It occurs at the onset of radiation therapy (acute radiation enteritis) and may also reappear after completion of the radiation treatment (chronic enteritis).

Causes

Radiation enteritis occurs because the large and small intestines are sensitive to all forms of ionizing radiation. Some areas of the gastrointestinal tract are more sensitive to radiation than others; the colon is more sensitive to the effects of radiation than the small intestine, for example. Although the probability of tumor control increases with the radiation therapy dose, so does the probability of damage to normal, healthy tissues. Since the doses required to destroy many tumors are very high, acute side effects to the intestines also occur, chief among which is enteritis. Thus, the majority of patients undergoing radiation to the abdomen, pelvis, or rectum will show signs of acute enteritis.

Symptoms of the disorder are observed during the first course of radiation treatment and take about eight weeks to become acute. Chronic radiation enteritis may also occur months to years after a patient has undergone a course of radiation therapy. The symptoms include colicky abdominal pain, bloody **diarrhea**, tenesmus, **weight loss**, **nausea and vomiting**, bowel obstruction and rectal bleeding, sometimes very severe.

Several factors influencing the occurrence and extent of radiation enteritis have been identified. They include the dose of radiation given to the patient, the size of the tumor being treated, the concomitant prescription of **chemotherapy** and the general state of the patient's health. For example, enteritis will be more severe in patients with a history of hypertension, diabetes or inadequate nutrition.

Treatments

Some symptoms of radiation enteritis are caused by an overgrowth of bacteria, and, in these cases, **antibiotics** may be prescribed. Patients who develop acute enteritis report nausea, vomiting, abdominal cramping, and diarrhea. Diarrhea impairs the digestive and absorptive functions of the gastrointestinal tract, resulting in malabsorption of fat, lactose, bile salts, and vitamin B12. Patients also complain about rectal pain and bleeding.

KEY TERMS

Acute—Medical condition which has a short and relatively severe course.

Chronic—Medical condition persisting over a long period of time.

Gastrointestinal tract—The gastrointestinal tract starts with the oral cavity (mouth) and proceeds to the esophagus, the stomach, the duodenum, the small intestine, the large intestine, the rectum and the anus.

Intestinal villi—Microscopic finger-like projections located on the lining of the small intestine which are responsible for the absorption of nutrients.

Ionizing radiation—Radiation sufficiently energetic so as to remove electrons from an atom. Examples are x rays, gamma rays, beta radiation (electrons) and alpha radiation (helium nuclei) as well as the radiation emitted by heavier elements. The higher the energy of ionizing radiation, the more likely the tissue or cell damage.

Lactose—The major sugar present in human and bovine milk.

Tenesmus —Painful straining to pass stool or to urinate.

Treatment of acute enteritis accordingly includes treating diarrhea, dehydration and abdominal and rectal pain or discomfort. Antidiarrheal drugs are usually prescribed, such as Kaopectate, Lomotil, Paregoric or Imodium. Additionally, bile salt–retaining drugs may also be indicated, such as cholestyramine. Bowel cramps may be alleviated with antispamodic drugs, such as Donnatal.

Approximately 5%–10% of patients having received radiation therapy for abdominal or pelvic cancers develop chronic enteritis. In some cases, surgery may be indicated. There is at present no agreement as to the proper timing and choice of surgical intervention in such cases. Surgery is thus only undertaken after careful assessment of individual patient conditions and health status.

Surgery may also be indicated for patients who have developed radiation enteritis–induced strictures. (Strictures are narrowing of passages or canals.)

Alternative and complementary therapies

An important complementary therapy is nutrition management. Another side effect of radiation is to destroy the intestinal villi, which impairs the body's capacity to absorb nutrients and also destroys enzymes required for digestion, such as lactase, required to digest milk and dairy products. Thus a lactose-free diet is often recommended.

Besides milk and dairy products, it is often recommended to avoid foods such as whole bran bread and cereals, nuts, seeds and coconuts, fried and greasy foods, fruit and some fruit juices (prune juice especially), uncooked vegetables, potato chips, pretzels, strong spices and herbs, chocolate, coffee, tea, alcohol and tobacco.

Recommended foods include fish, poultry, and cooked, broiled, or roasted meat, bananas, apple sauce, peeled apples, apple and grape juices, white bread, noodles, baked, boiled, or mashed potatoes, cooked vegetables such as asparagus tips, green and waxed beans, carrots, spinach, mild processed cheese, eggs, smooth peanut butter, buttermilk, yogurt and nutmeg.

Additionally, it is recommended to ingest food at room temperature and to drink plenty of water every day. Carbonated sodas should be allowed to lose their carbonation prior to drinking.

Monique Laberge, Ph.D.

Environmental factors in cancer development

Definition

Environment as a cause of cancer is a complex and often misunderstood topic. The term environment has several different meanings when referring to causation of cancer. Originally, the term "environmental cause of cancer" was used to refer to all cancers that were not caused by hereditary or inherited factors. This definition included all cancers caused by lifestyle practices such as diet and tobacco use, viruses, and many other causes. For purposes of clarification, the term "environment" has been further defined by adding the labels "personal environment" and "external environment" when referring to causes of cancer.

By this definition, causes of cancer related to an individual's personal environment includes lifestyle choices such as diet, use of tobacco, and other factors which may place the individual at high risk for the development of cancer. External environmental causes of cancer refer to factors in the environment such as environmental pollutants that increase risk for cancer. Up to 85%

of cancer is due to lifestyle choices made by individuals, which places them at higher risk for the development of cancer. For example, tobacco is directly related to more than 30% of cancer deaths. Considering more than half a million deaths per year are caused by tobacco alone, risk for cancer development due to external environmental factors pales in comparison.

Epidemiologists are scientists who research and identify factors which are common to cancer patients' histories and lifestyles, and then evaluate those factors within the context of current biological and disease causation theories. Eventually, evidence may persuade epidemiologists to conclude that one or more factors or characteristics shared by a study group "caused" a disease such as a type of cancer. The science of epidemiology enables researchers to determine causes of diseases such as specific types of cancer, and also to estimate or project numbers of deaths that can be attributed to the cause on an annual basis.

Personal environment/Lifestyle choices

Tobacco use

Tobacco is known as the one of the most potent carcinogens in humans. Tobacco causes more than 148,000 deaths each year in the form of various cancers such as lung, trachea, bronchus, larynx, pharynx, oral cavity, and esophagus. Other cancers linked to tobacco use include cancers of the pancreas, kidney, bladder, and cervix. Cigarette smoking is more common among men; however, because of the increase in the number of women who smoke, more women die from lung cancer each year than from **breast cancer**. The life span of an individual who smokes is shortened by an average of 12 years.

Diet and nutrition

According to the American Cancer Society, the single most important dietary intervention to lower risk for cancer is eating five or more servings of fruits and vegetables daily. Consuming a diet rich in plant sources provides phytochemicals that are non-nutritive substances in plants that possess health protective benefits. A diet rich in foods from plant sources reduces the risk for development of cancers of the gastrointestinal tract, respiratory tract, and colon. Increased consumption of fruits and vegetables is also associated with decreased risk for lung cancer.

Diets high in fat have been associated with increased risk for colon, rectal, prostate, and endometrial cancers. The association between high-fat diets and the development of breast cancer is much weaker. Specific recommendations are to replace high-fat foods with fruits and vegetables, eat smaller portions of high fat foods, and limit consumption of meats—especially those that are considered high fat. Foods from animal sources remain a staple in American diets. Consumption of meat, especially red meats such as beef, pork, and lamb, have been associated with increased risk of colon and **prostate cancer**.

Obesity is often the result of meat-based, high-fat diets. Obesity has been linked to cancers at several sites including colon and rectum, prostate, kidney, endometrium, as well as breast cancer in postmenopausal women.

Alcohol use

Drinking alcohol increases the risk of developing cancers of the mouth, esophagus, pharynx, larynx, and liver in men and women; and increases the risk of breast cancer in women. Cancer risk increases as the amount of alcohol consumed increases. An individual who both smokes and drinks alcohol greatly increases the risk of developing cancer when compared to either smoking or drinking alone.

Physical activity

Current recommendations related to physical exercise include engaging in moderate levels of activity for at least 30 minutes on most days of the week. Studies have revealed an association between physical activity and a reduced risk of the development of certain types of cancers, including colon, breast, and prostate cancer.

Radiation exposure

Only high frequency radiation such as ultraviolet (UV) radiation and ionizing radiation (IR) has been proven to cause cancer in humans. A source of UV radiation is sunlight. Prolonged exposure to UV radiation is the major cause of basal and squamous cell skin cancers. UV radiation is also a major cause of **melanoma**.

IR has cancer-causing capability, as proven by studies on atomic bomb survivors and other groups. Virtually any part of the body can by affected by IR, but the areas most affected are the bone marrow and the thyroid gland. IR is released in very low levels from diagnostic equipment such as medical and dental X-ray equipment. Much higher levels of IR are released from machines delivering **radiation therapy** to patients. Great precautions are taken not to expose patients or staff unnecessarily to the effects of IR.

Exposure to radon, a form of IR, can increase risk for lung cancer, especially among smokers. Radon is a naturally occurring radioactive gas formed by the decay of uranium in rocks and soil. The gas is odorless, colorless, tasteless and cannot be detected by sight. Radon seeps up through the ground and is released into the air. Radon gas exists at harmless levels outdoors. In areas where there is poor ventilation, such as underground mines, radon can accumulate to levels that pose a risk for the development of lung cancer. Radon causes cancer by emitting radioactive particles as it decays. These particles damage the lining of the lung when the radon is inhaled. Individuals at highest risk for the development of cancer from radon exposure include uranium miners and those individuals who live in well-insulated, tightly sealed homes built on uranium-rich soil. Testing for radon is the only way to determine if a home has elevated radon levels.

Reproductive and gynecologic factors

Lifestyle choices linked to breast cancer include diet, **alcohol consumption**, oral contraceptives, estrogen replacement therapy, postmenopausal obesity, and nulliparity (a woman who has never had a child). The relationship between dietary fats and breast cancer continues to be studied. Women who consume more than two alcoholic drinks per day are at higher risk. Oral contraceptive use has been linked to the development of breast cancer. Nulliparous women who began using oral contraceptives prior to the age of 18 years and continued uninterrupted use for more than eight years have a minimally increased risk. Risk related to use of estrogen replacement therapy seems to be most significant for those women who used hormone replacement therapy prior to 1958, who used replacement therapy for eight years or more, and for who also used oral contraceptives. Weight gain in early adulthood seems to increase risk for breast cancer, especially if the gain occurred in the third decade of life. The highest risk related to obesity and the development of breast cancer is in postmenopausal women.

Full-term pregnancy seems to exert a deterrent effect on the development of breast cancer. Women who become pregnant after the age of 30 years, or who never become pregnant, are at higher risk. Historically, lactation and breast-feeding have been recognized as protective mechanisms for breast cancer development. A correlation between the development of breast cancer and abortion has been documented in several studies conducted in the United States. A large study conducted in Denmark to investigate the correlation found no increased risk of breast cancer among women who had undergone abortions.

Precancerous and cancerous lesions of the cervix are associated with many personal risk factors, including a higher incidence in women who become sexually active prior to age 17, have many sex partners, and are multiparous (have borne at least one living child). An association has also been described between type of employment and increased **cervical cancer** mortality. Women with higher mortality rates include women once employed in farm work, manufacturing, personal services, or who worked as nurses' aides. Women who are infected with the human immunodeficiency virus (HIV) are at higher risk for the development of squamous intraepithelial lesions of the cervix. Cervical cancer is not often diagnosed in women who are nulliparous, those who are lifetime celibates, or who are lifetime monogamous (having sex with only one person).

KEY TERMS

Carcinogen—A cancer-causing agent.

Lactation—The process of synthesis and secretion of milk from the breasts for nourishment of an infant or child.

Mulitparous—A woman who has given birth to at least one child.

Nulliparous—A woman who has not given birth to a living infant.

Psychological stress

Stress is known to activate the body's endocrine or hormonal system which in turn causes changes in the immune system. There is no specific evidence that changes in the immune system caused by stress directly cause cancer. However, the relationship between stress and the development of breast cancer has been recently studied. Some studies report significantly higher rates of breast cancer in women who experienced stressful life events and losses in the years immediately preceding the diagnosis of breast cancer. Other studies do not support the association between stress and breast cancer development.

Cellular phone use

Studies in the United States and Denmark in 2000 and 2001 revealed there is no link between cellular telephone use and tumors of the brain, salivary gland, leukemia, or other cancers. The type of telephone, the duration of the cell phone use, or age of the phone user had no effect on cancer risk.

External environment

Chemicals and other substances

Exposure to certain chemicals, pesticides, and metals can increase an individual's risk for cancer. Carcinogens in this category include nickel, cadmium, vinyl chloride, and benzene. These carcinogens may act alone or in combination with another carcinogen, such as cigarette smoke, to increase risk for cancer.

Environmental tobacco smoke (secondhand smoke)

Environmental tobacco smoke (ETS) is a combination of two forms of smoke from tobacco products—sidestream smoke and mainstream smoke. Sidestream smoke is smoke released between puffs of a burning cigarette, cigar, or pipe. Mainstream smoke is the smoke that is exhaled by the smoker. Sidestream smoke contains essentially the same compounds as those in the mainstream smoke inhaled by the smoker. Tobacco smoke is known to contain at least 60 different carcinogens. Nonsmokers who are exposed to ETS absorb nicotine and other harmful compounds from the smoke. ETS can cause lung cancer in healthy adults who are nonsmokers and there is a 20% increased risk of lung cancer in nonsmokers exposed to ETS. ETS has been linked to other cancers, including cancers of the nasal cavity, cervix, breast, and bladder. In 1992, the U.S. Environmental Protection Agency classified ETS as a Group A carcinogen. Group A is reserved by the EPA to categorize only the most dangerous cancer-causing agents to humans.

Asbestos exposure

Asbestos is a group of minerals which occur naturally as strong, flexible fibers that can be separated into threads and then woven. Asbestos fibers cannot conduct electricity and are not affected by heat or chemicals. Because of these properties there have been many industrial applications of asbestos. Some of the applications include insulation, fireproofing, and absorption of sound. Serious health risks related to asbestos occur as a result of exposure to the dust that is formed when the fibers break into tiny particles. These asbestos particles can then be inhaled or swallowed. Exposure to asbestos can lead to lung, larynx, and gastrointestinal tract cancers, as well as to the rare cancer—**mesothelioma**. Individuals at highest risk include those with the combination of asbestos exposure and smoking. Smoking increases risk for lung cancer by 10 times more than for the nonsmoker also exposed to asbestos. Due to government regulations and public concerns about the health hazards from asbestos exposure, the use of asbestos in the United States has declined significantly. Workplace practices involving asbestos are highly regulated by industry and government to minimize worker exposure.

Electric and magnetic field (EMF) exposure

EMFs are emitted from devices that produce, transmit, or use electric power and arise from the motion of electrical charges. Examples of these devices include power lines, transmitters, and household products such as microwave ovens, electric blankets, televisions, and computers. EMFs are considered forms of nonionizing radiation. According to the National Cancer Institute (NCI), public concern has increased over the health effects of EMFs, particularly in relation to the risk of developing cancer in both children and adults exposed to EMFs. Numerous studies have been conducted in the past 15 years to evaluate risk of cancer from exposure to EMFs. As of 2001, the results have been inconsistent according to the NCI. One large NCI/Children's Cancer Group study sought to determine whether exposure to magnetic fields contributed to the development of acute lymphoblastic leukemia (ALL) in children under the age of 15 years. The results of this study revealed little evidence of a relationship between risk for ALL in children and exposure to magnetic fields.

Other studies focused on determining links between magnetic fields and central nervous system (CNS) tumors such as brain cancers continue to be actively researched. To date, expert panels that have reviewed the existing data have concluded that data are insufficient to support the conclusion that magnetic fields cause cancer.

Nuclear facility exposure

An NCI study published in 1991 concluded there was no general increased risk of death from cancer for people living in more than 100 U.S. counties containing, or closely adjacent to, nuclear facilities. A British survey of cancer mortality in areas around nuclear facilities in the United Kingdom did report an increase in deaths from childhood leukemia near some of the facilities. Other smaller surveys of cancer deaths around nuclear facilities in both countries yielded conflicting results.

See Also Cigarettes; Occupational exposures and cancer; Cancer prevention

Resources

BOOKS

Yarbro, J. W., "Carcinogenesis" In *Cancer Nursing Principles and Practice* edited by C. H. Yarbro, M. H. Frogge, M. Goodman, and S. L. Groenwald. Boston: Jones and Bartlett, 2000, pp.48-59.

Yupsa, S. H., and P. G. Shields. "Etiology of Cancer: Chemical Factors" In *Cancer: Principles and Practice of Oncology* edited by V. T. DeVita, S. Hellman, and S. A. Rosenberg. Philadelphia: Lippincott, 1997, pp.185-202.

PERIODICALS

Ballard-Barbash, R., M. R. Forman, and V. Kipnis. "Dietary Fat, Serum Estrogen Levels, and Breast Cancer Risk." *Journal of the National Cancer Institute* 91(1999): 492-494.

Franco, E. L., T. E. Rohan, and L. L. Villa. "Epidemiologic Evidence and Human Papillomavirus Infection as a Necessary Cause of Cervical Cancer." *Journal of the National Cancer Institute* 91(1999): 506-511.

Heath, C. W. "Electromagnetic Field Exposure and Cancer: A Review of Epidemiologic Evidence. " *A Cancer Journal for Clincians* 46 (1996): 29-44.

OTHER

"Lifestyle and Environmental Risk Factors for Breast Cancer." *The Komen Foundation* 2000, Breast Health. 22 April 2001, 1 July 2001 <http://www.breastcancerinfo.com/bhealth/html/environmental_risk_factors.html>

"Cancer." *CancerNet* 2000, National Cancer Institute. 22 April 2001, 1 July 2001 <http://www.cancernet.nci.nih.gov/wyntk_pubs/cancer.htm.>

"Environmental Factors and Cancer." *OncoLink* 1994-2001, The Trustees of the University of Pennsylvania. 3 April 2001, 1 July 2001 <http://www.oncolink.upenn.edu/causeprevent/environment.>

Melinda Granger Oberleitner, R.N., D.N.S.

Ependymoma

Definition

An ependymoma is a rare type of primary brain tumor that develops from the ependymal cells lining the ventricles of the brain and the central canal of the spinal cord. Ependymomas can be found anywhere in the brain or spine but are usually located in the main part of the brain, the cerebrum, and may spread from the brain to the spinal cord via the cerebrospinal fluid (CSF).

Description

Most brain tumors are named after the cells in which they are found, thus the name ependymoma for a tumor of ependymal cells. Ependymomas are classified as either supratentorial (located in the top part of the head) or infratentorial (located in the back of the head). In children, most ependymomas are of the infratentorial type and occur in or close to the fourth ventricle of the brain. Ependymomas may block the flow of cerebrospinal fluid out of the ventricles causing them to enlarge—a condition called hydrocephalus. Unlike other types of brain tumors, ependymomas as a rule do not spread into healthy brain tissue or outside the brain or spinal cord. As a result, it is often the case that they can be removed and cured by surgery, especially spinal cord ependymomas.

Demographics

Ependymomas are infrequent tumors, representing 2% to 8% of all brain tumors. However, ependymomas are the third most common brain tumor in childhood (5% to 10%) and are diagnosed in about 75 to 150 children each year in the United States. More than 50% of all ependymomas are diagnosed during childhood. In adults, ependymomas of the spine account for over half of all spinal tumors. The occurrence of ependymomas is equal among all races.

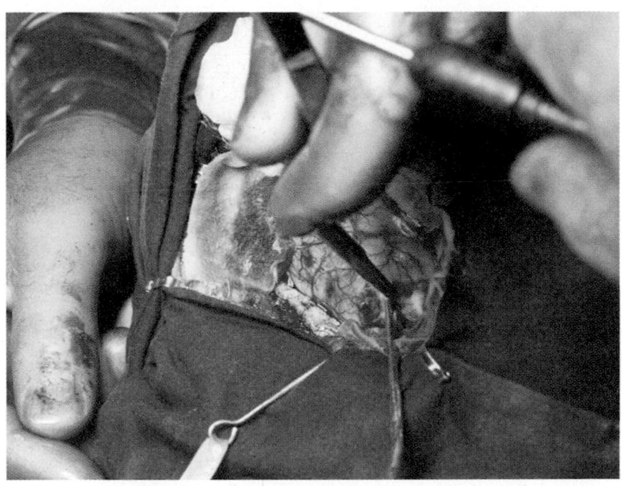

A brain surgery in progress. When possible, surgery is the first form of treatment for ependymoma. *(Custom Medical Stock Photo. Reproduced by permission.)*

Causes and symptoms

As is the case for most brain tumors, the cause of ependymoma is unknown. Ependymal cells usually grow in an orderly and controlled way, but if for some reason this process is disrupted, the cells continue to divide and form a tumor. Research is being carried out to identify possible contributing factors. Little is known, but researchers have begun to make progress in the areas of genetic, hereditary, and environmental causes.

The first symptoms of any type of brain tumor are usually due to increased pressure within the skull. This may be the result of a blockage in the ventricles of the brain causing a buildup of CSF or may be induced by swelling around the tumor itself. The increased pressure can cause headaches, vomiting and visual problems. Symptoms specific to ependymomas include swelling of the optic nerve, rapid and jerky eye movements, neck pain and irritability. Seizures, fits and personality changes are also general symptoms associated with a brain tumor. About 25% of children with ependymomas have seizures. Other ependymoma symptoms depend on which area of the brain is affected.

- If located in the frontal lobe of the brain, ependymomas may cause mood swings, personality changes, and paralysis on one side of the body.

KEY TERMS

Brain—One of the two parts of the central nervous system (CNS). It is responsible for the control of body activities and the interpretation of information obtained from the senses. The brain is the center of thoughts and emotions.

Brain ventricles—Four connected hollow cavities in the brain.

Central nervous system (CNS)—In humans, the CNS consists of the brain, cranial nerves, and spinal cord.

Cerebrospinal fluid (CSF)—A clear, colorless fluid that fills the ventricles of the brain and contains small quantities of glucose and proteins. It bathes the brain and spinal cord.

Cerebellum—Part of the brain responsible for somatic motor function, the control of muscle tone and maintenance of balance.

Cerebrum—Part of the brain where thought and higher functions reside.

Ependymal cells—These cells line the ventricles within the central part of the brain, and thus form part of the pathway through which cerebrospinal fluid travels.

Frontal lobe—Part of the brain responsible for higher thought processes.

Metatastis—The transfer of cancer from one location or organ to another one not directly related to it.

Metatastic brain cancer—Tumors that start in other organs and then spread to the brain.

Primary brain cancer—Cancers that start in the brain.

Parietal lobe—One of two brain hemispheres responsible for associative processes.

Spinal cord—Elongated part of the central nervous system of vertebrates that lies in the vertebral canal and from which the spinal nerves emerge.

Temporal lobe—Part of the brain located below the cerebrum and responsible for auditory (hearing) and receptive processes.

- If occurring on the temporal lobe of the brain, coordination, speech, and memory problems may result.
- If located on the parietal lobe of the brain, the condition may affect writing and related tasks.
- If located in the cerebellum, ependymomas may cause unsteady gait and problems with coordination and balance.

Diagnosis

To plan treatment, doctors need to find out as much as they can about the type, location, and size of the ependymoma. A number of diagnostic tests and examinations are scheduled. The first test is a neurological examination to evaluate any effect the tumor may have had on the nervous system. Every patient with ependymoma is usually subjected to diagnostic imaging of the spinal cord and brain. The most sensitive method available for evaluating spinal cord **metastasis** is spinal **magnetic resonance imaging** (MRI) performed with gadolinium, a contrast agent injected into the patient before the procedure. Other imaging studies—such as a CT scan—may also be performed to find the exact location and size of the ependymoma. To confirm the diagnosis, a **biopsy** will be perfomed and an ependymoma specimen will be examined under a microscope. Ependymomas sometimes spread from their original location through the CSF. An additional test called a myelogram may be done to check for this condition and to see if the tumor has spread to the spinal cord.

Treatment team

The primary physician will recommend one or more types of treatment based on the ependymoma diagnosis (size, location, type) and on the patient's medical history, age, and overall health. As a rule, the treatment team includes a neurosurgeon, a neurologist, a radiation oncologist and a medical oncologist.

Clinical staging, treatments, and prognosis

There is no formal staging system for ependymomas. They are divided into supratentorial and infratentorial tumors and treated accordingly. Treatment will proceed depending on a number of factors such as the patient's general health and age, the size and location of the ependymoma, and whether it has spread. Before any treatment is given for ependymoma, it will be important to reduce the pressure in the skull if this has occurred. If it is due to a buildup of CSF, a shunt may be inserted to drain off the excess fluid. Steroid drugs may also be prescribed to reduce swelling around the ependymoma.

When possible, surgery is the first form of treatment for ependymoma. The purpose of surgery is to remove as much of the tumor as possible without damaging the healthy brain tissue. However, it may not be possible to remove it entirely and follow-up treatment may be required. One approach is to prescribe repeated surgery in patients who still have ependymoma remaining after a first surgery and **radiation therapy**.

Radiation therapy, or the use of high-energy rays to destroy the cancer cells, is often used after surgery to destroy any remaining cancer cells. It may also be used alone to treat ependymomas that cannot be reached by surgery. Since ependymomas may spread to the spinal cord, radiation therapy is sometimes given to both the brain and spinal cord. Radiation oncologists are also using focal radiation techniques, meaning that they give a single large dose of radiation so as to kill residual cancer cells after regular radiation therapy in patients who have significant tumor tissue remaining after surgery.

Chemotherapy, or the use of anti-cancer drugs to destroy cancer cells, is another form of treatment indicated for ependymomas. It may be given alone or in conjunction with surgery and radiation therapy. Newer and improved chemotherapeutic drugs are now being used after surgery, with the goal of shrinking the ependymoma before radiation therapy.

Postoperative radiation therapy has definitely been shown to improve chances of recovery, but results of chemotherapy are considered somewhat disappointing. Age is also a factor in recovery. Usually, the younger the patient, the less favorable the prognosis. The best recoveries usually occur in patients who have no visible tumor after surgery.

Alternative and complementary therapies

In a search for less toxic therapies and improved quality of life, patients with primary brain tumors are increasingly considering complementary and alternative treatments. The American Brain Tumor Association provides a list of therapies such as acupuncture, antioxidant therapy, acupressure, meditation, etc. However, the association does not officially endorse any of them. The treatment team will be able to offer the best advice as to whether alternative and/or complementary treatments are indicated.

Coping with cancer treatment

Learning to live with ependymoma can be difficult for both patient and family. Several national associations exist to educate, support and advocate for families of children with cancer, survivors of childhood cancer, and the health professionals who care for them. These organizations offer contacts with peer-support groups and distribute a wealth of cancer-related brochures and publications.

Clinical trials

In 2001, the National Cancer Institute supported over 33 ependymoma **clinical trials** to evaluate a variety of new treatments. The National Cancer Institute monitors clinical trials and should be contacted for up-to-date information.

Prevention

A large, coordinated investigation recently carried out in Europe, Israel, and North America studied the factors that might affect the occurrence of primary brain tumors in infants and children under the age of 20. Conclusions were that women taking vitamin supplements containing C, A, E, and/or folate during the entire period of their pregnancy were half as likely to have their child develop a brain tumor before age 5, as compared to those who did not take **vitamins**.

Special concerns

Recurrence of an ependymoma is very dependent upon the extent of surgical removal as well as on the success of the treatment course following the initial diagnosis. Most recurrent ependymomas occur in the vicinity of the cavity from which the original tumor was surgically removed. Treatment options for an individual with a recurrent ependymoma usually include more surgery, chemotherapy, and further radiotherapy. An ependymoma can also metastasize into adjacent areas of the brain or, less commonly, to distant parts of the central nervous system. Approximately 12% of patients will have evidence of metastasis at the time of diagnosis. In these situations, more extensive treatment is used to treat the disease.

Children diagnosed with ependymomas are the object of special concern because of their vulnerability to radiation therapy. The organs in children are, generally speaking, significantly more sensitive to radiation than those of adults. Thus, radiation doses delivered to a child may have devastating side effects and must therefore be designed so as to address the issues of toxicity as well as that of treatment efficiency.

When the ependymoma causes blockage of CSF flow and leads to hydrocephalus, a special tubing called a ventriculo-peritoneal shunt (VP shunt) can be surgically implanted in the brain ventricles to drain the excess CSF into the abdomen. This procedure allows the fluid to

QUESTIONS TO ASK THE DOCTOR

- Where is the ependymoma located?
- What is the next step? Are more tests necessary
- What kinds of specialists should I seek out for treatment?
- What medication is necessary, and what is it for? What are the side-effects?
- Considering age and the extent of the ependymoma, what is the current prognosis?

bypass the tumor blockage and relieves the pain and symptoms of hydrocephalus.

See Also Imaging studies; Brain/Central nervous system tumors; Childhood cancers; Computed tomography; Spinal cord compression

Resources

BOOKS

Carachi, R.*Surgery of Childhood Tumors.*New York: Oxford University Press, 1999.

Greenberg, H. *Brain Tumors.* New York: Oxford University Press, 1999.

Poirer, J., et al.*Manual of Basic Neuropathology.* Philadelphia: W. Saunders & Co., 1990.

PERIODICALS

Smyth, M., B. Horn, C. Russo, and M. Berger. "Intracranial Ependymomas of Childhood: Current Management Strategies."*Pediatric Neurosurgery* 33 (September 2000): 138-50.

Verstegen, M. J., D. Bosch, and D. Troost. "Treatment of Ependymomas. Clinical and Non-clinical Factors Influencing Prognosis: a Review."*British Journal of Neurosurgery* 11 (December 1997): 542-53.

Duffau, H., M. Gazzaz, M. Kujas, and D. Fohanno. "Primary Intradural Extramedullary Ependymoma: Case Report and Review of the Literature."*Spine* 25 (August 2000): 1993-35

Ashby, L. S., E. A. Obbens, W. R. Shapiro. "Brain Tumors."*Cancer Chemotherapy and Biological Response Modification* 18 (1999): 498-549

ORGANIZATIONS

American Cancer Society. 1599 Clifton Road N.E., Atlanta, GA 30329. (800) 227-2345. <http://www.cancer.org>.

Cancer Research Institute. 681 Fifth Avenue, New York, NY 10022. (800)992-2623. <http://www.cancerresearch.org>.

American Brain Tumor Association. 2720 River Rd., Des Plaines, IL 60018. (800) 886-2282. <http://www.abta.org>.

National Cancer Institute's Cancer Information Service. (800) 4-CANCER.

Brain Surgery Information Center. <http://www.brain-surgery.com>.

Candlelighters Childhood Cancer Foundation. (800) 366-2223. <http://www.candlelighters.org>

OTHER

Dictionary for Brain Tumor Patients. ABTA Publication. 21 June 2001 <http://www131.rapidsite.net/abtaor/information/dictionary.htm>.

The National Cancer Institute Treatment Summary for Patients: Childhood Ependymoma. December 1999. 21 June 2001 <http://cancernet.nci.nih.gov>.

Monique Laberge, Ph.D.

Epirubicin

Definition

Epirubicin is a semi-synthetic anthracycline-based anticancer (or antineoplastic) drug derived from **doxorubicin**. It is also known by its trade name Ellence.

Purpose

Epirubicin is used as the **chemotherapy** agent for adjuvant therapy in patients diagnosed with **breast cancer**, and, as determined by the attending oncologist, epirubicin may be used in the treatment of lung, gastric, and pancreatic cancers.

Description

It has been used extensively since the mid-1980s for both early stage and metastatic breast cancer. Epirubicin received Federal Drug Administration approval in the fall of 1999 for adjuvant therapy in patients with node-positive breast cancer. Like other DNA- interactive antineoplastic family members, epirubicin binds to DNA to inhibit DNA, RNA, and protein synthesis resulting in cell death. It has been demonstrated that epirubicin also acts to block cell growth and to increase the production of cytotoxic free radicals. For breast cancer treatment, epirubicin has proved a highly effective chemotherapy agent when administered as a single agent in a sequential regimen. Epirubicin may be given in combination with **cyclophosphamide**, and 5-fluorouracil; however, currently there is no clinical evidence to suggest that long-term survival is greater in the combination regimen than with epirubicin alone. Indeed, the lower toxicity associated with epirubicin treatment promotes better quality of life for the patient.

Recommended dosage

Epirubicin is administered as a red fluid via intravenous injection (IV) into a cannula placed into the vein or through a central line inserted under the skin into a vein near the collarbone. The dose of epirubicin prescribed will vary among patients, correlated with patient body size, the purpose of the dose, whether the epirubicin will be used as a single agent or in combination, and the stage and aggressiveness of the cancer type. A starting dose of 50 $mg/m^2$of body surface per dose cycle of epirubicin is an appropriate regimen. Treatment cycles may be given weekly, or with higher doses, cycles may be reduced to only two to three times per month. The maximum cumulative dose for anthracyclines is defined by cardiotoxicity. Studies on epirubicin have only been conducted on adult patients; therefore, with the associated risk of cardiotoxicity there are no recommendations for dosage on young children or the elderly.

Precautions

To maximize treatment effects, patients receiving epirubicin should observe certain guidelines. Along with any specific modifications given by the oncologist, these guidelines should include monitoring the area surrounding the injection site, and regular laboratory testing for white blood cell count, and kidney, liver, and bone marrow function. In order to reduce the possibility of immunosupression, immunizations not approved or prescribed by the oncologist should be avoided. Avoid contact with individuals taking, or that have recently taken, oral polio vaccine or individuals that have an active infection. When necessary wear a protective facemask. Ask for specific instructions on oral hygiene procedures to reduce the risk of gum abrasion, and avoid touching the eye and nasal areas unless hands have been properly washed immediately prior to contact. To reduce bleeding and bruising complications, patients should exercise extreme caution when handling sharp instruments and decline participation in contact sports. The oncologist may suggest increased fluid intake to prevent kidney problems and to assure proper kidney function.

Prior to treatment, the patient's medical history should be thoroughly reviewed to avoid complications that might arise from previous conditions such as bone marrow depression; viral, fungal, or bacterial infection; heart, kidney disease, or liver disease; or tumor cell infiltration of bone marrow. The oncologist should also be made aware if the patient is pregnant, if there is the possibility the patient might be pregnant, or if the patient is a breast-feeding mother. Only prescribed medications or over the counter (OTC) drugs approved by the oncologist should be taken by a patient receiving epirubicin

KEY TERMS

Adjuvant therapy—Treatment that is prescribed to increase the effectiveness of a primary treatment.

Anthracycline—Drugs that have a characteristic four-ring structure that are linked, via a glycosidic bond, to daunosamine, an amino sugar, which are used in leukemia therapy to prevent cell division by disrupting the structure of the DNA.

Antineoplastic—Agents that inhibit or prevent the maturation and proliferation of malignant cells.

Cytotoxic—A term that refers to chemicals that are directly toxic to a cell, preventing the growth or reproduction of the cell.

Doxorubicin—An extremely effective anticancer drug isolated from the *Streptomyces peucetius* bacteria.

Free radicals—Highly reactive molecules that act as agents of tissue damage.

Oncologist—A physician who specializes in the diagnosis and treatment of cancer patients.

Side effects

Along with the desired anticancer effects from epirubicin treatment, less desirable side effects are to be anticipated. All presenting side effects should be discussed with the oncologist. Some side effects may occur that do not require medical attention, but nonetheless concern the patient. These commonly include hair loss (**alopecia**), lack of menstrual periods, discolored urine, **nausea and vomiting**, occasional **diarrhea**, hot flashes, and temporary decrease of bone marrow function. Less frequently, the patient may also experience loss of appetite with accompanying **weight loss**, darkening of the soles of the feet, palms, or nails, and cardiotoxicity. Most of these side effects disappear with the end of treatment or may be eased during treatment with prescribed intervention from the oncologist.

Other side effects from epirubicin treatment do require immediate attention from a healthcare professional. These indicators of potentially life-threatening conditions or medical overdose frequently include bleeding and brusing; the presence of ulcers, sores, or redness in the mouth, throat, or on the lips; a cough or hoarseness; pain or difficulty in urination; **fever** or chills; lower back or side pain; black tarry stools; redness or drainage from the eyes or eye-area; pinpoint red spots on the skin; and red streaks around the injected vein. More rare, but no less critical side effects may include wheezing or shortness of breath; joint pain; fast or irregular heartbeat; skin rash or **itching**; discoloration, redness, or warmth at the site of the injection; swelling in feet, legs, and abdomen; and tenderness of the abdomen or lymph nodes.

Interactions

Over 70 regularly prescribed drugs are known to have interactive effects with epirubicin. A complete and exhaustive list should be documented in the patient's history prior to treatment. In particular, the patient should be made aware of specific drugs that, when given concurrently with epirubicin, produce increased problems and risks in the following areas:

- liver problems
- blood disorders
- risk of infection
- risk of heart damage and heart failure
- extended clearance time of epirubicin from the body
- risk of secondary leukemia

Jane Taylor-Jones, Research Associate, M.S.

Epoietin alfa *see* **Erythropoietin**

Epstein-Barr virus

Definition

Epstein-Barr Virus, or EBV, is the name given to a member of the herpesvirus family that is associated with a variety of illnesses—from infectious mononucleosis (IM), to nasal-pharyngeal cancer, and **Burkitt's lymphoma**.

Description

Herpesviruses have long been known. The name actually comes from the Greek adjective *herpestes*, which means creeping. Many herpesvirus species appear to establish a life-long presence in the human body, remaining dormant for long periods and becoming active for some, often inexplicable, reason. EBV is only one of several members of the Herpesvirus family that have similar traits. Others include varicella zoster virus—the cause of both chickenpox and shingles—, and the **herpes simplex** virus responsible for both cold sores and genital herpes. EBV is usually transmitted through saliva but not blood, and is not normally an airborne infection.

EBV occurs in nearly all regions of the world, and is considered among the most common infectious viruses known to humankind. In the United States, the Center for Disease Control (CDC) estimates that 95% of adult Americans between the ages of 35 and 40 years have been infected, but it is less prevalent in children and teenagers. This pattern of infecting adults more than children persists throughout other prosperous western countries, but does not hold true in underdeveloped regions such as Africa and Asia. In Africa, most children have been infected by EBV by the age of three years

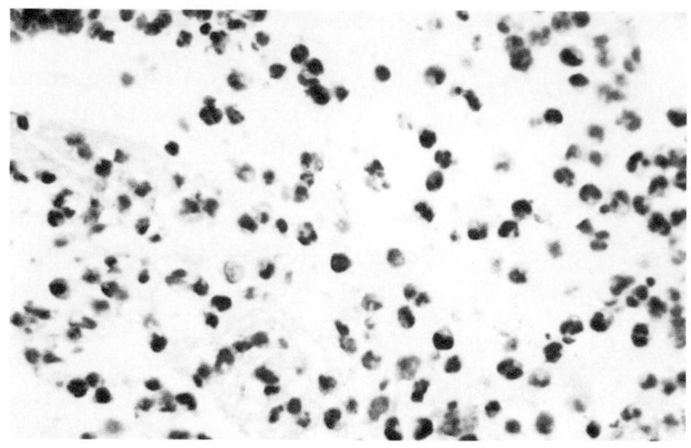

Epstein-Barr virus in situ. *(Custom Medical Stock Photo. Reproduced by permission.)*

Individuals with EBV infections typically show some elevation in the white blood cell count and a noticeable increase in lymphocytes—white blood cells associated with the **immune response** of the body. IM is a time-limited infection that usually lasts from one to two months. Symptoms include **fever**, malaise, sore throat, swollen glands and (sometimes) swollen spleen and/or liver. EBV infections that lead to Burkitt's lymphoma in Africa typically affect the jaw and mouth area, while the (very rare) incidences of Burkitt's lymphoma found in developed countries are more apt to manifest tumors in the abdominal region. **Nasopharyngeal cancer** is uncommon in the West but more prevalent in the Far East. It affects more men than women, and usually occurs between the ages of 40 and 50 years.

Causes

EBV has been linked to IM in the Western world for decades. It has also become associated consistently with nasopharyngeal cancers in Asia (especially China) and Burkitt's lymphoma in Africa and Papua New Guinea. According to the CDC, EBV is not the sole cause of these two malignancies, but does play an important role in the development of both cancers. The mechanism that allows Epstein-Barr Virus to at least help in producing such diverse illnesses in diverse regions of the world has been the subject of increasing research and scrutiny.

KEY TERMS

Lymphocyte—Any of a group of white blood cells of crucial importance to the immune system's production of a tailor-made defense against specific invading organisms.

Lymphoma—A group of cancers in which the cells of tissue usually found in the lymph nodes or spleen multiply abnormally.

Malaria—A serious disease prevalent in the tropics. It is caused by parasites and produces severe fever and sometimes complications affecting the kidneys, liver, brain, and blood. It is spread by the Anopheles mosquito and can be fatal.

Nasopharyngeal—Affecting the passage connecting the nasal cavity behind the nose to the top of the throat behind the soft palate.

It is known that, once it infects a person, EBV is one of the herpesviruses that remain in the human body for life. Under certain, still not-understood conditions, it alters white blood cells normally associated with the immune system, changing B lymphocytes (those normally associated with making antibodies), and causing them to reproduce rampantly. EBV can bind to these white blood cells to produce a solid mass made up of B lymphocytes—called Burkitt's lymphoma—or to the mucous membranes of the mouth and nose and cause nasopharyngeal cancer. Since Burkitt's lymphoma typically occurs in people living in moist, tropical climates, the same regions where people usually contract malaria, it has been speculated that the immune system is altered by its response to malaria. When EBV infection occurs, the altered immune system's reaction is the production of a tumor.

Special concerns

Though studies about the hereditary tendency of abnormal cell development after EBV infection are incomplete, some studies have shown it to be a hereditary trait based upon the X chromosome.

Treatments

Because EBV infections are viral in origin, **antibiotics** are ineffective against them. Much research is geared toward the development of a **vaccines** effective against both the virus and cancer.

Anticancer drugs, such as **cyclophosphamide**, or **radiation therapy** have been shown to be effective against Burkitt's lymphoma in four out of five cases.

QUESTIONS TO ASK THE DOCTOR

- What tests can be done if Epstein-Barr Virus infection is suspected?
- Have any vaccines against Epstein-Barr Virus been developed?

Alternative and complementary therapies

The goal of alternative treatment is to lower the white blood cell count to normal levels. Treatment often includes nutritional supplements such as flaxseed oil or shark cartilage, vitamins—including **vitamins** C and K, and mineral supplements containing magnesium and potassium. Well-conducted randomized **clinical trials** have not yet been conducted to prove efficacy of these therapies.

Resources

BOOKS

Clayman, Charles. *The American Medical Association Home Medical Encyclopedia* New York: Random House, 1989

Cotran, R. S., et al.*Robbins Pathologic Basis of Disease.* 5th ed. Philadelphia: W. B. Saunders, 1994.

Diamond, John W., W. Lee Cowden, and Burton Goldberg. *An Alternative Medicine Definitive Guide to Cancer* Puyallup, WA:: Future Medicine Publishing, Inc., 1997.

ORGANIZATIONS

Queensland Institute of Medical Research <http:www.web master@qimr.edu.au> 12/7/99

Center for Disease Control, National Center for Infectious Diseases *Epstein-Barr Virus and Infectious Mononucleosis* <http://www.cdc.gov.org> 3/26/01

Joan Schonbeck, R.N.

ERCP *see* **Endoscopic retrograde cholangiopancreatography**

ERCP stenting *see* **Stenting**

Erythropoietin

Definition

Erythropoietin, which is also referred to by the names Epogen, Procrit, erythropoietin alfa, and EPO, is a medicine used to treat a low red blood cell count.

Purpose

Erythropoietin is a drug approved by the Food and Drug Administration (FDA) to treat low red blood cell counts called **anemia**. This anemia can be caused by cancer **chemotherapy** treatment, kidney failure, or a drug used to treat AIDs. Erythropoietin has also been used to increase the red blood cell count in patients who are anemic and scheduled to have surgery. This can decrease the risk of needing blood transfusions.

Description

Erythropoietin is a natural substance made by the kidneys in the body. Sometimes the body cannot make enough erythropoietin to cause red blood cells to be produced. The synthetic drug erythropoietin can be given to act like the natural erythropoietin and increase red blood cells.

Chemotherapy drugs destroy cancer cells, but they also destroy normal cells in the bone marrow. Oxygen, which is need by the body to make energy, is carried to cells by the red blood cells. The destruction of the red blood cells causes anemia, which can make patients feel tired or dizzy.

Erythropoietin acts to stimulate the bone marrow to make more red blood cells. Patients need an adequate supply of iron in the body for erythropoietin to work best. If a patient's iron is low, the doctor may recommend oral iron tablets to keep the level of iron up. The increase in red blood cell levels should be seen in two to six weeks after beginning therapy in cancer-related anemia patients. When the red blood cell count rises, patients generally feel better.

Recommended dosage

Erythropoietin is a clear, colorless liquid that must be kept refrigerated. It is administered as an intravenous injection or an injection directly underneath the skin, referred to as a subcutaneous injection. There are several dosing schedules used to treat patients with anemia.

To treat cancer-related anemia

Erythropoietin is dosed in units per kilogram of body weight, starting at 150 units per kilograms of body weight administered three times per week. This dosage can be increased to 300 units per kilogram of body weight three times per week.

A common, but not FDA-approved, dosing schedule for cancer patients includes erythropoietin 10,000 units up to 60,000 units given as an injection under the skin once a week.

KEY TERMS

Anemia—A red blood cell count that is lower than normal.

Blood transfusion—The transfer of stored blood into a patient through a vein.

Chemotherapy—Specific drugs used to treat cancer.

Food and Drug Administration—A government agency that oversees public safety in relation to drugs and medical devices. The FDA gives approval to pharmaceutical companies for commercial marketing of their products

Intravenous—To enter the body through a vein.

Subcutaneous—Underneath the initial layer of skin.

Synthetic—Artificially made; not natural.

To treat patients with renal failure

Erythropoietin starting dose is 50-100 units per kilogram of body weight three times a week. This would be adjusted based on blood work and patient response.

To treat AIDS patients on the drug zidovudine

Erythropoietin starting dose is 100 units per kilogram of body weight three times per week for 8 weeks. This would be adjusted based on blood counts and patient response.

To treat patients prior to surgery

Erythropoietin starting dose is 300 units per kilogram of body weight per day for 10 days prior to surgery, the day of surgery, and four days after surgery.

An alternate schedule is erythropoietin 600 units per kilogram of body weight administered once weekly beginning three weeks before surgery, then a fourth dose on the day of surgery.

Surgery patients need to take iron replacement with the start of erythropoietin injections.

Precautions

Blood counts will be monitored before receiving erythropoietin and regularly while on the drug erythropoietin. This allows the doctor to determine if patients are candidates for this treatment and if the dose the patient is receiving needs to be increased or decreased.

Blood pressure should also be monitored regularly while on erythropoietin. Patients who have high blood pressure that is not under control should not use erythropoietin.

Patients may be instructed to take oral iron tablets while on erythropoietin to increase the drug's effectiveness.

It is not recommended to give erythropoietin to patients who have cancer, such as leukemias, arising from their bone marrow.

Patients with a known previous allergic reaction to erythropoietin or the drug albumin should tell their doctor.

Patients who may be pregnant or trying to become pregnant should tell their doctor before receiving erythropoietin.

Side effects

A common side effect due to erythropoietin administration is pain or burning at the site of the injection. This can be decreased by making sure that the erythropoietin is at room temperature before giving the infection. Ice can be placed in the area of injection to numb it before receiving the shot, and the site of injection should be changed with each shot.

Common side effects of patients that receive erythropoietin included **diarrhea** and swelling.

Less common side effects in cancer patients include **fever**, **nausea and vomiting**, **fatigue**, shortness of breath, and weakness.

Seizures have been reported in patients with kidney failure who are taking erythropoietin.

Erythropoietin can cause an increase in blood pressure, but this is uncommon in cancer patients. Blood pressure should be monitored while on this medicine.

Interactions

In clinical studies erythropoietin did not have any drug interactions.

In addition to taking oral iron replacement, patients should increase their intake of iron in their diet. This would include eating foods such as red meats, green vegetables, and eggs.

Patients should tell their doctors if they have a known allergic reaction to erythropoietin or any other medications or substances, such as foods and preservatives. Before taking any new medications, including nonprescription medications, **vitamins**, and herbal medications, the patients should notify their doctors.

Nancy J. Beaulieu, RPh.,BCOP

Esophageal cancer

Definition

Esophageal cancer is a malignancy that develops in tissues of the hollow, muscular canal (esophagus) along which food and liquid travel from the throat to the stomach.

Description

Esophageal cancer usually originates in the inner layers of the lining of the esophagus and grows outward. In time, the tumor can obstruct the passage of food and liquid, making swallowing painful and difficult. Since most patients are not diagnosed until the late stages of the disease, esophageal cancer is associated with poor quality of life and low survival rates.

Squamous cell **carcinoma** is the most common type of esophageal cancer, accounting for 95% of all esophageal cancers worldwide. The esophagus is normally lined with thin, flat squamous cells that resemble tiny roof shingles. Squamous cell carcinoma can develop at any point along the esophagus but is most common in the middle portion.

Adenocarcinoma has been increasing, and, among white males in the U.S., incidence of adenocarcinoma is almost equal to that of squamous cell carcinoma. Adenocarcinoma originates in glandular tissue not normally present in the lining of the esophagus. Before adenocarcinoma can develop, glandular cells must replace a section of squamous cells. This occurs in **Barrett's esophagus**, a precancerous condition in which chronic acid reflux from the stomach stimulates a transformation in cell type in the lower portion of the esophagus.

A very small fraction of esophageal cancers are melanomas, **sarcomas**, or lymphomas.

Demographics

There is great variability in the incidence of esophageal cancer with regard to geography, ethnicity, and gender. The overall incidence is increasing. About 13,000 new cases of esophageal cancer are diagnosed in the United States each year. During the same 12-month period, 12,000 people die of this disease. It strikes between five and ten North Americans per 100,000. In some areas of China the cancer is endemic.

Squamous cell carcinoma usually occurs in the sixth or seventh decade of life, with a greater incidence in African-Americans than in others. Adenocarcinoma develops earlier and is much more common in white

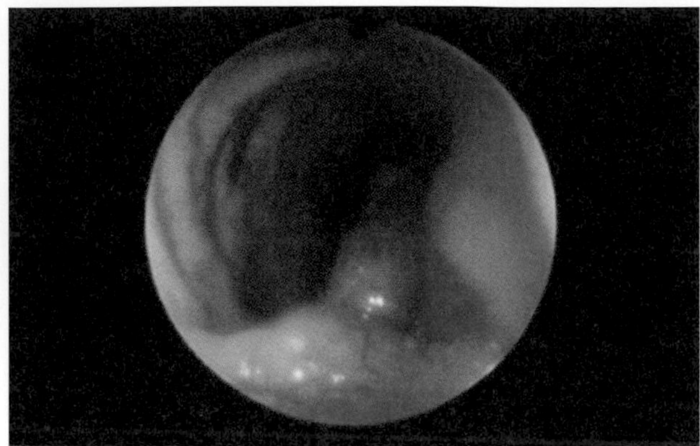

A close-up view of a cancerous esophageal tumor. *(© S. Benjamin. Custom Medical Stock Photo. Reproduced by permission.)*

patients. In general, esophageal cancer occurs more frequently in men than in women.

Causes and symptoms

Causes

The exact cause of esophageal cancer is unknown, although many investigators believe that chronic irritation of the esophagus is a major culprit. Most of the identified risk factors represent a form of chronic irritation. However, the wide variance in the distribution of esophageal cancer among different demographic groups raises the possibility that genetic factors also play a role.

Several risk factors are associated with esophageal cancer.

- Tobacco and **alcohol consumption** are the major risk factors, especially for squamous cell carcinoma. Smoking and alcohol abuse each increase the risk of squamous cell carcinoma by five-fold. The effects of the two are synergistic, in that the combination of smoking and alchohol increases the risk by 25- to 100- fold. It is estimated that drinking about 13 ounces of alcohol every day for an extended period of time raises the risk of developing esophageal cancer by 18%. That likelihood increases to 44% in individuals who also smoke one or two packs of **cigarettes** a day. Smokeless tobacco also increases the risk for esophageal cancer.
- Gastroesophageal reflux is a condition in which acid from the stomach refluxes backwards into the lower portion of the esophagus, sometimes causing symptoms of heartburn. In some cases of gastroesophageal reflux, the chronic exposure to acid causes the inner lining of the lower esophagus to change from squamous cells to glandular cells. This is called Barrett's esophagus. Patients with Barrett's esophagus are roughly 30 to 40 times more likely than the general population to develop adenocarcinoma of the esophagus.
- A diet low in fruits, vegetables, zinc, riboflavin, and other **vitamins** can increase risk of developing to esophageal cancer.
- Caustic injury to the esophagus inflicted by swallowing lye or other substances that damage esophageal cells can lead to the development of squamous cell esophageal cancer in later life.
- Achalasia is a condition in which the lower esophageal sphincter (muscle) cannot relax enough to let food pass into the stomach. Squamous cell esophageal cancer develops in about 6% of patients with achalasia.
- Tylosis is a rare inherited disease characterized by excess skin on the palms and soles. Affected patients have a much higher probability of developing esophageal cancer than the general population. They should have regular screenings to detect the disease in its early, most curable stages.
- Esophageal webs, which are protrusions of tissue into the esophagus, and diverticula, which are outpouchings of the wall of the esophagus, are associated with a higher incidence of esophageal cancer.

Symptoms

Unfortunately, symptoms generally don't appear until the tumor has grown so large that the patient cannot be cured. Dysphagia (trouble swallowing or a sensation of having food stuck in the throat or chest) is the most common symptom. Swallowing problems may occur occasionally at first, and patients often react by eating more slowly and chewing their food more carefully and, as the tumor grows, switching to soft foods or a liquid diet. Without treatment, the tumor will eventually prevent even liquid from passing into the stomach. A sensation of burning or slight mid-chest pressure is a rare, often-disregarded symptom of esophageal cancer. Painful swallowing is usually a symptom of a large tumor obstructing the opening of the esophagus. It can lead to regurgitation of food, **weight loss**, physical wasting, and malnutrition. Anyone who has trouble swallowing, loses a significant amount of weight without dieting, or cannot eat solid food because it is too painful to swallow should see a doctor.

Diagnosis

A barium swallow is usually the first test performed on a patient whose symptoms suggest esophageal cancer. After the patient swallows a small amount of barium, a series of x rays can highlight any bumps or flat raised areas on the normally smooth surface of the esophageal wall. It can also detect large, irregular areas that narrow the esophagus in patients with advanced cancer, but it cannot provide information about disease that has spread beyond the esophagus. A double contrast study is a barium swallow with air blown into the esophagus to improve the way the barium coats the esophageal lining. Endoscopy is a diagnostic procedure in which a thin lighted tube (endoscope) is passed through the mouth, down the throat, and into the esophagus. Cells that appear abnormal are removed for **biopsy**. Once a diagnosis of esophageal cancer has been confirmed through biopsy, staging tests are performed to determine whether the disease has spread (metastasized) to tissues or organs near the original tumor or in other parts of the body. These tests may include **computed tomography**, endoscopic ultrasound, **thoracoscopy**, **laparoscopy**, and **positron emission tomography**.

Treatment team

The treatment team includes the surgeon, radiologist, radiation therapist, and oncologist. Nutrition therapists are also vital in optimizing a diet that the patient can swallow easily.

Clinical staging, treatments, and prognosis

Staging

Stage 0 is the earliest stage of the disease. Cancer cells are confined to the innermost lining of the esophagus. Stage I esophageal cancer has spread slightly deeper, but still has not extended to nearby tissues, lymph nodes, or other organs. In Stage IIA, cancer has invaded the thick, muscular layer of the esophagus that propels food into the stomach and may involve connective tissue covering the outside of the esophagus. In Stage IIB, cancer has spread to lymph nodes near the esophagus and may have invaded deeper layers of esophageal tissue. Stage III esophageal cancer has spread to tissues or lymph nodes near the esophagus or to the trachea (windpipe) or other organs near the esophagus. Stage IV cancer has spread to distant organs like the liver, bones, and brain. Recurrent esophageal cancer is disease that develops in the esophagus or another part of the body after initial treatment.

Treatment

Treatment for esophageal cancer is determined by the stage of the disease and the patient's general health. The most important distinction to make is whether the cancer is curable. If the cancer is in the early stages, cure may be possible. If the cancer is advanced or if the patient will not tolerate major surgery, treatment is usually directed at palliation (relief of symptoms only) instead of cure.

KEY TERMS

Computed tomography—A radiology test by which images of cross-sectional planes of the body are obtained.

Endoscopic ultrasound—A radiology test utilizing high frequency sound waves, conducted via an endoscope.

Laparoscopy—Examination of the contents of the abdomen through a thin, lighted tube passed through a small incision.

Positron emission tomography—A radiology test by which images of cross-sectional planes of the body are obtained, utilizing the properties of the positron. The positron is a subatomic particle of equal mass to the electron, but of opposite charge.

Synergistic—The combined action of two or more processes is greater than the sum of each acting separately.

Thoracoscopy—Examination of the contents of the chest through a thin, lighted tube passed through a small incision.

SURGERY. The most common operations for the treatment of esophageal cancer are esophagectomy and esophagogastrectomy. Esophagectomy is the removal of the cancerous part of the esophagus and nearby lymph nodes. This procedure is performed only on patients with very early cancer that has not spread to the stomach. Esophagogastrectomy is the removal of the cancerous part of the esophagus, nearby lymph nodes, and the upper part of the stomach. The resected esophagus is replaced with the stomach or parts of intestine so the patient can swallow. These procedures can significantly relieve symptoms and improve the nutritional status of more than 80% of patients with dysphagia. Although surgery can cure some patients whose disease has not spread beyond the esophagus, but more than 75% of esophageal cancers have spread to other organs before being diagnosed. Less extensive surgical procedures can be used for palliation.

CHEMOTHERAPY. Oral or intravenous **chemotherapy** alone will not cure esophageal cancer, but pre-operative treatments can shrink tumors and increase the probability that cancer can be surgically eradicated. Palliative chemotherapy can relieve symptoms of advanced cancer but will not alter the outcome of the disease.

RADIATION. External beam or internal radiation, delivered by machine or implanted near cancer cells inside the body, is only rarely used as the primary form of treatment. Post-operative radiation is sometimes used to kill cancer cells that couldn't be surgically removed. Palliative radiation is effective in relieving dysphagia in patients who cannot be cured. However, radiation is most useful when combined with chemotherapy as either the definitive treatment or preoperative treatment.

Palliation

In addition to surgery, chemotherapy, and radiation, other palliative measures can provide symptomatic relief. Dilatation of the narrowed portion of the esophagus with soft tubes can provide short-term relief of dysphagia. Placement of a flexible, self-expanding stent within the narrowed portion is also useful in allowing more food intake.

Follow-up treatments

Regular barium swallows and other **imaging studies** are necessary to detect recurrence or spread of disease or new tumor development.

Prognosis

Since most patients are diagnosed when the cancer has spread to lymph nodes or other structures, the prognosis for esophageal cancer is poor. Generally, no more than half of all patients are candidates for curative treatment. Even if cure is attempted, the cancer can recur.

Alternative and complementary therapies

Photodynamic therapy (PDT) involves intravenously injecting a drug that is absorbed by cancer cells and kills them after they are exposed to specific laser beams. PDT can be used for palliation, but it also cured some early esophageal cancers during preliminary studies. Researchers are comparing its benefits with those of more established therapies.

Endoscopic laser therapy involves delivering short, powerful laser treatments to the tumor through an endoscope. It can improve dysphagia, but multiple treatments are required, and the benefit is seldom long-lasting.

Coping with cancer treatment

Many cancer patients have found it helpful to discuss cancer and treatment with other cancer patients and survivors in support groups. Guidance from a nutritionist may be helpful to maintain a balanced diet and to ensure that the patient is receiving adequate **nutritional support**. The hospital staff and treatment team may be valuable resources for locating support groups and other community resources.

Clinical trials

Researchers are searching more effective chemotherapeutic agents and radiation treatment regimens. Many studies are aimed at defining the most beneficial combination of surgery, chemotherapy, and radiation in the treatment of esophageal cancer.

Prevention

There is no known way to prevent esophageal cancer.

Resources

BOOKS

Heitmiller, Richard F., Arlene A. Forastiere, Lawrence R. Kleinberg. "Esophagus." In *Clinical Oncology*, edited by Martin D. Abeloff, second ed. New York: Churchill Livingstone, 2000, pp.1517–1539.

Zwischenberger, Joseph B., Scott K. Alpard, and Mark B. Orringer. "Esophageal Cancer." In *Sabiston Textbook of Surgery*, edited by Courtney Townsend Jr., 16th ed. Philadelphia: W.B. Saunders Company, 2001, pp.731–749.

ORGANIZATIONS

American Cancer Society. "Esophageal Cancer." <http://www3.cancer.org> 6 July 2001.

National Coalition for Cancer Survivorship. 1010 Wayne Avenue, 5th Floor, Suite 300, Silver Spring, MD 20910. Telephone: 1-888-650-9127.

Kevin O. Hwang, M.D.

Estramustine

Definition

Estramustine is a combination of two drugs, estradiol and **mechlorethamine**, that is used to slow growth and kill malignant cells in **prostate cancer**. It is also known by the brand names Emcyt and Estracyte.

Purpose

Estramustine is used in the palliative treatment of metastatic or progressive cancer of the prostate. Palliative treatment helps to relieve symptoms, but does not cure the cancer.

Description

Estramustine is classified as an antineoplastic drug. Estramustine is a combination of two drugs: estradiol, a potent female hormone (estrogen), and mechlorethamine, a nitrogen mustard. Its action is to decrease **testosterone**, increase estrogen level, and suppress cell growth. Estramustine is approved by the United States Food and Drug Administration (FDA) for the palliative treatment of metastatic or progressive cancer of the prostate.

Recommended dosage

As with many cancer-fighting drugs, the dose of estramustine a patient receives is individualized and depends on the patient's body weight and general health, as well as what other **chemotherapy** drugs are being used. A standard dose of estramustine is 14 mg per kg of body weight per day, divided into three or four doses. This is equivalent to one 140 mg capsule for each 22 lbs (10 kg) of body weight. It takes one to three months for estramustine to start to work. The therapy is continued as long as the patient has a favorable response. Some patients have successfully taken this drug for as long as three years.

Precautions

Estramustine should not be used by men who have a history of problems with blood clots, a blood clotting disorder, or allergic reactions to estrogen or nitrogen mustard.

Estramustine must be taken more than one hour before or more than two hours after meals. It should not be taken with dairy products, calcium supplements, of any food that is high in calcium.

Patients taking estramustine should avoid having any vaccinations while taking the drug, and should consult their doctor immediately if exposed to chicken pox or measles, as this drug may make them more susceptible to these diseases.

Side effects

Nausea and vomiting can occur within 2 hours of taking estramustine. This side effect is mild and patients will respond to **antiemetics** to control the nausea and vomiting. **Diarrhea** and flatulence can occur while taking this drug. Patients taking estramustine also have an increased risk of developing blood clots, congestive heart failure, and heart attacks, although these side effects are rare. Therefore, men with a history of blood clots and heart disease require frequent monitoring while receiving this drug. Estramustine also decreases the glucose (sugar) tolerance in people with diabetes, and frequent blood sugar monitoring is recommended in this patient population. Blood pressure may also be increased with estramustine, and monitoring of blood pressure is recommended, especially in patients with a history of high blood pressure. Men receiving estramustine may also experience enlargement of their breasts due to the estrogen component in the drug combination. Patients may also experience decreased sexual drive, although this side effect is reversible. If sexually active, the patient should use a contraceptive method (even if he is impotent) prior to initiating therapy, because estramustine may reverse impotency while on the drug. Estramustine may also cause genetic mutations. Therefore, use of contraceptive measures is advisable. Other side effects include lethargy, rash, **itching**, dry skin, easy bruising, flushing, and thinning hair. If any of the above side effects occur, patients should alert their physician to these side effects immdediately.

Serious side effects that require immediate medical attention include:

- sudden or severe headaches
- sudden shortness of breath or difficulty breathing
- increased weight gain or swelling of the feet or legs
- pain in the chest
- sudden pain or cramping in the legs or calves
- weakness or numbness in the legs or arms

Interactions

Dairy products and other foods containing calcium interfere with the absorption of estramustine. Prior to treatment, patients should notify their physician about any medications they are taking and of any known allergies.

Tish Davidson, A.M.

KEY TERMS

Malignant—Cancerous. Cells tend to reproduce without normal controls on growth and form tumors or invade other tissues.

Metastatic—Spreading of cells from the original site of the cancer to other parts of the body where secondary tumors are formed.

Etidronate *see* **Bisphosphonates**

Etoposide

Definition

Etoposide is a **chemotherapy** medicine used to treat cancer by destroying cancerous cells. Etoposide is also known as the brand name VePesid.

Purpose

Etoposide is approved by the Food and Drug Administration (FDA) to treat refractory **testicular cancer** and small cell lung cancer. It has also been useful for other types of cancer, including non-small cell cancer, leukemia (**acute myelocytic leukemia**), Hodgkin's and non-Hodgkin's **lymphoma**, muscle, brain tumors, bladder, stomach, **Kaposi's sarcoma**, **Ewing's sarcoma**, **Wilms' tumor**, **multiple myeloma**, hepatoma, uterine carcinoma, myeloblastoma, **mycosis fungoides**, **neuroblastoma**, and **prostate cancer**.

Description

Etoposide is a clear liquid for infusion into a vein and it is also available as a pink capsule form to be taken by mouth. It may also be referred to as VP-16, VP-16-213, and epipodophyllotoxin. Etopophos is a different formulation of the intravenous form of etoposide. Etoposide was originally derived from a plant and has been made for longer than 20 years. Etoposide is a member of the group of chemotherapy drugs known as topoisomerase II inhibitors. Topoisomerase II inhibitors cause breaks in the genetic material (DNA) inside the cancer cells and prevent them from further dividing and multiplying. Then the cells die.

Recommended dosage

An etoposide dose can be determined using a mathematical calculation that measures a person's body surface area (BSA). This number is dependent upon a patient's height and weight. The larger the person, the greater the body surface area. BSA is measured in the units known as square meter (m^2). The body surface area is calculated and then multiplied by the drug dosage in milligrams per square meter (mg/m^2). This calculates the actual dose a patient is to receive.

To treat refractory testicular cancer

Etoposide injection dosed at the range of 50–100 mg per square meter per day given into a vein over 30–60 minutes daily for 5 consecutive days, every 3–4 weeks. This is done in combination with other chemotherapy drugs, **cisplatin** and **bleomycin**.

Etoposide can also be dosed at 100 mg per square meter per day injected into a vein over 30–60 minutes on day 1, day 3, and day 5.

To treat lung cancer

Etoposide injection dosed at the range of 35 mg per square meter per day is given into a vein infused over 30–60 minutes for 4 consecutive days. It is dosed up to 50 mg per square meter per day given into a vein infused over 30–60 minutes for 5 days in a row. This is usually in combination with other chemotherapy drugs such as cisplatin or **carboplatin**.

Etoposide phosphate formulation is dosed the same as etoposide, but administered over a shorter period of time. The formulation is often used in transplant patients because it does not need to be mixed in large amounts of intravenous fluid and can be administered over less than 30 minutes, unlike regular etoposide.

Oral etoposide 50mg capsules for lung cancer are dosed by doubling the intravenous dose and rounding the number to the nearest 50 mg.

Patients with kidneys problems may receive smaller doses of etoposide than patients with kidneys that are normal. The doctor will monitor a patient's kidney function prior to therapy by checking certain blood counts. Patients with liver abnormalities may also need dose adjustments of the etoposide.

Precautions

Blood counts will be monitored regularly while on etoposide therapy. During a certain time period after receiving etoposide, there is an increased risk of getting infections. Caution should be taken to avoid unnecessary exposure to crowds and people with infections.

Patients with a known previous allergic reaction to chemotherapy drugs should tell their doctor.

Patients who may be pregnant or are trying to become pregnant should tell their doctor before receiving etoposide. Chemotherapy can cause men and women to be sterile, or unable to have children.

Patients should check with their doctors before receiving live virus **vaccines** while on chemotherapy.

Side effects

The most common side effect from etoposide is low blood counts (**myelosuppression**). When the white blood cell count is low (**neutropenia**), patients are at an increased risk for developing a **fever** and infections. Etoposide also causes the platelet count to fall. Platelets are blood cells in the body that allow for the formation of clots. When the platelet count is low, patients are at an increased risk for bruising and bleeding. Low red blood cell counts (**anemia**), may also occur due to etoposide administration. Low red counts may make patients feel tired, dizzy, and lacking in energy.

Etoposide infusions, if given too quickly into the vein, can cause a significant drop in blood pressure. This

KEY TERMS

Anemia—A red blood cell count that is lower than normal.

Chemotherapy—Specific drugs used to treat cancer.

Deoxynucleic acid (DNA)—Genetic material inside of cells that carries the information to make proteins that are necessary to run the cells and keep the body functioning smoothly.

Food and Drug Administration (FDA)—The government agency that oversees public safety in relation to drugs and medical devices, and gives the approval to pharmaceutical companies for commercial marketing of their products.

Intravenous—To enter the body through a vein.

Neutropenia—A white blood cell count that is lower than normal.

Refractory cancer—Cancer that is not responding to treatment.

can usually be avoided by administering the etoposide over a time period of at least 30–60 minutes. A patient's blood pressure may be taken when receiving an etoposide infusion.

Etoposide can cause mild to moderate **nausea and vomiting**. This is more common in patients taking the oral capsules. Patients will be given **antiemetics** before receiving etoposide to help prevent or decrease this side effect. Hair loss (**alopecia**) is common with etoposide administration. **Diarrhea**, loss of appetite (**anorexia**) and mouth sores are less common but have been reported to occur.

Liver problems may occur due to etoposide administration, though they are mild. The liver returns to normal when the drug is stopped. This side effect is more common with higher etoposide doses.

Less common neurological side effects caused by etoposide include tingling and numbness of the fingers and toes, dizziness, headache, sleepiness, visual disturbances, and confusion.

Other less common side effects caused by etoposide include rash, **itching**, sores in the mouth, darkening skin, fever, development of another type of cancer or leukemia, redness and pain at the site of injection into the vein, and irregular heart rate.

Rare side effects from using etoposide are allergic, or anaphylactic-type, reactions, which include fever, chills, tongue swelling, shortness of breath, low blood pressure, and increased heart rate.

Interactions

Etoposide, if given with the oral drug **warfarin** (also known as coumadin), can increase bleeding.

Nancy J. Beaulieu, R.Ph., B.C.O.P.

Ewing's sarcoma

Definition

Ewing's sarcoma is a cancer that affects children, teens, and less often, young adults. It begins in developing bone cells. Ewing's sarcoma cells grow uncontrollably and form masses or lumps called tumors. They can start in any bone in the body but about half of all cases involve flat bones such as the pelvic bones and the long bones in the leg—the tibia, fibula, and femur.

Description

Ewing's sarcoma is the second most common bone tumor among children and teens. It accounts for about 1% of all **childhood cancers**. This cancer is named for James Ewing, the researcher who first described the tumor in 1921. There are some rare cases of Ewing's sarcoma that do not begin in bones. These tumors are thought to start in nerve or other soft tissues.

Demographics

Ewing's sarcoma occurs most frequently in children ages 11 to 15 years old. Slightly more males than females develop Ewing's sarcomas, and like **osteosarcoma**, the most common bone cancer found in children, it is more often diagnosed in taller teens. The disease is rarely diagnosed in children younger than 5 or adults older than 30. It affects primarily Caucasians, and rarely occurs in African Americans and native Chinese.

Causes and symptoms

The causes of Ewing's sarcoma are not known. It is possible that certain inherited conditions increase the risk of developing this cancer.

About two–thirds of patients with Ewing's sarcoma have a painful swelling or lump that can be felt in the affected bone. Along with tenderness, the area of

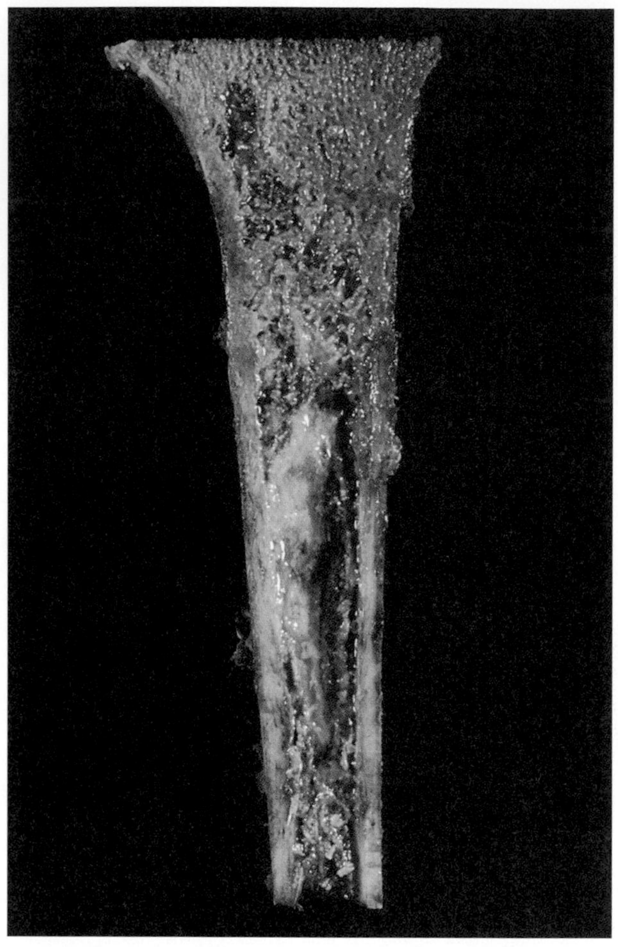

A femur of a patient diagnosed with Ewing's sarcoma. Ewing's sarcoma is the second most common bone tumor among children and teens, and half of all cases involve flat or long bones, such as the femur. *(Custom Medical Stock Photo. Reproduced by permission.)*

swelling may be hot. The symptoms depend on the site of the tumor and whether it has spread. For example, a tumor on a rib may cause painful breathing. When Ewing's sarcoma has spread, patients may have other symptoms such as **fatigue**, **weight loss**, and **fever**.

Diagnosis

Most patients who have Ewing's sarcomas go to the doctor because they have discovered a lump or mass or swelling on or near a bone. Others have symptoms related to the part of the body that is affected by the tumor, such as pressure on the bladder from a tumor on a pelvic bone.

The patient's doctor will take a detailed medical history to find out about the symptoms. The history is followed by a complete physical examination with special attention to the suspicious symptom or body part.

Depending on the location of the tumor (mass or lump), the doctor will order **imaging studies** such as **x ray**, **computed tomography** (CT) scans and **magnetic resonance imaging** (MRI) to help determine the size, shape and exact location of the tumor. The doctor will also order a chest x ray to find out if the tumor has spread to the lungs, and bone scans to determine if the tumor has spread to bones. Blood tests will be done and an examination of the bone marrow will be performed to see if the marrow is involved.

A **biopsy** of the tumor is necessary to make a diagnosis of Ewing's sarcoma. During a biopsy, some tissue from the tumor is removed. The tissue sample is examined by a pathologist, a doctor who specializes in the study of diseased tissue.

Types of biopsy

The type of biopsy done depends on the location of the tumor. For some small tumors, such as those on the arm or leg, the doctor may perform an excisional biopsy, removing the entire tumor and a margin of surrounding normal tissue. Most often, the doctor will perform an incisional biopsy, a procedure that involves cutting out only a piece of the tumor. This biopsy provides a core of tissue from the tumor that is used to confirm the diagnosis of Ewing's sarcoma.

Treatment team

Like other cancer patients, teens and young adults with Ewing's sarcoma are usually cared for by a multidisciplinary team of health professionals. The patient's pediatrician, family physician, or primary care doctor may refer the patient to other physician specialists, such as surgeons and oncologists (doctors who specialize in cancer medicine). Radiologic technicians perform x ray, CT and MRI scans and nurses and laboratory technicians may obtain samples of blood, urine and other laboratory tests.

Before and after any surgical procedures, including biopsies, specially trained nurses will explain the procedures and help to prepare patients and families. Depending on the tumor location and treatment plan, patients may also benefit from rehabilitation therapy with physical therapists and nutritional counseling from dieticians.

Clinical staging, treatments, and prognosis

Staging

The purpose of staging a tumor is to determine how far it has advanced. This is important because treatment varies depending on the stage. Generally, stage is determined by the size of the tumor, whether the tumor has spread to nearby lymph nodes, whether the tumor has spread elsewhere in the body, and what the cells look like under the microscope.

There is no commonly accepted system for staging Ewing's sarcomas. As is the case with other cancers, patients with metastases (spread) tend to have worse outlooks than patients whose tumors have not spread.

Between one quarter to one third of patients with Ewing's sarcoma have metastases when they are first diagnosed. Patients with tumors closer to the trunk of the body or in the pelvic bones are more likely to have metastases than patients with tumors located on the lower leg or foot. The most common sites for spread of Ewing's sarcoma are to the lungs or bones.

Treatment

Treatment for Ewing's sarcoma varies depending on the location of the tumor, its size and grade, and the extent of its spread. For most patients, the goals of treatment are to remove or control the tumor and combat the spread of the cancer.

Generally, when removing the tumor will not sharply reduce function, Ewing's sarcoma tumors are surgically removed. The goal of removing as much tumor as possible is to reduce the amount of radiation needed after surgery. The part of the body where the tumor was removed is treated with radiation to destroy remaining tumor cells. Most patients also receive **chemotherapy**, powerful anti–cancer drugs to destroy remaining cancer cells.

When the disease has spread throughout the body, there may be no benefit from surgical removal of the tumor. These patients, who have widespread metastases, are treated with radiation and chemotherapy.

SIDE EFFECTS. The surgical treatment of Ewing's sarcoma carries risks related to the surgical site, such as loss of function resulting from loss of a long bone in the leg. There also are the medical risks associated with any surgical procedure, such as reactions to general anesthesia or infection after surgery.

The side effects of **radiation therapy** depend on the site being radiated. Radiation therapy can produce side effects such as fatigue, skin rashes, nausea and **diarrhea**. Most of the side effects lessen or disappear completely after the radiation therapy has been completed.

The side effects of chemotherapy vary depending on the medication, or combination of anticancer drugs, used. Chemotherapy drugs often given to combat Ewing's sarcoma are **cyclophosphamide**, **doxorubicin**, **vincristine**, and **dactinomycin**.

KEY TERMS

Biopsy—The surgical removal and microscopic examination of living tissue for diagnostic purposes.

Chemotherapy—Treatment of cancer with synthetic drugs that destroy the tumor either by inhibiting the growth of cancerous cells or by killing them.

Metastasize—The spread of cancer cells from a primary site to distant parts of the body.

Oncologist—A doctor who specializes in cancer medicine.

Pathologist—A doctor who specializes in the diagnosis of disease by studying cells and tissues under a microscope.

Radiation therapy—Treatment using high energy radiation from x–ray machines, cobalt, radium, or other sources.

Stage—A term used to describe the size and extent of spread of cancer.

For patients with widespread disease, chemotherapy may be given along with bone marrow transplant and radiation to the entire body. **Nausea and vomiting**, **anemia**, lower resistance to infection, and hair loss (**alopecia**) are common side effects of chemotherapy. Medication may be given to reduce the unpleasant side effects of chemotherapy.

Alternative and complementary therapies

Many patients find that alternative and complementary therapies help to reduce the stress associated with illness, improve immune function and feel better. While there is no evidence that these therapies specifically combat disease, activities such as biofeedback, relaxation, therapeutic touch, massage therapy and guided imagery have been reported to enhance well–being.

Prognosis

The outlook for patients with Ewing's sarcoma varies, depending on the size and volume of the tumor, its stage, and the extent of its spread. Patients with large tumors do not fare as well as those with smaller tumors. Patients with tumors in certain sites, such as the bones of the pelvis and spinal column also seem to have poor outlooks because by the time these tumors are discovered they have already spread.

Ewing's sarcoma may spread locally to areas near the tumor and it can spread to nearby lymph glands. To

QUESTIONS TO ASK THE DOCTOR

- How big is the tumor?
- Has the Ewing's sarcoma spread?
- What are the recommended treatments?
- What are the side effects of the recommended treatments?
- Is treatment expected to cure the disease or only to prolong life?

spread to distant parts of the body, the cancer cells travel in the blood, bone marrow or through the lymph glands. In general, tumors that have spread widely throughout the body are not associated with favorable survival rates.

Nearly three quarters of patients diagnosed before the cancer has spread are disease free for five years after treatment. Patients with tumors that do not respond to treatment and those who suffer recurrences have poor outlooks for long–term survival.

Coping with cancer treatment

Teens undergoing cancer treatment have special needs. The diagnosis of a life–threatening illness, surgery and radiation or chemotherapy may cause fear, anxiety, **depression** and loss of self–esteem. Disruption of normal routines and discomfort from diagnostic tests and treatment may also cause anxiety. There are additional social problems including making up missed school work, explaining the illness and treatment to friends, and coping with physical limitations or disability.

Teens with serious illnesses and disabilities face emotional conflicts and psychological challenges. One conflict is between the teen's growing desire for independence and the reality of dependence on others for the activities of daily living. It is important for teens to be fully informed about their disease and treatment plan and involved in treatment decision making. Many teens benefit from continuing contact with friends, classmates, teachers, and family during hospital stays and recovery at home.

Depression, emotional distress, and anxiety associated with the disease and its treatment may respond to counseling from a mental health professional. Individual and group therapy often help teens and young adults to reveal and express their feelings about illness and treatment. Many cancer patients and their families find participation in mutual aid and group support programs help to relieve feelings of isolation and loneliness. By sharing problems with others who have lived through similar difficulties patients and families can exchange ideas and coping strategies.

Clinical trials

More than 25 clinical studies were underway during 2001. For example, at John Hopkins Oncology Center and other cancer centers across the United States, patients with recurring or widespread Ewing's sarcoma were being given chemotherapy to stop tumor cells from dividing as well as stem cells (**bone marrow transplantation**) to replace immune cells killed by chemotherapy.

Other **clinical trials** compare different combinations of drugs used for chemotherapy or combinations of chemotherapy and radiation to find out which combination is more effective. For example, in one study, patients with Ewing's sarcoma were randomly assigned to two different treatment groups. One group received chemotherapy followed by surgery and radiation therapy. The other group received radiation therapy during chemotherapy.

Other types of clinical research study individuals and families at high risk of cancer to help identify cancer genes. To learn more about clinical trials visit the National Cancer Institute (NCI) web site at http://cancertrials.nci.nih.gov or the Pediatric Oncology Branch of the National Cancer Institute web site at http://www–dcs.nci.nih.gov/pedonc/

Prevention

Since the causes of Ewing's sarcoma are not known, there are no recommendations about how to prevent its development. Among families with an inherited tendency to develop soft tissue sarcomas, careful monitoring may help to ensure early diagnosis and treatment of the disease.

Special concerns

Ewing's sarcoma, like other cancer diagnoses, may produce a range of emotional reactions in patients and families. Education, counseling and participation in group support programs can help to reduce feelings of guilt, fear, anxiety and hopelessness. For many parents suffering from spiritual distress, visits with clergy members and participation in organized prayer may offer comfort.

Resources

BOOKS

Murphy, Gerald P. et al. *American Cancer Society Textbook of Clinical Oncology, Second Edition.* Atlanta, GA: The American Cancer Society, Inc. 1995, pp.544–545.

Otto, Shirley E. *Oncology Nursing.* St. Louis, MO: Mosby, 1997 pp.400–401.

Pelletier, Kenneth R. *The Best of Alternative Medicine.* New York, NY: Simon & Schuster, 2000.

PERIODICALS

Arndt, Carola A.R. and William M. Crist. "Medical Progress: Common Musculoskeletal Tumors of Childhood and Adolescence." *New England Journal of Medicine.* 29 July 1999:342–352.

ORGANIZATIONS

American Cancer Society. 1599 Clifton Road, N.E., Atlanta, GA 30329. (800)227–2345.

Cancer Research Institute. 681 Fifth Avenue, New York, NY 10022. (800)992–2623.

National Cancer Institute (National Institutes of Health). 9000 Rockville Pike, Bethesda, MD 20892. (800)422–6237.

National Cancer Institute Clinical Cancer Trials <http://cancertrials.nci.nih.gov>.

The Pediatric Oncology Branch of the National Cancer Institute. (877) 624–4878 or (301)496–4256. <http://www- dcs.nci.nih.gov/pedonc/>.

Barbara Wexler, M.P.H.

Exemestane *see* **Aromatase inhibitors**

Exenteration

Definition

An exenteration is a major operation during which all the contents of a body cavity are removed. Pelvic exenteration refers to the removal of all the organs and adjacent structures of the pelvis, and orbital exenteration refers to the removal of the entire contents of the ocular orbit, sometimes including the eyelids as well.

Purpose

The pelvis is the basin-shaped cavity that contains the bladder, rectum and reproductive organs. (The reproductive organs include the ovaries, uterus and cervix for women and the prostate for men.) Pelvic exenteration is performed to surgically remove cancer that involves these organs and that has not responded well to other types of treatment. For example, pelvic exenteration might be performed for primary **rectal cancer** because 5%–10% of primary rectal cancers spread to nearby pelvic organs. Pelvic exenteration is also indicated when cancer returns after an earlier treatment, as rectal cancer does in some 20% of cases. In women, the operation is additionally performed mostly for advanced and invasive cases of endometrial, ovarian, vulvar, vaginal and **cervical cancer**, and in men for aggressive **prostate cancer**.

Similarly, orbital exenteration is performed to remove the eye and surrounding tissues when cancer of the orbital contents cannot be controlled by simple removal or irradiation. It is often the only course of treatment for advanced **basal cell carcinoma** of the eyelids, for cancers that have spread to the optic nerve, or retinoblastomas larger than 1/4 inch (0.6 cm), as well as for large tumors of the eyeball.

Exenteration is not only a major operation for a patient to undergo, it is also technically very challenging, because it involves elaborate **reconstructive surgery**. It is a radical surgical procedure, but it often provides the only opportunity available for patients to eliminate the cancer and to prevent cancer from recurring.

Precautions

Pelvic exenterations should not be performed on patients diagnosed with inflammation of the roots of spinal nerves, sciatica, lymphedema, liver cancer, extrapelvic disease, and obstructions of the urinary tract.

All precautions applying to major surgery apply to exenterations, whether pelvic or ocular.

After pelvic exenteration, sexual intercourse should be avoided as directed by the surgeon. This is to allow the wound to heal properly.

Description

Pelvic exenteration

There are three types of pelvic exenterations.

ANTERIOR EXENTERATION. This operation usually removes in women the uterus, bladder, vagina, and entire urethra. Patients selected for this operation have cancers that are located so as to allow the rectum to be spared. Vaginal reconstruction is performed afterwards if required. It is called anterior because it removes organs toward the front or in front of the pelvis.

POSTERIOR EXENTERATION. This operation removes in women the uterus, ovaries, Fallopian tubes, anus, supporting muscles and ligaments, and all the vagina except a portion of the wall that supports the urethra. In men, the bladder is also removed. It is called posterior because it removes organs located in the back part of the pelvis.

TOTAL PELVIC EXENTERATION. This operation removes the bladder, rectum and anus, supporting muscles and ligaments, together with either the prostate in men or the gynecologic (reproductive) organs in women. Total pelvic exenteration is performed when

KEY TERMS

Anus—The terminal orifice of the gastrointestinal (GI) or digestive tract which includes all organs responsible for getting food in and out of the body.

Catheter—Long thin tubes that carry urine from the kidneys to the bladder.

Conjunctiva—A clear membrane that covers the inside of the eyelids and the outer surface of the eye.

Cyst—Any closed cavity surrounded by a wall made up of cells joined by cementing substances and that contains liquid or semi-solid material.

General anesthesia—Method used to stop pain from being felt during an operation. General anesthesia is the most powerful type and is generally used only for major operations, such as brain, neck, chest, abdomen, and pelvis surgery.

Ocular orbit—Bony cavity containing the eyeball.

Resection—The complete or partial removal of an organ or tissue.

Rectum—The last part of the large intestine (colon) that connects it to the anus.

there is no opportunity to perform a less extensive operation, because of the location and size of the cancer. For women, vaginal reconstruction is performed, which also helps reconstruction of the pelvic area. In both anterior and total pelvic exenteration, a urinary tract can be constructed.

The exact surgical procedure followed depends on the type of exenteration, but generally, all pelvic exenterations start with an incision in the lower abdomen. Blood vessels are clamped and the organs specified by the procedure are removed. The site of incision is then stitched up.

Orbital exenteration

This operation removes the eyeball and surrounding tissues of the orbit. The eye is surrounded by bone, so orbital exenteration is easier to tolerate than pelvic exenteration and patients may even undergo the operation as outpatients. Orbital exenteration with partial preservation of eyelids and conjunctiva can sometimes be achieved. Within two weeks of surgery, patients are usually fitted with a temporary ocular prothesis (plastic eye). Later, facial prostheses are also attached to the facial skeleton.

Both pelvic and orbital exenterations are performed using general anesthesia.

Preparation

The evaluation of patients before pelvic exenteration includes a thorough physical exam with rectal and pelvic examination. **Endorectal ultrasound** and **imaging studies**, such as **computed tomography** scans (CT scans) and **magnetic resonance imaging** (MRI), are routinely used to obtain pictures of the abdominal and pelvic areas and evaluate the spread of the cancer.

Ocular ultrasound examination, CT scan and **angiography** evaluation is usually performed to prepare for ocular exenteration.

Preparing for the operation usually depends on the type of exenteration procedure selected. Most patients receive a combination of **radiation therapy** and **chemotherapy** before the operation. Surgery is typically performed approximately six weeks later.

In the case of pelvic exenteration, patients are required to clean as much waste as possible out of the large intestine, using various **laxatives** or enemas. This cleaning of the colon and rectum is required so as to eliminate stool and lower the level of bacteria, thus preventing infections after surgery. **Antibiotics** are also typically given to help sterilize the colon.

Aftercare

Pelvic exenteration

After a pelvic exenteration, a drainage tube is inserted at the site of the incision. There usually is some bleeding, discharge and considerable tenderness and pain for a few days. This is a major operation that requires at least a three- to five-day hospital stay. Side effects depend on the type of pelvic exenteration performed, but always include urination difficulty, especially if adjustment to a catheter is required, and a very painful lower abdomen.

Some exenterations require a temporary or permanent **colostomy**, meaning the creation of an opening (stoma) in the abdomen to allow solid waste to leave the body. Permanent colostomy may be needed, for example, if the rectum is removed. In such cases, the patient needs time to adjust and be taught how to irrigate, empty, clean and wear the colostomy bags.

Stitches are usually removed from the skin on the third day or before the patient is sent home. A prescription for pain medication is usually given as well as instructions for follow up care.

Ocular exenteration

After ocular exenteration, most patients have a headache for several days which goes away using medication such as tylenol. An eye ointment is also prescribed that contains antibiotics and steroids to help the healing process.

Risks

No surgical procedure is risk-free. Complications are always possible, especially if the operation is major. As with any operation, possible exenteration risks include possible complications due to the anesthetic and wound infection.

In the case of pelvic exenteration, the following complications are also possible:

- hemorrhage that may require a blood transfusion
- injury to the bowel
- urinary tract infection
- urinary retention requiring permanent use of a catheter
- bowel obstruction
- urinary tract infection

The following considerations also apply: after removal of the reproductive organs, women will no longer have monthly periods nor will they be able to become pregnant. For men, surgery involving the prostate and the nerves around the rectum may also result in the inability to produce sperm or to have an erection.

In the case of orbital exenteration, the following complications have been known to occur:

- growth of an orbital cyst (rare)
- chronic throbbing orbital pain
- sinusitis (nasal stuffiness)
- ear problems

See Also Adenocarcinoma; Cervical cancer; Endometrial cancer; Melanoma; Ovarian cancer; Vaginal cancer; Vulvar cancer

QUESTIONS TO ASK THE DOCTOR

- Why do I need the operation?
- What are the benefits of having the operation?
- What are the risks of having the operation?
- What if I don't have this operation?
- Where can I get a second opinion?
- What has been your experience in doing the operation?
- How long will it take me to recover?
- What are the surgeon's qualifications?

Resources

BOOKS

Deardorff, W. W. and J. Reeves. *Preparing for Surgery: A Mind-Body Approach to Enhance Healing and Recovery.* Oakland: New Harbinger, 1997.

Shields, J. A. *Diagnosis and Management of Orbital Tumors.* St. Louis: W. B. Saunders Publishing Company, 1989.

PERIODICALS

Kennedy, R. E., R. Frezzotti, R. Bonanni, A. Nuti, E. Polito, G. Bonavolonta, S. Evers, P. Soros, R. Brilla, H. Gerding, I. W. Husstedt, and K. W. Dolphin. "Indications and surgical techniques for orbital exenteration." *Advances in Ophthalmic Plastic Reconstructive Surgery* 9 (1992): 163-173.

Kersten, R. C., D. T. Tse, R. L. Anderson. "The role of orbital exenteration in choroidal melanomas." *Ophthalmology* 92(1985): 436-443.

Moffat, F. L. J. and R. E. Falk. "Radical surgery for extensive rectal cancer: is it worthwhile?" *Recent Results in Cancer Research* 146(1998): 71-83.

Petros, J. G., P. Augustinos, M. Lopez, J. S. Spratt, W. J. Temple, E. B. Saettler, R. E. Hautmann, D. Turns. "Pelvic exenteration for carcinoma of the colon and rectum." *Seminars in Surgical Oncology* 17(October-November 1999): 206-212.

Turns, D. "Psychosocial issues: pelvic exenterative surgery." *Journal of Surgical Oncology* 76 (March 2001): 224-236.

OTHER

Women's Health Matters. <http://www.womenshealthmatters.ca/centres/cancer/cervical/treatment/index.html>.

Information on eye cancer: Web sites: <http://www.EyeCancerBook.com/> and <http://eyecancerinfo.com/>.

Monique Laberge, Ph.D.

Extragonadal germ cell tumors

Definition

Germ cells are primitive cells within the body that normally mature into ova (egg) or sperm cells. More than 90% of all **germ cell tumors** are gonadal; that is, they develop in the ovaries or the testes (the gonads). The remaining 5–10% of germ cell tumors arise outside of the gonads: these are the extragonadal germ cell tumors. These tumors occur mostly in the chest, lower back, and head.

Description

Extragonadal germ cell tumors are related to developmental problems that occur prior to birth. In the growing embryo, germ cells migrate to the immature ovaries or testes. In some instances, these cells fail to move to the gonads and end up in the midchest area between the lungs (mediastinum), the lowest part of the back (presacral area), or near the pea-sized gland between the two hemispheres of the brain (pineal gland). When these germ cells grow in these extragonadal sites, they sometimes develop into tumors. These tumors can be benign (noncancerous) or malignant (cancerous).

Benign extragonadal germ cell tumors are called benign teratomas. Malignant extragonadal germ cell tumors are subdivided into seminoma and nonseminoma. The nonseminoma germ cell tumors include: embryonal **carcinoma**, malignant teratoma, endodermal sinus tumor, choriocarcinoma, and mixed germ cell tumors. The specific category of extragonadal germ cell tumor that is present has a major influence on both treatment and prognosis.

Demographics

Extragonadal germ cell tumors are quite rare. One new case is diagnosed annually for every 1 million people in the United States.

In young children, extragonadal germ cell tumors tend to occur primarily in the presacral area. The majority of these tumors are benign.

In adults, extragonadal germ cell tumors tend to be in the mediastinum. Of these, approximately 40% are malignant.

Malignant extragonadal germ cell tumors occur with equal frequency in boys and girls. But, they are approximately nine times more likely to occur in men than in women.

Extragonadal germ cell tumors occur with equal frequency in members of all races and ethnic groups. There does not appear to be any relationship of extragonadal germ cell tumors to any geographic region.

Causes and symptoms

The cause, or causes, of extragonadal germ cell tumors are not known.

The symptoms of an extragonadal germ cell tumor depend on the type and location of the tumor.

Mediastinum

Germ cell tumors of the mediastinum are primarily diagnosed in men between the ages of 20 and 30. Symptoms include:

KEY TERMS

Germ cells—Cells that are involved in reproduction. These cells are usually located in the gonads. Sometimes they fail to move to the gonads during embryonic development and cause tumors in other parts of the body.

Gonads—The reproductive organs: the testes and ovaries.

Mediastinum—The mid-chest area between the lungs.

Pineal gland—A pea-sized gland just below the brain.

Presacral area—The lowest part of the back.

- chest pain
- breathing problems
- cough
- fever

Presacral area

Presacral germ cell tumors are primarily diagnosed in children under the age of six. These are generally seen as a mass in the lower abdomen or buttocks. Because of the size and location of the tumor, the patient may have difficulty passing urine or having a bowel movement. Tumors detected in children under the age of six months are benign in 98% of cases. Tumors detected in children over the age of six months are malignant in approximately 65% of cases.

Pineal area

Almost all pineal germ cell tumors occur in people under the age of 40. Symptoms include:

- headache
- nausea
- vomiting
- lethargy
- difficulty walking
- memory loss
- an inability to look upward
- uncontrolled eye movement
- double vision

In some cases, a pineal germ cell tumor can begin to produce hormones that can cause a child to enter puberty at an abnormally young age (precocious puberty).

Diagnosis

The diagnosis of an extragonadal germ cell tumor usually begins with a thorough physical examination. In cases where a presacral tumor is suspected, this will include a rectal examination and a pelvic examination in women. In cases where a germ cell tumor of the pineal area is suspected, a complete neurological examination will be performed.

Mediastinum

The first test for a tumor of the mediastinum is a standard chest **x ray**. This will detect the tumor and show its location in 95% of cases. This will be followed by a **computed tomography** (CT) scan of the chest to determine the size of the tumor and by a CT scan of the abdomen to see if there has been a spread (**metastasis**) to the liver or other abdominal sites.

Diagnosis is generally confirmed by taking a needle **biopsy** of the tumor. In this procedure, a needle is injected directly into the tumor and a sample is removed.

Certain types of nonseminomas can be detected via blood tests for levels of alpha-fetoprotein (AFP) and beta-human chorionic gonadotropin (beta-hCG).

Presacral area

Germ cell tumors of the presacral area are diagnosed by either **magnetic resonance imaging** (MRI) or ultrasound imaging techniques. These techniques allow for the determination of both the location and the precise size of the tumor. To check for metastases, a bone scan, chest x rays, and a CT scan of the lungs should be performed. Sometimes a bone marrow biopsy is also ordered.

Diagnosis of a presacral germ cell tumor is confirmed by a direct biopsy of the tumor. This may be either an excisional biopsy, in which the tumor is first removed, then examined; or, a needle biopsy, in which only a sample of the tumor is removed for examination.

Pineal area

A CT scan of the head will usually show a pineal tumor. An MRI scan, using gadolinium as a tracer chemical, may also be ordered.

Blood tests for AFP and beta-hCG may help to diagnose pineal area germ cell tumors. Tests for these chemicals on the cerebrospinal fluid (**lumbar puncture**) may also be ordered.

The diagnosis of a pineal area germ cell tumor is usually confirmed upon biopsy of the tumor after it has been removed from the patient.

Treatment team

Treatment of an extragonadal germ cell tumor depends on the location of the tumor. Most tumors are treated with a combination of surgery, **chemotherapy**, and radiation treatments.

Germ cell tumors of the mediastinum are generally not surgically removed. They are treated with high-dose radiation and sometimes with chemotherapy. Germ cell tumors of the presacral area are treated with chemotherapy to shrink the tumor, then surgery to remove the tumor. This surgery is generally performed by a physician who specializes in tumor removal surgery of the lower abdomen and pelvis. Germ cell tumors of the pineal area are generally removed by a brain surgeon and then the patient is treated with radiation and/or chemotherapy.

Chemotherapy is administered under the direction of a physician who specializes in cancer (oncologist). Radiation therapies are generally administered by radiological technicians under the direction of an oncologist, a radiologist, a health physicist, and/or a medical radiation dosimetrist.

Clinical staging, treatments, and prognosis

The prognosis for patients with benign extragonadal germ cell tumors is excellent after surgery to remove the tumor is completed.

In the cases of malignant extragonadal germ cell tumors, the prognosis depends on the type and size of the tumor that is found.

Fifty-six percent of nonseminomas and 90% of seminomas have a good prognosis. Another 28% of nonseminomas and the remaining 10% of seminomas have an intermediate prognosis. While 16% of nonseminomas have a poor prognosis. A good prognosis is defined as a five-year survival rate above 85%. An intermediate prognosis is defined as a five-year survival rate between 50% and 85%. A poor prognosis is defined as a five year survival rate lower than 50%.

For both seminomas and nonseminomas, the prognosis is better if the tumors have not metastasized to other tissues. This is particularly true in the case of **mediastinal tumors**: those that have metastasized outside the general region of the lungs lead to particularly poor prognoses.

The prognosis for nonseminomas is based primarily on AFP and hCG concentrations found in the blood. The

QUESTIONS TO ASK THE DOCTOR

- Which type of extragonadal germ cell tumor do I have?
- Is my tumor operable?
- What are my treatment options?
- What is the likelihood of my type of tumor being successfully removed with a single surgery?
- What is the prognosis for my tumor type?
- How often should I seek follow-up examinations?

lower the levels of these two chemicals in the blood, the better the prognosis.

Alternative and complementary therapies

There are no effective alternative treatments for extragonadal germ cell tumors other than surgery, chemotherapy, and radiation.

Coping with cancer treatment

Most patients who undergo surgery to remove their tumors can resume their normal activities within a few days of the operation.

In some cases of presacral area germ cell tumors, it is difficult to remove the entire tumor in a single operation. In these cases, it is necessary for the patient to undergo a second course of chemotherapy prior to a second surgery to remove the remaining tumor.

When extensive chemotherapy is necessary, the patient may require counseling to help cope with the side effects of these treatments, such as loss of head and body hair, **weight loss**, nausea, **fatigue**, and changes in psychological well-being.

Clinical trials

There were 12 **clinical trials** underway, in early 2001, aimed at the treatment of extragonadal germ cell tumors. More information on these trials, including contact information, may be found by conducting a clinical trial search at the web site of the National Cancer Institute, CancerNet (<http://cancernet.nci.nih.gov>).

Prevention

Because the causes of extragonadal germ cell tumors are not known, there are no known preventions.

Special concerns

Repeat surgery may be necessary for extragonadal germ cell tumors, particularly those of the presacral area because these tumors are often difficult to remove completely. Careful monitoring by the medical team will be required.

See Also Bone marrow aspiration and biopsy; Nuclear medicine scan; Testicular cancer

Resources

BOOKS

Jones, W.G., I. Appleyard, P. Harnden, and J.K. Joffe, eds. *Germ Cell Tumors IV.* London: John Libbey & Company, Ltd., 1998.

PERIODICALS

Hainsworth, J.D., and F.A. Greco. "Extragonadal Germ Cell Tumors and Unrecognized Germ Gell Tumors." *Seminars in Oncology* (April 1992), 119–127.

ORGANIZATIONS

National Cancer Institute. Building 31, Room 10A03, 31 Center Dr., MSC 2580, Bethesda, MD 20892-2590. (800) 4-CANCER. <http://www.nci.nih.gov>.

OTHER

Extragonadal Germ Cell Cancer Articles and Links. 15 April 2001. 2 July 2001 <http://www.acor.org/TCRC/egc_links.html>.

Paul A. Johnson, Ed.M.

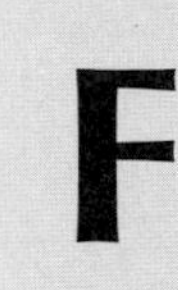

Famciclovir *see* **Antiviral therapy**

Familial cancer syndromes

Definition

Familial cancer syndrome is a genetic condition that causes an increased risk for specific types of cancers. Familial cancer syndromes account for only 5–10% of all cancers.

Description

Most cancer is not inherited. Cancer is common; in 2000, over 1.2 million new cancer cases were diagnosed. Many people have relatives who have had cancer, but most of the time this is due to chance or environmental factors. In a familial cancer syndrome, an inherited genetic mutation causes a person to be at increased risk for cancer and other physical symptoms. There are many different familial cancer syndromes, and each one has a specific set of characteristic cancers and physical symptoms associated with it. For example, BRCA1 and BRCA2 gene mutations are associated with an increased risk for breast and **ovarian cancer**. Examples of other familial cancer syndromes include **Von Hippel-Lindau syndrome**, **Peutz-Jeghers syndrome**, and **Li-Fraumeni syndrome**.

Features

Below is a list of "clues" in a family tree that make a familial cancer syndrome more suspicious:

- Two or more close relatives with the same type of cancer (on the same side of the family).
- Cancer diagnosed at an earlier age than usual.
- Cancer diagnosed more than once in the same person (more than one primary cancer, not a cancer recurrence).
- Cluster of cancers associated with a known familial cancer syndrome (such as breast and ovarian).
- Many cases of cancer in a family, more than can be accounted for by chance.
- Cancer in a person who also has birth defects.
- Evidence of autosomal dominant inheritance, which is when a gene from one parent overrides that of the other parent. When one parent has a dominant abnormal gene, offspring each have a 50% chance of inheriting that gene.

KEY TERMS

Gene—A unit of heredity that codes for the formation of a protein. Genes determine how we grow and develop.

Inherited—Qualities that are transmitted from parent to offspring in the genes.

Mutation—A change in a genetic code which may result in altered function of a gene.

Syndrome—The clustering of signs and symptoms that characterize a disease.

Diagnosis

The most important step in determining if a family has a familial cancer syndrome is gathering an accurate family history. The family history should include children, brothers and sisters, parents, aunts, uncles, grandparents, nieces, nephews and cousins on both sides of the family. For a person who has had cancer, the type of cancer and age at diagnosis should be listed for each cancer. It may be necessary to obtain medical records to confirm what type of cancer a person had since family members may not always be aware of specific information. Birth defects, unusual skin findings, benign tumors, and spe-

Suppressor genes that, when deleted, predispose families to cancers

Gene	Consequence of gene loss
Rb	Retinoblastoma and osteosarcoma
TP53	Li-Fraumeni syndrome
Wt1	Wilms' tumor
VHL	von Hippel-Lindau syndrome; renal cell carcinoma
NF1	von Recklinghausen's disease; neurofibromatosis type 1; schwannoma and glioma
NF2	Neurofibromatosis type 2; acoustic neuroma and meningiomas
APC	Familial adenomatous polyposis; colorectal tumors
MMR	Hereditary nonpolyposis-colorectal cancer

cial screening tests (such as **colonoscopy** to look for colon polyps) should also be noted. When this type of family information is unavailable, it may be possible to look for clues in one or a small number of family members. Many hospitals have a "familial cancer clinic," which is a team of health professionals with expertise in familial cancer syndromes. Geneticists, genetic counselors, oncologists and social workers assist individuals and families by providing risk assessment, support, screening and prevention recommendations, and **genetic testing** options (if available).

Inheritance

Some familial cancer syndromes show autosomal dominant inheritance, which means that an affected person has a 50% chance of passing on the genetic mutation to each of his/her children. Other familial cancer syndromes show autosomal recessive inheritance, which means that both parents are usually not affected, but are carriers of a mutation for the condition. In autosomal recessive inheritance, each child born to parents who are carriers has a 25% chance of having the condition. When a person is diagnosed with a familial cancer syndrome, relatives should be examined for signs of the syndrome. Sometimes a person identified as having a familial cancer syndrome is the first person in the family to be affected. That person is able to pass the condition on to his or her children, but the parents and siblings are not affected. Depending on the syndrome, genetics professionals can determine who in the family is at risk.

Risks

Different familial cancer syndromes have different risks for cancer and associated symptoms. In general, a person who inherits the syndrome has a higher risk of developing the cancer associated with the syndrome than the general population, but this is not a guarantee that cancer will ever develop. On the other hand, someone who does not inherit the syndrome is not at increased risk for cancer above that of the general population, but this is no guarantee that cancer will not develop, and screening guidelines for the general population should be followed.

Genetic Testing

Although genetic testing is available for many familial cancer syndromes, there are genes that have yet to be discovered. Each syndrome has special issues surrounding genetic testing; for example, what age should the test be done? How would the results change medical management? Does insurance cover the test? How will the information affect the family? Health professionals familiar with familial cancer syndromes keep up to date with advances in **cancer genetics**, and work with families to discuss the risks, benefits and limitations of genetic testing.

Resources

BOOKS

Offit, K. *Clinical Cancer Genetics: Risk Counseling and Management.* New York: Wiley-Liss, 1998.

PERIODICALS

Cummings, S. "The Genetic Testing Process: How Much Counseling Is Needed?" *Journal of Clinical Oncology* 18 (1 Nov Supplement 2000): 60–4.

Elsas, L. J., and A. Trepanier. "Cancer genetics in primary care: When is genetic screening an option and when is it the standard of care?" *Postgraduate Medicine* 107 (April 2000): 191–208.

Lindor, N. M., and M. H. Greene. "The Concise Handbook of Family Cancer Syndromes." *Journal of the National Cancer Institute* 90 (15 July 1998): 1039–71.

Lynch, H., et al. "Clinical Impact of Molecular Genetic Diagnosis, Genetic Counseling, and Management of Hereditary Cancer: Part I: Studies of Cancer in Families." *Cancer* 86 (1999): 2449–56.

OTHER

"Autosomal Dominant Genes." *WebMD* June 2001. 27 June 2001 <http://my.webmd.com/content/asset/adam_image page_9084>.

"Statistics." *American Cancer Society* June 2001. 27 June 2001 <http://www3.cancer.org/cancerinfo/>.

Laura L. Stein, M.S., C.G.C.

Famotidine *see* **Histamine 2 antagonists**

Fanconi anemia

Definition

Fanconi anemia is an inherited form of aplastic anemia characterized by an abnormally low number of cellular components in the blood due to failing bone marrow.

Description

Fanconi anemia (FA) is a rare genetic disease caused by mutations or alterations in one of seven different genes. The disease is an autosomal recessive condition, meaning that the genes are not located on the sex chromosomes and a mutated gene copy must be inherited from both parents in order for a person to be affected. Test results of cells from FA patients suggest that the genetic defects of FA reduce the cell's ability to repair damaged deoxyribonucleic acid (DNA), the primary chemical component of chromosomes. Five of the seven genes associated with FA have been isolated.

Demographics

With only approximately 1000 cases documented in the literature, FA is a rare disease with varied frequency in different ethnic groups. It is particularly prevalent in the Ashkenazi Jewish population, where carriers are 1 in 89 persons, compared to an overall carrier frequency of 1 in 100 to 600. A carrier is a person unaffected by the disease who has one mutated and one normal gene in their genome. Both parents must be carriers in order to produce a child with FA.

Causes and symptoms

FA is caused by inheriting two abnormal copies of one of seven different genes, all thought to be involved in DNA repair. About 67% of children with FA are born with some sort of congenital defect. The problems seen include:

- short stature
- abnormalities of the thumb or arm
- other skeletal abnormalities such as of the hip or ribs

KEY TERMS

Aplastic anemia—A disease in which the bone marrow stops producing all three types of cells of the blood: red blood cells, white blood cells, and platelets.

Fludarabine—A drug that inhibits a blood cell's ability to produce DNA, eliminating native cells from FA patients so they can undergo BMT.

Myelodysplastic syndrome—A disease where the bone marrow stops producing healthy blood cells and the cells that are produced function poorly. This syndrome sometimes develops into leukemia.

Neutrophil—A type of white blood cells important in the defense of the body against infection.

- kidney malformations
- skin discoloration
- small eyes or head
- mental retardation
- low birth weight and failure to thrive
- abnormalities of the digestive system
- heart defects

The defining characteristic of FA is progressive pancytopenia, a gradual reduction of the cellular components of the blood. A reduction in red blood cells is typically noted first, then white blood cells, and finally, platelets. Complete bone marrow failure in FA patients is usually seen between the ages of three and twelve, with a median of seven.

Later in life, FA patients have delayed sexual maturity and an increased probability of developing cancer. For FA patients surviving into adulthood, 50% develop leukemia (a malignancy of the white blood cells) and/or myelodysplastic syndrome (MDS, a pre-leukemic state). Persons with FA also have an elevated chance of developing squamous cell cancers (originating in the outer layer of the skin), particularly gynecological cancers (for females); head, neck and throat cancers; **gastrointestinal cancers**; and liver cancers.

Diagnosis

Diagnosis can be made upon the appearance of the characteristic congenital defects, but is more common upon development of aplastic anemia (when the bone marrow fails to produce normal numbers of blood cells).

QUESTIONS TO ASK THE DOCTOR

- Which FA gene is responsible for my child's illness?
- Are growth factor or gene therapies appropriate for my child?
- When should bone marrow transplantation be considered as an appropriate treatment?

Definitive diagnosis involves a showing of an unusual level of chromosome breakage when cells are exposed to DNA damaging agents. Additionally, with five of the seven genes associated with FA isolated, genetic engineering techniques can often be used to determine exactly what gene mutation is responsible for the disease. An estimated 90% of FA patients have mutations within the FANCA, FANCC and FANCG genes, all of which have been isolated.

Treatment team

FA is usually treated by pediatricians, hematologists, and, if a bone marrow transplant (BMT) is performed, a specialized teams of physicians, nurses, and medical assistants who are experienced in BMT.

Clinical staging, treatments, and prognosis

There is no clinical staging system for FA.

BMT and androgen therapy are two long-term non-experimental treatments for FA. BMT involves the suppression of the patient's own marrow and replacement with stem cells of the donor. The effectiveness of BMT is highly dependent on the existence of a donor that is closely matched to the patient. For sibling match (full match) transplants, the two-year survival rate is about 80%, compared to about 37% for less than a full match. The difference is due the prevalence of **graft-versus-host disease** (GVHD), where the recipient's body rejects the donor cells. The use of T-cell (a type of immune cell) depletion before transplantation and the drug **fludarabine** have significantly reduced the occurrence of GVHD. BMT does not alter the tendency of FA patients to develop other malignancies later in life, however.

Androgen therapy involves the administration of male hormones to stimulate the production of blood cells. Most FA patients respond for at least a time to this therapy. The cell increase lasts a few years at most, however, and the hormones have serious side effects, including masculinization of female patients and liver disease.

Clinical trials

Growth factor therapy and gene therapy are two treatments being tested in **clinical trials**. Two growth factors—granulocyte/macrophage colony stimulating factor (GM-CSF) and granulocyte colony stimulating factor (G-CSF)—were shown to increase blood cell production. Patients with low neutrophil counts particularly benefit from this treatment.

A clinical trial for gene therapy of FA patients is ongoing. The normal copy of the mutated gene is introduced into the patient's own bone marrow stem cells using a viral vector. When the virus infects the stem cells, the normal FANC gene is integrated into the stem cell's DNA. This therapy will, theoretically, correct the defect in the stem cells and prevent their premature death, curing the aplastic anemia seen in FA patients. As with BMT, however, this gene therapy will not reduce the development of other cancers in FA patients.

Prevention

The only known method of prevention of this disease is prenatal diagnosis and termination of pregnancies for affected embryos. Preimplantation genetic diagnosis, where one or two cells are tested from *in vitro* fertilized embryos, is also available. This method avoids the need for abortion, but carries more risk.

Special concerns

Because FA can be present without any outward symptoms, it is essential that any potential sibling donor for BMT be carefully tested for the disease using white blood cell exposure to DNA damaging agents or direct examination of their FANC gene copies before the transplant.

See Also Bone marrow transplantation; Genetic testing

Resources

BOOKS

Frohnmeyer, Lynn, and Dave Frohnmeyer. *Fanconi Anemia: A Handbook for Families and Their Physicians.* Eugene, Oregon: Fanconi Anemia Research Fund, Inc., 2000.

PERIODICALS

de Winter, J.P., et al. "The Fanconi anemia protein FANCF forms a nuclear complex with FANCA, FANCC and FANCG." *Human Molecular Genetics* 9 (November 2000): 2665-74.

Garcia-Higuera, I., et al. "Interaction of the Fanconi anemia proteins and BRCA1 in a common pathway." *Molecular Cell* 7 (February 2001): 249-62.

ORGANIZATIONS

Fanconi Anemia Research Fund, Inc. 1801 Willamette St., Suite 200, Eugene, OR 97401. (800) 828-4891. <www.fanconi.org>.

OTHER

Online Mendelian Inheritance in Man (OMIM). John Hopkins University, Baltimore, MD. MIM Nos. 602956, 603467, 227645, 227646, 227650. April 2001. 25 June 2001 <http://www.ncbi.nlm.nih.gov/omim/>.

Michelle Johnson, M.S., J.D.

Fatigue

Description

Fatigue is a feeling of exhaustion or loss of strength. The duration of fatigue for a patient with cancer has been found to last from one to two times the length of time between diagnosis and completion of treatment, so it is common for fatigue to persist beyond a patient's treatment regimen.

Causes

Many people experience fatigue as a side effect of cancer treatment. Both **chemotherapy** and **radiation therapy** are associated with fatigue. Scientists believe fatigue also occurs because the body is devoting so much of its energy fighting the cancer that it has little left over for daily life. Often the feelings of exhaustion are more intense immediately following a cancer treatment, but they gradually ease over time as the body gains strength.

During chemotherapy, anti-cancer drugs kill both cancer cells and healthy cells, including red blood cells. This can lead to **anemia**, or low red blood cell counts, which causes fatigue. Chemotherapy agents also attack white blood cells, weakening the immune system.

Medications, pain, **depression**, and the stress of the diagnosis and treatment are other factors that result in fatigue.

Treatments

If anemia is a problem, physicians may prescribe iron supplements or drugs, such as **erythropoietin**, to stimulate blood cell growth. In some cases, blood transfusions may be necessary.

KEY TERMS

Anemia—A condition that occurs when the body has low red blood cell counts. It can cause fatigue.

Erythropoietin—A drug used to stimulate blood cell growth when a person has anemia.

Many people with cancer find that they must pace themselves, alternating periods of activity with small naps. Going to bed earlier also seems to help.

Research has shown that people who exercise experience less cancer-related fatigue. Walking or using an exercise bicycle are good choices. For those who have severe weakness, even a few minutes of gentle stretching in bed can make a difference.

Eating nutritious food is another way to get an energy boost to better fight cancer. Include a variety of fruits and vegetables, whole grains and plenty of protein, if **nausea and vomiting** are not a problem. High-calorie liquid meals can help offset severe **weight loss** for those who cannot tolerate solid foods. Drinking plenty of water also helps prevent **diarrhea** and dehydration, which add to fatigue.

Alternative and complementary therapies

Yoga has proven to be highly effective in reducing stress, thereby increasing energy and helping people to relax and sleep better.

Marijuana has been used to help ease nausea in cancer patients. Since a loss of appetite can cause weakness and fatigue, marijuana may help indirectly. Most states do not permit the use of marijuana for medical reasons. Physicians will be aware of these regulations.

Other complementary therapies, such as massage, aromatherapy, meditation, or prayer, help people with cancer relax, easing their worries and ultimately combatting fatigue.

See Also Complementary cancer therapies

Resources

BOOKS

Clegg, Holly B., and Gerald Miletello, MD. *Eating Well Through Cancer.* Baton Rouge: Holly B. Clegg Inc., 2001.

Hassett Dahm, Nancy, and Robert Schirmer. *Mind, Body and Soul: A Guide to Living with Cancer.* New York: Taylor Hill Publishing, 2000.

PERIODICALS

Dimeo, F. C. et al. "Effects of Physical Activity on the Fatigue and Psychologic Status of Cancer Patients During Chemotherapy." *Cancer* 85, no. 10 (May 15, 1999): 2273–7.

ORGANIZATIONS

American Cancer Society. 1599 Clifton Road, Atlanta, GA 30329. (800) ACS-2345. <http://www.cancer.org>.

CancerFatigue.org. Oncology Nursing Society, 501 Holiday Dr., Pittsburgh, PA 15220. (412) 921-7373. <http://www.cancerfatigue.org>.

OTHER

"Fatigue." *American Cancer Society* June 2001. 28 June 2001 <http://www3.cancer.org/cancerinfo/>.

Melissa Knopper, M.S.

Fecal occult blood test

Definition

The fecal occult blood test (FOBT) is performed as part of the routine physical examination during the examination of the rectum. It is used to detect microscopic blood in the stool and is a screening tool for colorectal cancer.

Purpose

FOBT uses chemical indicators on stool samples to detect the presence of blood not otherwise visible. (The word "occult" in the test's name means that the blood is hidden from view.) Blood originating from or passing through the gastrointestinal tract can signal many conditions requiring further diagnostic procedures and, possibly, medical intervention. These conditions may be benign or malignant and some of them include:

- colorectal and gastric (stomach) cancers
- ulcers
- hemorrhoids
- polyps
- inflammatory bowel disease
- irritations or lesions of the gastrointestinal tract caused by medications (such as **nonsteroidal anti-inflammatory drugs,** also called NSAIDs)
- irritations or lesions of the gastrointestinal tract caused by stomach acid disorders, such as reflux esophagitis

The FOBT is used routinely (in conjunction with a rectal examination performed by a physician) to screen for colorectal cancer, particularly after age 50. The ordering of this test should not be taken as an indication that cancer is suspected. The FOBT must be combined with regular screening endoscopy (such as a **sigmoidoscopy**) to detect cancers at an early stage.

Precautions

Certain foods and medicines can influence the test results. Some fruits contain chemicals that prevent the guaiac, the chemical in which the test paper is soaked, from reacting with the blood. Aspirin and some NSAIDs irritate the stomach, resulting in bleeding and should be avoided prior to the examination, along with red meat and many vegetables and fruits containing vitamin C. All of these factors could result in a false-positive test.

Description

Feces for the stool samples is obtained either by the physician at the rectal examination or by the patient at home, using a small spatula or a collection device. In most cases, the collection of stool samples can easily be done at home, using a kit supplied by the physician. The standard kit contains a specially prepared card on which a small sample of stool will be spread, using a stick provided in the kit. The sample is placed in a special envelope and either mailed or brought in for analysis. When the physician applies hydrogen peroxide to the back of the sample, the paper will turn blue if an abnormal amount of blood is present.

Types of fecal occult blood tests

Hemoccult is one type of fecal occult blood test, and it is the most commonly used. The Hemoccult test takes less than five minutes to perform and may be performed in the physician's office or in the laboratory. The Hemoccult blood test can detect bleeding from the colon as low as 0.5 mg per day.

Tests that use anti-hemoglobin antibodies (or immunochemical tests) to detect blood in the stool are also used. Immunochemical tests can detect up to 0.7 mg of hemoglobin in the stool and do not require dietary restrictions. Immunochemical tests

- are not accurate for screening for stomach cancer
- are more sensitive than Hemoccult tests in detecting colorectal cancer
- are more expensive than Hemoccult tests

Hemoquant, another fecal occult blood test, is used to detect as much as 500 mg/g of blood in the stool. Like the Hemoccult, the Hemoquant test is affected by red meat. It is not affected by chemicals in vegetables.

Fecal blood may also be measured by measuring the chromium in the red blood cells in the feces. The stool is collected for three to ten days. The test is used in cases where the exact amount of the blood loss is required and it is the only test that can exclude blood loss from the gastrointestines with accuracy.

KEY TERMS

Occult—Not visible or easily detected.

Preparation

For 72 hours prior to collecting samples, patients should avoid red meats, NSAIDs (including aspirin), antacids, steroids, iron supplements, and vitamin C, including citrus fruits and other foods containing large amounts of vitamin C. Foods like uncooked broccoli, uncooked turnips, cauliflower, uncooked cantaloupe, uncooked radish and horseradish and parsnips should be avoided and not eaten during the 72 hours prior to the examination. Fish, chicken, pork, fruits (other than melons) and many cooked vegetables are permitted in the diet.

Results

Many factors can result in false-positive and false-negative findings.

Positive results

It is important to note that a true-positive finding only signifies the presence of blood—it is not an indication of cancer. The National Cancer Institute states that, in its experience, less than 10% of all positive results were caused by cancer. The FOBT is positive in 1%–5% of the unscreened population and 2%–10% of those are found to have cancer. The physician will want to follow up on a positive result with further tests, as indicated by other factors in the patient's history or condition.

Negative results

Alternatively, a negative result (meaning no blood was detected) does not guarantee the absence of **colon cancer**, which may bleed only occasionally or not at all. (Only 50% of colon cancers are FOBT-positive.)

Conclusions

Screening using the FOBT has been demonstrated to reduce colorectal cancer. However, because only half of colorectal cancers are FOBT-positive, FOBT must be combined with regular screening endoscopy to increase the detection of pre-malignant colorectal polyps and cancers.

QUESTIONS TO ASK THE DOCTOR

- What kinds of foods should I avoid prior to the FOBT?
- How much stool should I collect for the stool samples?
- What is the next step if my test is postive?

Resources

BOOKS

DeVita, Vincent, Samuel Hellman, and Steven Rosenburg. *Cancer:Principles and Practices of Oncology.* Philadelphia:Lippincott Williams & Wilkins, 2001.

Yamada, Tadetaka, Ed. *Textbook of Gastroenterology Volumes One and Two.* Philadelphia:Lippincott Williams & Wilkins, 2001.

PERIODICALS

From the Centers for Disease Control and Prevention. "Trends in screening for colorectal cancer—United States, 1997 and 1999." *Journal of the American Medical Association* 28 (March 2001):12.

ORGANIZATIONS

American Cancer Society. Phone: 1-800-ACS-2345. Web site: <http://www.cancer.org>

National Cancer Institute (NCI). 1-800-4-CANCER (1-800-422-6237), TTY: 1-800-332-8615. Web site: <http: //rex.nci.nih.gov>

OTHER

"ColorectalCancer Screening." *WebMD* <http://my.webmd.com/content/article/2955.291>.

"Fecal Occult Bood Test." *Virtual Health Fair.* Copyright 1997-2000. 10 July 2001 <http://vfair.com/resources/lab/fecal.htm>

"Colon and Rectum Cancer." *American Cancer Society.* Copyright 2000. 10 July 2001 <http://www.cancer.org>

Jill S. Lasker
Cheryl Branche, M.D.

Fentanyl *see* **Opioids**

Fertility issues

Overview

Any procedure or medication that interferes with the functioning of the testes or ovaries affects fertility. The choices made before cancer treatment begins can determine whether the patient will remain fertile after treatment. Prior to deciding on a treatment plan, it is important for the patient to discuss the issue of fertility with the treatment team so that all options, with their associated risks, can be considered.

Conventional cancer treatments and their effects on fertility

Cancer is usually treated with surgery, **chemotherapy**, and/or radiation, with the type and stage of the cancer dictating the treatment regimen recommended. While some physicians may routinely take into consideration alternatives to spare a patient's fertility, others may not, feeling that to differ from the treatment norm may compromise the patient's best chances for survival. Patients for whom fertility preservation is important, or for whom fertility-sparing measures could compromise treatment outcome, must discuss this issue fully with their treatment team.

Surgery

Surgery for cancer usually involves removal of the cancerous area, with some sampling of the adjacent area and lymph nodes to check for **metastasis**. If surgery must involve the removal of both of the testes or ovaries, the man will not be able to provide his own sperm, and the woman her own egg, towards the development of a biologic child. (A couple may be able to use donated sperm or egg when attempting a future pregnancy, however.) Fertility-sparing surgery may be an option for some individuals, depending on the type and stage of their cancer. For example, a woman with **ovarian cancer** contained to one ovary may be able to have just that one removed. The same is true for a man with **testicular cancer** contained to one testicle. In the case of testicular cancer, removal of retroperitoneal lymph nodes during surgery may damage the nerves affecting ejaculation. Men may wish to discuss nerve-sparing surgery and their concerns for fertility with their surgeon prior to surgery.

Chemotherapy

Chemotherapy affects the whole body, but certain drugs are less harmful to the reproductive tract than others. The drugs used in chemotherapy are highly toxic, in order to kill any cancer cell. However, they are not very selective, meaning that in addition to cancerous cells, normal cells are killed as well. It may take a few years after chemotherapy has finished to understand its temporary or permanent effect on fertility. It is generally recommended that women wait about two years after chemotherapy before attempting to become pregnant, to avoid the risk of a pregnancy that may end in miscarriage or a fetal malformation. Men who have had chemotherapy can have their sperm analyzed after treatment has finished to check sperm counts and motility.

There is a concern that individuals may delay treatment in order to undergo various fertility-preserving measures, such as sperm banking or egg retrieval and cryopreservation, and that this delay could result in a poorer treatment outcome. Some women undergo attempts at egg retrieval and embryo cryopreservation after an initial dose of chemotherapy. Some treatment centers offer the option of doing the chemotherapy in stages. The first stage of chemotherapy uses medications that are considered less toxic. Then the more intensive treatment follows after the harvesting of egg or sperm. However, it is still not yet clear what kind of damage may have been endured by tissue harvested right after some chemotherapy.

Radiation

Radiation is known to damage the highly sensitive sperm and eggs. Just as chemotherapy attacks healthy cells, so does radiation. However, radiation technology is able to focus very tightly on the cancerous area, which decreases risk to healthy tissue. When radiation for cancer does not involve the pelvic area, it may be possible to successfully shield the reproductive organs to preserve fertility. If the area needing irradiation is the pelvis, the reproductive organs are at great risk of damage.

When radiation is done to the pelvic area, women often experience a pause in menstruation, along with other symptoms of menopause. There may also be vaginal dryness, **itching**, and burning. Radiation may affect sexual desire as well. Men may experience a decrease in sperm count and motility, and difficulty in having or maintaining an erection. These changes may be temporary or permanent, and it may take up to a few years to determine if the effects were temporary or permanent. Sperm banking or cryopreservation of eggs may allow the individual reproductive success in the future.

Since radiation can be harmful to the fetus, pregnancy during **radiation therapy** is contraindicated, and because the full effect of the radiation on fertility cannot be predicted, individuals should use contraception during sexual relations while receiving radiation therapy.

Bone marrow transplant

A bone marrow transplant (BMT) may be part of the suggested treatment regimen. If so, patients need to understand its potential impact on future fertility. While the actual BMT does not jeopardize fertility, chemotherapy or radiation done prior to the BMT in preparation for the body's receiving of the new marrow can damage fertility. This pretreatment can destroy cells in the reproductive organs, rendering the individual infertile. While each case is unique, patients may wish to discuss the impact of their treatment on their reproductive future, and consider sperm banking or egg cryopreservation.

Children's cancers and future fertility

In the case of children, chemotherapy and radiation for childhood cancer can cause permanent damage to the ovaries or testes. In boys who have become sexually mature, sperm banking may provide future reproductive options. Options such as sperm aspiration, and cryopreservation of female ova are still considered experimental in children. While they may be effective, researchers are concerned that parents and their children may be unrealistic in their hopes for future fertility, and that the reintroduction of the harvested tissue may return latent cancer cells into the body. While research may bring new options, obtaining true informed consent involving children and their parents is an issue of moral and practical concern.

Alternative and complementary therapies

Individuals undergoing cancer treatment may turn to alternative therapies for a number of reasons. Techniques such as meditation, therapeutic touch, yoga, t'ai chi, and guided imagery can be very helpful in reducing stress and its effects on the body. Acupuncture has been shown through research studies to be effective in reducing the **nausea and vomiting** associated with chemotherapy. However, a study reported in the March 1999 issue of the medical journal *Fertility and Sterility* investigated several herbal remedies and their effect on sperm and ova. While this study was involved in animal research, the finding that high concentrations of St. John's wort, an herbal supplement used for mild to moderate **depression**, Echinacea, and ginkgo biloba damaged reproductive cells raises concern for its effect on humans. In particular, St. John's wort was found to be mutagenic to sperm cells.

Special concerns

Some cancers, such as testicular cancer, affect primarily young men. Most men diagnosed with testicular cancer are between the ages of 15 and 40. Sperm banking is highly recommended for these men. The method intracytoplasmic sperm injection uses just one sperm to fertilize one egg, by injecting the sperm directly into the egg. This can result in a fertilized egg for insemination, even when the sperm has decreased motility. It has a success rate of 30%.

Fertility issues and the development of cancer

Fertility issues can also play a role in the development of cancer. For example, women having their first child after 30 are at slightly higher risk of developing ovarian cancer than those having their first child before age 30. The number of ovulatory cycles a woman experiences also appears to affect her risk for ovarian cancer. A longer reproductive period (early menarche and late menopause) appears to raise the risk, while having children (there is no ovulation during pregnancy), breastfeeding (there is some suppression of ovulation during breastfeeding), and the use of oral contraceptives for at least five years decreases the risk.

Women who used the infertility medication clomiphene citrate without becoming pregnant were found in some studies to have a greater risk of developing a low malignancy potential ovarian cancer. In a November 1999 issue of the medical journal *Lancet*, researchers reported that women whose infertility remained unexplained were found to have more ovarian and uterine cancers, irrespective of whether or not they had been treated for the infertility. Also, more breast cancers were detected in the first year after treatment for infertility terminated than was expected. The lead author of the study speculated that these cancer diagnoses may be due to closer medical supervision that resulted in early detection. In some cases it was believed that the infertility was a symptom of the undiagnosed cancer.

KEY TERMS

Cryopreservation—The process of freezing sperm, ova, or embryos to preserve them for future use.

Oocyte retrieval—The process of obtaining eggs from a woman's ovary for future reproduction.

Sperm banking—Sperm banking is a process of freezing, or cryopreserving, sperm for use in the future. The sperm may be obtained via ejaculation, or by aspiration. The process of sperm banking may take one to two weeks to complete. The method of aspirating the sperm directly from the testicle is called testicular semen aspiration.

Treatment team—An interdisciplinary group of professionals whose focus is to collaborate on and coordinate the care of the patient. For the cancer patient this team might be comprised of a surgeon, oncologist, radiologist, gynecologic oncologist, urologic oncologist, nurse specialists, and social workers.

Resources

BOOKS

Coleman, C. Norman. *Understanding Cancer.* Baltimore, Maryland: The Johns Hopkins University Press, 1998.

QUESTIONS TO ASK THE DOCTOR

- What is the type and stage of my cancer?
- What treatment options do I have that would retain my fertility?
- Is my survival compromised if I choose fertility-sparing treatment?
- Would the health of future child/children be compromised if I undergo this treatment?
- Can you provide me with research studies of others who had this treatment and went on to have children?
- How long should I wait after treatment before attempting a pregnancy?
- If treatment is successful, what can I expect in terms of survival and quality of life?
- If treatment is unsuccessful, what can I expect in terms of survival and quality of life?
- What is the type and stage of my child's cancer?
- Does the treatment of this cancer have a risk of developing another cancer later on?
- How will this treatment affect my child's development during puberty?
- What effect will this treatment have on my child's future fertility?

McGinn, Kerry A. and Pamela J. Haylock. *Women's Cancers: How to prevent them, how to treat them, how to beat them.* Alameda, California: Hunter House, 1998.

Runowicz, Carolyn D., Jeanne A. Petrek, and Ted S. Gansler. *The American Cancer Society: Women and Cancer.* New York: Villard Book, 1999.

Schover, Leslie R., Ph.D. *Sexuality and Fertility After Cancer.* New York: John Wiley & Sons, Inc., 1997.

Teeley, Peter and Philip Bashe. *The Complete Cancer Survival Guide.* New York: Doubleday, 2000.

PERIODICALS

Venn, Alison et al. "Risk of cancer after use of fertility drugs with in-vitro fertilization." *The Lancet.* (November 6, 1999):190.

ORGANIZATIONS

American Cancer Society. (800) ACS-2345. <http://www.cancer.org>.

Esther Csapo Rastegari, R.N., B.S.N., Ed.M.

Fever

Description

Normal body temperature varies somewhat from one individual to another but displays a general range and pattern around the "normal" temperature of 98.6°F. Early morning body temperature may be as low as 97°F, and as high as 99.3°F in the afternoon hours yet still be considered normal. Higher temperatures may be observed in healthy people, but an abnormal elevation (pyrexia) is classified as **hyperthermia**, or fever. Fever results from a failure in the body's ability to regulate and dissipate heat. Any fever presents an unpleasant and uncomfortable state for the patient. Fever may cause the patient to experience **fatigue**, chills, sweats, nausea, and—in some cases—life-threatening conditions. When fevers occur in the elderly or the very young, the effects can be more harmful than in individuals who fall between those two age groups. The elderly may experience poor blood circulation, heart failure, an irregular heartbeat, or mental episodes. Children may lapse into fever-induced seizures. It is possible to treat fever with lukewarm sponge baths or bathing, removing excess clothing or bedding, and increasing the patient's fluid intake; however an important treatment is medication that lowers the body temperature to its normal range.

Causes

Fever associated with cancer can generally be categorized into four major causal groups: infection, tumors, allergic reactions to a drug, or allergic reaction to blood components in transfusion therapies. For cancer patients, fever should be considered a result of infection until an alternative cause is diagnosed. When a fever develops in a cancer patient, the individual must be thoroughly examined to determine the cause. A comprehensive physical examination should be administered by the physician and blood drawn for laboratory analysis.

Once a diagnosis has been made and treatment initiated, it is important to address problems created by the fever itself. It may be necessary to increase fluids and nutritional supplements. Because fever places increased demands on the body, this can be critical in restoring normal health for patients who may already be nutritionally compromised. Fever in a patient with **neutropenia** (low white blood cell count) represents the potential for a critical, life-threatening situation, and treatment should begin as quickly as the patient can reach the emergency room.

Physicians do not fully understand how tumors can cause fever, but certain correlations are well documented. Fever spikes may indicate that a tumor has grown or spread to other areas of the body, or that the tumor has produced some type of blockage. The fever associated with a tumor tends to be cyclic, and subsides with tumor treatment and recurs when the tumor returns or increases in size. In the case of drug-associated fever, the fever is an allergic-type reaction to a particular medication or combination of medications. Similarly, an **immune response** to donor blood cells is the typical cause of fever associated with blood components.

Treatments

Each of the major causes for fever associated with cancer has recommended conventional treatment procedures. For infection-related fever, broad-spectrum **antibiotics**, given orally, rectally, or intravenously, are the principle method of control. Some antibiotics may be started before a definitive diagnosis is made to retard additional complications caused by the infection. Treatment typically is administered for five to seven days as long as the fever and infection show a positive response.

Fever from a tumor is best treated by treating the tumor itself. Supplemental treatment for the fever may include the use of **nonsteroidal anti-inflammatory drugs** (NSAIDs) and acetaminophen. Aspirin should only be used in patients with no risk of bleeding problems. The allergic responses manifesting in drug- or blood-associated fever may be treated by various methods: antihistamines and acetaminophen may be administered prior to drug therapy or blood **transfusion therapy**; discontinuing the present drug and choosing alternate medication may be required; blood may require irradiation or removal of white blood cells from the donor blood.

Alternative and complementary therapies

Some patients are investigating and adhering to the use of alternative treatments and complementary therapies. These choices may include holistic healing or herbal medication, and therapy utilizing biofeedback, relaxation therapy, and imagery techniques. Patients maintain that these alternative and complementary therapies add a sense of control to their life during a period when they have little control over anything. No conclusive data exists on the effectiveness of the therapies used alone; however in conjunction with conventional methods of fever management, they do not appear to hinder therapy and may provide the patient increased goodwill and a positive outlook.

KEY TERMS

Acetaminophen—The generic name for a common nonprescription medication useful in the treatment of mild pain or fever.

Antibiotic—A drug that fights infection.

Antihistamine—A drug that counteracts allergic responses.

Biofeedback—A process by which a person learns to influence two kinds of physiologic responses: those that are not ordinarily under voluntary control; and those that are easily regulated but for which regulation has broken down because of trauma or disease.

Immune response—An alteration in the reactivity of the body's immune system in response to a foreign substance.

Neutropenia—Lowered blood cell counts, especially in white blood cells, chiefly the neutrophils that aid in fighting infection.

Nonsteroidal anti-inflammatory drugs (NSAIDs)—A family of anti-inflammatory drugs that work by inhibiting the production of prostaglandins (a group of compounds that affect diverse bodily processes).

Resources

PERIODICALS

Kern, Winfried., et al. "Oral versus Intravenous Empirical Antimicrobial Therapy for Fever in Patients with Granulocytopenia Who Are Receiving Cancer Chemotherapy." *The New England Journal of Medicine* 341, no. 5 (29 July 1999): 312-318

OTHER

Herbs for Relieving Cancer. *InnerSelf* 2000 Copyright. 21 April 2001, 1 July 2001 <http://www.innerself.com>

Jane Taylor-Jones, M.S.

Fibrocystic breast disease *see* **Fibrocystic condition of the breast**

Fibrocystic condition of the breast

Definition

Fibrocystic condition of the breast is a term that may refer to a variety of symptoms: breast lumpiness or tenderness, microscopic breast tissue, and/or the x-ray or

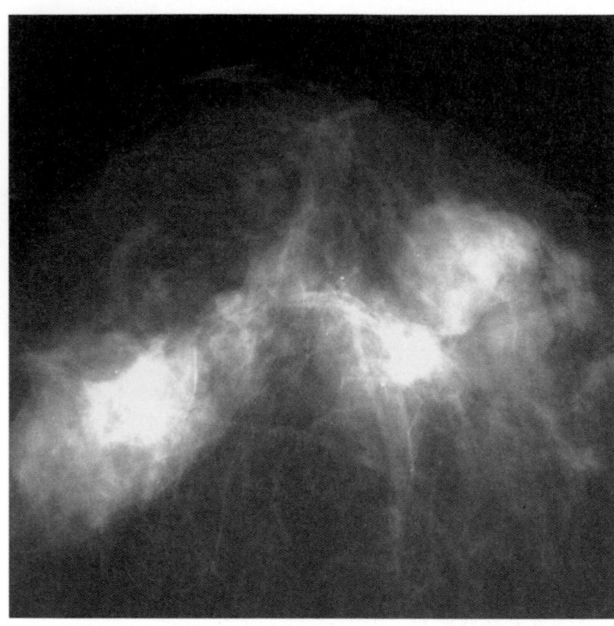

A mammogram of a female breast indicating multiple cysts. *(Custom Medical Stock Photo. Reproduced by permission.)*

ultrasound picture of the breast. It has been called a "wastebasket" diagnosis because a wide range of vaguely defined benign breast conditions may be labeled as fibrocystic condition. It is not a cancer, and the majority of types of fibrocystic conditions do not increase the risk of **breast cancer**.

Description

There is no such thing as a normal or typical female breast. Breasts come in all shapes and sizes, with varying textures from smooth to extremely lumpy. The tissues of the female breast change in response to hormone levels, normal aging, nursing (lactation), weight fluctuations, and injury. To further complicate matters, the breast has several types of tissue; each of these tissue types may respond differently to changes in body chemistry.

Fibrocystic breast condition may be called fibrocystic disease, although it is clearly not a single, specific disease process. Variations or changes in the way the breast feels or looks on **x ray** may cause the condition to be called "fibrocystic change." Other names have been used to refer to this imprecise and ill-defined term: mammary dysplasia, mastopathy, chronic cystic mastitis, indurative mastopathy, mastalgia, lumpy breasts, or physiologic nodularity.

Estimates vary, but 40–90% of all women have some evidence of "fibrocystic" condition, change, or disease. It is most common among women between the ages 30 and 50, but may be seen at other ages.

Causes and symptoms

Fibrocystic condition of the breast refers to technical findings on diagnostic testing (signs); however, this discussion focuses on symptoms that may fall under the general category of the fibrocystic condition. First, a brief review of the structure and function of the breast may be useful.

The breast is not supposed to be a soft, smooth organ. It is actually a type of sweat gland. Milk, the breasts' version of sweat, is secreted when the breast receives appropriate hormonal and environmental stimulation.

The normal breast contains milk glands, with their accompanying ducts, or pipelines, for transporting the milk. These complex structures may not only alter in size, but can increase or decrease in number as needed. Fibrous connective tissue, fatty tissue, nerves, blood and lymph vessels, and lymph nodes, with their different shapes and textures, lie among the ever-changing milk glands. It is no wonder that a woman's breasts may not feel uniform in texture and that the "lumpiness" may wax and wane.

The fibrocystic condition refers to the tenderness, enlargement, and/or changing "lumpiness" that many women encounter just before or during their menstrual periods. At this time, female hormones are preparing the breasts for pregnancy, by stimulating the milk-producing cells, and storing fluid. Each breast may contain as much as three to six teaspoons of excess fluid. Swelling, with increased sensitivity or pain, may result. If pregnancy does not occur, the body reabsorbs the fluid, and the engorgement and discomfort are relieved.

Symptoms of fibrocystic breast condition range from mildly annoying in some women to extremely painful in others. The severity of discomfort may vary from month to month in the same woman. Although sometimes distressing, this experience is the body's normal response to routine hormonal changes.

This cycle of breast sensitivity, pain and/or enlargement, can also result from medications. Some hormone replacement therapies (estrogen and progesterone) used for postmenopausal women can produce these effects. Other medications, primarily, but not exclusively those with hormones may also provoke these symptoms.

Breast pain unrelated to hormone shifts is called "noncyclic" pain. "Trigger-zone breast pain" is a term that may also be used to describe this area-specific pain. This type of pain may be continuous, or it may be felt intermittently. Trauma, such as a blow to the chest area, a prior breast **biopsy**, or sensitivity to certain medications may also underlie this type of pain. Fibrocystic condition of the breast may be cited as the cause of otherwise unexplained breast pain.

Lumps, apart from those clearly associated with hormone cycles, may also be placed under the heading of fibrocystic condition. These lumps stand out from enlarged general breast tissue. Although noncancerous lumps may occur, the obvious concern with such lumps is cancer.

Noncancerous breast lumps include:

- Adenosis. This condition refers to the enlargement of breast lobules, which contain a greater number of glands than usual. If a group of lobules are found near each other, the affected area may be large enough to be felt.
- Cysts. These are fluid-filled sacs in the breast and probably develop as ducts that become clogged with old cells in the process of normal emptying and filling. Cysts usually feel soft and round or oval. However a cyst deep within the breast may feel hard, as it pushes up against firmer breast tissue. A woman with a cyst may experience pain, especially if it increases in size before her menstrual cycle, as is often the case. Women between the age of 30 and 50 are most likely to develop cysts.
- Epithelial hyperplasia. Also called proliferative breast disease, this condition refers to an overgrowth of cells lining either the ducts or the lobules.
- Fibroadenomas. These are tumors that form in the tissues outside the milk ducts. The cause of fibroadenomas is unknown. They generally feel smooth and firm, with a somewhat rubber-like texture. Typically a fibroadenoma is not attached to surrounding tissue and moves slightly when touched. They are most commonly found in adolescents and women in their early twenties but can occur at any age.
- Fibrosis. Sometimes one area of breast tissue persistently feels thicker or more prominent than the rest of the breast. This feeling may be caused by old hardened scar tissue and/or dead fat tissue as a result of surgery or trauma. Often the cause of this type of breast tissue is unknown.
- Miscellaneous disorders. A number of other benign (noncancerous) breast problems may be placed under the heading of "fibrocystic condition." These problems include disorders that may lead to breast inflammation (mastitis), infection, and/or nipple discharge.

Atypical ductal hyperplasia

The condition known as atypical ductal hyperplasia (ADH) is a condition in which the cells lining the milk ducts of the breast are growing abnormally. This condition may appear as spots of calcium, or calcifications, on the mammogram. A biopsy removed from the breast would confirm the diagnosis. Atypical ductal hyperplasia is not a cancer. In most women, this condition will cause no problems. However, for some women, especially women with family histories of breast cancer, the risk of developing breast cancer is increased. (One study with over 3,000 female participants indicated that about 20% of the participants with atypical hyperplasia and a family history of breast cancer developed breast cancer, as compared to the 8% of participants who developed the disease with atypical hyperplasia and no family history of breast cancer.) For women with ADH and a family history of breast cancer, more frequent mammograms and closer monitoring may be required.

Diagnosis

Breast cancer is the most common concern of women who feel a breast lump or experience an abnormal breast symptom. For peace of mind, and to rule out any possibility of cancer, any newly discovered breast lumps should be brought to the attention of a family physician or an obstetrician-gynecologist. He or she will obtain a history and conduct thorough physical examination of the area. Depending on the findings on physical examination, the patient is usually referred for tests. The most common of these tests include:

- **Mammography**. A mammogram is an x-ray examination of the breasts. The two major types of abnormalities doctors look for are masses and calcifications; either abnormality may be benign or malignant. The size, shape, and edges of these masses help doctors determine whether or not cancer is present. Sometimes, however, this test may be difficult to interpret, however, due to dense breast tissue.
- Ultrasonography. If a suspicious lump is detected during mammography, an ultrasound (the use of high-frequency sound waves to outline the shape of various organs and tissues in the body) is useful (although not definitive) in distinguishing benign from cancerous growths.
- Ductography. A **ductogram** (also called a galactogram) is a test that is sometimes useful in evaluating nipple discharge. A very fine tube is threaded into the opening of the duct onto the nipple. A small amount of dye is injected, outlining the shape of the duct on an x ray, and indicates whether or not there is a mass in the duct.
- Biopsy. If a lump cannot be proven benign by mammography and ultrasound, a breast biopsy may be considered. Usually a tissue sample is removed through a needle (fine-needle aspiration biopsy, or FNAB) to obtain a sample of the lump. The sample is examined under the microscope by a pathologist, and a detailed diagnosis regarding the type of benign lesion or cancer is established. In some cases, however, FNAB may not provide a clear diagnosis, and another type of biopsy (such as a surgical biopsy, core-needle biopsy, or other stereotactic

biopsy methods—such as the Mammotome or Advanced Breast Biopsy Instrument) may be required.

Other breast conditions such as inflammation or infection are usually recognized on the basis of suspicious history, breastfeeding, or characteristic symptoms such as pain, redness, and swelling. A positive response to appropriate therapies often confirms the diagnosis.

Treatment

Once a specific disorder within the broad category of fibrocystic condition is identified, treatment can be prescribed. There are a number of treatment options for women with a lump that has been diagnosed as benign. If it is not causing a great deal of pain, the growth may be left in the breast. However, some women may choose to have a lump such as a fibroadenoma surgically removed, especially if it is large. Another option to relieve the discomfort of a painful benign lump is to have the cyst suctioned, or drained. If there is any uncertainty regarding diagnosis, the fluid may be sent to the lab for analysis.

Symptoms of cycle breast sensitivity and engorgement may also be treated with diet, medication, and/or physical modifications. For example,

- Although there is no scientific data to support this claim, many women have reported relief of symptoms when caffeine was reduced or eliminated from their diets. Decreasing salt before and during the period when breasts are most sensitive may also ease swelling and discomfort. Low-fat diets and elimination of dairy products also appear to decrease soreness for some women. However, it may take several months to realize the effects of these various treatments.
- Over-the-counter analgesics such as acetaminophen (Tylenol) or ibuprofen (Advil) may be recommended. In some cases, treatment with prescription drugs such as hormones or hormone blockers may prove successful. Oral contraceptives may also be prescribed.
- Warm soaks or ice packs may provide comfort. A well-fitted support bra can minimize physical movement and do much to relieve breast discomfort. Breast massage may promote removal of excess fluid from tissues and alleviate symptoms. Massaging the breast with castor oil, straight or infused with herbs or essential oils, can help reduce and dissipate fibroadenomas as well as keep women in touch with changes in their breast tissue.
- Infections are often treated with warm compresses and **antibiotics**. Lactating women are encouraged to continue breastfeeding because it promotes drainage and healing. However, a serious infection may progress to form an abscess that may need surgical drainage.
- Some studies of alternative or complementary treatments, although controversial, have indicated that **vitamins** A, B complex and E, and mineral supplements may reduce the risk of developing fibrocystic condition of the breast. Evening primrose oil (*Oenothera biennis*), flaxseed oil, and fish oils have been reported to be effective in relieving cyclic breast pain for some women.

KEY TERMS

Advanced Breast Biopsy Instrument (ABBI)—Uses a rotating circular knife and thin heated electrical wire to remove a large cylinder of abnormal breast tissue.

Lobules—A small lobe or subdivision of a lobe (often on a gland) that may be seen on the surface of the gland by bumps or bulges.

Lymph nodes—Rounded, encapsulated bodies consisting of an accumulation of lymphatic tissue.

Mammotome—A method for removing breast biopsies using suction to draw tissue into an opening in the side of a cylinder inserted into the breast tissue. A rotating knife then cuts tissue samples from the rest of the breast; also known as a vacuum-assisted biopsy.

Stereotactic biopsy—A biopsy taken by precisely locating areas of abnormal growth through the use of delicate instruments.

Prognosis

Most benign breast conditions carry no increased risk for the development of breast cancer. However, a small percentage of biopsies uncover overgrowth of tissue in a particular pattern in some women; this pattern indicates a 15–20% increased risk of breast cancer over the next 20 years. Strict attention to early detection measures, such as annual mammograms, is especially important for these women.

Prevention

There is no proven method of preventing the various manifestations of fibrocystic condition from occurring. Some alternative health care practitioners believe that eliminating foods high in methyl xanthines (primarily coffee and chocolate) can decrease or reverse fibrocystic breast changes.

QUESTIONS TO ASK THE DOCTOR

- How common is this condition?
- Do cysts show up on mammography?
- Can fibrocystic condition of the breast lead to cancer?
- How can I tell the difference between cysts and cancer when I perform my breast self-exam?
- Can I do anything to prevent this condition?
- What are my treatment options?
- Will I have this condition forever?

Resources

BOOKS

Goldmann, David R., and David A. Horowitz, eds. *The American College of Physicians Home Medical Guide: Breast Problems.* New York: Dorling Kindersley, 2000.

Kneece, Judy C. *Finding a Lump In Your Breast.* Columbia, SC: EduCare Publishing, 1996.

Love, Susan M., with Karen Lindsey. *Dr. Susan Love's Breast Book, 3rd rev. ed.* Reading, MA.: Addison-Wesley, 2000.

Singer, Sydney Ross. *Get It Off! Understanding the Cause of Breast Pain, Cysts, and Cancer.* Pahoa, HI: ISCD Press, 2000.

PERIODICALS

"Benign Conditions." *Harvard Women's Health Watch* 5 (May 1998): 4-5.

Duijm, Lucien E.M., et al. "Value of Breast Imaging in Women With Painful Breasts: Observational Follow Up Study." *British Medical Journal* 317 (November 1998): 1492-1495.

Horner, N.K. and J.W. Lampe. "Potential Mechanisms of Diet Therapy for Fibrocystic Breast Conditions Show Inadequate Evidence of Effectiveness." *Journal of the American Dietetic Association* 100 (November 2000):1368-1380.

Mannello, F., M. Malatesta, and G. Gazzanelli. "Breast Cancer in Women With Palpable Breast Cysts." *Lancet* 354 (August 1999): 677- 678.

Morrow, Monica. "The Evaluation of Common Breast Problems." *American Family Physician* 61 (April 15, 2000): 2371-2378, 2385.

ORGANIZATIONS

American Cancer Society. 1599 Clifton Rd. NE, Atlanta, GA 30329. 1-800-ACS-2345 <http://www.cancer.org>

American College of Obstetricians and Gynecologists. 409 12th St., S.W., P.O. Box 96920, Washington, DC 20090-6920. <http://www.acog.org>

Cancer Information Service (CIS). 9000 Rockville Pike, Building 31, Suite 10A18, Bethesda, MD 20892. Phone: 1-800-4-CANCER. Free telephone service provided by the National Cancer Institute.

OTHER

National Cancer Institute. *Understanding Breast Changes: A Health Guide for All Women.* 10 July 2001 <http://rex.nci.nih.gov/MAMMOG_WEB/PUBS_POSTERS/UNDR STNDNG/UNDER_STANDING_CHANGE.html>.

Ellen S. Weber
Genevieve Slomski, Ph.D.

Fibrosarcoma

Definition

Fibrosarcoma is a malignant tumor that arises from fibroblasts (cells that produce connective tissue). This is a type of sarcoma that is predominantly found in the area around bones or in soft tissue.

Description

Fibrosarcomas are the result of fibroblasts, which produce connective tissue such as collagen. Fibrosarcoma tumors are consequently rich in collagen fibers. The immature, proliferating fibroblasts take on an interlacing, or herringbone, pattern.

Fibrosarcomas can form from fibroblasts in soft tissue such as muscles, connective tissues, blood vessels, joints, and fat. Soft tissue fibrosarcoma normally occurs in fibrous tissue of the body's trunk and the extremities such as the arms and legs. Soft tissue fibrosarcomas are extremely rare, with approximately 500 new cases reported each year.

Sarcomas of the bone

Fibrosarcoma can also occur in bones. While a bone is made up of inorganic molecules such as calcium phosphate, it also has an organic element made up of 95% collagen, similar to the collagen found in the skin. Fibrosarcomas of the bone usually occur in long bones in the bone marrow cavity where collagen is formed. The bones that predominantly yield fibrosarcomas are those in the legs, arms, pelvis, and hip.

Sarcomas of the bone are rare and represent about 0.2 percent of all new cancer cases each year. The two most common forms of bone cancer are **osteosarcoma** and **Ewing's sarcoma**. Among the less common are **chondrosarcoma**, fibrosarcoma, and **malignant fibrous histiocytoma**, all of which arise from spindle cell neoplasms.

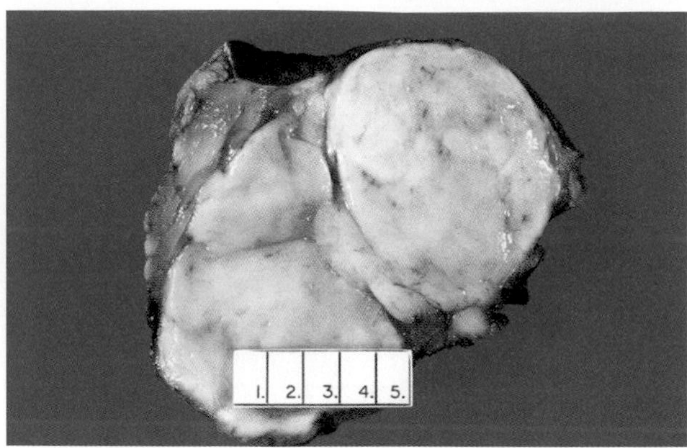

Excised specimen of a skin tumor known as a fibrosarcoma, sliced open (white). *(© Dr. E. Walker, Science Source/Photo Researchers, Inc. Reproduced by permission.)*

Demographics

Fibrosarcomas typically develop in people between the ages of 25–79. The peak age of occurrence is 55–69 years. Generally, fibrosarcomas develop equally in men and women, though they are rare in children.

Infantile fibrosarcoma, also known as congenital fibrosarcoma or juvenile fibrosarcoma, is unique. Under microscopic examination, it is similar to fibrosarcomas seen in adults. However, infantile fibrosarcomas have a more positive prognosis with a post-treatment, five-year survival rate of 83% to 94%.

Causes and symptoms

Fibrosarcomas of the bone are sometimes connected with underlying benign bone tumors. Both fibrosarcomas of soft tissue and of the bone can develop as a result of exposure to radiation. This can result as a side effect from previous **radiation therapy** for unrelated primary cancer treatment. Individuals with other bone diseases, such as Paget's disease and osteomyelitis, are at a higher risk for developing fibrosarcomas.

There are many symptoms associated with the onset of fibrosarcomas. The following is a list of the main symptoms that may be present:

- pain
- swelling
- firm lump just under the skin or on a bone
- broken bone
- impeded normal range of motion
- neurologic symptoms
- gastrointestinal bleeding (seen in soft tissue abdominal fibrosarcomas)
- urinary frequency (seen in pelvic fibrosarcomas)
- urinary obstruction (seen in pelvic fibrosarcomas)

Diagnosis

In order to diagnose fibrosarcoma, a doctor will take the patient's medical history and will conduct a thorough physical exam. Blood tests will be performed to rule out other conditions and to identify cancer markers.

The most revealing initial exam is an **x ray**. It can show the location, size, and shape of the tumor. If a malignant tumor is present, the x ray will expose a soft tissue mass with ill-defined edges. This procedure takes less than an hour and can be performed in the doctor's office.

Once there is evidence of a tumor, one or more of several other procedures may be performed, including **computed tomography** (CT) scans, **magnetic resonance imaging** (MRI), angiograms, and biopsies.

Treatment team

The patient's primary care physician may perform the initial diagnostic tests. However, in order to comprehensively diagnose and treat fibrosarcomas, the primary care physician will refer the patient to an oncologist (cancer specialist). Radiologists, pathologists, and surgeons will also be involved to read x rays, examine tissue samples, and, if needed, remove the tumor.

Other individuals might be involved with the treatment of fibrosarcoma, including nurses, dieticians, and physical or vocational therapists.

Clinical staging, treatments, and prognosis

After the physician makes the diagnosis, it is important to determine the stage of the cancer. This will help reveal how far the cancer has progressed and how much tissue has been affected.

The American Joint Committee on Cancer developed the most widely used staging system for fibrosarcomas. The foremost categories of this system include grade (G), size of the tumor (T), lymph node involvement (N), and presence of metastases (M). Low grade and high grade are designated G1 and G3, respectively. The size of the tumor can be less than 5 centimeters (2 inches), designated as T1, or greater than 5 centimeters, designated as T2. If the lymph nodes are involved, N1 is designated, while no lymph involvement is designated N0. Finally, there may be a presence of distant metastases (M1), or no metastases (M0). The following is a list of stages and their indications:

- Stage IA: (G1, T1, N0, M0)
- Stage IB: (G1, T2, N0, M0)
- Stage IIA: (G2, T1, N0, M0)
- Stage IIB: (G2, T2, N0, M0)
- Stage IIIA: (G3, T1, N0, M0)
- Stage IIIB: (G3, T2, N0, M0)
- Stage IVA: (Any G, any T, N1, M0)
- Stage IVB: (Any G, any T, N1, M1)

Tumors with lower stage numbers, such as IA and IB, contain cells that look very similar to normal cells, while tumors with higher stage designations are composed of cells that appear very different from normal cells. In higher staged tumors, the cells appear undifferentiated.

Physicians can employ several courses of treatment to remove fibrosarcomas. The most effective treatment is surgical removal; this is used as a primary treatment for all stages of fibrosarcoma. When performing the surgery, the surgeon will remove the tumor and some healthy soft tissue or bone around it to ensure that the tumor does not recur near the original site.

Prior to surgery, large tumors (greater than 5 centimeters, or 2 inches) may be treated with **chemotherapy** or radiation in order to shrink them, thus rendering the surgical procedure more effective.

Even individuals with low-grade fibrosarcoma who have undergone surgery experience a moderate risk of local recurrence. To combat recurrence, adjuvant chemotherapy (the use of one or more cancer-killing drugs) and radiation therapy (the use of high-energy rays), such as irradiation and brachytherapy, are also used to complement surgery. Employing chemotherapy or radiation therapy individually without surgery is much less effective.

After therapy, low-stage fibrosarcomas (stages IA and IB) have greater five-year survival rates than high stages (Stages IVA and IVB). Because high-grade tumors are more aggressive and more highly metastatic than lower grade tumors, patients with high-grade tumors have a lower survival rate. Not only is the grade of the tumor (the estimate of its aggressiveness) important in determining prognosis, the age of the patient is also crucial. Generally, fibrosarcomas that occur in childhood and infancy have a lower mortality rate than those that occur in adults. Additionally, patients with fibrosarcomas that occur in the extremities have a better survival rate than those with fibrosarcomas in the visceral region.

Metastases appear later in the development of fibrosarcomas. The lungs are the primary sites of **metastasis** for fibrosarcomas that develop in the extremities. Once metastasis to the lungs has occurred, the chances of survival are significantly decreased.

KEY TERMS

Adjuvant—A treatment that has been added to a curative treatment to combat recurrence.

Brachytherapy—Radiotherapy that places the source of radiation close to the surface of the body or within a body cavity.

Carcinogen—An agent that is capable of causing cancer.

Epiphysis—The end of long tubular bones such as femur in the leg and the humerus in the arm.

Spindle cell—Cells shaped like a spindle, typically found in connective tissue.

Undifferentiated—Cells that have not matured normally, and do not function properly.

Visceral—Having to do with an organ in the human torso.

Alternative and complementary therapies

Many individuals choose to supplement traditional therapy with complementary methods. Often, these methods improve the tolerance of side effects and symptoms, as well as enrich the quality of life. The American Cancer Society recommends that patients talk to their doctor to ensure that the methods they choose are safely supplementing their traditional therapy. Some **complementary cancer therapies** include the following:

- yoga
- meditation
- religious practices and prayer
- music therapy
- art therapy
- massage therapy
- aromatherapy

Coping with cancer treatment

Chemotherapy often results in several side effects, depending on the drug used and the patient's individual tolerance. Patients may have to deal with nausea, vomiting, loss of appetite (**anorexia**), and hair loss (**alopecia**). Many times, chemotherapy as well as radiation therapy are better handled if patients are eating well. Nurses and dieticians can aid patients in choosing healthful foods to incorporate into their diet.

QUESTIONS TO ASK THE DOCTOR

- What diagnostic procedures are best for the location and type of tumor suspected?
- What treatments are best for the location and type of tumor suspected?
- What kinds of side effects will this course of treatment cause?
- Are there support services available?
- What treatments are currently in clinical trials?
- What treatments will my health care insurance cover?
- What alternative treatments are safe?

If the fibrosarcoma necessitated a limb **amputation**, then patients will need to learn how to cope with a prosthetic device. Both physical and vocational therapists can effectively help patients adjust and learn how to use the prosthetic device to perform their daily activities.

Clinical trials

Fibrosarcomas are rare, but advances are being made in both diagnostic and curative procedures. Although surgery is the most effective treatment, both pre- and post-operative adjuvant therapies are being researched to complement surgery.

Exploring the results of chemotherapy trials uncovers a trend of improved results with more intense regimens—meaning higher and more prolonged doses of drug therapy. Drugs that are being studied in 2001 include **cyclophosphamide**, **doxorubicin**, **methotrexate**, **vincristine**, **dacarbazine**, **dactinomycin**, or a combination of two or three of these.

Patients should consult with their physicians or contact the American Cancer Society to learn what procedures are currently being investigated in **clinical trials**. In some cases, insurance companies will not cover procedures that are part of clinical trials. Patients should talk with their doctor and insurance company to determine which procedures are covered.

Prevention

The prevention of cancer can be assisted by avoiding known chemical carcinogens such as alpha-naphthylamine, carbon tetrachloride, and benzene. Another way to avoid developing cancer is to minimize exposure to penetrating radiation such as x rays and radioactive elements. Medical x rays revolutionized the field of medicine and are used to detect and treat many diseases. In most cases, the benefits of medical x rays outweigh the risks.

Special concerns

Treatment, especially surgical amputation, can take a physical and psychological toll on cancer patients and their families. To deal with the psychological impact, there are many different support groups and psychotherapists that can help. Some therapists will consider amputation a posttraumatic stress disorder, and treat it accordingly. To deal with their condition, relying on faith practices can also be beneficial for cancer patients. Patients should discuss all options with their physician to determine what is available.

Once the cancer has been treated, patients should make sure to schedule follow-up appointments with their physicians. Physicians will want to monitor the patient for side effects or possible recurrence that may develop years after treatment.

Resources

BOOKS

Cordon-Cardo, Carlos. "Sarcomas of the Soft Tissues and Bone." In *Cancer Principles and Practice of Oncology.*, edited by Vincent T. DeVita, Jr. et al. New York: Lippincott-Raven Publishers, 1997, pp.1731-82.

Rosen, Gerald. "Sarcomas of Nonosseous Tissues." In *Cancer Medicine*, edited by Robert C. Bast Jr. et al. London: BC Decker, Inc., 2000, pp.1901-1921.

PERIODICALS

Palumbo, Joseph S., et al. "Soft Tissue Sarcomas of Infancy." *Seminars in Perinatology* (August 1999): 299-309.

ORGANIZATION

American Cancer Society (National Headquarters). 1599 Clifton Road, N.E. Atlanta, GA 30329. (800) 227-2345. <http://www.cancer.org>.

Cancer Research Institute (National Headquarters). 681 Fifth Avenue, New York, NY 10022. (800) 992-2623. <http://www.cancerresearch.org>.

Sally C. McFarlane-Parrott

Filgrastim

Definition

Filgrastim is a medicine used to increase the white blood cell count in the body, which will help prevent infection. Filgrastim is known by the brand name Neupogen.

Purpose

Filgrastim is a drug approved by the Food and Drug Administration (FDA) to increase white blood cell counts. If a patient has a lower than normal white blood cell count it is referred to as **neutropenia**.

Filgrastim can be used to treat neutropenia caused by cancer **chemotherapy** treatment. In these patients the filgrastim increases the recovery of white blood cells after chemotherapy. Filgrastim can also be used to treat patients who have a neutropenia not related to chemotherapy. In both cases, the filgrastim decreases the risk of **fever** and infection.

Filgrastim is not usually used in leukemia patients. However, in patients with the disease known as **acute myelcytic leukemia** it is approved for use after chemotherapy. Filgrastim can increase the recovery of the white blood cell count thereby decreasing the length of time a patient may have a fever associated with a low white count.

Filgrastim can also be used after **bone marrow transplantation**. Once the new healthy bone marrow has been given back to a patient, filgrastim can be administered to help increase the white blood cell count and decrease the risk of fever and infection.

Filgrastim can be used for patients who will receive a peripheral blood stem cell transplant. Patients will receive the filgrastim before the transplant. The filgrastim in these patients causes young, non-developed blood cells, known as stem or progenitor cells, to move from the bone marrow to the blood where they will then be removed from a patient by the process of apheresis. These blood cells are stored until after the patient receives larges doses of chemotherapy that destroy the bone marrow and the cancer. The patient then receives these stored cells back by an intravenous infusion. The stored cells repopulate the bone marrow and develop into the many types of functioning blood cells.

Description

Filgrastim has been available to cancer patients since the 1990s, and is highly effective at decreasing neutropenia. Filgrastim may be referred to as G-CSF, granulocyte colony stimulating factor, colony stimulating factor. This compound is manufactured by recombinant DNA methods using E. coli as the host organism. Chemotherapy destroys white blood cells temporarily. These white blood cells will grow again, but during the time that the levels are low, patients are at an increased risk of developing fevers and infection. Filgrastim acts to stimulate the bone marrow to make more white blood cells, which can either prevent the white count from dropping below normal or decrease the time that the level is low. By effectively avoiding fevers and infections, patients are able to receive their next doses of chemotherapy without delay.

Recommended dosage

Filgrastim is a clear colorless liquid that is dosed on body weight in kilograms. It is kept refrigerated until ready to use, and it is administered to patients as a subcutaneous injection (directly underneath the skin) It is usually administered in the back of the arms, upper legs, or stomach area. Filgrastim can also be given to patients as a short intravenous infusion into a vein over 15 to 30 minutes.

Chemotherapy-caused neutropenia

The starting dose for patients who have just finished chemotherapy is 5 micrograms per kilogram of body weight per day. This is given as a subcutaneous injection under the skin daily for up to 14 consecutive days, and sometimes longer. The doctor will inform the patient when it is time to stop the filgrastim.

Bone marrow transplants

The recommended dose is 10 micrograms per kilogram per day. This can be administered as a 4- to 24-hour infusion intravenously, or as a 24-hour subcutaneous infusion.

Peripheral blood stem cell transplant

The recommended dose is 10 micrograms per kilogram per day. This can be given either as a under the skin injection, intravenously, or as a continuous infusion over 24 hours. This dosing should begin four days before the first apheresis collection process and continue until the last day of collection.

Other neutropenia

The dose recommendation is variable based on the reason for neutropenia. The range of filgrastim doses has been from 5 micrograms per kilogram per day up to 100 microgram per kilogram per day. Doctors may increase the filgrastim dose based on how the white blood cell count responds to the treatment. Other factors that play a role in filgrastim dosing include how low the white blood cell count is and the length of time the white blood cell count remains low.

Precautions

Filgrastim should not be received by a patient in the 24-hour time frame before or after receiving chemotherapy or reinfusion of bone marrow or stem cells.

KEY TERMS

Food and Drug Administration (FDA)—A government agency that oversees public safety in relation to drugs and medical devices. The FDA gives the approval to pharmaceutical companies for commercial marketing of their products.

Chemotherapy—Specific drugs used to treat cancer.

Subcutaneous—Underneath the initial layer of skin.

Intravenous—To enter the body through a vein.

Reinfusion—The transfer through a vein of healthy stem cells or bone marrow to a patient that had received larges doses of chemotherapy used to destroy cancer cells.

Neutropenia—Low white blood cell count.

Recovery—Blood counts that are returning back to normal levels.

Apheresis—The process of removing and collecting specific cells from the blood through a machine.

Peripheral blood stem cell transplant—A procedure that collects and stores healthy young and non-developed blood stem cells. These are then given back to a patient to help them recovery from high doses of chemotherapy that they received to destroy their cancer.

Bone marrow transplant—A procedure that destroys all of a patients' diseased bone marrow and replaces it with healthy bone marrow.

Blood counts will be monitored while on the drug filgrastim. This allows the doctor to determine if the drug is working and when to stop the drug.

It is not recommended to give filgrastim to patients who have certain types leukemias.

Patients with a known previous allergic reaction to filgrastim or to any other substance that derived from the bacteria *E-Coli* should not take filgrastim.

Patients who may be pregnant, or trying to become pregnant, should tell their doctor before receiving filgrastim.

Side effects

The most common side effect from the filgrastim is **bone pain**. The filgrastim causes the bone marrow to produce more white blood cells, and, as a result, patients may experience pain in their bones. Tylenol, an over-the-counter pain reliever, can usually control mild to moderate pain that occurs with standard dosed filgrastim. Larger doses of filgrastim, like those given for bone marrow transplant patients, can cause severe bone pain that may need a prescription pain reliever to ease the pain.

Another common side effect due to filgrastim administration is pain or burning at the site of the injection. This can be decreased by bringing the filgrastim to room temperature before administering the injection, icing the area of injection to numb it before receiving the injection, and moving the site of the injection with each dose.

Patients who have received filgrastim after cancer chemotherapy have reported fever, **nausea and vomiting**, muscle pain, **diarrhea**, hair loss (**alopecia**), mouth sores, fatigue, shortness of breath, weakness, headache, cough, rash, constipation, and pain. These side effects may be due to the chemotherapy administration.

Interactions

Filgrastim should not be given at the same time as chemotherapy or **radiation therapy**. Dosing should begin at least 24 hours after the last dose of treatment.

Patients on the drug lithium should tell their doctor before starting filgrastim therapy.

Filgrastim use for delayed **myelosuppression** has not been studied after the use of the chemotherapy agents **mitomycin-C**, and nitrosoureas, or after the drug **fluorouracil**.

Nancy J. Beaulieu, RPh., BCOP

Flow cytometry

Definition

Flow cytometry, is a method of sorting and measuring types of cells by fluorescent labeling of markers on the surface of the cells. It is sometimes referred to as FACS (Fluorescent Activated Cell Sorting) analysis.

Purpose

Flow cytometric analysis is most often clinically used to help determine the type of leukemia or **lymphoma** a patient has and to assess the prognosis. Flow cytometry is quite sensitive; it is able to detect rare cell types and residual levels of disease.

KEY TERMS

Antibody—A protein formed by the immune system (white blood cells) which reacts with a specific antigen.

Cytometer—An instrument that measures cells.

Fluorescence—Light absorbed at one wavelength and emitted at another. That is, it glows.

QUESTIONS TO ASK THE DOCTOR

- What type of information do you expect to learn from this test?
- Are there any alternatives to doing this test?
- Are there any risks or complications?
- Are there any special preparations required?
- Is it possible that the test may give unclear or inaccurate results?
- Is this the best way to tell if, or what type of cancer I have?

Precautions

Drugs, such as steroids, that suppress the immune system will affect the number of white blood cells in the patient's sample.

Description

The physician will select a sample based on the type of cancer the patient is thought to have. In the case of lymphoma, the sample may be collected by fine needle aspiration **biopsy**, then the tissue sample will be separated into single cells. Analysis of leukemia will require a patient to give a blood sample. The patient's blood sample will be separated and the red blood cells removed. The sample will be mixed with a variety of different antibodies that can interact with markers on the surface of the cells. Different types of cells have characteristic markers on their cell surfaces, so a particular cell type can be identified by the antibodies that bind to it. The antibodies are labeled so that they will give off fluorescent light (glow) as they pass through the laser beam in the cytometer. The cytometer also measures the size of the cell and some information about the interior of the cell. The physician uses this information to determine the specific type of leukemia, such as myelogenous or lymphocytic, which in turn, helps to determine the type of treatment that will be best suited to the patient.

Sample analysis may also be performed using a more complex type of flow cytometer combined with a microscope, called a laser-scanning cytometer. This instrument is similar to a regular flow cytometer, but is better able to analyze solid tumor samples.

Preparation

Flow cytometry is usually performed on blood, body fluids, or bone marrow. In most cases, no special preparation is required. If bone marrow aspiration is necessary or a biopsy is required from a solid tumor, the patient should be appropriately prepared for these procedures. However, the flow cytometry itself does not require any additional preparation on the part of the patient.

Aftercare and Risks

The only aftercare and risks associated with flow cytometric analysis are those associated with the sample collection procedure. The cell analysis itself requires no effort or risk from the patient.

Normal results

A normal result will indicate that there is no increase in the number of any particular type of immune cell. The pathologist will see several different types of cells, but no one type will be present in increased numbers.

Abnormal results

If the results are abnormal, the pathologist will observe an unusually large number of one particular cell type. The types of marker present on the cell will give further information about the type of leukemia or lymphoma and may indicate the patient's prognosis. For example, leukemic cells that have markers that are normally found on less mature cell types may suggest a poorer prognosis, and therefore more aggressive therapy may be recommended.

See Also Tumor grading

Resources

BOOKS

Javois, Lorette C.*Immunocytochemical Methods and Protocols* Totowa, NJ: Humana Press, 1999.

PERIODICALS

Rew, David A. et al. "Laser-scanning Cytometry." In *The Lancet* 353: (23 January 1999): 255–56.

Rosen, Shara, "Flow Cytometry: an Underexploited Diagnostic Power."*Medical Laboratory Observer* 30(March 1998): 52–58.

OTHER

"FACS Laboratory."*Imperial Cancer Research Fund* <http://www.icnet.uk> 5 July 2001.

"Flow Cytometry Core Educational Links."*University of Florida* <http://www.biotech.ufl.edu/~fccl/flow_edu.html> 6 July 2001.

Racquel Baert, M.S.

Floxuridine

Definition

Floxuridine is an anti-cancer drug that is injected directly into the artery that carries blood to the liver or the abdominal cavity. The brand names of floxuridine are Fluorodeoxyuridine, FUDR, and Floxuridine For Injection USP. The generic name product may be available in the United States.

Purpose

Floxuridine is used to treat **gastrointestinal cancers** that have metastasized, or spread, to the liver. These cancers include **rectal cancer** and Stage IV **colon cancer**. Floxuridine also has been used to treat cancerous gastrointestinal tumors; however the response rate is poor and usually the drug is used only to relieve symptoms.

Description

Floxuridine is approved by the United States Food and Drug Administration.

Floxuridine is a type of medicine called an antimetabolite because it interferes with the metabolism and growth of cells. Floxuridine prevents the production of DNA in cells. The cells cannot reproduce and eventually they die.

Floxuridine sometimes is used in conjunction with the drugs **fluorouracil** (5-FU), **cisplatin**, and/or **leucovorin**. Leucovorin increases the activity of floxuridine. In general, floxuridine is more effective than other chemotherapies against liver metastases, but its use does not improve overall survival rates. Ongoing studies are comparing floxuridine with other chemotherapies. The drug may be used in conjunction with surgery. Its use in conjunction with **radiation therapy** is being evaluated.

Recommended dosage

Floxuridine is injected directly into the liver. This is called hepatic intra-arterial infusion, or **hepatic arterial infusion**. A special pump delivers the drug through an implanted infusion port or catheter into an artery that goes to the liver. Injection of floxuridine into a vein is being evaluated. Floxuridine also may be injected into the abdominal cavity (intraperitoneal therapy). The dosage of floxuridine depends on a number of factors including body weight, type of cancer, and any other medicines that are being used.

Precautions

Floxuridine may lower the number of white blood cells and, therefore, reduce the body's ability to fight infection. Immunizations (vaccinations) should be avoided during or after treatment with floxuridine because of the risk of infection. It also is important to avoid contact with individuals who have recently taken an oral polio vaccine. Treatment with floxuridine may cause chicken pox or shingles (**Herpes zoster**) to become very severe and spread to other parts of the body.

Kidney or liver diseases may increase the effects of floxuridine, since the drug may be removed from the body at a slower rate. Floxuridine also may put an individual at an increased risk for hepatitis.

Floxuridine can cause birth defects in animals. Therefore this drug should not be taken by pregnant women or by either the man or the woman at the time of conception. Women usually are advised against breastfeeding while receiving this drug.

Side effects

Since floxuridine may affect the growth of normal cells as well as cancer cells, side effects may occur during or after drug treatment. Some effects may occur months or even years after the drug is administered. Floxuridine increases the risk of later developing certain types of cancer, such as leukemia.

The more common side effects of floxuridine include:

- **diarrhea**
- loss of appetite (**anorexia**)
- sores in the mouth or on the lips
- stomach pain or cramps
- numbness or tingling in the hands and feet

Less common side effects of floxuridine include:

- **nausea and vomiting**
- black, tar-like stools
- heartburn
- redness or scaling of the hands or feet
- sore, swollen tongue
- skin rash or itching
- temporary thinning of hair (**alopecia**)
- bleeding at the site of the catheter
- infection from the catheter
- closing off of the catheter

Other, rare side effects of floxuridine include:

- blood in urine or stools
- hiccups
- hoarseness or coughing
- fever or chills
- sore throat
- difficulty swallowing
- blurred vision
- lower back or side pain
- painful or difficult urination
- small red skin spots
- difficulty walking
- bleeding or bruising
- yellow eyes or skin
- seizures
- **depression**

In addition to lowering the white blood cell count, increasing the risk of infection, floxuridine may reduce the level of blood platelets that are necessary for normal blood clotting. This can increase the risk of bleeding. The drug also may lead to abnormalities in liver function. Intraperitoneal floxuridine therapy has been associated with the development of fibrous masses in the abdomen.

Interactions

Previous treatment with radiation or other anti-cancer drugs can increase the effects of floxuridine on the blood.

Drugs that may interact with floxuridine include:

- amphotericin B (Fungizone)
- antithyroid drugs that are used to treat an overactive thyroid
- **azathioprine** (Imuran)
- chloramphenicol (Chloromycetin)
- colchicine
- flucytosine (Ancobon)
- ganciclovir (Cytovene)
- interferon (Intron A, Roferon-A)
- plicamycin (Mithracin)
- zidovudine (AZT, Retrovir)

Margaret Alic, Ph.D.

KEY TERMS

Catheter—Tube used to inject medicine into the body.

Hepatic intra-arterial infusion—Injection of medicine into the artery to the liver.

Intraperitoneal—Within the abdominal cavity.

Metastasis—Spread of cancer from its point of origin to other parts of the body.

Fluconazole *see* **Antifungal therapy**

Fludarabine

Definition

Fludarabine is a **chemotherapy** medicine used to treat certain types of cancer by destroying cancerous cells. It is known as the brand name Fludara. Fludarabine may also be referred to as Fludarabine phosphate, 2-fluoroadenine aribinoside 5-phosphate, and FAMP.

Purpose

Fludarabine is approved by the Food and Drug Administration (FDA) to treat refractory **chronic lymphocytic leukemia** (CLL). Patients must have a disease that did not respond to other treatment or a disease that became worse during other treatment. Fludarabine has also been used to treat Hodgkin's and non-Hodgkin's **lymphoma**, **cutaneous T-cell lymphoma**, macroglobulinemic lymphoma, **mycosis fungoides**, and **hairy cell leukemia**.

KEY TERMS

Anemia—A red blood cell count that is lower than normal.

Chemotherapy—Specific drugs used to treat cancer.

Deoxynucleic acid (DNA)—Genetic material inside of cells that carries the information to make proteins that are necessary to run the cells and keep the body functioning smoothly.

Electrolytes—Elements normally found in the body (sodium, potassium, calcium, magnesium, phosphorus, chloride, and acetate) that are important to maintain the many cellular functions and growth.

Food and Drug Administration (FDA)—The government agency that oversees public safety in relation to drugs and medical devices, and gives the approval to pharmaceutical companies for commercial marketing of their products.

Gout—A disease caused by the build up of uric acid in the joints causing swelling and pain.

Intravenous—To enter the body through a vein.

Neutropenia—A white blood cell count that is lower than normal.

Refractory—Cancer that no longer responds to treatment.

Description

Fludarabine has been available for use since the early 1990s, and is a member of the group of chemotherapy drugs known as antimetabolites. Antimetabolites interfere with the genetic material (DNA) inside the cancer cells and prevent them from further dividing and growing more cancer cells.

Recommended dosage

Fludarabine is a clear solution that is administered through a vein.

A fludarabine dose can be determined using a mathematical calculation that measures a person's body surface area (BSA). This number is dependent upon a patient's height and weight. The larger the person, the greater the body surface area. BSA is measured in the units known as square meter (m^2). The body surface area is calculated and then multiplied by the drug dosage in milligrams per square meter (mg/m^2). This calculates the actual dose a patient is to receive.

The approved dose for chronic lymphocytic leukemia is 25 milligrams per square meter per day for 5 days in a row. The fludarabine is given intravenously into a vein over a 30-minute to 2-hour time period. This 5-day cycle is repeated every 4 weeks.

The dose of fludarabine may need to be decreased in patients who have kidney problems.

Precautions

Blood counts will be monitored regularly while on fludarabine therapy. During a certain time period after receiving fludarabine, there is an increased risk of getting infections. Caution should be taken to avoid unnecessary exposure to crowds and people with infections.

Patients with a known previous allergic reaction to chemotherapy drugs should tell their doctor.

Patients who may be pregnant or are trying to become pregnant should tell their doctor before receiving fludarabine. Chemotherapy can cause men and women to be sterile, or unable to have children. It is unknown if fludarabine has this effect on humans.

Patients should check with their doctors before receiving live virus **vaccines** while on chemotherapy.

Side effects

The most common side effect expected from taking fludarabine is low blood counts (**myelosuppression**). When the white blood cell count is lower than normal (**neutropenia**), patients are at an increased risk of developing a **fever** and infections. Patients may need to be treated with **antibiotics** at this point. The platelet blood count can also be decreased due to fludarabine administration, but generally returns to normal within 2 weeks after the end of the infusion. Platelets are blood cells that cause clots to form to stop bleeding. When the platelet count is low, patients are at an increased risk for bruising and bleeding. Fludarabine causes low red blood cell counts (**anemia**). Low red counts make people feel tired and dizzy.

Fludarabine can cause the development of autoimmune **hemolytic anemia**, which occurs when the body begins to destroy its own red blood cells. It is an uncommon side effect, but very serious when it occurs.

Common side effects from fludarabine include **nausea and vomiting**. If nausea and vomiting are a problem, patients can be given **antiemetics** before receiving fludarabine. This medication helps prevent or decrease these side effects. Other common side effects include **fever**, chills, joint pain, fluid gain, fatigue, sleepiness, pain, muscle ache, weakness, and infection. Other less common side effects include loss of appetite (**anorexia**), **diarrhea**, abnormal touch sensation, cough, **pneumonia**, and shortness of breath.

Damage to the nerves and nervous system tissues can occur with fludarabine. Side effects due to this nerve damage include sleepiness, confusion, weakness, fatigue, irritability, numbness or tingling in the hands and feet, visual changes, and difficulty walking.

Infrequent side effects of fludarabine are skin rashes, pain, **itching**, fever, lung problems, insomnia, headache, muscle and joint aches, swelling, and decreased blood pressure.

Rare side effects of fludarabine include mouth sores, constipation and abdominal cramping, bleeding from the bladder, hair loss (**alopecia**), hearing problems, and liver and kidney problems.

Fludarabine can cause the rapid breakdown of cancer cells. Patients that have large numbers of cancer cells in their blood stream can develop a problem known as **tumor lysis syndrome**. The symptoms of this syndrome include pain in the lower back and blood in the urine. A patient can develop high or low levels of electrolytes and high levels of uric acid, which can lead to gout and kidney damage. The drug **allopurinol** may be given to patients prior to fludarabine treatment to prevent this from occurring. Drinking an increased amount of liquids also may help prevent the kidney damage.

All side effects a patient experiences should be reported to the doctor.

Interactions

Fludarabine should not be used in combination with the drug **pentostatin**. The combination causes severe lung damage.

Nancy J. Beaulieu, R.Ph., B.C.O.P.

Fluorouracil

Definition

Fluorouracil is a medication that kills cancer cells. It is also known as 5-FU or 5-fluourouracil, and as the brand name Adrucil.

Purpose

5-FU may be used in combination with other **chemotherapy** agents to treat cancers of the breast, stomach, colon, rectum, and pancreas.

KEY TERMS

Cytotoxic drug—A medicine that kills (cancer) cells.

DNA—A molecule found in all living cells that contains tiny bits of genetic information.

Infusion therapy—Administration of a medication as a liquid through an intravenous (IV) device.

RNA—A molecule found in all living cells that plays a role in transmitting information from the DNA to the protein-forming system of the cell.

Description

5-FU is a cytotoxic drug. This means that it kills cancer cells. 5-FU kills cells by interfering with the activities of DNA and RNA, which are molecules in the cells important in expressing genetic material.

Recommended dosage

Most frequently, 5-FU is given as an injection into the vein (intravaneous injection or IV). Many different doses and regimens are used depending on the cancer diagnosis, and patients should discuss with their physician the dose based on the individual protocol used. A sample dose is 500 to 1,000 mg per square meter of body surface area given as a 24-hour infusion for four to five days every three weeks. A dose of 425 mg per square meter of body surface area per day for five days given along with the drug **leucovorin** is also common.

Precautions

Patients with allergic reaction to 5-FU should not be administered this drug. It is also inadvisable for pregnant women. 5-FU should be administered with caution to patients with impaired liver or kidney function, or in patients with a history of heart problems.

Side effects

The amount of drug given and the duration of which it is given during a single session greatly influences the side effects seen. For example, when given as a 24-hour continuous infusion, the most common side effects are **diarrhea** and mouth ulcers. If 5-FU is given as a bolus infusion (a high quantity of the drug all at once), the most common side effect is bone marrow suppression; this results in a decrease of the white blood cells responsible for fighting infections, the platelets responsible for blood clotting, and the red blood cells responsible for providing oxygen to the cells of the body.

The severity of the side effects is increased when 5-FU is given with the drug leucovorin. Vomiting, diarrhea, nausea, and loss of appetite (**anorexia**) may occur regardless of how 5-FU is administered. The diarrhea side effect may be severe in some patients, and it is important for them to alert their doctor immediately so that appropriate medications for the diarrhea can be prescribed.

5-FU may cause rashes, increased sensitivity to sunlight, changes in skin color, changes to the fingernails, and redness and swelling in the palms of the hands and soles of the feet. Patients who have had heart disease before starting therapy with 5-FU may have problems with blood flow to the heart. Rarely, 5-FU may cause an allergic reaction, dry eyes, sleepiness, confusion, headache, changes in walking gait, involuntary rapid movement of the eyes, and difficulty speaking. When 5-FU is applied directly on the skin, there are usually no side effects except for those to the skin itself. These may include burning sensations, pain, and darkening of the skin color.

Some authorities recommend discontinuation of 5-FU therapy as soon as mild side effects are observed as a way of reducing the extent of injury to the digestive tract. Administration may then be restarted at a lower dose after the side effects have stopped.

Interactions

People taking fluorouracil should consult their doctor before taking any other prescription drug, over-the-counter drug, or herbal remedy.

Bob Kirsch

Fluoxymesterone

Definition

Fluoxymesterone is a synthetic male hormone used to treat women with hormone-dependent **breast cancer**, and may also be used as a **testosterone** replacement for men. Fluoxymesterone is sold as Halotestin, Android-F, and Ora-Testryl.

Purpose

Fluoxymesterone is used to manage metastatic breast cancer in menopausal women who have hormone receptor–positive tumors. It may also be used as a supplement to **chemotherapy** for metastatic breast cancer, or as a hormone replacement for men. Additionally, it is sometimes used to treat **anemia**.

Description

Fluoxymesterone is a synthetic androgen, or male hormone, similar in action to testosterone. Fluoxymesterone works by attaching itself to androgen receptors; this causes it to interact with the parts of the cell involved in the making of proteins. It may cause an increase in the synthesis of some proteins or a decrease in the synthesis of others. These proteins have a variety of effects, including blocking the growth of some types of breast cancer cells, stimulating cells that cause male sexual characteristics, and stimulating the production of red blood cells.

When used as a breast cancer treatment, this drug blocks the growth of tumor cells that are dependent on female hormones to grow. It can only be used on female breast cancer patients who have reached menopause one to five years earlier, or as a result of surgery. It may be used in addition to other chemotherapeutic drugs, such as **tamoxifen** or **cyclophosphamide**, **doxorubicin**, and **fluorouracil**.

Fluoxymesterone may be used to treat men; it replaces male hormones which are not being released in the body as a result of tumors, radiation, or surgery affecting the pituitary or hypothalamus.

Recommended dosage

The recommended dosage will depend on the age, sex, and diagnosis of the patient, as well as the response to treatment and occurrence of side effects. Treatment is usually with a full therapeutic dose initially, then adjusted to the individual needs of the patient.

Women being treated for breast cancer usually take 10 to 40 mg per day orally, divided into several doses. Up to three months may be required for a response to treatment.

Androgen replacement therapy for men is usually started at 5 to 20 mg per day, taken orally in divided doses.

If a dose is missed, it should be taken as soon as it is remembered, unless it is more than two hours late. If it is more than two hours late, the patient should skip that dose and continue to follow the normal dosing schedule.

Precautions

Fluoxymesterone may be taken with food if it causes stomach upset. Patients taking this medication should ensure that they see their physician regularly during treatment and receive appropriate laboratory tests. Liver function should be monitored and cholesterol and red blood cell levels may need to be examined during treatment. Female breast cancer patients should have their serum and urine calcium levels checked. Prepubescent males will require x rays to determine the rate of their bone maturation. Diabetics should be aware that this medication may affect blood sugar levels.

Fluoxymesterone should not be taken by pregnant women as it will affect the sexual development of the fetus. The hormone may also pass into the milk of nursing mothers, affecting sexual development of the infant. Fluoxymesterone should not be taken by people with liver, kidney, heart or blood vessel disease, prostate problems, or sensitivity to the dye tartrazine. Patients with migraines or epilepsy should discuss these conditions with their physician before using the drug. Elderly male patients using fluoxymesterone have an increased risk of prostate enlargement.

Patients should consult their physician before discontinuing the drug.

Side effects

Patients who use fluoxymesterone have an increased risk of developing liver disease, and should report symptoms such as yellowing of the eyes and skin to their physicians immediately. Women being treated for breast cancer and patients who are immobilized may develop **hypercalcemia**. Other side effects which may occur include the following:

- fluid retention
- **nausea and vomiting**
- **diarrhea**
- anxiety
- **depression**
- changes in sex drive
- dizziness
- suppression of blood clotting factors II, V, VII, and X
- headache
- **itching**
- reduction in number of white blood cells
- increase in number of red blood cells

Women who take this medication may also experience menstrual irregularities, acne, enlarged clitoris, and masculine characteristics such as deepening of the voice, increased hair growth, and male pattern baldness. Some of these changes may go away if the medication is stopped, while others may remain.

Men taking fluoxymesterone may experience breast growth, erections of excessive frequency and duration, impotence, decreased ejaculatory volume, and bladder irritation.

KEY TERMS

Androgen—a male hormone

Hypercalcemia—high levels of calcium in the blood

Interactions

A large number of medications may cause interactions with fluoxymesterone, including acetaminophen, anabolic steroids, anticoagulants, antidiabetic agents, and many others. Patients should notify their physicians of any medications they are taking before using fluoxymesterone.

Racquel Baert, M.Sc.

Flutamide *see* **Antiandrogens**

Folic acid

Definition

Folic acid is a water-soluble B vitamin essential in the human diet. It is an important cofactor in the synthesis of DNA and RNA of dividing cells, particularly during pregnancy and infancy when there is an increase in cell division and growth.

Purpose

Folic acid is important to the field of oncology in two ways. First, prior to neoplasm formation, folic acid is important in the synthesis of DNA and RNA and the repair of damaged DNA. Second, after a tumor develops, a form of folic acid is used to counter the side effects of **methotrexate** and **fluorouracil**.

Description

Prior to tumor formation

Since folic acid is a cofactor in DNA replication and biosynthesis of purines and also in DNA repair, there is an increasing amount of research (epidemiological, clinical, and experimental) that suggests a folic acid deficien-

KEY TERMS

Folic acid antagonist—a drug that interferes with the action of folic acid

Neoplasm—abnormal tissue growth that is not controlled by normal stimuli and lacks normal structural organization

Purines—a substance that is part of the structure of guanine and adenine, molecules that combine to form DNA

cy might be a factor that predisposes the formation of tumors in normal epithelial tissue. There is an inverse relationship associated with low folate diets and an increase in DNA breakage and mutation that is unable to be effectively repaired. The preventative influence of dietary folic acid on the formation of **colon cancer** is currently under heavy research. Although a correlation is observed, it has not yet been proven to show cause and effect. However, there is enough evidence to encourage consuming minimal daily dietary requirements of folic acid to potentially reduce the risk. When choosing supplements, other names for folic acid that may be encountered are folate and folacin.

After tumors form

Once a neoplasm forms, folic acid levels need to be decreased. In neoplasms, DNA replication and cell division are both occurring in an uncontrolled manner. Folate, which assists in this process, needs to be inhibited, causing an interruption in DNA synthesis and slowing the growth of the tumor. Chemotherapeutic agents called antimetabolites, or folic acid antagonists, such as methotrexate and 5-fluorouracil (5-FU), inhibit the enzymatic pathways for biosynthesis of nucleic acids by substituting for folic acid and sabotaging the reaction. Unfortunately, drugs that inhibit the biosynthesis of cancer cells also inhibit the biosynthesis of normal cells, resulting in extremely toxic side effects. To counter the side effects, a drug called **leucovorin** (a form of folate also known as Wellcovorin, Citrovorum and folinic acid) opposes the toxic effects of methotrexate on normal tissue. Leucovorin also increases the anticancer effect of 5-FU.

Recommended dosage

Non-cancer individuals supplementing their diet with folic acid may reduce the risk of cancer. Supplemental folic acid can be purchased over the counter and is also fortified in breakfast cereals and whole grain products produced in the United States. The recommended intake for adults is 400 micrograms (mcg) each day. While the risk of upper limit toxicity is low, adult men and women should not exceed the advised upper limit of 1,000 mcg per day. It is especially important that individuals diagnosed with cancer seek the advice of medical professionals before commencing or continuing supplemental folic acid use because it may interact with **chemotherapy**.

Cancer patients treated with methotrexate may be given leucovorin as a "rescue" treatment approximately 24 hours later to counteract the toxic side effects on normal tissues of the gastrointestinal system and bone marrow. Leucovorin is only available by prescription. It is a systemic drug available in oral form (tablets) or via injections. The dosage varies from person to person and is based on body size.

Precautions

Patients should inform their physician of the following conditions before they begin to take leucovorin:

- Pregnancy or breast-feeding.
- Pernicious anemia.
- Allergies to leucovorin or any other drugs.
- Vitamin B_{12} deficiency. Folic acid may mask hematologic signs of B_{12} deficiency while neurologic damage progresses.

Side effects

Folic acid in general and specifically leucovorin are usually well-tolerated. However, there are some uncommon side effects that include skin rashes, **itching**, vomiting, nausea, **diarrhea**, and difficulty breathing. Although extremely rare, seizures have occurred in some patients taking leucovorin. Since leucovorin is taken with chemotherapeutic drugs, some side effects may be due to drug interaction.

Interactions

Supplemental folic acid can interact with anti-convulsant medications such as dilantin, **phenytoin**, and primidone. It also complicates the effects of metformin (used in individuals with type 2 diabetes), sulfasalazine (used in individuals with Crohn's disease), and triamterene (a diuretic).

Leucovorin enhances the effects of 5-FU and antagonizes the effects of methotrexate. It additionally interacts with barbiturate medications that may be taken by people with sleep disorders.

Sally C. McFarlane-Parrott

Foscarnet *see* **Antiviral therapy**

G

Gabapentin

Definition

Gabapentin is indicated to be used in combination with other anti-seizure (anticonvulsant) drugs for the management of partial seizure types. Gabapentin should not be used alone for the treatment of seizures unless the patient cannot tolerate other anticonvulsant drugs. This medication can also be used for the treatment of certain syndromes associated with nerve (neuropathic) pain (diabetic **neuropathy**, postherpetic neuralgia), pain associated with multiple sclerosis, neuropathic cancer pain, trigeminal neuralgia, and bipolar mood disorder. Gabapentin is also known as Neurontin.

Description

Gabapentin was introduced in 1994 as an anticonvulsant medication. Other medications in the anticonvulsant class include **phenytoin**, **carbamazepine**, phenobarbital, valproic acid, topiramate, and lamotrigine. Gabapentin's structure is similar to that of gamma-aminobutiric acid (GABA), which is a chemical found in the central nervous system (brain and spinal cord) that decreases firing of neurons leading to a decrease in seizure activity. Despite this structural similarity, gabapentin does not interact with GABA receptors and its exact mechanism of action for either epilepsy or pain is not known.

Gabapentin is a relatively recent addition to the arsenal of drugs used in the treatment of neuropathic pain. Traditionally, tricyclic antidepressants (**amitriptyline**, nortriptyline, desipramine) have been used as first-line agents. It takes one to three weeks for either gabapentin or tricyclic antidepressants (TCAs) to provide relief of pain after starting treatment. Gabapentin appears to be a safer agent to use than TCAs, especially in elderly patients and patients on multiple other medications. One of the disadvantages of gabapentin over TCAs is its higher cost.

Recommended Dosage

Adults and children over 12 years of age

MANAGEMENT OF PARTIAL SEIZURE TYPES. Therapy should be started at a dose of 300 mg, three times daily. The dose can be increased to 1,800 mg/day in three divided doses. Some patients may need even higher doses to control their seizures. Doses up to 3,600 mg per day have been well tolerated in research studies.

TREATMENT OF NEUROPATHIC PAIN. Dosages of 300-3,600 mg/day have been effective in research studies. However, optimal dosage appears to be 1,200-2,400 mg/day divided in three doses.

TREATMENT OF BIPOLAR DISORDER. Optimal dose has not been well established. Doses up to 4,800 mg/day have been used.

Children less than 12 years of age

Dosage varies due to the child's size, weight, and extent of condition. Parents should ask their physician about appropriate dosage levels for their child.

Administration

To minimize side effects, the first dose should be taken at bedtime. Capsules should not be chewed or crushed. Patients should avoid taking antacids (Mylanta, Maalox) at the same time as gabapentin. Doses should be taken at even intervals, and if a dose is missed, it should be taken as soon as remembered. However, double-doses can be hazardous, and should be avoided.

Precautions

Gabapentin should be used with caution by breast-feeding mothers, children under 12 years of age (because of a lack of safety and efficacy studies in this population), and patients with impaired kidney function.

KEY TERMS

Bipolar disorder—Recurrent mood disorder equally common among men and women, in which patients have extreme mood alterations between depression and mania or a mix of both. During manic episodes patients may have elevated mood, decreased need for sleep, rapid speech, extreme involvement in pleasurable activities, and may be easily distracted. The drugs commonly used in treatment of bipolar disorder include lithium, carbamazepine, valproic acid, and antidepressants.

Diabetic neuropathy—A chronic complication of diabetes that can take two forms, peripheral and autonomic. Patients with peripheral neuropathy experience dullness of sensation of pain, temperature, and pressure, especially in lower legs and feet. Autonomic neuropathy can cause alteration in bowel habits, impotence, and decreased heart function. The peripheral type can be treated with medications such as amitriptyline or gabapentin, while the autonomic type is more resistant to treatment.

Multiple sclerosis—A disorder of central nervous system, causing patches of plaques in brain and spinal cord and usually affecting young adults. Patients may experience visual changes, weakness, numbing or tingling of the hands or feet, changes in bladder and mood patterns.

Postherpetic neuralgia—Severe stabbing or throbbing pain associated with herpes zoster infection (shingles), resulting from the inflammation of nerve endings where the herpes vesicles erupt.

Trigeminal neuralgia—Severe, sudden bursts of throbbing and stabbing pain in one of the branches of trigeminal nerve located on the face. The pain can affect any area of the face, teeth, or tongue, and is often caused by some trigger points around the mouth.

Gabapentin has resulted in fetal abnormalities in mice, rats, and rabbit offsprings. There are no current studies on gabapentin use in pregnant women. This drug should only be used during pregnancy if potential benefits justify the risk to the baby.

This medication should not be discontinued suddenly because of the possibility of increased frequency of seizures. Gabapentin doses should be decreased gradually over a period of at least one week.

Gabapentin may cause drowsiness and dizziness. Alcoholic beverages may intensify these effects and their intake should be limited. Patients should use caution when driving, operating dangerous machinery, or performing activities requiring alertness.

A patient experiencing any of the following should contact their physician or pharmacist immediately:

- mental or mood changes
- tingling or numbness of hands or feet
- swelling of ankles
- vision problems
- fever or unusual bleeding

Side effects

This medication is usually well tolerated. Nervous system side effects are the most common, including drowsiness, dizziness, unsteadiness when walking, **fatigue**, and vision changes (double-vision, blurred vision). These side effects appear to be dose-related, and some patients may develop tolerance to these effects after the first several weeks of therapy. If these side effects persist or worsen, a physician should be notified. Other side effects that occur less frequently are irritability, dyspepsia, mood changes, memory loss, difficulty concentrating, slurred speech, and impotence. Elderly patients may be more sensitive to the side effects of gabapentin.

Interactions

One of the advantages of gabapentin is that it is not broken down in the body and does not have a lot of drug interaction. Antacids may interfere with the absorption of this medication in the body; they should be taken at least two hours apart. Gabapentin does not effect other commonly used anticonvulsants (for example, phenytoin, carbamazepine, valproic acid, and phenobarbital).

Olga Bessmertny, Pharm.D.

Gallbladder cancer

Definition

Cancer of the gallbladder is cancer of the pear-shaped organ that lies on the undersurface of the liver.

Description

Bile from the liver is funneled into the gallbladder by way of the cystic duct. Between meals, the gallbladder stores a large amount of bile. To do this, it must absorb much of the water and electrolytes from the bile. In fact, the inner surface of the gallbladder is the most absorptive surface in the body. After a meal, the gallbladder's muscular walls contract to deliver the bile back through the cystic duct and eventually into the small intestine, where the bile can help digest food.

Demographics

About 5,000 people are diagnosed with gallbladder cancer each year in the United States, making it the fifth most common gastrointestinal cancer. It is more common in females than males and most patients are elderly. Southwest American Indians have a particularly high incidence—6 times that of the general population.

Causes and symptoms

Gallstones are the most significant risk factor for the development of gallbladder cancer. Roughly 75 to 90 percent of patients with gallbladder cancer also have gallstones. Larger gallstones are associated with a higher chance of developing gallbladder cancer. Chronic inflammation of the gallbladder from infection also increases the risk for gallbladder cancer.

Unfortunately, sometimes cancer of the gallbladder does not produce symptoms until late in the disease. When symptoms are evident, the most common is pain in the upper right portion of the abdomen, underneath the right ribcage. Patients with gallbladder cancer may also report symptoms such as nausea, vomiting, weakness, jaundice, skin **itching**, **fever**, chills, poor appetite, and **weight loss**.

Diagnosis

Gallbladder cancer is often misdiagnosed because it mimics other more common conditions, such as gallstones, cholecystitis, and pancreatitis. But the imaging tests that are utilized to evaluate these other conditions can also detect gallbladder cancer. For example, ultrasound is a quick, noninvasive imaging test that reliably diagnoses gallstones and cholecystitis. It can also detect the presence of gallbladder cancer as well as show how far the cancer has spread. If cancer is suspected, a **computed tomography** scan is useful in confirming the presence of an abnormal mass and further demonstrating the size and extent of the tumor. Cholangiography, usually performed to evaluate a patient with jaundice, can also detect gallbladder cancer.

There are no specific laboratory tests for gallbladder cancer. Tumors can obstruct the normal flow of bile from the liver to the small intestine. Bilirubin, a component of bile, builds up within the liver and is absorbed into the bloodstream in excess amounts. This can be detected in a blood test, but it can also manifest clinically as jaundice. Elevated bilirubin levels and clinical jaundice can also occur with other conditions, such as gallstones.

On occasion, gallbladder cancer is diagnosed incidentally. About one percent of all patients who have their gallbladder removed for symptomatic gallstones are found to have gallbladder cancer. The cancer is found either by the surgeon or by the pathologist who inspects the gallbladder with a microscope.

Treatment team

The main member of the treatment team is the surgeon, since surgical removal of the cancer is the only measure that offers a significant chance of cure. Sometimes the cancer is too advanced such that surgery would be of no benefit. But the patient might suffer from jaundice or blockage of the stomach. In this case, the gastroenterologist or interventional radiologist may be able to provide non-surgical alternatives to address these complications. In limited scenarios, the oncologist or radiation therapist may treat the patient with **chemotherapy** or **radiation therapy**.

Clinical staging, treatments, and prognosis

Staging of gallbladder cancer is determined by the how far the cancer has spread. The effectiveness of treatment declines as the stage progresses. Stage I cancer is confined to the wall of the gallbladder. Approximately 25% of cancers are at this stage at the time of diagnosis. Stage II cancer has penetrated the full thickness of the wall, but has not spread to nearby lymph nodes or invaded adjacent organs. Stage III cancer has spread to nearby lymph nodes or has invaded the liver, stomach, colon, small intestine, or large intestine. Stage IV disease has invaded very deeply into two or more adjacent organs or has spread to distant lymph nodes or organs by way of **metastasis**.

Early Stage I cancers involving only the innermost layer of the gallbladder wall can be cured by simple removal of the gallbladder. Cancers at this stage are sometimes found incidentally when the gallbladder is removed in the treatment of gallstones or cholecystitis. The majority of patients have good survival rates. Late Stage I cancers, which involve the outer muscular layers of the gallbladder wall, are generally treated in the same way as Stage II or III cancers. Removal of the gallbladder is not sufficient for these stages. The surgeon also removes nearby lymph nodes as well as a portion of the adjacent liver (radical

KEY TERMS

Cholangiography—Radiographic examination of the bile ducts after injection with a special dye

Cholecystitis—Inflammation of the gallbladder, usually due to infection

Computed tomography—A radiology test by which images of cross-sectional planes of the body are obtained

Jaundice—Yellowish staining of the skin and eyes due to excess bilirubin in the bloodstream

Metastasis—The spread of tumor cells from one part of the body to another through blood vessels or lymphatic vessels

Pancreatitis—Inflammation of the pancreas

Stent—Slender hollow catheter or rod placed within a vessel or duct to provide support or maintain patency

Ultrasound—A radiology test utilizing high frequency sound waves

surgery). Survival rates for these patients are considerably worse than for those with early Stage I disease. Patients with early Stage IV disease may benefit from radical surgery, but the issue is controversial. Late Stage IV cancer has spread too extensively to allow complete excision. Surgery is not an option for these patients.

Other therapies

When long-term survival is not likely, the focus of therapy shifts to improving quality of life. Jaundice and blockage of the stomach are two problems faced by patients with advanced cancer of the gallbladder. These can be treated with surgery, or alternatively, by special interventional techniques employed by the gastroenterologist or radiologist. A stent can be placed across the bile ducts in order to re-establish the flow of bile and relieve jaundice. A small feeding tube can be placed in the small intestine to allow feeding when the stomach is blocked. Pain may be treated with conventional pain medicines or a celiac ganglion nerve block.

Current chemotherapy or **radiation therapy** cannot cure gallbladder cancer, but they may offer some benefit in certain patients. For cancer that is too advanced for surgical cure, treatment with chemotherapeutic agents such as 5-**fluorouracil** may lengthen survival for a few months. The limited benefit of chemotherapy must be weighed carefully against its side effects. Radiation therapy is sometimes used after attempted surgical resection of the cancer to extend survival for a few months or relieve jaundice.

Coping with cancer treatment

After cancer treatment, many patients find that good nutrition, and a strong support system (which may include a support group) improve their quality of life. Treatment team members or hospital social workers can often recommend local resources that can be of assistance to the patient.

Clinical trials

More **clinical trials** are needed to define the role of chemotherapy and radiation therapy after attempted surgical resection of Stage II and III cancer. Some investigators are conducting trials to assess whether extremely radical surgery is beneficial in early Stage IV disease.

Special concerns

After the removal of the gallbladder, patients may experience a temporary change in bowel habits. The bowel movements may be more frequent or more liquid than before surgery. This situation usually resolves within about six months.

Resources

BOOKS

Ahrendt, Steven A. and Henry A. Pitt. "Biliary Tract." In *Sabiston Textbook of Surgery*, edited by Courtney Townsend Jr., 16th ed. Philadelphia: W.B. Saunders Company, 2001, pp. 1076-1111.

Corsetti, Ralph L. and Harold J. Wanebo. "Bile Duct Cancer." In *Current Surgical Therapy*, edited by John L. Cameron, sixth ed. St Louis: Mosby, 1998, pp.462-468.

"Gallbladder Carcinoma." In *Clinical Oncology*, edited by Abeloff, Martin D., second ed. New York: Churchill Livingstone, 2000, pp.1730-1737.

OTHER

National Cancer Institute Cancer Trials web site. <http://cancer trials.nci.nih.gov/system>. <http://www.cancertrials.com>.

Kevin O. Hwang, M.D.

Gallium nitrate

Definition

Gallium nitrate is a drug that is used to treat **hypercalcemia**, or too much calcium in the blood. This condition may occur when individuals develop various types of cancer. Gallium nitrate is also known by the common brand name Ganite.

Purpose

The purpose of gallium nitrate is to reduce the level of calcium in a patient's blood. It is a liquid medication that is injected into a person's vein.

Description

Due to the fact that hypercalcemia is a serious condition that can be fatal, it is very important that it is effectively treated. Hypercalcemia is a common complication of cancer, affecting approximately 10–20% of all cancer patients. This condition can affect many systems of the body and has various signs and symptoms. Sometimes, these symptoms may be thought to be associated with the cancer, and therefore the hypercalcemia itself may go undiagnosed.

Symptoms of hypercalcemia include frequent urination, thirst, dizziness, constipation, nausea, vomiting, and disruptions in cardiac rhythm. If severe, this complication can lead to seizure, cardiac arrest, coma, or death.

Hypercalcemia should first be treated with fluids. Doctors should make sure that their patients are properly hydrated, meaning that they have enough fluid in their body. However, fluid treatment alone is usually not effective to treat this condition. Therefore, some physicians may recommend that their patients take gallium nitrate to establish a normal balance of calcium in the blood.

Recommended dosage

The recommended dosage of gallium nitrate differs depending on the patient, and should be determined by a physician. For adults and teenagers, the dosage of this medication is based on body weight/size, and must be calculated by a doctor. The medication is injected into a patient's vein at a slow pace for 24 hours over a period of five days. If a patient's calcium level is still too high, this process can be repeated in two to four weeks. For younger children, up to the age of 12, there are no specific studies to determine the effects of gallium nitrate. Therefore, use and dosage of this medication must be determined by the young cancer patient's personal physician.

While undergoing treatment with gallium nitrate, patients' doctors should check calcium levels at regular intervals. Even if a patient's condition has improved, he or she may still need to be followed closely to make sure that they do not develop hypercalcemia again.

KEY TERMS

Cancer—One cell that grows out of control in the body and subsequently invades nearby cells and tissue.

Ganite—The commonly used brand name for gallium nitrate.

Hypercalcemia—Excessive or increased calcium in the blood. Often a complication of cancer.

Precautions

Before taking gallium nitrate, there are specific precautions that should be taken to avoid potential complications. Patients should let their physician know if they are allergic to any foods, preservatives or dyes. In addition, patients with certain medical problems, specifically kidney disease, should make sure that their prescribing physician is aware of this, as use of gallium nitrate can exacerbate this condition. Adequate hydration may minimize toxic effects on the kidney.

In addition, use of gallium nitrate has not been studied in pregnant animals or humans. It is not recommended for women who are pregnant or breast-feeding, as it may cause negative side effects.

With regard to children, as stated, there are no studies of gallium nitrate in younger populations. There are also no studies of this medication in the elderly. However, it is not thought that the use of gallium nitrate would cause very different side effects in older people versus younger adults.

Side effects

Individuals who are considering taking gallium nitrate should discuss its use in detail with their physician. This includes talking about the potential benefits versus any potential side effects. Some individuals may experience all, some, or none of these side effects. Some of these side effects may lessen as a person's body gets used to the medication. However, it is important to be aware of these potential side effects because some of them may require medical interventions.

More common side effects:

- blood in the urine
- pain in the bones
- change in urination frequency
- feeling thirsty

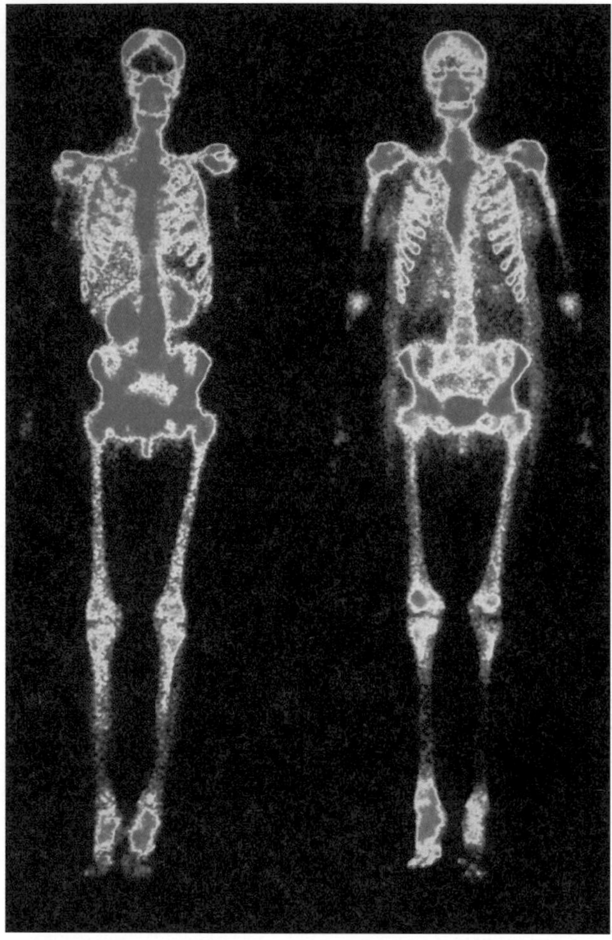

Nuclear medicine scan of the skeleton. A radioisotope, like gallium, is used to produce this image. This scan reveals that lung cancer has spread to ribs and there is osteomyelitis in ankle. *(© Scott Camazine and Sue Trainor, Science Source/ Photo Researchers, Inc. Reproduced by permission.)*

- loss of appetite (**anorexia**)
- weakness of muscles
- feeling nauseous
- **diarrhea**
- metallic taste in the mouth
- **nausea and vomiting**
- decrease of phosphate levels in the blood

Less common side effects:

- cramps in the abdomen
- a feeling of confusion
- muscle spasms

Rare side effects:

- excessive **fatigue** or weakness

Interactions

Patients should tell their physician if they are taking any other medications on a regular basis, especially the ones listed below, as they could cause a negative interaction if taken with gallium nitrate.

- certain medications taken for infections
- **cisplatin**
- medications for pain that contain acetaminophen or aspirin
- **cyclosporine**
- deferoxamine
- some medications for treatment of arthritis
- lithium
- **methotrexate**
- pencillamine
- gentamicin
- amphotericin B
- "nephrotoxic agents"

Tiffani A. DeMarco, MS

Gallium scan

Definition

A gallium scan of the body is a nuclear medicine test that is conducted using a camera that detects gallium, a form of radionuclide, or radioactive chemical substance.

Purpose

Most gallium scans are ordered to detect cancerous tumors, infections, or areas of inflammation in the body. Gallium is known to accumulate in inflamed, infected, or cancerous tissues. The scans are used to determine whether a patient with an unexplained **fever** has an infection and the site of the infection, if present. Gallium scans also may be used to evaluate cancer following **chemotherapy** or **radiation therapy**.

Precautions

Children and women who are pregnant or breast-feeding are only given gallium scans if the potential diagnostic benefits will outweigh the risks.

Description

The patient will usually be asked to come to the testing facility 24–48 hours before the procedure to receive the injection of gallium. Sometimes, the injection will be given only four to six hours before the study or as long as 72 hours before the procedure. The timeframe is based on the area or organs of the body being studied.

For the study itself, the patient lies very still for approximately 30–60 minutes. A camera is moved across the patient's body to detect and capture images of concentrations of the gallium. The camera picks up signals from any accumulated areas of the radionuclide. In most cases, the patient is lying down throughout the procedure. Back (posterior) and front (anterior) views will usually be taken, and sometimes a side (lateral) view is used. The camera may occasionally touch the patient's skin, but will not cause any discomfort. A clicking noise may be heard throughout the procedure; this is only the sound of the scanner registering radiation.

Preparation

The intravenous injection of gallium is done in a separate appointment prior to the procedure. Generally, no special dietary requirements are necessary. Sometimes the physician will ask that the patient have light or clear meals within a day or less of the procedure. Many patients will be given **laxatives** or an enema prior to the scan to eliminate any residual gallium from the bowels.

Aftercare

There is generally no aftercare required following a gallium scan. However, women who are breastfeeding who have a scan will be cautioned against breastfeeding for four weeks following the exam.

Risks

There is a minimal risk of exposure to radiation from the gallium injection, but the exposure from one gallium scan is generally less than exposure from x rays.

Normal results

A radiologist trained in nuclear medicine or a nuclear medicine specialist will interpret the exam results and compare them to other diagnostic tests. It is normal for gallium to accumulate in the liver, spleen, bones, breast tissue, and large bowel.

Abnormal results

An abnormal concentration of gallium in areas other than those where it normally concentrates may indicate the presence of disease. Concentrations may be due to inflammation, infection, or the presence of tumor tissue. Often, additional tests are required to determine if the tumors are malignant (cancerous) or benign.

Even though gallium normally concentrates in organs such as the liver or spleen, abnormally high concentrations will suggest certain diseases and conditions. For example, Hodgkin's or non-Hodgkin's **lymphoma** may be diagnosed or staged if there is abnormal gallium activity in the lymph nodes. After a patient receives cancer treatment, such as radiation therapy or chemotherapy, a gallium scan may help to find new or recurring tumors or to record regression of a treated tumor. Physicians can narrow causes of liver problems by noting abnormal gallium activity in the liver. Gallium scans also may be used to diagnose lung diseases or a disease called sarcoidosis, in the chest.

KEY TERMS

Benign—Not cancerous. Benign tumors are not considered immediate threats, but may still require some form of treatment.

Gallium—A form of radionuclide that is used to help locate tumors and inflammation (specifically referred to as GA67 citrate).

Malignant—This term, usually used to describe a tumor, means cancerous, becoming worse and possibly growing.

Nuclear medicine—A subspecialty of radiology used to show the function and anatomy of body organs. Very small amounts of radioactive substances, or tracers, are detected with a special camera as they accumulate in certain organs and tissues.

Radionuclide—A chemical substance, called an isotope, that exhibits radioactivity. A gamma camera, used in nuclear medicine procedures, will pick up the radioactive signals as the substance gathers in an organ or tissue. They are sometimes referred to as tracers.

Resources

BOOKS

Fischbach, Frances T. *A Manual of Laboratory and Diagnostic Tests.* Philadelphia, PA: Lippincott-Raven Publishers, 1996.

Illustrated Guide to Diagnostic Tests. Springhouse, PA: Springhouse Corporation, 1998.

ORGANIZATIONS

American Cancer Society. 1599 Clifton Road NE, Atlanta, GA 30329. (404) 320-3333. <http://www.cancer.org>.

American College of Nuclear Medicine. PO Box 175, Landisville, PA 31906. (717) 898-6006.

American Liver Foundation. 1425 Pompton Avenue, Cedar Grove NJ 07009. (800) GO LIVER (465-4837). <http://www.liverfoundation.org>

Society of Nuclear Medicine. 1850 Samuel Morse Drive, Reston, VA 10016. (703) 708-9000. <http://www.snm.org>.

OTHER

"A Patient's Guide to Nuclear Medicine." *University of Iowa Virtual Hospital.* <http://www.vh.org/Patients/IHB/Rad/NucMed/PatGuideNucMed/PatGuideNucMed.html>. 2 July 2001.

Teresa G. Norris

Ganciclovir *see* **Antiviral therapy**

Gastric cancer *see* **Stomach cancer**

Gastrinoma *see* **Zollinger-Ellison syndrome**

Gastrointestinal cancers

Definition

Gastrointestinal (GI) cancers include cancer of the esophagus, stomach, small intestine, colon, rectum, and anus as well as cancers of the liver, pancreas, gallbladder, and biliary system.

Description

The GI tract, or digestive tract, starts from the oral cavity (mouth) and proceeds to the esophagus, the stomach, the duodenum, the small intestine, the large intestine (colon and rectum), and the anus. It processes all the food consumed. Along the way through the tract, food is digested, nutrients and water are extracted, and waste is eliminated from the body in the form of stool and urine. Cancer can affect any of the gastrointestinal organs. The National Cancer Institute estimates that 25% of all cancers are gastrointestinal, with the majority of these occurring in the colon and rectum (colorectal cancers). The next sites most commonly affected by GI cancers are the pancreas, stomach, liver, and esophagus. A brief overview of GI cancers follows; the reader should refer to other specific encyclopedia entries shown in bold for more comprehensive information on these cancers and their treatment. The reader should also note that the overview below does not discuss oral cavity cancers. Those cancers are also discussed in individual entries.

Types of cancers

Esophageal cancer

The esophagus is a muscular, hollow tube that carries food from the oropharynx (area behind mouth and soft palate) to the stomach. It consists of several layers. **Esophageal cancer** usually develops in the inner layer cells and grows outward. There are two major types of esophageal cancer. The first occurs in the cells found in the lining of the esophagus (squamous cells), and the cancer is called squamous cell carcinoma. It can develop anywhere along the entire length of the esophagus and represents approximately half of all reported esophageal cancers. The second type of cancer known to occur in the esophagus is an adenocarcinoma, which is cancer of the glandular cells that line the inside of organs. Adenocarcinoma occurs near the stomach entrance and may be associated with a condition known as **Barrett's esophagus**. This is a disorder in which the lining of the esophagus undergoes cellular changes as a result of chronic irritation and inflammation resulting from a backwash of acidic stomach gastric juices. Esophageal **adenocarcinomas** cannot develop unless squamous cells have been transformed by the acid reflux of the stomach juices. The American Cancer Society (ACS) predicted the occurrence of approximately 12,300 new cases of esophageal cancer in 2000 which will result in some 12,100 deaths in the United States.

Stomach cancer

Stomach cancer is also called gastric cancer. The stomach is located in the upper abdomen under the ribs. It is the most expandable organ of the digestive system. Food reaches the stomach from the esophagus and is broken down by gastric juices secreted by the stomach. After leaving the stomach, partially broken down food passes into the small intestine and afterwards into the colon (first part of the large intestine). In cancer of the stomach, cancerous cells are found in the tissues of the stomach and this cancer can develop anywhere in the organ. It may grow along the stomach wall into other organs such as the esophagus or small intestine. Or it may go through the stomach wall and invade the nearby lymph nodes or organs such as the liver, pancreas, and colon. And it may also spread to more distant organs, such as the lungs, the lymph nodes located above the collar bone, and the ovaries. The major type of stomach cancer is adenocarcinoma (90%). Approximately 24,000 new cases of stomach cancer are diagnosed per year in the US. The number of cases, as well as the death rate, have declined significantly over the past several decades, but it is still the sev-

KEY TERMS

Abdomen—A part of the body which lies between the thorax and the pelvis. It contains a cavity (abdominal cavity) which holds organs such as the pancreas, stomach, intestines, liver, gallbladder. It is enclosed by the abdominal muscles and the vertebral column (backbone).

Bile—A greenish-yellow fluid produced by the liver and stored in the gallbladder.

Bile ducts—Passages external to the liver for the transport of bile.

Digestion—The conversion of food in the stomach and in the intestines into substances capable of being absorbed by the blood.

Digestive system—Organs and paths responsible for processing food in the body. These are the mouth, the esophagus, the stomach, the liver, the gallbladder, the pancreas, the small intestine, the colon and the rectum.

Gastric juice—An acidic secretion of the stomach that breaks down the proteins contained in the ingested food, prior to digestion.

Gland—An organ that produces and releases substances for use in the body, such as fluids or hormones.

Lymph nodes—Small, bean-shaped organs surrounded by a capsule of connective tissue. Also called lymph glands. Lymph nodes are spread out along lymphatic vessels and store special cells (lymphocytes), which filter the lymphatic fluid (lymph).

Lymphatic system—The tissues and organs that produce, store, and carry white blood cells that fight infection. It includes the bone marrow, spleen, thymus, and lymph nodes as well as a network of thin vessels (lymphatic vessels) that carry lymph and white blood cells into all the tissues of the body.

Metastasis—The transfer of cancer from one location or organ to another one not directly related to it.

Ovary—One of two small oval-shaped organs located on either side of the uterus. They are female reproductive glands in which the ova (eggs) are formed.

Small intestine—The part of the digestive tract located between the stomach and the large intestine.

Squamous cells—Flat, thin cells, such as found on the outer layer of the skin.

Stage—The extent to which a cancer has spread from its original site to other parts of the body. A Stage 1 cancer is less advanced than a Stage 4 cancer.

enth leading cause of cancer deaths. A cure is possible if the cancer is found before spreading to other organs. Unfortunately, the early symptoms are not very noticeable, and by the time stomach cancer is diagnosed, it has in many cases already metastasized.

Liver cancer

The liver is one of the largest organs in the body. In normal adults, it weighs about three pounds and is located in the upper right side of the abdomen, under the right lung and rib cage. It plays a major role in digestion, in the transformation of food into energy and in filtering and storing blood. It is also responsible for processing nutrients and drugs, producing bile, controlling the level of glucose (sugar) in the blood, detoxifying blood, and regulating blood clotting. In cancer of the liver, cancerous cells are found in the tissues of the liver. Primary liver cancer is cancer that starts in the liver. As such, it is different from cancer that starts somewhere else and spreads to the liver. Liver cancer is a rare form of GI cancer in the United States with only about 15,000 new cases diagnosed in 2000. Primary cancers of the liver and of the bile ducts are far more common in Africa and Asia than in America, where they only represent 1.5% of all cancer cases. The highest occurrence rate is in Vietnamese men (41.8 per 100,000), probably a result of the high incidence of viral hepatitis infections in their country. Asian-American groups also have higher liver cancer incidence rates than the Caucasian population. Liver cancer mortality rates calculated for populations for which statistics are available are highest in China.

There are four main types of liver cancer: angiosarcoma, a rare type of cancer that starts in the blood vessels of the liver; hepatoblastoma, another rare type of liver cancer occurring chiefly in young children; cholangiocarcinoma, which starts in the bile ducts and accounts for approximately 13% of liver cancers; and finally, hepatocellular carcinoma, also known as hepatoma. The most common liver cancer is hepatocellular carcinoma which accounts for approximately 84% of liver cancers. As is the case with stomach cancer, liver cancer is hard to diagnose early because there are seldom any clear-cut symptoms.

Gastrointestinal cancers

Cancer	Types
Esophageal cancer	Squamous cell carcinoma Adenocarcinoma
Stomach cancer	Adenocarcinoma
Liver cancer	Angiosarcoma Hepatoblastoma Cholangiocarcinoma Hepatocellular carcinoma (hepatoma)
Gallbladder cancer	Adenocarcinoma Squamous cell carcinoma Carcinosarcoma Small cell (oat cell) carcinoma
Pancreatic cancer	Adenocarcinoma Insulinoma Gastrinoma Glucagonoma Vipoma Somatostinoma Acinar cell carcinoma Cystic tumors Papillary tumors Pancreatoblastoma
Colorectal cancer	Adenocarcinoma Carcinoid tumors Gastroinstestinal stromal tumors Lymphomas
Anal cancer	Squamous cell carcinoma Basal cell carcinoma Melanoma Adenocarcinoma

However, some diseases have been identified as liable to increase a person's risk of getting liver cancer. They include: hepatitis B, hepatitis C, cirrhosis of the liver, exposure to certain chemicals such as aflatoxin (a substance made by a fungus in tropical regions and that can infect wheat, peanuts, soybeans, corn, and rice), vinyl chloride, thorium dioxide, anabolic steroids, arsenic, and birth control pills (of a type no longer prescribed).

Gallbladder cancer

The gallbladder is a pear-shaped organ located just under the liver in the upper abdomen. Its role in digestion is to store and release the bile produced by the liver into the stomach to help break down fat. In **gallbladder cancer**, the cancer cells develop in the tissues of the gallbladder. Several types of cancer can occur, such as adenocarcinoma, squamous cell carcinoma, carcinosarcoma and small cell (oat cell) carcinoma, all of them uncommon. Approximately 6,000 to 7,000 new cases are diagnosed per year in the U. S., affecting women twice as often as men and occurring mostly in the elderly.

Pancreatic cancer

The pancreas is a tongue-shaped glandular organ lying below and behind the stomach. It consists of two areas, the exocrine and endocrine regions. The endocrine pancreas secretes the hormones insulin and glucagon, which regulate blood sugar. The exocrine pancreas secretes pancreatic juice into the small intestine. The juice contains enzymes that break down fats and proteins so that the body can use them. In pancreatic cancer, the cancer can develop either in the cells that secrete the pancreatic juice (exocrine pancreatic cancer) or in the cells that release the hormones (endocrine pancreatic cancer). Exocrine pancreatic cancer is much more common than endocrine. Several types can develop, the majority being various types of carcinomas. The American Cancer Society predicted that, in 2000, about 28,300 people in the U. S. will be diagnosed with this type of cancer and that approximately 28,200 will die of the disease. Pancreatic cancer is the fourth leading cause of cancer death in men and women. Because the pancreas is located deep inside the body, it cannot be felt during a routine physical exam, and no tests are presently available to allow early detection.

Colorectal cancers

The colon, the first part of the large intestine, extends from the end of the small intestine to the rectum. The colon has four major divisions. The first is called the ascending colon, it starts where the small intestine attaches and extends upward on the right side of the abdomen. The second part is the transverse colon and it extends across the body to the left side where it joins the third section, called the descending colon, which continues downward on the left side. The fourth part of the colon is the sigmoid colon, which joins the rectum. The rectum joins the anus, where stool passes out of the body.

Each of the divisions of the colon and rectum has several layers of tissue. Colorectal cancers usually start in the innermost layer and can grow through some or all of the other layers. Colorectal cancers are common, and occur more frequently in people over the age of 50. The ACS estimated that in 2001 in the U. S., about 46,000 new cases of **colon cancer** will be diagnosed in men, and about 52,000 cases in women. For rectal cancers, the ACS estimates that about 21,000 men and 16,000 women will be diagnosed in 2001. The number of new colorectal cancer cases and reported deaths have declined in recent years due to improved screening and diagnostic methods. Colorectal cancers are highly treatable when detected early, but the symptoms are often not obvious in early stages.

Over 95% of colorectal cancers are adenocarcinomas. Other, less common types of colorectal cancers are: carcinoid tumors, which develop from the hormone-producing cells of the intestine, gastrointestinal stromal tumors, which start in the connective tissue and muscle layers located in the wall of the colon and rectum, and lymphomas, which are cancers of the immune system cells that usually occur in the lymph nodes but may also start in the colon.

Anal cancer

The anus has several types of tissues. Each type of tissue also contains several types of cells and cancer can develop in each of these kinds of tissues. Approximately half are squamous cell carcinomas. This type of cancer is found in the surface cells that line the anus and most of the anal canal. Another 15% of anal cancers consist of adenocarcinomas and usually start in glands found in the anus area. The remaining anal cancers are accounted for by basal cell carcinomas and malignant melanomas. **Anal cancer** is usually diagnosed in people over 50. People who have the human papillomavirus (HPV) also have a greater chance of developing anal cancer as well as men who practice anal sex. How treatable the cancer is depends partly on where it starts.

See Also Bile duct cancer; Carcinoid tumors, gastrointestinal; Human papilloma virus; Laryngeal cancer; Liver cancer, primary; Melanoma; Pancreatic cancer, endocrine; Pancreatic cancer, exocrine; Small intestinal cancer; Upper gastrointestinal endoscopy

Resources

BOOKS

Daly, J. *Management of Upper Gastrointestinal Cancer.* St. Louis: W. B. Saunders, 1999.

Feczko, P. *Gastrointestinal Imaging: Case Review.* New York: Mosby-Yearbook Inc., 2000.

Tahara, E. *Molecular Pathology of Gastrointestinal Cancer: Applications to Clinical Practice.* New York:Springer-Verlag, 1997.

Wanebo, H. *Surgery for Gastrointestinal Cancer: A multidisciplinary Approach.* New York: Lippincott, Williams & Wilkins, 1997.

PERIODICALS

Catalano, V., A. M. Baldelli, P. Giordani, S. Cascinu. "Molecular markers predictive of response to chemotherapy in gastrointestinal tumors." *Critical Reviews of Oncology and Hematology* 38 (May 2001): 93-104.

Lunn, J. A., W. M. Weinstein. "Gastric biopsy." *Gastrointestinal Endoscopic Clinicology of North America* 10 (October 2000):723-38.

Nishida, T., S. Hirota. "Biological and clinical review of stromal tumors in the gastrointestinal tract." *Histology and Histopathology* 15 (October 2000):1293-301.

Royce, M. E., P. M. Hoff, R. Pazdur. "Progress in colorectal cancer chemotherapy: how far have we come, how far to go?" *Drugs and Aging* 17 (September 2000):201-16.

Zock, P. L. "Dietary fats and cancer." *Current Opinions in Lipidology* 12 (February 2001):5-10.

ORGANIZATIONS

American Cancer Society (National Headquarters). 1599 Clifton Road, N.E., Atlanta, GA 30329.(800) 227-2345. Web site: <http://www.cancer.org>.

Cancer Research Institute (National Headquarters). 681 Fifth Avenue, New York, NY 10022. (800)992-2623. Web site: <http:://www.cancerresearch.org>.

National Cancer Institute's Cancer Information Service: 1-800-4-CANCER.

OTHER

University of Michigan Gastrointestinal Cancer Clinic Web site: <http://www.cancer.med.umich.edu/clinic/giclinic.htm>.

Monique Laberge, Ph.D.

G-CSF *see* **Filgrastim**

Gemcitabine

Definition

Gemcitabine is a drug that is used to treat advanced stages of pancreatic, lung, and other cancers. Its brand name is Gemzar.

Purpose

Gemcitabine is used to treat pancreatic cancer, particularly when it has metastasized, or spread to other parts of the body (Stage IVB). In combination with the drug **cisplatin**, gemcitabine is the first-line treatment for inoperable, metastasized non-small cell lung cancer. Sometimes it is used to treat cancers of the bladder or breast, or epithelial **ovarian cancer**.

Description

Gemcitabine is a relatively new anti-cancer drug. It is a type of medicine called a pyrimidine antimetabolite because it interferes with the metabolism and growth of cells. It does this by replacing the pyrimidine deoxycytidine in DNA, thereby preventing the DNA from being manufactured or repaired. As a result, cells cannot reproduce and eventually die.

Gemcitabine is approved by the U.S. Food and Drug Administration. It may relieve pain and other symptoms of advanced pancreatic cancer and increase survival time by several weeks to two months. Clinical studies of pancreatic cancer are comparing the effectiveness of combination treatments using gemcitabine with 5-**fluorouracil**, cisplatin, **streptozocin**, or **radiation**

KEY TERMS

Deoxycytidine—Component of DNA, the genetic material of a cell, that is similar in structure to gemcitabine.

Metastasis—Spread of cancer from its point of origin to other parts of the body.

Platelet—Blood component that aids in clotting.

Pyrimidine—Class of molecules that includes gemcitabine and deoxycytidine.

therapy. Gemcitabine has activity against metastatic **bladder cancer** and recurrent ovarian cancer, and further **clinical trials** are underway. Gemcitabine is being evaluated for its effectiveness in the treatment of uterine, stomach, laryngeal and hypopharyngeal, and colon and rectal cancers.

Recommended dosage

Gemcitabine is administered by injection over a period of 30 minutes. The dosage and number of administrations depend on a variety of factors, including the type of cancer, body size, and other concurrent treatments.

Precautions

Gemcitabine may temporarily reduce the number of white blood cells, particularly during the first 10-14 days after administration. A low white blood cell count reduces the body's ability to fight infection. Thus, it is very important to avoid exposure to infections and to receive prompt medical treatment. Immunizations (vaccinations) should be avoided during or after treatment with gemcitabine. It also is important to avoid contact with individuals who have recently taken an oral polio vaccine. Treatment with gemcitabine may cause chicken pox or shingles (**herpes zoster**) to become very severe and spread to other parts of the body.

Gemcitabine also may lower the blood platelet count. Platelets are necessary for normal blood clotting. The risk of bleeding may be reduced by using caution when cleaning teeth, avoiding dental work, and avoiding cuts, bruises, or other injuries.

Gemcitabine can cause birth defects and fetal death in animals. Therefore, this drug should not be taken by pregnant women or by either the man or woman at the time of conception. Women usually are advised against breast-feeding while taking this drug.

Side effects

Gemcitabine affects normal cells as well as cancer cells, resulting in various side effects. The most common side effects are related to reduction in red and white blood cells and blood platelets. These side effects may include symptoms of infection or unusual bleeding or bruising. Older patients are more likely to suffer from low blood cell counts after treatment.

Flu-like symptoms are common following the first treatment with gemcitabine. Other common side effects of gemcitabine may include:

- nausea
- vomiting
- chills and fever
- constipation
- diarrhea
- loss of appetite (**anorexia**)
- headache
- muscle pain
- weakness or fatigue
- shortness of breath
- blood in urine or stools
- skin rash
- swelling of the hands, feet, legs, or face
- insomnia

Less common side effects of gemcitabine may include:

- cough or hoarseness
- lower back or side pain
- painful or difficult urination
- chest, arm, or back pain
- difficulty with speech
- fast or irregular heartbeat
- high blood pressure
- pain or redness at the site of injection
- numbness or tingling in hands or feet
- sores or white spots on lips and in mouth
- hair loss (**alopecia**)
- **itching**

Some of these side effects may occur, or continue, after treatment with gemcitabine has ended. Itching, hives, swelling, or a skin rash, particularly if accompanied by breathing problems, may indicate an allergic reaction to gemcitabine.

Additional side effects of gemcitabine may be symptoms associated with liver or kidney malfunction. Furthermore, kidney or liver disease may cause gemcitabine to be removed from the body at a slower rate, thus increasing the effects of the drug.

Interactions

Previous treatment with radiation or other anti-cancer drugs can increase the risk of very low blood counts with gemcitabine. Serious problems may develop in areas previously treated with radiation.

Drugs that may interact with gemcitabine, or that may increase the risk of infections while being treated with gemcitabine, include live **vaccines** and **warfarin**. Because some other medications have a tendency to interact with gemcitabine, patients should alert their doctor to any drugs they are taking.

It is also important not to take any medicines containing aspirin during treatment with gemcitabine, since aspirin can increase the chances of excessive bleeding.

Margaret Alic, Ph.D.

Gemtuzumab

Definition

Gemtuzumab ozogamicin is a humanized monoclonal antibody produced by recombinant DNA technology that binds specifically to CD33, a protein that is found on the cell surface of most leukemic blasts, the abnormal, cancerous cells in acute myeloid leukemia (also known as **acute myelocytic leukemia**, or AML). It is marketed in the United States under the brand name Mylotarg.

Purpose

Gemtuzumab is a monoclonal antibody used to treat AML that is characterized by expression of the CD33 protein on the cancerous cells, called leukemic blasts. The CD33 protein is found on the surface of the leukemic blasts of about 80% of AML patients. After the gemtuzumab antibody is produced in the laboratory, a chemical reaction is used to link it to an antitumor drug called calicheamicin. About half of the antibody succeeds in acquiring the antitumor drug.

When the antibody-calicheamicin molecule binds to the cancerous cells, both the antibody and the drug are taken into the cell. There the drug binds to the cell's genetic material (deoxyribose nucleic acid or DNA) inducing breaks in the molecule and killing it. Because the antibody carries and delivers the toxic drug to the leukemic blasts targets, gemtuzumab treatment is called antibody-targeted **chemotherapy**.

Gemtuzumab can also be used to induce remission (remove cancerous cells) in AML patients to prepare them for stem-cell transplantation. It is indicated for refractory AML (AML that does not readily yield to treatment). The use of antibody-targeted chemotherapy has been shown to have fewer side effects than traditional chemotherapy courses and does improve the disease-free survival time after transplantation.

Description

Gemtuzumab is a genetically engineered monoclonal antibody linked to an antitumor antibiotic. It was approved by the FDA in 2000 as a method of treating relapsed AML in older patients (over 60 years of age) that are not candidates for other cytotoxic chemotherapy. About 75% of all patients with AML experience a relapse after initial treatment. In **clinical trials** focusing on the treatment of older patients with relapsed AML, gemtuzumab had an overall response rate of 30%, with 16% having a complete response.

Most of the gemtuzumab sequence is derived from human sequences, while about 2% are from mice. The human sequences were derived from the constant domains of human IgG4 (called "constant" because it is essentially the same for all IgG antibodies) and the variable framework regions of a human antibody. These areas do not bind to the CD33 protein. Using human sequences in this part of the antibody helps to reduce patient **immune response** to the antibody itself and is called humanization. The actual binding site of gemtuzumab to the CD33 protein is from a mouse anti-CD33 antibody. The antibiotic antitumor drug calcheamicin is linked to the antibody in a way that does not interfere with the ability of the antibody to bind CD33.

Gemtuzumab is not currently approved for use in combination with other chemotherapy drugs or treatments. However, clinical trials that combine the drug with **cytarabine**, **fludarabine**, total-body irradiation, as well as other cancer treatments, are ongoing.

Recommended dosage

Gemtuzumab is administered intravenously. In the pivotal clinical trial, the drug was given at a dose of 9 mg/m^2 for two doses that were fourteen days apart.

Precautions

Extreme caution should be used when using gemtuzumab to treat patients with existent liver problems.

KEY TERMS

Antibody—A protective protein made by the immune system in response to an antigen, also called an immunoglobulin.

Blasts—A type of immature cell that lacks some of the outward characteristics of the mature cell. In AML, the cancerous cells are leukemic blasts.

Calicheamicin—An anti-tumor drug that binds to DNA within the tumor cells, causing breaks in the strands and killing the cell.

IgG—Immunoglobulin type gamma, the most common type found in the blood and tissue fluids.

Humanization—Fusing the constant and variable framework region of one or more human immunoglobulins with the binding region of an animal immunoglobulin, done to reduce human reaction against the fusion antibody.

Monoclonal—Genetically engineered antibodies specific for one antigen.

Myelosuppression—Reduction in the number of the cells of the bone marrow, which leads to reduction of many other circulating blood cells that are produced by the marrow.

Animal studies showed that the drug can cause significant harm to the development of a fetus, so it is likely the drug should not be used during pregnancy, and women of childbearing age should avoid pregnancy while on the drug. Because of the adverse effects of calicheamicin on DNA, the drug greatly reduced fertility in animal studies for males, but not females.

Side effects

A severe side effect of gemtuzumab treatment is a depletion of various types of cells in the bone marrow, including those that make white and red blood cells, a condition known as myelosuppression. Because CD33 is expressed on a patient's normal bone marrow cells, as well as on the surface of the abnormal leukemic blasts, the treatment eliminates both normal and cancerous cells. This results in severe reduction of the circulating blood cells normally produced by the bone marrow, including red blood cells (**anemia**), white blood cells (**neutropenia**), and clotting cells (**thromboccytopenia**). These conditions are treated with blood transfusions. However, the population of all these cells will rebound after clearance of gemtuzumab because the precursor to cells of the bone marrow, called pluripotent hematopoietic stem cells, do not express CD33 and will restore the various cell populations.

Gemtuzumab can produce a postinfusion symptom complex of **fever** and chills, and less commonly, low blood pressure and labored breathing during the first 24 hours after administration. Some patients developed severe liver function abnormalities, which were generally transient and reversible. The most common side effects were fever, chills, nausea, vomiting, thrombocytopenia, neutropenia, asthenia (loss of strength or energy), **diarrhea**, abdominal pain, headache, and **stomatitis** (inflammation of the lining of the mouth).

Interactions

There have been no formal drug interaction studies done for gemtuzumab.

See Also Monoclonal antibodies

Michelle Johnson, M.S., J.D.

Genetic testing

Definition

Genetic testing is a process which involves examining individuals' genetic material for the presence of a change that indicates why they may have developed a disease or disorder. Genetic testing may also tell patients if they are at increased risk for developing a disease such as cancer in the future, but currently do not have any symptoms of that particular disease.

Description

Genetic testing is usually done by taking a sample of a person's blood. The changes in the genetic material that can be detected by this testing vary in size. Sometimes parts or even entire chromosomes may be altered or missing completely. Other times, a mutation is present on a gene that causes it to malfunction. One type of mutation is known as a hereditary mutation. Hereditary mutations may also be called germline mutations because they are found in all the cells of a person's body, including the reproductive or germ cells, the sperm for a male and the egg for a female. This is why hereditary mutations can be inherited, or passed from a parent to a child. Genetic testing often looks for the presence or absence of these types of mutations in genes.

Genes and cancer

Cancer is defined as one cell that grows out of control and subsequently invades nearby cells and tissue. There are several steps involved in the process that causes a normal cell to become malignant (cancerous). It is believed that different genes play a role in this specialized process. Oncogenes typically promote or encourage cell growth. However, if they are overexpressed or mutated, they may cause cancer to arise. Tumor-suppressor genes, when working properly, prevent cells from growing too quickly or out of control. They are often compared to brakes in a car. If these genes cannot perform their function because of the presence of a mutation, cells may grow out of control and become cancerous. Finally, cancer may also be caused by faulty DNA repair genes. These genes usually correct the common mistakes that are made by the body as the DNA copies itself, a normally occurring process. However, if these genes can't correct mistakes, the mistakes may accumulate and lead to cancer.

It is very important to remember that while all cancer is genetic, or caused by changes in genes, just a small amount of cancer is hereditary, or passed from parent to child. It is thought that only about 5-10% of cancer falls into this category. Therefore, the majority of cancer is not hereditary. Most cancer is due to other causes, such as environmental exposures. Usually it is very difficult to determine the exact cause of cancer that is not known to be the result of an altered gene.

Identifying at-risk individuals and families for hereditary cancer

Although scientists have identified genetic tests for common cancers, like breast and **colon cancer**, genetic testing is not an option that should be offered to all people with cancer, or even to those who may have cancer in their family. This is primarily due to the fact that most cancer does not run in families. Therefore, genetic testing will not be helpful for many people. In order to determine those who may benefit from undergoing genetic testing for cancer, health care providers need to be aware of certain aspects of an individual's personal and family history of cancer.

A person who is thinking about having a genetic test for cancer often meets with a genetic counselor, a specially trained health care provider. When a patient meets with a genetic counselor, the counselor will ask the patient about their personal and family history of cancer. The counselor will also draw a very detailed family tree, also known as a pedigree. The counselor will then examine the family tree to determine if there are certain "clues" that the cancer may be hereditary.

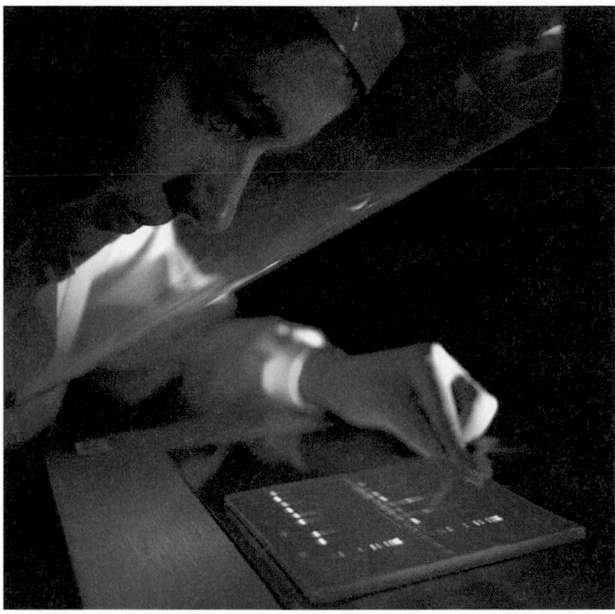

Researcher examining the genetic code of a sequenced sample of neuroblastoma DNA. *(© Colin Cuthbert, Science Source, Photo Researchers, Inc. Reproduced by permission.)*

The clues that may be observed in a family tree are listed below, with **breast cancer** used as an example.

- Multiple relatives in more than one generation with the same type of cancer, or related cancers. For example, a grandmother, mother and daughter with breast cancer. Or, relatives with both breast and **ovarian cancer**.
- Cancer occurring in the family at younger ages than is typically observed in the general population. For example, breast cancer usually occurs in women as they get older, most commonly in their 60's to 70's. However, in families that may have an alteration in a gene increasing their risk for developing breast cancer, the disease may occur in women at much younger ages.
- Cancer that occurs in paired organs. For example, breast cancer that occurs in both of a woman's breasts. This is also called bilateral breast cancer.
- Development of more than one type of related cancer in the same person within a family. For example, a female relative with both breast and ovarian cancer diagnosed at young ages.
- Specific ethnic background. Mutations in certain cancer susceptibility genes may be more likely to occur in individuals of specific ethnic backgrounds. For this reason, it is very important that a complete family tree includes the country where a person's relatives originally lived.

If a genetic counselor or other health care provider observes one or more of the above features in an individual's family tree, he or she may talk about the option of genetic testing with the patient. In the case of cancer genetic testing, it is only offered to a patient if there are options available to screen for the certain cancer and detect it early, or to possibly prevent it from occurring at all.

The process of genetic testing

The process of genetic testing for genes that may increase risk for cancer is different from other medical tests. Genes involved in cancer are called cancer susceptibility genes. If a mutation is identified in one of these genes, it does not reveal that a person has cancer, but rather whether an individual has an increased risk to develop cancer in the future. In addition, if the person undergoing genetic testing has already had cancer, genetic testing may tell them whether they are at increased risk for developing cancer again. However, the risk for developing cancer is not 100%. The likelihood that a person will develop cancer if they carry an altered gene is called penetrance. Penetrance may differ even among relatives in the same family, and the reasons are not well understood. For example, a mother with a mutation in a cancer susceptibility gene may never develop cancer, but may pass this mutation on to her daughter, who is then diagnosed with cancer at a young age.

For a family in which an inherited mutation has not been previously identified, it is best to begin genetic testing by obtaining a blood sample from a person who has had cancer at a young age. From this blood sample, scientists will be able to extract some DNA. There are a number of different ways that they can then look at the DNA to determine if a mutation is present. The most common is known as sequencing, whereby the chemical sequence of a patient's DNA is compared to DNA that is known to be normal. Scientists will look for any differences, such as missing or extra pieces of DNA in the patient's gene.

Testing can be very expensive and it may take several weeks or months to obtain results. Also, insurance companies will sometimes not cover the cost of testing. Some families are able to participate in research studies where genetic counseling and testing is offered at a lower cost or free of charge.

Categories of results

A positive result indicates the presence of a genetic mutation that is known to be associated with an increased risk for developing cancer. Once this kind of mutation has been found in an individual, it is possible to test this person's relatives, like their children, for the presence or absence of that particular mutation. This testing can be done in a relatively short period of time and provides results that are clearly positive or negative for a particular mutation.

If a relative in a family is tested for a mutation in a cancer susceptibility gene that was previously identified in their family, and they are not found to have this mutation, this type of test result is called a true negative. This means that they did not inherit the mutation in the gene that is the reason why their relative(s)developed cancer. If a person receives a true negative test result, their risk for developing cancer is generally considered to be reduced to that of someone in the general population. Also, because they did not inherit the mutation, they cannot pass it down to any of their children. The term true negative is used to distinguish this test result from a negative or indeterminate result, which is described below.

If the first person tested within a family is not found to have an alteration in a cancer susceptibility gene, this result is negative. However, this result is often called indeterminate. This is because a negative test result cannot completely rule out the possibility of hereditary cancer still being present within a family. The interpretation of this type of result can be very complex. For example, a negative result may mean that the method used to detect mutations may not be sensitive enough to identify all mutations in the gene, or perhaps the mutation is in a part of the gene that is difficult to analyze. It may also mean that a person has a mutation in another cancer susceptibility gene that has not yet been discovered or is very rare. Finally, a negative result could mean that the person tested does not have an increased risk for developing cancer because of a mutation in a single cancer susceptibility gene.

Finally, sometimes mutations are identified in cancer genes and scientists do not know what they mean. They do not know if these types of mutations affect the functioning of the gene and thereby increase a person's risk for cancer, or if they are normal changes in the DNA that just make one person's gene a little bit different from another person's. When this occurs, the genetic counselor may work with the laboratory to determine if future research can be done to find out the meaning of the patient's test result.

In general, a genetic counselor will help a patient to understand the meaning of his or her genetic test result, whether positive, negative, or indeterminate.

Benefits and limitations of undergoing genetic testing for cancer susceptibility genes

There are potential benefits for patients who undergo genetic testing, but there are also possible limitations

KEY TERMS

Cancer—The process by which cells grow out of control and subsequently invade nearby cells and tissue.

Cancer susceptibility gene—The type of genes involved in cancer. If a mutation is identified in this type of gene it does not reveal whether or not a person has cancer, but rather whether an individual has an increased risk (is susceptible) to develop cancer (or develop cancer again) in the future.

Colonoscopy—A screening test performed with a tube called a colonoscope that allows a doctor to view a patient's entire colon and rectum.

Chromosome—Structures found in the center of a human cell on which genes are located.

DNA repair genes—A type of gene that usually corrects the common mistakes that are made by the body as DNA copies itself. If these genes are mutated and cannot correct these mistakes they may accumulate and lead to cancer.

Gene—Packages of DNA that control the growth, development and normal function of the body.

Genetic counselor—A specially trained health care provider who helps individuals understand if a disease (such as cancer)is running in their family and their risk for inheriting this disease. Genetic counselors also discuss the benefits, risks and limitations of genetic testing with patients.

Hepatoblastoma—A cancerous tumor of the liver. Individuals with FAP have an increased risk for developing this type of tumor at a young age.

Mammogram—A screening test that uses X-rays to look at a woman's breasts for any abnormalities, such as cancer.

Mutation—An alteration in the number or order of the DNA sequence of a gene.

Oncogene—Genes that typically promote cell growth. If mutated, they may encourage cancer to develop.

Pedigree—A family tree. Often used by a genetic counselor to determine if a disease may be passed from a parent to a child.

Penetrance—The likelihood that a person will develop a disease (such as cancer), if they have a mutation in a gene that increases their risk for developing that disorder.

Polyp—A growth that may develop in the colon. These growths may be benign or cancerous.

Prophylactic surgery—The preventive removal of an organ or tissue before a disease such as cancer develops.

Sequencing—A method of performing genetic testing where the chemical order of a patient's DNA is compared to that of normal DNA.

Sigmoidoscopy—A screening test performed with a flexible scope called a sigmoidoscope, that allows a doctor to view a limited portion of a patient's colon or rectum for the presence of polyps.

Tumor suppressor gene—Genes that typically prevent cells from growing out of control and forming tumors that may be cancerous.

and risks regarding the information that is obtained. A genetic counselor will discuss these issues in detail with a patient. Before undergoing genetic testing, a patient will also sign a consent form. This is a written agreement indicating that the patient understands the benefits and risks of genetic testing and has made an independent decision to undergo the testing. The informed consent process is a very important part of genetic counseling and testing. With the exception of FAP, where polyps and subsequently colon cancer can occur at young ages or in the teens, the cancers associated with carrying an altered breast or colon cancer susceptibility gene do not typically occur at very young ages. Therefore, genetic testing for mutations in these genes is usually only offered to those men and women who are 18 years of age or older. In addition, individuals who are 18 or older are considered legally able to provide informed consent.

Benefits of participating in genetic testing for alterations in cancer susceptibility genes:

- Results of genetic testing may provide additional information about the increased risk for developing cancer in the future. It may also provide relief from anxiety if a person learns that they do not carry an altered gene.
- If a person finds out that they are at increased risk for developing cancer, they may choose to be screened for this cancer at a younger age and more often than someone without an altered cancer susceptibility gene.

Results may also help men and women decide about prophylactic surgery.

- Testing may provide information about cancer risks for children, brothers and sisters, and other relatives.
- Genetic testing may help a person understand why they and/or their family members developed cancer. This may relieve a person from the emotional burden surrounding their cancer diagnosis.

Limitations and risks of participating in genetic testing for cancer susceptibility genes:

- It is possible that the results of genetic testing may be difficult to interpret. Even if a patient receives a positive test result, this does not mean that he/she will definitely develop cancer.
- During the process of undergoing genetic testing, a person may learn information about themselves or their family members. For example, they may learn about an adoption or that an individual is not the biological father of a child. This kind of information may cause strained relationships among relatives.
- Some patients may become sad, angry or anxious if they learn that they have a mutation in a cancer susceptibility gene. If these feelings are very intense, psychological counseling may be helpful.
- Results of genetic testing may place a person at risk for discrimination by health or life insurers, or their employer. There are some laws in effect that provide limited protection to people who undergo genetic testing. The completion of the Human Genome Project, which has mapped all the genes in the human body, will increase the number of genetic tests that are available. Therefore, additional laws need to be passed to completely protect all people who undergo genetic testing from any type of discrimination.

Genes and cancer types

As of 2001,genes have been discovered that are associated with or responsible for several types of cancer, including **Chronic myelocytic leukemia**, **Burkitt's lymphoma**, **retinoblastoma**, **Wilms' tumor**, and breast and colon cancers. The remainder of this entry will focus only on genetic testing for two of the most common cancers, breast and colon cancer.

Breast cancer genetic testing

Breast and ovarian cancer statistics

All women have a risk for developing breast and ovarian cancer during their lifetime. While breast cancer is a common cancer among women in the United States, ovarian cancer is not. Most women are diagnosed with breast or ovarian cancer after the age of 50, and the great majority of cases are not hereditary. But, of the 5-10% of breast and ovarian cancer that does run in families, most is due to mutations in two genes, the BReast CAncer–1 gene (BRCA1) and the BReast CAncer–2 gene (BRCA2). The BRCA1 gene is located on chromosome 17, and was discovered in 1994. The BRCA2 gene is on chromosome 13, and was discovered in 1995.

BRCA1 and BRCA2 genes

BRCA1 and BRCA2 genes are tumor suppressor genes and are inherited in a dominant fashion. This means that children of a parent with a mutation in one of the breast cancer genes have a 50% chance to inherit this mutation. These mutations can be passed from either mother or father, and can be inherited by both males and females. The mutations may be detected by performing genetic testing on a patient's blood sample.

Mutations in these genes are more common in people who are Ashkenazi (Eastern or Central European) Jewish. While these mutations may be more common in this specific population, they can be identified in a person of any ethnic background.

Cancer risks

Females who inherit a mutation in the BRCA1 or the BRCA2 gene have an increased risk for developing breast and/or ovarian cancer over their lifetime. The lifetime risk for breast cancer may be as high as 85%, as compared to about 13% in the general population. The lifetime risk for developing ovarian cancer may be as high as 60%, as compared to 1.5% in the general population. Males who inherit a mutation in one of these genes are also at increased risk for developing certain cancers, including prostate, colon and breast cancer.

Men and women who inherit an alteration in the BRCA2 gene also have an increased risk to develop more rare cancers, such as pancreatic and **stomach cancer**. However, these risks are much lower than those observed for breast, ovarian, and **prostate cancer**.

Screening and prevention options

It is recommended that individuals who are at increased risk for developing breast cancer undergo increased surveillance. This means that they may choose to see their physicians for medical screening tests at an earlier age and more often than they would if they did not have an altered gene. For example, it is recommended that women with an altered BRCA1 or BRCA2 gene undergo mammograms at a younger age than is recommended in the general population. It is also recommended that these women see their doctors more often to do a breast exam and also perform breast self-exams regularly. Because women who have a mutation in BRCA1 or BRCA2 are also at increased risk for developing ovarian cancer, they may also choose to be screened closely for this cancer. This screening involves undergoing a test, called a CA-125, which looks for protein levels in a woman's blood. Women may also undergo a pelvic ultrasound to look at the size and shape of the ovaries to determine if cancer may be growing in that area. It is important to mention that ovarian cancer is a difficult cancer to detect, and these screening methods may not be able to find the cancer at an early stage when a woman can undergo successful treatment.

Men with an altered BRCA1 or BRCA2 gene may also choose to be screened earlier and more frequently for the cancers they are at increased risk to develop. Prostate screening consists of a test called prostate specific antigen (PSA) that looks for protein levels in a man's blood. Men may also undergo an examination by a physician. There are no standard screening recommendations for males who are at increased risk for breast cancer. It is usually recommended that they learn to do breast self-exams and talk with their doctors if they find any changes in their breast tissue.

Some women at increased risk for developing breast or ovarian cancer may decide to have prophylactic or preventive surgery. This means that they may choose to have their healthy breasts or ovaries removed before cancer develops. However, even the very best surgeon cannot remove all of the breast or ovarian tissue. Therefore, even if a woman has her breasts or ovaries removed preventively, she may still develop cancer in the remaining tissue, but this risk is believed to be small.

Finally, some healthy women who are at increased risk for breast or ovarian cancer may decide to take certain medications that have been shown to reduce risk. As some of these medications have been studied only in the general population, further research is underway to find out how effective these medications are for women with an inherited risk for developing cancer.

Colon cancer genetic testing

Colon cancer statistics

Males and females in the general population have a 6% risk for developing colon cancer over their lifetime, and the average individual is diagnosed in their 60s to 70s. Similar to breast and ovarian cancer, most colon cancer does not run in families. However, some colon cancer is hereditary, and may be due to a mutation in a colon cancer susceptibility gene. Three of the more common hereditary colon cancer syndromes are described below.

Familial Adenomatous Polyposis (FAP)

FAP is a syndrome in which individuals develop numerous polyps (growths) in their colon or rectum. This disorder may also be called familial polyposis or Gardner's syndrome. Males or females with FAP often have hundreds of precancerous polyps at young ages, such as when they are teenagers or young adults.

FAP is due to a mutation in a gene called APC. Mutations in this gene are dominantly inherited. In about 80% of families genetic testing performed on a blood sample can find the alteration in the APC gene that is causing this disorder. It is believed that 2/3 of the people with FAP have inherited a mutated gene from their parent. The other 1/3 of individuals with FAP are believed to be new (sporadic) mutations, meaning that the alteration in the APC gene was not inherited from a parent. Individuals with sporadic mutations can pass the mutation on to their children.

Cancer risks

Due to the fact that individuals with FAP develop so many polyps in their colon, there is a very high risk that these polyps, if not removed, will develop into colon cancer. Individuals with FAP may also develop precancerous polyps in other organs, such as their stomach or small intestine. Young people with FAP may also be at increased risk for developing a tumor in the liver, known as a hepatoblastoma. They are also at increased risk for developing tumors in other parts of the body, such as the thyroid gland or pancreas. Males or females with FAP may also have other manifestations of the disease. For example, they may have cysts or bumps on their skin or on the bones of their legs or arms, or freckle-like spots in their eyes.

APC I1307K mutation

In 1997 scientists identified another mutation on the APC gene, known as I1307K. This mutation is found only in individuals who are of Ashkenazi Jewish descent. It is estimated that about 6% of individuals who are Jewish have this particular mutation. The I1307K mutation itself does not cause an increased risk for colon cancer, but rather makes the APC gene more likely to undergo other genetic changes. These other genetic changes increase a person's risk for developing colon cancer. Genetic testing can be performed on a blood sample to determine if an individual carries the I1307K mutation. A person with this mutation has a 50% chance of passing it on to his/her children.

QUESTIONS TO ASK THE DOCTOR

- What is the likelihood that the cancer in my family is due to a mutation in a cancer susceptibility gene?
- If the cancer in my family is hereditary, what is the chance that I carry a mutation in a cancer susceptibility gene?
- What are the benefits, limitations and risks of undergoing genetic testing?
- What is the cost of genetic testing and how long will it take to obtain results?
- If I undergo genetic testing, will my insurance company pay for testing? If so, will I want to share my results with them?
- What does a positive test result mean for me?
- What does a negative test result mean for me?
- If I test positive for a mutation in a cancer susceptibility gene, what are the best options available for screening and prevention? What research studies may I be eligible to participate in?
- What legislation is in effect to protect me against discrimination by my insurer or employer?

Cancer risks

Individuals who carry the I1307K mutation have an 18%-30% risk for developing colon cancer over their lifetime. Research is ongoing to determine if individuals with this mutation may also be at risk for developing other types of cancer, such as breast cancer.

Hereditary Non-Polyposis Colorectal Cancer (HNPCC)

HNPCC, also known as Lynch Syndrome, is a condition in which individuals have an increased risk for developing colon cancer, even if there are very few or no polyps present in the colon. It is believed that mutations in one of five cancer susceptibility genes are associated with most cases of HNPCC. These genes are known as hMSH2, hPMS1, MSH6 (all on chromosome 2), hMLH1 (chromosome 1) and hPMS2 (chromosome 7). It is possible that other genes may be found which are also associated with HNPCC. Mutations in these genes are dominantly inherited, and may be able to be detected through genetic testing performed on a patient's blood sample.

Cancer risks

Individuals with an altered HNPCC gene have a much higher risk for developing colon cancer, often at a younger age (less than 50) than people in the general population. Those with an HNPCC mutation are at increased risk for developing other types of cancer, including stomach, urinary tract, bile duct, uterine and ovarian cancer. It is recommended that men and women also be screened closely for these cancers.

Screening and prevention options

It is recommended that all individuals who are at increased risk for developing colon cancer undergo screening for this cancer. Screening for colon cancer consists of two main types of tests. The first test is called a **sigmoidoscopy**. It is performed by inserting a flexible tube, called a sigmoidoscope into the anus to look at the rectum and the lower colon. The doctor can use the scope to see whether polyps may be present, but these growths can not be removed with this test. The second test is known as a **colonoscopy**. While it is very similar to a sigmoidoscopy, it allows a doctor to see the entire colon. Also, with the use of a colonoscope a polyp can be easily removed at the same time a person is undergoing the test. However, because a colonoscopy is a more invasive test, patients have to be sedated. For patients who are at increased risk for developing colon cancer, it is recommended that they undergo this screening at younger ages and more often then individuals in the general population. For example, because cancer can occur at such young ages for individuals with FAP, it is recommended that they have a sigmoidoscopy beginning at age 11.

Finally, men and women with a mutation in a colon cancer susceptibility gene may take certain medications that have been approved for use in individuals with an increased risk for developing colon cancer.

The only way to prevent colon cancer from developing is to remove the colon entirely. If a person with FAP, HNPCC or the I1307K mutation develops colon cancer he/she may choose to have the colon removed. In addition, if an individual is very anxious about developing colon cancer he or she may choose to have the colon removed before cancer develops. There are several different procedures for removing the colon that allow a person to function normally. Women with an HNPCC mutation may also consider prophylactic removal of their ovaries and uterus.

See Also Cancer genetics; Familial cancer syndromes

Resources

BOOKS

Offitt, Kenneth, M.D.,M.P.H., *Clinical Cancer Genetics.* New York:Wiley Liss Inc.,1998.

PERIODICALS

Burke, W., et al. "Recommendations for Follow-up Care of Individuals With an Inherited Predisposition to Cancer-Hereditary Nonpolyposis Colon Cancer." *Journal of the American Medical Association* 277 (March 1997): 915-19.

Burke,W., et al. "Recommendations for Follow-up Care of Individuals With an Inherited Predisposition to Cancer-BRCA1 and BRCA2." *Journal of the American Medical Association* 277 (March 1997): 997-03.

Cummings, S., and O. Olopade. "Predisposition Testing for Inherited Breast Cancer." *Oncology* 12 (August 1998): 1227-41.

Laken, S.J., et al. "Familial Colorectal Cancer in Ashkenazim due to a hymermutable tract in APC." *Nature Genetics* 17 (1997): 79-83.

Lindor, N.M., et al. "The Concise Handbook of Family Cancer Syndromes." *Journal of the National Cancer Institute* 90 (July 1998): 1039-71.

ORGANIZATIONS

American Cancer Society. 1599 Clifton Road, NE, Atlanta, GA 30329. (800)ACS-2345.<http://www.cancer.org>.

National Cancer Institute. 31 Center Drive, MSC 2580 Bethesda, MD 20892-2580. (800)4-CANCER.<http://www.nci.nih.gov>.

National Society of Genetic Counselors. 233 Canterbury Drive, Wallingford, PA 19086-6617. (610) 872-7608. <http://www.nsgc.og>.

OTHER

Johns Hopkins Hereditary Colorectal Cancer Resources. 23 March 2001 <http://www.hopkins-coloncancer.org/>.

Genetic Health. 27 March 2001 <http://www.genetichealth.com/>.

Tiffani A. DeMarco, M.S.

Genetics of cancer *see* **Cancer genetics**

Gentamicin *see* **Antibiotics**

Germ cell tumors

Definition

Germ cell tumors are tumors that begin in cells that, in a developing fetus, become sperm or egg cells. Because of the way a baby develops in the womb, these kinds of tumors are found in the ovaries and testes, and in other sites along the midline of the body, such as the brain, the center of the chest, and the center back wall of the abdominal cavity. They can also be found in the center parts of the pelvis, cervix, and uterus, in the vagina or prostate, in the oral or nasal cavities, or on the lips. These tumors are usually discovered either during the first few years of life, or shortly after puberty (when an increase in hormone levels may initiate cancer formation).

Description

Germ cell tumors are a diverse group of tumors that all begin in germ cells, the cells in the developing fetus that become sperm or egg cells. Incidence in the United States is 2–3 cases/million live births. They can occur in the ovaries or testes or outside the reproductive organs in many other locations along the middle of the body. Some are very malignant and some are almost always benign; most require surgery, although some kinds are also treated with additional radiation or **chemotherapy**. Some typically appear in infancy, others are more common in adolescents. The treatment and prognosis will depend on the kinds of tissues present in the tumor and on the location.

Germ cell tumors are divided into two types: germinomas, which contain only immature germ cells; and embryonic tumors, which contain some cells that have started to develop into other tissues (as would happen in normal development of a fetus). Embryonic types of tumor commonly include endodermal sinus tumors, embryonal **carcinoma**, choriocarcinoma and teratoma. Gonadoblastoma and polyembryoma are rare types of embryonic germ cell tumors. Many tumors are mixed, containing more than one cell type.

Generally, any kind of germ cell tumor can appear at any germ cell tumor site, although some types are significantly more common at some locations. For example, about 40% of all germ cell tumors are teratomas in the area of the tailbone, which are typically diagnosed in the first month or two of life. Germinomas and endodermal sinus tumors are most common in the ovaries. Embryonal carcinomas are most common in the testes, usually mixed with endodermal sinus tumors or choriocarcinoma.

Demographics

Like other features of this diverse group of tumors, demographics of this cancer vary with the site and type. The peak in incidence of germ cell tumors during the first few years of life is primarily due to the high numbers of teratomas in the tailbone area, which are about 4 times more common in girls than in boys. The second peak, however, in adolescents reflects a significant number of testicular cancers in teenage and young adult males. Other common childhood germ cell tumors are tumors of the abdomen, vagina and testicles in infants, brain tumors in childhood, and ovarian tumors in early teens. Adult germ cell tumors in adults are usually in the testes or ovaries. Germ cell tumors are found in all populations of the world in approximately equal numbers.

Causes and symptoms

The causes of germ cell tumors are not well understood, although events at puberty—probably increases in certain hormone level—are thought to play a role in tumors of the ovaries and testicles that occur in adolescents or early teens. Some germ cell tumors have a high percentage of certain genetic sequences, thought to be a possible cause of those types of cancers, while some have a high frequency of abnormal chromosome numbers. Some types of germ cell tumors do tend to run in families. Since germ cell tumors are made up of several different types of cancers, there are probably at least several different causes.

The most common symptom of germ cell tumors is a mass along the midline of the body. This mass may be accompanied by abdominal pain or bloating. Other possible symptoms include:

- constipation
- enuresis (involuntary discharge of urine)
- early entry into puberty
- vaginal bleeding
- late onset of menstruation
- menstrual problems
- excessive hair growth
- weakness in legs
- need to urinate often
- shortness of breath, other breathing problems
- diabetes
- hormonal abnormalities
- stunted growth
- headaches or vision problems

Diagnosis

Most germ cell cancers are initially identified by the discovery of lump in the testicles or somewhere else along the midline of the body. When a lump is identified, often the person's physician will arrange for a **biopsy** of the lump. During a biopsy, a small piece of the lump is removed and cut into thin sections. A specialist examines these sections under a microscope, looking for abnormal kinds of cells. How much the biopsied tissue is different from healthy tissue is a good indication of how severe the disease will probably be, and the results of biopsies are used to give tumors a grade that indicates the patient's chances of survival.

Tests that give a doctor pictures of the tumor are also used, such as x rays, **computed tomography** (CT) scans, or ultrasound. X rays can show the doctors where calcium deposits have occurred in normally soft tissues (an indication of disease). Ultrasound and CT scanning give more details with regard to a specific tumor, such as its site of origin, whether it is solid or cystic, and how well defined its borders are. Well-defined borders have a better chance of complete surgical removal.

Another type of useful test which is specific to germ cell tumors is the measurement of several **tumor markers**. Tumor markers are proteins, often identified in blood samples, that are produced by tumor cells. Two main tumor markers are commonly seen to suggest a germ cell tumor, alpha-fetoprotein (AFP) and ß-Human Chorionic Gonadotropin (ß-HCG). Germ cell tumors which produce elevated levels of AFP include endodermal sinus tumors and teratoma, although high levels of AFP are also produced by normal infants. ß-HCG is usually associated with tumors which contain elements of the choriocarinoma or embryonic carcinoma types of germ cell tumors. These markers are also used as a measure of the success of surgery or other therapies, and to monitor patients for a recurrence of the disease.

Treatment team

As the understanding of cancer grows and new treatment approach are developed, the complexity of cancer treatment also increases. Today, a multi-disciplinary approach to cancer treatment is considered necessary for effective patient care. People involved in the treatment of a germ cell cancer will typically include the referring physician (often a gynecologist or pediatrician), a gynecological oncologist, a pathologist, and a nurse. If **radiation therapy** is pursued, a radiation oncologist, radiation therapist, radiation nurse, radiation physicist, and a dosimetrist will also be involved. Treatment may also include a psychologist, nutritionist, social worker and chaplain.

Clinical staging, treatments, and prognosis

Staging

Staging and grading tumors is a way of predicting the severity of the disease. Tumor grades are based on the types of tissues present in the tumor; stages indicate the cancer's spread. Separate staging systems exist for both adult and childhood ovarian cancers and adult and childhood testicular cancers. These are developed separately by groups of pediatric and adult oncologists.

OVARIAN CANCERS. Pediatric ovarian cancers are usually graded according to the following scheme: Grade 0 contains only mature tissues (tissues which have already become specific kinds of tissues, rather than primitive developing cells. Grade 1 contains mostly mature tissues, with some immature cells present. Grade 2 contains a moderate amount of immature cells, and in Grade 3, numerous immature cells are present.

Adult **ovarian cancer** is usually staged, with Stage I being found only in the ovaries. Stage II in adult ovarian cancer means that the cancer has spread to the uterus or the fallopian tubes, or other structures in the pelvic area. Stage III tumors are those which have spread to the lymph nodes or outer parts of abdominal organs. Stage IV tumors have spread to the interior of abdominal organs such as the liver or the intestines.

TESTICULAR CANCERS. Pediatric testicular cancers are typically staged in a manner similar to adult ovarian cancers: Stage I tumors are limited to the testes, with normal postoperative tumor markers. Stage II tumors have spread to the abdominal lymph nodes and have elevated tumor markers; Stage III have greater involvement of the abdominal lymph nodes. Stage IV tumors have spread to other organs such as the lung.

Adult testicular cancers are commonly staged according to a simplified TNM system. Stage T (with several levels described) indicates a tumor that is localized, N means a tumor that has spread to local lymph nodes, and M means a tumor that has spread to distant lymph nodes and organs.

Treatment

The treatment choice in any specific germ cell tumor depends mainly on the type of tumor and the stage at diagnosis, although the age of the patient and whether or not future childbearing is an issue will also influence treatment choices. Treatment of most germ cell tumors involves surgical removal of the tumor. Advanced cancers normally will be followed by chemotherapy. For some tumors, it may not be possible to completely remove the cancerous tissues. In those cancers, "debulking" surgery will be performed in order to reduce the size of the tumor in order for chemotherapy (or radiation) to be most effective.

Chemotherapy can be given through pills taken by mouth, by injections or through IVs. Chemotherapy works by killing cancerous cells, and can kill cancer cells that have traveled away from the initial site. Therefore, in more advanced stages of disease, chemotherapy will sometimes be the primary treatment. Possibly another surgery will be performed after radiation therapy or chemotherapy is finished. This surgery (second-look surgery) allows the doctor to confirm that cancerous tissues have been eradicated.

Chemotherapy usually involves a platinum-based drug such as **cisplatin** in combination with one or two other anti-cancer medications. These drugs are used in combination because, since they each have different side effects, high doses can be given without increasing the risk of a serious drug reaction. Using combinations also decreases the chance that a cancer will develop resistance to any particular drug. Different combinations of drugs are used to treat different types of tumors.

The treatment of some types of germ cell cancers may follow a slightly different pattern. Germinomas are especially sensitive to radiation. This may be the primary treatment mode for those kinds of tumors. Radiation is used to shrink the size of tumors, and even in ovarian cancers usually involves only external irradiation. The only type of germ cell tumor in children in which radiation is regularly used is germinomas occurring in the brain.

When first-line treatments fail, stronger combinations of drugs may be given, or different, sometimes experimental therapies may be tried. These kinds of therapies includes immune system products like **interferons** that have been shown to destroy cancerous cells and new drugs being developed that decrease blood flow to tumors. Therapies like immunotoxins, which include anti-cancer drugs attached to antibodies specific to tumor cells, and other ways of making drugs more specific for tumor cells, are also being investigated. Many **clinical trials** for germ cell cancers are evaluating a therapy called "peripheral stem cell rescue," in which the patient's red blood cells are removed before high-dose chemotherapy is given, then replaced after the

KEY TERMS

Choriocarcinoma—A highly aggressive malignant germ cell tumor made up of tissue derived from the outer membrane which covers the fetus.

Embryonic carcinoma—A highly malignant germ cell tumor made up of tissues derived from the embryo.

Endodermal sinus tumor—A more aggressive germ cell tumor made up of tissue originating in the nutrient sac of the embryo.

Germinoma—A tumor that develops purely from primitive germ cells.

Gonadoblastoma—A rare and almost always benign form of cancer highly associated with abnormal development of reproductive organs.

Polyembryoma—A very rare, aggressive form of germ cell tumor usually found in the ovaries.

chemotherapy is complete. This decreases the side effects of the medications and improves the patient's chances of successful treatment.

The prognosis for germ cell tumors depends greatly on the type of germ cell tumor involved and the location in which it is found. Generally, about 90% of patients diagnosed with only localized tumors survive, compared to 50–70% of those who are diagnosed with tumors which have already spread. There is wide variation in the cure rates, depending on the tumor types involved. Mature teratomas of the ovaries, which are by far the most common type of ovarian tumor, are almost always benign, unless mixed with other, more malignant germ cell tumor types. Choriocarcinomas and embryonal carcinomas, on the other hand, are especially malignant, with an average survival time without treatment of only a few months. Since ovarian cancers are the most difficult to catch early, ovarian cancers of types more malignant than the mature teratoma have the worst prognosis among the germ cell tumors. With modern treatment methods, most often including chemotherapy after surgical removal, survival rates have greatly improved. If caught early, most germ cell tumors have good cure rates.

Alternative and complementary therapies

Alternative and complementary therapies are therapies which fall outside the scope of traditional, first-line therapies like surgery, chemotherapy and radiation. Complementary therapies are meant to supplement those traditional therapies with the objective of relieving symptoms. Alternative therapies are nontraditional, unproven attempts to cure the disease.

Common complementary therapies in germ cell disease include aromatherapy, art therapy, massage, meditation, music therapy, prayer, t'ai chi, yoga, and other forms of exercise. These therapies have the objective of reducing anxiety and increasing a patient's feeling of well-being.

Numerous alternative therapies exist in cancer treatment. Laetril, a product of apricot seeds, is probably one of the most well known. Laetril contains a form of cyanide that may be released by tumor enzymes and may act to kill cancerous cells. However, the product is not approved for use in the United States, and the National Cancer Institute sponsored two clinical trials for the drug in the late 1970s and early 1980s, and decided that no further investigation into the drug was necessary. **Vitamins** and other nutritional elements like vitamins A, C, and E, and selenium are thought to act as **antioxidants**. Vitamin E, melatonin, aloe vera, and a compound called beta-1,3-glucan are thought to stimulate the immune system. Natural substances like garlic, ginger, and shark cartilage are also commonly held to shrink tumors, with less defined modes of action. Antineoplastons are believed by some to be another alternative approach to a cancer cure. Antineoplastons are small proteins which may act as molecular messengers and which may be absent from the urine and blood of many cancer patients. Replacing these proteins may have beneficial effects. After some proposed clinical trials were not completed, the National Cancer Institute draws no definitive conclusions about the effectiveness of antineoplaston therapy. Patients should discuss any supplements with their treating physicians.

Coping with cancer treatment

The use of chemotherapy and radiation therapy in addition to surgery has greatly increased the numbers of germ cell tumor patients that survive; but both of these treatments unavoidably result in damage to some healthy tissues and other undesirable side effects. Some of the more common side effects of chemotherapy include:

- hair loss (**alopecia**)
- **fatigue** and weakness
- **nausea and vomiting**
- bed wetting

Hair loss is a very common side effect of many drugs used to treat cancer. Getting a sample of hair before hair loss begins is desirable in case a wig is desired after hair loss begins. The patient's hair color and texture could then be more closely matched. Hair may thin out gradually or it may come out in big clumps. To slow down the rate of hair loss, avoid any unnecessary sources of damage to the hair, like curling, blow-drying, or chemical treatments.

Hair loss is a difficult part of dealing with cancer for all patients past infancy, especially for teenage patients. Children should be given the right to choose their own way of coping and their choices should be supported. Children may choose to remain bald, or may want to choose hats or scarves instead of wigs. Schools may need to be persuaded to allow a child to wear some kind of head covering. It is important to assure the child that loss of hair is a sign that the medication is doing its job, and that hair loss is temporary.

Hair usually begins regrowth within a few months of the end of intensive chemotherapy, although it may begin to thin out again during the course of maintenance drugs. Sometimes hair comes in a different color or texture than the original hair. It may be a good idea to prepare a child for that possibility.

Fatigue and weakness are other common side effects of chemotherapy. Side effects of the chemotherapy medications, along with the natural depletion of the body's resources as it fights off the disease and normal psychological consequences of the disease such as **depression** combine to make fatigue a very significant part of coping with cancer treatment.

The best way to deal with these symptoms is to cut back on activities and allow plenty of time for resting to let the body heal. Patients should avoid as much extra stress as possible, limiting visitors if necessary in order to avoid being overtired. Children should not be forced into the role of invalid. Children must be allowed to pursue normal activities and hobbies as much as possible. Parents can best manage this by helping to select those activities that the child considers most important, and by providing a backup plan for times when the child does become too fatigued, such as alternate means of mobility (for example, a stroller, wheel chair or other acceptable and safe vehicle). It is also important to make sure that a well-balanced diet is provided.

Nausea and vomiting are also fairly common side effects of many chemotherapy drugs. Radiation to the brain or the GI tract can also cause nause and vomiting. After a few courses of chemotherapy drugs, some patients will become nauseated just from the thought of an upcoming treatment, or from smelling certain odors that act as nausea triggers. Drugs that combat nausea and vomiting can be prescribed, but are often not effective for anticipatory nausea. There are self-help measures that can be tried. If nausea and vomiting are a problem, heavy, regular meals should be avoided in favor of small, frequent snacks made up of light but nourishing foods like soup. Avoiding food smells and other strong odors may help.

Desensitization, hypnosis, guided imagery, and relaxation techniques may be used if nausea and vomiting are severe. These techniques help to identify the causes which trigger the nausea and vomiting, decrease patient anxiety, and distract the patient from thinking about getting sick. In children, activities like playing video games can be offered as very effective means of distraction.

Bedwetting is another common side effect of anticancer drugs, and one which can be especially distressing for older children. A child who experiences this problem should be reassured that the problem is temporary and will go away when the drug treatment is over. Parents can help the child cope by keeping extra linens ready or covering the wet spot with towels kept handy and most of all, by conveying an attitude that wetting the bed is not a big deal. Children should never be punished. It may also help to limit drinks for a couple of hours before bedtime, or to wake the child at regular intervals overnight to use the bathroom.

The biggest problem for those undergoing radiation therapy is the development of dry, sore, "burned" skin in the area being treated. Radiation does not hurt during treatment and does not make the person radioactive. Skin in the treatment area will become red, get itchy and sore, and may blister and peel, becoming painful. Patients with fair skin, or those who have undergone previous chemotherapy have a greater risk of more serious reactions. Dry, itchy or sore skin is temporary; but affected skin may be more sensitive to sun exposure for the rest of the patient's lifetime, so a good sunscreen should be used whenever affected skin is exposed to sunlight.

Fear and anxiety are major factors in coping with cancer, including cancer treatments. The feelings are completely normal. Some patients find that concentrating on restful, pleasurable activities like hobbies, prayer, or meditation is helpful in decreasing negative emotions. Support groups are another useful tool, since they provide an environment where fears can be freely expressed and understood.

Clinical trials

Nearly a hundred clinical trials testing new treatments for germ cell tumors are ongoing. New approaches being evaluated emphasize new combinations of existing chemotherapy drugs, peripheral stem cell therapies to supplement chemotherapy, alternative therapies like antineoplastons, and new drug delivery approaches such as immunotoxins.

Therapies being evaluated in clinical trials are usually considered experimental and some, like peripheral stem cell rescue, can be very expensive. Most insurance companies do not cover the costs of experimental therapies.

To find an ongoing clinical trial for a specific kind of germ cell tumor, call the National Cancer Institute at 1-800-4-CANCER.

Prevention

Since the causes of germ cell tumors are not well understood, few identified risk factors exist, thus providing little information on the possibility of preventing these kinds of cancers. However, there are ways of improving prognosis with regards to germ cell tumors. Ovarian cancers are difficult to catch in early stages; women who get regular gynecological check-ups are more likely to have ovarian cancer diagnosed in more treatable stages. Males who have had **testicular cancer** can improve their chances of catching recurrences in early stages by doing regular self-exams.

QUESTIONS TO ASK THE DOCTOR

- Can you explain what kind of cancer I have?
- Is it a benign or aggressive form of germ cell tumor? Can you explain the grade and stage of my cancer? What are the chances that it will come back?
- How was this cancer diagnosed?
- What is my prognosis?
- What treatments are we going to pursue? What happens if these don't work?
- Do you have experience in treating this type of cancer?
- Is there anything I can do to optimize treatment? Are there any particular side effects I should expect?
- Are there complementary therapies that you would recommend? Any other things that would help me cope with the diagnosis or treatment?

Special concerns

A special concern in germ cell tumor patients, especially since most patients are children or young adults, is maintaining these patients' ability to bear children. Unfortunately, all of the common treatments can have a negative effect on future fertility. Radiation, especially, destroys fertility and is avoided in children except for germinomas of the brain. Patients whose reproductive organs must be removed suffer major psychological consequences of the loss of childbearing potential and often, as well, suffer from altered feelings of **sexuality**. The treatment team will attempt to choose treatment options that will preserve the patient's childbearing ability to the best of medical capabilities.

See Also Ovarian cancer; Testicular cancer; Extragondal germ cell tumors; Gynecological cancers; Childhood cancers

Resources

BOOKS

Cook, Allan R., ed.*The New Cancer Sourcebook.* New York: Omnigraphics, Inc.,1996.

Pizzo and Poplack, ed. *Principles and Practice of Pediatric Oncology.* Philadelphia: Lippincott-Raven, 1997.

Buckman, R. *What You Really Need to Know About Cancer.* Baltimore: Johns Hopkins University Press, 1999

Pinkerton, C.R., and P.N. Plowman. ed.*Pediatric Oncology.* Chapman and Hall Medical, 1998.

ORGANIZATIONS

American Cancer Society, 1599 Clifton Road, NE, Atlanta, GA 30329-4251. (800)586-4872 <http://www.cancer.org> 29 June 2001.

National Cancer Institute, 9000 rockville Pike, Bethesda, Maryland, 20892. (800)422-6237. <http:www.nci.nih.gov.> 29 June 2001.

The Wellness Community, 10921 Reed Harman Highway, Cincinnati, Ohio, 45242 (888)793-9355. "A free program of emotional support, education and hope for people with cancer and their loved ones." <http://www.wellness-community.org> 29 June 2001.

OTHER

QUACKWATCH "Your Guide to Health Fraud, Quackery and Intelligent Decisions." <http://www.quackwatch.com>

Wendy Wippel, M.S.

Gestational trophoblastic tumors

Definition

A gestational trophoblastic tumor (GTT) is a rare cancer that develops in tissues formed when a sperm fertilizes an egg but does not create a fetus.

Description

Also known as gestational trophoblastic neoplasms (GTN), these highly curable malignancies originate inside the uterus, in cells (trophoblasts) that make up one layer of the placenta. The most common types of GTT are hydatidiform mole (molar pregnancy) and choriocarcinoma. Placental-site trophoblastic tumor is an extremely rare type of GTT. It originates at the place where the placenta was attached to the wall of the uterus.

Hydatidiform mole

A hydatidiform mole forms when sperm and egg cells unite but do not create a fetus. Cells that form the placenta continue to grow until they look like drops of rain or clusters of grapes. Also known as molar pregnancy, a hydatidiform mole does not spread beyond the uterus.

Choriocarcinoma

Characterized by rapid growth and heavy bleeding, this aggressive, invasive tumor is considered a medical emergency and requires immediate medical attention. Although choriocarcinoma usually originates in a hydatidiform mole, it can also develop in tissue that remains in the uterus following a normal delivery, an abortion, or an ectopic pregnancy.

A malignancy of the trophoblastic cells that form the lining of the uterus (epithelium), choriocarcinoma can spread (metastasize) to any part of the body. **Metastasis** begins at an early stage of the disease and usually involves the lungs, vagina, pelvis, brain, and/or liver. Symptoms of lung metastasis include severe shortness of breath (respiratory insufficiency) and coughing up blood. Irregular, abnormal bleeding can indicate that choriocarcinoma has invaded the vagina. The central nervous system (CNS) is rarely affected unless the disease has spread to one or both lungs; a patient whose brain does become involved may experience headaches, seizures, and stroke-like symptoms. More rarely, choriocarcinoma may spread to the kidneys, spleen, and/or gastrointestinal tract.

Demographics

GTTs occur only in women of childbearing age. These tumors are most common:

- before the age of 16
- after the age of 40
- in women who have had them before
- among women who are poor

Accounting for only 1% of all gynecologic malignancies, GTTs are five times more common in Africa and Asia than in Europe and North America. In the United States, hydatidiform mole occurs in only one of every 1,500 to 2,000 pregnancies.

Causes and symptoms

The cause of GTTs is unknown. A woman's chance of developing a second GTT, while still very low, is about twice as great as her risk of developing a first one.

Symptoms of hydatidiform mole

The most common symptoms of hydatidiform mole are vaginal bleeding and severe morning sickness during the first trimester of pregnancy. Other symptoms that suggest a hydatidiform mole include:

- a uterus larger than expected at a particular stage of pregnancy
- a uterus enlarged on only one side
- a fetus not visible on a sonogram
- absence of fetal heart sounds
- passage of clots with the color and consistency of prune juice or of finger-like structures containing fetal blood cells (villi)
- toxemia
- ovarian cysts
- hyperthyroidism

Recurrent bleeding often causes iron deficiency **anemia** in women who have had a hydatidiform mole. Although molar pregnancy is almost always diagnosed during the first trimester, it is often difficult to distinguish this condition from the early stages of a normal pregnancy. A woman should see her doctor if she experiences abnormal bleeding or cannot feel her baby move when she should.

Symptoms of choriocarcinoma

This GTT occurs in 4% of women whose hydatidiform mole was surgically removed or treated with **radiation therapy**. Following term pregnancies or abortion, the incidence of choriocarcinoma is 1 in 40,000.

A doctor should always consider choriocarcinoma when vaginal bleeding persists after a woman has given birth. Other abnormalities commonly associated with choriocarcinoma are unusual and unexplained neurological symptoms in women of childbearing age and lesions that can be seen on a chest **x ray** but do not cause shortness of breath or other symptoms.

Diagnosis

The process of diagnosing GTT usually begins with an internal pelvic examination that allows the doctor to detect lumps or abnormalities in the size or shape of the uterus. **Imaging studies** such as **computed tomography** (CT) scans, **magnetic resonance imaging** (MRI), and ultrasound may be used to locate tumors. Blood and urine tests measure levels of beta human chorionic gonadotropin (HCG). This hormone is normally produced during pregnancy but is abnormally elevated in the blood and urine of a woman with GTT. HCG is a sensitive marker of the presence of GTT before, during, and after treatment.

After diagnosing GTT, the doctor will perform a regular blood test (every week), pelvic exam (every other week), and chest x ray (every four to six weeks) until the level of HCG in the patient's blood has returned to normal. Once the patient's HCG levels have normalized, medical monitoring includes blood tests with decreasing frequency for the next three years.

KEY TERMS

Ectopic pregnancy—An abnormal pregnancy in which the fertilized egg becomes implanted outside the uterus.

Ovarian cyst—A fluid-filled or semi-solid sac that may be painful or malignant.

Placenta—The organ that develops in the uterus during pregnancy and connects the mother's blood supply with the baby.

Remission—Disappearance or lessening of symptoms.

Salvage surgery—An operation used to treat a patient who has not responded to any other therapy.

Systemic—Affecting the whole body.

Toxemia—An abnormal pregnancy-related condition characterized by high blood pressure, swelling and fluid retention, and proteins in the urine.

Treatment team

GTT is typically treated by a treatment team of gynecologists, gynecologic oncologists, and medical oncologists. A patient who has a poor prognosis should be treated at a specialized trophoblastic disease center by a doctor experienced in caring for high-risk GTT patients.

Clinical staging, treatments, and prognosis

A common system used in U.S. cancer centers to describe the extent (stage) of GTT classifies patients into different prognostic groups. These groups include:

- Nonmetastatic disease: Cancer cells have not invaded tissues outside of the uterus. Cancer found in the muscle of the uterus is called invasive mole or choriocarcinoma destruens.
- Metastatic disease, good prognosis: Cancer cells have invaded tissues outside of the uterus but have not spread to the liver or brain; levels of HCG in the blood are low and the last pregnancy was less than four months ago. No **chemotherapy** treatment has been initiated.
- Metastatic disease, poor prognosis: Cancer cells have invaded tissues outside of the uterus, including the liver or brain; levels of HCG in the blood are high and/or the last pregnancy was more than four months ago. Chemotherapy treatment has been given but was not successful.

Treatment options

Because GTT cells respond well to chemotherapy drugs and HCG blood tests are a reliable means of determining whether cancer cells are still present and if therapy should continue, this disease is one of the most curable cancers of the female reproductive system.

Doctors usually treat GTT with surgery to remove the tumor, followed by chemotherapy taken in pill form or administered intravenously to kill any cancer cells still present after surgery. Radiation therapy is sometimes used to treat GTT that has spread to other parts of the body. Radiation used to treat GTT may be provided by:

- machine (external-beam radiation)
- radiation-producing pellets (radioisotopes) inserted into the area of the body where cancer cells have been found

Choice of treatment is determined by the following factors:

- patient's age and general health
- tumor type
- stage of disease
- areas of the body to which GTT has spread
- HCG levels in the patient's blood
- how much time elapsed between conception and start of treatment
- prior pregnancy-related problems
- extent of treatment for prior pregnancy-related problems
- whether the patient wants to become pregnant in the future

HYDATIDIFORM MOLE. Hydatidiform mole is 100% curable with surgery. If the patient wants to become pregnant in the future, the doctor performs **dilatation and curettage** (D&C) with suction evacuation. This procedure involves:

- stretching the opening of the uterus (cervix)
- using a small vacuum-like device to remove material from inside the uterus
- gently scraping the walls of the uterus to remove any remaining material.

If the patient does not wish to become pregnant in the future, the doctor removes her uterus (hysterectomy).

Following either of these operations, the doctor carefully monitors the level of HCG in the patient's blood. Chemotherapy is initiated when:

- HCG levels continue to rise for a period of two weeks or remain constant for a period of three weeks

- HCG levels become elevated after having fallen to normal value
- analysis of tissue removed during surgery indicates the presence of invasive disease (choriocarcinoma)
- heavy, unexplained bleeding occurs after material has been evacuated from the uterus

PLACENTAL-SITE GTT. Hysterectomy is usually performed to remove cancer cells that have developed where the placenta was attached to the wall of the uterus. Although placental-site GTTs do not generally spread to other parts of the body, they do not respond well to chemotherapy and can be fatal.

NONMETASTATIC DISEASE. The most common form of GTT, nonmetastatic disease does not spread beyond the uterus, where its cells develop from tissue remaining after treatment for hydatidiform mole, normal delivery, or abortion. Treatment for nonmetastatic disease consists of single-agent chemotherapy. Hysterectomy is sometimes performed if the patient does not want to become pregnant in the future.

METASTATIC DISEASE, GOOD PROGNOSIS. This type of GTT originates as nonmetastatic disease but spreads from the uterus to other parts of the body. The likelihood of cure (prognosis) is considered good if:

- less than four months has elapsed since the patient's previous pregnancy
- HCG blood levels are low
- cancer cells have not spread to the liver or brain
- the patient has not previously received chemotherapy

Doctors may treat metastatic disease with good prognosis with chemotherapy alone, hysterectomy followed by chemotherapy, or chemotherapy followed by hysterectomy. These patients must be carefully monitored. Almost all of these cases can be cured, but between 40% and 50% will develop resistance to the first chemotherapy drug used in treatment.

METASTATIC DISEASE, POOR PROGNOSIS. The prognosis for metastatic disease is considered poor if:

- more than four months has elapsed since the patient's previous pregnancy
- HCG blood levels are high
- cancer cells have spread to the liver or brain
- previous chemotherapy treatments did not eradicate the patient's disease

Treatment for this type of GTT must be started immediately and should be performed in a specialized medical center or by a doctor experienced in treating this disease. Treatment usually consists of combination chemotherapy but may include surgery and radiation to parts of the body that cancer cells have invaded.

Metastatic GTT is can also be described as low-risk, medium-risk, or high-risk. This classification enables doctors to identify patients who should be treated with the strongest, most effective combination of chemotherapy drugs. Factors used to determine a woman's risk include:

- age
- prior pregnancy experience
- how much time elapsed between conception and start of treatment
- HGC levels in her blood
- the size of her largest tumor
- where and to how many locations the cancer has spread
- whether she has previously been treated with chemotherapy

RECURRENT DISEASE. GTT that recurs after a woman has been treated may reappear in the uterus or in another part of her body. One study indicates that GTT recurs in:

- 2.5% of patients treated for nonmetastatic disease
- 3.7% of patients treated for metastatic disease, good prognosis
- 13% of patients treated for metastatic disease, poor prognosis

All these recurrences happened within 36 months of the disappearance of symptoms of the initial disease (remission), while 85% occurred within 18 months of remission.

A woman who develops one or more new GTTs after having been treated with chemotherapy is considered to be a high-risk patient and is categorized as having

QUESTIONS TO ASK THE DOCTOR

- What should I do if I am not sure my pregnancy is proceeding normally?
- Why is it important for me to see my doctor as soon as I realize something might be wrong?
- Will GTT affect my ability to have other children?
- Why must I wait so long before becoming pregnant?

a poor prognosis. She should subsequently be treated with aggressive chemotherapy. If surgery is not successful in eradicating the cancer, treatment with single-agent chemotherapy is usually indicated unless one or more risk factors indicate that she should receive multiple-drug therapy. When recurrent disease spreads to the central nervous system, whole brain radiation and systemic chemotherapy are given at the same time. About half (50% to 60%) of patients receiving this treatment experience sustained remission. Combination chemotherapy may also be used to treat a woman whose recurrent GTT has spread to the brain.

The prognosis is poor for a woman whose recurrent GTT has spread to her liver; in this case radiation does not improve survival and may make chemotherapy less effective. The prognosis is even poorer if both the liver and brain are affected. "Salvage" surgery is sometimes used to treat patients whose disease has not responded to any other available form of treatment.

Disease outcomes

Although very rare in North America, GTT is an important disease because of its life-threatening potential and high curability rates with early, specialized treatment. The probability of cure is high even when the disease has spread far from the uterus. About 70% of patients with high-risk disease go into remission, while the cure rates for properly managed molar pregnancy and vigorously treated nonmetastatic GTT are nearly 100%. About 80% of patients with widely metastasized disease are cured when treated with prompt, aggressive chemotherapy sometimes combined with surgery and radiation.

Combination chemotherapy achieves results in nearly three out of four patients (74%) who have not responded to other forms of treatment, and more than three out of four high-risk patients (76%) who have not previously been treated with chemotherapy. More than half of patients (57%) whose earlier treatment did not eradicate the disease also achieve good results with combination chemotherapy. The survival rate for patients treated with combination chemotherapy is 84%.

Clinical trials

Researchers throughout the United States are currently investigating the following concerns:

- How effective are certain chemotherapy drugs in treating GTT that has not responded to other therapies or that has recurred after treatment?
- At what dosages do specific chemotherapy drugs become toxic?
- How does the frequency of chemotherapy treatments affect a patient's prognosis?
- What is the relationship between the start of chemotherapy and an immediate drop in a patient's HCG levels?

Prevention

The cause of GTT is not known, but the risk is higher than normal for a woman who belongs to blood group A and whose partner belongs to blood group O.

Special concerns

Medical oncologists emphasize the importance of the following treatment factors:

- Chemotherapy should be started as early in the course of the disease as possible.
- Chemotherapy should be administered every 14 to 21 days until HCG blood levels drop to normal.
- High-risk patients should be treated with combination chemotherapy regardless of the stage of their disease.
- Monthly blood tests should be continued for one year after HCG levels drop to normal.
- A woman who has been treated for GTT should wait at least a year before becoming pregnant and see her doctor as soon as she becomes or thinks she might be pregnant.

See Pregnancy and cancer

Resources

BOOKS

DeVita, Vincent T. Jr., et al, eds. *Cancer: Principles & Practice of Oncology, 5th ed.* Philadelphia: Lippinott-Raven, 1997, pp. 1499-1501.

Kirkwood, John M., et al, eds. *Current Cancer Therapeutics, 3rd ed.* Philadelphia:Current Medicine, Inc., 1998, pp. 252-254.

ORGANIZATIONS

American College of Obstetricians and Gynecologists. 409 12th St. SW, PO Box 96920, Washington, DC 20090-6920. (202) 863-2518. <http://www.acog.org>.

National Cancer Institute. 31 Center Dr., MSC 2580, Bethesda, MD 20892-2580. (800) 4-CANCER. <http://cancernet.nci.nih.gov>.

OTHER

"Gestational Trophoblastic Disease." *American Cancer Society.* 27 March 2000. 5 July 2001. <http://www3.cancer.org/cancerinfo/load_cont.asp?st=ds&ct=49>.

"Gestational Trophoblastic Disease." *OBGYN.net Publications.* 2001. 3 July 2001. <http://www.obgyn.net/women/articles/rich/gest.htm>.

"Gestational Trophoblastic Tumor." *National Cancer Institute.* May 2001. 3 July 2001. <http://cancernet.nci.nih.gov/cancer_Types/Gestational_Trophoblastic_Tumor.shtml>.

Maureen Haggerty

Giant cell tumors

Definition

Giant cell tumor generally refers to a bone tumor and is typically found in the end of arm and leg bones.

Description

Giant cell tumor of the bone is also referred to as an osteoclastoma as it contains a large number of giant cells resembling a type of bone cells called osteoclasts. Half of all giant cell tumors occurs in the knee, at the lower end of femur (thigh bone) or upper tibia (one of the bones of the lower leg). The tumor is usually located eccentrically and often causes expansion of the bone end. The tumor destroys the bony structure and thus could lead to fractures, even in the absence of stress. Other giant cell tumors can occur in virtually any other bone, including the sacrum, pelvis, and small bones of hands and feet. The growth of this tumor is variable and unpredictable. It is considered to be benign, but can recur following surgical removal. It can also have pulmonary metastases that are mostly curable. Some of the giant cell tumors may change into malignant **sarcomas**, especially when they recur after high-dose radiation treatment.

Giant cell tumor of tendon sheath

Giant cell tumor of tendon sheath is also referred to a localized nodular tenosynovitis. It usually occurs as single, painless mass that grows slowly. It is mainly found in the wrist and fingers. These are benign growths that can be easily excised (surgically removed). This type is not discussed further in this entry.

Demographics

Giant cell tumor of bone is mostly seen in adults between the ages of 20 and 40 years. It is slightly more common among women than men and is seen in Asians more than other ethnic groups. It is very uncommon in children.

Causes and symptoms

The cause of giant cell tumors of bone is unknown.

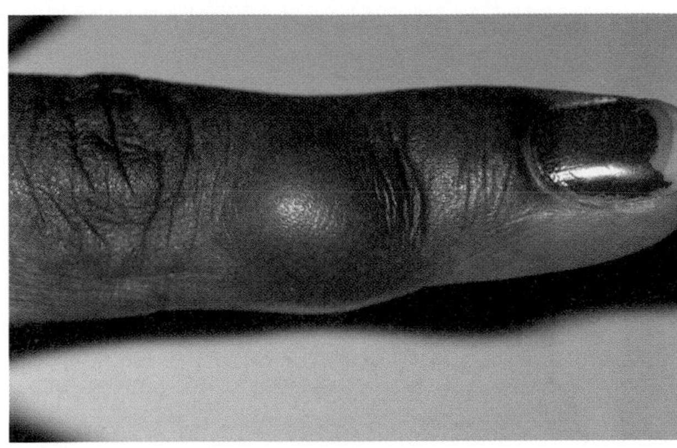

Giant cell tumor of a tendon in a woman's finger. *(Custom Medical Stock Photo. Reproduced by permission.)*

The following symptoms may be seen in patients with giant cell tumors:

- Pain: As this tumors mainly occurs in the joints, arthritic pain is usually the first symptom.
- Swelling: Giant cell tumor causes enlargement of the bone and, as it grows, the patient may find a swelling at the site of the tumor.
- Fracture: Giant cell tumors destroy the surrounding bone and, unlike other bone cancers, fractures are common as the tumor grows. Initially the patient may have a sore or painful joint and the fracture could make it suddenly, severely painful.

Diagnosis

Typically the patient with giant cell tumor will go to the doctor because of pain. The doctor will perform routine physical tests and test the affected area for tenderness, swelling, warmth, redness, and mobility. An **x ray** of the affected area will be obtained. Certain other imaging tests could be done, including **magnetic resonance imaging** (MRI) and **computed tomography** (CT scan) to see extent of growth. CT scan of the chest will also be done to test for **metastasis** to the lungs. An isotope scan may be also done to test for extent of damage. These techniques are noninvasive and can be performed within a day. A surgical **biopsy** is always done either before or during surgical removal of the tumor. The biopsy determines whether the tumor is malignant and identifies the stage of the tumor. This may done under either local or general anesthesia, depending upon the location of the tumor and the condition and age of the patient.

Treatment team

The treatment team will consist primarily of radiation oncologist, orthopedic oncologist, and oncology

KEY TERMS

Computed tomography—Commonly known as CT or CAT scan. It uses a rotating beam of x ray to get internal images of the body from different angles. During this test a harmless dye may be injected to increase contrast between normal and abnormal tissues.

Curettage—Surgical method in which a tumor is scraped away from the healthy tissue.

Magnetic resonance imaging—Also referred to as MRI. A procedure using a powerful magnetic field and radio waves to produce images of internal organs. MRI images can be used to look at soft tissues like muscle and fat.

Sarcoma—Uncommon, malignant tumors that begin in bones, or soft tissues such as muscle or fat.

nurse. Following surgical removal of the tumor, recovery may be aided by physical therapists.

Clinical staging, treatments, and prognosis

As of 2001 no satisfactory method for grading the tumor into either benign or malignant was available. Most giant cell tumors are initially classified as benign (grade 0). The tumor may progress in three stages. Stage 1, or latent stage, consists of a very slow growing tumor. It is well demarcated and there is little destruction of the outer surface of the bone. Stage 2, or the active stage, is the most commonly found stage. In this stage the tumor grows more steadily and the cortex (or outer layer of the bone) is lost. Stage 3 is the aggressive stage and accounts for about 20% of all giant cell tumors. In this stage the tumor grows rapidly and extends beyond the bone into the soft tissue. This stage is also associated more frequently with fractures.

Treatment of giant cell tumors is mainly surgical. Most stage 1 and 2 and some stage 3 tumors are treated by aggressive curettage, and the bone may be treated chemically and filled with cement. In some stage 2 and most stage 3 lesions the affected section of the bone may have to be removed (en bloc resection). In very rare cases the tumor may be so expanded that **amputation** may be necessary. Radiation is used to treat giant cell tumors in a location difficult to treat surgically. **Chemotherapy** has not been shown to be effective against giant cell tumors.

Prognosis following resection is excellent, with less than 5% chance of recurrence. When the tumor is removed by curettage followed by aggressive chemical treatment, there is a 5-10% chance of local recurrence. When the tumors recur locally it is usually within three years of surgical removal and the patient needs to be monitored closely during this time. A small percentage of giant cell tumors can metastasize to the lungs. The metastases can be removed surgically and most can be cured.

When a rare case of malignant sarcoma develops from a giant cell tumor, it is treated aggressively by surgery. In these cases prognosis is poor and long-term survival rate is as low as 20-30%.

Alternative and complementary therapies

There are no alternative or complementary therapies available for giant cell tumors.

Coping with cancer treatment

As the treatment for giant cell tumors is mainly surgical, physical therapy with strengthening exercises to restore range of motion is extremely important. If amputation is required resulting psychological effects will also have to be addressed, especially as this disease occurs in adults who are physically and sexually active.

Clinical trials

As of 2001 there were no ongoing **clinical trials** by any major agencies specifically for treatment of giant cell tumors.

Prevention

As the cause of giant cell tumors is not known, there is no known method for prevention. When adults in the age group of 20-40 years notice pain and swelling in the joints, prompt radiological evaluation could identify giant cell tumors in early stages and lead to a complete cure.

Special concerns

Whenever a giant cell tumor is suspected, a chest CT scan should also be performed to check for metastasis to the lungs. During pregnancy the tumor can grow more rapidly, in which case it may be better to wait to perform surgery until the baby can be safely delivered by induction. If a patient with giant cell tumor suffers a fracture at the affected area, it may be best to wait until the fracture is healed before performing the surgery.

Resources

BOOKS

Campanacci, Mario. *Bone and soft tissue tumors.* New York:Springer-Verlag Wien Publishing, 1999.

QUESTIONS TO ASK THE DOCTOR

- What kind of surgery will need to be done for removal of the tumor?
- What will be the limitations after the removal of the tumor?
- Did you find any metastasis in the lungs?
- Is curettage instead of resection a possibility?

DeVita, Vincent T., Samuel Hellman., and Steven A. Rosenberg, eds. *Cancer, Principles and Practice of Oncology.* Philadelphia: J. B. Lippincott Company, 1993.

PERIODICALS

Blackley, H. R. et al., "Treatment of giant cell tumors with curettage and bone grafting." *Journal of Bone and Joint Surgery,* American, 81, no. 6: (1999) 811-20.

ORGANIZATIONS

The American Academy of Orthopaedic Surgeons. 6300 N. River Road, Suite 200, Rosemont, IL 60018. (847) 823-8125. <http://www.aaos.org>

Malini Vashishtha, Ph.D.

Gliomas *see* **Brain and central nervous system tumors**

GM-CSF *see* **Sargramostim**

Gonadal dysfunction *see* **Fertility issues;** also **Sexuality**

Goserelin acetate

Definition

Goserelin acetate is a synthetic (man-made) hormone that acts similarly to the naturally occurring gonadotropin-releasing hormone (GnRH). It is available in the United States under the tradename Zoladex.

Purpose

Goserelin acetate is used primarily to counter the symptoms of late-stage **prostate cancer** in men or is offered as an alternative to treat prostate cancer when surgery to remove the testes or estrogen therapy is not an option or is unacceptable for the patient. Goserelin is also given as combination therapy with the drug flutamide to manage prostate cancer that is locally confined and not widespread. It is often used to ease the pain and discomfort of women suffering from endometrosis and to relieve symptoms in women with advanced **breast cancer**.

Description

Goserelin acetate is a man-made protein that mimics many of the actions of gonadotropin-releasing hormone (GnRH). In men, this results in decreased blood levels of the male hormone **testosterone**. In women, it decreases blood levels of the female hormone estrogen.

Recommended dosage

Goserelin acetate is given in the form of an implant containing 3.6 mg of the medication. This implant is placed just under the skin of the upper abdominal wall. The drug lasts for 28 days, after which a new implant has to be placed. Goserelin is also available in a dose of 10.8 mg, in which case the drugs lasts for three months.

Precautions

If a woman becomes pregnant while taking this drug, goserelin acetate may cause birth defects or the loss of the pregnancy. It is not known if goserelin is passed into breast milk; therefore, it is not recommended to breast feed while on this drug.

Goserelin acetate will also interfere with the chemical actions of birth control pills. For this reason, sexually active women who do not wish to become pregnant should use some form of birth control other than birth control pills during treatment with goserelin acetate and for at least 12 weeks after the completion of treatment.

Goserelin acetate will cause sterility in men, at least for the duration of the treatment.

Side effects

In patients of both sexes, common side effects of goserelin acetate include:

- sweating accompanied by feelings of warmth (hot flashes)
- a decrease in sex drive
- depression or other mood changes
- headache
- tumor flare, which is exhibited as **bone pain** (this is due to a temporary initial increase in testosterone/estrogen before its production is finally decreased)

Other common side effects in men include:

KEY TERMS

Endometrial tissue—The tissue lining the uterus that is sloughed off during a woman's menstrual period.

Gonadotropin releasing hormone (GnRH)—A hormone produced in the brain that controls the release of other hormones that are responsible for reproductive function.

Prostate gland—A small gland in the male genitals that contributes to the production of seminal fluid.

- impotence (erectile dysfunction)
- sterility
- breast enlargement

Other common side effects in women include:

- light, irregular, vaginal bleeding
- no menstrual period
- vaginal dryness and/or itching
- emotional instability
- **depression**
- change in breast size
- an increase in facial or body hair
- deepening of the voice

Less common side effects, in patients of either sex, include:

- **nausea and vomiting**
- insomnia
- weight gain
- swollen feet or lower legs
- acne or other skin rashes
- abdominal pain
- increased appetite

A doctor should be consulted immediately if the patient experiences any of the above symptoms.

Interactions

There are no known interactions of goserelin acetate with any food or beverage.

Patients taking goserelin acetate should consult their physician before taking any other prescription, over-the-counter, or herbal medication. Patients taking any other hormone or steroid-based medications should not take goserelin acetate without first consulting their physician.

See Also Endometrial cancer; Ovarian cancer

Paul A. Johnson, Ed.M.

Graft-vs.-host disease

Description

Graft-vs.-host disease is a response by the immune system that occurs when cells from a blood or bone marrow donor attack those of the recipient. The only transplanted tissues that contain enough immune cells to cause graft-vs.-host disease are the blood and the bone marrow. Blood transfusions are used every day in hospitals for many reasons. Bone marrow transplants are used to replace blood-forming cells and immune cells in cancer patients whose own bone marrow has been destroyed by **radiation therapy** or **chemotherapy**.

Blood transfusion graft-vs.-host disease affects mostly the blood. Blood cells perform three functions: carrying oxygen, fighting infections, and clotting. All of these functions are decreased in a transfusion graft-vs.-host reaction, leading to **anemia** (lack of red blood cells in the blood), reduced resistance to infections, and increased bleeding. The reaction occurs 4–30 days after the transfusion.

The tissues most affected by bone marrow graft-vs.-host disease are the skin, the liver, and the intestines. One of these forms of tissue is affected in nearly half of the patients who receive bone marrow transplants.

Bone marrow graft-vs.-host disease comes in both an acute and a chronic form. The acute form appears within two months of the transplant, while the chronic form usually appears within three months. The acute disease produces a skin rash, liver abnormalities, and **diarrhea** that can be bloody. The skin rash is primarily a patchy thickening of the skin. Chronic disease can produce a similar skin rash, a tightening or an inflammation of the skin, lesions in the mouth, drying of the eyes and mouth, hair loss (**alopecia**), liver damage, lung damage, and indigestion. The symptoms are similar to an autoimmune disease called scleroderma.

Both forms of graft-vs.-host disease bring with them an increased risk of infections, either because of the process itself or its treatment with cortisone-like drugs and immunosuppressives that inhibit the **immune response**. Patients can die of liver failure, infection, or other severe disturbances of their system.

Causes

Cells from the donor who has an active immune system may be transplanted along with the organ or tissue into the host who has a suppressed immune system. These transplanted cells attack the host's body, causing graft-vs.-host disease. Substances made in the body called cytokines are thought to play a role in the development of this reaction. Cytokines are protein substances made by cells that affect other cells.

Even if the donor and recipient are well matched, graft-vs.-host disease can still occur. There are many different components involved in generating immune reactions, and all people (except identical twins) are different. Testing can often find donors who match all the major components, but there are many minor ones that will always be different. Making a match between a donor and recipient depends upon the urgency of the need for a transplant and the chance that a suitable donor will be found.

Treatments

Both the acute and the chronic diseases are treated with cortisone-like drugs, immunosuppressive agents, or with **antibiotics** and immune chemicals from donated blood (gamma globulin). **Cyclosporine** and prednisone are two immunosuppressive drugs that are often used, and **methotrexate** may enhance efficacy. Another way to prevent graft-vs.-host disease is, before transplantation, rid donor bone marrow of the immune cells (T cells) that would attack the recipient's body. Another possibility to avoid complications in **bone marrow transplantation** is to cleanse the bone marrow of cancer cells and use the patient's own cells to grow more bone marrow. Cancer cells that reside in the bone marrow may be removed, leaving behind only those cells that are needed to grow new blood cells (stem cells). These stem cells from the patient can be grown and returned back to the patient.

For recipients of blood transfusions who are especially likely to have graft-vs.-host reactions, the red blood cells can safely be irradiated (using x rays) to kill all the immune cells. The red blood cells are less sensitive to radiation and are not harmed by this treatment.

New directions in research may help to solve the problem of graft-vs.-host disease. A potential source for new stem cells is the umbilical cord. Cells from this area do not give such strong immune reactions and may be useful for re-establishing cell populations. Another potential is to use genetically engineered cells to correct genetic defects in stem cells within the marrow.

KEY TERMS

Anemia—Too few red blood cells, or too little hemoglobin in them.

Immunoglobulin—Chemicals in the blood that defend against infections.

Immunosuppressive—A chemical that suppresses an immune response.

Lesion—Localized disease or damage.

Scleroderma—Progressive disease of the connective tissue of the skin and internal organs.

Alternative and complementary therapies

Alternative and complementary therapies range from herbal remedies, vitamin supplements, and special diets to spiritual practices, acupuncture, massage, and similar treatments. When these therapies are used in addition to conventional medicine, they are called complementary therapies. When they are used instead of conventional medicine, they are called alternative therapies.

Complementary or alternative therapies are widely used by people suffering with illness. Good nutrition and activities, such as yoga, meditation, and massage, that reduce stress and promote a positive view of life have no unwanted side effects and appear to be beneficial. Alternative and experimental treatments are normally not covered by insurance.

Special concerns

If graft-vs.-host disease is suspected as a complication to a cancer treatment, a skin punch **biopsy** may be performed to confirm this diagnosis. This is a relatively minor procedure in which the skin is anesthetized in a local area and a small piece is removed for testing in the laboratory.

Infection with one particular virus, called cytomegalovirus (CMV), is so likely a complication of graft-vs.-host disease that some experts recommend treating it in advance, using ganciclovir or valacyclovir.

It is an interesting observation that patients with leukemia who develop graft-vs.-host disease are less likely to have a recurrence of the leukemia that was being treated. This phenomenon is called graft-vs.-leukemia.

Bone marrow transplant patients who do not have a graft-vs.-host reaction gradually return to normal immune function in a year. A graft-vs.-host reaction may prolong the diminished immune capacity indefinitely, requiring supplemental treatment with immunoglobulins (gamma globulin). The grafted cells develop a tolerance to the recipient's body after 6–12 months, and the medications can be gradually withdrawn.

Graft-vs.-host disease is not the only complication of blood transfusion or bone marrow transplantation. Host-vs.-graft disease, or rejection, occurs when the recipient's immune system is strong enough to attack the transplant. This is also a common occurrence and may require a repeat transplant with another donor organ. Infections are a constant threat in bone marrow transplant because of the disease being treated, the prior radiation or chemotherapy and the medications used to treat the transplant.

See also Bone marrow transplantation; Transfusion therapy

Resources

BOOKS

Anderson, William L. *Immunology.*Madison, CT: Fence Creek Publishing, 1999.

Armitage, James O. "Bone Marrow Transplantation." In *Harrison's Principles of Internal Medicine*, edited by Kurt Isselbacher, et al. New York: McGraw-Hill, 1998, pp.726-727.

Janeway, Charles A., et al. *Immunobiology:The Immune System in Health and Disease.* New York, NY: Current Biology Publications; London, England: Elsevier Science London/Garland Publishing, 1999.

Menitove, Jay E. "Blood Transfusion." In *Cecil Textbook of Medicine*, edited by J. Claude Bennett and Fred Plum. Philadelphia: W. B. Saunders, 1996, p. 896.

Rappeport, Joel. "Bone Marrow Transplantation." In *Cecil Textbook of Medicine*, edited by J. Claude Bennett and Fred Plum. Philadelphia: W. B. Saunders, 1996, p.975.

Roitt, Ivan and Arthur Rabson. *Really Essential Medical Immunology.* Malden, MA: Blackwell Science, 2000.

Ruscetti, Francis W., Jonathan R. Keller, and Dan L. Longo. "Hematopoiesis." In *Harrison's Principles of Internal Medicine*, edited by Kurt Isselbacher, et al. New York: McGraw-Hill, 1998.

Widmann, Frances K., and Carol A. Itatani. *An Introduction to Clinical Immunology and Serology.* Philadelphia, PA: F.A. Davis Company, 1998.

Wier, Donald M. and John Stewart. *Immunology.* New York, NY: Churchill Livingston, Inc., 1997.

OTHER

Complementary and Alternative Medicine Web site for the American Cancer Society. <http:cancer.org/alt_therapy/index.html>.

University of Michigan Patient Education Resource Center (PERC). <http://www.cancer.med.umich.edu htm>.

University of Michigan Transplant Center. <http://www.med.umich.edu/trans/public/>.

J. Ricker Polsdorfer, M.D.
Jill Granger, M.S.

Granisetron *see* **Antiemetics**

Gynecologic cancers

Definition

Gynecologic cancers are malignant tumors within the female reproductive organs.

Description

Gynecologic cancers account for approximately 13% of all cancers that affect women. They are responsible for 10% of the cancer deaths among women.

The female reproductive tract is comprised of the ovaries, fallopian tubes, uterus, cervix, vagina, and vulva. Together, these organs allow a woman to become pregnant, protect and nourish an unborn baby, and to give birth. An understanding of each organ and its role in reproduction may help the patient to understand her particular gynecologic cancer. There are two ovaries, which are the internal organs dedicated to producing eggs. Released eggs are captured by the fallopian tubes, through which the egg (or fertilized egg) travels to the womb (uterus). The lining of the uterus (endometrium) responds to female hormones, such as estrogen, and becomes thickened to allow for implantation of a fertilized egg. The cervix is the opening of the uterus which opens (dilates) during labor to allow for passage of the baby. The vagina is a short tube that extends from the outer female genitalia (vulva) to the cervix.

Gynecologic cancers are defined not solely by the organ affected but also by the type of cancerous cells in the tumor. The type of cancer depends on the cell types that make up an organ. Adenocarcinomas are cancers that contain primarily cells originating from glands or ducts. Squamous cell carcinomas are tumors that arose from squamous cells, the main cell type found in skin. Sarcomas are cancers that originated from cells of basic connective tissue (mesenchymal cells). Sarcomas are comprised of cells that have become specialized (differentiated) and are named according to the predominant cell type. Endometroid tumors are those that originated from the endometrium. Clear-cell **carcinoma** is a rare gynecologic tumor that contains cells from the mullerian duct, which gives rise to the uterus, vagina, and fallopian tubes during development.

Because the reproductive organs are interconnected, spread of cancer from one organ to another (direct extension) is not uncommon. Gynecologic cancer carries the

Gynecologic cancers

Cancer type	Occurs in	Tumor types
Endometrial cancer	Uterus	Endometrioid tumors Clear-cell carcinomas Papillary serous Sarcomas Mixed tumors
Fallopian tube cancer	Fallopian tubes, but frequently spreads	Serous carcinomas Mucinous tumors Endometrioid tumors
Cervical cancer	Cervix	Squamous cell carcinomas Adenocarcinomas Clear-cell carcinoma Serous carcinoma Glassy-cell carcinoma
Ovarian cancer	Ovaries	Serous carcinomas Mucinous tumors Endometrioid tumors
Vaginal cancer	Vagina	Squamous cell carcinoma Adenocarcinoma Melanoma Sarcoma
Vulvar cancer	Vulva	Squamous cell carcinomas Melanoma Basal cell carcinoma Paget's disease Adenocarcinomas

name of the organ where the cancer originated (primary cancer site). For example, a tumor restricted to the vagina would be "primary vaginal cancer," whereas one that has extended from the cervix to the vagina would be "primary cervical cancer."

Types of cancers

Ovarian cancer is the second most common cancer of the female reproductive organs. It accounts for 30% of all gynecologic cancers and 53% of the deaths in this group. The high death rate associated with ovarian cancer is due to the fact that most women are not diagnosed until the cancer has progressed to an advanced stage. The average age at diagnosis is 63 years. Serous carcinomas are the most common type of ovarian cancer. Other common types of ovarian cancer include mucinous tumors and endometroid tumors.

Fallopian tube cancers, as primary cancers, are very rare. They frequently spread widely within the abdominal cavity. Although often diagnosed earlier than ovarian cancer, fallopian tube cancer produces similar symptoms and originates from similar cell types as ovarian cancer.

Uterine cancer, also called **endometrial cancer**, is the most common gynecologic cancer and accounts for 46% of the cases. Endometrial cancer primarily affects postmenopausal women, however, 25% of cases are in premenopausal women. There are two types of endometrial cancer: estrogen-dependent and non-estrogen-dependent. Estrogen-dependent cancers are usually comprised of well-differentiated cells and are associated with a good outcome and a long survival time. Non-estrogen-dependent cancers are usually made up of poorly-differentiated cells and are invasive and associated with a poor prognosis. Uterine tumors are most frequently endometroid tumors, usually adenocarcinomas. Clear-cell carcinomas, papillary serous, sarcomas, and mixed tumors also occur.

Cervical cancer is the third most common cancer of the female reproductive tract. It accounts for 17% of the gynecologic cancers. Although cervical cancer can affect any adult woman, there are peaks of occurrence around the ages of 37 years and 62 years. Between 60% and 80% of the cases of cervical cancer are squamous cell carcinomas with the remainder being adenocarcinomas. Clear-cell carcinoma, serous carcinoma, and glassy-cell carcinoma are less frequent cervical cancers. Cervical cancer is very strongly associated with **human papilloma virus**.

Vaginal cancer is rare and accounts for just 3% of the gynecologic cancers. It most often strikes women in their sixties. Greater than 90% of the vaginal cancers are squamous cell carcinomas. Adenocarcinoma, **melanoma**, and sarcoma account for the remaining cases. There is an association between vaginal cancer and human papilloma virus.

KEY TERMS

Differentiated—A term describing cells that have become specialized and have matured normally, such as muscle cells.

Direct extension—The spread of cancer directly from one organ to a neighboring organ, such as from the cervix to the vagina.

Glassy cell carcinoma—Tumorous cells that have a glass-like appearance

Human papilloma virus (HPV)—A sexually-transmitted virus that causes genital warts. It is associated with certain gynecologic cancers.

Mucinous tumors—Adenocarcinomas that produce significant amounts of the complex sugar molecule known as mucin.

Papillary serous carcinoma—A serous carcinoma with papillary (nipple-like) outgrowths.

Primary cancer (or tumor)—The organ in which a cancerous tumor originated.

Serous carcinoma—A carcinoma that produces or contains serum, the liquid portion of blood.

Vulvar cancer is rare and accounts for 4% of the gynecologic cancers. It most often strikes women in their sixties. Squamous cell carcinoma is the most common type and melanoma is the second most common type of vulvar cancer. Other types of vulvar cancer include **basal cell carcinoma**, Paget's disease, and adenocarcinomas (arising from the Bartholin's, Skene's, or sweat glands). There is an association between vulvar cancer and human papilloma virus.

Resources

BOOKS

Fields, A., J. Jones, G. Thomas, and C. Runowicz. "Gynecologic Cancer." In *Clinical Oncology.* Lenhard, Raymond, Robert Osteen, and Ted Gansler, eds. Atlanta: American Cancer Society, 2000.

PERIODICALS

Brown, Jean, and Anne Cloutier. "Gynecologic Cancers." *American Journal of Nursing* 100 (April 2000): 32-5.

Zanotti, Kristine, and Alexander Kennedy. "Screening for Gynecologic Cancer." *Medical Clinics of North America* 83, no. 6 (November 1999): 1467- 87.

ORGANIZATIONS

American Cancer Society. 1599 Clifton Rd. NE, Atlanta, GA 30329. (800) ACS-2345. <http://www.cancer.org>.

Cancer Research Institute, National Headquarters. 681 Fifth Ave., New York, NY 10022. (800) 992-2623. <http://www.cancerresearch.org>.

Gynecologic Cancer Foundation. 401 N. Michigan Ave., Chicago, IL 60611. (800) 444-4441 or (312) 644-6610. <http://www.wcn.org/gcf>.

National Institutes of Health. National Cancer Institute. 9000 Rockville Pike, Bethesda, MD 20982. (800) 4-CANCER. <http://cancernet.nci.nih.gov>.

Belinda Rowland, Ph.D.

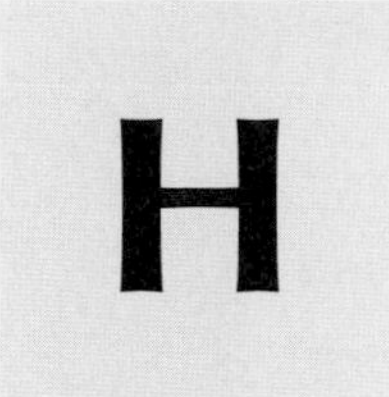

Hair loss *see* **Alopecia**

Hairy cell leukemia

Definition

Hairy cell leukemia is a disease in which a type of white blood cell called the lymphocyte, present in the blood and bone marrow, becomes malignant and proliferates. It is called hairy cell leukemia because the cells have tiny hair-like projections when viewed under the microscope.

Description

Hairy cell leukemia (HCL) is a rare cancer. It was first described in 1958 as *leukemic reticuloendotheliosis*, erroneously referring to a red blood cell because researchers were unsure of the cell of origin. It became more easily identifiable in the 1970s. There are approximately 600 new cases diagnosed every year in the United States, making up about 2% of the adult cases of leukemia each year.

HCL is found in cells located in the blood. There are three types of cells found in the blood: the red blood cells that carry oxygen to all the parts of the body; the white blood cells that are responsible for fighting infection and protecting the body from diseases; and the platelets that help in the clotting of blood. Hairy cell leukemia affects a type of white blood cell called the lymphocyte. Lymphocytes are made in the bone marrow, spleen, lymph nodes, and other organs. It specifically affects B-lymphocytes, which mature in the bone marrow. However, extremely rare variants of HCL have been discovered developing from T-lymphocytes, which mature in the thymus.

When hairy cell leukemia develops, the white blood cells become abnormal both in the way they appear (by acquiring hairy projections) and in the way they act (by proliferating without the normal control mechanisms). Further, the cells tend to accumulate in the spleen, causing it to become enlarged. The cells may also collect in the bone marrow and prevent it from producing normal blood cells. As a result, there may not be enough normal white blood cells in the blood to fight infection.

Demographics

The median age at which people develop HCL is 52 years. Though it occurs in all ages, HCL more commonly develops in the older population. Men are four times more likely to develop HCL than women. There have been reports of familial aggregation of disease, with higher occurrences in Ashkenazi Jewish men. A potential genetic link is undergoing further investigation.

Causes and symptoms

The cause of hairy cell leukemia is not specifically known. However, exposure to radiation is a known cause of leukemia in general. Familial involvement is another theory, suggesting that there is a genetic component associated with this disease.

HCL is a chronic (slowly progressing) disease, and the patients may not show any symptoms for many years. As the disease advances, the patients may suffer from one or more of the following symptoms:

- weakness
- **fatigue**
- recurrent infections
- **fever**
- **anemia**
- bruising
- pain or discomfort in the abdominal area
- **weight loss** (uncommon)
- **night sweats** (uncommon)

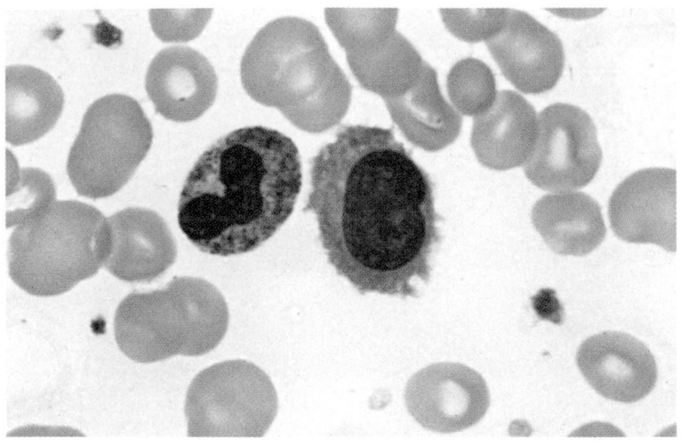

A magnified image of white blood cells with "hairy" projections. *(Photograph by M. Abbey, Photo Researchers, Inc. Reproduced by permission.)*

Pain and discomfort are caused by an enlarged spleen, which results from the accumulation of the abnormal hairy cells in the spleen. Blood tests may show abnormal counts of all the different types of cells. This happens because the cancerous cells invade the bone marrow as well and prevent it from producing normal blood cells. Because of the low white cell count in the blood, the patient may have frequent infections. Fever often accompanies the infections. The patient is most susceptible to bacterial infections, but infections of any kind are the major cause of death. The low red cell count may cause anemia, fatigue, and weakness, and the low platelet count may cause the person to bruise and bleed easily.

Diagnosis

When a patient suffers from the above symptoms, the doctor will palpate (examine with fingers) the abdomen and may order scans to see if the spleen is enlarged (splenomegaly). An enlarged spleen is present in 80% of patients. An enlarged liver is less common, but can occur.

If the spleen is enlarged, the doctor may order several blood tests. In these tests, the total numbers of each of the different types of blood cells (CBC) are reported. Sixty to eighty percent of patients suffer from pancytopenia, which is a dramatic reduction in the number of red blood cells, white blood cells, and platelets circulating in the blood.

If the blood tests are abnormal, the doctor may order a **bone marrow aspiration and biopsy**. In order to establish a diagnosis, hairy cells must be present in the bone marrow.

Treatment team

If the patient is seeing a primary care provider, the provider may perform the initial diagnostic tests. However, in order to diagnose and treat HCL comprehensively, the primary care provider will refer the patient to an oncologist (cancer specialist). Radiologists and pathologists will also be involved to read scans and examine tissue samples. Other specialists involved with the treatment of hairy cell leukemia will be nurses and dieticians who are available to explain side effects of treatment and offer suggestions on eating healthy meals that may help fight the side effects.

Clinical staging, treatments, and prognosis

When physicians perform blood tests, they will determine the level of hemoglobin (the oxygen-transporting molecule of red blood cells). Serum hemoglobin levels and the size of the spleen, which can be measured on exam and by using an **x ray**, are proposed criteria for determining the stage of HCL. The following are the three proposed stages and their criteria:

- Stage I: Hemoglobin greater than 12 g/dL (1 g = approximately 0.02 pint and 1 dL = approximately 0.33 ounce) and spleen less than or equal to 10 cm (3.9 inches).
- Stage II: Hemoglobin between 8.5 and 12 g/dL and spleen greater than 10 cm (3.9 inches).
- Stage III: Hemoglobin less than 8.5 g/dL and spleen greater than 10 cm (3.9 inches).

Since there is generally no accepted staging system, another method for evaluating the progression of HCL is to group patients into two categories: untreated HCL and progressive HCL, in which hairy cells are present after therapy has been administered.

Some people with hairy cell leukemia have very few or no symptoms at all, and it is reasonable to expect that 10% of patients may not need any treatment. However, if the patient is symptomatic and needs intervention, HCL is especially responsive to treatment.

There are three main courses of treatment: **chemotherapy**, **splenectomy** (surgical removal of the spleen), and immunotherapy. Once a patient meets treatment criteria, purine analogues, particularly the drugs, **pentostatin** and **cladribine**, are the first-line therapy. Pentostatin is administered at $5mg/m^2$ for two days every other week until total remission is achieved. Patients may experience side effects such as fever, **nausea and vomiting**, photosensitivity, and keratoconjuctivitis. However, follow-up studies estimate a relapse-free survival rate at 76%. Cladribine (2-CdA) taken at 0.1mg/kg/day for seven days also has an impressive response. Eighty-six percent of patients experience complete remission after treatment, while 16% experience partial remission. Fever is the principal side effect of 2-CdA.

Biological therapy or **immunologic therapy**, where the body's own immune cells are used to fight cancer, is also being investigated in **clinical trials** for hairy cell leukemia. A substance called interferon that is produced by the white blood cells of the body was the first systemic treatment that showed consistent results in fighting HCL. The FDA approved interferon-alpha (INF-alpha) to fight HCL. The mechanism by which INF-alpha works is not clearly understood. However, it is known that **interferons** stimulate the body's natural killer cells that are suppressed during HCL. The standard dosage is 2 MU/m^2 three times a week for 12 months. Side effects include fever, myalgia, malaise, rashes, and gastrointestinal complaints.

If the spleen is enlarged, it may be removed in a surgical procedure known as splenectomy. This usually causes a remission of the disease. However, 50% of patients that undergo splenectomy require some type of systemic treatment such as chemotherapy or immunotherapy. Splenectomy is not the most widely used course of treatment as it was many years ago. Although the spleen is not an indispensable organ, it is responsible for helping the body fight infection. Therefore, other therapies are preferred in order to salvage the spleen and its functions.

Most patients have excellent prognosis and can expect to live 10 years or longer. The disease may remain silent for years with treatment. Continual follow-up is necessary to monitor the patient for relapse and determine true cure rates.

Alternative and complementary therapies

Many individuals choose to supplement traditional therapy with complementary methods. Often, these methods improve the tolerance of side effects and symptoms as well as enrich the quality of life. The American Cancer Society recommends that patients talk to their doctor to ensure that the methods they are using are safely supplementing traditional therapy. Some complementary treatments include the following:

- yoga
- meditation
- religious practices and prayer
- music therapy
- art therapy
- massage therapy
- aromatherapy

Coping with cancer treatment

The treatment and the disease interfere with the patient's ability to produce red blood cells, white blood cells, and platelets, causing the patient to be vulnerable to anemia and life-threatening infection and bleeding. Transfusions can be given to patients in order to increase the number of red blood cells and platelets in the blood. In addition, colony-stimulating factors are being studied. These increase the number of the patient's own white blood cells.

Nausea and vomiting can result from chemotherapy and are often controlled by prescription drugs called **antiemetics**. Patients can also curb nausea and vomiting by eating slowly and avoiding large meals. Drinking water an hour before meals and staying away from foods that are sweet or fried is also helpful. Many times, chemotherapy is handled better if the patient is eating

KEY TERMS

Anemia—A condition in which there is low iron in the blood due to a deficiency of red blood cells.

Bone marrow—The spongy tissue inside the large bones in the body that is responsible for making the red blood cells, white blood cells, and platelets.

Bone marrow aspiration and biopsy—A procedure in which a needle is inserted into the large bones of the hip or spine and a small piece of marrow is removed for microscopic examination.

Immunotherapy—A mode of cancer treatment in which the immune system is stimulated to fight the cancer.

Leukemia—A disease in which the cells that constitute the blood become cancerous or abnormal.

Lymph nodes—Oval-shaped organs that are the size of peas, located throughout the body, and contain clusters of cells called lymphocytes. They filter out and destroy bacteria, foreign particles, and cancerous cells from the blood.

Malignant—Cells that have the ability to invade locally, cause destruction of surrounding tissue, and travel to other sites in the body.

Keratoconjunctivitis—Inflammation of the conjunctiva and cornea of the eye.

Spleen—An organ that lies next to the stomach. Its function is to remove the worn-out blood cells and foreign materials from the blood stream.

Splenectomy—A surgical procedure that involves the surgical removal of the spleen.

QUESTIONS TO ASK THE DOCTOR

- How long will this course of treatment take?
- How long will the side effects last after treatment ends?
- What kinds of side effects will this course of treatment cause?
- Are there support services available?
- What treatments are currently in clinical trials?
- What treatments will my health care insurance cover?
- What alternative or complementary treatments are safe and effective?
- Why is this type of treatment being used?

well. Nurses and dieticians can aid patients in choosing healthful foods to incorporate into their diet.

Patients can fight anemia and fatigue by getting plenty of rest and minimizing strenuous activities. A well-balanced diet can also counter anemia and fatigue.

Although physicians will do everything possible to keep a patient's blood count high, there are precautions that can be taken by patients in order to reduce their risk of infection. Patients should regularly wash their hands, especially before and after eating meals and after using the restroom. Patients should avoid individuals who are contagious with colds, the flu, or the chicken pox. It is also helpful if patients do not cut themselves or do anything to expose deeper layers of the skin where bacteria can contaminate and cause infection. Finally, patients should avoid large crowds.

Clinical trials

Clinical trials are being performed to improve the effectiveness of treatment and to minimize the side effects. Patients may choose to volunteer for a clinical trial if they do not respond to standard therapy or if they want to reduce side effects. Clinical trials for the treatment of HCL involving purine analogues were being researched in 2001. Clinical trials are being performed all over the United States, and patients should discuss options with their doctors or contact the Cancer Information Service at (800) 4-CANCER (800-422-6237).

In many cases, insurance companies will not cover procedures that are part of clinical trials. Patients should talk with their doctor and insurance company to determine which procedures are covered.

Prevention

Since the cause for the disease is unknown and there are no specific risk factors, there is no known prevention.

Special concerns

Cancer treatments and their side effects can take a physical and psychological toll on cancer patients and their families. To deal with the psychological impact, there are many different support groups and psychotherapists that can help. Psychiatrists can prescribe medication to help with **depression**. Support groups can encourage and strengthen the psyche by relating to one another through shared experiences and success stories. Relying on faith practices is also beneficial for cancer patients to deal with their condition. Patients should discuss all options with their physician to determine what is available to them.

See Also Tumor staging

Resources

BOOKS

Bast, Robert C. *Cancer Medicine.* Lewiston, NY: B.C. Decker Inc., 2000.

Cook, Allan R. *The New Cancer Sourcebook.* Detroit, MI: Omnigraphics, Inc., 1996.

DeVita, Vincent T.*Cancer Principles and Practice of Oncology, 5th Edition, Vol. 2.* Philadelphia: PA: Lippincott Williams & Wilkins, 1997.

Dollinger, Malin. *Everyone's Guide to Cancer Therapy.* Kansas City: Somerville House Books Limited, 1994.

Haskell, Charles M. *Cancer Treatment, 5th Edition.* Philadephia: W.B. Saunders Company, 2001.

Murphy, Gerald P. *Informed Decisions: The Complete book of Cancer Diagnosis, Treatment and Recovery.* Atlanta, GA: American Cancer Society, 1997.

ORGANIZATIONS

American Cancer Society (National Headquarters). 1599 Clifton Road, N.E. Atlanta, Georgia 30329. (800) 227-2345. <http://www.cancer.org>.

Cancer Research Institute (National Headquarters). 681 Fifth Avenue, New York, N.Y. 10022. (800) 992-2623. <http://www.cancerresearch.org>.

Hairy Cell Leukemia Research Foundation. 2345 County Farm Lane, Schaumburg, IL 60194. (800) 693-6173.

Leukemia Society of America, Inc. National Office, 600 Third Avenue, 4th Floor, New York, NY 10016. (800) 955-4LSA.

National Cancer Institute. 9000 Rockville Pike, Building 31, Room 10A16, Bethesda, Maryland, 20892. (800) 422-6237. <http://wwwicic.nci.nih.gov>.

Oncolink. University of Pennsylvania Cancer Center. <http://cancer.med.upenn.edu>.

OTHER

NCI/PDQ Patient Statement, "Hairy cell leukemia." National Cancer Institute, 2001.

"Coping With Side Effects." *National Cancer Institute.* 2 July 2001. <http://cancernet.nci.nih.gov/chemotherapy/chemoside.html>.

Lata Cherath, Ph.D.
Sally C. McFarlane-Parrott

Haloperidol *see* **Antiemetics**

Hand-foot syndrome

Description

Hand-foot syndrome (HFS), also called palmar-plantar erythrodysesthesia syndrome (PPES), is a relatively common side effect associated with high dosage **chemotherapy** treatments involving **fluorouracil** (5-FU) and drugs belonging to the chemical class called anthracyclines.

Anthracyclines have been widely used since the 1960s as dose-limited chemotherapy drugs for a variety of cancers, particularly leukemia, metastatic **breast cancer**, **ovarian cancer**, and colorectal cancer. The most familiar anthracyclines are **capecitabine** (Xeloda), **daunorubicin** (Cerubidine), **doxorubicin** (Adriamycin), **idarubicin** (Idamycin), and **vinorelbine** (Navelbine). Each of these drugs is broken down into 5-FU by chemicals inside the cancer cells.

A dose-limited drug is a drug for which the maximum dose is determined by the reactions of an individual patient. Symptoms of HFS usually indicate that a patient is receiving too much 5-FU or a particular anthracycline. In such a case, the dosage of the drug that is causing HFS is usually decreased until these symptoms either disappear completely or become tolerable to the patient.

The primary symptom of HFS is a tingling sensation and/or numbness of the skin, particularly on the palms of the hands or the soles of the feet. Swelling and redness (erythema) often accompany this symptom. In severe cases, the skin may peel, develop ulcerations or blisters, and cause severe pain. In the most extreme cases, symptoms of HFS may make it difficult, or impossible, for the patient to grasp small objects, walk, or conduct other normal daily activities.

KEY TERMS

Dose-limited drug—A drug for which the proper dosage is determined by the reaction of each individual patient to the drug.

Causes

The symptoms of HFS are believed to be caused by some of the chemicals that 5-FU is broken down into by the natural biochemical processes of the body. Since all anthracycline drugs chemically breakdown into 5-FU, these drugs will all eventually be broken down into the chemicals that can cause the symptoms of HFS. For reasons that are not clear, some patients seem more prone to developing symptoms of HFS than other patients.

Treatments

The symptoms of HFS are usually alleviated by lowering the dosage of the drug that the patient is receiving. In severe cases of HFS, it may be necessary to discontinue the use of the drug that is causing these symptoms. In some, but not all, patients the symptoms of HFS are reduced by treatment with steroid-containing skin creams, such as hydrocortisone.

Alternative and complementary therapies

Treatment of the hands and feet with an aloe vera-containing skin cream may help to alleviate some of the symptoms of HFS. Topical treatment of the skin with dimethyl sulfoxide (DMSO) has also been suggested as an alternative treatment.

Resources

PERIODICALS

"Capecitabine gives new life to fluorouracil in treatment of breast cancer." *Drugs and Therapy Perspectives* 16 (26 September 2000): 1-5.

"Daunorubicin liposomal: First report of palmar-plantar erythrodysesthesia syndrome." *Reactions* (25 November 2000): 829.

Hui, Yuk Fung and Jorge E. Cortes. "Palmar-Plantar Erythrodysesthesia Syndrome Associated with Liposomal Daunorubicin." *Pharmacotherapy* 20 (2000): 1221-23.

Markman, M., A. Kennedy, K. Webster, G. Peterson, B. Kulp, and J. Belinson. "Phase 2 trial of liposomal doxorubicin (40 mg/m(2)) in Platinum/Paclitaxel-refractory ovarian and fallopian tube cancers and primary carcinoma of the peritoneum." *Gynecologic Oncology* 78 (September 2000): 369-72.

OTHER

Abushullaih, Samer, Everardo Saad, and Paulo M. Hoff. "Characterizing hand-foot syndrome (HFS) caused by capecitabine." *ASCO OnLine.* 2000. 4 July 2001. <http://www.asco.org/prof/me/html/00abstracts/sm/m_2403.htm>.

"Clinical aspects of Xeloda." *Roche Laboratories.* 2000. 4 July 2001. <http://www.xeloda.com/clinical/index.html>.

Hoff, P. M., V. Valero, N. Ibrahim, J. Willey, and G. N. Hortobagyi. "Prolonged infusion of vinorelbine causing hand-foot syndrome." *ASCO OnLine.* 1997. 4 July 2001. <http://www.asco.org/prof/me/html/abstracts/cp/m_840.htm>.

"Prevention and management of Doxil-related side effects: Basic strategies." *ASCO OnLine.* 1998. 5 July 2001. <http://www.asco.org/prof/me/html/98abstracts/asc/m_281.htm>.

Titgan, M. A. "Prevention of palmar-plantar erythrodysesthesia associated with liposomal-encapsulated doxorubicin by oral dexamethasone." *ASCO OnLine.* 1997. 5 July 2001. <http://www.asco.org/prof/me/html/abstracts/asc/m_288.htm>.

Vail, D. M., R. Chun, D. H. Thamm, L. D. Garrett, A. J. Cooley, and J. E. Obradovich. "Efficacy of pyridoxine to ameliorate the cutaneous toxicity associated with Doxil: A randomized, double-blind clinical trial using a canine model." *ASCO OnLine.* 1998. 5 July 2001. <http://www.asco.org/prof/me/html/98abstracts/cp/m_878.htm>.

Paul A. Johnson, Ed.M.

Head and neck cancers

Definition

The group of cancers found in the head and neck region, excluding tumors of the eyes and brain.

Description

The tumors associated with head and neck cancers are found in several regions, including the lips, tongue, mouth, nasal passages, pharynx, larynx (voice box), salivary glands, thyroid gland, and parathyroid glands. Many head and neck cancers interfere with the functions of eating and breathing. **Laryngeal cancer** affects speech. Loss of any of these functions is significant. Therefore, early detection and appropriate treatment is of utmost importance.

Roughly 5% of all cancers are related to the head and the neck. It is estimated that more than 59,000 Americans will develop cancer of the head and neck in 2001, and 13,000 will die from the disease.

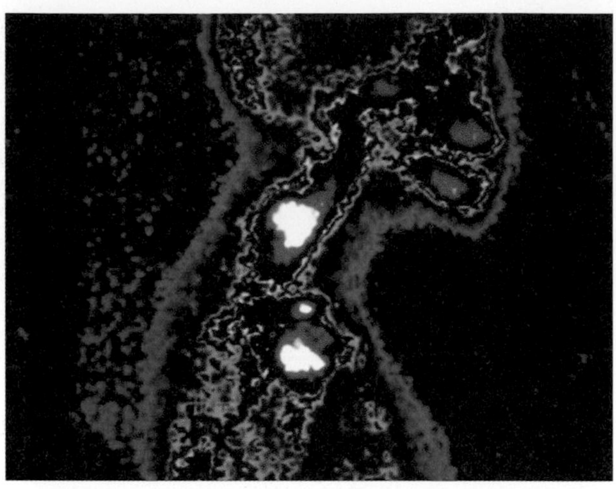

False color scintigram (gamma camera scan) showing metastatic (secondary) cancer affecting the cervical (neck) vertebrae (white area). *(© CNRI, Science Source/Photo Researchers, Inc. Reproduced by permission.)*

The common cancers of the head and neck area are **oral cancers**, **thyroid cancer**, and laryngeal cancer. Half of all head and neck cancers occur in the oral cavity and pharynx, a third are thyroid cancer, and almost 20% are found in the larynx. The American Cancer Society estimates that in 2001 approximately 10,000 new cases of laryngeal cancer will be diagnosed and 4,000 people will die of this disease. New cases of thyroid cancer in 2001 will likely reach over 19,000 and result in 1,300 deaths. Oral cancer is the tenth most common cancer in the United States, reaching nearly 30,000 new cases each year and causing at least 7,800 deaths.

The survival rates for head and neck cancers varies from good to poor, depending on the specific cancer. About 54% of the patients diagnosed with oral cancer will survive five years or more after the initial diagnosis. Laryngeal cancer has a 5-year survival rate of nearly 65%. Among the different cancers, thyroid cancer has one of the better 5-year survival rates, approaching 95%. The poorer survival rates for some head and neck cancers result because the early signs of these cancers are frequently ignored. Hence, when first diagnosed, they are often in an advanced stage and not very amenable to treatment.

Tobacco is regarded as the single greatest risk factor contributing to the occurrence of oral and laryngeal cancer: 75% to 80% of these patients are smokers. Heavy alcohol use has also been included as a risk factor. A combination of tobacco and alcohol use increases the risk for oral cancer by 6 to 15 times more than for users of either substance alone. Exposure to asbestos appears to increase the risk of developing laryngeal cancer. The chance for developing certain types of thyroid cancer is linked to an exposure to radiation.

The risk for both oral cancer and laryngeal cancer seems to increase with age. Most of the cases occur in individuals over 40 years of age, and the average age at diagnosis is 60. While oral cancer strikes men twice as often as it does women, laryngeal cancer is four times more common in men than in women. Both diseases are more common in African-Americans than among whites. Thyroid cancer is three times more common in women than in men and is usually diagnosed between the ages of 30 and 50.

Types of cancers

There are many types of head and neck cancers. These are classified by where the cancer is found:

- Oral cancers occur in the mouth, or oral cavity, which includes the lips, the lining inside the lips and cheeks, the front two-thirds of the tongue, the teeth, the gums, the floor of the mouth (under the tongue), the roof of the mouth, and the small area behind the wisdom teeth. Symptoms and signs include a mouth sore that does not heal within two weeks, unusual bleeding from the teeth or gums, or a lump in the gums, mouth, or tongue.
- **Lip cancers** occur on the inside or outside surface of the lips. Signs of this cancer include a lump on the inside of the lip or a sore on the outside, which is usually a form of skin cancer.
- **Oropharyngeal cancer** is found on the back one-third of the tongue, the upper section of the pharynx, and the area around the tonsils. Symptoms include a lump in the back of the mouth or throat, ear pain, or difficulty swallowing.
- **Nasopharyngeal cancer** is found in the area behind the nose and the upper section of the pharynx, the area just behind the mouth. Symptoms include difficulty breathing or speaking, pain or ringing in ears, frequent headaches, or trouble hearing.
- Hypopharyngeal cancer is found only in the bottom section of the pharynx. Symptoms include a sore throat that does not subside, difficulty swallowing, a lump in the neck, or ear pain.
- Laryngeal cancer starts in the larynx, which is located in front of the neck, in the region of the Adam's apple. Symptoms include pain when swallowing, a sore throat that does not subside, a change in voice, or ear pain.
- Paranasal sinus cancer and **nasal cancer** develop in the small, hollow spaces in the nose called the sinuses and in the nasal cavity, which is the passageway for air moving to the throat during breathing. Symptoms include frequent sinus infections, nosebleeds, a sore inside the nose that does not heal, or pain in the sinus area.

Cancers of the head and neck

Cancer types	Cancer occurs in
Hypopharyngeal cancer	Lowest section of the pharynx (region behind mouth)
Laryngeal cancer	Larynx (front of neck, near Adam's apple)
Nasopharyngeal cancer	Behind nose Pharynx
Oral cancer	Lips Lining of lips and cheeks Front two-thirds of tongue Teeth Gums Under tongue
Oropharyngeal cancer	Back one-third of tongue Upper section of pharynx Area around tonsils
Parathyroid cancer	Parathyroid glands (found behind or next to the thyroid gland)
Thyroid cancer	Thyroid gland (found at front of neck, below the Adam's apple)

- **Salivary gland tumors** form in the salivary glands, which produce saliva to help prevent the mouth from drying out and aids with digestion. They are located under the jaw, in front of the ears, underneath the tongue, and in other regions of the digestive tract. Symptoms include swelling under the chin or around the jawbone, facial numbness, muscles in the face that will not move, or persistent pain in the face, chin, or neck.
- Thyroid cancer is found on the thyroid gland, which is located in the front of neck and secretes hormones that help regulate body temperature and metabolism. Symptoms include a lump on the neck, pain in the neck region, a cough with bleeding, or difficulty swallowing or breathing.
- **Parathyroid cancer** is found on one or on all four of the small parathyroid glands, which secrete a hormone that controls the level of calcium in the blood. They are located in neck area, with a pair on either side of the thyroid gland. Symptoms include **bone pain**, a lump in the neck, weak muscles, or nausea.

See Also Cigarettes; Laryngeal nerve palsy; Squamous cell carcinoma of the skin; Alcohol consumption

Resources

BOOKS

Cummings, C.W., J.M. Fredrickson, L.A. Harker, et al. *Otolaryngology – Head and Neck Surgery.* St. Louis: Mosby–Year Book, Inc., 1998.

Fraker, D.L., M. Skarulis, and V. Livolsi. "Thyroid Tumors." In *Cancer: Principles and Practice of Oncology* 5th ed. DeVita, V. Jr., et al, eds. Philadelphia: Lippincott–Raven Publishers, 1997.

KEY TERMS

Larynx—The voice box or sound-producing organ in the body, located in the upper section of the trachea (windpipe). The movement of the muscles of this organ alters the sounds emitted by the vocal cords.

Pharynx—The space behind the mouth that connects to the trachea and the esophagus (swallowing tube). It serves as a passageway for food and air.

Risk factor—Anything that increases a person's chance of developing a disease.

PERIODICALS

Greenlee, R., M. Hill-Harmon, T. Murray, and M. Thun. "Cancer Statistics, 2001." *CA: A Cancer Journal for Clinicians* 51 (2001): 15-36.

OTHER

"PDQ: A Cancer Information Database." *CancerNet* 2 July 2001 <http://www.nci.nih.gov>

Lata Cherath, Ph.D.
Monica McGee, M.S.

Health insurance

Definition

Health insurance is insurance that pays for all or part of a person's health care bills. The types of health insurance are group health plans, individual plans, workers' compensation, and government health plans such as Medicare and Medicaid.

Health insurance can be further classified into fee-for-service (traditional insurance) and managed care. Both group and individual insurance plans can be either fee-for-service or managed care plans.

The following are types of managed care plans:

- Health Maintenance Organization (HMO)
- Preferred Provider Organization (PPO)

Purpose

The purpose of health insurance is to help people cover their health care costs. Health care costs include doctor visits, hospital stays, surgery, procedures, tests, home care, and other treatments and services.

Description

Health insurance is available to groups as well as individuals. Government plans, such as Medicare, are offered to people who meet certain criteria.

Group and individual plans can be further classified as either fee-for-service or managed care. Cancer patients may have specific concerns, such as the freedom to select specialists, that play a factor in choosing a health care plan. Fee-for-service plans traditionally offer greater freedom when choosing a health care professional. Managed care often limits a patient to health care professionals listed by the managed care insurance company.

Group health plans

A group health plan offers health care coverage for employers, student organizations, professional associations, religious organizations, and other groups. Many employers offer group health plans to employees and their dependents as a benefit of working with that particular employer (medical benefits). The employer may pay for part or all of the insurance cost (premium).

When an employee leaves a job he or she may be eligible for continued health insurance as a result of the Consolidated Omnibus Budget Reconciliation Act of 1986 (COBRA). This federal law protects employees and their families in certain situations by allowing them to keep their health insurance for a specified amount of time. The individual must, however, pay a premium to keep their insurance plan in effect It is important to note that COBRA only applies under certain conditions, such as job loss, death, divorce, or other life events. The COBRA law usually applies to group health plans offered by companies with more than 20 employees. Some states have laws that require employers to offer continued health care coverage for people who do not qualify for COBRA. Each state's insurance board can provide additional information.

Individual plans

These type of health care plans are sold directly to individuals.

Fee-for-service

Fee-for-service is traditional health insurance in which the insurance company reimburses the doctor, hospital, or other health care provider for all or part of the fees charged. Fee-for-service plans may be offered to groups or individuals. This type of plan gives people the highest level of freedom to choose a doctor, hospital, or other health care provider. A person may be able to receive medical care anywhere in the United States and, often, in the world.

Under this type of insurance a premium is paid and there is usually a yearly deductible, which means benefits do not begin until this deductible is met. After the person has paid the deductible (an amount specified by the terms of the insurance policy) the insurance company pays a portion of covered medical services. For example, the deductible may be $250 so the patient pays the first $250 of yearly covered medical expenses. After that he or she may pay 20% of covered services while the insurance company pays 80%. The exact percentages and deductibles will vary with each policy. The person may have to fill out forms (claims) and send them to the insurance company to have their claims paid.

People who have cancer may be attracted to the freedom of choice that traditional fee-for-service plans offer. However, they will most likely have higher out-of-pocket costs than they would in a managed care plan.

Managed care

Managed care plans are also sold to both groups and individuals. In these plans a person's health care is managed by the insurance company. Approvals are needed for some services, including visits to specialist doctors, medical tests, or surgical procedures. In order for people to receive the highest level of coverage they must obtain services from the doctors, hospitals, labs, imaging centers, and other providers affiliated with their managed care plan.

People with cancer who are considering a managed care plan should check with the plan regarding coverage for services outside of the plan's list of participating providers. For example, if a person wants to travel to a cancer center for treatment, he or she should find out what coverage will be available. In these plans coverage is usually much less if a person receives treatment from doctors and hospitals not affiliated with the plan.

HEALTH MAINTENANCE ORGANIZATION (HMO). An HMO is a type of managed care called a prepaid plan. This type of coverage was designed initially to help keep people healthy by covering the cost of preventive care, such as medical checkups. The patient selects a primary care doctor, such as a family physician, from an HMO list. This doctor coordinates the patient's care and determines if referrals to specialist doctors are needed. People pay a premium, usually every month, and receive their health care services (doctor visits, hospital care, lab work, emergency services, etc.) when they pay a small fee called a copayment. The HMO has arrangements with caregivers and hospitals and the copayment only applies to those caregivers and facilities affiliated with the HMO. This type of coverage offers less freedom than fee-for-service, but out-of-pocket health care costs are generally lower and more predictable. A person's out-of-pocket costs will be much higher if he or she receives care outside of the HMO unless prior approval from the HMO is received.

PREFERRED PROVIDER ORGANIZATION (PPO). A PPO combines the benefits of fee-for-service with the features of an HMO. If patients use health care providers (doctors, hospitals, etc.) who are part of the PPO network, they will receive coverage for most of their bills after a deductible and, perhaps a copayment, is met. Some PPOs require people to choose a primary care physician who will coordinate care and arrange referrals to specialists when needed. Other PPOs allow patients to choose specialists on their own. A PPO may offer lower levels of coverage for care given by doctors and other professionals not affiliated with the PPO. In these cases the patient may have to fill out claim forms to receive coverage.

Government health plans

Medicare and Medicaid are two health plans offered by the U.S. government. They are available to individuals who meet certain age, income, or disability criteria. TRICARE Standard, formerly called CHAMPUS, is the health plan for U.S. military personnel.

MEDICARE. Medicare, created in 1965 under Title 18 of the Social Security Act, is available to people who meet certain age and disability criteria. Eligible people include:

- those who are age 65 years and older
- some younger individuals who have disabilities
- those who have end-stage renal disease (permanent kidney failure)

KEY TERMS

Clinical trial—A study to determine the efficacy and safety of a drug or medical procedure. This type of study is often called an experimental or investigational procedure.

Health care provider—A doctor, hospital, lab, or other professional person or facility offering health care services.

Health insurance claim—A bill for health care services that is turned in to the health insurance company for payment.

> **QUESTIONS TO ASK THE DOCTOR**
>
> - What types of insurance do you accept?
> - Does your office file claims for patients?
> - Will your office get pre-authorization for procedures where it is required?
> - Do you have a list of providers for my type of insurance in case a referral is necessary?
> - If an experimental procedure is recommended, what costs will be involved?

Medicare has two parts: Part A and Part B. Part A is hospital insurance and helps cover the costs of inpatient hospital stays, skilled nursing centers, **home health services**, and **hospice care**. Part B helps cover medical services such as doctors' bills, ambulances, outpatient therapy, and a host of other services, supplies, and equipment that Part A does not cover.

MEDICAID. Medicaid, created in 1965 under Title 19 of the Social Security Act, is designed for people receiving federal government aid such as Aid to Families with Dependent Children. This program covers hospitalization, doctors' visits, lab tests, and x rays. Some other services may be partially covered.

TRICARE. Eligible military families may enroll in TRICARE Prime, which is an HMO; TRICARE Extra, which offers an expanded choice of providers; or TRICARE Standard, which is the new name for CHAMPUS.

Supplemental insurance

Supplemental insurance covers expenses that are not paid for by a person's health insurance. Cancer insurance is a specific form of supplemental insurance that covers expenses that are not normally covered by health insurance but are specifically related to cancer treatments.

Workers' compensation

Workers' compensation covers health care costs for an injury or illness related to a person's job. Medical conditions that are unrelated to work are not covered under this plan. In some cases an evaluation is done to determine whether or not the medical condition is truly related to a person's employment.

Special concerns

There are a variety of special concerns that people with cancer have regarding health insurance.

Waiting period

Insurance may not take effect immediately upon signing up for a policy. Sometimes a waiting period exists, during which time premiums are not paid and benefits are not available. Health care services received during this period are not covered.

Preexisting condition

A preexisting condition, such as cancer, is a concern when choosing insurance. If a person received medical advice or treatment for a medical problem within six months of enrolling in new insurance, this condition is called preexisting, and it can be excluded from the new coverage. The six-month time lapse before a person enrolls in a new health insurance policy is called the look-back period. If a person received medical advice, recommendations, prescription drugs, diagnosis, or treatment for a health problem during the look-back period, he or she is considered to have a preexisting condition. People should check with their state insurance boards to determine preexisting condition rules.

Coverage renewal

Some people with diseases such as cancer worry about group health plans renewing their coverage. As long as the person meets the plan's eligibility requirements and the plan covers similar cases, the coverage must be offered. Coverage cannot be cancelled for health reasons.

Experimental/investigational treatments

Experimental/investigational treatments are often a concern for people with cancer. These treatments may or may not be covered by a person's health insurance. Some states mandate coverage for investigational treatments. People should check with their insurance plan and state insurance board to determine if coverage is available.

A clinical trial is a type of investigational treatment. Costs involved include patient care costs and research costs. Usual patient care costs that may be covered by insurance are visits to the doctor, stays in the hospital, tests, and other procedures that occur whether a person is part of an experiment or is receiving traditional care. Extra patient care costs that may or may not be covered by insurance are the special tests required as part of the research study.

Health insurance plans have policies regarding coverage for **clinical trials**. People should determine their level of health insurance coverage for clinical trials, and they should learn about the costs associated with a particular study.

In 2000, Medicare began covering certain clinical trials. The trials must meet specific criteria in order to be covered. In eligible trials treatments and services such as tests, procedures, and doctor visits that are normally covered by Medicare are covered. Some items may not be covered including investigational items like the experimental drug itself or items that are used only for data collection in the clinical trial. Patients should check to see if the clinical trial sponsor is providing the **investigational drug** at no charge.

Complementary therapies

Complementary cancer therapies are another coverage consideration. A cancer patient undergoing this type of therapy should check with his or her insurance policy regarding coverage.

Cancer screening coverage

Cancer screening coverage is an important consideration. As of 2000, 44 states mandate insurance coverage of screenings for at least one of these cancers: breast, cervical, prostate, and colorectal. **Breast cancer** screening coverage is most commonly mandated. Most mandates refer to screenings that follow the American Cancer Society guidelines. A Women's Health Initiative Observational Study investigated the use of cancer screenings by more than 55,000 women between September 1994 and February 1997. The study found that the type of insurance a woman had was linked with the number of cancer screenings she reported. Women age 65 years and older who had Medicare plus prepaid insurance were more likely to report that they had screenings than those who had Medicare alone.

Health care regulations

The Health Insurance Portability and Accountability Act (HIPAA), passed by the U.S. Congress in 1996, offers people rights and protections regarding their health care plans. Because of HIPAA there are limits on preexisting condition exclusions, people cannot be discriminated because of health factors, there are special enrollment requirements for people who lose other group plans or have new dependents, small employers are guaranteed group health plan availability, and all group plans have guaranteed renewal if the employer wishes to renew. In summary these rights and protections include:

- Portability. This is the ability for a person to get new health insurance if a change is desired or needed.
- Availability. This refers to whether or not health insurance must be offered to a person and his or her dependents.
- Renewability. This refers to whether or not a person is able to renew his or her health plan.

The Women's Health and Cancer Rights Act of 1998 requires health insurance plans to cover breast reconstruction related to a **mastectomy** if the patient chooses to have reconstruction and if the health plan covered the mastectomy. The law became effective for different health plans on different dates, with the earliest date of effect being October 21, 1998.

Resources

BOOKS

Schwartz, Alan N. *Getting the best from your doctor.* Minneapolis, MN: Chronimed Publishing, 1998.

PERIODICALS

Hsia, Judith et al., "The Importance of Health Insurance as a Determinant of Cancer Screening: Evidence from the Women's Health Initiative." *Preventive Medicine* (September 2000): 261-70

Rathore, Saif S. et al., "Mandated Coverage for Cancer-Screening Services: Whose Guidelines Do States Follow?" *American Journal of Preventive Medicine* (August 2000): 71-8

ORGANIZATIONS

Agency for Health Care Research and Quality, *Checkup on Health Insurance Choices* 27 March 2001 <http://www.ahcpr.gov/consumer/insuranc.htm>

National Cancer Institute, *Cancer Trials and Insurance Coverage: A Resource Guide* 4 May 2001 <http://cancertrials.nci.nih.gov/understanding/indepth/insurance>

Health Care Choices *Our Newsletter: Better Health Choices* (January 1999) 9 May 2001 <http://www.healthcarechoices.org/newslet/news199brreconst.htm>

Health Care Financing Administration *HIPAA Online* 27 March 2001 <http://www.hcfa.gov>

TRICARE *The History of CHAMPUS and its Evolving Role* 9 May 2001 <http://www.tricare.osd.mil/factsheets/history.pdf>

OTHER

"Supplemental Insurance Policies May Be Offered Under a Flex Plan, IRS Says" In *Flex Plan Handbook: November 1999* 9 May 2001 5 July 2001 <http://207.226.10.52/tpg/pen_ben/flex/flexnov99.html>

Rhonda Cloos, R.N.

Hemolytic anemia

Description

Red blood cells (erythrocytes) transport oxygen and carbon dioxide in the bloodstream, maintain a normal acid-base balance, and determine how thick or thin the blood is. Hemolytic anemia refers to the premature,

KEY TERMS

Erythrocytes—Red blood cells.

Erythropoietin—A glyco-protein hormone secreted by the kidney in the adult and by the liver in the fetus, which acts on stem cells of the bone marrow to stimulate red blood cell production (erythropoiesis).

Hemolysis—The rupture of red blood cells with the release of hemoglobin into the plasma.

Thalassemia—A hereditary hemolytic anemia marked by a decreased rate of synthesis of hemoglobin chains.

Spherocytosis—The presence of small, round erythrocytes that have a smaller surface area than normal and carry less oxygen as a result.

Stem cells—Any precursor cell having the ability to both replicate and differentiate and give rise to other precursors of different blood cell lines.

increased destruction of erythrocytes. Hemolysis is the rupture of these erythrocytes with the release of hemoglobin into the plasma, and anemia is a reduced delivery of oxygen to the tissues. Some of the symptoms of hemolytic anemia include nosebleeds, bleeding gums, shortness of breath, **fatigue**, rapid heartbeat, pale skin color or yellow skin color (jaundice), chills, and dark-colored urine.

Causes

Erythrocyte (red blood cell) formation takes place in the red bone marrow in an adult and in the liver, spleen, and bone marrow of the fetus. Their formation requires an adequate supply of iron, cobalt, copper, amino acids, and certain **vitamins**. When the bone marrow loses its ability to compensate for the destruction of the erythrocytes by increasing their production, hemolytic anemia occurs. There are many types of hemolytic anemia, which are classified according to the location of this inability to produce red blood cells. If the problem lies within the red blood cell itself, it is referred to as an intrinsic factor, and if the problem is outside the red blood cell, it is referred to as an extrinsic factor. The overall incidence of hemolytic anemia is approximately 4 per 100,000 people.

Rh factor incompatibility refers to genetically determined substances capable of producing an **immune response** (antigens). This can cause hemolytic anemia not only during pregnancy when the mother is Rh negative and the fetus is Rh positive, but in mismatched blood transfusions as well. There are a number of industrial poisons that produce hemolytic anemia. These include:

- antimalarial agents
- organic solvents (benzene)
- certain chemotherapies
- hypersensitivity to certain antibiotics
- metals (chromium, platinum salts, nickel, lead, copper)
- Pyridium
- arsenic
- intravenous (IV) water (an IV that is not normal or half-normal saline)
- snake bites (if the venom contains hemolytic toxins)

These are all factors external to the red blood cell and thus are extrinsic in nature.

One important extrinsic factor in the cause of hemolytic anemia is in the course of widespread cancer, leukemia, **Hodgkin's disease**, acute alcoholism and liver disease. Many of the **chemotherapy** agents (**cisplatin**, **carboplatin** and nonplatinum drugs) utilized in treating various cancers have side effects that cause a suppression of bone marrow activity, which results in severe hemolytic anemia. In essence, an individual is not only anemic as a result of cancer, but this anemia is worsened by the treatment. Since nausea, vomiting, and lack of appetite are also side effects of chemotherapy, it is extremely difficult for the patient to overcome this anemia with diet and supplements. Eventually, severe hemolytic anemia is the end result.

Intrinsic factors would include disorders in the immune response and genetically inherited disorders such as glucose-6-phosphate dehydrogenase deficiency, an essential enzyme. People with this disorder do not display any symptoms until exposed to certain medications or stress. Aspirin and non-steroidal anti-inflammatory drugs (NSAIDs) can precipitate this reaction. This disorder is more common among African-American males, with approximately 10% to 14% of the population being affected. Other genetic disorders include sickle cell anemia, thalassemia, and spherocytosis. All of these produce structurally abnormal red blood cells to varying degrees.

Treatments

The treatment depends upon the cause and severity of the anemia. Medicines like **folic acid** and **corticosteroids** may be used to treat the anemia if it is not severe. Severe hemolytic anemia may be very quickly fatal and immediate hospitalization is required for transfusion of washed and packed red blood cells. Severe anemias can aggravate pre-existing heart disease, lung disease and cerebrovascular disease.

Frequently with cancer treatments, a patient may undergo numerous blood transfusions to accomodate for the severe anemia suffered as a result of chemotherapy. Researchers, investigating ways to enhance the quality of life for chemotherapy patients, have primarily looked at controlling pain and loss of appetite (**anorexia**). Recent studies, however, have examined the use of **erythropoietin** (a protein hormone that stimulates red blood cell production) in improving fatigue symptoms and enhancing overall quality of life. Once-weekly therapy with erythropoietin was found to increase hemoglobin levels, decrease transfusion requirements, and improve quality of life in patients with cancer and anemia undergoing chemotherapy.

Alternative and complementary therapies

Since there is no known prevention for hemolytic anemia, there is relatively little that can be done except to be aware of the risk factors and know the potential for genetic disorders within the family. Avoiding exposure to chemicals that precipitate the reaction, eating natural, whole grain foods, avoiding stress, and taking vitamin supplements can be helpful. With cancer patients, yoga and meditation provide a means of enhancing relaxation, reducing stress, and incorporating visualization for healing. Those patients who attend and participate in support groups have an increased quality of life with better outcomes from treatments.

Resources

BOOKS

Jarvis, Carolyn.*Physical Examination and Health Assessment.* Philadelphia: W.B. Saunders Company, 2000.

Hoffman, Matthew, ed.*The Doctors Book of Food Remedies.* New York: St. Martin's Press, 1998.

PERIODICALS

Gabrilove, J.L., C.S. Cleeland, R.B. Livingston, et al. "Once-Weekly Dosing of Epoetin Alfa in Chemotherapy Patients."*Journal of Clinical Oncology* 19 (2001): 2875–82.

Mantovani, L., G. Lentini, B. Hentschel, et al. "Treatment of Anaemia in Myelodysplastic Syndromes."*British Journal of Haematology* 109 (2000): 367–75.

Osoba, D. "Health-Related Quality-of-Life Assessment in Clinical Trials."*Support Care Cancer* 8 (2000): 84–8.

Parsons, S.K., "Hematopoietic Growth Factors for Children With Cancer."*Current Opinions in Pediatrics* 12 (2000): 10–7.

Linda K. Bennington, C.N.S., M.S.N.

Hemoptysis

Description

Hemoptysis is the coughing up of blood or bloody sputum from the respiratory tract. The blood can come from the nose, mouth, throat, airway passages leading from the lungs, or the lungs.

Hemoptysis can range from small quantities of blood-stained sputum to life-threatening amounts of blood. Massive hemoptysis is defined as the spitting up of so much blood that it interferes with the patient's breathing. Generally, this is 200 to 600 or more milliliters of blood coughed up within a 24 hour period. Massive hemoptysis is considered a medical emergency. Up to 75 percent of patients with massive hemoptysis die from asphyxiation (lack of oxygen) caused by too much blood in the airways.

Hemoptysis refers specifically to the spitting up of blood that comes from the respiratory tract. Often when persons spit up blood, they are not spitting up blood from the respiratory tract, but from somewhere else. When the blood comes from somewhere other than the respiratory tract, such as from a bloody nose or from the gastrointestinal tract, this is called pseudohemoptysis. Vomiting up blood from the gastrointestinal tract, called hematemesis, is one type of pseudohemoptysis. It is important to distinguish between true hemoptysis and pseudohemoptysis because they often involve very different parts of the body and the treatments are radically different.

Causes

Hemoptysis is caused by a variety of medical conditions including tuberculosis, bronchitis, bronchiectasis, **pneumonia**, and respiratory tract trauma. It is also caused by many forms of lung and respiratory tract cancers, such as: bronchial **carcinoma**, bronchial **adenoma**, respiratory tract hemangioma, and occasionally by metastatic cancer to the lungs.

Treatments

The goal of treatment for patients with hemoptysis is to stop the bleeding as soon as possible while also treating the cancer or other underlying disorder that is causing the hemoptysis.

Hemoptysis generally will stop spontaneously and no treatment is necessary, apart from reassurance of the patient that this condition will resolve on its own. Therefore, the general treatment for hemoptysis is to keep the patient calm and to ensure complete bed rest.

If the coughing that accompanies the hemoptysis is troublesome or aggravating the condition, cough suppressants may be recommended.

In cases of massive hemoptysis, the placement of a tube in the respiratory tract (intubation) may be necessary to allow for adequate airflow into and out of the res-

KEY TERMS

Bronchial carcinoma—Cancer arising from the bronchi, the major vessels that convey air to and from the lungs to the mouth and nose.

Bronchial adenoma—A tumor arising in the linings of the bronchi.

Hemangioma—A tumor of the blood vessels that is usually present at birth. When these occur on a visible portion of the skin, they are called "birthmarks." When they occur within the respiratory tract, they may lead to hemoptysis.

Sputum—Material ejected from the lungs, bronchi, or trachea, through the mouth.

piratory tract. A **bronchoscopy** may be performed, not only to clear the airway of blood, but also to assist in diagnosing the endobronchial cause of the hemoptysis. When large amounts of blood have been lost, the patient may also require intravenous (IV) fluids and/or a blood transfusion.

In the most severe cases of hemoptysis, surgery to remove the cancer that is causing the spitting up of blood may be necessary to relieve the symptoms of hemoptysis. Other treatment modalities include PDT (photodynamic therapy).

Alternative and complementary therapies

Inhalation of the fumes of a tea made from the bark of the wild cherry (*Prunus virginiana*) tree has been an herbal remedy for many respiratory tract ailments, including tuberculosis and hemoptysis among the Native Americans for centuries.

Hydrazine sulfate, a naturally occurring monoamine oxidase inhibitor (MAOI), has also been suggested as a treatment for hemoptysis.

Resources

BOOKS

Idell, Steven."Hemoptysis" In *Current Diagnosis 9*, edited by Rex B. Conn, et al. Philadelphia: W. B. Saunders Company, 1997.

ORGANIZATIONS

The Alliance for Lung Cancer (ALCASE). 1601 Lincoln Avenue, P. O. Box 849, Vancouver, WA 98666. Telephone 1-800-298-2436. Fax 360-735-1305. Internet <http://www.alcase.org>

American Lung Association (ALA). 1740 Broadway, New York, NY 10019. Telephone 1-212-315-8700. Internet <http://www.lungusa.org>

Paul A. Johnson, Ed.M.

Heparin

Definition

Heparin is a drug that helps prevent blood clots from forming and belongs to the family of drugs called anticoagulants (blood thinners), although it does not actually thin the blood. It is sold in the U.S. under the brand names of Calciparine, Liquaemin, Calciparine, Hepalean, and Heparin Leo, and Calcilean in Canada.

Purpose

Heparin is used to decrease the clotting ability of the blood and to help prevent harmful clots from forming in the blood vessels. Heparin will not dissolve blood clots that have already formed, but it may prevent the clots from becoming larger and causing more serious problems. Heparin possesses several antithrombotic mechanisms. It is often used as a treatment for certain blood vessel, heart, and lung conditions and is also used to prevent blood clotting during open-heart surgery, bypass surgery, and dialysis. Heparin is used in low doses to prevent the formation of blood clots in certain patients, especially those who must have certain types of surgery or who must remain in bed for a long time. It is also used for the long-term treatment of thromboembolic disease, a common side effect of cancer.

One of the most common hematological complications is disordered coagulation. Approximately 15% of all cancer patients are affected by thromboembolic disease, which is the second leading cause of death for cancer patients. However, thromboembolic disease may represent only one of many complications in end-stage patients. Thromboembolic disease includes superficial and deep venous thrombosis, pulmonary emboli, thrombosis of venous access devices, arterial thrombosis, and embolism. The cancer itself or cancer treatments may induce coagulation. For example, **chemotherapy** can increase the risk of thromboembolic disease. An increased risk for arterial thrombosis has been observed with chemotherapy treatment.

Cancer and its treatment can affect all three causes of thromboembolic disease, including the alteration of blood flow, damage to endothelial cells (the cells in blood vessels), and enhancing procoagulants (causing the blood to clot). Cancer can affect blood flow by mechanically affecting blood vessels close to a tumor. In addition, tumors cause angiogenesis, which may create complexes of blood vessels that have a disordered appearance and flow (varying in magnitude and direction). Chemotherapy or tumors may directly damage endothelial cells. Procoagulants may be secreted into the blood stream by cancer cells or can be increased on the surface of cancer cells.

Description

Heparin is the most common anticoagulant used and the generic name product may be available in the U.S. and Canada.

Mechanisms of action:

Heparin increases the release of specific proteins, like tissue plasminogen activator and tissue factor pathway inhibitor (TFPI), into the blood in order to inhibit blood coagulation. It can also increase the activity of these proteins. Heparin augments the activity of antithrombin III, a natural compound that inhibits activated clotting factors from contributing to more coagulation. Furthermore, heparin has been found to inhibit substances that may contribute to angiogenesis, including vascular endothelial growth factor, tissue factor, and platelet-activating factor.

Whether anticoagulants like heparin may also improve cancer survival rates independent of their effect on thromboembolism has been investigated. In fact, experimental and clinical data have demonstrated that heparin is an effective compound in preventing metastases. Many investigators have shown that heparin inhibits tumor **metastasis** in experimental animals; a few **clinical trials** also suggest a positive effect in humans with cancer.

Recommended dosage

Heparin is available only with a doctor's prescription, in parenteral and injection (U.S. and Canada) dosage forms. A doctor will need to prescribe a specific dose for an individual's based on the type of heparin, as well as the patient's medical condition and body weight.

Dosing schedule

Heparin should be taken under the doctor's direction and at the same time every day. If a dose is missed, take it as soon as possible. However, if a dose is missed until the following day, patients should not double-dose, but just take the usual daily dose. Double-dosing may cause bleeding.

KEY TERMS

Angiogenesis—The formation of new blood vessels that occurs naturally under certain circumstances, for example, in the healing of a cut.

Anticoagulant—Anticoagulants are nonhabit-forming medications that prevent the formation of new blood clots and keep existing blood clots from growing larger.

Blood clot—A clump of blood that forms in or around a vessel as a result of coagulation. The formation of blood clots when the body has been cut is essential because without blood clots to cease the bleeding, a person would bleed to death from a relatively small wound.

Coagulation—The blood's natural tendency to clump and stick.

Embolism—An embolism occurs when a clump of material such as a broken-off piece of plaque, a blood clot, or air travels through the bloodstream and becomes lodged in a blood vessel.

Endothelial cells—The cells lining the inside of blood vessels.

Parenteral—Medications administered through intravenous, subcutaneous, or intramuscular injection.

Procoagulants —Inducing the blood to clot.

Thromboembolism—Another word for embolism (see embolism).

Thrombosis—The formation of a blood clot in an artery or vein that may be accompanied by inflammation. If untreated in arteries, thrombosis can lead to death of the nearby tissue.

Precautions

Some medications should not be combined. Over-the-counter medicines, **vitamins**, and herbal products may cause interactions when combined with heparin, so the patient should check with the doctor monitoring the heparin medication before taking any new medication, even when prescribed by another doctor.

Patients who are pregnant, breastfeeding, have given birth recently, or using an IUD for birth control should consult their doctor. The doctor should also be notified if radiation treatments, surgery, or a fall or other injury has recently occurred.

The presence of other medical problems may affect the use of heparin. Patients should be sure to tell their doctor about any other medical problems, in particular:

- allergies or asthma (or history of)
- blood disease or bleeding problems
- colitis or stomach ulcer (or history of)
- diabetes mellitus
- high blood pressure (hypertension)
- kidney disease
- liver disease
- tuberculosis (active)

Side effects

The doctor should be contacted immediately if any of these side effects are present:

- wheezing or trouble breathing
- skin rash, **itching**, or hives
- red or "coffee ground" vomit
- unexplained nosebleeds
- swelling in the face, lips, or tongue
- blood in urine or stools
- black tarry stools

Interactions

Using any of the following medicines together with heparin may increase the risk of bleeding. Again, candidates for heparin should alert their physicians if they are taking any of these medications:

- aspirin
- persantine
- carbenicillin by injection (e.g., Geopen)
- cefamandole (e.g., Mandol)
- cefoperazone (e.g., Cefobid)
- cefotetan (e.g., Cefotan)
- dipyridamole (e.g., Persantine)
- divalproex (e.g., Depakote)
- medicine for inflammation or pain (Motrin, Aleve), except narcotics
- medicine for overactive thyroid
- pentoxifylline (e.g., Trental)
- plicamycin (e.g., Mithracin)
- probenecid (e.g., Benemid)
- sulfinpyrazone (e.g., Anturane)
- ticarcillin (e.g., Ticar)
- valproic acid (e.g., Depakene)
- medicines via intramuscular injection

See Also Low molecular weight heparin; Warfarin

Crystal Heather Kaczkowski, MSc.

Hepatic arterial infusion

Definition

Hepatic arterial infusion (HAI) therapy, delivers chemotherapeutic agents directly to the liver through a catheter placed in the hepatic artery. The hepatic artery is the main route of blood supply to liver tumors. HAI is also known as regional **chemotherapy**.

Purpose

Approximately 160,000 patients are diagnosed with **colon cancer** in the U.S. each year. The cancer spreads to the liver in about 70 percent of those patients. For patients with colorectal liver metastases, tumor progression within the liver is typically the primary cause of death.

Systemic chemotherapy using various agents has some efficacy, but the side effects can have a profound negative impact on the patient's quality of life during treatment. HAI therapy may be an effective option because it delivers chemotherapy medication directly to the site of the tumor, making it appropriate as an alternative or adjuvant treatment to systemic chemotherapy. When metastases is limited to the liver, HAI with **floxuridine** (FUDR) or radioactive microspheres through an implantable pump under the skin or an external pump worn on the belt may be a better option than systemic chemotherapy.

HAI may extend life expectancy and reduce the chance that more liver tumors will develop.

Precautions

- Strict aseptic techniques should be used to prevent infection during all procedures.
- Pump flow rate will vary depending on factors such as body temperature, altitude, arterial pressure at the catheter tip, and solution viscosity.
- Patients should not attempt to resterilize the pump.
- The manufacturer's instructions should be followed regarding drug preparation, dosage, and administration.
- FUDR should be used with added caution in patients with impaired liver or kidney function.

Systemic therapy should be considered for patients with disease known to extend beyond the area capable of being infused.

Description

HAI enhances cancer therapy by increasing drug delivery directly to the site of the tumor (the liver) while minimizing systemic drug exposure and side effects.

Development of fully implanted infusion systems have allowed for long-term delivery of hepatic regional chemotherapy.

Benefits of HAI therapy:

- yields higher tumor response rates and delays cancer progression
- trend toward increased survival rates
- enhances quality of life
- reduced systemic side effects

Preparation

Patient selection criteria

Successful results depend on careful patient selection.

Candidates for HAI therapy should:

- have primary liver cancer or liver metastases from primary colorectal cancer
- show an absence of tumors outside the liver
- have demonstrated portal vein patency
- be a suitable surgical candidate
- show no evidence of infection
- be willing to participate in frequent pump refill appointments

Studies have demonstrated that patients with metastatic colorectal cancer who had liver disease only, had less than 70% of their liver involved with metastases, and had a good performance status responded best to HAI. When metastases are also located outside of the liver, HAI does not offer an advantage over systemic chemotherapy.

Aftercare

During the course of treatment, pump pocket infections occur rarely. At the first sign of infection at the pump pocket, systemic **antibiotics** need to be started. The pump needs to be moved to a new location in a newly created pocket if the infection does not resolve itself. The old pocket should be opened and drained.

Risks

The major problems with HAI are not surgical. They include gastritis, duodenitis, and biliary sclerosis.

Drug toxicity and medication side effects may occur. The most commonly reported side effects for FUDR are **nausea and vomiting**, **diarrhea**, and intestinal inflammation.

Other possible complications include:

- arterial thromboses
- catheter dislodgement
- the catheter may erode through the wall of the duodenum when the pump has been in place for more than a year.
- overdose or underdose of medication if certain conditions affect the rate at which the pump delivers medication, i.e. pump damage due to strenuous activity, high heat, or a change in air pressure.
- disruption in therapy if the pump is damaged by improper handling or filling.

Normal results

Morbidity or mortality occurring as a result of this procedure should be close to zero. Appropriate selection of patients and new combinations of chemotherapy should provide at least a 70% response rate from HAI for the treatment of hepatic metastases from colorectal primary tumors. This response rate is at least twice that of current systemic chemotherapies.

KEY TERMS

Adjuvant treatment—A treatment that is added to increase effectiveness of the first treatment.

Cancer—A term for diseases in which abnormal cells divide without control. Cancer cells can invade nearby tissues and can spread through the bloodstream and lymphatic system to other parts of the body.

Catheter—A flexible tube used to administer or withdraw fluids. During a course of chemotherapy, an indwelling catheter can be placed in a vein to administer intravenous fluids and chemotherapy. Catheters can stay in place for several weeks or months with proper care.

Chemotherapy—A cancer treatment using medicines.

Hepatic—Refers to the liver.

Implant—A device inserted into the body to either treat cancer or to replace or substitute for a lost part or ability.

Metastases—The spread of cancer to other body parts.

Tumor—An abnormal mass of tissue that serves no purpose. Tumors may be either benign (non-cancerous) or malignant (cancerous).

When used in conjunction with traditional chemotherapy, HAI therapy has been shown to extend life expectancy and reduce recurrence of liver tumors after two years for certain patients.

Abnormal results

Complications that can occur with surgery:

- infection
- fluid build up around the implant site
- skin erosion over the site of the implant
- incision breakdown
- drugs may be delivered to organs other than the liver

Resources

PERIODICALS

Henderson, C.W. "Combined Criteria Predict Response to Hepatic Arterial Infusion Chemotherapy." *Cancer Weekly* (1 August 2000).

Venook, Alan, Betsy Althaus, et al. " Hepatic Arterial Infusion of Chemotherapy for Metastatic Colorectal Cancer." *New England Journal of Medicine* 342 no. 20 (18 May 2000): 1524.

Link, Karl H., Marko Kornmann, et al. " Thymidylate Synthase Quantitation and In Vitro Chemosensitivity Testing Predicts Responses and Survival of Patients with Isolated Nonresectable Liver Tumors Receiving Hepatic Arterial Infusion Chemotherapy." *Cancer* 89, no 12 (15 July 2000): 288–9.

Crystal Heather Kaczkowski, M.S.

Hepatocellular carcinoma *see* **Liver cancer, primary**

Herpes simplex

Description

Herpes simples virus (HSV, or herpesvirus) is a virus that causes infection of skin and mucous membrane and rarely infects other parts of the body. However, in the immunosuppressed patient, HSV may cause **pneumonia** and other more severe infections. When the infection occurs in the mouth it is commonly referred to as cold sores. An outbreak of HSV infection can be very painful. There are two distinct types of HSV: type 1 and type 2. It was believed that HSV-1 mostly caused oral herpes (herpes labialis), while HSV-2 generally caused genital herpes that typically affects the penis, vulva, and rectum. This is not completely true. Both type 1 and type 2 can cause herpes lesions on the lips or genitals. The first symptoms occur within 2-20 days after contact with an infected person.

Symptoms of the primary infection are usually more severe than those of recurrent infections. The primary infection can cause symptoms like those experienced in other viral infections, including lack of energy, headache, **fever**, and swollen lymph nodes in the neck. The first sign of infection is formation of fluid-filled blisters that may last up to two weeks. However, the pain in the area may last much longer. Once HSV enters the body it spreads to nearby mucosal areas through nerve cells. Once it infects the body the virus remains latent for the life of that individual. During the period of latency there are no symptoms. At times the infected person may shed the virus, even in the absence of visible symptoms, and infect others. Individuals infected with the virus can have recurrent infections; however, normally, recurrent infections are milder and shorter. However, cancer patients can have severe recurrences.

Typically, 50–80% of persons with oral herpes experience a prodrome (symptoms of oncoming disease) of pain, burning, **itching**, or tingling at the site where blisters will form. This prodrome stage may last anywhere from a few hours to one to two days. The herpes infection prodrome occurs in both the primary infection and recurrent infections.

Causes

Everyone with cancer has a higher risk of catching viral infections of any type. This is because the cancer itself, and the methods used to treat it, affect the immune defense mechanisms that fight infection. Normally the mucous membrane is one of the first lines of defense against infectious organisms. However, **chemotherapy** and radiation can damage this very important barrier. The barrier that skin provides is also compromised because of needles used for drawing blood or injecting drugs. Radiation and chemotherapy also suppress the immune system. Certain cancers like **Hodgkin's disease**, lymphoma, and T-cell leukemia cause defects in cellular immunity, which is a primary defense mechanism against viral infections. Thus cancer patients, especially those who are undergoing chemotherapy or radiation treatments, are at greater risk of primary and secondary herpes infections.

Oral herpes simplex infections are more common in children than adults following chemotherapy. Patients who have the virus latent in the system have a higher chance of recurrent infection. Primary infection generally causes gingivitis (inflammation of the gums, vesicles on the mucosa (blisters on the lining of the mouth), and a coated tongue (white covering on tongue). Women with genital herpes can have severe recurrence following chemotherapy because of immunosuppression.

Treatment

There is no cure for HSV infection although there are antiviral drugs available that have some effect in lessening the symptoms and decreasing the length of herpes outbreaks. There is evidence that some of these drugs may also prevent future outbreaks. For the best results drug treatment should begin during the prodrome stage before blisters are visible. Depending upon the length of the outbreak, drug treatment could continue up to 10 days.

Acyclovir (Zovirax) is the drug of choice for herpes infection and can be given intravenously or taken by mouth. It can be applied directly to sores as an ointment but is not very useful in this form. A liquid form for children is also available. Acyclovir is effective in treating both the primary infection and recurrent outbreaks. When taken by mouth to prevent an outbreak, acyclovir reduces the frequency of herpes outbreaks.

Alternative and complementary therapies

A number of steps can relieve the symptoms of herpes infections. It is important to keep the blisters or sores clean and dry with an agent like cornstarch. One should avoid touching the sores, and wash hands frequently. Local application of ice may relieve the pain. Over-the-counter medication for fever, pain, and inflammation—such as aspirin, acetaminophen, or ibuprofen—may help. Children should never be given aspirin. Sexual intercourse should be avoided during both the active stage and the prodrome stages. During an outbreak of cold sores salty foods, citrus foods (oranges etc.), and other foods that irritate the sores should be avoided. Over-the-counter lip products that contain the chemical "phenol" (such as Blistex Medicated Lip Ointment) and numbing ointments (such as Anbesol) help to relieve the pain of cold sores. A bandage may be placed over the sores to protect them and prevent spreading the virus to other sites on the lips or face.

A diet rich in the amino acid lysine may help prevent recurrences of cold sores. Foods that contain high levels of lysine include most vegetables, legumes, fish, turkey, and chicken. Oral lysine supplements in the amount of 1000 mg per day may help sores heal faster. There is a belief that foods with high lysine-to-arginine ratio will help prevent outbreaks of herpes simplex. That has not been proven, and it is important to include foods that have a low lysine-to-arginine ratio also, such as nuts, onion, garlic, and green vegetables. It is also suggested that the amount of arginine in the diet be limited as there is a belief that arginine is needed for herpesvirus growth. This amino acid is found in peanuts, beer, chocolate, gelatin, and raisins.

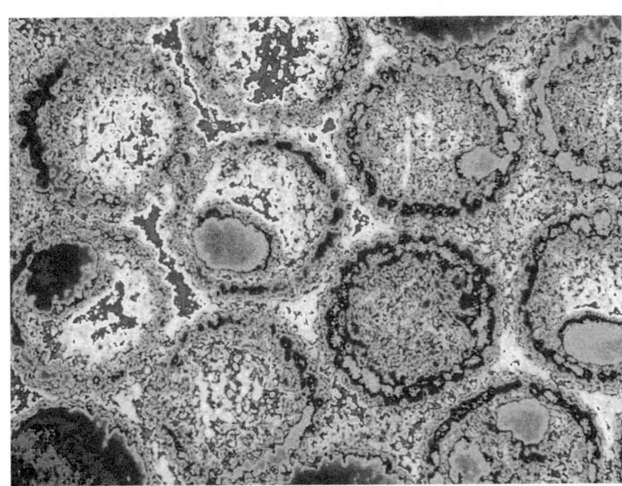

Color digitized electron micrograph image of herpes simplex virus. Cancer patients, especially those who are undergoing chemotherapy or radiation treatments, are at greater risk of herpes infections. *(Custom Medical Stock Photo. Reproduced by permission.)*

Resources

BOOKS

Noskin, Gary A. *Management of Infectious Complications in Cancer Patients.* Norwell: Kluwer Academic Publishers, 1998.

PERIODICALS

Whitley, Richard J., and Bernard Roizman. "Herpes Simplex Virus Infections." *The Lancet* 357 (12 May 2001) 1513.

ORGANIZATIONS

American Herpes Foundation. (201) 342-4441. <http://www.herpes-foundation.org>.

Belinda M. Rowland, Ph.D.
Malini Vashishtha, Ph.D.

Herpes zoster

Description

Herpes zoster, also called shingles, and referred to as "zosteer", gets its name from both the Latin and French words for belt or girdle and refers to belt-like skin eruptions that may occur on the trunk of the body. The virus

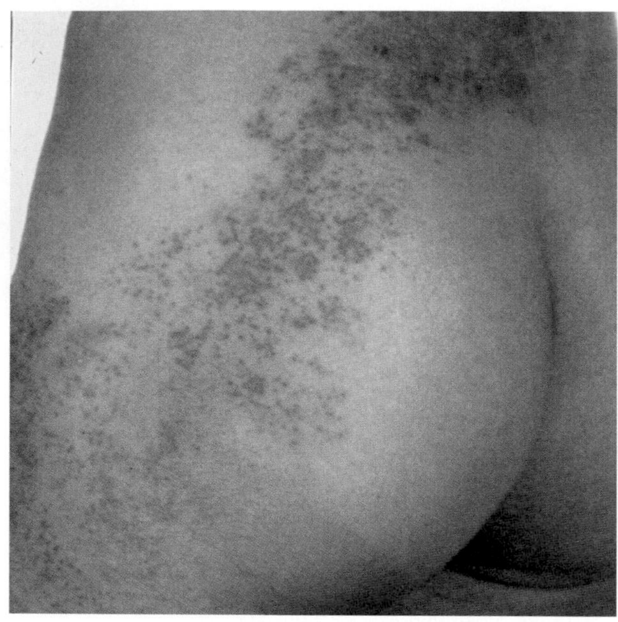

Shingles, or herpes zoster, on patient's buttocks and thigh. *(Custom Medical Stock Photo. Reproduced by permission.)*

that causes chickenpox, the varicella zoster virus (VSV), can become dormant in nerve cells after an episode of chickenpox and later re-emerge as shingles. Any individual who has had chickenpox can develop shingles. People of all ages, even children, can be affected, but the incidence increases with age. There are many other conditions which can predispose to developing shingles. These include: newborn infants, bone marrow and other transplant recipients, and individuals with immune systems weakened by diseases like HIV or cancer, or drugs, such as those used in **chemotherapy**.

Shingles erupts along the course of the affected nerve, producing lesions anywhere on the body and may cause severe nerve pain. The most common areas to be affected are the face and trunk, which correspond to the areas where the chickenpox rash is most concentrated. The disease is caused by a reactivation of the chickenpox virus that has been dormant in certain nerves following an episode of chickenpox. Exactly how or why this reactivation occurs is not clear; however, it is believed that the reactivation is triggered when the immune system becomes weakened as in the examples described above. Early signs of shingles are often vague and can easily be mistaken for other illnesses. The condition may begin with **fever** and malaise (a vague feeling of weakness or discomfort). Within two to four days, severe pain, **itching**, and numbness/tingling (paresthesia) or extreme sensitivity to touch (hyperesthesia) can develop, usually on the trunk and occasionally on the arms and legs. Pain may be continuous or intermittent, usually lasting from one to four weeks. It may occur at the time of the eruption, but can precede the eruption by days, occasionally making the diagnosis difficult. Signs and symptoms may include the following:

- itching, tingling, or severe burning pain
- red patches that develop into blisters
- grouped, dense, deep, small blisters that ooze and crust
- swollen lymph nodes

Immunocompromised patients usually have a more severe course that is frequently prolonged for weeks to months. They develop shingles frequently and the infection can spread to the skin, lungs, liver, gastrointestinal tract, brain, or other vital organs.

Potentially serious complications can result from herpes zoster. Many individuals continue to experience persistent pain long after the blisters heal. This pain, called post-herpatic neuralgia, can be severe and debilitating. Post-herpetic neuralgia can persist for months or years after the lesions have disappeared.

Other complications include a secondary bacterial infection, and rarely, potentially fatal inflammation of the brain (encephalitis) and the spread of an infection throughout the body. These rare, but extremely serious, complications are more likely to occur in those individuals who have weakened immune systems (immunocompromised).

Causes

Herpes zoster has been reported in patients with many different types of cancer. However, the cancers that affect an individual's immune system, such as leukemia or **lymphoma**, are the types that place people at particular risk. Herpes zoster is also a particular problem after the various forms of cancer therapy. A study performed in 1998 looked at 766 episodes of herpes zoster infection at a large cancer center from 1972 to 1980. The highest risk of infection was present among patients with lymphoma and leukemia. In those who received radiation treatment and then developed herpes zoster, half of them developed this within seven months. They developed zoster on the area of their body where the radiation was given. This study showed that a period of months can pass before developing zoster as a consequence of radiation. In those who developed zoster after being treated with chemotherapy, half of them developed zoster within a month.

A study in 1999 looked at 215 consecutive patients who had received high-dose chemotherapy and autologous stem cell rescue to help determine what the incidence and severity of herpes zoster infection was. Herpes zoster was developed in 40 people. Over 80% of these infections occurred within six months of receiving the autologous stem cell rescue. Similar rates of herpes zoster have been seen in patients who received bone marrow transplants. A 1996 study looked at 107 children who had received bone marrow transplants for various malignancies. Thirty-three percent of these children developed herpes zoster. Approximately 90% of the cases developed within one year from the time of bone marrow transplant.

Treatments

Shingles almost always resolves spontaneously and may not require any treatment except for the relief of symptoms. In most people, the condition clears on its own in one or two weeks and seldom recurs. The antiviral drugs acyclovir, valacyclovir, and famciclovir can be used to treat shingles. These drugs may shorten the course of the illness. Their use results in more rapid healing of the blisters when drug therapy is started within 72 hours of the onset of the rash. In fact, the earlier the drugs are administered, the better, because early cases can sometimes be stopped. If taken later, these drugs are less effective but may still lessen the pain. Antiviral drug treatment does not seem to reduce the incidence of post-herpetic neuralgia, but recent studies suggest famciclovir may cut the duration of post-herpetic neuralgia in half. Side effects of typical oral doses of these antiviral drugs are minor with headache and nausea reported by 8-20% of patients. Severely immunocompromised individuals, such as those with cancer, may require intravenous administration of antiviral drugs. Preventive administration of acyclovir to seropositive patients (people who have evidence in their blood of past infection with varicella) who undergo leukemia induction or bone marrow transplant not only effectively prevents herpes zoster recurrence but also reduces the severity of chemotherapy-induced **mucositis**. Therefore, acyclovir prophylaxis should be considered in seropositive patients, especially if they have had a recurrence during previous chemotherapy cycles.

Alternative and complementary therapies

Cool, wet compresses may help reduce pain. If there are blisters or crusting, applying compresses made with diluted vinegar will make the patient more comfortable. The patient can mix one-quarter cup of white vinegar in two quarts of lukewarm water, and use the compress twice each day for 10 minutes. The patient should stop using the compresses when the blisters have dried up.

Soothing baths and lotions such as colloidal oatmeal baths, starch baths or lotions, and calamine lotion may help to relieve itching and discomfort. The skin should be kept clean, and contaminated items should not be re-used. While the lesions continue to ooze, the person should be isolated to prevent infecting other susceptible individuals.

KEY TERMS

Acyclovir—An antiviral drug that is available under the trade name Zovirax, in oral, intravenous, and topical forms. The drug blocks the replication of the varicella zoster virus.

Antibody—A specific protein produced by the immune system in response to a specific foreign protein or particle called an antigen.

Famciclovir—An oral antiviral drug that is available under the trade name Famvir. The drug blocks the replication of the varicella zoster virus.

Immunocompromised —A state in which the immune system is suppressed or not functioning properly.

Post-herpetic neuralgia—The term used to describe the pain after the rash associated with herpes zoster is gone.

Valacyclovir—An oral antiviral drug that is available under the trade name Valtrex. The drug blocks the replication of the varicella zoster virus.

Later, when the crusts and scabs are separating, the skin may become dry, tight, and cracked. If that happens, the patient can rub on a small amount of plain petroleum jelly three or four times a day.

There are non-medical methods of prevention and treatment that may speed recovery. For example, getting lots of rest, eating a healthy diet, exercising regularly, and minimizing stress are always helpful in preventing disease. Supplementation with vitamin B_{12} during the first one to two days and continued supplementation with vitamin B complex, high levels of vitamin C with bioflavonoids, and calcium, are recommended to boost the immune system. Herbal antivirals such as echinacea can be effective in fighting infection and boosting the immune system. Patients should consult physician before taking supplements.

Although no single alternative approach, technique, or remedy has yet been proven to reduce the pain, there are a few options which may be helpful. For example, topical applications of lemon balm (*Melissa officinalis*) or licorice (*Glycyrrhiza glabra*) and peppermint (*Mentha piperita*) may reduce pain and blistering. Homeopathic remedies include *Rhus toxicodendron* for blisters, *Mezereum* and *Arsenicum album* for pain, and *Ranunculus* for itching. Practitioners of Eastern medicine recommend self-hypnosis, acupressure, and acupuncture to alleviate pain. All of these or similar alternative therapies should be discussed with the treating physician before using.

See Also Antiviral therapy

Resources

BOOKS

Berger, Joseph.*Cecil Textbook of Medicine,* 21st Ed. Philadelphia: W.B. Saunders Company, 2000.

Lockie, Andrew. *The Family Guide to Homeopathy: Symptoms and Natural Solutions.* Prentice Hall Press, 1989.

Thomsen, Thomas Carl. *Shingles.* Cross River Press, 1990.

PERIODICALS

Balfour, Henry H. "Varicella Zoster Virus Infections in Immunocompromised Hosts." *American Journal of Medicine* 85 (29 August 1988): 68–72.

Bilgrami, S. et al. "Varicella zoster virus infection associated with high-dose chemotherapy and autologous stem-cell rescue."*Bone Marrow Transplant* 23 (March 1999): 469–74.

Kawasaki, H. et al. "Herpes zoster infection after bone marrow transplantation in children." *Journal of Pediatrics* 128 (March 1996):353–58.

Rusthoven, J. J. et al. "Varicella-zoster infection in adult cancer patients. A population study." *Archives of Internal Medicine* 148 (July 1988):1561–1566.

Perren, Timothy J., et al. "Prevention of Herpes Zoster in Patients by Long-Term Oral Acyclovir After Allogeneic Bone Marrow Transplantation." *American Journal of Medicine* 85 (29 August 1988): 99–101.

Wood, Martin J., et al. "Efficacy of Oral Acyclovir Treatment of Acute Herpes Zoster." *American Journal of Medicine* 85 (August 29, 1988): 79–83.

ORGANIZATION

American Academy of Dermatology. 930 N. Meacham Road, PO Box 4014, Schaumberg, IL 60168-4014. (708) 330-0230. http://www.aad.org. 29 June 2001.

David Greenberg, M.D.

Hickman lines *see* **Vascular access**

Histamine 2 antagonists

Definition

Histamine 2 antagonists are drugs that block the production of acid in the stomach.

Purpose

Histamine 2 antagonists are used to treat the precancerous condition of **Barrett's esophagus**. They are also used to treat **Zollinger-Ellison syndrome** and multiple endocrine neoplasia, rare cancerous conditions in which the stomach makes too much acid and to prevent the development of gastric (stomach) and duodenal (upper part of the small intestine) ulcers.

Description

Histamine 2 blockers are familiar to most people as the over-the counter heartburn medications Tagamet (cimetidine), Pepcid, (famotidine), and Zantac (ranitidine). Axid (nizatidine) is less well known. These drugs also come in prescription strengths. Histamine 2 blockers work by reducing the amount of acid the stomach produces.

The esophagus is a tube 10–13 inches long and about 1 inch wide that carries food from the mouth to the stomach. Normally, the esophagus is lined with cells that are similar to skin cells and look smooth and pinkish-white.

The stomach makes acid to help digest food. A different type of cell that is resistant to acid lines the stomach. These cells look red and velvety. At the place where the esophagus meets the stomach, there is a ring of muscle called a sphincter that normally keeps acid stomach juices from backflowing into the esophagus. When this sphincter is not working correctly, stomach acid enters the bottom portion of the esophagus. This backflow is called reflux or heartburn. When reflux occurs frequently over an extended period of time, it is called gastroesophageal reflux disease (GERD).

Barrett's esophagus is pre-cancerous condition in which normal cells lining the esophagus are repeatedly exposed to stomach acid and are replaced with abnormal cells that, in some people, develop into a type of cancer of the esophagus called **adenocarcinoma**. Histamine 2 blockers are given to reduce acid in the stomach and eliminate exposure of the esophagus cells to acid.

Histamine 2 blockers are also used to treat two rare cancerous conditions: multiple endocrine neoplasia (MEN) and Zollinger-Ellison syndrome, both of which can cause the stomach to produce too much acid. In MEN, an inherited form of cancer, tumors form in more than one gland. Depending on which glands are affected, the stomach may be stimulated to produce excess acid. In Zollinger-Ellison syndrome, a tumor in the digestive tract secretes a hormone called gastrin that stimulates the production of stomach acid. These tumors are malignant (cancerous) in 50% to 65% of people with Zollinger-Ellison syndrome.

Histamine 2 blockers are sometimes given in advance of **chemotherapy** to help reduce the gastrointestinal side effects of chemotherapy drugs. Cimetidine was the first histamine 2 blocker approved by the United States Food and Drug Administration (FDA) in 1976.

KEY TERMS

Esophagus—The canal between the pharynx and stomach that allows passage of food and liquids.

Gastrointestinal—Pertaining to the stomach and intestine.

Recommended dosage

Recommended dose varies depending on how much stomach acid is produced. Histamine 2 blockers are available in low doses without a prescription and in higher doses with a prescription. They are available in tablet, chewable tablet, liquid, and injectable liquid form. If histamine 2 inhibitors are unsuccessful in controlling acid reflux, proton pump inhibitors (Prevacid, Prilosec) are usually given as an alternative.

Precautions

People who have trouble with heartburn should stay away from acidic foods such as orange, grapefruit, and tomato juice, coffee, and carbonated drinks (sodas) because these all increase stomach acid. Although animal studies show that histamine 2 blockers appear to be safe during pregnancy, these drugs do pass into breast milk and should not be taken by nursing mothers.

Side effects

Histamine 2 blockers have few side effects. These drugs are excreted by the kidney, and may slow the excretion of other drugs excreted by the kidney. People with reduced kidney function may need a reduced dose of histamine 2 blockers.

Rare cases of irregular heart rhythms and high blood pressure have been reported when histamine 2 blockers are given intravenously (IV, injected directly into a vein). Mild **diarrhea** has been reported by some people taking these drugs.

Interactions

Histamine 2 blockers are reported to have few interactions with other drugs. However, because they reduce the level of acid in the stomach, they may inhibit the uptake of drugs such as ketoconazole that depend on an acid environment in the stomach to work. These drugs should be administered at least two hours before histamine 2 blockers are taken. Prior to starting any over-the-counter medications, herbal medications, or new medications, patients should notify their physician and check with their pharmacists for any potential drug interactions.

Tish Davidson, A.M.

Histiocytosis X

Definition

Histiocytosis X is a generic term that refers to an increase in the number of histiocytes, a type of white blood cell, that act as scavengers to remove foreign material from the blood and tissues. Since recent research demonstrated Langerhans cell involvement as well as histiocytes, this led to a proposal that the term Langerhans Cell Histiocytosis (LCH) be used in place of histiocytosis X. Either term refers to three separate illnesses (listed in order of increasing severity): eosinophilic granuloma, Hand-Schuller-Christian disease and Letterer-Siwe disease.

Description

Epidermal (skin) Langerhans cells (a form of dendritic cell) accumulate with other immune cells in various parts of the body and cause damage by the release of chemicals. Normally, Langerhans cells recognize foreign material, including bacteria, and stimulate the immune system to react to them. Langerhans cells are usually found in skin, lymph nodes, lungs, and the gastrointestinal tract. Under abnormal conditions these cells affect skin, bone, and the pituitary gland as well as the lungs, intestines, liver, spleen, bone marrow, and brain. Therefore, the disease is not confined to areas where Langerhans cells are normally found. The disease is more common in children than adults and tends to be most severe in very young children.

Histiocytosis X or LCH is a family of related conditions characterized by a distinct inflammatory and proliferative process but differs from each other in which parts of the body are involved. The least severe of the histiocytosis X/LCH family is eosinophilic granuloma. Approximately 60–80% of all diagnosed cases are in this classification, which usually occurs in children aged 5–10 years. The bones are involved 50–75% of the time, which includes the skull or mandible, and the long bones. If the bone marrow is involved, **anemia** can result. With skull involvement, growths can occur behind the eyes, bulging them forward. The lungs are involved less than 10% of the time, and this involvement signals the worst prognosis.

Next in severity is Hand-Schuller-Christian disease, a chronic, scattered form of histiocytosis. It occurs most

KEY TERMS

Anemia—Abnormally low level of red blood cells in the blood.

Biopsy—Surgical removal of tissue for examination.

CT or CAT—Computed tomography, a radiologic imaging that uses computer processing to generate an image of tissue density in slices through the patient's body.

Cytokines—The term used to include all protein messengers that regulate immune responses.

Dendritic—Branched like a tree.

Eosinophils—A leukocyte with coarse, round granules present.

Epidermal—The outermost layer of the skin.

Inflammatory—A localized protective response of the body caused by injury or destruction of tissues.

MRI—Magnetic resonance imaging, a noninvasive nuclear procedure for imaging tissues of high fat and water content that cannot be seen with other radiologic techniques.

Pituitary gland—The master gland located in the middle of the head that controls the endocrine glands and affects most bodily functions.

Prostaglandins—A group of nine naturally occurring chemicals in the body that affect smooth muscles.

Serous—Thin and watery, like serum.

commonly from the age of one to three years and is a slowly progressive disease that affects the softened areas of the skull, other flat bones, the eyes, and skin. Letterer-Siwe disease is the acute form of this series of diseases. It is generally found from the time of birth to one year of age. It causes an enlarged liver, bruising and skin lesions, anemia, enlarged lymph glands, other organ involvement, and extensive skull lesions.

Causes and symptoms

This is a rare disorder affecting approximately 1 in 200,000 children or adults each year. Because it is so rare, little research has been done to determine the cause. Over time, it may lessen in its assault on the body but there are still problems from damage to the tissues. There are no apparent inheritance patterns in these diseases with the exception of a form involving the lymphatic system.

The symptoms of histiocytosis are caused by substances called cytokines and prostaglandins, which are normally produced by histiocytes and act as messengers between cells. When these chemicals are produced in excess amounts and in the wrong places, they cause tissue swelling and abnormal growth. Thus, symptoms may include painful lumps in the skull and limbs as well as rashes on the skin. General symptoms may include: poor appetite, failure to gain weight, recurrent **fever**, and irritability. Symptoms from other possible sites of involvement include:

- Gums: swelling, usually without significant discomfort.
- Ear: chronic discharge.
- Liver or spleen: abdominal discomfort or swelling.
- Pituitary: This gland at the base of the brain is affected at some stage in approximately 20%–30% of children causing a disturbance in water balance to produce thirst and frequent urination.
- Eyes: Due to the bony disease, behind-the-eye bulging may occur (exophthalmos).
- Lungs: Breathing problems.

Diagnosis

The diagnosis can only be made by performing a **biopsy**, that is, taking a tissue sample under anesthesia from a site in the patient thought to be involved. Blood and urine tests, chest and other x rays, **magnetic resonance imaging** (MRI) and **computed tomography** scans (CAT scans) (to check the extent of involvement), and possibly bone marrow or breathing tests may be required to confirm the diagnosis.

Treatments and Prognosis

Although this disease is not cancer, most patients are treated in cancer clinics. There are two reasons for this:

- Historically, cancer specialists treated it before the cause was known.
- The treatment requires the use of drugs typically required to treat cancer.

Any cancer drugs utilized are usually given in smaller doses, which diminishes the severity of their side effects. **Radiation therapy** is rarely used, and special drugs may be prescribed for skin symptoms. If there is only one organ affected, steroids may be injected locally, or a drug called indomethacin may be used. Indomethacin is an anti-inflammatory medication that may achieve a similar response with less severe side effects.

The disease fluctuates markedly. If only one system is involved, the disease often resolves by itself. Multisystem disease usually needs treatment although it may disappear spontaneously. The disease is not normally fatal unless organs vital to life are damaged. In general, the younger the child at diagnosis and the more organs involved, the poorer the outlook. If the condition resolves, there could still be long-term complications because of the damage done while the disease was active.

Resources

BOOKS

Behrman, Richard E., Robert Kliegman, and Hal B. Jenson, eds. *Nelson Textbook of Pediatrics,* Philadelphia: W. B. Saunders, 2000.

PERIODICALS

Kobyahsi, M., O. Yamamoto, Y. Suenaga, and M. Asahi. "Electron Microscopic Study of Langerhans Cell Histiocytosis." *Journal of Dermatology* (July 27, 2000): 453–7.

Kusumakumary, P., F. V. James, V. G. Chellam, K. Ratheesan, and M. K. Nair. "Disseminated Langerhans Cell Histiocytosis in Children: Treatment Outcome." *American Journal of Clinical Oncology,* (April 2, 1999): 180–83.

ORGANIZATIONS

Histiocytosis Association of America, 302 North Broadway, Pitman, NJ 08071. 800–548–2758 (USA and Canada). <http://www.histio.org>.

OTHER

"Immunity Disorders." *Nurse Minerva.* 26 June 2001. <http://nurseminerva.co.uk/immunity.htm>.

Linda K. Bennington, C.N.S., M.S.N.

Hodgkin's disease

Definition

Hodgkin's disease is a rare **lymphoma**, a cancer of the lymphatic system.

Description

Hodgkin's disease, or Hodgkin's lymphoma, was first described in 1832 by Thomas Hodgkin, a British physician. Hodgkin clearly differentiated between this disease and the much more common **non-Hodgkin's lymphomas**. Prior to 1970, few individuals survived Hodgkin's disease. Now, however, the majority of individuals with this cancer can be cured.

The lymphatic system

The lymphatic system is part of the body's immune system, for fighting disease, and a part of the blood-producing system. It includes the lymph vessels and nodes, and the spleen, bone marrow, and thymus. The narrow lymphatic vessels carry lymphatic fluid from throughout the body. The lymph nodes are small organs that filter the lymphatic fluid and trap foreign substances, including viruses, bacteria, and cancer cells. The spleen, in the upper left abdomen, removes old cells and debris from the blood. The bone marrow, the tissue inside the bones, produces new red and white blood cells.

Lymphocytes are white blood cells that recognize and destroy disease-causing organisms. Lymphocytes are produced in the lymph nodes, spleen, and bone marrow. They circulate throughout the body in the blood and lymphatic fluid. Clusters of immune cells also exist in major organs.

Hodgkin's lymphoma

Hodgkin's disease is a type of lymphoma in which antibody-producing cells of the lymphatic system begin to grow abnormally. It usually begins in a lymph node and progresses slowly, in a fairly predictable way, spreading via the lymphatic vessels from one group of lymph nodes to the next. Sometimes it invades organs that are adjacent to the lymph nodes. If the cancer cells spread to the blood, the disease can reach almost any site in the body. Advanced cases of Hodgkin's disease may involve the spleen, liver, bone marrow, and lungs.

There are different subtypes of Hodgkin's disease:

- nodular sclerosis (30–60% of cases)
- mixed cellularity (20–40% of cases)
- lymphocyte predominant (5–10% of cases)
- lymphocyte depleted (less than 5% of cases)
- unclassified

Demographics

The American Cancer Society estimates that there will be 7,400 new cases of Hodgkin's disease in the United States in 2001—3,500 in females and 3,900 in males. It is estimated that 700 men and 600 women in the United States will die of the disease in 2001.

Hodgkin's disease can occur at any age. However, the majority of cases develop in early adulthood (ages 15–40) and late adulthood (after age 55). Approximately 10–15% of cases are in children under age 17. It is more common in boys than in girls under the age of 10. The disease is very rare in children under five.

Causes and symptoms

The cause of Hodgkin's disease is not known. It is suspected that some interaction between an individual's genetic makeup, environmental exposures, and infectious agents may be responsible. Immune system deficiencies also may be involved.

Early symptoms of Hodgkin's disease may be similar to those of the flu:

- fevers, **night sweats**, chills
- **fatigue**
- loss of appetite (**anorexia**)
- **weight loss**
- itching
- pain after drinking alcoholic beverages
- swelling of one or more lymph nodes

Sudden or emergency symptoms of Hodgkin's disease include:

- sudden high fever
- loss of bladder and/or bowel control
- numbness in the arms and legs and a loss of strength

As lymph nodes swell, they may push on other structures, causing a variety of symptoms:

- pain due to pressure on nerve roots
- loss of function in muscle groups served by compressed nerves
- coughing or shortness of breath due to compression of the windpipe and/or airways, by swollen lymph nodes in the chest
- kidney failure from compression of the ureters, the tubes that carry urine from the kidneys to the bladder
- swelling in the face, neck, or legs, due to pressure on veins
- paralysis in the legs due to pressure on the spinal cord

As Hodgkin's disease progresses, the immune system becomes less effective at fighting infection. Thus, patients with Hodgkin's lymphoma become more susceptible to both common infections caused by bacteria and unusual (opportunistic) infections. Later symptoms of Hodgkin's disease include the formation of tumors.

Significantly, as many as 75% of individuals with Hodgkin's disease do not have any typical symptoms.

Diagnosis

As with many forms of cancer, diagnosis of Hodgkin's disease has two major components.

- identification of Hodgkin's lymphoma as the cause of the patient's disease
- staging of the disease to determine how far the cancer has spread

The initial diagnosis of Hodgkin's disease often results from abnormalities in a chest **x ray** that was performed because of nonspecific symptoms. The physician then takes a medical history to check for the presence of symptoms and conducts a complete physical examination.

Lymph node biopsy

The size, tenderness, firmness, and location of swollen lymph nodes are determined and correlated with any signs of infection. In particular, lymph nodes that do not shrink after treatment with **antibiotics** may be a cause for concern. The lymph nodes that are most often affected by Hodgkin's disease include those of the neck, above the collarbone, under the arms, and in the chest above the diaphragm.

Diagnosis of Hodgkin's disease requires either the removal of an entire enlarged lymph node (an excisional **biopsy**) or an incisional biopsy, in which only a small part of a large tumor is removed. If the node is near the skin, the biopsy is performed with a local anesthetic. However, if it is inside the chest or abdomen, general anesthesia is required.

The sample of biopsied tissue is examined under a microscope. Giant cells called Reed-Sternberg cells must be present to confirm a diagnosis of Hodgkin's disease. These cells, which usually contain two or more nuclei, are named for the two pathologists who discovered them. Normal cells have only one nucleus (the organelle within the cell that contains the genetic material). Affected lymph nodes may contain only a few Reed-Sternberg cells and they may be difficult to recognize. Characteristics of other types of cells in the biopsied tissue help to diagnose the subtype of Hodgkin's disease.

A fine needle aspiration (FNA) biopsy, in which a thin needle and syringe are used to remove a small amount of fluid and bits of tissue from a tumor, has the advantage of not requiring surgery. An FNA may be performed prior to an excisional or incisional biopsy, to check for infection or for the spread of cancer from another organ. However an FNA biopsy does not provide enough tissue to diagnose Hodgkin's disease.

Occasionally, additional biopsies are required to diagnose Hodgkin's disease. In rare instances, other tests, that detect certain substances on the surfaces of cancer cells or changes in the DNA of cells, are used to distinguish Hodgkin's disease from non-Hodgkin's lymphoma.

Clinical staging

Staging is very important in Hodgkin's disease. This is because the cancer usually spreads in a predictable pattern, without skipping sets of lymph nodes until late in the progression of the disease.

IMAGING. Imaging of the abdomen, chest, and pelvis is used to identify areas of enlarged lymph nodes and abnormalities in the spleen or other organs. **Computed tomography** (CT or CAT) scans use a rotating x ray beam to obtain pictures. **Magnetic resonance imaging** (MRI) uses magnetic fields and radio waves to produce images of the body. Chest x rays also may be taken. These images will reveal rounded lumps called nodules in the affected lymph nodes and other organs.

Another imaging technique for Hodgkin's disease is a **gallium scan**, in which the radioactive element gallium is injected into a vein. The cancer cells take up the gallium and a special camera that detects the gallium is used to determine the location and size of tumors. Gallium scans are used when Hodgkin's disease is in the chest and may be hard to detect by other methods. Gallium scans also are used to monitor progress during treatment.

A lymphangiogram, a radiograph of the lymphatic vessels, involves injecting a dye into a lymphatic vessel in the foot. Tracking of the dye locates the disease in the abdomen and pelvis. This method is used less frequently and is usually not used with children.

Positron emission tomography (PET) scans are an extremely accurate method for staging Hodgkin's disease. A very low dose of radioactive glucose, a sugar, is injected into the body. The glucose travels to metabolically active sites, including cancerous regions that require large amounts of glucose. The PET scan detects the radioactivity and produces images of the entire body that distinguish between cancerous and non-cancerous tissues.

BONE MARROW. **Anemia** (a low red-blood-cell count), fevers, or night sweats are indications that Hodgkin's disease may be in the bone marrow. In these cases, a **bone marrow aspiration and biopsy** may be ordered. In biopsy, a large needle is used to remove a narrow, cylindrical piece of bone. Alternatively, an aspiration, in which a needle is used to remove small bits of bone marrow, may be used. The marrow usually is removed from the back of the hip or other large bone. This procedure may help to determine cancer spread.

Pathological staging

Sometimes further staging, called pathological staging or a staging laparotomy, is used for Hodgkin's disease. In this operation, a surgeon checks the abdominal lymph nodes and other organs for cancer and removes small pieces of tissue. A pathologist examines the tissue samples for Hodgkin's disease cells. Usually the spleen is removed (a **splenectomy**) during the laparotomy. The splenectomy helps with staging Hodgkin's disease, as well as removing a disease site.

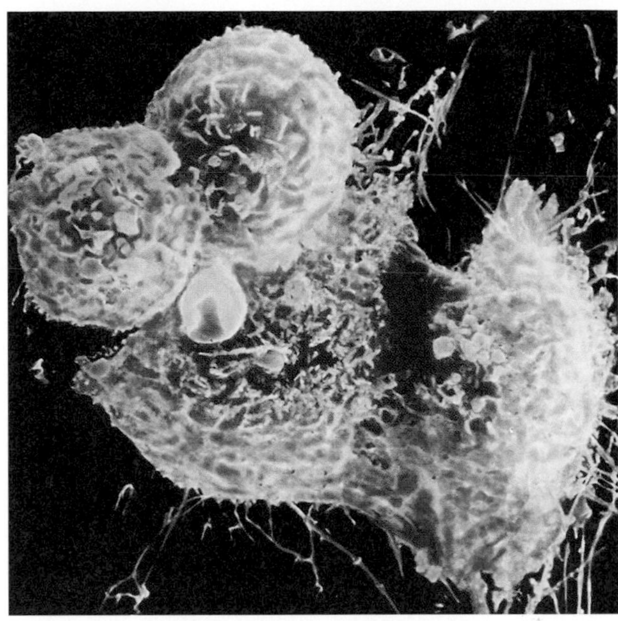

A scanning electron micrograph (SEM) image of dividing Hodgkin's cells from the pleural effusions (abnormal accumulations of fluid in the lungs) of a 55-year-old male patient. *(Photograph by Dr. Andrejs Liepins, National Audubon Society Collection/Photo Researchers, Inc. Reproduced by permission.)*

Treatment team

The cancer care team for Hodgkin's disease includes a medical oncologist (a physician specializing in cancer), oncology nurses, technicians, and social workers. A surgeon performs the biopsies, as well as the laparotomy and splenectomy if required. Pathologists examine the biopsy specimens for the presence of Reed-Sternberg and other abnormal cells.

In the United States, most children with Hodgkin's disease are treated at children's cancer centers. Here, the treatment team includes psychologists, child life specialists, nutritionists, and educators, as well as a pediatric oncologist.

Clinical staging, treatments, and prognosis

The stages

All of the available treatments for Hodgkin's disease have serious side effects, both short and long-term. However, with accurate staging, physicians and patients often can choose the minimum treatment that will cure the disease. The staging system for Hodgkin's disease is the Ann Arbor Staging Classification, also called the Cotswold System or the Revised Ann Arbor System.

Hodgkin's disease is divided into four stages, with additional substages:

- Stage I: The disease is confined to one lymph node area
- Stage IE: The disease extends from the one lymph node area to adjacent regions
- Stage II: The disease is in two or more lymph node areas on one side of the diaphragm (the muscle below the lungs)
- Stage IIE: The disease extends to adjacent regions of at least one of these nodes
- Stage III: The disease is in lymph node areas on both sides of the diaphragm
- Stage IIIE/IIISE: The disease extends into adjacent areas or organs (IIIE) and/or the spleen (IIISE)
- Stage IV: The disease has spread from the lymphatic system to one or more other organs, such as the bone marrow or liver

Treatment for Hodgkin's disease depends both on the stage of the disease and whether or not symptoms are present. Stages are labeled with an A if no symptoms are present. If symptoms are present, the stage is labeled with a B. These symptoms include:

- loss of more than 10% of body weight over the previous six months
- fevers above 100 degrees F
- drenching night sweats

Treatments

RADIATION THERAPY. **Radiation therapy** and/or **chemotherapy** (drug therapy) are the standard treatments for Hodgkin's disease. If the disease is confined to one area of the body, radiotherapy is usually used. This treatment, with x rays or other high-energy rays, also is used when the disease is in bulky areas such as the chest, where chemotherapeutic drugs cannot reach all of the cancer. External-beam radiation, a focused beam from an external machine, is used to irradiate only the affected lymph nodes. This procedure is called involved field radiation.

More advanced stages of Hodgkin's disease may be treated with mantle field radiation, in which the lymph nodes of the neck, chest, and underarms are irradiated. Inverted Y field radiation is used to irradiate the spleen and the lymph nodes in the upper abdomen and pelvis. Total nodal irradiation includes both mantle field and inverted Y field radiation.

Since external-beam radiation damages healthy tissue near the cancer cells, the temporary side effects of radiotherapy can include sunburn-like skin damage, fatigue, nausea, and **diarrhea**. Other temporary side effects may include a sore throat and difficulty swallowing. Long-term side effects depend on the dose and the location of the radiation and the age of the patient. Since radiation of the ovaries causes permanent sterility (the inability to have offspring), the ovaries of girls and young women are protected during radiotherapy. Sometimes the ovaries are surgically moved from the region to be irradiated.

CHEMOTHERAPY. If the Hodgkin's disease has progressed to additional lymph nodes or other organs, or if there is a recurrence of the disease within two years of radiation treatment, chemotherapy is used.

Chemotherapy utilizes a combination of drugs, each of which kills cancer cells in a different way. The most common chemotherapy regimens for Hodgkin's disease are MOPP (either **mechlorethamine** or **methotrexate** with Oncovin, **procarbazine**, prednisone) and ABVD (Adriamycin or **doxorubicin**, **bleomycin**, **vincristine**, **dacarbazine**). Each of these consists of four different drugs. ABVD is used more frequently than MOPP because it has fewer severe side effects. However MOPP is used for individuals who are at risk for heart failure. The chemotherapeutic drugs may be injected into a vein or muscle, or taken orally, as a pill or liquid.

Children who are sexually mature when they develop Hodgkin's disease, and whose muscle and bone mass are almost completely developed, usually receive the same treatment as adults. Younger children usually are treated with chemotherapy, since radiation will adversely affect bone and muscle growth. However, radiation may be used in low dosages, in combination with chemotherapy. The chemotherapy for children with Hodgkin's disease usually includes more drugs than ABVD and MOPP.

The side effects of chemotherapy for Hodgkin's disease depend on the dose of drugs and the length of time they are taken. Since these drugs target rapidly dividing cancer cells, they also affect normal cells that grow rapidly. These include the cells of the bone marrow, the linings of the mouth and intestines, and hair follicles. Damage to bone marrow leads to lower white blood cell counts and lower resistance to infection. It also leads to lower red blood cell counts can result in fatigue and easy bleeding and bruising. Damage to intestinal cells leads to a loss of appetite (**anorexia**), nausea, and vomiting. Mouth sores and hair loss (**alopecia**)also are common side effects of chemotherapy. These side effects disappear when the chemotherapy is discontinued. Some drugs can reduce or prevent the **nausea and vomiting**.

Chemotherapy for Hodgkin's disease may lead to long-term complications. The drugs may damage the heart, lungs, kidneys, and liver. In children, growth may be impeded. Some chemotherapy can cause sterility, so men may choose to have their sperm frozen prior to treatment. Women may stop ovulating and menstruating during chemotherapy. This may or may not be permanent.

Treatment for higher-stage Hodgkin's disease often involves a combination of radiotherapy and chemotherapy. Following three or four chemotherapy regimens, involved field radiation may be directed at the most affected areas of the body. The long-term side effects often are more severe when radiation and chemotherapy are used in combination.

The development of a second type of cancer is the most serious risk from radiation and chemotherapy treatment for Hodgkin's disease. In particular, there is a risk of developing leukemia, **breast cancer**, bone cancer, or **thyroid cancer**. Chemotherapy, particularly MOPP, or chemotherapy in conjunction with radiotherapy, significantly increases the risk for leukemia.

RESISTANT, PROGRESSIVE, AND RECURRENT HODGKIN'S DISEASE. Following treatment, the original diagnostic tests for Hodgkin's disease are repeated, to determine whether all traces of the cancer have been eliminated and to check for long-term side effects of treatment. In resistant Hodgkin's disease, some cancer cells remain following treatment. If the cancer continues to spread during treatment, it is called progressive Hodgkin's disease. If the disease returns after treatment, it is known as recurrent Hodgkin's disease. It may recur in the area where it first started or elsewhere in the body. It may recur immediately after treatment or many years later.

Additional treatment is necessary with these types of Hodgkin's disease. If the initial treatment was radiation therapy alone, chemotherapy may be used, or vice versa. Chemotherapy with different drugs, or higher doses, may be used to treat recurrent Hodgkin's. However, radiation to the same area is never repeated.

BONE MARROW AND PERIPHERAL BLOOD STEM CELL TRANSPLANTATIONS. An autologous bone marrow and/or a peripheral blood stem cell transplantation (PBSCT) often is recommended for treating resistant or recurrent Hodgkin's disease, particularly if the disease recurs within a few months of a chemotherapy-induced remission. These transplants are autologous because they utilize the individual's own cells. The patient's bone marrow cells or peripheral blood stem cells (immature bone marrow cells found in the blood) are collected and frozen prior to high-dosage chemotherapy, which destroys bone marrow cells. A procedure called leukapheresis is used to collect the stem cells. Following the high-dosage chemotherapy, and possibly radiation, the bone marrow cells or stem cells are reinjected into the individual.

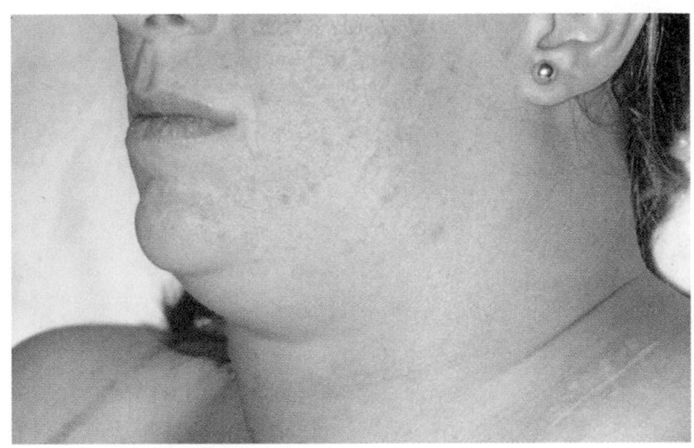

Swollen lymph nodes of a Hodgkin's disease patient. *(Custom Medical Stock Photo. Reproduced by permission.)*

Alternative and complementary therapies

Most complementary therapies for Hodgkin's disease are designed to stimulate the immune system to destroy cancer cells and repair normal cells that have been damaged by treatment. These therapies are used in conjunction with standard treatment.

Immunologic therapies, also known as immunotherapies, biological therapies, or biological response modifier therapies, utilize substances that are produced by the immune system. These include interferon (an immune system protein), **monoclonal antibodies** (specially engineered antibodies), colony-stimulating (growth) factors (such as **filgrastim**), and **vaccines**. Many immunotherapies for Hodgkin's disease are experimental and available only through **clinical trials**. These biological agents may have side effects.

Coenzyme Q10 (CoQ10) and polysaccharide K (PSK) are being evaluated for their ability to stimulate the immune system and protect healthy tissue, as well as possible anti-cancer activities. Camphor, also known as 714-X, green tea, and hoxsey (which is a mixture of a number of substances), have been promoted as immune system enhancers. However there is no evidence that they are effective against Hodgkin's disease. Hoxsey, in particular, can produce serious side effects.

Prognosis

Hodgkin's disease, particularly in children, is one of the most curable forms of cancer. Approximately 90% of individuals are cured of the disease with chemotherapy and/or radiation.

KEY TERMS

Antibody—An immune system protein that recognizes a specific foreign molecule.

Biopsy—The removal of a small sample of tissue for examination under a microscope; used for the diagnosis of cancer and to check for infection.

Bone marrow—Tissue inside the bones that produce red and white blood cells.

Chemotherapy—Treatment with various combinations of chemicals or drugs, particularly for the treatment of cancer.

Epstein-Barr virus (EBV)—Very common virus that infects immune cells and can cause mononucleosis.

Interferon—A potent immune-defense protein produced by viral-infected cells; used as an anti-cancer and anti-viral drug.

Interleukins—A family of potent immune-defense molecules; used in various medical therapies.

Laparotomy—A surgical incision of the abdomen.

Leukapheresis—A technique that uses a machine to remove stem cells from the blood; the cells are frozen and then returned to the patient following treatment that has destroyed the bone marrow.

Lymph nodes—Small round glands, located throughout the body and containing lymphocytes that remove foreign organisms and debris from the lymphatic fluid.

Lymphatic system—The vessels, lymph nodes, and organs, including the bone marrow, spleen, and thymus, that produce and carry white blood cells to fight disease.

Lymphocyte—White blood cells that produce antibodies and other agents for fighting disease.

PBSCT—Peripheral blood stem cell transplant; a method for replacing blood-forming cells that are destroyed by cancer treatment.

Radiotherapy—Disease treatment involving exposure to x rays or other types of radiation.

Reed-Sternberg cells—An abnormal lymphocyte that is characteristic of Hodgkin's disease.

Spleen—An organ of the lymphatic system, on the left side of the abdomen near the stomach; it produces and stores lymphocytes, filters the blood, and destroys old blood cells.

Splenectomy—Surgical removal of the spleen.

Staging—The use of various diagnostic methods to accurately determine the extent of disease; used to select the appropriate type and amount of treatment and to predict the outcome of treatment.

Stem cells—The cells from which all blood cells are derived.

Thymus—An organ of the lymphatic system, located behind the breast bone, that produces the T lymphocytes of the immune system.

Thyroid—A gland in the throat that produces hormones that regulate growth and metabolism.

The one-year relative survival rate following treatment for Hodgkin's disease is 93%. Relative survival rates do not include individuals who die of causes other than Hodgkin's disease. The percentage of individuals who have not died of Hodgkin's disease within five years of diagnosis is 90–95% for those with stage I or stage II disease. The figure is 85–90% for those diagnosed with stage III Hodgkin's and approximately 80% for those diagnosed with stage IV disease. The 15-year relative survival rate is 63%. Approximately 75% of children are alive and cancer free 20 years after the original diagnosis of Hodgkin's.

Acute myelocytic leukemia, a very serious cancer, may develop in as many as 2–6% of individuals receiving certain types of treatment for Hodgkin's disease. Women under the age of 30 who are treated with radiation to the chest have a much higher risk for developing breast cancer. Both men and women are at higher risk for developing lung or thyroid cancers as a result of chest irradiation.

Individuals with the type of Hodgkin's disease known as nodular lymphocytic predominance have a 2% chance of developing non-Hodgkin's lymphoma. Apparently, this is a result of the Hodgkin's disease itself and not the treatment.

Coping with cancer treatment

Sufficient rest and good nutrition are important for relieving the side effects of treatment for Hodgkin's disease. As strength returns, a weekly exercise routine should be initiated. Support groups can be beneficial for helping with emotional problems that may arise during treatment.

Clinical trials

As of 2001, at least 115 clinical trials for the treatment of Hodgkin's disease were recruiting or planning to recruit participants. A number of these studies are directed at treating resistant (refractory) or recurrent (relapsed) Hodgkin's disease in both children and adults. Some are aimed at specific stages or subtypes of Hodgkin's disease. Some trials are for previously treated individuals and others are for those who have not yet received treatment.

Clinical trials of new treatments for Hodgkin's disease include:

- new drugs
- new chemotherapies
- monoclonal antibody therapy
- interferon, interleukin-2, and interleukin-12
- a vaccine made from cancer cells that contain the **Epstein-Barr virus**
- bone marrow and umbilical cord blood transplantations
- PBSCT
- various combinations of treatments

There also are ongoing genetic studies of children and adults with Hodgkin's disease and quality-of-life studies of children who are undergoing treatment.

Prevention

There are very few known risk factors for Hodgkin's disease. A family history of the disease and the presence of the Epstein-Barr virus are associated with an increased risk. Individuals with acquired immunodeficiency syndrome (AIDS) are particularly susceptible to Hodgkin's disease.

Special concerns

Follow-up examinations continue for many years following treatment for Hodgkin's disease. Women who have had chest irradiation must have frequent mammograms and clinical and breast self examinations for early detection of breast cancer. Frequent physical exams and chest x rays may help to detect lung or thyroid cancer. Treatment with mantle field radiation causes hyperthyroidism, which requires thyroid medication and annual thyroid function tests.

Individuals with Hodgkin's disease do not have normal immune system function, a problem that can be intensified by chemotherapy, radiation, and removal of the spleen. Therefore, vaccinations and prompt treatment of infections are very important.

See Also Amenorrhea; Bone marrow transplantation; Childhood cancers; Fertility and cancer; Imaging studies; Immune response

QUESTIONS TO ASK THE DOCTOR

- What type of Hodgkin's disease do I have?
- What is the stage of my disease?
- What are the choices for treatment and what do you recommend?
- Should I obtain a second opinion?
- What are the short-term side effects of the treatment and what can be done about them?
- What are the possible long-term side effects of the treatment?
- Are there other risks from the treatment?
- How should I prepare for the treatment?
- How long will the treatment continue?
- What is the recovery time following the treatment?
- What are the chances of success?
- Are there clinical trials which may be appropriate for me?
- Are there complementary or alternative therapies that may be helpful?
- What is the likelihood that the cancer will return? How will a recurrence be diagnosed?
- Is a recurrence more likely with one treatment than with another?

Resources

BOOKS

Dollinger, Malin, et al. *Everyone's Guide to Cancer Therapy.* Kansas City: Andrews McKeel Publishing, 1997.

Freedman, Arnold S., and Lee M. Nadler. "Hodgkin's Disease." In *Harrison's Principles of Internal Medicine,* edited by Anthony S. Fauci, et al. New York: McGraw-Hill, 1998.

Mauch, Peter M., et al., eds. *Hodgkin's Disease.* Philadelphia: Lippincott Williams & Wilkins, 1999.

Murphy, Gerald P., et al. *Informed Decisions.* New York: Viking, 1997.

Sutcliffe, Simon B., ed. *Lymphoma and You: A Guide for Patients Living with Hodgkin's Disease and Non-Hodgkin's Lymphoma.* Toronto: The Medicine Group Ltd., 1998.

PERIODICALS

Bhatia, S., L. L. Robison, O. Oberlin, M. Greenberg, G. Bunin, F. Fossati-Bellani, and A. T. Meadows. "Breast Cancer and Other Second Neoplasms after Childhood Hodgkin's

Disease." *New England Journal of Medicine* 334, no. 12 (1996): 745-51.

Stoval, Ellen. "A Cancer Survivor Discusses Her Experiences." *Washington Post* 118 (February 14, 1995): WH15+.

ORGANIZATIONS

American Cancer Society. (800) ACS-2345. <http://www.cancer.org>. Provides information, funds for cancer research, prevention programs, and patient services, including education and support programs for patients and families, temporary accommodations for patients, and camps for children with cancer.

ClinicalTrials.gov. U. S. National Library of Medicine. National Institutes of Health. 8600 Rockville Pike, Bethesda, MD 20894. <http://clinicaltrials.gov/ct/gui/c/a1b/screen/BrowseAny/action/GetStudy?JServSessionIdcs_current=mgdpq4z7pm>. Information about clinical trials involving Hodgkin's disease.

Cure for Lymphoma Foundation. 215 Lexington Avenue, New York, NY 10016. (212) 213-9595. (800)-CFL-6848. infocfl@cfl.org. <http://www.cfl.org/home.html>. An advocacy organization that provides education and support programs, research grants, and information on clinical trials for Hodgkin's and non-Hodgkin's lymphomas.

The Leukemia and Lymphoma Society. 600 Third Avenue, New York, NY 10016. (800) 955-4572. (914) 949-5213. <http://www.leukemia-lymphoma.org> Provides information, support, and guidance to patients and health care professionals.

The Lymphoma Research Foundation of America, Inc. 8800 Venice Boulevard, Suite 207, Los Angeles, CA 90034. (310) 204-7040). <http://www.lymphoma.org>. Supports research into treatments for lymphoma and provides educational and emotional support programs for patients and families.

National Cancer Institute. Public Inquiries Office, Building 31, Room 10A31, 31 Center Drive, MSC 2580, Bethesda, MD 20892-2580. (800)-4-CANCER. <http://www.nci.nih.gov/>. <http://cancernet.nci.nih.gov>. Provides information on cancer and on clinical trials; conducts cancer research.

OTHER

FS-8 - Complementary and Alternative Therapies for Leukemia, Lymphoma, Hodgkin's Disease, and Myeloma. The Leukemia and Lymphoma Society. 27 Mar. 2001. <http://www.leukemia-lymphoma.org>.

"Hodgkin's Disease." *Cancer Resource Center.* 10 Dec. 1999. American Cancer Society. 27 Mar. 2001. <http://www3.cancer.org>.

"Hodgkin's Disease." *CancerNet.* 12 Dec. 2000. National Cancer Institute. NIH Publication No. 99-1555. 27 Mar. 2001. > http://cancernet.nci.nih.gov/wyntk_pubs/hodgkins.htm>.

"Hodgkin's Lymphoma." *Diseases & Conditions.* 13 Mar. 2001. MayoClinic.com. 27 Mar. 2001. <http://www.mayohealth.org>.

National Cancer Society. "NCI/PDQ Patient Statement: Adult Hodgkin's Disease." *Oncolink.* Nov. 2000. University of Pennsylvania Cancer Center. 27 Mar. 2001. <http://www.oncolink.upenn.edu/pdq_html/2/engl/200003.html>.

National Cancer Society. "NCI/PDQ Patient Statement: Childhood Hodgkin's Disease." *Oncolink.* Feb. 2001. University of Pennsylvania Cancer Center. 27 Mar. 2001 <http://www.oncolink.upenn.edu/pdq_html/2/engl/203043.html>.

"PET Scans Help Doctors Treat Hodgkin's Disease." *ACS News Today.* 13 Mar. 2001. American Cancer Society. 27 Mar. 2001 <http://www2.cancer.org>.

Rosalyn S. Carson-DeWitt, M.D.
Margaret Alic, Ph.D.

Home health services

Definition

Home health services refers to those health care services provided to the patient in his or her own home.

Description

Home health services can vary depending on the insurance coverage, but usually include nursing, physical therapy, occupational therapy, speech therapy, home health aides, social work, nutritional education, infusion therapy, blood drawing, and other laboratory services. Such services may also include bringing medical equipment into the home for patient use. Home health services do not provide around-the-clock care, but rely on the patient having other caregivers, such as family members, friends, or other community resources.

Home care services can be provided by many different organizations, such as the Visiting Nurses Association (VNA), home health agencies (which vary in the range of services provided), hospice organizations, providers of home medical equipment, and pharmacies with delivery services. Patients requiring a range of specialized services may find more continuity of care if one agency is able to provide all, or almost all, of the services they need. **Hospice care** is care provided to patients who are terminally ill. Most hospices care for their clients within the home. The goal of hospice is to help the client and their family deal with the physical, emotional, and spiritual issues associated with dying. Excellent pain management is a priority.

Nursing care

Skilled nursing care provides the backbone for home care. Visits may include wound and ostomy care; infusion therapy such as home **chemotherapy**, **antibiotics**, or home parenteral nutrition (HPN); patient and caregiver teaching; ongoing assessment of the client's physical and emotional condition and progress; pain control; psychological support; and supervision of home health aides. The nurse may function as a case manager and coordinate the various other services the client is receiving. The nurse assesses the home environment for safety and for appropriateness of continued home care.

Physical therapy

Physical therapists develop a plan for the client to restore (as much as possible) the physical condition lost following surgery or as a result of a decline due to the disease process. They also teach patients how to prevent further injury or deterioration and how to maintain gains made.

Occupational therapy

Occupational therapists assist patients in restoring or enhancing their ability to perform their tasks of daily living. Patients may need to learn how to use adaptive equipment such as a prosthesis. The goal is to achieve the highest level of functioning possible.

Speech therapy

Speech therapists work with clients who have difficulty swallowing or clearly communicating.

Home health aides

Home health aides function under the supervision of a registered nurse. They provide care with personal hygiene, such as bathing and dressing, feeding, and ambulating. They may assist a nurse in providing patient care. They may provide homemaking services and companionship, or those tasks may be covered by a homemaker or attendant.

Social work

Social workers may assist clients in accessing the services that are available to them based on their insurance, and in learning what community resources exist. They may also facilitate the referral process, and provide counseling and patient advocacy.

Nutritional education

Nutritionists and registered dieticians may educate clients on their nutritional needs, and on how to go about attaining them. They may also be involved if HPN is required.

Infusion therapy

Some patients may receive their chemotherapy or antibiotics at home, or may require infusion of liquid nutrition (HPN). While these services may be provided by a nurse, a separate agency or company may provide the equipment and products.

KEY TERMS

Home parenteral nutrition (HPN)—HPN provides liquid nutrition via infusion for patients who are malnourished, or who have had surgery altering the usual process of chewing, swallowing, or digesting food.

Meditation—Meditation is a technique in which the individual focuses on a word or phrase to the exclusion of other thoughts. It has been shown to lower blood pressure and reduce stress.

T'ai chi—An Asian practice of breathing and slow physical movements that develops strength and reduces stress.

Laboratory work

Blood drawing and other laboratory services may be provided by a nurse, a phlebotomist, or a laboratory technician.

Home medical equipment

Following surgery or treatment in a hospital, patients may need the delivery and servicing of items such as special beds, wheelchairs, walkers, catheters, and wound care and ostomy supplies.

Volunteers

Volunteers may provide a range of assistance such as respite care for the primary caregiver(s), caring for the home, cooking, cleaning, emotional support, companionship, running errands, making telephone calls, child care, elder care, and providing transportation. They may come from the patient's circle of friends or religious organization, or from agencies such as Meals on Wheels.

Causes

Many individuals with conditions that do not necessitate care in a hospital setting often require short-term or long-term home care. They may need care to assist them in regaining their health similar to that prior to their illness, or may need ongoing care as their condition deteriorates due to metastatic disease.

QUESTIONS TO ASK THE DOCTOR

- What kind of home care will I need?
- For how long will I need the different services?
- What happens if my condition worsens?
- Will my insurance cover the services you are prescribing?
- What kind of care is available to help my family care for me?
- Are there alternative therapies that would help my condition?
- Are any of these therapies covered by my insurance?
- Are there any side effects to these therapies?
- Who is in charge of making sure my pain is well controlled?

Special concerns

Insurance coverage plays a major role in funding home health care. In organizing home care the patient must fully understand which services will be fully covered, covered but with a co-payment, or not covered at all. Insurance coverage may vary depending on whether the service provider is within a specified approved network. It must also be clear how often and for how long the services will be needed, and whether the insurance benefits cover the entire time period of anticipated care. The patient's safety must always remain a priority. The patient and the caregiver(s) may suffer from isolation and **depression**. Primary caregivers may become overwhelmed with caring for the patient, and there may come a point at which the level of care needed may no longer be able to be provided in the home setting. The health of the primary caregiver must periodically be assessed.

Treatments

Treatments provided in the home include wound and ostomy care, intravenous (IV) chemotherapy or antibiotics, HPN, and physical, occupational, and speech therapy.

Alternative and complementary therapies

Clients may contract to have home acupuncture or massage therapy. On their own they may engage in yoga, t'ai chi, meditation, guided imagery, visualization, or other stress-reducing techniques that help them better cope with their situation. They may also choose to investigate herbal supplements and medications; all supplemental medications should be approved by a physician before use.

Resources

BOOKS

Dollinger, Malin, Ernest H. Rosenbaum, and Greg Cable. *Everyone's Guide to Cancer Therapy, Revised Third Edition.* Kansas City, MO: Somerville House Books Limited, 1997.

Levin, Bernard. *American Cancer Society: Colorectal Cancer.* New York: Villard Books, 1999.

Runowicz, Carolyn D., Jeanne A. Petrek, and Ted S. Gansler. *American Cancer Society: Women and Cancer.* New York: Villard Books/Random House, 1999.

Teeley, Peter and Philip Bashe. *The Complete Cancer Survival Guide.* New York: Doubleday, 2000.

ORGANIZATIONS

The American Cancer Society. 800–ACS–2345. <http://www.cancer.org>.

National Association for Home Care. 228 7th Street, S.E. Washington, D.C. 20003. 202–547–7424. <http://www.nahc.org>.

National Cancer Institute. Building 31, Room 10A31, 31 Center Drive, MSC 2580, Bethesda, MD 20892–2580. 301–435–3848. <http://www.nci.nih.gov>.

National Center for Complementary and Alternative Medicine. NCCAM Clearinghouse, P.O. Box 8218, Silver Spring, MD 20907–8218. 888–644–6226. <http://nccam.nih.gov>.

Visiting Nurse Association of America. 11 Beacon Street, Suite 910; Boston, MA 02108. 617–523–4042. Fax: 617–227–4843. <http://www.vnaa.org>.

Esther Csapo Rastegari, R.N., B.S.N., Ed.M.

Horner's syndrome

Description

William Edmonds Horner (1793-1853) first described a small muscle at the angle of the eyelid (tensor tarsi) as well as a description of an ingenious operation to correct problems with the lower lid in 1824 in the American Journal of the Medical Sciences. Since that time, his name has been associated with the syndrome of a small, regular pupil, drooping of the eyelid on the same side and occasional loss of sweat formation on the forehead of the affected eye. In appearance, it occurs on one side of the face with a sinking in of the eyeball (enophthalmos), drooping upper eyelid (ptosis), slight elevation of the lower lid, excessive contraction of the pupil of the eye (miosis), narrowing of the eyelid, and an absence of facial sweat on the affected side (anhidrosis). Other symptoms may include a variation in eye color of the iris and changes in the consistency of tears.

Causes

Horner's syndrome is caused by damage or interruption of the sympathetic nerve to the eye. There are two major divisions of the nervous system: the voluntary (conscious control) and involuntary (without conscious control). The involuntary (autonomic nervous system) itself has two divisions: sympathetic and parasympathetic nervous systems. Under normal conditions, there is a fine balance between sympathetic and parasympathetic stimulation. If an individual is threatened by a situation, the pupils dilate, blood is shifted to the muscles and the heart beats faster as the person prepare to fight or flee. This is sympathetic stimulation. The eye has both sympathetic (responds to challenges) and parasympathetic (slows the body down) innervation. The nerve that carries the sympathetic innervation travels down the spinal cord from the brain (hypothalamus), emerges in the chest cavity, and then finds it way up the neck along with the carotid artery and jugular vein through the middle ear and into the eye. If these sympathetic impulses were blocked, the eye would have an overbalance of parasympathetic supply, which would result in a constriction of the pupil, relaxation of all the muscles around the eye and a sinking of the eye into the orbit—Horner's syndrome. Thus, damage that occurs anywhere along the course of this nerve's route from the brain to the eye can evoke this syndrome.

If the syndrome exists from birth (congenital), it is typically noted around the age of two years with the presence of a variation in the color of the iris and the lack of a crease in the drooping eye. Since eye color is completed by the age of two, a variation in color is an uncommon finding in Horner's syndrome acquired later in life.

The common causes of acquired Horner's syndrome include aortic dissection (a tear in the wall of the aorta to create a false channel where blood becomes trapped), carotid dissection, tuberculosis, Pancoast tumor (a tumor in the upper end of the lung), brain tumors, spinal cord injury in the neck, trauma to the cervical or thoracic portions of the spinal cord, cluster migraine headache, vertebrae destruction or collapse, compression of the spinal cord by enlarged lymph nodes, and neck or thyroid surgery.

The diagnosis and localization of this disorder is made with the use of pharmacological testing by an ophthalmologist. Topically placing drops of a 10% liquid cocaine into the eyes blocks the parasympathetic nerves so the sympathetic nervous system can be evaluated. After thirty minutes, the dilation of the pupils is noted and a Horner's pupil dilates poorly. A positive cocaine test does not, however, localize the area of the damage. After waiting for 48 hours, other medications are used to determine where the nerve interruption occurs. An individual's urine can test positive for cocaine up to two days following the initial test.

KEY TERMS

Congenital—Present at and existing from the time of birth.

Hypothalamus—That part of the third ventricle in the brain which anatomically contains the optic nerves.

Neuroblastoma—A tumor of nervous system origin composed chiefly of neruoblasts (embryonic nerve cells), affecting mostly infants and children up to 10 years of age, usually arising in the autonomic nervous system.

Pancoast tumor—A tumor or growth in the pointed end of the lung.

Treatments

Treatment for congenital cases

Children who are diagnosed with Horner's syndrome of a congenital origin may undergo surgical correction to strengthen the muscle of the eyelid and give it an appearance similar to the unaffected eye. The surgery improves the appearance of the child but does not alleviate the syndrome. For these cases a plastic surgeon may be preferred. Occasionally Horner's syndrome may be seen in a newborn with a **neuroblastoma** (tumor originating from nerve cells). This is almost always a sign of a localized tumor and is associated a relatively good prognosis. In these cases, a neurologist may be consulted for treatment since their specialty is the nervous system.

Treatment for acquired cases

The treatment for acquired Horner's syndrome depends upon the cause and is focused toward eliminating the disease that produces the syndrome. Frequently, there is no treatment that improves or reverses the condition, but recognition of the signs and symptoms is extremely important for early diagnosis and treatment. Early detection of the syndrome may facilitate treatment related to those caused by tumors as they can be removed before extensive damage is done. Causes related to an interruption in nerve transmission once the nerve leaves the spinal cord are usually related to blood circulation and are easier to treat. Any numbness or paralysis on one side of the body means the problem is within the spinal cord or brain and is more difficult to treat. Some acquired Horner's may be corrected slightly by plastic surgery for appearance changes.

Alternative and complementary therapies

Acupuncture may be utilized to enhance disruptions in nerve transmissions and herbs or supplements that improve circulation may benefit some cases of acquired syndrome. These herbs and supplements would include Gingko biloba and vitamin E. As with any complementary treatment, patients should notify their physician of any herbal or over-the-counter medications they are taking.

Resources

BOOKS

Jarvis, Carolyn.*Physical Examination and Health Assessment* Philadelphia: W.B. Saunders Company, 2000.

Hoffman, Matthew, ed.*The Doctors Book of Food Remedies* USA: St. Martin's Press, 1998.

OTHER

Handbook of Ocular Disease Management 6 July 2001 <http://www.revoptom.com>

Linda K. Bennington, C.N.S., M.S.N.

Hospice care

Definition

Hospice care is palliative care given to individuals who are terminally ill, with an expected survival of six months or less. The focus of hospice care is on meeting the physical, emotional, and spiritual needs of the dying individual, while fostering the highest quality of life possible.

Description

Hospice services provide palliative care to individuals with a life expectancy of six months or less. Most hospice care is provided in the home, but may take place in a hospice home or a hospice/palliative care area within a medical facility. Requesting hospice care may be the first time that individuals, or their families, acknowledge that their condition is not treatable. It may be the first time that they have to deal with their death as a reality taking place within a few months. The emotional journey to be able to deal with these issues may take a while, and therefore may delay the time when the person begins to receive hospice care.

The focus of hospice is not on treatment, but on pain and symptom management, comfort measures, acknowledging that the individual will die, supporting the family, and trying to provide the best quality of life for the time remaining. Hospice functions under the philosophy that although some terminally ill patients may no longer receive treatment, they still require and deserve care.

Hospice care is interdisciplinary in nature, providing the services of physicians, nurses, social workers, physical, speech, or occupational therapists, clergy or other spiritual guides, health care aides, and volunteers. Home hospice care relies on the family and friends of the patient to provide most of the daily care. Nursing and other services are provided daily or weekly, but with 24 hours, 7 days a week on-call access. Addressing the spiritual needs of the hospice client is a fundamental aspect of hospice care.

Some studies about hospice care have gleaned the following:

- When asked their preference, about two-thirds of cancer patients said they preferred to die in their own home.
- The majority of patients still die in the hospital.
- When surveyed, about 95% of families who received hospice care said that it had been helpful.
- Although satisfied with hospice care, caregivers report the job of caregiving as having a negative impact on their own quality of life, and felt the job was burdensome.
- When compared to a control group of noncaregivers, caregivers had higher levels of **depression**, anxiety, anger, and health problems. Caregivers had a higher rate of deteriorating health, social, and occupational functioning.
- Quality of life was influenced by the individual's spiritual well-being.
- Hospice patients expressed feelings of conflict between a hope for living, and "living in hope," being able to reconcile with others and coming to terms with death.
- Although hospice is focused on helping people in the last six months of their life, most hospice patients only receive about one month of hospice care prior to their death.
- Only 20% of physicians' prognoses about a patient's survival was accurate. Sixty-three percent were overly optimistic, and 17% were overly pessimistic. The more experience the physicians had, the better their accuracy of prognosis.

Causes

Hospice care was first established in the United States in 1974 in Connecticut. In 1969, the book "On Death and Dying", by Dr. Elizabeth Kugler-Ross identified five stages that a terminally ill person goes through. In the book, Dr. Kubler-Ross addressed the importance of patients having a role in the decisions affecting the quality of their life and death. In 1972 she testified at the first U.S. Senate national hearing on dying with dignity.

Deciding on hospice care is a choice made by the terminally ill individual. To be eligible, one's physician needs to document that the individual's survival is expected to be six months or less. Should the patient recover, and the prognosis change, the relationship with hospice is terminated, but can be reestablished when needed at a later date. Not all patients will choose hospice. If only home hospice care is available, individuals who would be eligible may decide that hospice is not a good choice for them. Reasons for not choosing home hospice include:

- The patient lives alone, with little or no family support available.
- The patient has a need for 24-hour nursing care.
- The patient has family, but they are unable to provide the supportive care required.
- The patient is concerned about being a burden to the caregiver.
- The patient feels more secure in a hospital environment.

Special concerns

A study looking at the communication between physicians and their dying patients found these issues to be very important:

- Being honest and straightforward with patients.
- A willingness to talk about dying.
- Being sensitive when conveying bad news.
- Listening to patients.
- Encouraging patients to ask questions.
- Finding a balance between being honest without discouraging hope.

A November 15, 2000 *Journal of the American Medical Association* article found that patients at the end of their life expressed these issues as important:

- being mentally aware
- not being a burden
- having their funeral arrangements planned
- helping others
- coming to peace with God
- freedom from pain
- talking about the meaning of death
- Among nine issues, dying at home was rated the least important.

Because time is limited for patients in hospice, patients and their caregivers need to act swiftly on areas of dissatisfaction, such as quality of care being provided or insufficient symptom management.

KEY TERMS

Meditation—Meditation is a technique in which the individual focuses on a word or phrase to the exclusion of other thoughts. It has been shown to reduce stress and anxiety.

Palliative care—Care focused on providing comfort, not cure.

T'ai chi—An Asian practice of breathing and slow physical movements that develops strength and reduces stress.

Treatments

Curative treatments are not a part of hospice care. However, hospice places great importance on minimizing or alleviating pain and symptoms such as appetite loss (**anorexia**), **fatigue**, weakness, constipation, difficulty breathing, confusion, **nausea and vomiting**, cough, and dry or sore mouth. For many with advanced cancer, fatigue may be their worst symptom. Research has shown that a tailored exercise program can increase activity tolerance without increasing fatigue. In addition, patients reported an increase in quality of life and decreased anxiety. Patients who expressed the most fatigue showed the most decrease in fatigue with the exercise program. Many hospice patients have breakthrough pain in addition to their chronic pain. Research using a subcutaneous needle for pain control showed 88% pain control with this method when pain was not well controlled with oral medications. Chronic pain requires ongoing pain relief, such as might be handled with a pump or patch. Good pain control may mean waking the patient up at night for oral medication to prevent the pain from mounting during sleep.

Alternative and complementary therapies

Dealing with the issues of death may be addressed through talking with others, writing in a journal, creative

QUESTIONS TO ASK THE DOCTOR

- What do you think is my prognosis?
- What choices are there to manage my pain and other symptoms?
- What level of symptom management can I expect to receive?
- What types of care, conventional or alternative, would improve the quality of the time I have left?
- Will my insurance cover the care you suggest?
- If I choose hospice care, how will that affect my relationship with my doctors and treatment team?
- What kind of support is there for my family, both until I die and afterwards?

expression such as painting, writing a poem, or composing music. Meditation may be beneficial to some patients. Gentle body movements such as with t'ai chi or yoga may be helpful, depending on the patient's activity tolerance.

Resources

BOOKS

Dollinger, Malin, Ernest H. Rosenbaum, and Greg Cable. *Everyone's Guide to Cancer Therapy, Revised Third Edition.* Kansas City, MO: Somerville House Books Limited, 1997.

Teeley, Peter and Philip Bashe. *The Complete Cancer Survival Guide.* New York: Doubleday, 2000.

PERIODICALS

Steinhauser, K. E. et al. "Factors Considered Important at the End of Life by Patients, Family, Physicians, and Other Care Providers." *Journal of the American Medical Association.* (Nov 15, 2000):2476–482.

ORGANIZATIONS

American Cancer Society. 800–ACS–2345. <http://www.cancer.org>.

American Pain Society. 4700 W. Lake Ave., Glenview, IL 60025. 847–375–4715. <http://ampainsoc.org>.

Hospice Association of America. 228 Seventh Street, SE; Washington, DC 20003. 202–546–4759. Fax: 202–547–9559. <www.hospice-america.org>.

National Association for Home Care. 228 7th Street, S.E. Washington, D.C. 20003. 202–547–7424. <http://www.nahc.org>.

National Cancer Institute. Building 31, Room 10A31, 31 Center Drive, MSC 2580, Bethesda, MD 20892–2580. 301–435–3848. <http://www.nci.nih.gov>.

National Center for Complementary and Alternative Medicine. NCCAM Clearinghouse, P.O. Box 8218, Silver Spring, MD 20907–8218. 888–644–6226. <http://nccam.nih.gov>.

OTHER

Cancer Resources. 457 West 22nd Street, Suite B, New York, NY 10011. 800–401–2233. Fax: 212–243–1063. e-mail: info@cancerresources.com. <http://www.cancerresouces. com>.

Esther Csapo Rastegari, R.N., B.S.N., Ed.M.

HPV *see* **Human papilloma virus**

Human growth factors

Definition

Human growth factors are compounds made by the body that function to regulate cell division and cell survival. Some growth factors are also produced in the laboratory by genetic engineering and are used in biological therapy.

Description

Human tumors express large amounts of growth factors and their receptors. A tumor will not grow beyond the size of a pinhead without new blood vessels to supply oxygen and nutrients. Growth factors are significant because they can induce angiogenesis, the formation of blood vessels around a tumor. These growth factors also encourage cell proliferation, differentiation, and migration on the surfaces of the endothelial cells—cells found inside the lining of blood vessels. Of the approximately 20 proteins that activate endothelial cell growth, two growth factors in particular, vascular endothelial growth factor (VEGF) and basic fibroblast growth factor (bFGF), are expressed by many tumors and appear important in contributing to tumor growth and promoting tumor spread throughout the body. Several compounds that block VEGF or its receptor are now in **clinical trials**.

See also Angiogenesis inhibitors

Crystal Heather Kaczkowski, MSc.

Human papilloma virus

Definition

Human papilloma viruses (HPV) are a large group or related viruses, some of which play a part in the devel-

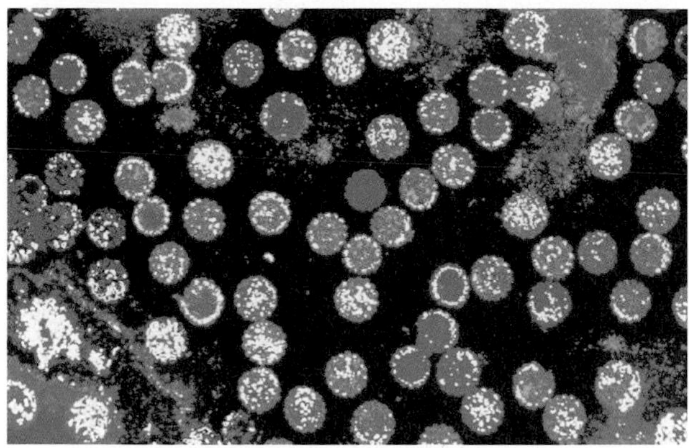

Transmission electron micrograph of human papilloma virus, magnified 40,000 times. HPV is the cause of warts, including genital warts, and has been implicated in cervical cancer. *(Custom Medical Stock Photo. Reproduced by permission.)*

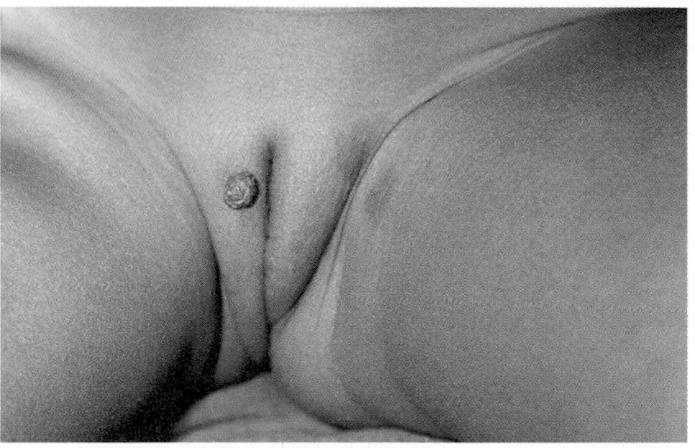

Large brown genital wart of a female. *(Custom Medical Stock Photo. Reproduced by permission.)*

opment of cervical epithelial cancers. HPV is also associated with skin cancer, oral and anal cancers.

Description

The family of human papilloma viruses includes a large number of genetically related viruses. Many of these cause warts, including the warts commonly found on the skin. Another group of HPV preferentially infect the mucosal surfaces of the genitals, including the penis, vagina, vulva, and cervix. These are spread sexually in adults. One group of HPV that infect the genitals causes soft warts, often designated condyloma acuminata. These genital warts are quite common and rarely, if ever, become cancerous. The most common of these low-risk HPV types are designated HPV 6 and 11. The second group of viruses, termed high-risk HPV types, is associated with the development of **cervical cancer**. Individuals infected with these viruses are at higher risk for the development of precancerous lesions. Typically, infection with these viruses is common in adolescents and women in their twenties, and usually do not result in cancerous growth. The most common high-risk HPV is type 16. The appearance of abnormal cells containing high-risk HPV types is seen most frequently in women over the age of 30 who have abnormal Pap smears.

HPV infections are very common. At some point in their lives, greater than 75% of people are infected with HPV, making HPV the most common sexually transmitted disease. In general, HPV infections do not cause any obvious symptoms increasing the likelihood of sexual transmission. Genital warts will occur in 1 or 2 of every 100 people. Abnormal Pap smears with atypical cells due to HPV can occur in 2–5% of women. If untreated, these women are at increased risk to develop cervical cancer. Virtually all cases of cervical cancer involve high-risk HPV types. It is believed that most cervical cancers take about five years to progress from early cellular changes to an invasive, life-threatening cervical cancer. It is not fully understood why most infections with high-risk HPV are of short duration, while a small percentage persist and eventually transform cervical cells to a state of cancerous growth.

The relationship among HPV, precancerous cellular changes, and cervical cancer have led to the suggestion that testing for the presence of HPV can be a useful addition to Pap smears. Pap smears involve microscopic analysis of cells removed from the cervix. The results of these tests are generally reported as normal, or consistent with the presence of cancer or a precancerous condition. Patients receiving the latter diagnosis usually are treated, either by excisional or ablative therapy surgery or some other means, in order to remove the tumor or precancerous lesion. In some cases the cytologist or pathologist examining a Pap smear reports a "borderline" result when abnormal cells are observed; but it is not possible to distinguish whether the changes seen are due to early precancerous changes, or inflammation caused by some infectious agent or irritant. In these cases, some physicians and scientists believe that testing for the presence of HPV can help to identify those women who should be closely followed for the development of early cancerous lesions, or who should undergo colposcopy, a procedure to examine the cervix for precancerous lesions. These cancer precursors, termed cervical intraepithelial neoplasia (CIN) when identified early, before they have become invasive, can almost always be completely removed by minor surgery, essentially curing the patient before the cancer has had a chance to develop. The cervical tissue removed, which includes the precancerous tissue, is

KEY TERMS

Ablative—Also known as "Ablation" and referring to the surgical removal of lesions associated with HPV.

Biopsy—The removal of a small bit of tissue for diagnostic examination

Cervical intra-epithelial neoplasia (CIN)—A pre-cancerous condition in which a group of cells grow abnormally on the cervix but do not extend into the deeper layers of this tissue.

Colposcopy—Procedure in which the cervix is examined using a special microscope.

Epithelial—Referring to the epithelium, the layer of cells forming the epidermis of the skin and the surface layer of mucous membranes.

High-risk HPV type—A member of the HPV family of viruses that is associated with the development of cervical cancer and precancerous growths.

Pap smear—A test that checks for abnormal cells that can lead to cervical cancer.

examined as part of a **biopsy** to confirm the diagnosis, and if requested by a doctor, can be tested for the presence of high-risk HPV types. This does not occur often.

Treatments

In 2001 the only accepted treatment for HPV-related lesions is removal or eradication. Since the incidence of latent and recurrent infections is high, the eradication of HPV is not always 100% effective. It is essential to be aware that HPV is a sexually transmitted disease and women must engage in safe sex practices to decrease the risk of spreading the virus or becoming re-infected. The development of an HPV vaccine that would render individuals resistant to infection by at least some of the high-risk HPV types is a matter of considerable interest. It is possible that by 2010 such a vaccine will be available.

Resources

PERIODICALS

Cuzick J. "Human papillomavirus testing for primary cervical cancer screening."*JAMA* 283(January 2000):108–9

Cox J.T. "Evaluating the role of HPV testing for women with equivocal Papanicolaou test findings."*JAMA* 281(May 1999):1645–7.

QUESTIONS TO ASK THE DOCTOR

- If my Pap smear is abnormal, do you think I should have an HPV test?
- Based upon my Pap smear result and HPV testing, when should I have my next Pap smear?
- What can I do to decrease my risk of becoming (re)infected with HPV?

ORGANIZATIONS

National HPV and Cervical Cancer Prevention Resource Center. <http:www.ashastd.org> June 2001.

Herpes.Org. <http:www.herpes.org> June 2001.

OTHER

"HPV - The culprit behind cervical cancer."*Mayo Health* <http://www.mayohealth.org/home?id=HQ00889> 29 June 2001.

Antopia's HPV Page.<http:www.antopia.com/hpv> 29 June 2001.

Warren Maltzman, Ph.D.

Hydrocodone *see* **Opioids**

Hydrocortisone *see* **Corticosteroids**

Hydromorphone *see* **Opioids**

Hydroxyurea

Definition

Hydroxyurea, also known by its trade name Hydrea, is an antineoplastic agent, meaning it is used to treat cancer. It is taken orally.

Purpose

Hydroxyurea is used to treat the following conditions:

- **Melanoma**
- **Chronic myelocytic leukemia** that is resistant to other therapies
- **Ovarian cancer** that is recurrent, metastatic or inoperable.
- Squamous cell carcinoma of the head and neck, excluding the lip. (In this case, it is treated with radiation therapy.)

- Sickle cell anemia
- Other: Hydroxyurea has shown promise in the management of thrombocytosis, a condition in which platelet levels are abnormally high

Description

Hydroxyurea belongs to antimetabolites, a group of compounds that interfere with the production of nucleic acids. Hydroxyurea exerts its anticancer activity by inhibiting ribonucleotide reductase, an enzyme required for DNA synthesis. When used in conjunction with **radiation therapy**, the effectiveness of hydroxyurea increases because it also inhibits the ability of cells damaged by radiation to repair themselves.

KEY TERMS

Mucositis—A painful inflammation of the mucous membranes.

Mutagen—An agent capable of causing DNA changes.

Myelosuppression—Diminished bone marrow activity resulting in decreased red blood cells, white blood cells, and platelets.

Plateletpheresis—A procedure in which platelets are removed from whole blood.

Recommended dosage

Hydroxyurea dosages are calculated based on a person's weight as milligrams per kilogram (mg/kg). Doctors will usually use whichever value is lowest—the patient's actual weight or the patient's ideal weight—to calculate dosages. The drug is not given if white blood cell levels drop below 2500 mm^3, or if red blood cell levels drop below 100,000 mm^3. Usually, bone marrow recovery is rapid, and few doses are missed. Hydroxyurea is usually given for six weeks before its effectiveness can be adequately evaluated.

Hydroxyurea is administered in a capsule form, each containing 500 mg of the drug. If a patient is unable to swallow the capsule, its contents can be dissolved in a glass of water and swallowed immediately. The drug will not completely dissolve in water. Dosages have not been established for children in part because the cancers for which hydroxyurea is useful do not normally occur in that age group.

In the treatment of solid tumors, such as ovarian cancers, patients are usually given 80 mg/kg once every three days. Alternatively, a dose of 20–30 mg/kg may be given every day.

In **head and neck cancers** also treated with radiation, 80 mg/kg of hydroxyurea is given once every three days. The drug should be started a week before radiation therapy begins, and should continue for some time after radiation therapy.

When it is used to treat resistant chronic myelocytic leukemia, hydroxyurea is given in the dosage of 20–30 mg/kg once a day.

In thrombocytosis, doses of 15–30 mg/kg taken once a day are usually effective. Platelet levels return to a normal level within two to six weeks of therapy. In more severe cases, doses of 1.5–3.0 grams per day have been given with plateletpheresis, a procedure that removes platelets from the blood.

Precautions

This drug should not be administered to a person who has had a previous allergic reaction to it. Liver and kidney function should be evaluated prior to, and during, treatment. The drug may interfere with certain lab tests. For example, creatinine levels may be elevated. Patients taking hydroxyurea should stay well-hydrated, drinking up to 12 glasses per day of water or other fluids.

Hydroxyurea is potentially mutagenic, meaning that it causes mutations in DNA. Patients taking the drug should discuss the potential effects on their future conception plans. Hydroxyurea should not be administered to pregnant women, and women taking the drug should use birth control methods to prevent pregnancy. Hydroxyurea is excreted in breast milk; therefore, women taking the drug should not breast-feed.

Side effects

Hydroxyurea and radiation therapy each cause adverse side effects. When they are used together, the incidence and severity of side effects may increase.

Bone marrow suppression is the major side effect of hyroxyurea therapy, and may develop within two days of the first dose. Blood tests are performed routinely to monitor for changes. Usually, leukopenia (decreased white blood cells) develops first. Reduced red blood cells and platelets can also occur, but generally not as frequently. If anemia develops, it should be corrected with whole blood transfusions. Hydroxyurea causes red blood cell abnormalities that are not severe and that do not reduce the red blood cell survival time.

Gastrointestinal symptoms are not as common as **myelosuppression** and are usually mild. These symptoms may include nausea, vomiting, **diarrhea**, and constipation. Usually, medications can control **nausea and vomiting**. **Mucositis**, a painful swelling of the mucous membranes, may also develop, especially if the patient is undergoing radiation treatment to the head and neck. Mucositis can be managed with medicated mouthwashes, good oral hygiene, and hydration to keep the mouth moist.

Headache and dizziness may occur. With long-term use, skin changes, such as hyperpigmentation of the skin and nails, have also been reported.

Interactions

Patients at risk for bone marrow suppression should inform their doctor about all medications they are taking, both prescription and non-prescription. Many over-the-counter medications contain aspirin, which acts as a blood-thinner, increasing the potential for bleeding. Patients with reduced platelets should not take aspirin.

Tamara Brown, R.N.

Hypercalcemia

Description

Hypercalcemia is an abnormally high level of calcium in the blood, usually more than 10.5 milligrams per deciliter of blood. It is the most common life-threatening metabolic disorder associated with cancer.

Calcium plays an important role in the development and maintenance of bones in the body. It is also needed in tooth formation and is important in other body functions. As much as 99% of the body's calcium is stored in bone tissue. A healthy person experiences a constant turnover of calcium as bone tissue is built and reshaped. The remaining 1% of the body's calcium circulates in the blood and other body fluids. Calcium in the blood plays an important role in the control of many body functions, including blood clotting, transmission of nerve impulses, muscle contraction, and other metabolic activities.

Cancer-caused hypercalcemia produces a disruption in the body's ability to maintain a normal level of calcium. This abnormally high level of calcium in the blood develops because of increased bone breakdown and release of calcium from the bone. The disorder occurs in approximately 10-20% of all cancer cases. The most common cancers associated with hypercalcemia are breast, prostate, and lung cancer, as well as **multiple myeloma** or other tumors with extensive **metastasis** to the bone. It may also occur in patients with head and neck cancer, cancer of unknown primary, **lymphoma**, leukemia, kidney cancer, and gastrointestinal cancer. Hypercalcemia most commonly develops as a late complication of cancer, and its appearance constitutes an emergency.

Several clinical symptoms are associated with cancer-related hypercalcemia. Symptoms may appear gradually and often look like signs of other cancers and diseases. The symptoms of hypercalcemia are not only related to the elevated level of calcium in the blood, but—more importantly—to how rapidly the hypercalcemia develops. The severity of the symptoms is often dependent upon factors such as previous cancer treatment, reactions to medications, or other illnesses a patient may have. Most patients do not experience all of the symptoms of hypercalcemia, and some may not have any signs at all. Rapid diagnosis of hypercalcemia may be complicated because the symptoms are often nonspecific and are easily ascribed to other factors. These symptoms include:

- decreased muscle tone and muscle weakness
- delirium, disorientation, incoherent speech, and psychotic symptoms such as hallucinations and delusion
- constipation
- **fatigue**
- poor appetite, nausea and/or vomiting
- frequency of urination and increased thirst
- pain

Causes

The fundamental cause of cancer-related hypercalcemia is increased movement of calcium out of the bones and into the bloodstream, and secondarily, an inadequate ability of the kidneys to get rid of higher calcium levels. Normally, healthy kidneys are able to filter out large amounts of calcium from the blood, getting rid of the excess that is unneeded by the body and keeping the amount of the calcium the body does need. However, the high levels of calcium in the body caused by cancer-related hypercalcemia may cause the kidneys to become overworked, thus making them unable to excrete the excess. Another problem is that some tumors produce a substance that may cause the kidneys to get rid of too little calcium.

Two types of cancer-caused hypercalcemia have been identified: osteolytic and humoral. Osteolytic occurs because of direct bone destruction by a primary or metastatic tumor. Humoral is caused by certain factors secreted by malignant cells, which ultimately cause calcium loss from the bones. Certain types of hormonal therapy may precipitate hypercalcemia and the use of some diuretics may contribute to the disorder.

Because immobility causes an increase in the loss of calcium from bone, cancer patients who are weak and spend most of their time in bed are more prone to hypercalcemia. Cancer patients are often dehydrated because they take in inadequate amounts of food and fluids and often suffer from **nausea and vomiting**. Dehydration reduces the ability of the kidneys to remove excess calcium from the body, and therefore is another contributing factor in the development of hypercalcemia in cancer patients.

Treatments

Individuals at risk for developing hypercalcemia may be the first to recognize symptoms, such as fatigue. The patient and family should be aware of the signs and symptoms so that a health care professional can be notified as early as possible should they occur. Patients can take several preventative measures like ensuring adequate fluid intake, controlling nausea and vomiting, maintaining the highest possible mobility, and avoiding drugs that affect the functioning of the kidneys. This includes avoiding those medications containing calcium, vitamin D, or vitamin A. Since absorption of calcium is usually decreased in individuals with hypercalcemia, dietary calcium restriction is unnecessary.

The mortality rate for untreated hypercalcemia is quite high. Early diagnosis and prompt treatment are essential. The magnitude of hypercalcemia and the severity of symptoms is usually the basis for determining what type of treatment is indicated.

For those patients who have mild hypercalcemia, are experiencing no symptoms, and have cancer that is responsive to treatment, giving intravenous fluids and observing the patient may be all that is necessary to treat the condition. If the patient is experiencing symptoms or has a cancer that is expected to respond poorly to treatment, then medication to treat the hypercalcemia should be initiated. Additional treatment focuses on controlling nausea and vomiting, encouraging activity, and avoiding any medication that causes drowsiness.

In treating moderate or severe hypercalcemia, replacing fluids is the first treatment intervention. Though providing fluid replacement will not restore normal calcium levels in all patients, it is still the most important initial step. Improvement in mental status and nausea and vomiting is usually apparent within 24 hours for most patients. However, rehydration is only a temporary measure. If the cancer is not treated, then drugs that will help to control the hypercalcemia are necessary. Many drugs are used to treat hypercalcemia, including **calcitonin**, **plicamycin** (formerly mithramycin), **gallium nitrate**, and **bisphosphonates**. Bisphosphonates are some of the most effective drugs for controlling hypercalcemia. Loop diuretics like furosemide are often given because they help to increase the excretion of excess serum calcium. For severe hypercalcemia that is complicated by kidney failure, dialysis is an option. Because of the large amounts of intravenous fluids given to treat hypercalcemia, the health care team will carefully observe for any signs of overhydration or other electrolyte imbalances.

The severity of hypercalcemia determines the amount of treatment necessary. Severe hypercalcemia should be treated immediately and aggressively. Less severe hypercalcemia should be treated according to the symptoms. A positive response to the treatment is exhibited by the disappearance of the symptoms and a decreased level of calcium in the blood. Mild hypercalcemia does not usually need to be treated aggressively. After calcium levels return to normal, urine and blood should continue to be checked often to make certain the treatment is still working.

Alternative and complementary therapies

There are no known proven alternative treatments for cancer-related hypercalcemia. Some of the medications used are more effective than others, and the patient and family should discuss which ones are the most appropriate for the patient's needs.

Hypercalcemia usually develops as a late complication of cancer, and its appearance is very serious. The outlook is often quite grim. However, it is not clear if death occurs because of the hypercalcemia cri-

KEY TERMS

Calcium—A silvery-yellow metal that is the most abundant mineral in the human body. Calcium and phosphorous combine as calcium phosphate, the hard material of bones and teeth.

Humoral hypercalcemia—An abnormally elevated blood calcium level caused by factors released from cancer cells, ultimately causing the loss of calcium from bone.

Osteolytic hypercalcemia—An abnormally elevated blood calcium level caused by destruction of bone by a primary or metastatic tumor.

sis or because of the advanced cancer. Because hypercalcemia is often a complication that occurs in the final stages of cancer, the decision to treat it depends upon the overall goals of treatment determined by the patient, family, and physician. The natural course of untreated hypercalcemia will progress to loss of consciousness and coma. Some patients may prefer this at the end of life rather than have unrelieved suffering and/or untreatable symptoms. It is therefore important for the patient and caregivers to discuss what supportive care measures are wanted.

Resources

BOOKS

Prucha, Edward J., ed. *Cancer Sourcebook.* Detroit: Omnigraphics, 2000.

PERIODICALS

Falk, Stephen, and Marie Fallon. "Emergencies." *British Medical Journal* (December 6, 1997): 1525

OTHER

National Cancer Institute. Building 31, Room 10A31, 31 Center Drive, MSC 2580, Bethesda, MD 20892-2580. (800) 4-CANCER 5 July 2001<http://www.nci.nih.gov>

Deanna Swartout-Corbeil, R.N.

Hypercoagulation disorders

Description

Hypercoagulation disorders (or hypercoagulable states or disorders) cause an increased tendency for clotting of the blood. In normal hemostasis (the stoppage of bleeding) clots form at the site of the blood vessel's injury. However, in hypercoagulation disorders the clots can develop in circulating blood. This may put a patient at risk for obstruction of veins and arteries (phlebitis, thrombosis, or thrombophlebitis). The hypercoagulable state and thrombophlebitis is common cases of cancer involving solid tumors such as pancreatic, breast, ovarian, and **prostate cancer**.

Hypercoagulation disorders can cause clots throughout the body's blood vessels, a condition known as thromboembolic disease. Thromboembolic disease can lead to infarction (death of tissue as a result of blocked blood supply to the tissue). Other serious results of hypercoagulation make this a dangerous condition. Clotting (thrombosis) in the veins and arteries leading to the lungs can prevent blood flow, causing sudden and severe loss of breath and chest pain. These clots, called pulmonary embolisms, are potentially fatal. Clots in the blood vessels of the brain can result in a stroke, and clots in the heart's blood vessels can result in a heart attack.

Symptoms of hypercoagulation disorders include swelling or discoloration of the limbs, pain or tenderness of the skin, visible obstructions in the surface veins, and ulcers of the lower parts of the legs.

The diagnosis of hypercoagulation disorders is completed with a combination of physical examination, **imaging studies**, and blood tests. The presence of deep clots can be determined using Doppler ultrasound examination—special x-ray techniques called venography or arteriography (in which a solution is injected into the blood vessel to aid in imaging), or a specific type of blood pressure test called plethysmography. There are a number of blood tests that can determine the presence or absence of proteins, clotting factors, and platelet counts in the blood. Among the tests used to detect hypercoagulation is the Antithrombin III assay. Protein C and Protein S concentrations can be diagnosed with immunoassay or plasma antigen level tests.

KEY TERMS

Antithrombin—Any substance that counters the effect of thrombin. Thrombin is an enzyme that converts fibrinogen into fibrin, leading to blood coagulation.

Congenital—A condition or disorder present at birth.

Hemostasis—The arrest of bleeding.

Heparin—An anticoagulant, or blood clot dissolver.

Phlebitis—Inflammation of a vein.

Polycythemia—A condition characterized by an overabundance of red blood cells.

Thrombophlebitis—Inflammation of the vein with the formation of a thrombosis (blood clot).

Thrombosis—Formation of a clot in the blood that either blocks, or partially blocks, a blood vessel. The thrombus may lead to infarction (death of tissue due to a blocked blood supply).

Causes

Hypercoagulation disorders are associated with cancer of the pancreas. About half of patients with pancreatic cancer experience incidence of thrombosis. Approximately 10% of patients with pancreatic cancer develop a specific type of hypercoagulation disorder known as migratory thrombophlebitis, or Trousseau's syndrome. In Trousseau's syndrome the blood vessels become inflamed and clots in the blood vessels spontaneously appear and disappear. Other types of cancer may also result in hypercoagulation disorders.

In order for blood coagulation to occur, platelets (small, round fragments in the blood) help contract blood vessels to lessen blood loss and also to help plug damaged blood vessels. The conversion of platelets into actual clots is a complicated process involving proteins that are identified clotting factors. The factors are carried in the plasma, or liquid portion, of the blood. Proteins C and S are two of the clotting factors that are present in the plasma to help regulate or activate parts of the clotting process. It is believed that pancreatic tumors produce chemicals that promote clotting, or coagulation, of the blood (procoagulants), or that they activate platelet function. It is also possible that tumors interfere with the functions of proteins C and S.

Treatments

The treatment for patients with hypercoagulation disorders varies depending upon the severity of the clotting and the other conditions it may have caused. Medications may include blood thinners (anticoagulants) such as **heparin** and **warfarin**, which prevent the formation of new blood clots; antiplatelet drugs such as aspirin; or thrombolytic drugs to dissolve existing clots. Pain medications and nonsteroidal anti-inflammatory medications may be given to reduce pain and swelling. **Antibiotics** will be prescribed if infection has occurred.

Resources

BOOKS

Deloughery, Thomas G. *Hemostasis and Thrombosis.* Georgetown, TX: Landes Bioscience, 1999.

Goodnight, Scott H., and William E. Goodnight. *Disorders of Hemostasis and Thrombosis,* 2nd ed. New York: McGraw-Hill, 2000.

ORGANIZATIONS

National Heart, Lung and Blood Institute. Building 31, Room 4A21, Bethesda, MD 20892. (301) 496-4236. <http://www.nhlbi.nih.gov>

National Hemophilia Foundation. 116 West 32nd St., 11th Floor, New York, NY 10001. 800-42-HANDI. <http://www.hemophilia.org>

OTHER

American Academy of Family Physicians. *Hypercoagulation: Excessive Blood Clotting.* <http://familydoctor.org/handouts/244.html> (15 April 2001) 5 July 2001

Paul A. Johnson, Ed.M.

Hyperthermia

Definition

Hyperthermia is the use of therapeutic heat to treat various cancers on and inside the body.

Purpose

The purpose of hyperthermia is to shrink and hopefully destroy cancer without harming noncancerous cells. It can be used to treat cancer in many areas of the body, including the brain, thyroid, lung, breast, and prostate. It is thought that high temperatures, up to 106 degrees Fahrenheit, can help shrink cancerous tumors. Hyperthermia is starting to be more widely used because it does not have side effects like other forms of cancer treatment such as radiation or **chemotherapy**. In some instances, hyperthermia is used at the same time with other forms of cancer therapy.

Through years of research, it has been found that the effectiveness of some forms of **radiation therapy** and chemotherapy are enhanced when combined with hyperthermia.

Although the treatment was considered experimental 15–20 years ago, its proponents believe that the treatment has been accepted by many physicians, and that use of hyperthermia will increase as more cancer centers install the high-tech equipment necessary for regional and whole body hyperthermia. (Currently, cancer care centers offering this treatment are limited.) In 2001, the American Cancer Society acknowledges that hyperthermia can make the cancer cells of some cancers more responsive to treatment, but still considers the treatment experimental, especially in whole-body form. The National Institutes of Health are sponsoring ongoing **clinical trials** studying hyperthermia.

Precautions

Patients who have extensive **metastasis** (spreading of the cancer throughout their body) may not be good candidates for hyperthermia. Patients need to be free of major infections and able to tolerate the high temperatures of the treatment. Caution must be used when areas of the body are heated with external heat sources such as heating pads to avoid potentially dangerous burns.

Description

Hyperthermia can be used on the body from very small areas of the body to the entire body itself. Local hyperthermia refers to heating just one area of body, usually where the tumor is located. Heat can be applied from outside the body using microwaves or high-frequency radio waves. Heat can be applied from inside the body or even inside the tumor itself by the use of thin, heated wires, small tubes filled with hot water, or implanted microwave antennae.

If heat is used to treat an entire organ or limb, it is referred to as regional hyperthermia. High-energy magnets or other devices that produce high energy, and thus heat, are placed over the larger areas to be heated. Another method of regional hyperthermia is the use of perfusion. Hyperthermia perfusion uses the patient's own blood; the blood is removed, heated outside the body, then pumped back into the area that contains the cancer.

For treatment of cancers that have spread throughout the body, whole-body hyperthermia can be considered. Various methods are used to heat up a patient's entire body, including warm-water or electric blankets, hot wax, or thermal chambers which are very much like incubators used to warm newborn babies, except much larger.

Preparation

There are generally no advance preparations needed for a patient considering the use of hyperthermia.

Risks

The major risks of hyperthermia use are pain and external burns. Heat applied directly to the skin can cause minor discomfort to significant pain, especially when high temperatures are used. Blistering and actual burning of the skin can also occur at higher temperatures, although with careful application of the hyperthermia, these side effects are very rare.

Normal Results

The goal of hyperthermia is to control the growth and shrink hyperthermia-sensitive tumors. As stated earlier, hyperthermia can also be used to help sensitize tumors to other cancer treatment modalities such as radiation and chemotherapy.

Abnormal Results

There are generally no abnormal results seen with the use of hyperthermia. Side effects, such as pain and burning from external heat sources, can be minimized with careful application of the heat.

Resources

BOOKS

Abeloff, D. Martin, James O. Armitage, Allen S. Lichter, and John E. Niederhuber. *Clinical Oncology.* New York: Churchill Livingstone, 2000.

Bicher, I. Haim, John R. McLaren, and Giuseppe M. Pigliucci, ed. *Consensus on Hyperthermia for the 1990s.* New York: Plenum Press, 1990.

Freeman, L. Michael and Kurt J. Henle. "Hyperthermia." In *Encyclopedia of Cancer,* Volume II. Academic Press, 1997: 888-900.

Edward R. Rosick, D.O., M.P.H.

I

Idarubicin

Definition

Idarubicin is a medication that kills cancer cells.

Purpose

As of 2001, idarubicin is approved to treat only one single cancer, **acute myelocytic leukemia** (AML) in adults. Recent research suggests that using idarubicin rather than the more traditional **daunorubicin** in treating AML results in higher rates of complete remission (CR) and longer survival for patients. CR is the total elimination of all diseased cells detectable following therapy. The Food and Drug Administration (FDA) has not approved idarubicin as treatment for **acute lymphocytic leukemia** (ALL).

Much research involving idarubicin is now being conducted. Some of this has involved acute lymphocytic leukemia (ALL) as well as AML. For example, a recent study was conducted in patients with either AML or ALL who had received **bone marrow transplantation** and then relapsed. Patients received a combination of **cytarabine**, idarubicin, and **etoposide**, as well as a medicine called G-CSF (**filgrastim**). This treatment achieved a high CR rate in these patients.

Another recent study looked at the use of idarubicin in children with AML. All of the children received cytarabine and etoposide. In addition, some of the children received idarubicin, while some received daunorubicin. Overall, patients in both groups fared equally well in terms of survival length. However, patients who had larger numbers of cells known as blasts (immature cells) tended to do better if they received idarubicin rather than daunorubicin. In addition, high-risk patients tended to do better with idarubicin than with daunorubicin. No subgroup of patients achieved better outcomes with daunorubicin than with idarubicin.

KEY TERMS

Bilirubin—A pigment produced when the liver processes waste products. A high bilirubin level causes yellowing of the skin.

Blasts—Immature cells

Complete remission (CR)—Complete remission is the total elimination of all diseased cells detectable following therapy.

Necrosis—The sum of the morphological changes indicative of cell death. It may affect groups of cells or part of a structure or an organ.

Description

Idarubicin is an antibiotic, although doctors do not use this drug to attack infections. Its only use is to kill cancer cells. It does so by affecting how the DNA of cancer cells work.

Recommended dosage

In the treatment of AML, 12 mg of idarubicin per square meter may be given over a period of two to three days every three weeks in combination with other medications. Patients with liver problems may be given lower doses than other patients receive. Idarubicin is not typically given by mouth, as an insufficient amount of the medication would be transported through the stomach wall if this were done. Rather, this medication is usually administered through an intravenous (IV) procedure. During this time, it circulates widely throughout the body.

A new formulation of idarubicin has been developed. This permits idarubicin to be taken orally. However, this formulation is currently available only in France and only for older patients who are not good candidates for intensive intravenous treatment. There is little information currently available on the effectiveness of this oral formulation. The studies that have been performed suggest that it is less effective than other formulations of idarubicin.

Precautions

Idarubicin may be associated with excessive toxicity in patients with congestive heart failure, liver function characterized by a high bilirubin level, or prior chest radiation to the heart.

Side effects

Like daunorubicin and **doxorubicin**, idarubicin may adversely affect the patient's heart. However, doctors are not certain how much of the drug it takes to cause such harm and, therefore, how to limit dosage so that such harm is not caused. However, idarubicin appears to be less likely to cause heart damage than similar drugs such as daunorubicin and doxorubicin. Another serious side effect that limits how much of the drug is given to patients is its potential adverse effect upon the bone marrow, where blood cells are produced.

Idarubicin may cause **nausea and vomiting**, baldness (**alopecia**), and stomach problems. In addition, idarubicin may cause blistering if extravasation occurs. Extravasation is when **chemotherapy** gets outside of the vein during infusion. If this occurs, the drug may cause severe local pain, swelling, or tissue necrosis that may require plastic surgery.

Patients receiving idarubicin in conjunction with certain other anticancer drugs may develop a type of leukemia. However, this is extremely rare.

In the few studies that have been conducted on the oral formulation of idarubicin, the most prominent side effects seen are low blood cell counts, nausea, vomiting, **diarrhea**, and hair loss.

Bob Kirsch

Ifosfamide

Definition

Ifosfamide is an anticancer (antineoplastic) agent. It also acts as a suppressor of the immune system. It is available under the brand name IFEX.

Purpose

Ifosfamide is approved by the Food and Drug Administration (FDA) to treat germ cell **testicular cancer**. It is generally prescribed in combination with another medicine (**mesna**), which is used to prevent the bladder problems that may be caused by ifosfamide alone.

Ifosfamide also has activity against other cancers and is prescribed in practice for these cancer types:

- pancreatic cancer
- **stomach cancer**
- soft-tissue sarcoma
- **Ewing's sarcoma**
- acute and **chronic lymphocytic leukemia**
- **bladder cancer**
- bone cancer
- **breast cancer**
- **cervical cancer**
- **head and neck cancers**
- lung cancer
- **lymphomas**
- **neuroblastomas**
- **ovarian cancer**
- **Wilms' tumor**

Description

Ifosfamide chemically interferes with the synthesis of the genetic material (DNA and RNA) of cancer cells by cross-linking of DNA strands, which prevents these cells from being able to reproduce and continue the growth of the cancer.

Recommended dosage

Ifosfamide may only be taken as an injection into the vein. The dosage prescribed varies widely depending on the patient, the cancer being treated, and whether or not other medications are also being taken. Examples of common doses for adults are: 50 mg per kg per day, or 700 to 2000 mg per square meter of body surface area for five days every three to four weeks. Another alternative regimen is 2400 mg per square meter of body surface area for three days or 5000 mg per square meter of body surface area as a single dose every three to four weeks. Examples of common dosing regimens for children are: 1200 to 1800 mg per square meter of body surface area per day for three to five days every 21 to 28 days; 5000 mg per square meter of body surface area once every 21 to 28 days; or 3000 mg per square meter of body surface area for two days every 21 to 28 days.

Precautions

Ifosfamide can cause an allergic reaction in some people. Patients with a prior allergic reaction to ifosfamide should not take this drug.

Ifosfamide should always be taken with plenty of fluids.

Ifosfamide can cause serious birth defects if either the man or the woman is taking this drug at the time of conception or if the woman is taking this drug during pregnancy. Contraceptive measures should be taken by both men and women while on this drug. Because ifosfamide is easily passed from mother to child through breast milk, breast feeding is not recommended during treatment.

Ifosfamide suppresses the immune system, and its excretion from the body is dependent on a normal functioning kidney and liver. For these reasons, it is important that the prescribing physician is aware of any of the following pre-existing medical conditions:

- a current case of, or recent exposure to, chicken pox
- herpes zoster (shingles)
- all current infections
- kidney disease
- liver disease

Also, because ifosfamide is such a potent immunosuppressant, patients taking this drug must exercise extreme caution to avoid contracting any new infections.

Side effects

Inflammation and irritation of the bladder, causing blood in the urine, is the most common and severe side effect of ifosfamide. However, this side effect can be prevented and controlled with the administration of the bladder protectant drug mesna and vigorous hydration with intravenous fluids before, during, and after **chemotherapy**. Patients should also urinate frequently (at least every 2 hours) to enhance removal of the drug from the body, and drink 2 to 3 liters of fluids a day for 2 to 3 days after discontinuation of the chemotherapy.

Other common side effects of ifosfamide are:

- confusion
- hallucinations
- drowsiness
- dizziness
- temporary hair loss (**alopecia**)
- increased susceptibility to infection
- increased risk of bleeding (due to a decrease of the platelets involved in the clotting process)
- **nausea and vomiting** (can be prevented with prescribed antiemetics)

Less common side effects include:

- increased coloration (pigmentation) of the skin and fingernails
- loss of appetite (**anorexia**)
- **diarrhea**
- nasal stuffiness
- skin rash, **itching**, or hives

A doctor should be consulted immediately if the patient experiences any of these side effects:

- painful or difficult urination
- increase in frequency or feeling of urgency to urinate
- blood in the urine
- blood in the stool
- severe diarrhea
- mental status changes such as confusion, drowsiness, or hallucinations
- signs of infection such as cough, sore throat, **fever** and chills
- shortness of breath
- chest or abdominal pain
- pain in the lower back or sides
- unusual bleeding or bruising
- tiny red dots on the skin

Interactions

Ifosfamide should not be taken in combination with any prescription drug, over-the-counter drug, or herbal remedy without prior consultation with a physician.

Paul A. Johnson, Ed.M.

KEY TERMS

Antineoplastic—A drug that prevents the growth of a neoplasm by interfering with the maturation or proliferation of the cells of the neoplasm.

Neoplasm—New abnormal growth of tissue.

Imaging studies

Definition

Imaging studies are tests performed with a variety of techniques that produce pictures of the inside of a patient's body. They have become indispensable tools in cancer screening and detection.

Description

Imaging tests are performed using sound waves, radioactive particles, magnetic fields, or x rays that are detected and converted into images after passing through body tissues. Dyes are sometimes used as contrasting agents with x-ray tests so that organs or tissues not seen with conventional x rays can be enhanced. The operating principle of the various techniques is based on the fact that rays and particles interact differently with various types of tissues, especially when cancerous growths are present. In this way, the interior of the body can be visualized and pictures are provided of normal structure and function as well as of abnormalities.

Imaging tests differ from endoscopic tests, which are carried out with a flexible, lighted piece of tubing connected to a viewing lens or camera.

Imaging studies are used to detect cancer in its early stages in a procedure called screening. Screening is performed in patients who have no obvious cancer symptoms. Imaging studies are also used to locate tumors in patients who have symptoms which the physician may wish to investigate further so as to distinguish between benign growths or cancerous tumors. They are also used to determine the extent of a cancer and indicate how a given treatment is unfolding. As such, they represent crucial tools for cancer diagnosis and management.

Major imaging techniques

Computed tomography scan (CT scan)

Computed tomography scans show a cross-section of a part of the body. In this technique, a thin beam is used to produce a series of exposures detected at different angles. The exposures are fed into a computer which overlaps them so as to yield a single image analogous to a slice of the organ or body part being scanned. A dye is often injected into the patient so as to improve contrast and obtain images that are clearer than images obtained with x rays.

Magnetic resonance imaging (MRI)

Magnetic resonance imaging also produces cross-sectional images of the body using powerful magnetic fields instead of radiation. MRI is especially useful to detect and locate cancers of the liver and the central nervous system, which occur in the brain or the spinal cord. It uses a cylinder housing a magnet which will induce the required magnetic field. The patient lies on a platform inside the scanner. The magnetic field aligns the hydrogen atoms present in the tissue being scanned in a given direction. Following a burst of radio-frequency radiation, the atoms flip back to their original orientation while emitting signals which a fed into a computer for conversion into a two- or three-dimensional image. Dyes can also be injected into patients to produce clearer images.

Mammography

Mammography is an x-ray examination of the breast. It is often used as a screening tool to detect breast abnormalities and cancers before they can be felt. Mammograms (the image produced) are acquired using an x-ray machine working at lower radiation levels than conventional **x ray**. The breast is compressed between two plates so as to allow the low-level x-ray radiation to produce a film.

Nuclear scan

Nuclear scans, also called radionuclide imaging or scintigraphy, use substances called tracers or radionuclides that release low levels of radioactivity. The test is based on the principle that the tracers will be absorbed to a different degree by different tissues, thus allowing to distinguish between normal and cancerous tissues. Common **nuclear medicine scans** for cancer patients to receive are bone scans; liver, spleen, and thyroid scans are also frequently performed.

Position emission tomography (PET)

Positron emission tomography uses a form of sugar that contains a radioactive atom which emits particles called positrons. The positrons are absorbed to a different extent by cells varying in their metabolic rate. PET scans are especially useful for brain imaging studies and are widely applied to the assessment of the spread of cancers in the lungs. PET scans are also being used experimentally in the assessment of breast, colon, rectum, and ovarian cancers.

X rays

X rays produce shallow images of certain specific organs or tissues. X rays are a form of high-energy radiation and tissues of the body can absorb it to varying degrees. For example, bones absorb less x rays than soft tissue. After passing through the body, the x rays are directed on a film, where the dense tissue appears as a white shadow, thus providing contrast with the soft tissue, which produces a darker impression on the film. X rays produce a single image.

Chest x rays are used to detect lung and bronchial cancers, and also to evaluate a patient's symptoms, such as shortness of breath. Other types of x rays, such as abdominal x rays, may also be ordered to assess a patient's symptoms, but are not used as cancer screening tools as chest x rays may be used.

X rays with dye studies

Dye studies are usually performed by injecting the contrasting agent in the patient's circulatory system or in the target organ. These studies are used to produce angiograms, cystograms, myelograms, lymphangiograms and fistulograms.

ANGIOGRAM. An angiogram is an examination of the blood vessels using x rays. It is usually performed with intravenous injection of fluorescein dye followed by multiframe photography. The doctor inserts a small tube (catheter) into the blood vessel and then injects the dye that makes the vessels visible when the x-ray pictures are acquired.

CYSTOGRAM. A cystogram is a scan of the bladder and ureters. The ureters are passages that lead from the kidneys to the bladder. A catheter is inserted into the bladder or a radioactive material, called a radioisotope, is introduced into the bladder. An oral cholecystogram (OCG) is an x-ray examination of the gallbladder, the organ that helps release bile into the small intestine for the digestion of fats. The gallbladder is not seen well on conventional x-ray pictures and special tablets are ingested by mouth to enhance contrast.

MYELOGRAM. A myelogram is an x ray of the spine and spinal cord. The spinal cord is the nerve tissue enclosed in the vertebral column that goes from the bottom of the brain to halfway down the back. During a myelogram, x-ray dye is injected into the spinal fluid and mixes with it, flowing around the spinal cord which can then be seen and recorded on x-ray film.

LYMPHANGIOGRAM. A lymphangiogram is an x ray of the lymphatic system, also carried out with dye injection for contrasting purposes. It is used to screen for lymph node involvement in cancer.

FISTULOGRAM. A fistula is an abnormal passage within body tissue. For example, a fistula may connect two organs inside the body that are not normally connected. A fistula may also lead from an internal organ inside the body to the surface outside. Examples are: between the skin and the bowel (enterocutaneous fistula), between the stomach and the colon (gastrocolic fistula). A fistulogram is an x-ray examination of this abnormal passage. The contrasting agent is injected directly into the fistula so that it will show up on x-ray pictures.

Fluoroscopy

Fluoroscopy is one of the oldest areas of diagnostic radiology. It is similar to x ray in that a small dose of x rays is directed through a body part but the image obtained is displayed on a monitor rather than on the conventional x-ray film. The fluoroscope provides images of internal body parts as they move, similar to a movie. A continuous x-ray beam is passed through the body part being examined, and is transmitted to an image-intensifying tube, which is a TV-like monitor so that the body part and its motion can be seen in detail.

During fluoroscopy, the patient is placed between the x-ray source and the monitor. The live images generated by the x-ray source strike the image-intensifying tube and allow doctors to see the size, shape, and structure of a patient's internal structures. Because the radiation is blocked more effectively by dense tissue, such as that of a tumor, the result is a dark shadow of the tumor on the screen, against a light background. Most fluoroscopy devices include television or video cameras attached to the image-intensifier tube. The camera output can be digitized and sent through a computer for image enhancement.

In fluoroscopic studies, the radiologist can either insert an intravenous (IV) catheter (hollow tube inserted into blood vessels or into an organ) to **biopsy** a tumor or he can use a contrast agent to visualize the organ or area of interest. The contrast agent allows the image to be viewed more clearly. Contrast agents may be introduced into the patient's body by injection, swallowing, or an enema. Fluoroscopic exams include the following types of tests: barium swallow, **barium enema**, and intravenous pyelography, also called **intravenous urography**.

BARIUM SWALLOW. Used for GI series. The patient drinks a chalky, milkshake-like concoction containing barium, which coats the esophagus and stomach. The barium absorbs the x rays so that the lining of the upper digestive tract can be clearly seen. In barium x rays, fluoroscopy allows the physician to see the movement of the intestines as the barium moves through them.

BARIUM ENEMA. In a lower GI series, the patient receives a barium enema, which coats the intestines and rectum. A gap in the image in the stomach or small intestine could indicate an ulcer and bubbles in the normally smooth large intestinal lining may be abnormal growths.

INTRAVENOUS PYELOGRAPHY (IVP). Pyelography, also called urography, consists of several x rays of all the

KEY TERMS

Cancer screening—A procedure designed to detect cancer even though a person has no symptoms, usually performed using an imaging technique.

CT scan—An imaging technique that uses a computer to combine multiple x-ray images into a two-dimensional cross-sectional image

Mammography—An imaging technique producing x-ray pictures of the breast called mammograms.

MRI—A special imaging technique used to image internal parts of the body, especially soft tissues.

PET—A highly specialized imaging technique using radioactive substances to identify active tumors.

Radionuclide imaging—An imaging technique in which a radionuclide is injected through tissue and a display is obtained from a scanner device.

urinary system, meaning kidneys, ureter, bladder and urethra. A contrast agent is injected through a vein, to make the organs visible for the x rays.

See Also Screening test; Ultrasonography

Resources

BOOKS

Seeram, E. *Computed Tomography: Physical Principles, Clinical Applications and Quality Control.* Philadelphia: W. B. Saunders & Co., 2001.

von Schulthess, G. K., ed. *Clinical Positron Emission Tomography* Philadelphia: Lippincott, Williams & Wilkins, 1999.

Webb, W. Richard, William E. Brant, Clyde A. Helms, and others, eds. *Fundamentals of Body CT.* Philadelphia: W. B. Saunders Company, 1997.

Westbrook, C. *Handbook of MRI Techniques.* Malden, MA: Blackwell Science, 1999.

PERIODICALS

Frassica, F. J., J. A. Khanna, E. F. McCarthy. "The role of MR imaging in soft tissue tumor evaluation:perspective of the orthopedic oncologist and musculoskeletal pathologist." *Magnetic Resonance Imaging, Clin. N. Am.* 8 (November 2000):915-27.

Hopper, K. D., K. Singapuri, A. Finkel. "Body CT and oncologic imaging." *Radiology* 215 (April 2000):27-40.

Jain, P., A. C. Arroliga. "Spiral CT for lung cancer screening: is it ready for prime time?" *Cleveland Clinical Journal of Medicine* 68 (January 2001):74-81.

Pomper, M. G., J. D. Port. "New techniques in MR imaging of brain tumors." *Magnetic Resonance Imaging, Clin. N. Am.* 8 (November 2000):691-713.

Roelcke, U., K. L. Leenders. "PET in neuro-oncology." *Journal of Cancer Research and Clinical Oncology* 127 (January 2001):2-8.

ORGANIZATIONS

National Cancer Information Center:1-800-ACS-2345

National Cancer Institute, Public Inquiries Office, Building 31, Room 10A31, 31 Center Drive, MSC 2580, Bethesda, MD 20892-2580. (301)435-2848. Imaging Information and data sheets: <http://search.nci.nih.gov/search97cgi/s97_cgi>.

OTHER

"Imaging Information." *American Cancer Society.* 15 October 1999. 11 July 2001 <http://www3.cancer.org/cancerinfo/load_cont.asp?ct=1&doc=66>.

Monique Laberge, Ph.D.

Imatinib mesylate

Definition

Imatinib mesylate is an enzyme inhibitor used for cancer therapy. Imatinib mesylate is also known as STI571 and is sold under the brand name, Gleevec. It was given the name STI571 during early development. STI stands for signal transduction inhibitor.

Purpose

Imatinib mesylate is approved by the U. S. Food and Drug Administration to treat a rare cancer called chronic myeloid leukemia (CML). (CML is also called chronic myelogenous leukemia or **chronic myelocytic leukemia**, as well.)

Description

Imatinib mesylate is the first drug of its kind developed. It fights cancer by turning off an enzyme called tyrosine kinase that causes CML cells to lose their ability to die so they can multiply at an abnormal rate. Its function is different from other cancer drugs because it specifically targets an enzyme that allows the growth of CML cells. This drug has been shown to significantly reduce the number of cancer cells in the blood and bone marrow of treated patients.

Patients who are diagnosed with CML in the three phases of disease can be treated with imatinib mesylate. Chronic myeloid leukemia appears to respond within one to three months following administration of this drug.

Recommended dosage

A doctor experienced in the treatment of patients with CML should initiate therapy.

To minimize the risk of gastrointestinal irritation, imatinib mesylate should be taken with food and a large glass of water. The recommended dosage varies according to clinical circumstances and phase of disease, but generally ranges between 300 and 600 mg per day. As long as the patient continues to benefit, treatment should be continued.

Precautions

Studies have not been performed with imatinib mesylate to determine if it is a carcinogen (cancer-causing); therefore it is not known whether this drug may cause mutations or may have cancer-causing effects. In addition, imatinib mesylate's safety and effectiveness has not been established in pediatric patients.

- Fluid retention and edema. If patients experience swelling or weight gain from water retention, they should inform their doctor and should be closely monitored. Signs and symptoms of fluid retention should be closely monitored and patients should be weighed regularly. Appropriate treatment must be provided if an unexpected rapid weight gain occurs. The likelihood of edema is increased with higher doses and in those over age 65 years.
- gastrointestinal irritation
- hematologic toxicity (toxicity of the blood)
- hepatotoxicity (toxicity of the liver)
- toxicities from long-term use

Side effects

Commonly reported side effects include **nausea and vomiting**, muscle cramps, edema (water retention), skin rash, **diarrhea**, heartburn, and headache. Serious side effects occur less frequently, but if they occur may include: severe edema liver toxicity, and the potential for bleeding especially in the elderly.

Interactions

Imatinib mesylate interacts with many other drugs. In some cases, side effects may be increased because imatinib mesylate might increase blood levels of certain drugs. Alternatively, imatinib mesylate may decrease blood levels of the drugs, thus reducing their effectiveness. In addition, the blood levels of imatinib mesylate may rise or fall because of other drugs. Therefore, side effects of imatinib mesylate may be increased or effectiveness may be reduced. The patient must discuss all of their medications with their doctor due to many potential drug-drug interactions.

CYP3A4 is an enzyme that is predominately responsible for the metabolism of imatinib mesylate.

The following drugs or families of drugs may interact with imatinib mesylate:

- Inhibitors of the CYP3A4 family, such as ketoconazole, itraconazole, erythromycin.
- Co-medications that induce CYP3A4, such as **dexamethasone**, **phenytoin**, **carbamazepine**, rifampicin, phenobarbital or St. John's Wort). No formal studies have been conducted on these medications and imatinib mesylate together.
- CYP3A4 substrates, such as **cyclosporine** or pimozide.
- CYP3A4 metabolized drugs, such as certain HMG-CoA reductase inhibitors, triazolo-benzodiazepines, and dihydropyridine calcium channel blockers.
- **Warfarin**. Patients needing anticoagulant therapy while taking imatinib mesylate should be prescribed low-molecular weight or standard **heparin**.

This list is not all-inclusive of all possible interactions. Patients must inform their doctors of any drugs they are taking in order to avoid drug interactions.

KEY TERMS

CYP3A4—An enzyme that is predominately responsible for the metabolism of imatinib mesylate.

Enzyme—Any protein that acts as a catalyst, increasing the rate of a chemical reaction.

Kinase—An enzyme.

Leukemia—A type of cancer in which the bone marrow produces an excessive number of abnormal (leukemic) white blood cells. White blood cells protect the body against infection but the abnormal cells suppress the production of normal white blood cells.

Tumor—An abnormal mass of tissue that serves no purpose. Tumors may be either benign (non-cancerous) or malignant (cancerous).

Tyrosine—A non-essential amino acid. Amino acids are the building blocks of protein. They are the raw materials used by the body to make protein. Tyrosine is labeled "nonessential" because, when the amino acids are lacking in the diet, they can be manufactured in the body.

See Also Low molecular weight heparins

Crystal Heather Kaczkowski, MSc.

Immune globulin

Definition

Immune globulin is a concentrated solution of antibodies, pooled from donated blood, which is sometimes given to cancer patients whose own immune systems are either not working or are suppressed as a side effect of treatment. Immune globulin can also be called gamma globulin; in the United States some of the brand names are Gamimune, Gammagard, Gammar-P, Iveegam, Polygam, Sandoglobulin, and Venoglobulin.

Purpose

A healthy human body produces proteins called antibodies that act to destroy microorganisms (bacteria and viruses) that invade the body. Some cancer patients, due to the illness itself or side effects of treatment, become depleted of these proteins and therefore susceptible to serious infections. Immune globulin is given to these patients to restore their body's immunity. The use of immune globulin in this way is also called passive immunization. For example, immune globulin is given to bone marrow transplant recipients to prevent the development of severe bacterial infections while their own immune system is not functioning, and **chronic lymphocytic leukemia** patients (of the type whose antibody-producing cells are the malignant cells) are given immune globulin to prevent the recurrent infections these patients sometimes suffer. Use in this disorder also allows the use of aggressive **chemotherapy** that will destroy the patient's own cancerous antibody-producing cells.

Immune globulin is also used to treat other diseases such as **Eaton-Lambert Syndrome**, a rare neurological disorder that sometimes occurs in association with small cell lung cancer called Eaton-Lambert syndrome, an autoimmune disease in which a patient's own antibodies attack nerve cells. The use of immune globulin appears to cause the body to reduce its own production of antibody, thereby improving the neurological disorder.

Description

Immune globulin primarily consists of antibody proteins of the type called IgG or gamma, although the solution may contain small amounts of other antibody types as well as sugars, proteins, and salt.

It is produced by pooling donated blood from at least 1000 people who have been tested to be free of blood-borne diseases like HIV or hepatitis. The antibody proteins are then separated out of the whole blood, and the pH of the immune globulin solution is adjusted to match the normal pH of blood. The preparation is also treated to remove any contaminants, including infectious bacteria or viruses.

Recommended dosage

The dose of immune globulin used varies with the specific problem that it is being used for. When immune gobulin is used in patients with Eaton-Lambert Syndrome, the effective dose is usually about 1 g/kg of body weight/day. (One gram equals 0.035274 ounce; one kilogram equals 2.2046 pounds.) When used to counteract immunodeficiency, the dose is designed to produce an antibody level that stays at an effective threshold over a period of time.

When immune globulin is given to bone marrow transplant recipients, it is usually begun at the time of the transplant and continued for 100 days thereafter, with the objective of maintaining the level of IgG in the patient's blood above 400 mg per deciliter. (A deciliter equals 3.38 fluid ounces.) In patients with chronic lymphocytic leukemia (B-cell type) the target threshold for antibodies in the patient's blood is usually about 600 mg/dL. Although the amount required to maintain these levels varies from patient to patient (because different patients metabolize the drug at different rates) a dose between 10 and 200 mg/kg of body weight, given every 3-4 weeks, is usually sufficient.

Immune globulin is usually given intravenously, although intramuscular shots are available.

Precautions

Some people may have experienced severe reactions, including allergy-type reactions, to other antibody preparations. Generally these people should not be given intravenous immune globulin. Patients with deficiency of antibody IgA, specifically, should also avoid the use of immune globulin. People with a tendency to form blood clots, or those with kidney problems should also avoid the use of this product, especially if elderly. While many pregnant women have been treated with immune globulin for different problems that have occurred during their pregnancy, since the method of action and specific effects on the fetus are not completely understood, pregnant women should avoid the use of immune globlulin

KEY TERMS

Autoimmune disease—A disease in which the body produces an immunologic reaction against itself.

Epinephrine—A medication used to treat heart failure and severe allergic reactions.

Immunoglobulins—An antibody of a specific type. Five main types are produced, known as IgA, IgD, IgE, Ig G, and IgM. Most antibody in the blood is IgG.

Intramuscular administration—A shot usually in the hip or arm, in which medication is delivered into a muscle.

Intravenous administration—Introduction of medication straight into a vein (commonly called IV).

Neurologic—Involving the nervous system.

unless it is clearly necessary. Any patient who is given immune globulin should be watched carefully, and epinephrine should be kept available in case a severe allergic reaction is experienced. Immune globulin which was made to be given through intramuscular injection should never be administered intravenously.

Side effects

Administration of intramuscular immune globulin may result in tenderness, swelling, and possibly hives at the site of the injection.

Intravenous immune globulin may cause more severe reactions related to rapid introduction into the blood system. Possible side effects include headache, backache, aching muscles, **fever**, low blood pressure, and chest pain. More commonly, fever accompanied by chills or **nausea and vomiting** may be experienced. If these side effects occur, they are usually related to the immune globulin being administered too rapidly. If the rate of infusion is reduced, or if the infusion is stopped temporarily, negative effects will generally disappear. Rare, but potentially serious, side effects observed have been kidney failure and aseptic meningitis.

Interactions

Use of immune globulin may reduce the effectiveness of vaccinations (for example, measles, mumps, and rubella) for a few months following the use of the immune globulin preparation. Patients who have been given immune globulin should notify their doctors before any vaccinations are given. In addition, in some situations patients may need to have antibody levels measured to determine whether or not they have had previous infection with a specific microorganism. Use of immune globulin can create the false impression of prior exposure to the organism due to the donated antibodies in their blood.

See Also Immunologic therapies

Wendy Wippel, M.S.

Immune response

Definition

The ability of any given cell in the body to distinguish self from nonself is called the immune response.

All cells in the body are recognized as self. Any microorganism (for example, a foreign body or tumor) that invades or attacks the cells is recognized as nonself—or foreign—requiring the immune system to mount a combat against the nonself.

Immune system

The immune system is comprised of a network of immune cells that are generated in the bone marrow stem cell (a cell whose daughter cells may develop into other types of cells). From stem cells different types of immune cells originate that can handle specific immune functions. Phagocytes (cell eaters), serve as the first line of defense, engulfing dead cells, debris, virus, and bacteria. Macrophages are an important type of phagocyte, often presenting the antigen—which is usually a foreign protein—to other immune cells and thus are also called "antigen-presenting cells" (APC). T and B lymphocytes, important immune-system cells, are also capable of recognizing the antigen and become activated. T lymphocytes are classified into two subtypes: killer T cells (also called cytotoxic T cells) and helper T cells. Killer T cells recognize and kill the infected or cancer cells that contain the antigen or the foreign protein. Helper T cells release cytokines (chemical messengers) upon activation that either directly destroy the tumor or stimulate other cells to kill the target (tumor). B lymphocytes produce antibodies after recognizing the antigens. The antibodies, which help protect the body from the antigen, are normally specific to that particular antigen. In cases of tumor the specific antibodies attach to tumor cells and,

KEY TERMS

Antigen—Molecules or fragments of molecules that belong to a foreign invader that can elicit an immune response. These may include germs, toxins, and tissues from another person used in organ transplantation.

Cytokines—Proteins (chemical messengers) that are predominantly released by immune cells upon activation or stimulation that help bring about tumor cell death.

Stem cell—A cell whose daughter cells may differentiate (develop into other cell types).

through various mechanisms, impair the functions of the tumor, ultimately leading to the death of the cancer cell.

In addition to these lymphocytes are natural killer (NK) cells that particularly perform the task of eliminating foreign cells. Natural killer cells differ from killer T cells in that they target tumor cells and do not have to recognize an antigen before activation. These cells have been shown to be of potential use in treating cancer.

Immune system and cancer

The immune system serves as one of the primary defenses against cancer. When normal tissue becomes a tumor or cancerous tissue, new antigens develop on their surface. These antigens send a signal to immune cells such as the cytotoxic T lymphocytes, NK cells, and macrophages, which in turn directly kill the tumor cells or release substances like cytokines that may bring about tumor cell death. Thus, under normal circumstances, the immune system provides continued surveillance and eliminates cells that become cancers. However, tumors may survive by hiding or disguising their tumor antigens, or by producing substances that allow suppressor T cells (cells that block cytotoxic, or killer T cells that would normally attack the tumor) to proliferate (multiply).

Biological response modifiers in cancer therapy

Researchers have been working on stimulating the immune cells during cancer with substances broadly classified as biological response modifiers. Cytokines are one such substance. These are proteins that are predominantly released by immune cells upon activation or stimulation. During the 1990s the number of cytokines identified increased enormously and the functions associated with them are of immense potential in diagnostics and immune therapy. Some of the key cytokines that have proven therapeutic value in cancer are interleukin-2 (IL-2), Interferon gamma, and interleukin-12 (IL-12). Cytokines are normally injected directly to cancer patients; however, there are other cases where a cancer patient's own lymphocytes are modified under laboratory conditions and injected back into the patient. Examples of these are lymphokine-activated killer (LAK) cells and tumor-infiltrating lymphocytes (TILs). These modified cells are capable of devouring cancer cells.

Immunoprevention of cancer

Immunotherapy is emerging as one of the management strategies for cancer. However, established tumors or large masses of tumor do not respond well to immunotherapy. There is clinical evidence, however, that suggests that patients with minimal residual cancer cells (a few cells left after other forms of cancer treatment) are potential candidates for effective immunotherapy. In these cases immunotherapy often results in a prolonged tumor-free survival. Thus, immune responses can be manipulated to prevent recurrence, even though it does not destroy large tumors. Based on results of immunotherapy trials, most immune therapies are geared towards designing immunoprotective strategies such as cancer **vaccines**.

Cancer vaccines

Cancer vaccines can be made either with whole, inactivated tumor cells, or with fragments or cell surface substances (called cell-surface antigens) present in the tumors. In addition to the whole cell or antigen vaccines, biological modifiers, like cytokines, serve as substances that boost immune response in cancer patients.

Since cancer vaccines are still under clinical evaluation, caution should be exercised while choosing them as the mode of therapy. The cancer care team will provide further insight on whether or not cancer vaccine or cytokine therapy will be beneficial after they assess the patient's stage and the various modes of treatments available.

Kausalya Santhanam, Ph.D.

Resources

BOOKS

DeVita, Vincent T., Samuel Hellman, and Steven A. Rosenberg, eds. *Cancer: Principles and Practice of Oncology.* Philadelphia: J. B. Lippincott Company, 1997.

PERIODICALS

"Immunoprevention of Cancer: Is the Time Ripe?" *Cancer Research* (15 May 2000) 60: 2571-2575

"Therapies of the Future: Immunotherapy for Cancer." *Scientific American* (October 1996).

"Genetic Vaccines." *Scientific American* (July 1999).

OTHER

"Treating Cancer with Vaccine Therapy." *National Cancer Institute.* 2000. 5 July 2001 <http://cancertrials.nci.nih.gov/news/features/vaccine/html/page05.html>.

Immunoelectrophoresis

Definition

Immunoelectrophoresis, also called gamma globulin electrophoresis, or immunoglobulin electrophoresis, is a method of determining the blood levels of three major immunoglobulins: immunoglobulin M (IgM), immunoglobulin G (IgG), and immunoglobulin A (IgA).

Purpose

Immunoelectrophoresis is a powerful analytical technique with high resolving power as it combines separation of antigens by electrophoresis with immunodiffusion against an antiserum. The increased resolution is of benefit in the immunological examination of serum proteins. Immunoelectrophoresis aids in the diagnosis and evaluation of the therapeutic response in many disease states affecting the immune system. It is usually requested when a different type of electrophoresis, called a serum **protein electrophoresis**, has indicated a rise at the immunoglobulin level. Immunoelectrophoresis is also used frequently to diagnose **multiple myeloma**, a disease affecting the bone marrow.

Precautions

Drugs that may cause increased immunoglobulin levels include therapeutic gamma globulin, hydralazine, isoniazid, **phenytoin** (Dilantin), procainamide, oral contraceptives, methadone, steroids, and tetanus toxoid and antitoxin. The laboratory should be notified if the patient has received any vaccinations or immunizations in the six months before the test. This is mainly because prior immunizations lead to the increased immunoglobulin levels resulting in false positive results.

It should be noted that, because immunoelectrophoresis is not quantitative, it is being replaced by a procedure called immunofixation, which is more sensitive and easier to interpret.

Description

Serum proteins separate in agar gels under the influence of an electric field into albumin, alpha 1, alpha 2, and beta and gamma globulins. Immunoelectrophoresis is performed by placing serum on a slide containing a gel designed specifically for the test. An electric current is then passed through the gel, and immunoglobulins, which contain an electric charge, migrate through the gel according to the difference in their individual electric charges. Antiserum is placed alongside the slide to identify the specific type of immunoglobulin present. The results are used to identify different disease entities, and to aid in monitoring the course of the disease and the therapeutic response of the patient with such conditions as immune deficiencies, autoimmune disease, chronic infections, chronic viral infections, intrauterine fetal infections, multiple myeloma, and monoclonal gammopathy of undetermined significance.

There are five classes of antibodies: IgM, IgG, IgA, IgE, and IgD.

IgM is produced upon initial exposure to an antigen. For example, when a person receives the first tetanus vaccination, antitetanus antibodies of the IgM class are produced 10 to 14 days later. IgM is abundant in the blood but is not normally present in organs or tissues. IgM is primarily responsible for ABO blood grouping and rheumatoid factor, yet is involved in the immunologic reaction to other infections, such as hepatitis. Since IgM does not cross the placenta, an elevation of this immunoglobulin in the newborn indicates intrauterine infection such as rubella, cytomegalovirus (CMV) or a sexually transmitted disease (STD).

IgG is the most prevalent type of antibody, comprising approximately 75% of the serum immunoglobulins. IgG is produced upon subsequent exposure to an antigen. As an example, after receiving a second tetanus shot, or booster, a person produces IgG antibodies in five to seven days. IgG is present in both the blood and tissues, and is the only antibody to cross the placenta from the mother to the fetus. Maternal IgG protects the newborn for the first months of life, until the infant's immune system produces its own antibodies.

IgA constitutes approximately 15% of the immunoglobulins within the body. Although it is found to some degree in the blood, it is present primarily in the secretions of the respiratory and gastrointestinal tract, in saliva, colostrum (the yellowish fluid produced by the breasts during late pregnancy and the first few days after childbirth), and in tears. IgA plays an important role in defending the body against invasion of germs through the mucous membrane-lined organs.

KEY TERMS

Antibody—A protein manufactured by the white blood cells to neutralize an antigen in the body. In some cases, excessive formation of antibodies leads to illness, allergy, or autoimmune disorders.

Antigen—A substance that can cause an immune response, resulting in production of an antibody, as part of the body's defense against infection and disease. Many antigens are foreign proteins not found naturally in the body, and include germs, toxins, and tissues from another person used in organ transplantation.

Autoimmune disorder—A condition in which antibodies are formed against the body's own tissues, for example, in some forms of arthritis.

IgE is the antibody that causes acute allergic reactions; it is measured to detect allergic conditions. IgD, which constitutes the smallest portion of the immunoglobulins, is rarely evaluated or detected, and its function is not well understood.

Preparation

This test requires a blood sample.

Aftercare

Because this test is ordered when either very low or very high levels of immunoglobulins are suspected, the patient should be alert for any signs of infection after the test, including **fever**, chills, rash, or skin ulcers. Any **bone pain** or tenderness should also be immediately reported to the physician.

Risks

Risks for this test are minimal, but may include slight bleeding from the blood-drawing site, fainting or feeling lightheaded after venipuncture, or bruising.

Normal results

Reference ranges vary from laboratory to laboratory and depend upon the method used. For adults, normal values are usually found within the following ranges (1 mg = approximately.000035 oz. and 1 dL = approximately 0.33 fluid oz.):

- IgM: 60–290 mg/dL
- IgG: 700–1,800 mg/dL
- IgA: 70–440 mg/dL

Abnormal results

Increased IgM levels can indicate **Waldenström's macroglobulinemia**, a malignancy caused by secretion of IgM at high levels by malignant lymphoplasma cells. Increased IgM levels can also indicate chronic infections, such as hepatitis or mononucleosis and autoimmune diseases, like rheumatoid arthritis.

Decreased IgM levels can be indicative of AIDS, immunosuppression caused by certain drugs like steroids or dextran, or leukemia.

Increased levels of IgG can indicate chronic liver disease, autoimmune diseases, hyperimmunization reactions, or certain chronic infections, such as tuberculosis or sarcoidosis.

Decreased levels of IgG can indicate Wiskott-Aldrich syndrome, a genetic deficiency caused by inadequate synthesis of IgG and other immunoglobulins. Decreased IgG can also be seen with AIDS and leukemia.

Increased levels of IgA can indicate chronic liver disease, chronic infections, or inflammatory bowel disease.

Decreased levels of IgA can be found in ataxia, a condition affecting balance and gait, limb or eye movements, speech, and telangiectasia, an increase in the size and number of the small blood vessels in an area of skin, causing redness. Decreased IgA levels are also seen in conditions of low blood protein (hypoproteinemia), and drug immunosuppression.

Resources

BOOKS

Fischbach, Frances T. *A Manual of Laboratory Diagnostic Tests.* Philadelphia: Lippincott Williams & Wilkins, 1999.

Pagana, Kathleen D., and Timothy J. Pagana. *Mosby's Manual of Diagnostic and Laboratory Tests.* St. Louis, MO: Mosby, Inc., 1999.

Janis O. Flores

Immunohistochemistry

Definition

Immunohistochemistry is a method of analyzing and identifying cell types based on the binding of antibodies to specific components of the cell. It is sometimes referred to as immunocytochemistry.

Purpose

Immunohistochemistry (IHC) is used to diagnose the type of cancer and to help determine the patient's prognosis. In cases such as metastases or **carcinoma of unknown primary** origin, where it may be difficult to determine the type of cell from which the tumor originated, immunohistochemistry can identify cells by the characteristic markers on the cell surface. IHC can also help distinguish between benign and malignant tumors.

Description

Immunohistochemistry requires a sample of tissue from a **biopsy**; usually the tissue sample is examined fresh, but frozen or chemically preserved material can be used. A blood sample or bone marrow may also be examined. The tissue sample is sliced extremely thinly, so that it is approximately one cell thick, then the sample is fixed onto a glass slide. The tumor cells in the sample have characteristic markers, or antigens, on their cell surfaces which can be used to help identify the specific type of tumor cell. Antibodies against these characteristic antigens are added to the sample on the slide, and the antibodies bind wherever the antigens are present. Excess antibody is then washed away. The antibodies that remain bound to the cell have labels on them that either fluoresce (glow) or undergo a chemical reaction that makes them visible by microscope. The pathologist is able to see the specially labeled tumor antigens as they appear in the patient's tissue.

The pathologist will try to assess the level of maturity of the tumor cells, which will help him to determine their origin. He will be checking for cell types that are found in an inappropriate part of the body, for example prostate cells in a lymph node. He will also look for cell characteristics that will indicate if the tumor is benign or malignant. Proteins involved in the replication of genetic material and cell growth may be present in greater amounts; for example, antibodies against the antigen Ki-67 are used to evaluate malignant melanomas, breast carcinomas, and **non-Hodgkin's lymphomas**. Hormone receptors may also be examined. The presence of receptors to estrogen and progesterone indicate a good prognosis for **breast cancer** patients. Pathologists may also look for an increase in tumor suppressor proteins. A wide variety of antibodies are available to help determine the origin of the tumor, whether it is growing rapidly, and whether it is a type of tumor that responds well to particular treatments.

Preparation

The physician will choose the type of sample to be taken based on the type of tumor. If the patient has a solid tumor, a tissue sample may be biopsied; if the entire tumor is being removed a biopsy may be taken during surgery. In this case the patient should prepare for the surgery or the biopsy as the physician suggests. A routine blood sample may also be required; in most cases, no additional preparation is required.

KEY TERMS

Antibody—A protein formed by the immune system to react with a specific antigen.

Antigen—Any protein that elicits a unique immune response.

Biopsy—A sample of tissue taken from a tumor to compare with other normal tissue.

Histology—The study of tissues.

Aftercare

The only aftercare that might be required is from the sample collection process.

Risks

The risks associated with IHC are the risks associated with the sample collection, either the biopsy of the tumor or the drawing of blood. The only other concern is the possibility that the test could yield unclear results.

Normal results

Normal results will simply look like normal cells. The cells will have a high level of maturity and be located only in sites appropriate to their cell type. For example, analysis of lymph nodes will show only the cells that belong there, not cells that would normally be present in the breast. No specific tumor antigens will be present in increased numbers.

Abnormal results

An abnormal result would consist of cells which appear immature or poorly differentiated, or that are found in an inappropriate tissue for their cell type. The pathologist may test for the presence of a particular antigen, such as Ki-67, carcinoembryonic antigen (CEA), or prostate specific antigen (PSA). In this case, there may be a numerical standard value to compare normal to abnormal results and help the physician in determining prognosis.

See Also Receptor analysis; Tumor markers

QUESTIONS TO ASK THE DOCTOR

- What do you expect to learn from this test?
- What are the alternatives to this test?
- Are there any risks or complications?
- Are any special preparations required?
- Is hospitalization required?
- Is it possible that the test may give a false positive, a false negative, or unclear results?

Resources

BOOKS

Javois, Lorette C. *Immunocytochemical Methods and Protocols* Totowa, NJ:Humana Press Inc., 1999.

Polak, J.M., and S. Van Noorden. *Introduction to Immunocytochemistry* New York: Springer-Verlag, 1997.

PERIODICALS

Bendayan, Moise. "Worth Its Weight in Gold." In *Science* 291(16 February 2001): 1363–1365.

Cote, RJ et al. "Role of Immunohistochemical Detection of Lymph-Node Metastases in Management of Breast Cancer." In *The Lancet* 354:(11 September 1999): 896–900.

Elledge, Richard M. and C Kent Osborne. "Oestrogen Receptors and Breast Cancer."*British Medical Journal* 314:(28 June 1997): 1843–1845.

Gastl, Gunther et al. "Ep-CAM Overexpression in Breast Cancer as a Predictor of Survival." In *The Lancet* 356:(9 December 2000) 1981–1982.

Racquel Baert, M.S.

Immunologic therapies

Definition

Immunologic therapy is the treatment of disease using medicines that boost the body's natural **immune response**.

Purpose

Immunologic therapy is used to improve the immune system's natural ability to fight diseases such as cancer, hepatitis and AIDS. These drugs may also be used to help the body recover from immunosuppression resulting from treatments such as **chemotherapy** or **radiation therapy**.

Description

Most drugs in this category are synthetic versions of substances produced naturally in the body. In their natural forms, these substances help defend the body against disease. For example, **aldesleukin** (Proleukin) is an artificially-made form of interleukin-2, which helps white blood cells work. Aldesleukin is administered to patients with kidney cancers and skin cancers that have spread to other parts of the body. **Filgrastim** (Neupogen) and **sargramostim** (Leukine) are versions of natural substances called colony stimulating factors, which drive the bone marrow to make new white blood cells. Another type of drug, epoetin (Epogen, Procrit), is a synthetic version of human **erythropoietin** that stimulates the bone marrow to make new red blood cells. **Thrombopoietin** stimulates the production of platelets, disk-shaped bodies in the blood that are important in clotting. **Interferons** are substances the body produces naturally using immune cells to fight infections and tumors. The synthetic interferons carry brand names such as Alferon, Roferon or Intron A. Some of the interferons that are currently in use as drugs are Recombinant Interferon Alfa-2a, Recombinant Interferon Alfa-2b, interferon alfa-n1 and Interferon Alfa-n3. Alfa interferons are used to treat **hairy cell leukemia**, malignant **melanoma** and AIDs-related **Kaposi's sarcoma**. In addition interferons are also used for other conditions such as laryngeal papillomatosis, genital warts and certain types of hepatitis.

Recommended dosage

The recommended dosage depends on the type of immunologic therapy. For some medicines, the physician will decide the dosage for each patient, taking into account a patient's weight and whether he/she is taking other medicines. Some drugs used in immunologic therapy are given only in a hospital, under a physician's supervision. For those that patients may give themselves, check with the physician who prescribed the medicine or the pharmacist who filled the prescription for the correct dosage.

Most of these drugs come in injectable form. These drugs are generally administered by the cancer care provider.

Precautions

Aldesleukin

This medicine may temporarily increase the chance of getting infections. It may also lower the number of platelets in the blood, and thus possibly interfering with the blood's ability to clot. Taking these precautions may reduce the chance of such problems:

- Avoid people with infections, if possible.
- Be alert to signs of infection, such as **fever**, chills, sore throat, pain in the lower back or side, cough, hoarseness, or painful or difficulty with urination. If any of these symptoms occur, get in touch with a physician immediately.
- Be alert to signs of bleeding problems, such as black, tarry stools, iny red spots on the skin, blood in the urine or stools, or any other unusual bleeding or bruising.
- Take care to avoid cuts or other injuries. Be especially careful when using knives, razors, nail clippers and other sharp objects. Check with a dentist for the best ways to clean the teeth and mouth without injuring the gums. Do not have dental work done without checking with a physician.
- Wash hands frequently, and avoid touching the eyes or inside of the nose unless the hands have just been washed.

Aldesleukin may make some medical conditions worse, such as chickenpox, shingles (**herpes zoster**), liver disease, lung disease, heart disease, underactive thyroid, psoriasis, immune system problems and mental problems. The medicine may increase the chance of seizures (convulsions) in people who are prone to having them. Also, the drug's effects may be greater in people with kidney disease, because their kidneys are slow to clear the medicine from their bodies.

Colony stimulating factors

Certain drugs used in treating cancer reduce the body's ability to fight infections. Although colony stimulating factors help restore the body's natural defenses, the process takes time. Getting prompt treatment for infections is important, even while taking this medicine. Call the physician at the first sign of illness or infection, such as a sore throat, fever or chills.

People with certain medical conditions could have problems if they take colony stimulating factors. People who have kidney disease, liver disease or conditions caused by inflammation or immune system problems can worsen these problems with colony stimulating factors. Those who have heart disease may be more likely to experience side effects such as water retention and heart rhythm problems while taking these drugs. Finally, patients who have lung disease might increase their chances of suffering from shortness of breath. Those who have any of these medical conditions should check with their personal physicians before using colony stimulating factors.

Epoetin

Epoetin is a medicine that may cause seizures (convulsions), especially in people who are prone to having them. No one who takes these drugs should drive, use machines or do anything considered dangerous in case of a seizure.

Epoetin helps the body make new red blood cells, but it is not effective unless there is adequate iron in the body. The physician may recommend taking iron supplements or certain **vitamins** that help supply the body with iron. It is necessary to follow the physician's advice in this instance —recommendations for iron in this case, as with any supplements should only come from a physician.

In studies of laboratory animals, epoetin taken during pregnancy caused birth defects, including damage to the bones and spine. However, the drug has not been reported to cause problems in human babies whose mothers take it. Women who are pregnant or who may become pregnant should check with their physicians for the most up-to-date information on the safety of taking this medicine during pregnancy.

People with certain medical conditions may have problems if they take this medicine. For example, the chance of side effects may be greater in people with high blood pressure, heart or blood vessel disease or a history of blood clots. Epoetin may not work properly in people who have bone problems or sickle cell anemia.

Interferons

Interferons can add to the effects of alcohol and other drugs that slow down the central nervous system, such as antihistamines, cold medicine, allergy medicine, sleep aids, medicine for seizures, tranquilizers, some pain relievers, and muscle relaxants. They may also add to the effects of anesthetics, including those used for dental procedures. Those taking interferons should check with their physicians before taking any of the above.

Some people experience dizziness, unusual fatigue, or become less alert than usual while being treated with these drugs. Because of these possible problems, anyone who takes these drugs should not drive, use machines or do anything else considered dangerous until they have determined how the drugs affect them.

Interferons often cause flu-like symptoms, including fever and chills. The physician who prescribes this medicine may recommend taking acetaminophen (Tylenol) before—and sometimes after—each dose to keep the fever from getting too high. If the physician recommends this, follow instructions carefully.

Like aldesleukin, interferons may temporarily increase the chance of getting infections and lower the number of platelets in the blood, leading to clotting problems. To help prevent these problems, follow the precautions for reducing the risk of infection and bleeding listed for aldesleukin.

People who have certain medical conditions may have problems if they take interferons. For example, the drugs may worsen some medical conditions, including heart disease, kidney disease, liver disease, lung disease, diabetes, bleeding problems and mental problems. In people who have overactive immune systems, these drugs can even increase the activity of the immune system. People who have shingles or chickenpox, or who have recently been exposed to chickenpox may increase their risk of developing severe problems in other parts of the body if they take interferons. People with a history of seizures or mental problems could at risk if taking interferon.

In teenage women, interferons may cause changes in the menstrual cycle. Young women should discuss this possibility with their physicians. Older people may be more sensitive to the effects of interferons. This may increase the chance of side effects.

These drugs are not known to cause fetal death, birth defects or other problems in humans when taken during pregnancy. Women who are pregnant or who may become pregnant should ask their physicians for the latest information on the safety of taking these drugs during pregnancy.

Women who are breastfeeding their babies may need to stop while taking this medicine. Whether interferons pass into breast milk is not known. Because of the chance of serious side effects to the baby, breast-feeding while taking interferon is discouraged. Check with a physician for advice.

General precautions for all types of immunologic therapy

Regular physician visits are necessary during immunologic therapy treatment. This gives the physician a chance to make sure the medicine is working and to check for unwanted side effects.

Anyone who has had unusual reactions to drugs used in immunologic therapy should let the physician know before resuming the drugs. Any allergies to foods, dyes, preservatives, or other substances should also be reported.

Side effects

Aldesleukin

In addition to its helpful effects, this medicine may cause serious side effects. Generally, it is given only in a hospital, where medical professionals can watch for early signs of problems. Medical tests might be performed to check for unwanted effects.

Anyone who has breathing problems, fever or chills while being given aldesleukin should check with a physician immediately.

Other side effects should be brought to a physician's attention as soon as possible:

- dizziness
- drowsiness
- confusion
- agitation
- **depression**
- **nausea and vomiting**
- **diarrhea**
- sores in the mouth and on the lips
- tingling of hands or feet
- decrease in urination
- unexplained weight gain of five or more pounds

Some side effects are usually temporary and do not need medical attention unless they are bothersome. These include dry skin; itchy or burning skin rash or redness followed by peeling; loss of appetite; and a general feeling of illness or discomfort.

Colony stimulating factors

As this medicine starts to work, the patient might experience mild pain in the lower back or hips. This is nothing to cause undue concern, and will usually go away within a few days. If the pain is intense or causes discomfort, the physician may prescribe a painkiller.

Other possible side effects include headache, joint or muscle pain and skin rash or **itching**. These side effects tend to disappear as the body adjusts to the medicine, and do not need medical treatment. If they continue, or they interfere with normal activities, check with a physician.

Epoetin

This medicine may cause flu-like symptoms, such as muscle aches, **bone pain**, fever, chills, shivering, and sweating, within a few hours after it is taken. These symptoms usually go away within 12 hours. If they do not, or if they are troubling, check with a physician. Other possible side effects that do not need medical attention are diarrhea, nausea or vomiting and fatigue or weakness.

Certain side effects should be brought to a physician's attention as soon as possible. These include headache, vision problems, increased blood pressure, fast heartbeat, weight gain and swelling of the face, fingers, lower legs, ankles or feet.

Anyone who has chest pain or seizures after taking epoetin should seek professional emergency medical attention immediately.

KEY TERMS

AIDS—Acquired immunodeficiency syndrome. A disease caused by infection with the human immunodeficiency virus (HIV). In people with this disease, the immune system breaks down, increasing vulnerability to other infections and some types of cancer.

Bone marrow—Soft tissue that fills the hollow centers of bones. Blood cells and platelets (disk-shaped bodies in the blood that are important in clotting) are produced in the bone marrow.

Chemotherapy—Treatment of an illness with chemical agents. The term is usually used to describe the treatment of cancer with drugs.

Clot—A hard mass that forms when blood gels.

Fetus—A developing baby inside the womb.

Hepatitis—Inflammation of the liver caused by a virus, chemical, or drug.

Immune response—The body's natural, protective reaction to disease and infection.

Immune system—The system that protects the body against disease and infection through immune responses.

Inflammation—Pain, redness, swelling, and heat that usually develop in response to injury or illness.

Psoriasis—A skin disease that manifests itself with itchy, scaly, red patches on the skin.

Seizure—A sudden attack, spasm, or convulsion.

Shingles—A disease caused by an infection with the Herpes zoster virus—the same virus that causes chickenpox. Symptoms of shingles include pain and blisters along one nerve, usually on the face, chest, stomach, or back.

Sickle cell anemia—An inherited disorder in which red blood cells contain an abnormal form of hemoglobin, a protein that carries oxygen. The abnormal form of hemoglobin causes the red cells to become sickle-shaped. The misshapen cells may clog blood vessels, preventing oxygen from reaching tissues and leading to pain, blood clots and other problems. Sickle cell anemia is most common in people of African descent and in people from Italy, Greece, India, and the Middle East.

Interferons

This medicine may cause temporary hair loss (**alopecia**). While upsetting, it is not a sign that something is seriously wrong. The hair should grow back normally after treatment ends.

As the body adjusts to the medicine many other side effects usually go away during treatment. These include flu-like symptoms, **taste alteration**, loss of appetite (**anorexia**), nausea and vomiting, skin rash, and unusual fatigue. If these problems persist, or if they interfere with normal life, check with a physician.

A few more serious side effects should be brought to a physician's attention as soon as possible:

- confusion
- difficulty thinking or concentrating
- nervousness
- depression
- sleep problems
- numbness or tingling in the fingers, toes and face

General caution regarding side effects for all types of immunologic therapy

Other side effects are possible with any type of immunologic therapy. Anyone who has unusual symptoms during or after treatment with these drugs should should contact the physician immediately.

Interactions

Anyone who has immunologic therapy should let the physician know all other medicines being taken. Some combinations of drugs may interact, that can increase or decrease the effects of one or both drugs or can increase the likelihood of side effects. Consultation with a physician is highly recommended to get the insight on whether the possible interactions can interfere with drug therapy or cause harmful effects.

Immunoprevention

Considering that most of the biological modifiers such as cytokines elicit immune response that inhibit incipient tumors before they are clinically evident, immunoprevention has been proposed as a recent strategy for combating cancer. Treatment involving immune molecules (such as cytokines) prepared synthetically or that are not produced by the patients themselves is called as passive immunotherapy. Conversely, a vaccine is a form of active immune therapy because it elicits an immune response in patients. A cancer vaccine may be made of whole tumor cell or of substances or fragments contained in the tumor called as antigens.

Adoptive Immunotherapy

Adoptive immunotherapy involves stimulating T lymphocytes by exposing them to tumor antigens. These modified cells are grown in the laboratory and then injected into patients. Since the cells taken from a different individual for this purpose often results in rejection, patients serve both as donor and recipient of their own T cells. Adoptive immunotherapy is particularly effective in patients who have received massive doses of radiation and chemotherapy. In such patients, therapy results in immunosuppression (weakened immune systems), making them vulnerable to viral infections. For example, CMV-specific T cells can reduce the risk of cytomegalovirus (CMV) infection in transplant patients.

Resources

BOOKS

Reiger, Paula T. *Biotherapy: A Comprehensive Overview.* Sudbury: Jones and Bartley, Inc. 2000.

Stern, Peter L., P.C. Beverley, M. Carroll. *Cancer Vaccines and Immunotherapy.* New York: Cambridge University Press, 2000.

PERIODICALS

National Cancer Institute. *Treating Cancer with Vaccine therapy* <http://cancertrials.nci.nih.gov/news/features/vaccine/html/page05.htm> 2000. 29 June 2001.

"Immunoprevention of Cancer: Is the time Ripe?" *Cancer Research* 60: 2571–2575, May 15, 2000.

MEDLINE plus Drug information *Aldesleukin (Systemic)* <http://www.nlm.nih.gov/ medlineplus/druginfo/aldesleukinsystemic202669.html> June 1998. 29 June 2001.

MEDLINE plus Drug information *Interferons, Alpha (Systemic)* <http://www.nlm.nih.gov/medlineplus/druginfo/interferonsalphasystemic202299.html> July 1998; 29 June 2001.

Rosenberg, S. A. "Progress in human tumor immunology and immunotherapy." *Nature* 411, no. 6835 (2001): 380-385.

Nancy Ross-Flanigan
Kausalya Santhanam, Ph.D.

Immunotherapy *see* **Immunologic therapies**

Implantable subcutaneous ports *see* **Vascular access**

Incontinence

Description

Incontinence is the loss of normal control of the bowel or bladder. Incontinence can involve the involuntary voiding of urine (urinary incontinence) or of stool and gas (fecal or bowel incontinence). There are several types of urinary incontinence. Those most frequently seen as side effects of cancer include overflow incontinence, urge incontinence, and stress incontinence. In rare cases incontinence occurs as the result of cancer, but more commonly it is a side effect of treatment. Because the subjects of bowel and bladder control are perceived as socially unacceptable, those affected with incontinence often feel ashamed or embarrassed by the problem. Instead of seeking medical attention, these individuals try to hide the problem or manage it themselves. For this reason, incontinence is sometimes referred to as "the silent affliction." Impacts of incontinence include low self-esteem, social withdrawal and isolation, and **depression**. In most cases incontinence can be successfully treated, so affected individuals should discuss the problem with a doctor.

Causes

Incontinence can result from damage to the muscle, nerves, or the structure of the body parts involved in the control of voiding. Complex systems of hollow organs (such as the bladder) and tube-shaped structures (such as the rectum and urethra) work together to store and release waste. Special muscles, including sphincters, are especially important in maintaining the tight seals that hold in waste. When physical damage to muscle or organ structure occurs, the system can no longer maintain these tight seals, and waste can leak out.

Nerves carry messages between the brain and the bowel and bladder systems. Injury to these nerves, or the related part of the brain, interferes with the delivery of these messages, which can prevent the body from recognizing the signals telling it when to void. Without these signals and messages, an individual cannot coordinate the brain with the bowel and bladder systems, and incontinence results.

Several types of cancer and its treatments are associated with incontinence. Usually, it is the treatment of cancer that causes incontinence, rather than the cancer itself.

Prostate cancer

The treatment of **prostate cancer** is one of the most common causes of cancer-related urinary incontinence, largely because the prostate is located so closely to the nerves, muscles, and structures involved in urine control. Surgical removal of the prostate, or **prostatectomy**, carries the highest risk of urinary incontinence as a side effect; the risk from **radiation therapy** is somewhat lower. The incontinence (typically stress or urge incontinence) is often temporary, but in a small percentage of men it may be long lasting.

Prostate cancer itself seldom causes incontinence. However, this depends on the location and size of the cancer; a large cancerous prostate can interfere with the flow of urine and result in overflow incontinence.

Bladder cancer

Incontinence is only occasionally the direct result of **bladder cancer**, but it is a common side effect of some treatments. For early-stage cancer where treatment does not require the bladder to be removed, incontinence almost never occurs. But removal of the bladder and surrounding structures is often necessary to treat more advanced cancer. This requires creation of an artificial system for storing and releasing urine and carries a risk of long-term incontinence.

Colon cancer and rectal cancer

Muscles in the anal and rectal region largely control bowel evacuation, with the colon storing stool and gas. When these regions are removed or damaged during cancer treatment, or if injury to the related nerves occurs, fecal incontinence can result. Fecal incontinence is most commonly a side effect of surgery. Weakening of bowel muscles or damaging of nerves by radiation therapy can also cause incontinence, but this type is more likely to be mild and temporary, and will often improve as these areas heal. However, in some patients, radiation causes permanent and severe fecal incontinence.

Other causes

Loss of voluntary bowel and bladder control is less commonly associated with other cancers of the genital and urinary systems, mainly as a side effect of treatment. Incontinence can also result from cancer or treatment damage in the brain and spinal cord. Other cancers indirectly cause incontinence; for example, constant coughing from lung cancer can lead to stress incontinence. Very rarely, incontinence can be a side effect of certain medications.

KEY TERMS

Evacuation—Release of stool or gas from the bowel system.

Overflow incontinence—Slow leaking or dripping of urine from an overfilled bladder that may be unable to empty completely.

Sphincter—A circular muscle that relaxes and tightens to control the storage and release of bodily waste.

Stress incontinence—Involuntary loss of waste resulting from sudden pressure or force, such as by coughing, sneezing, laughing, or lifting an object.

Urethra—A tube-like structure allowing the passage of urine between the bladder and the outside of the body.

Urge incontinence—Involuntary loss of waste after feeling a strong, sudden need to void, without enough time to get to a toilet.

Voiding—Release of urine from the bladder system.

Treatments and complementary therapies

The method of treatment depends on the cause and type of incontinence. Surgical treatment is usually reserved for severe or long-lasting incontinence. An artificial pouch for storing urine or stool can be placed inside the body as a substitute for a removed bladder, colon, or rectum. Placement of an artificial sphincter successfully treats other cases. For mild or temporary incontinence, treatment may include medications, dietary changes, muscle-strengthening exercises, or behavioral training, such as establishing a time pattern for voiding. A small group of patients, however, requires a permanent **colostomy** or **urostomy**.

Electrical stimulation therapy, which targets involved muscles with low-current electricity, can be used to treat either urinary or fecal incontinence. Biofeedback uses electronic or mechanical devices to improve bladder or bowel control by teaching an individual how to recognize and respond to certain body signals.

Embarrassment may lead some people to manage the symptoms of incontinence themselves by wearing absorbent pads to prevent the soiling of their clothes. However, many treatments exist to successfully restore or improve control of bowel and bladder function, so individuals experiencing incontinence should speak to a doctor or nurse.

Resources

BOOKS

Walsh, Patrick C., and Alan B. Retik. *Campbell's Urology* Seventh edition. Philadelphia: W. B. Saunders Co., 1998.

PERIODICALS

Jackson, Susan L., Tracy L. Hull. "Fecal Incontinence in Women." *Obstetrical and Gynecological Survey* Vol. 53, no. 12 (December, 1998): pp. 741–747.

Kamm, Michael. "Fortnightly Review:Faecal Incontinence." *British Medical Journal* Vol. 316, no. 7130: pp. 528–532.

Kunkel, Elisabeth J. S., M.D., Jennifer R. Bakker, Ronald E. Meyers, Ph.D., Olo Oyesanmi, M.D., and Leonard Gomella, M.D. "Biopsychosocial Aspects of Prostate Cancer." *Psychosomatics* Vol. 42, no. 2 (March/April 2000): pp.85–94.

Scientific Committee of the First International Consultation on Incontinence. "Assessment and treatment of urinary incontinence." *The Lancet* Vol. 355, no. 9221 (June 17, 2000): pp. 2153–2158.

Smith, Dorothy B., RN, MS, CETN, FAAN. "Urinary Continence Issues in Oncology." *Clinical Journal of Oncology Nursing* Vol. 3, No. 4: 161–167.

Stefanie B. N. Dugan, M.S.

Infection and sepsis

Description

Infection is characterized by an inflammatory response to the presence of microorganisms in the body. This response may include **fever**, chills, redness, swelling, pus formation and other responses. The most common cause of illness and death in patients with cancer is infection. Patients with cancer who are treated with **chemotherapy**, **radiation therapy**, and/or surgery are at increased risk of developing an infection. Mortality, or death, from infection in cancer patients decreased during the late 1900s due to the development of new types of **antibiotics**, the use of hematopoietic growth factors (HGFs) which activate proliferation (multiplication) and maturation of blood cell lines, and due to the prophylactic (preventive) use of antifungal and antiviral agents. Blood cell lines, markedly decreased due to chemotherapy, are required to fight infections. Most infections in cancer patients are due to bacteria; however, fungal infections are usually the cause of fatal infections.

If left untreated, or if inadequately treated, infection can progress to sepsis. Sepsis is defined as a systemic (total body) inflammatory response to the presence of microorganisms in the body. Several conditions indicate sepsis, including a temperature of greater than 38 degrees Centigrade (100.4 Fahrenheit) or less than 36 degrees Centigrade (96.8 Fahrenheit), heart rate greater than 90 beats per minutes, and respiratory rate greater than 20 breaths per minute. The incidence rate of sepsis in cancer patients is estimated at 45%. Mortality rates from sepsis in cancer patients exceed 30%.

Causes

There are many possible causes of infection in the patient with cancer. For example, certain cancers interfere with the body's immune system response, which results in increased risk of infection to the patient. These cancer types include **acute leukemia**, **chronic lymphocytic leukemia**, **multiple myeloma**, **Hodgkin's disease**, and non-Hodgkin's lymphoma. Certain therapies used to treat cancer, such as chemotherapy (which interrupts bone marrow production of white blood cells, red blood cells, and platelets), radiation therapy, **bone marrow transplantation**, and treatments using **corticosteroids**, can lead to infection in the patient with cancer. The protein-calorie malnutrition that some cancer patients experience can result in suppression of the immune system, which results in increased risk for infection. Many cancer patients develop infections from procedures which break the integrity of the skin, which then leads to the introduction of microorganisms into the body. These procedures include common interventions in the care of cancer patients such as venipunctures, biopsies, insertion of urinary catheters, and use of long-term central venous catheters. Infection rates associated with long-term central venous catheter use in cancer patients is estimated to be as high as 60%. If the cancer patient's immune system is severely compromised, infection can occur from food sources, plants, and/or air the patient comes in contact with.

Myelosuppression is the term used to describe the decrease in numbers of circulating white blood cells (WBC), red blood cells (RBC), and platelets. Myelosuppression is often a side effect of treatment with chemotherapy and/or radiation therapy. Blood counts usually begin to fall one to three weeks after treatment with chemotherapy, depending upon the type of chemotherapy and the lifespan of the blood cell. The counts generally begin to recover to normal levels within two to three weeks. The neutrophil, which is a component of the white blood cells, is the body's first line of defense against infection caused by bacteria. When neutrophils are decreased a state of **neutropenia** exits. Neutropenia is the single greatest predictor of infection in patients with cancer. Three key factors are important in predicting the potential of a patient to experience an infectious episode when myelosuppressed. These factors include: 1) the degree of neutropenia, i.e., the lower the neutrophil count the more likely the patient will become infected, 2) the duration of the neutropenia, i.e., the longer a patient is neutropenic, the greater the likelihood of infection, and 3) the rate at which neutropenia develops the greater the risk of infection.

Bacterial infections in cancer patients develop quickly, especially in the neutropenic patient, and account for 85-90% of the microorganisms associated with neutropenia accompanied by fever. The most serious episodes occur from infections attributed to gram-negative organisms such as *Enterobacteriaceae* or *Pseudomonas aeruginosa*. However, infections from gram-positive organisms such as *Staphylococcus, Streptococcus, Corynebacteria*, and *Clostridia* have increased in the 1990s, probably due to the increased use of implanted central venous catheters and prophylactic antibiotics (to which these organisms develop an immunity). Other organisms that cause infections in the immunocompromised cancer patient include herpesvirus infections such as **herpes simplex** virus 1 and 2 (HSV-1, HSV-2), varicella zoster virus (VZV), cytomegalovirus (CMV), and **Epstein-Barr virus** (EBV). Sources of secondary infections include the fungal infection, *Candida albicans*. Common causes of secondary infection in severely immunosuppressed patients include CMV, and the filamentous fungi, *Aspergillus*.

The incidence of sepsis and septic shock increases when the patient remains neutropenic for longer than seven days. Other factors that put the cancer patient at high risk for the development of sepsis include infection with a gram-negative organism, presence of a central venous catheter, history of prior infection, malnutrition, history of frequent hospitalization, increased age of patient, and concurrent (at the same time) presence of other diseases such as diabetes, cardiovascular, gastrointestinal, hepatic, pulmonary, and/or renal disease. Sites of infection that most often lead to sepsis include infection of the lungs, invasive lines, and urinary tract.

Sepsis manifests (develops) with both local and systemic symptoms that involve the neurologic, endocrine, immunologic, and cardiovascular systems. Signs of sepsis and septic shock include changes in blood pressure, heart rate and respiratory rate, among others. If left untreated, the patient can progress to septic shock which may result in death even if the shock episode is treated.

Prevention

Strategies that can be used to prevent or minimize infection in the neutropenic patient include:

- Identification of patients at highest risk for infection.
- Avoiding practices by health care team members that increase colonization of microorganisms.
- Implementation of fewer invasive procedures when possible.

KEY TERMS

Corticosteroids—Adrenal cortex steroids.

Central venous catheters—Devices used for access to the blood stream. The distal tip of the catheter after insertion is located in the superior vena cava, or above the junction of the right atrium. May be used for blood sampling and for the infusion of any type of fluids, medications, nutritional supplements, and blood components.

Gram-negative—Types of bacteria that do not retain gram stain.

Gram-positive—Types of bacteria that retain gram stain.

Specific interventions in the hospital setting that can be used to prevent or minimize infection include:

- scrupulous handwashing by patient, staff, and visitors.
- good personal hygiene, including an oral care protocol by the patient.
- ambulation (movement).
- aggressive efforts to promote lung expansion.
- elimination of uncooked fruits and vegetables from the diet.
- removal of plants and other sources of stagnant water from the patient's room.
- screening and minimizing outside visitors to avoid those with infection

In addition, the hospitalized patient is assessed by the staff at least every four hours and laboratory results are collected and analyzed to determine risk for and presence of neutropenia.

A newer method to prevent infection in the cancer patient works by decreasing the duration of neutropenia. This method decreases the period of maximum risk for infection by using hematopoietic growth factors (HGFs). These growth factors are administered daily beginning 24 hours after chemotherapy, and shorten the duration and severity of neutropenia. Therefore, the period of risk for infection is shortened. HGFs work by activating the production and maturation of RBCs, WBCs, and platelet cell lines. Specific HGFs stimulate the production and maturation of aggressive neutrophils and macrophages, which are effective in destroying pathogens (bacteria or viruses that cause infection or disease).

Sepsis can be avoided by preventing infection in immunocompromised patients and by recognizing risk factors and altering those factors whenever possible.

Treatment

Empiric antibiotic therapy is the mainstay of treatment for infection in the cancer patient. Empiric therapy refers to initiation of antibiotic therapy prior to the identification of the infecting organism. Broad-spectrum antibiotics, antibiotics effective against both gram-negative and gram-positive organisms, are administered. Commonly used agents include aminoglycosides, fluoroquinolones, glycopeptides, and beta-lactams such as penicillins, cephalosporins, carbapenems, and monobactams. Empiric **antifungal therapy** is initiated five to seven days after empiric antibiotic therapy has been started if the patient remains febrile (with a fever). Antiviral agents may be administered if there is evidence of a viral infection. The Infectious Diseases Society of America recommends a minimum of five to seven days further treatment with parenteral (introduced in other ways than intestinal absorption) antibiotic therapy after the fever resolves (returns to normal). Continued monitoring of bacterial and fungal culture results is essential. This allows the use of more tailored antibiotics for the specific infectious agents.

The neutropenic patient with fever can progress quickly to sepsis and septic shock if left untreated. The patient may also progress to septic shock if empiric antibiotic coverage is inadequate. The most common cause of septic shock in cancer patients is infection with gram-negative bacteria. The management of sepsis and septic shock is considered an emergency situation and includes treatment with broad-spectrum antibacterial coverage and maintenance of ventilation, oxygenation, fluid volume, and cardiac output.

See Also Vascular access

Resources

BOOKS

Freifeld, A. G., T. J. Walsh, and P. A. APizzo. "Infections in the Cancer Patient." In *Cancer: Principles and Practice of Oncology.* DeVita, V.T., S. Hellman, and S. A. Rosenberg. Philadelphia: Lippincott, 1997, pp.2659-2704.

Schaffer, S. D., L. S. Garzon, and D. L. Heroux, et al. *Infection Prevention and Safe Practice* St. Louis: Mosby, 1996.

Wujcik, D. "Infection." In *Cancer Symptom Management* Boston: Jones and Bartlett, 1999, pp. 307-321.

PERIODICALS

Shelton, B. "Sepsis." *Seminars in Oncology Nursing* 15 (August 1999): 209-221.

Toney, J. F., and M. M. Parker. "New Perspectives on the Management of Septic Shock in the Cancer Patient." *Infectious Diseases Clinics of North America* 10 (1996): 239-253.

Yoshida, M. "Infections in Patients with Hematological Diseases: Recent Advances in Serological Diagnosis and Empiric Therapy." *International Journal of Hematology* 66(1997): 279-289.

OTHER

"Supportive Care for Patients - Fever, Chills, and Sweats." *National Cancer Institute CancerNet* 16 April 2001 <http://cancernet.nci.nih.gov/coping.html>

Melinda Granger Oberleitner, R.N., D.N.S.

Infertility *see* **Fertility issues**

Interferons

Definition

Interferons are small, natural or synthetic protein and glycoprotein cytokines that are produced by leucocytes, T-lymphocytes, and fibroblasts in response to infection and other biological stimuli. In cancer treatment, they are used as immunotherapy against the proliferation of cancer cells.

Purpose

The goal of interferon use is to activate tumor-specific cytotoxic T-lymphocytes. T-lymphocytes are cells of the immune system that destroy foreign cells. Thus, tumor cells would be destroyed based on immunotherapy.

Description

Interferons attach to special receptors on the surface of cell membranes. They have a variety of functions, including enhancing or inhibiting enzymes, decreasing cell proliferation, or enhancing the activity of macrophages and T-lymphocytes. There are several different classes of interferons, including alpha, beta, gamma, tau, and omega. The classes can be further broken into subclasses and classified using Arabic numerals and letters. Cancer therapy research primarily focuses on alpha interferons.

In 1957 researchers discovered that the immune system produced a substance in response to a viral infection that acted as an anti-viral agent. They called that substance "interferon." Since then, recombinant DNA technology has provided a larger supply of interferons and has allowed extensive research regarding interferon's therapeutic properties against cancer.

Alpha interferons are used to treat cancers such as **hairy cell leukemia**, malignant **melanoma**, and **Kaposi's sarcoma** (an AIDS-related cancer). Off the label, alpha interferons are used to treat many other cancers including **bladder cancer**, **chronic myelocytic leukemia**, kidney cancer, carcinoid tumors, **non-Hodgkin's lymphomas**, **ovarian cancer**, and skin cancers. Alpha interferons can be combined with other chemotherapeutic drugs such as **doxorubicin**.

In the United States alpha interferons are sold under the brand names Roferon-A (Interferon Alfa-2a, recombinant) and Intron A (Interferon Alfa-2b, recombinant). There are no generic forms of these drugs.

Recommended dosage

Alpha interferons are only available by prescription and are given parenterally. A physician will determine dosage based on several factors such as what type of cancer is being treated, the patient's weight, and what other types of medications the patient is taking. Therefore, the dose will vary from patient to patient.

Patients can inject this drug themselves. Their physician may recommend that they drink extra water to avoid low blood pressure while on this medication. Since this drug can have flu-like side effects, it is recommended that patients inject the drug prior to bedtime so that they are sleeping during the worst part of the side effects.

Precautions

Alpha interferons have not been shown to cause problems in the fetus of pregnant women. Because it is not known whether this drug can cross over into breast milk, it is not recommended for use in women who are breast-feeding. Before this drug is given, patients should notify their doctors if they are allergic to immunoglobulins or egg whites.

There are several medical conditions that should be considered prior to deciding whether to use alpha interferons. There can be an increase in the following disorders: bleeding problems, mental problems, convulsions, diabetes mellitus, heart attack, heart disease, liver disease, kidney disease, and lung disease. People with an overactive immune system could also have this disorder exacerbated when using alpha interferons.

Caution should be taken when using alpha interferons because they can depress the number of white blood cells. This can make patients more susceptible to infection. Therefore, they should avoid contact with others who have infections and should contact their physician immediately if they think they are developing an infection. Patients should take care not to cut themselves, should not touch their eyes or inside of their nose with unwashed hands, and should take care when brushing their teeth so as not to cause bleeding.

KEY TERMS

Cytokines—Molecules released by cells to regulate the length and intensity of an immune response and to mediate intercellular communication.

Glycoprotein—A protein that has a carbohydrate group attached.

Immunotherapy—Treating cancer using molecules that are intended to stimulate the patient's own immune system to fight the disease.

Macrophages—A type of white blood cell that produces antibodies and molecules for cell-to-cell immune responses.

Parenteral—Medications that are administered by some means other than through the gastrointestinal tract, including through intravenous, subcutaneous, or intramuscular injection.

T-lymphocytes—A part of the immune system that fights foreign cells.

The effects of alcohol can be exaggerated while taking alpha interferons. Alcohol should only be used by permission from a physician.

Side effects

Alpha interferons can have side effects that range from minor and irritating to major and severe, needing immediate attention. Some of the less serious side effects are muscle aches, unusual metallic taste in the mouth, **fever** and chills, and general flu-like symptoms such as headache, loss of appetite (**anorexia**), **nausea and vomiting**, and **fatigue**. To reduce the flu-like symptoms physicians may suggest that the patient take acetaminophen (e.g., Tylenol) before each dosage.

Other side effects may need medical attention. Any changes with the central nervous system such as confusion, trouble thinking and focusing, mental **depression**, nervousness, or numbness or tingling of fingers, toes and face require immediate medical attention.

The side effects are dependent on the dose. As a result, the physician may modify the dose if the side effects are severe.

Interactions

Alpha interferons can interact with several different drugs, increasing their effects. Most drugs that interact with alpha interferons are those used with disorders of the central nervous system. Some of the depressants include antihistamines, sedatives, tranquilizers, sleeping medications, prescription pain medicines, seizure medications, muscle relaxants, narcotics, and barbiturates. Prior to treatment, the doctor should be notified if the patient is taking any of these medications because this could impact the dosage prescribed.

Sally C. McFarlane-Parrott

Interleukin-2 *see* **Aldesleukin**

Intimacy *see* **Sexuality**

Intravenous pyelography *see* **Intravenous urography**

Intravenous urography

Definition

Intravenous urography is a test that x rays the urinary system using intravenous dye for diagnostic purposes.

The kidneys excrete the dye into the urine. X rays can then create pictures of every structure (kidney, renal pelvis, ureter, bladder, urethra) through which the urine passes.

The procedure has several variations and many names:

- Intravenous pyelography (IVP)
- Urography
- Excretory urography
- Pyelography
- Antegrade pyelography differentiates this procedure from "retrograde pyelography," which injects dye into the lower end of the system, therefore flowing backward or "retrograde." Retrograde pyelography is better able to define problems in the lower parts of the system and is the only way to get x rays if the kidneys are not working well.
- Nephrotomography is somewhat different in that the x rays are taken by a moving **x ray** source onto a film moving in the opposite direction. By accurately coordinating the movement, all but a single plane of tissue is blurred, and that plane is seen without overlying shadows.

Every method available gives good pictures of this system, and the question becomes one of choosing among many excellent alternatives. Each condition has special requirements, while each technique has distinctive benefits and drawbacks.

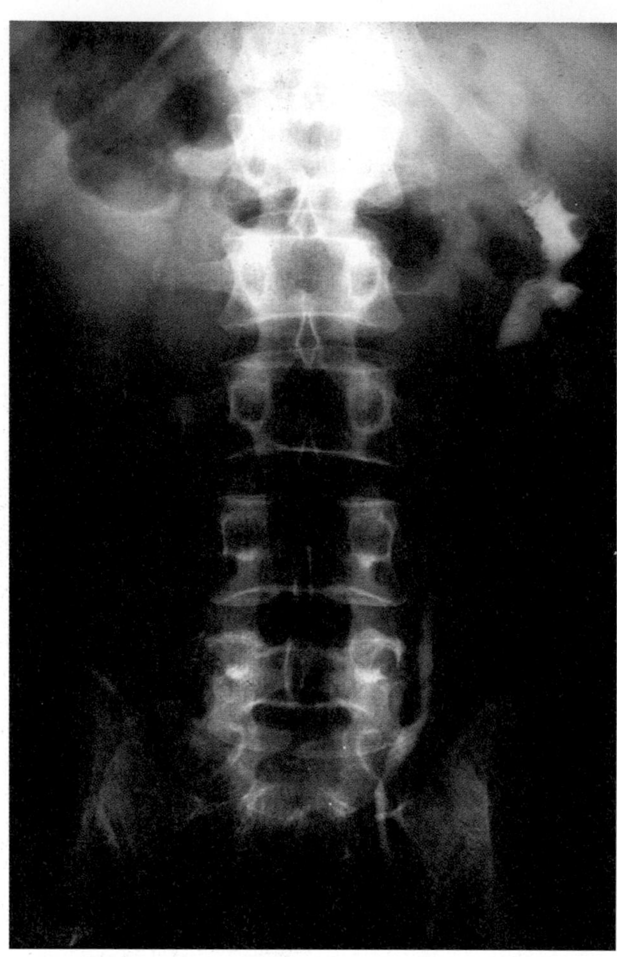

Intravenous urography showing contrast in distal ureter. Ureter is the narrow tube shown at the lower right of the image, and the dye has traveled from the kidney (above) and is traveling to the bladder. *(Custom Medical Stock Photo. Reproduced by permission.)*

- **Nuclear medicine scans** rely on the radiation given off by certain atoms. Chemicals containing such atoms are injected into the bloodstream. They reach the kidneys, where images are constructed by measuring the radiation emitted. The radiation is no more dangerous than standard x rays. The images require considerable training to interpret, but unique information (e.g. blood flow, kidney function, etc.) is often available using this technology. Different chemicals can concentrate the radiation in different types of tissue. This technique may require several days for the chemical to concentrate at its destination. It also requires a special detector to create the image.
- Ultrasound is a quick, safe, simple, and inexpensive way to obtain views of internal organs. Although less

detailed than other methods, it may be sufficient, especially to detect obstructions.

- Retrograde pyelography is better able to define problems in the lower parts of the system and is the only way to get x rays if the kidneys are not working well. Dye is usually injected through an instrument (cystoscope) passed into the bladder through the urethra.
- A **computed tomography** scan (CT or CAT scanning) uses the same kind of radiation used in x rays, but it collects information by computer in such a way that three dimensional images can be constructed, eliminating interference from nearby structures. CT scanning requires a special apparatus, but often gives better information on masses within the kidney.
- **Magnetic resonance imaging** (MRI) uses magnetic fields and radio frequency signals, instead of ionizing radiation, to create computerized images. This form of energy is entirely safe as long as the patient does not have any implanted metal such as artificial joints, aneurysm clips, etc. The technique is far more versatile than CT scanning as it can not only demonstrate masses, but also look at the blood vessels. However, MRI requires special apparatus and, because of the powerful magnets needed, even a special, separate building. It is quite expensive and only occasionally is this degree of detail required.

Purpose

IVP will provide information concerning most diseases of the kidneys, ureters, and bladder. The procedure is comprised of two phases. First, it requires a functioning kidney to filter the dye out of the blood into the urine. The time required for the dye to appear on x rays correlates accurately with kidney function. The second phase gives detailed anatomical images of the urinary tract. Within the first few minutes the dye "lights up" the kidneys, a phase called the nephrogram. Subsequent pictures follow the dye down the ureters and into the bladder. A final film taken after urinating reveals how well the bladder empties.

IVPs are most often done to assess structural abnormalities or obstruction to urine flow. If kidney function is at issue, more films are taken sooner to catch the earliest phase of the process.

- Stones, tumors and congenital malformations account for many of the findings.
- Kidney cysts and cancers can be seen.
- Displacement of a kidney or ureter suggests a space-occupying lesion (like a cancer of the colon, rectum, or gynecological organs) pushing it out of the way.

KEY TERMS

Contrast agent—Any substance that causes shadows on x rays; also known as contrast dye or medium.

Intravenous—Into a vein.

- Bad valves where the ureters enter the bladder will often show up.
- Bladder cancers and other abnormalities are often outlined by the dye in the bladder.
- An enlarged prostate gland will show up as incomplete bladder emptying and a bump at the bottom of the bladder.

Precautions

The only serious complication of an IVP is allergy to the iodine-containing dye that is used. Such an allergy is rare, but it can be dramatic and even lethal. Emergency measures taken immediately are usually effective.

Description

IVPs are usually done in the morning. In the x ray suite, the patient undresses and lies down. There are two methods of injecting the dye. An intravenous line can be established, through which the dye is consistently fed through the body during the procedure. The other method is to give the dye all at once through a needle that is immediately withdrawn. X rays are taken until the dye has reached the bladder, an interval of half an hour or less. The patient is asked to empty the bladder before one last x ray. A compression device (a wide belt containing 2 balloons that can be inflated) may be used to keep the contrast material in the kidneys. The patient needs to urinate after the compression device is removed. Another picture is taken after the bladder is emptied to see how empty the bladder is.

In the past, of the many ways to obtain images of the urinary system, the intravenous injection of a contrast agent has been considered the best. Recent studies are showing, however, that while intravenous urography is a useful technique, there may be other imaging techniques, such as B mode ultrasound, Doppler ultrasound, renal scintigraphy with angiotensin-converting enzyme inhibitors, intra-venous and intra-arterial catheter **angiography**, computed tomographic angiog-

QUESTIONS TO ASK THE DOCTOR

- What should I feel when I am being imaged?
- Why do you recommend intravenous urography rather than another imaging technique?

raphy, and magnetic resonance angiography, that are better or less costly.

Preparation

Emptying the bowel with **laxatives** or enemas prevents bowel shadows from obscuring the details of the urinary system. An empty stomach prevents the complication of vomiting, a rare effect of the contrast agent. Therefore, the night before the IVP the patient is asked to evacuate the bowels and to drink sparingly.

Preparation for infants and children depends on the age of the infant or child.

Aftercare

Feeling weak, nauseous, and/or lightheaded for a short time after the procedure is a possibility.

Risks

Allergy to the contrast agent is the only risk. Anyone with a possible iodine allergy, a previous reaction to x ray dye, or an allergy to shellfish must be particularly careful to inform the x ray personnel.

Exposure to x ray radiation should be noted. Most experts agree that the risk of exposure to low radiation is low compared to the benefits. Pregnant women and children are more sensitive to the risks of x rays.

Normal results

X-ray images of the kidney and bladder structures appear normal.

Abnormal results

An abnormal intravenous urography result may indicate kidney disease, birth defect, tumor, kidney stone, and/or inflammation caused by infections.

Resources

BOOKS

Ballinger, Philip W., and Eugene D. Frank. *Merrill's Atlas of Radiographic Positions and Radiologic Procedures.* 9th ed. St. Louis, MO: Year Book Medical Publishers, 1999.

PERIODICALS

Aitchson, F., and A. Page. "Diagnostic Imaging of Renal Artery Stenosis" *Journal of Human Hypertension* (September 1999): 595–603.

Dalla–Palma, L. "What is Left of I.V. Urography?" *European Radiology* (March 2001): 931–939.

Hession, P., et al."Intravenous Urography in Urinary Tract Surveillance in Carcinoma of the Bladder." *Clinical Radiology* (July 1999): 465–467.

Little, M. A., et al."The Diagnostic Yield of Intravenous Urography" *Nephrology Dialysis Transplantation* (February 2000): 200–204.

ORGANIZATIONS

American Cancer Society (National Headquarters). 1599 Clifton Road, N.E., Atlanta, GA 30329. (800) 227-2345. <http://www.cancer.org>.

Cancer Research Institute (National Headquarters). 681 Fifth Avenue, New York, NY 10022. (800) 992-2623. <http://www.cancerresearch.org>.

Kidney Cancer Association. 1234 Sherman Avenue, Suite 203, Evanston, IL 60202-1375. (800) 850-9132. <http://www.kidneycancerassociation.org>.

National Cancer Institute. 9000 Rockville Pike, Building 31, Room 10A16, Bethesda, MD 20892. (800) 422-6237. <http://www.nci.nih.gov>.

National Kidney Cancer Association. 1234 Sherman Avenue, Suite 203, Evanston, IL 60202-1375. (800) 850-9132.

National Kidney Foundation. 30 East 33rd Street, New York, NY 10016. (800) 622-9010. <http://www.kidney.org>.

J. Ricker Polsdorfer, M.D.
Laura Ruth, Ph.D.

Investigational drugs

Definition

Investigational drugs is the term that refers to drugs that have received FDA approval for human testing, including those drugs still undergoing **clinical trials**, but are not approved for marketing to the general public.

Description

Investigational drugs represent interesting and novel new agents in the fight against cancer. These agents include **chemotherapy** designed to treat specific cancers, to provide palliative therapy for pain and symptoms, and to reduce invasive cancers in high-risk patients. The challenge faced by private and commercial investigators is to reduce the lag time in bringing an investigational drug to market without compromising drug quality or patient safety. The guidelines that insure

KEY TERMS

Oncologist—A physician who specializes in the diagnosis and treatment of cancer patients.

Palliative—Therapy or medication designed to provide relief but does not affect a cure for the condition.

the correct procedures are being followed in the process of drug development and approval fall under the direction of the Food and Drug Administration (FDA).

At present, the cycle of investigational drug research and development, to clinical trials, to FDA approval can easily cover a period of 10-12 years. Under exceptional circumstances, provisions can be made for patient use of investigational drugs under the guidance of specially trained and registered oncologists. These specific investigational drugs are classified as "Group C" drugs, and have demonstrated a high level of reproducible activity in pre-clinical testing. There is also the route of "Accelerated FDA Approval" for some investigational drugs. Accelerated approval relies on specific indicators that suggest that a particular investigational drug is likely to have beneficial effects before the benefits have been clinically verified. All investigational drugs that have been granted accelerated approval must undergo follow-up testing in order to receive final FDA approval. Some researchers are presently working on a format to combine traditional clinical testing of investigational drugs with a global database of drug information. This integrated system would give FDA monitoring agencies and healthcare providers access to the most comprehensive source of archived data available on investigational drugs. This combined approach is another attempt to reduce approval time for investigational drugs and make these agents available to the cancer patient for treatment.

Resources

PERIODICALS

Chopra, Ian. "Research and development of antibacterial agents." *Current Opinions in Microbiology* 1998(1):495-501.

Johnson, Dale E. and Grushenka H.I. Wolfgang. "Predicting human safety: screening and computational approaches." *Drug Discovery Today* 5:10 (October 2000): 445-454

OTHER

Preclinical Development of Investigational Agents: The Developmental Therapeutics Program *CTEP* Feb. 2001 Info CTEP. 08 May 2001 <http://www.CTEP.info.nih.gov>

Understanding the Approval Process for New Cancer Drugs. *Understanding Trials.* July 1999 NCI Cancer Trials.18 May 2001 <http://www.cancertrials.nci.nih.gov>

Jane Taylor-Jones, Research Associate, M.S.

Irinotecan

Definition

Irinotecan is a drug used to treat certain types of cancer. Irinotecan, also known as CPT-11, is available under the trade name Camptosar, and may also be referred to as irinotecan hydrochloride or camptothecin-11.

Purpose

Irinotecan is an antineoplastic agent used to treat cancers of the colon or rectum that have recurred or progressed while on 5-FU (**fluourouracil**) therapy, or it can be given as first line therapy with 5-FU and **leucovorin** for patients with metastatic colon or **rectal cancer**. Other uses for irinotecan include treatment of small cell lung cancer, **ovarian cancer**, **stomach cancer**, **breast cancer**, pancreatic cancer, leukemia, **lymphoma**, and **cervical cancer**.

Description

Irinotecan is a synthetic derivative of the naturally-occurring compound camptothecin. Camptothecin belongs to a group of chemicals called alkaloids and is extracted from plants such as *camptotheca acuminata.* Captothecin was initially investigated as a chemotherapeutic agent due to its anti-cancer activity in laboratory studies. The chemical structure and biological action of irinotecan is similar to that of camptothecin and **topotecan**.

Irinotecan inhibits the normal functioning of the enzyme topoisomerase I. The normal role of topoisomerase I is to aid in the replication, recombination, and repair of deoxyribonucleic acid (DNA). Higher levels of topoisomerase I have been found in certain cancer tumors compared to healthy tissue. Inhibiting topoisomerase I causes DNA damage. This damage leads to apoptosis, or programmed cell death.

Recommended dosage

Patients should be carefully monitored during irinotecan treatment for toxicity. Irinotecan is given at a dose of 125 mg per square meter of body surface area per week for four weeks, followed by a two week rest period. Other dosing schedules include 100 mg per square meter of body surface area per day for three days every three

KEY TERMS

Alkaloid—A nitrogen-containing compound occurring in plants.

Anorexia—Loss of appetite and the inability to eat.

Apoptosis—An active process in which a cell dies due to a chemical signal. Programmed cell death.

Diuretic—An agent that increases the amount of urine the body produces.

Inflammation—A response to injury, irritation or illness characterized by redness, pain, swelling, and heat.

Metastatic—Spread of a disease from the organ or tissue of origin to other parts of the body.

weeks, or 100-115 mg per square meter of body surface area per week, or 200-350 mg per square meter of body surface area every 3 weeks. The drug is administered through the vein over 90 minutes. The initial dose of irinotecan may be adjusted downward depending on patient tolerance to the toxic side effects of irinotecan.

Treatment may be continued as long as intolerable side effects do not develop and patients continue to benefit from the treatment.

Precautions

Irinotecan should only be used under the supervision of a physician experienced in the use of cancer chemotherapeutic agents. Special caution, especially in those 65 years and older, should be taken to monitor the toxic effects of irinotecan, particularly **diarrhea**, nausea, and vomiting. Because irinotecan is administered intravenously, the site of infusion should be monitored for signs of inflammation. Should inflammation occur, flushing the site with sterile water and applying ice are recommended. Irinotecan may cause **nausea and vomiting**, and premedication with antiemetic agents is recommended.

Neither the effects of irinotecan in patients with significant liver dysfunction nor the safety of irinotecan in children have been established. Irinotecan should not be administered to pregnant women. Women of child-bearing age are advised not to become pregnant during treatment with this drug.

Side effects

Early- or late-onset diarrhea are common side effects of irinotecan. Late-onset diarrhea, occurring more than 24 hours after irinotecan administration, can be life-threatening and should be treated promptly. Patients should immediately report diarrhea to their physician. Patients can also take the antidiarrheal drug loperamide as prescribed by their physician at the first sign of diarrhea. Suppression of bone marrow function is another serious side effect commonly observed in this treatment. Additional side effects, including nausea, vomiting, **anorexia** (loss of appetite), pain, **fatigue**, and hair loss (**alopecia**) may occur.

Interactions

Irradiation treatment during the course of irinotecan treatment is not recommended. Patients who have received prior pelvic or abdominal irradiation treatment should notify their physician. Since irinotecan may cause diarrhea, the use of **laxatives** should be avoided. The use of diuretics should be closely monitored. The adverse side effects caused by irinotecan may be increased by other **antineoplastic agents** having similar adverse effects and should generally be avoided.

Marc Scanio

Islet cell carcinoma *see* **Pancreatic cancer, endocrine**

Itching

Description

Itching, also called pruritus, is an unpleasant sensation of the skin that causes a person to scratch or rub the area to find relief. Itching can be confined to one spot (localized) or over the whole body (generalized). Severe scratching can injure the skin causing redness, bumps, and scratches. Injured skin is prone to infection.

Itching can profoundly affect quality of life. It can torment the patient and cause discomfort, stress, loss of sleep, concentration difficulty, and constant concern.

Causes

The biology underlying itching is not fully understood. It is believed that itching results from the interactions of several different chemical messengers. Although they are quite different sensations, itch and pain signals are sent along the same nerve pathways.

Itching is associated with a variety of factors including skin diseases, blood diseases, emotions, and drug reactions as well as by cancer and cancer treatments. Itching can be a symptom of cancer including **Hodgkin's disease**, **non-Hodgkin's lymphomas**, leukemia, **Bowen's disease**, **multiple myeloma**, central nervous system (brain and spinal cord) tumors, **germ cell tumors**, and invasive squamous cell carcinoma. The buildup of toxins in the blood, caused by kidney, gallbladder, and liver disease, can cause itching. Cancer treatments that are associated with itching are: **radiation therapy**, **chemotherapy**, and biological response modifiers (drugs that improve the patient's immune system). Skin reactions are more severe when both chemotherapy and radiation therapy are used. Patients treated with **bone marrow transplantation** may develop itching resulting from **graft-vs.-host disease**. Itching can be caused by infection.

General medications, which may be used by cancer patients, can cause itching. Itching can be caused by drug reactions from **antibiotics**, **corticosteroids**, hormones, and pain relievers (analgesics).

Itching can be a sign that the patient is very sensitive to a particular chemotherapy drug. Chemotherapy drugs and biological response modifiers that can cause itching include:

- **allopurinol**
- **aminoglutethimide**
- **bleomycin**
- **carmustine**
- **chlorambucil**
- **cyclophosphamide**
- **cytarabine**
- **daunorubicin**
- **doxorubicin**
- **hydroxyurea**
- **idarubicin**
- interleukin (**aldesleukin**)
- **mechlorethamine**
- **megestrol acetate**
- **mitomycin-C**
- **tamoxifen**

Itching commonly occurs during radiation therapy. Parts of the body that are particularly sensitive to radiation are the underarms, groin, abdomen, breasts, buttocks, and skin around the genitals (perineum) and anus (perianal). Itching is usually caused by skin dryness when the oil (sebaceous) glands are damaged by the radiation. Radiation also causes skin darkening, redness, and skin shedding, which can all cause itching.

Itching caused by cancer usually disappears once the cancer is in remission or cured. Chemotherapy-induced itching usually disappears within 30 to 90 minutes after the drug has been administered. Itching caused by radiation therapy will resolve once the injured skin has healed.

Treatments

There are three aspects in the treatment of itching: managing the underlying cancer, maintaining skin health, and relief of itching.

Patients should avoid the particular things that cause or worsen their itching. Also, patients can take measures to maintain skin health. Suggestions include:

- taking short baths in warm water
- using mild soaps and rinsing well
- applying bath oil or moisturizing cream after bathing
- avoiding use of cosmetics, perfumes, deodorants, and starch-based powders
- avoiding wool and other harsh fabrics
- using mild laundry detergents and rinsing thoroughly
- avoiding use of dryer anti-static sheets
- wearing loose-fitting cotton clothing
- avoiding high-friction garments such as belts, pantyhose, and bras
- maintaining a cool environment with a 30% to 40% humidity level
- using cotton sheets
- avoiding vigorous exercise (if sweating causes itching)
- avoiding skin products that are scented or contain alcohol or menthol

To reduce skin injury caused by scratching the patient should keep fingernails short, wear soft cotton mittens and socks at night, and keep the hands clean. Gently rubbing the skin around the itch or applying pressure or vibration to the itchy spot may reduce itching. Using a soft infant toothbrush to gently stroke the itchy area may relieve itching. Itching may be relieved by applying a cool washcloth or ice to the itchy area.

The most effective way to relieve itching is to treat the underlying disease. Sometimes, itching disappears as soon as a tumor is treated or removed.

Itching may be relieved by applying any of a variety of different products to the skin. The patient may need to try several before the most effective one is found. The patient's physician should be consulted before any anti-itch products are used. Topical treatments include:

KEY TERMS

Chemical messengers—Chemicals that transmit messages from one place to another.

Generalized itching—Itching that occurs over the whole body.

Histamine—A chemical messenger that can be associated with itching.

Localized itching—Itching that is confined to one spot.

- Corticosteroids, such as hydrocortisone, reduce inflammation and itching.
- Calamine lotions can cool and soothe itchy skin. These products can be drying, which may be helpful for weeping or oozing rashes.
- Antihistamine creams stop itching that is associated with the chemical messenger histamine.
- Moisturizers treat dry skin which helps to relieve itching. Moisturizers that are recommended to cancer patients include brand names Alpha Keri, Aquaphor, Eucerin, Lubriderm, Nivea, Prax, and Sarna. Moisturizers should be applied after bathing and at least two or three times daily.
- Gels that contain a numbing agent (e.g. lidocaine) can be used on some parts of the body.

Itching may be treated with whole-body medications. Some of these systemic treatments include:

- antihistamines
- tricyclic antidepressants
- sedatives or tranquilizers
- binding agents (such as cholestyramine which relieves itching associated with kidney or liver disease).
- aspirin
- cimetidine

Alternative and complementary therapies

A well-balanced diet that includes carbohydrates, fats, minerals, proteins, **vitamins**, and liquids will help to maintain skin health. Capsules that contain eicosapentaenoic acid, which is obtained from herring, mackerel, or salmon, may help to reduce itching. Vitamin A plays an important role in skin health. Vitamin E (capsules or ointment) may reduce itching. Patients should check with their treating physician before using supplements.

Baths containing oil with milk or oatmeal are effective at relieving localized itching. Evening primrose oil may soothe itching and may be as effective as corticosteroids. Calendula cream may relieve short-term itching.

Distraction, music therapy, relaxation techniques, and visualization may be useful in relieving itching. Ultraviolet light therapy may relieve itching associated with conditions of the skin, kidneys, blood, and gallbladder. There are some reports of the use of acupuncture and transcutaneous electrical nerve stimulators (TENS) to relieve itching.

Belinda Rowland, Ph.D.

Itraconazole *see* **Antifungal therapy**

IVP, *see* **Intravenous urography**

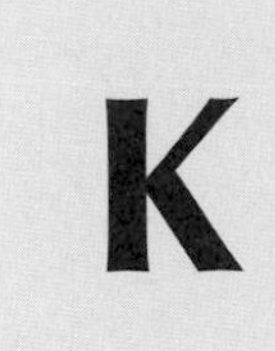

Kaposi's sarcoma

Definition

Kaposi's sarcoma (KS) is a cancer of the skin, mucous membranes, and blood vessels; it is the most common form of cancer in AIDS patients. It was named for Dr. Moritz Kaposi (1837-1902), a Hungarian dermatologist who first described it in 1872. As of 2001, researchers disagree as to whether KS is a true cancer or a disorder of the skin that develops as a reaction to infection by a herpesvirus.

Description

The formal medical term for Kaposi's sarcoma is multiple idiopathic hemorrhagic sarcoma. This term means that KS develops in many different sites on the patient's skin or internal organs; that its cause is unknown; and that it is characterized by bleeding. The lesions (areas of diseased or damaged skin), which are usually round or elliptical in shape and a quarter of an inch to an inch in size, derive their characteristic purple or brownish color from blood leaking out of capillaries (small blood vessels) in the skin. In KS, the capillaries begin to grow too rapidly and irregularly, which causes them to become leaky and eventually break. The lesions themselves may become enlarged and bleed, or cause the mucous membranes of the patient's internal organs to bleed.

There are three types of KS lesions, defined by their appearance:

- Nodular. These are reddish-purple, but are sometimes surrounded by a border of yellowish or brown pigment. Nodular lesions may appear to be dark brown rather than purple in patients with dark skin.
- Infiltrating. Infiltrating lesions may be large or have a raised surface. They typically grow downward under the skin.
- Lymphatic. These lesions are found in the lymph nodes and may be confused with other causes of swollen lymph nodes.

As of 2001, KS is classified into five types:

- Classic KS. This form of KS is sometimes called indolent KS because it is slow to develop. Classical KS is most commonly found in males between 50 and 70 years of age, of Italian or Eastern European Jewish descent.
- African KS. This form of the disease appears in both an indolent and an aggressive form in native populations in equatorial Africa. It accounts for almost 10% of all cancers in central Africa.
- Immunosuppressive treatment-related KS. The third form of KS occurs in kidney transplant patients who have been given drugs to suppress their immune systems-usually prednisone and **azathioprine**. This form of KS is sometimes called iatrogenic KS, which means that it is caused unintentionally by medical treatment.
- Epidemic KS. Epidemic KS was first reported in 1981 as part of the AIDS epidemic. Most cases of epidemic KS in the United States have been diagnosed in homosexual or bisexual men.
- Non-epidemic gay-related KS. This form of KS occurs in homosexual men who do not develop HIV infection. Non-epidemic gay-related KS is an indolent form of the disease that primarily affects the patient's skin.

Demographics

The demographic distribution of KS varies considerably across its five types:

- Classic KS. Classic KS is considered a rare disease, with a male/female ratio of 10:1 or 15:1. In North America and Europe, most patients are between 50 and 70 years old. Classic KS is more common in men from Mediterranean countries and in Ashkenazic Jews.
- African KS. African KS has the same male/female ratio as classic KS, although most patients with African KS

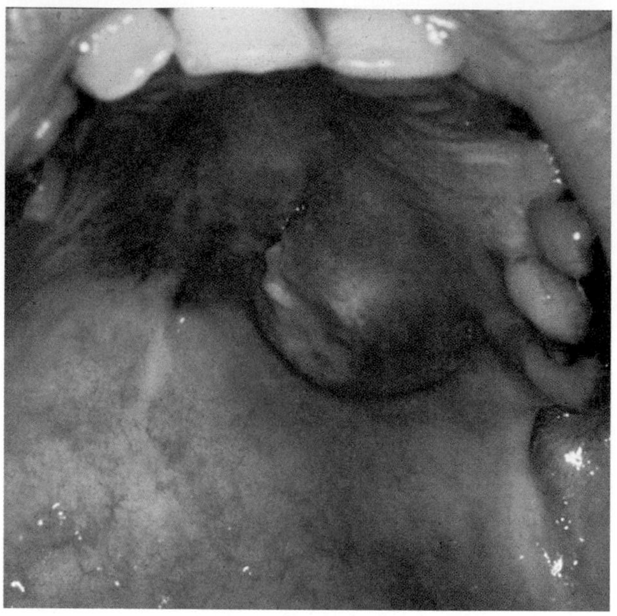

This HIV-positive patient is afflicted with Kaposi's sarcoma inside the mouth. The tumor is toward the back of the mouth, to the right. *(Custom Medical Stock Photo. Reproduced by permission.)*

are younger. A form of African KS that attacks the lymphatic system primarily affects children, with a male/female ratio of 3:1.

- Immunosuppresive treatment-related KS. This form of KS occurs mostly in kidney-transplant patients, at a rate of 150 to 200 times as often as in the general population. It represents 3% of all tumors that occur in kidney-transplant patients. The male/female ratio is 2:1.
- Epidemic KS. Epidemic KS is overwhelmingly a disease of adult homosexual or bisexual males. It is 20,000 times more common in people with AIDS than in those without HIV infection. According to the National Institutes of Health (NIH), 95% of all the cases of epidemic KS in the United States have been diagnosed in homosexual or bisexual males. Epidemic KS is far more prevalent among homosexual or bisexual males with AIDS than among hemophiliacs or intravenous drug users with AIDS. Prior to 1995, about 26% of all homosexual males with AIDS had KS as their first symptom or eventually developed KS, as compared with fewer than 3% of heterosexual intravenous drug users with AIDS. This clustering of KS cases among a subpopulation of AIDS patients led to the hypothesis that a blood factor transmitted by sexual contact is a partial cause of KS. The number of new cases of AIDS-related KS has declined in recent years, for reasons that are not yet clear. Some researchers think that the introduction of highly active antiretroviral therapy, or HAART, is related to the decline in the number of cases of epidemic KS. As of 2001, only about 12% of AIDS patients develop KS.
- Non-epidemic gay-related KS. This small group of KS patients is entirely male.

Causes and symptoms

Causes

GENETIC FACTORS. The role of genetic factors in KS varies across its five types. Classic KS is the only form associated with specific ethnic groups. In addition, patients with classic KS and immunosuppressive treatment-related KS have a higher incidence of a genetically determined immune factor called HLA-DR.

MALE HORMONES. The fact that all forms of KS affect men more often than women may indicate that androgens (male sex hormones) may be a factor in the development of KS.

IMMUNOSUPPRESSION. In addition to organ transplant patients receiving immunosuppressive drugs, patients who are taking high-dose **corticosteroids** are also at increased risk of developing KS.

INFECTIOUS AGENTS. Some researchers think that cytomegalovirus (CMV) and **human papilloma virus** (HPV) may be involved in the development of KS because fragments of these two types of virus have been found in KS tumor samples. The most likely candidate for an infectious agent, however, is human herpesvirus 8 (HHV-8), which is sometimes called KS-associated herpesvirus (KSHV). Fragments of the HHV-8 genome were first detected in 1994 by using a technique based on polymerase chain reaction (PCR) analysis. HHV-8 belongs to a group of herpesviruses called rhadinoviruses, and is the first herpesvirus of this subtype to be found in humans. HHV-8 is, however, closely related to the human herpesvirus called **Epstein-Barr virus** (EBV). EBV is known to cause infectious mononucleosis as well as tumors of the lymphatic system, and may be involved in other malignancies, including the African form of **Burkitt's lymphoma**, **Hodgkin's disease**, and **nasopharyngeal cancer**. HHV-8 has been found in tissue samples from patients with African KS, classic KS, and immunosuppression treatment-related KS as well as epidemic KS. HHV-8 is also associated with a rare non-cancerous disease called Castleman's disease, which affects the lymph nodes. Some KS patients have been found to have KS and Castleman's disease occurring together in the same lymph node.

OTHER CAUSES. Some practitioners of alternative medicine regard environmental toxins, psychological distress, and constitutional weaknesses as probable or partial causes of KS. These theories are discussed in more detail under the heading of alternative treatments.

Symptoms

CLASSIC KS. The symptoms of classic KS include one or more reddish or purplish patches or nodules on one or both legs, often on the ankles or soles of the feet. The lesions slowly enlarge over a period of 10-15 years, with additional lesions sometimes developing. It is rare for classic KS to involve the patient's internal organs, although bleeding from the digestive tract sometimes occurs. About 34% of patients with classic KS eventually develop non-Hodgkin's lymphoma or another primary cancer.

AFRICAN KS. The symptoms of the indolent form of African KS resemble those of classic KS. The aggressive form, however, produces tumors that may penetrate the tissue underneath the patient's skin, and even the underlying bone.

EPIDEMIC KS. Epidemic KS has more varied presentations than the four other types of KS. Its onset is usually, though not always, marked by the appearance of widespread lesions at many different points on the patient's skin and in the mouth. Most HIV-infected patients who develop KS skin and mouth lesions feel healthy and have no systemic symptoms. On the other hand, KS may affect the patient's lymph nodes or gastrointestinal tract prior to causing skin lesions.

Patients with epidemic KS almost always develop disseminated (widely spread) disease. The illness progesses from a few localized lesions to lymph node involvement and further spread to other organs. Disseminated KS is defined by the appearance of one or more of the following: a count of 25 or more external lesions; the appearance of 10 or more new lesions per month; and the appearance of visible lesions in the patient's lungs or stomach lining.

In some cases, disseminated KS causes painful swelling (edema) of the patient's feet and lower legs. The lesions may also cause the surrounding skin to ulcerate or develop secondary infections. The spread of KS to the lungs, called pleuropulmonary KS, usually occurs at a late stage of the disease. KS involvement of the lungs causes bleeding, coughing, shortness of breath, and eventual respiratory failure. Most patients who die directly of KS die from its pleuropulmonary form.

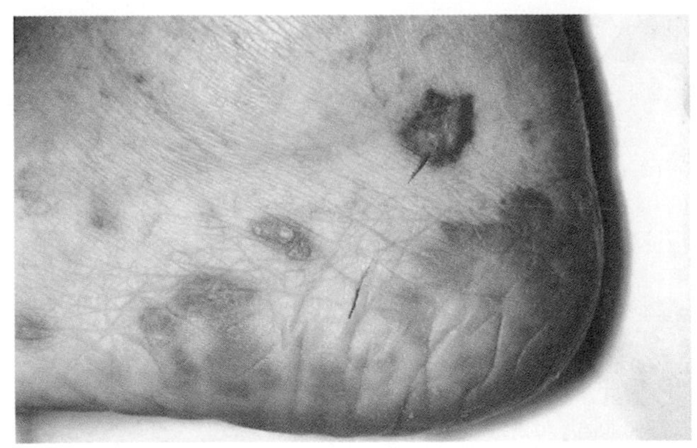

Purple-colored (violaceous) plaques of Kaposi's sarcoma on the heel and side of foot. *(Centers for Disease Control.)*

Diagnosis

Physical examination and patient history

The diagnosis of any form of KS requires a careful examination of all areas of the patient's skin. Even though the characteristic lesions of classic KS appear most frequently on the legs, all forms of KS can produce lesions on any area of the skin. An experienced doctor, who may be a dermatologist, an internist, or a primary care physician, can make a tentative diagnosis of KS on the basis of the external appearance of the skin lesions (size, shape, color, and location on the face or body), particularly when they are accompanied by evidence of lymph node involvement, internal bleeding, and other symptoms associated with disseminated KS. The doctor may touch or press on the lesions to find out whether they turn pale (blanch) ; KS plaques and nodules do not blanch under fingertip pressure. In addition, KS lesions are not painful when they first appear.

Other signs of KS may appear on the soft palate or the membrane covering the eye (conjunctiva). In addition, the doctor will press on the patient's abdomen in order to detect any masses in the liver or spleen.

A thorough history is necessary in order to determine whether the patient's ethnic background, lifestyle, or medical history places him or her in a high-risk category for KS.

Biopsy

A definitive diagnosis of KS requires a skin **biopsy** in order to rule out bacillary angiomatosis, a bacterial infection resembling cat-scratch disease. It is caused by a bacillus, *Bartonella henselae*. Collecting a tissue sample for a biopsy is not difficult if the patient has skin lesions, but can be complicated if the nodules are primarily internal. An endoscopy of the upper end of the digestive tract may be performed in order to obtain a tissue sample from an internal KS lesion.

Under the microscope, an AIDS-related KS lesion will show an unusually large number of spindle-shaped cells mixed together with small capillaries. The origin of the spindle-shaped cells is still unknown. The tumor cells in a KS lesion resemble smooth muscle cells or fibroblasts, which are cells that help to form the fibers in normal connective tissue.

If the patient's lymph nodes are enlarged, a biopsy may be done in order to rule out other causes of swollen lymph nodes.

Other tests

Other diagnostic tests may be performed if the patient appears to have disseminated KS. These tests include:

- Chest x rays. A radiograph of the patient's lungs will show patchy areas of involved tissue.
- **Gallium scan**. The results will be negative in KS.
- **Bronchoscopy**. This procedure allows the doctor to examine the patient's bronchial pathways for visible KS lesions. It is not, however, useful for obtaining tissue samples for biopsy.
- **Upper gastrointestinal endoscopy**. Examination of the patient's stomach allows the doctor to examine the mucous lining for KS lesions as well as to obtain a tissue sample.

Treatment team

KS patients may receive treatment for skin lesions from a dermatologist or radiologist as well as treatment for lung or lymphatic involvement from internists or primary care practitioners. A surgeon may be called in to remove lesions in the digestive tract if they are bleeding or blocking the passage of food. Children with KS may be treated by pediatricians or by primary care physicians who specialize in treating AIDS patients.

Clinical staging, treatments, and prognosis

Staging

The NIH recommends individualized staging of patients with classic KS, due to the age of most patients, the localized nature of the lesions, the slow progression of the disease, and the low risk of spread to the internal organs.

The criteria for staging epidemic KS have evolved over the past decade in response to changes in the treatment of HIV infection and to the recognition that KS does not fit well into standard categories of tumor assessment. Several different systems have been used to stage epidemic KS, but none is completely satisfactory.

NYU STAGING SYSTEM. One staging system that originated at New York University divides KS patients into four groups according to the following symptom clusters:

- Skin lesions that are indolent (slow-growing) and limited to relatively small areas of the body.
- Skin lesions limited to specific regions of the body but aggressive in growth. There may or may not be involvement of lymph nodes.
- General involvement of the skin and mucous membranes, with or without lymph node involvement.
- Involvement of the internal organs.

AIDS CLINICAL TRIALS GROUP (ACTG) STAGING SYSTEM. The ACTG Oncology Committee published a staging system for epidemic KS in 1989. This system was reevaluated in 1995 and is undergoing continued assessment. It is based on three criteria: extent of tumor; condition of the patient's immune system; and presence of systemic illness:

- Tumor (T): Good risk (0) is a tumor limited to the skin and/or lymph nodes and/or minimal oral disease (limited to the palate). Poor risk (1) is any of the following: edema associated with the tumor; widespread KS in the mouth; KS in the digestive tract; KS in other viscera.
- Immune system (I): Good risk (0) is a CD4 cell count greater than 200 per cubic millmeter. Poor risk (1) is a CD4 cell count lower than 200 per cubic millimeter.
- Systemic illness (S): Good risk (0) is no history of opportunistic infections (OI) or **thrush**; no "B" symptoms (unexplained **fever**, **night sweats**, **diarrhea** lasting more than 2 weeks, **weight loss** greater than 10%); performance status above 70 on the Karnofsky scale. Poor risk (1) is any of the following: history of OI or thrush; presence of "B" symptoms; Karnofsky score lower than 70; and other HIV-related illnesses.

Treatment

Treatment of KS depends on the form of the disease.

CLASSIC KS. Radiation therapy is usually quite effective if the patient has small lesions or lesions limited to a small area of skin. Low-voltage photon radiation or electron beam therapy give good results. Surgical removal of small lesions is sometimes done, but the lesions are likely to recur. The best results are obtained from surgical treatment when many small lesions are removed over a period of years.

For widespread skin disease, radiation treatment with electron beam therapy is recommended. Classic KS has not often been treated with **chemotherapy** in the United States, but some researchers report that treatment with **vinblastine** or **vincristine** has been effective. Disease that has spread to the lymph nodes or digestive tract is treated with a combination of chemotherapy and radiation treatment.

IMMUNOSUPPRESSIVE TREATMENT-RELATED KS. The standard pattern of therapy for this form of KS begins with discontinuing the immunosuppressive medications if they are not essential to the patient's care. Treatment of the KS itself may include radiation therapy if the disease is limited to the skin, or single- or multiple-drug chemotherapy.

EPIDEMIC KS. As of 2001, there is no cure for epidemic KS. Treatment is aimed at reducing the size of skin lesions and alleviating the discomfort of open ulcers or swollen tissue in the legs. There are no data that indicate that treatment prolongs the survival of patients with epidemic KS. In addition to treatment of the KS itself, these patients also need ongoing retroviral therapy and treatment of any opportunistic infections that may develop. An additional complication in treating epidemic KS is that highly active antiretroviral therapy, or HAART, is not the "magic bullet" that some had hoped when it was introduced in 1998. HAART uses three- or four-drug combinations to treat HIV infection. Problems with HAART include severe psychiatric as well as physical side effects, in addition to the patient's risk of developing a drug-resistant form of HIV if even one dose of medication is missed. The complex dosing schedules as well as the medication side effects make it difficult to assess the effectiveness of treatments aimed at the KS by itself.

Small KS lesions respond very well to radiation treatment. They can also be removed surgically or treated with **cryotherapy**, a technique that uses liquid nitrogen to freeze the lesion. Lesions inside the mouth (on the palate) can be treated with injections of vinblastine. In addition, the patient may be given topical alitretinoin (Panretin gel), which is applied directly to the lesions. Alitretinoin received FDA approval for treating KS in 1999.

Systemic treatments for epidemic KS consist of various combinations of anti-cancer drugs, including vincristine (Oncovin), vinblastine (Velban), **bleomycin** (Blenoxane), **doxorubicin** (Adriamycin), **daunorubicin** (DaunoXome), interferon-alpha (Intron A, Roferon-A), **etoposide** (VePesid), or **paclitaxel** (Taxol). The effectiveness of systemic treatments ranges from 50% for high-dose therapy with interferon-alpha to 80% for combinations of vincristine, vinblastine, bleomycin, doxorubicin, and etoposide. The drawbacks of systemic treatment include the toxicity of these drugs and their many side effects. Interferon-alpha can be given only to adult patients with relatively intact immune systems and no signs of lymphatic involvement. The side effects of systemic chemotherapy include hair loss (**alopecia**), **nausea and vomiting**, **fatigue**, diarrhea, headaches, loss of appetite (**anorexia**), allergic reactions, back pain, abdominal pain, and increased sweating.

As of 2001, the standard for first-line treatment of epidemic KS is one of the FDA-approved anthracyclines such as liposomal doxorubicin (Doxil) or liposomal daunorubicin (DaunoXome), rather than a combination drug regimen. Liposomes are small sacs consisting of an outer layer of fatty substances used to coat an inner core of

KEY TERMS

Angiogenesis—The formation of blood vessels. Some complex proteins found in shark cartilage appear to prevent angiogenesis in tumor cells in laboratory tests.

Cryotherapy—A form of treating KS lesions that involves freezing them with liquid nitrogen.

Disseminated—Widely distributed or spread. Epidemic KS almost always develops into a disseminated form, in which the disease spreads throughout the patient's body.

Highly active antiretroviral therapy (HAART)—A form of drug-combination treatment for HIV infection introduced in 1998. Most HAART regimens are combinations of three or four drugs, usually nucleoside analogs and protease inhibitors.

Iatrogenic—Caused unintentionally by medical treatment. Immunosuppressive treatment-related KS is sometimes called iatrogenic KS.

Immunosuppressive—Any form of treatment that inhibits the body's normal immune response.

Indolent—Relatively inactive or slow-spreading. Classic KS is usually an indolent disease.

Liposomes—Artificial sacs composed of fatty substances that are used to coat or encapsulate an inner core containing another drug. Some drugs used to treat epidemic KS are given in the form of liposomes.

Opportunistic infections (OI)—Diseases caused by organisms that multiply to the point of producing symptoms only when the body's immune system is impaired.

another medication. In addition to concentrating the drug's effects on the tumor, liposomes moderate the side effects.

In 1997 the FDA approved paclitaxel (Taxol) for epidemic KS resistant to treatment. Paclitaxel is a drug derived from the bark of the Pacific yew tree that prevents the growth of cancer cells by preventing the breakdown of normal cell structures called microtubules. After paclitaxel treatment, cancer cells become so clogged with microtubules that they cannot grow and divide. The drug has serious side effects, most notably suppression of the patient's bone marrow.

Experimental treatments for AIDS-related KS include retinoic acid, which is derived from vitamin A; and other drugs that inhibit the formation of new blood vessels (angiogenesis) in tumors. The reason for inhibiting angiogenesis is that new blood vessels keep a cancer supplied with oxygen and nutrients, which help the cancer grow and spread to other parts of the body. Antiangiogenic agents that have been proposed for treating KS include Fumagillin, SP-PG, and Platelet 4 factor. As of 2001, the effectiveness of these substances in humans is not yet known. Approval by the Food and Drug Administration will require several years after the test results are known.

Prognosis

The prognosis of KS varies depending on its form. Patients with classic KS often survive for many years after diagnosis; death is often caused by another cancer, such as non-Hodgkin's lymphoma, rather than the KS itself. The aggressive form of African KS has the poorest prognosis, with a fatality rate of 100% within three years of diagnosis. Patients with immunosuppressive treatment-related KS have variable prognoses; in many cases, however, the KS goes into remission once the immune-suppressing drug is discontinued. The prognosis of patients with epidemic KS also varies, depending on the patient's general level of health. As a rule, patients whose KS has spread to the lungs have the poorest prognosis.

Alternative and complementary therapies

SHARK CARTILAGE. The only alternative treatment for epidemic KS that has been evaluated by the NIH is shark cartilage. Shark cartilage products are widely available in the United States as over-the-counter (OTC) preparations that do not require FDA approval. A 1995 review of alternative therapies found more than 40 brand names of shark cartilage products for sale in the United States to treat arthritis and psoriasis as well as KS. The cartilage can be taken by mouth or by injection.

The use of shark cartilage to treat KS derives from a popular belief that sharks and other cartilaginous fish (skates and rays) do not get cancer. This belief is countered by findings from samples of captured sharks that they do in fact develop various kinds of tumors. There are three explanations of the role of shark cartilage in preventing KS. Some researchers have proposed that it kills cancer cells directly. A second explanation is that cartilage stimulates the human immune system. The third theory, which has more evidence in its favor than the first two, is that the cartilage slows down or prevents angiogenesis. Two complex proteins in shark cartilage, identified as U-995 and SCF2, have been shown to inhibit angiogenesis in laboratory studies. As of December 2000, only three studies using human subjects have been published; the results are inconclusive. The complete results of three other studies using shark cartilage in human subjects have not yet been published in complete form. Preliminary reports of NIH-sponsored **clinical trials** are also not yet available; however, all three studies being currently conducted have received the lowest rating (3iii) for the statistical strength of the study's design.

The side effects of treatment with shark cartilage include mild to moderate nausea, vomiting, abdominal cramps, constipation, low blood pressure, abnormally high levels of blood calcium (**hypercalcemia**), and general feelings of weakness.

OTHER ALTERNATIVE THERAPIES. Other alternative treatments for KS are aimed almost completely at epidemic KS. Most are based on assumptions that AIDS victims have had their immune systems weakened by such environmental toxins as lead and radioactive materials, or by psychological stress generated by societal disapproval of homosexuality. Naturopaths would add such life-style stresses as the use of tobacco and alcohol, as well as poor sleep patterns and nutritional deficiencies. Homeopaths believe that AIDS is the product of hereditary predispositions to disease called miasms, specifically two miasms related to syphilis and gonorrhea respectively.

Alternative topical treatments for the skin lesions of AIDS-related KS include homeopathic preparations made from periwinkle, mistletoe, or phytolacca (poke root). Other alternative skin preparations include a selenium solution made from aloe gels, selenium, and tincture of silica; a mixture of aloe vera and dried kelp (seaweed); and a mixture of aloe vera, tea tree oil, and tincture of St. John's wort. Alternative treatments for KS lesions on the internal organs include a mixture of warm wine and Yunnan Paiyao powder, a Chinese patent medicine made from ginseng; castor oil packs; or a three-to seven-day grape fast repeated every 120 days.

Alternative systemic treatments for AIDS-related KS include:

- Naturopathic remedies: High doses of vitamin C, zinc, echinacea, or goldenseal to improve immune function; or preparations of astragalis, osha root, or licorice to suppress the HIV virus.
- Homeopathic remedies: These include a homeopathic preparation of **cyclosporine** and another made from a dilution of killed typhoid virus.
- Ozone therapy: There are isolated reports from Europe and the United States of AIDS-related KS going into several months of remission after treatment with ozone given via rectal insufflation.

Alternative treatments aimed at improving the quality of life for KS patients include Reiki, reflexology, meditation, and chromatherapy.

Coping with cancer treatment

Studies of treatment side effects in patients with epidemic KS are complicated by the difficulty of distinguishing between side effects caused by treatment aimed at the HIV retrovirus itself and those caused by treatment for KS. Common problems related to KS treatment include damage to the bone marrow, hair loss, and nerve damage from medications.

Other treatment-related problems include weight loss due to poor appetite, and swelling of body tissues due to fluid retention. Patients may be given nutritional counseling, medications to stimulate the appetite, and radiation treatment or diuretics to reduce the level of fluid in the tissues.

Clinical trials

As of March 2001, there are thirteen open and active clinical trials being conducted for treatments for KS, twelve for epidemic KS and one for unspecified KS. Some of these are comparing the relative effectiveness of doxorubicin, daunorubicin, and paclitaxel. Others are studies of other agents, including interleukin-11, interleukin-12, cidofovir, and **filgrastim**. One is a study of the effects of HAART on AIDS-related KS. As of July 2000, the National Cancer Institute (NCI) reported that clinical trials of **thalidomide** indicated that the drug has some activity against epidemic KS. Updated information about the content of and patient participation in clinical trials can be obtained at the web site of the National Cancer Institute: http://cancertrials.nci.nih.gov.

Prevention

As of 2001, the only known preventive strategy for reducing one's risk for epidemic KS is abstinence from intercourse or modification of sexual habits. Homosexual or bisexual males can reduce their risk of developing KS by avoiding passive anal intercourse. Women can reduce their risk by avoiding vaginal or anal intercourse with bisexual males.

Kidney transplant patients who are at increased risk of developing KS as a result of taking prednisone or other immunosuppressive drugs should consult their primary physician about possible changes in dosage.

Special concerns

The two special concerns most likely to arise with epidemic KS are social isolation due to the disfigurement caused by KS lesions on the patient's face, and spiritual or psychological concerns related to the tumor's connection to AIDS and homosexuality. There are many local and regional support groups for cancer patients that can help patients deal with concerns about appearance. With regard to religious/spiritual issues, most major Christian and Jewish bodies in the United States and Canada have task forces or working groups dealing with AIDS-related concerns. The National Catholic AIDS Network (NCAN) maintains an information database and web site (http:// www.ncan.org) and accepts call-in referrals at (707) 874-3031.

Resources

BOOKS

The Burton Goldberg Group. *Alternative Medicine: The Definitive Guide.* Fife, WA: Future Medicine Publishing, Inc., 1995.

"Hematology and Oncology." Section 11 in *The Merck Manual of Diagnosis and Therapy*, edited by Mark H. Beers, MD, and Robert Berkow, MD. Whitehouse Station, NJ: Merck Research Laboratories, 1999.

James, Nicholas D., and Karol Sikora. "Immunotherapy of Tumors," in *Encyclopedia of Immunology*, v. 3, 2nd ed., edited by Peter J. Delves and Ivan M. Roitt. San Diego and London: Academic Press, 1998.

Kubota, Marshall K., MD. "Human Immunodeficiency Virus Infection and Its Complications," in *Conn's Current Therapy*, edited by Robert E. Rakel, MD. Philadelphia: W. B. Saunders Company, 2000.

Schulz, Thomas F. "Herpesvirus-8, Infection and Immunity," in *Encyclopedia of Immunology*, v. 2, 2nd ed., edited by Peter J. Delves and Ivan M. Roitt. San Diego and London: Academic Press, 1998.

Silverberg, Ivan J., MD. "Kaposi's Sarcoma." In Dollinger, Malin, MD, Ernest H. Rosenbaum, MD, and Greg Cable. *Cancer Therapy.* Kansas City, MO: Andrews and McMeel, 1994.

PERIODICALS

Correspondence: Kaposi's Sarcoma. *New England Journal of Medicine* 343 (8) (August 24, 2000).

San Francisco AIDS Foundation. *Bulletin of Experimental Treatments for AIDS.*

ORGANIZATIONS

AIDS Clinical Trials Group (ACTG). c/o William Duncan, Ph.D., National Institutes of Health. 6003 Executive Boulevard, Room 2A07, Bethesda, MD 20892.

American Cancer Society (ACS). 1599 Clifton Road, NE, Atlanta, GA 30329. (404) 320-3333 or (800) ACS-2345. Fax: (404) 329-7530. Web site: <http://www.cancer.org>

National Cancer Institute, Office of Cancer Communications. 31 Center Drive, MSC 2580, Bethesda, MD 20892-2580. (800) 4-CANCER (1-800-422-6237). TTY: (800) 332-8615. Web site: <http://www.nci.nih.gov>.

NIH National Center for Complementary and Alternative Medicine (NCCAM) Clearinghouse. P. O. Box 8218, Silver Spring, MD 20907-8218. TTY/TDY: (888) 644-6226. Fax: (301) 495-4957.

San Francisco AIDS Foundation (SFAF). 995 Market Street, #200, San Francisco, CA 94103. (415) 487-3000 or (800) 367-AIDS. Fax: (415) 487-3009. Web site: http://www.sfaf.org.

Rebecca J. Frey, Ph.D.

Ketoconazole *see* **Antifungal therapy**

Ki67

Definition

Ki67 is a molecule that can be easily detected in growing cells in order to gain an understanding of the rate at which the cells within a tumor are growing.

Purpose

Detection of Ki67 is carried out on biopsies, samples of tumor tissue. The goal of this assay is to evaluate an important characteristic of the cells within the tumor, the percentage of tumor cells that are actively dividing and giving rise to more cancer cells. The number obtained through this examination is termed the S-phase, growth, or proliferative fraction. This information can play an important part in deciding the best treatment for a cancer patient.

Precautions

This test is performed on tissue or cells that have been removed during the initial surgery or diagnostic procedure used to determine the precise nature of the cancer. It usually does not require any new surgery or blood draw on the patient and, so, does not entail any additional precautions for the patient.

KEY TERMS

Immunocytochemistry—Method for staining cells or tissues using antibodies so that the location of a target molecule can be determined

Nucleus—The part of the cell containing chromosomes

S phase—The part of the cell division cycle during which the genetic material, DNA, is duplicated

Description

Cancer is a group of diseases characterized by abnormal, or neoplastic, cellular growth in particular tissues. In many instances this growth is abnormal because cells are growing more rapidly than is normal. This unregulated growth is how a tumor is formed. A tumor is more or less a collection of cells that grow more rapidly than the surrounding normal tissue. Most importantly, this difference in growth rate is central to how many cancer drugs, termed cytotoxic agents, work. The ability of these drugs to eliminate cancer cells depends on their ability to kill cells that are actively proliferating, but do less damage to cells that are not actively dividing. This makes it useful to know how actively the cells in tumor are growing compared to the surrounding tissue. The measurement of Ki67 is one of the most common ways to measure the growth fraction of tumor cells. This molecule can be detected in the nucleus of only actively growing cells.

Analysis of Ki67 in tumors is accomplished by a pathologist who examines a piece of the tumor tissue using special techniques. The technique used is termed immunocytochemistry. This involves the preparation of a histologic section, a very thin piece of tumor tissue placed on a glass microscope slide. These kinds of tissue sections are used in the diagnosis of cancer. In the case of Ki67 assays, the section is incubated with antibodies that can react with the Ki67 molecule, and then treated with special reagents that cause a color to appear where antibody has bound. In this way, when the pathologist looks at the section using a microscope the fraction of growing cells, whose nuclei are stained for Ki67, can be determined for the tumor cells and compared with the normal tissue. In some instances, depending on the particular type of cancer, the pathologist might feel it more appropriate to use a different technique to assess the growth fraction for a specific tumor or leukemia.

QUESTIONS TO ASK THE DOCTOR

- How far from normal is the Ki-67 labeling index of my tumor?
- To what extent is this result influencing the treatment I will receive?
- In your experience, does the proliferative fraction of my tumor predict a good response to chemotherapy?

Preparation, Aftercare, and Risks

Because this test is performed on tissue or cells that had been removed during an initial **biopsy** or other diagnostic procedure, and because no new surgery or sample is required, no additional recommendations regarding preparation, aftercare, or risks are necessary.

Results

The proliferative or growth fraction as determined by Ki67 analysis is interpreted in view of what is normal for the tissue in which the tumor has been found or from which it originated. In the case of certain types of tissue—for example, brain—there is little cellular growth in normal tissue. In other cases, such as breast or the cells that line the colon, cellular growth is a normal part of the function of that tissue. The significance of an increased proliferative fraction is interpreted in light of the experience of the oncologist as well as the knowledge and experience of other clinicians as reported in the medical literature. The Ki67 result, often termed the "Ki67 labeling index," can be used in some cases as a prognostic indicator for some cancers. For example, for brain tumors, such as astrocytomas and glioblastomas, a high Ki67 labeling index is one factor that predicts a poor prognosis. For breast tumors, the clinician will consider the proliferative fraction in conjunction with other factors such as patient age, results of receptor assays, and whether or not there is evidence of spread of the disease to lymph nodes or other sites within the body. The value of Ki67 is not as firmly established for other cancers such as bladder or **pituitary tumors**.

Resources

PERIODICALS

Chassevent, A., et al. "S-Phase Fraction and DNA Ploidy in 633 T1T2 Breast Cancers: A Standardized Flow Cytometric Study." *Clinical Cancer Research* 7 (2001): 909-17.

Warren Maltzman, Ph.D.

Kidney cancer

Definition

Kidney cancer is a disease in which the cells in certain tissues of the kidney start to grow uncontrollably and form tumors. Renal cell **carcinoma**, sometimes referred to as hypernephroma, occurs in the cells lining the kidneys (epithelial cells). It is the most common type of kidney cancer. Eighty-five percent of all kidney tumors are renal cell carcinomas. **Wilms' tumor** is a rapidly developing cancer of the kidney most often found in children under four years of age.

Description

The kidneys are a pair of organs shaped like kidney beans that lie on either side of the spine just above the waist. Inside each kidney are tiny tubes (tubules) that filter and clean the blood, taking out the waste products and making urine. The urine that is made by the kidney passes through a tube called the ureter into the bladder. Urine is held in the bladder until it is discharged from the body. Renal cell carcinoma (RCC) generally develops in the lining of the tubules that filter and clean the blood. Cancer that develops in the central portion of the kidney (where the urine is collected and drained into the ureters) is known as **transitional cell carcinoma** of the renal pelvis. Transitional cell cancer is similar to **bladder cancer**. Wilms' tumor is the most common type of childhood kidney cancer and is distinct from kidney cancer in adults.

Demographics

Kidney cancer accounts for approximately 3% of all cancers. In the United States, kidney cancer is the tenth most common cancer and the incidence has increased by 43% since 1973; the death rate has increased by 16%. There are approximately 20,000 new cases of kidney cancer found each year. There are approximately 95,000 deaths per year worldwide due to kidney cancer. RCC accounts for 90–95% of malignant neoplasms that originate from the kidney.

Kidney cancer occurs most often in men over the age of 40. The median age of diagnosis is 65. Men are twice as likely as women are to have cancer of the kidney.

Causes and symptoms

The causes of kidney cancer are unknown, but there are many risk factors associated with kidney cancer. The risk factors listed from greatest to smallest include:

- von Hippel-Lindau disease (> 100)

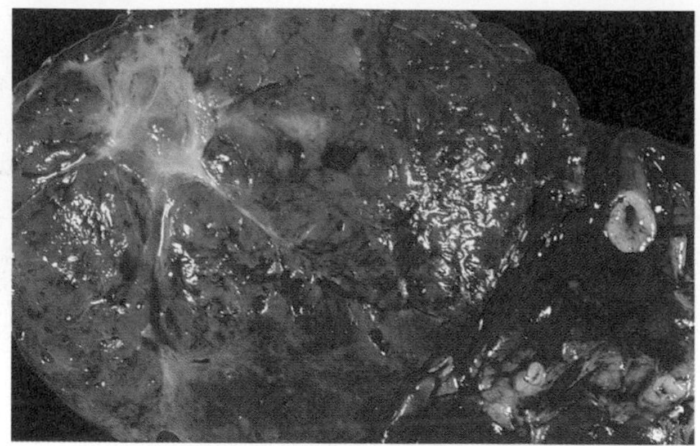

An extracted cancerous kidney. *(Photo by Robert Riedlinger. Custom Medical Stock Photo. Reproduced by permission.)*

- Chronic dialysis (32)
- Obesity (3.6)
- Tobacco use (**cigarettes**) (2.3)
- First-degree relative with kidney cancer (1.6)
- Hypertension (1.4)
- Dry-cleaning worker (1.4)
- Diuretics(non-hypertension use) (1.3)
- Trichloroethylene exposure (1.0)
- Heavy phenacetin use (1.1–6.0)
- Polycystic kidney disease (0.8–2.0)
- Cadmium exposure (1.0–3.9)
- Arsenic exposure (1.6)
- Asbestos (1.1–1.8)

The most common symptom of kidney cancer is blood in the urine (hematuria). Other symptoms include painful urination, pain in the lower back or on the sides, abdominal pain, a lump or hard mass that can be felt in the kidney area, unexplained **weight loss**, **fever**, weakness, **fatigue**, and high blood pressure.

Diagnosis

A diagnostic examination for kidney cancer includes taking a thorough medical history and making a complete physical examination in which the doctor will probe (palpate) the abdomen for lumps. Blood tests will be ordered to check for changes in blood chemistry caused by substances released by the tumor. Laboratory tests may show abnormal levels of iron in the blood. Either a low red blood cell count (**anemia**) or a high red blood cell count (erythrocytosis) may accompany kidney cancer. Occasionally, patients will have high calcium levels.

If the doctor suspects kidney cancer, an **intravenous urography** (also called pyelogram or IVP) may be ordered. An IVP is an x-ray test in which a dye is injected into a vein in the arm. The dye travels through the body, and when it is concentrated in the urine to be discharged, it outlines the kidneys, ureters, and the urinary bladder. On an x-ray image, the dye will reveal any abnormalities of the urinary tract. The IVP may miss small kidney cancers.

Renal ultrasound is a diagnostic test in which sound waves are used to form an image of the kidneys. Ultrasound is a painless and non-invasive procedure that can be used to detect even very small kidney tumors. Imaging tests such as **computed tomography** (CT) scans and **magnetic resonance imaging** (MRI) can be used to evaluate the kidneys and the surrounding organs. These tests are used to check whether the tumor has spread outside the kidney to other organs in the abdomen. If the patient complains of **bone pain**, a special **x ray** called a bone scan may be ordered to rule out spread to the bones. A chest x ray may be taken to rule out spread to the lungs.

A kidney **biopsy** is used to positively confirm the diagnosis of kidney cancer. During this procedure, a small piece of tissue is removed from the tumor and examined under a microscope. The biopsy will give information about the type of tumor, the cells that are involved, and the aggressiveness of the tumor (tumor stage).

Staging, treatment, and prognosis

Staging

Staging guidelines for kidney cancer are as follows (2.5 cm equals approximately 1 in):

- Stage I: Primary tumor is 5 cm or less in greatest dimension and is limited to the kidney, with no lymph node involvement.
- Stage II: Primary tumor is larger than 5 cm in greatest dimension and is limited to the kidney, with no lymph node involvement.
- Stage III: Primary tumor may extend into major veins or invade adrenal glands or perinephric tissues, but not beyond Gerota's fascia. There may be **metastasis** in a single lymph node.
- Stage IV: Primary tumor invades beyond Gerota's fascia. Metastasis in more than one lymph node. Possible metastasis to distant structures in the body.

Treatment

Each person's treatment is different and depends on several factors. The location, size, and extent of the tumor have to be considered in addition to the patient's age, general health, and medical history.

The primary treatment for kidney cancer that has not spread to other parts of the body, which is a Stage I, II, or III tumor, is surgical removal of the diseased kidney (nephrectomy). Because most cancers affect only one kidney, the patient can function well on the one remaining. Two types of surgical procedure are used. Radical nephrectomy removes the entire kidney and the surrounding tissue. Sometimes, the lymph nodes surrounding the kidney are also removed. Partial nephrectomy removes only part of the kidney along with the tumor. This procedure is used either when the tumor is very small or when it is not practical to remove the entire kidney. It is not practical to remove a kidney when the patient has only one kidney or when both kidneys have tumors. There is a small (5%) chance of missing some of the cancer. Nephrectomy can also be useful for Stage IV cancers, but alternative surgical procedures such as transarterial angioinfarction may be used.

Radiation therapy, which consists of exposing the cancer cells to high-energy gamma rays from an external source, generally destroys cancer cells with minimal damage to the normal tissue. Side effects are nausea, fatigue, and stomach upsets. These symptoms disappear when the treatment is over. In kidney cancer, radiation therapy has been shown to alleviate pain and bleeding, especially when the cancer is inoperable. However, it has not proven to be of much use in destroying the kidney cancer cells. Therefore radiation therapy is not used very often as a treatment for cancer or as a routine adjuvant to nephrectomy. Radiotherapy, however, is used to manage metastatic kidney cancer.

Treatment of kidney cancer with anti-cancer drugs (**chemotherapy**) has not produced good results. However, new drugs and new combinations of drugs continue to be tested in **clinical trials**.

Immunotherapy or **immunologic therapy**, a form of treatment in which the body's immune system is harnessed to help fight the cancer, is a new mode of therapy that is being tested for kidney cancer. Clinical trials with substances produced by the immune cells (**aldesleukin** and interferon) have shown some promise in destroying kidney cancer cells. These substances have been approved for use but they can be very toxic and produce severe side effects. The benefits derived from the treatment have to be weighed very carefully against the side effects in each case. Immunotherapy is the most promising systemic therapy for metastatic kidney cancer.

Prognosis

Because kidney cancer is often caught early and sometimes progresses slowly, the chances of a surgical cure are good. It is also one of the few cancers for which there are well-documented cases of spontaneous remission without therapy.

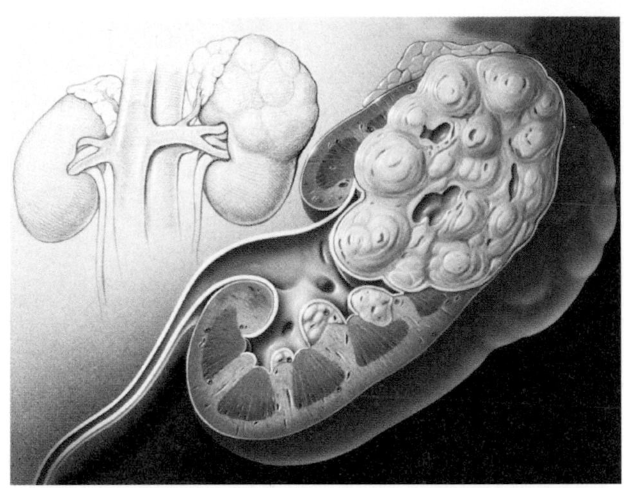

Background of illustration and to left: a pair of kidneys. One kidney is normal, while the other is cancerous. The foreground of the illustration and in color: a cutaway of the cancerous kidney. *(Custom Medical Stock Photo. Reproduced by permission.)*

Alternative and complementary therapies

There are several healing philosophies, approaches, and therapies that may be used as supplemental or instead of traditional treatments. All of the items listed may have varying effectiveness in boosting the immune system and/or treating a tumor. The efficacy of each treatment also varies from person to person. None of the treatments, however, have demonstrated safety or effectiveness on a consistent basis. Patients should research such treatments for any potential dangers (laetrile, for example, has caused death due to cyanide poisoning) and notify their physician before taking them.

- 714-X
- antineoplastons
- Cancell
- cartilage (bovine and shark)
- Coenzyme Q10
- Gerson Therapy
- Gonzalez Protocol
- Hydrazine sulfate
- immuno-augementative therapy
- Laetrile
- mistletoe

KEY TERMS

Biopsy—The surgical removal and microscopic examination of living tissue for diagnostic purposes.

Bone scan—An x-ray study in which patients are given an intravenous injection of a small amount of a radioactive material that travels in the blood. When it reaches the bones, it can be detected by x ray to make a picture of their internal structure.

Chemotherapy—Treatment with anticancer drugs.

Computed tomography (CT) scan—A medical procedure in which a series of x-ray images are made and put together by a computer to form detailed pictures of areas inside the body.

Hematuria—Blood in the urine.

Immunotherapy—Treatment of cancer by stimulating the body's immune defense system.

Intravenous pyelogram (IVP)—A procedure in which a dye is injected into a vein in the arm. The dye travels through the body and concentrates in the urine to be discharged. It outlines the kidneys, ureters, and the urinary bladder. An x-ray image is then made and any abnormalities of the urinary tract are revealed.

Magnetic resonance imaging (MRI)—A medical procedure used for diagnostic purposes in which pictures of areas inside the body can be created using a magnet linked to a computer.

Nephrectomy—A medical procedure in which the kidney is surgically removed.

Primary tumor—A cancer's origin or initial growth.

Radiation therapy—Treatment with high-energy radiation from x-ray machines, cobalt, radium, or other sources.

Renal ultrasound—A painless and non-invasive procedure in which sound waves are bounced off the kidneys. These sound waves produce a pattern of echoes that are then used by the computer to create pictures of areas inside the kidney (sonograms).

Coping with cancer treatment

Side effects of treatment, as well as nutrition, emotional well-being, and other complications, are all parts of coping with cancer. There are many possible side effects for a cancer treatment that include:

- constipation
- delirium
- fatigue
- fever, chills, sweats
- **nausea and vomiting**
- mouth sores, dry mouth, bleeding gums
- pruritus (**itching**)
- **sexuality**
- sleep disorders

Anxiety, **depression**, loss, post-traumatic stress disorder, sexuality, and substance abuse are all possible emotional side-effects. Nutrition and eating before, during, and after a treatment can also be of concern. Other complications of coping with cancer include fever and pain.

Clinical trials

There are many clinical trials in place studying new types of radiation therapy and chemotherapy, new drugs and drug combinations, biological therapies, ways of combining various types of treatment for kidney cancer, side effect reduction, and improving quality of life. Immunostimulatory agents and gene-therapy techniques that modify tumor cells, antiangiogenesis compounds, cyclin-dependent kinase inhibitors, and differentiating agents are all being investigated as possible therapies. Consult <http://ClinicalTrials.gov> and your doctor for a list of kidney cancer clinical trials.

Prevention

The exact cause of kidney cancer is not known, so it is not possible to prevent all cases. However, because a strong association between kidney cancer and tobacco has been shown, avoiding tobacco is the best way to lower one's risk of developing this cancer. Using care when working with cancer-causing agents such as asbestos and cadmium and eating a well-balanced diet may also help prevent kidney cancer.

See Also Renal pelvis tumors; Von Hippel-Lindau Syndrome

Resources

BOOKS

Berkow, Robert, ed. *The Merck Manual of Diagnosis and Therapy,* 16th ed. Rahway, NJ: Merck Research Laboratories, 1997.

QUESTIONS TO ASK THE DOCTOR

- What should I expect from a biopsy test?
- What type of kidney cancer do I have?
- What is the stage of the disease?
- What are the treatment choices? Which do you recommend? Why?
- What are the risks and possible side effects of each treatment?
- What are the chances that the treatment will be successful?
- What new treatments are being studied in clinical trials?
- How long will treatment last?
- Will I have to stay in the hospital?
- Will treatment affect my normal activities? If so, for how long?
- What is the treatment likely to cost?

Dollinger, Malin, Ernest H. Rosenbaum, and Greg Cable. *Everyone's Guide to Cancer Therapy. How Cancer Is Diagnosed, Treated, and Managed Day to Day.* Kansas City: Andrews McMeel, 1998.

Murphy, Gerald P., Lois B. Morris, and Dianne Lange. *Informed Decisions: The Complete Book of Cancer Diagnosis, Treatment and Recovery.* New York: Viking, 1997.

Scher, H.I., and R.J. Motzer. "Renal Cell Carcinoma." In*Harrison's Principles of Internal Medicine.* Fauci, Anthony, et al, eds. New York: McGraw–Hill, 1998.

PERIODICALS

Dutcher, J.P. "Immunotherapy: Are We Making a Difference?" *Current Opinion in Urology* (September 2000): 435–9.

Godley, P.A., and K.I. Ataga. "Renal Cell Carcinoma." *Current Opinion in Oncology* (May 2000): 260–4.

Halperin, E.C. "Kidney Cancer." *Lancet* (February 1999): 594.

Vogelzang, N.J., and W.M. Stadler. "Kidney Cancer." *Lancet* (November 1998): 1691–6.

ORGANIZATIONS

American Cancer Society (National Headquarters). 1599 Clifton Rd. NE, Atlanta, GA 30329. (800) 227-2345. <http://www.cancer.org.>

American Foundation for Urologic Disease. E-mail: admin@afud.org.

Cancer Research Institute (National Headquarters). 681 Fifth Ave., New York, NY 10022. (800) 992-2623. <http://www.cancerresearch.org>.

Kidney Cancer Association. 1234 Sherman Ave., Suite 203, Evanston, IL 60202-1375. (800) 850-9132. <http://www.kidneycancerassociation.org>.

National Cancer Institute. 9000 Rockville Pike, Building 31, Room 10A16, Bethesda, MD 20892. (800) 422-6237. <http://www.nci.nih.gov>.

National Kidney Cancer Association. 1234 Sherman Ave., Suite 203, Evanston, IL 60202-1375. (800) 850-9132.

National Kidney Foundation. 30 East 33rd St., New York, NY 10016. (800) 622-9010. <http://www.kidney.org>.

American Urological Association. 1120 N. Charles St., Baltimore, MD 21201. (410) 727-1100. <http://www.auanet.org/patient_info/find_urologist/index.cfm>.

Lata Cherath, Ph.D.
Laura Ruth, Ph.D.